GLAUCOMA

MEDICAL DIAGNOSIS & THERAPY

VOLUME ONE

Commissioning Editor: Russell Gabbedy
Development Editor: Sven Pinczewski
Editorial Assistant: Rachael Harrison, Kirsten Lowson
Project Manager: Alan Nicholson
Design: Sarah Russell, Stewart Larking
Illustration Manager: Kirsteen Wright, Gillian Richards
Illustrator: Martin Woodward
Marketing Manager(s) (UK/USA): John Canelon / Helena Mutak

GLAUCOMA

MEDICAL DIAGNOSIS & THERAPY

VOLUME ONE

TAREK M SHAARAWY MD MSc

Consultant Ophthalmologist and Head
Glaucoma Sector, Ophthalmology Service
Department of Clinical Neurosciences
University of Geneva
Geneva
Switzerland

MARK B SHERWOOD FRCP FRCOphth

Daniels Professor
Departments of Ophthalmology and Cell Biology
Director of Vision Research Center
University of Florida
Gainesville FL
USA

ROGER A HITCHINGS FRCOphth

Professor of Glaucoma and Allied Studies
Consultant Ophthalmologist
Glaucoma Unit
Moorfields Eye Hospital
London
UK

JONATHAN G CROWSTON PhD FRCOphth FRANZCO

Professor
Department of Ophthalmology
University of Melbourne
Centre for Eye Research Australia
Royal Victorian Eye & Ear Hospital
East Melbourne
Australia

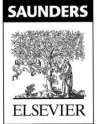

SAUNDERS

ELSEVIER

SAUNDERS
ELSEVIER

SAUNDERS is an imprint of Elsevier Limited

The following chapters are copyright of Moorefields Eye Hospital:
'Uveitic Glaucoma' by Avinash Kulkarni and Keith Barton
'Aqueous Shunts: Choice of Implant' by Keith Barton and Dale K Heuer
'Aqueous Shunts after Retinal Surgery' by Maria Papadopoulos and Keith Barton

First published 2009

ISBN (2-volume set): 978-0-7020-2976-9

ISBN (Volume 1): 978-0-7020-2977-6

ISBN (Volume 2): 978-0-7020-2978-3

British Library Cataloguing in Publication Data
A catalogue record for this book is available from the British Library

Library of Congress Cataloging in Publication Data
A catalog record for this book is available from the Library of Congress

Notice
Medical knowledge is constantly changing. Standard safety precautions must be followed, but as
new research and clinical experience broaden our knowledge, changes in treatment and drug therapy
may become necessary or appropriate. Readers are advised to check the most current product
information provided by the manufacturer of each drug to be administered to verify the recommended
dose, the method and duration of administration, and contraindications. It is the responsibility of
the practitioner, relying on experience and knowledge of the patient, to determine dosages and
the best treatment for each individual patient. Neither the Publisher nor the author assume any
liability for any injury and/or damage to persons or property arising from this publication.

The Publisher

Printed in China
Last digit is the print number: 9 8 7 6 5 4 3 2 1

CONTENTS

Foreword   xi
Preface   xiii
List of Contributors   xiv
Acknowledgements   xxv
Dedication   xxvi
The Editors   xxvii

VOLUME 1
MEDICAL DIAGNOSIS AND THERAPY

Section 1   Glaucoma in the World

1   Prevalence and Geographical Variations   3
    Winnie Nolan and Jennifer LY Yip
    Spotlight: Prevalence and Geographical Variations   12
    Harry A Quigley
    Spotlight: Clinical Epidemiology: Stimulating and
    Applying Glaucoma Research to the Patient   12
    R Thomas and R Parikh

2   Screening for Glaucoma   15
    Paul R Healey

3   Economics of Glaucoma Care   25
    Paul P Lee and David B Matchar

4   Practical Application of Glaucoma Care in
    Different Societies   33
    Alan L Robin, Donald L Budenz, Nathan
    G Congdon, and Ravilla D Thulasiraj

Section 2   Pathogenesis

5   Pathogenesis of Glaucomatous
    Optic Neuropathy   45
    James E Morgan

6   Aqueous Humor Dynamics and Intraocular
    Pressure Elevation   55
    Carol B Toris

7   Mechanical Strain and Restructuring of
    the Optic Nerve Head   67
    J Crawford Downs, Michael D Roberts, and
    Claude F Burgoyne

8   Role of Ocular Blood Flow in the
    Pathogenesis of Glaucoma   91
    Ali S Hafez and Mark R Lesk

Section 3   Diagnosis of Glaucoma

9   Tonometry and Intraocular
    Pressure Fluctuation   103
    Aachal Kotecha, K Sheng Lim, and David
    Garway-Heath

10 Visual Fields   115
    David P Crabb

11 Function-Specific Perimetry   133
    Felipe A Medeiros and Luciana M Alencar

12 Electrophysiology in Glaucoma Assessment   151
    Stuart L Graham and Brad Fortune

13 Gonioscopy   173
    John F Salmon

14 Ultrasound Biomicroscopy   185
    Giorgio Marchini, Robero Tosi, and
    Piero Ceruti

15 Angle Imaging: Ultrasound Biomicroscopy
    and Anterior Segment Optical Coherence
    Tomography   197
    Gus Gazzard and Winnie Nolan

16 The Impact of Central Corneal Thickness
    and Corneal Biomechanics on Tonometry   207
    James D Brandt, Cynthia J Roberts, Mark
    B Sherwood, and Clinton W Sheets

17 Optic Disc Photography in the Diagnosis of
    Glaucoma   213
    Jost B Jonas

18 Optic Disc Imaging   225
    Linda M Zangwill, Christopher Bowd, and
    Felipe A Medeiros

19 Retinal Nerve Fiber Layer Photography and
    Computer Analysis   239
    Neil T Choplin, E Randy Craven, Toni
    T Meyers, Nicolaas J Reus, and Hans G Lemij

20 Structure and Function Relationships
    in Glaucoma   251
    Marcelo Nicolela, Lesya M Shuba, and
    Bettina K Windisch

21 Techniques Used for Evaluation of
    Ocular Blood Flow   257
    Ali S Hafez and Mark R Lesk

22 Genetics of Glaucoma   269
    Mohammed K ElMallah and R Rand Allingham

CONTENTS

23 Genetic Epidemiology 277
Leonieke ME van Koolwijk, Catey Bunce, and Ananth C Viswanathan

Section 4   Types of Glaucoma

24 Definitions: What is Glaucoma Worldwide? 293
George L Spaeth

25 Ocular Hypertension 307
Thad Labbe and Michael A Kass

26 Primary Open-Angle Glaucoma 315
Albert S Khouri and Robert D Fechtner

27 Primary Angle-Closure Glaucoma 327
Paul J Foster and Sancy Low

28 Exfoliation Syndrome and Exfoliative Glaucoma 339
Robert Ritch, Anastasios GP Konstas, and Ursula Schlötzer-Schrehardt

29 Pigmentary Glaucoma 349
Stefano A Gandolfi, Nicola Ungaro, Paolo Mora, and Chiara Sangermani

30 Normal-Tension Glaucoma 361
Angelo P Tanna and Theodore Krupin

31 Congenital Glaucoma and other Childhood Glaucomas 369
Camille Hylton and Allen Beck

32 Secondary Angle-Closure Glaucoma 383
Syril K Dorairaj, Jeffrey M Liebmann, and Robert Ritch

33 Uveitic Glaucoma 393
Avinash Kulkarni and Keith Barton

34 Neovascular Glaucoma 409
Danny Kim, Arun D Singh, and Annapurna Singh

35 Other Secondary Glaucomas 419
Jody Piltz-Seymour and Tara A Uhler

36 Post-Traumatic Glaucoma 431
Sheila Bazzaz, L Jay Katz, and Jonathan S Myers

37 Glaucoma and Intraocular Tumors 441
Kathryn E Bollinger, Annapurna Singh, and Arun D Singh

Section 5   Principles of Management

38 Management of Ocular Hypertension and Primary Open-angle Glaucoma 451
Roger A Hitchings

39 An Overview of Angle-Closure Management 455
Chaiwat Teekhasaenee

40 Target Intraocular Pressure 463
Nitin Anand

41 Quality of Life 471
Alexander Spratt, Aachal Kotecha, and Ananth C Viswanathan

42 Optimizing Quality of Life: Low-vision Rehabilitation in Glaucoma 481
Jill E Keeffe

43 Adherence and Persistence 489
Gail F Schwartz

44 Outcomes 495
Ridia Lim and Ivan Goldberg

Spotlight: Principles of Management: Outcomes 505
Paul R Lichter

45 Benefit Versus Risk 509
Ravi Thomas and Rajul S Parikh

Section 6   Medical Therapy

46 Parasympathomimetics 517
Lineu Oto Shiroma and Vital P Costa

47 Beta-Blockers 525
Ann M Hoste

Spotlight: Beta-Blockers 534
Tony Realini and TJ Zimmerman

Spotlight: Beta-Blockers 535
Josef Flammer

48 Carbonic Anhydrase Inhibitors 539
Gábor Holló

49 Alpha Agonists 547
Adam C Reynolds

50 Prostaglandin Analogues 559
Norbert Pfeiffer and Hagen Thieme

51 Fixed-Combination Therapy in Glaucoma 565
Anastasios GP Konstas, Dimitrios Mikropoulos, and William C Stewart

Section 7   New Horizons

52 Neuroprotection and Neuroregeneration 579
Leonard A Levin

53 Interpreting Clinical Studies on Glaucoma Neuroprotection 591
Robert N Weinreb and Anne L Coleman

54 Stem Cells: A Future Glaucoma Therapy? 595
Thomas V Johnson, Natalie D Bull, and Keith R Martin

55 Gene Therapy in Glaucoma 605
Stuart J McKinnon

56 Ultrastructural Imaging 615
Aachal Kotecha and Frederick W Fitzke

Section 8   Emergency Care Management

57 Acute Intraocular Pressure Rise 625
Prin RojanaPongpun

58 Glaucoma Secondary to Trauma 637
Baha' N Noureddin and Karim Tomey

Index 653

VOLUME 2
SURGICAL MANAGEMENT

Section 9   Introduction

59 Economics of Surgery Worldwide:
Developed countries   3
Anja Tuulonen
Developing countries   13
Boateng Wiafe

60 When to Perform Glaucoma Surgery   17
George A Cioffi and E Michael Van Buskirk

61 Lowering Intraocular Pressure: Surgery versus
Medications   23
Clive Migdal

62 The Trabecular Meshwork Outflow Pathways:
Functional Morphology and Surgical Aspects   31
Ernst R Tamm

Section 10   Laser Therapy

63 Argon Laser Trabeculoplasty: a Proven, Effective
Option in the Treatment of Patients with
Glaucoma   47
Eve J Higginbotham and Ijeoma M Asota

64 Selective Laser Trabeculoplasty   53
*Syril K Dorairaj, Celso Tello, Jeffrey M
Liebmann, and Robert Ritch*

   Spotlight: Selective Laser Trabeculoplasty   58
   L Jay Katz

65 Peripheral Iridotomy for Angle-Closure
Glaucoma   61
*Dennis SC Lam , Clement CY Tham, and
Nathan G Congdon*

66 Laser Peripheral Iridoplasty   71
Chaiwat Teekhasaenee

Section 11   Trabeculectomy

67 Preoperative Evaluation and Diagnostic
Approach   81
Thierry Zeyen and Ingeborg Stalmans

   Spotlight: Risk Factors for Suprachoroidal
   Hemorrhage   84
   J Caprioli

   Spotlight: Local Anesthesia   84
   J Caprioli

   Spotlight: Surgery in Short Eyes   85
   J Caprioli

68 Preoperative Conjunctival Health and
Trabeculectomy Outcome   87
Matthew J Hawker and David C Broadway

69 Ophthalmic Anesthesia   95
Meenakashi Gupta and Douglas J Rhee

70 Trabeculectomy   111
Ronald Fellman

   Spotlight: Releasable Sutures   143
   Mark B Sherwood

71 Alternative Techniques   151
Fabian Lerner

72 The Ex-PRESS™ Miniature Glaucoma
Implant   157
Eli Dahan and André Mermoud

73 Intraoperative Complications of
Trabeculectomy   165
*Rajendra K Bansal, Daniel S Casper, and
James C Tsai*

74 Early Postoperative Increase in Intraocular
Pressure   175
Pratap Challa

75 Shallow Anterior Chamber   183
*Anil K Mandal, Debasis Chakrabarti, and
Raka Chakrabarti*

76 Choroidal Effusion and Hemorrhage   195
Carolyn D Quinn and David S Greenfield

77 Corneal Complications of Trabeculectomy   205
Magdy A Nofal and Fathi F El Sayyad

78 Aqueous Misdirection   211
Pradeep Y Ramulu and Steven J Gedde

79 Tenon's Cyst Formation, Wound Healing,
and Bleb Evaluation   223

   Part A: Tenon's Cyst Formation and
   Management   223
   Anthony Wells

   Part B: Wound Healing and Bleb Evaluation
   after Trabeculectomy   229
   *Anthony Wells, Tina Wong and Jonathan
   G Crowston*

80 Late Failure of Filtering Bleb   239
Robert L Stamper

81 Late Bleb Leaks   243
Jacob Wilensky

82 Blebitis and Endophthalmitis   247
Peter Shah, Mark Chiang, and Graham Lee

83 Late Hypotony   257
John Thygesen

84 Cataract Following Trabeculectomy   277
Alain Bron

Section 12   Nonpenetrating Glaucoma Surgery

85 Principle and Mechanism of Function   287
Rafael V Mérula and Ivan O Haefliger

86 Deep Sclerectomy   295
Sylvain Roy and André Mermoud

   Spotlight: Deep Sclerectomy   304
   Yury S Astakhov and Sergey Yu Astakhov

87 Viscocanalostomy   307
Roberto G Carassa

CONTENTS

Spotlight: Nonpenetrating Surgery: Evolution in Technique 312
Richard A Lewis

88 Complications of Nonpenetrating Glaucoma Surgery 315
Juan R Sampaolesi

89 Postoperative Management of Nonpenetrating Glaucoma Surgery 327
Corinne C Schnyder

90 Results 337
Daniel E Grigera, Jorge Acosta, and Virginia E Zanutigh

Section 13 Management of Coexisting Cataract and Glaucoma

91 Cataract Surgery in Patients with Functioning Filtering Blebs 349
Franz Grehn and Thomas Klink

92 One-site Combined Surgery/Two-site Combined Surgery 355
Yvonne M Buys

93 Combined Cataract Extraction and Glaucoma Drainage Implant Surgery 365
Vital P Costa

94 Combined Cataract and Nonpenetrating Glaucoma Surgery 369
Gema Rebolleda, Francisco J Muñoz-Negrete, and Javier Moreno-Montañes

95 Goniosynechialysis 383
Chaiwat Teekhasaenee

Section 14 Drainage Devices

96 Preoperative Evaluation of Patients Undergoing Drainage Implant Surgery 391
Jeffrey Freedman

97 Aqueous Shunts: Choice of Implant 395
Keith Barton and Dale K Heuer

98 Surgical Technique 1 (Molteno Glaucoma Implant) 403
Andrew M Thompson, Tui H Bevin, and Anthony CB Molteno

99 Surgical Technique 2 (Baerveldt Glaucoma Implant) 417
George Baerveldt

Spotlight: Anesthetic Considerations 422
Don Minckler

Spotlight: Operative Techniques and Potential Modifications 422
Don Minckler

100 Surgical Technique 3 (Ahmed Glaucoma Valve Drainage Implant) 425
John W Boyle IV and Peter A Netland

101 Other Glaucoma Implants 437
Remo Susanna, Mirko Babic, and Roberto M Vessani

102 Intraoperative Complications 445
Steven H McKinley, Peter T Chang, and Ronald L Gross

103 Postoperative Complications 453
Yara Paula Martin Catoira-Boyle, Darrell WuDunn, and Louis B Cantor

104 Results 467
Oscar Albis-Donado

105 Aqueous Shunts after Retinal Surgery 473
Maria Papadopoulos and Keith Barton

106 Aqueous Shunts and Penetrating Keratoplasty 483
Don Minckler

Section 15 Surgery for Congenital Glaucoma

107 Goniotomy and Trabeculotomy 493
Maria Papadopoulos and Peng Tee Khaw

108 Further Surgical Options in Children 501
Mark Werner and Alana Grajewski

Section 16 Modulation of Wound Healing

109 Indications 519
Arvind Neelakantan and Richard K Parrish II

110 Choice of Antifibrosis Therapies 525
Antoine Labbé and Christophe Baudouin

111 Technique 537
Ann Caroline Fisher, Amish Doshi, and Kuldev Singh

112 Complications Associated with Modulation of Wound Healing in Glaucoma Surgery 543
Herbert Fechter and Francisco Fantes

113 Biological Drivers of Postoperative Scarring 557
Sonal S Tuli, Douglas Esson, Mark B Sherwood, and Gregory S Schultz

114 Future Strategies 565
Peng Tee Khaw, Stelios Georgoulas, Annegret H Dahlmann, Qian Ru, Belen Martin and Stephen Brocchini

Section 17 Cyclodestructive Procedures

115 Cyclodestructive Techniques 577
Philip A Bloom, Anil K Negi

Spotlight: Cyclodestructive Procedures 578
Stephen A Vernon

Spotlight: Anesthetic Considerations 579
Stephen A Vernon

Spotlight: Operative Techniques 581
David Broadway

Spotlight: Operative Techniques 581
Jeremy Diamond

Spotlight: Postoperative Management and Interventions 582
David Broadway

Spotlight: Re-Treatment and Further
Postoperative Care   582
Stephen A Vernon

116 Complications of Cyclodestructive
Procedures   587
Malik Y Kahook and Joel S Schuman

117 Endophotocoagulation   591
Stanley J Berke

Section 18   New Procedures

118 New Procedures   601
Mark B Sherwood and Tarek M Shaarawy

Index   *611*

FOREWORD

In spite of the widespread use of the internet, there seems to be a need for a book that reports on the current philosophy of glaucoma and explores the boundaries of its many subjects. The Editors, who are among the leaders in glaucoma field, have demonstrated their competence by choosing some of the best people to write the chapters for both volumes. This first volume deals with the non-surgical aspects of glaucoma. Reading some of the chapters, I was not surprised by the advances that have occurred since the last book of this kind was compiled. The chapter on the molecular biology of our genetic knowledge is a good example of the explosion of our knowledge, but we are not anywhere near the time when the genetics of the elevated intraocular pressure are known and we are quite in the dark of the genetics of the many other risk factors at play in this multifactorial disease. Quoting from the book 'It is now clear that glaucoma has wide genetic heterogeneity with no single gene accounting for all cases of any single glaucoma phenotype. In other words, alterations in different genes can lead to the same phenotype while in other cases variants in the same gene may lead to different phenotypes.' We are still far away 'from the time when it will be possible to predict at birth what ailments we are prone to and whether glaucoma is on the cards for the individual.'

We are also much more aware of geographical differences in the disease and of the economic imperatives which affect many aspects of the disease. The philosophy of screening, the pathogenesis of the diseases, the role of the vascular factors, the definition of the disease and its diagnosis, the ever more sophisticated diagnostic tools available, the many types of glaucoma and their managements as well as the medical agents are all included.

The recognition that there are risk factors, in addition to intraocular pressure, for the development of glaucoma and its progression have not yet fully found their way into clinical practice. We remain surprised when patients with major reduction of their IOP either continue to progress or start to progress again later in their lives. I know that under these circumstances the further reduction of the pressure in the eye is usually contemplated before considering whether there are other risk factors responsible for the progression. It is often stated, that nothing can be done about these other, non pressure, risk factors. Some of these other risk factors can be controlled or treated at present providing they are looked for and recognized. We do not have evidence-based knowledge that their control and treatment favourably affects the disease. If we channeled a fraction of our effort and resources to the entire disease, instead of channeling them almost entirely to IOP and its control, rapid progress would be made.

Both of the controlled clinical trials, CNTGS and EMGT, which followed, for the first time, untreated glaucoma patients over fairly long periods of time make it clear that the course of untreated glaucoma is variable. Half of the untreated newly diagnosed patients with NTG showed no progression over a 5- to 8-year period. In the EMGT in patients with IOPs between 21 and 30 mmHg the number of untreated patients who did not progress was still 20%. It is not difficult to identify those patients in whom the disease progresses rapidly which would endanger their future visual well being. They clearly require appropriate treatment. On the other hand those in whom we can not identify current progression or find progression which is so slow as not to endanger their visual competence in their predicted life span probably require a different management. This is not currently widely practiced even though the information from the CNTGS and the EMGT have been in the public domain for quite a long time.

One of my former fellows often said 'everybody writes but nobody reads'. While this is an amusing exaggeration I know that this comprehensive book will deserve to be read widely.

Stephen M Drance, OC MD
Vancouver, April 2007

PREFACE

Glaucoma has been chosen as the title of this two volume book in order to emphasize the remit of the authors. In choosing this title we are mindful for earlier books bearing the same or similar name. In 1951 H Saul Sugar wrote 'The Glaucomas' a textbook devoted entirely to this subspecialty. In 1989 Ritch, Shields and Krupin co-authored a three volume text of the same name that brought our knowledge of the subspecialty up to date. With the second edition in 1996 they further collected together our knowledge under 'one roof'. Although there have also been excellent single volume texts (for example Kanski and Salmon (2003) and Shields' Textbook of Glaucoma (2004) they have been as single volumes less comprehensive and with recent advances in this field can also be said to be less than up to date.

We felt therefore that the time was right for an update of our knowledge about Glaucoma. There have been significant changes in medical, surgical and laser treatment, new knowledge about intraocular pressure, its measurement fluctuation and targets, as well as updated methods of analysing the anterior and posterior segment, both for diagnosis and for follow-up. Our knowledge about the paediatric and the secondary glaucomas has greatly increased, and we have had the benefit of long-term analysis of the two treatments and other long-term trials and surveys.

In 35 chapters we have looked at glaucoma from these points of view together with writers capable of providing the reader with individual texts (cross referenced where necessary) that give state of the art information. In many instances we have commissioned additional writers to create short essays (spotlights) highlighting one or more of the points made in the chapter.

Ophthalmology is a visual discipline, with diagnosis and management relying heavily on observed and measured change. The book recognises this, and is profusely illustrated, with the surgical chapters having the additional benefit of video clips used to emphasize technique.

Glaucoma is a global problem within our speciality; causes, diagnostic procedures and management possibilities vary considerably form continent to continent. We have recognised this, both by identifying regional and national differences in diagnosis and prevalence, but also in therapeutic possibilities. Even if a particular approach is not correct or even possible for the part of the world where you practice, there is always something to be learned by seeing how others address a particular problem.

As authors and with editorial responsibility, it has been our challenge to ensure conformity throughout the two volumes of this text. We acknowledge this responsibility; if you, the reader, feel that we have failed in that respect we would value feedback on this and any other quality aspects of the book. Our task in this regard has been greatly helped by Russell Gabbedy and Sven Pinczewski of Elsevier who have guided, encouraged and just occasionally harried us during the whole process. We are in their debt.

Tarek M Shaarawy
Mark B Sherwood
Roger A Hitchings
Jonathan G Crowston
2009

LIST OF CONTRIBUTORS

Jorge Acosta MD
Assistant Professor of Ophthalmology
University of CEMIC
Head, Ophthalmology Service
Hospital Rivadavia
Buenos Aires
Argentina

Oscar Albis-Donado MD
Assistant Professor of Glaucoma
Asociación Para Evitar la Ceguera en
Mexico
Universidad Nacional Autonoma de
Mexico
Coyoacan
Mexico DF
Mexico

Luciana M Alencar MD
Postdoctoral Fellow
Hamilton Glaucoma Center
Department of Ophthalmology
University of California San Diego
La Jolla CA, USA
and Glaucoma Unit
Department of Ophthalmology
University of São Paulo
São Paulo
Brazil

R Rand Allingham MD
Professor of Ophthalmology
Director, Glaucoma Service
Department of Ophthalmology
Duke University Eye Center
Durham NC
USA

**Nitin Anand MBBS MD (Ophth)
FRCSEd FRCOphth**
Glaucoma Specialist
Department of Ophthalmology
Calderdale and Huddersfield Royal
Infirmaries
Halifax
UK

Ijeoma M Asota MD
Post Doctoral Research Fellow
Department of Ophthalmology
Emory University
Atlanta GA
USA

Sergey Yu Astakhov MD
I P Pavlov Medical University
St Petersburg
Russia

Yury S Astakhov MD PhD
I P Pavlov Medical University
St Petersburg
Russia

Mirko Babic MD
Clinical and Research Fellow
Glaucoma Service
Department of Ophthalmology
University of São Paulo
São Paulo
Brazil

George Baerveldt MD
Irving H Leopold Professor and Chair
The Gavin S Herbert Eye Institute
University of California, Irvine
Irvine CA
USA

Rajendra K Bansal MD
Associate Clinical Professor of
Ophthalmology
Department of Ophthalmology
Columbia University Medical Center
New York NY
USA

**Keith Barton MD FRCP FRCS
FRCOphth**
Consultant Ophthalmologist
Glaucoma Service Director
Moorfields Eye Hospital NHS
Foundation Trust
London
UK

Christophe Baudouin MD PhD
Professor of Ophthalmology
Head, Department of Ophthalmology
III
Director, Laboratory of Ocular and
ImmunoPathology, Vision Institute
Quinze-Vingts National
Ophthalmology Hospital
University Paris 6, Pierre et Marie
Curie
Paris
France

Sheila Bazzaz MD
Clinical Fellow
Glaucoma Service
Wills Eye Institute
Philadelphia PA
USA

Allen Beck MD
Associate Professor
Department of Ophthalmology
Emory University
Atlanta GA
USA

Sonya L Bennett MBChB
Glaucoma Research Unit
Moorfields Eye Hospital
London
UK

Stanley J Berke MD FACS
Associate Clinical Professor of
Ophthalmology and Visual Sciences
Albert Einstein College of Medicine
Chief, Glaucoma Service
Nassau University Medical Center
Ophthalmic Consultants of Long
Island
Lynbrook NY
USA

Michael S Berlin MD
Director, Glaucoma Institute of
Beverly Hills
Professor of Clinical Ophthamology
Jules Stein Eye Institute–UCLA
Los Angeles
USA

Tui H Bevin MPH
Assistant Research Fellow in
Ophthalmology
Ophthalmology Section, Medical and
Surgical Sciences Department
University of Otago
Dunedin School of Medicine
Dunedin
New Zealand

**Philip A Bloom MBChB FRCS
FRCOphth**
Honorary Professor of Ophthalmology
Middlesex University
Honorary Senior Lecturer, Imperial
College
St Mary's, The Western Eye Hospital
London
UK

Kathryn E Bollinger
Glaucoma Fellow
Cole Eye Institute
Cleveland OH
USA

Christopher Bowd PhD
Associate Research Scientist
Hamilton Glaucoma Center
Department of Ophthalmology
University of California San Diego
La Jolla CA
USA

John W Boyle IV MD
Instructor
Department of Ophthalmology
Hamilton Eye Institute
University of Tennessee Health
Science Center
Memphis TN
USA

James D Brandt MD
Professor and Director, Glaucoma
Service
Department of Ophthalmology and
Vision Science
University of California, Davis
Sacramento CA
USA

**David C Broadway MBBS MD
FRCOphth DO (RCS)**
Consultant Ophthalmic Surgeon and
Honorary Senior Lecturer
Department of Ophthalmology
Norfolk and Norwich University
Hospital
University of East Anglia
Norwich
Norfolk
UK

Stephen Brocchini PhD
Professor of Pharmacology
The School of Pharmacy
University of London
National Institutes of Health Research
Biomedical Research Centre
Moorfields Eye Hospital and UCL
Institute of Ophthalmology
London
UK

Alain M Bron MD
Professor of Ophthalmology
Department of Ophthalmology
University Hospital
Dijon
France

Donald L Budenz MD MPH
Professor
Department of Ophthalmology,
Epidemiology, and Public Health
Bascom Palmer Eye Institute
Miller School of Medicine
University of Miami
Miami FL
USA

Natalie D Bull PhD
Research Associate
Centre for Brain Repair
University of Cambridge
Cambridge
UK

Catey Bunce MSc DSc
Research and Development
Moorfields Eye Hospital NHS
Foundation Trust
London
UK

Claude F Burgoyne
Van Buskirk Chair for Ophthalmic
Research
Senior Scientist and Research Director
Optic Nerve Head Research
Laboratory
Devers Eye Institute
Portland OR
USA

Yvonne M Buys MD FRCSC
Associate Professor
Department of Ophthalmology
University of Toronto
Toronto ON
Canada

Louis B Cantor MD
Chairman and Professor of
Ophthalmology
Jay C and Lucile L Kahn Professor of
Glaucoma Research and Education
Director of Glaucoma Service
Eugene and Marilyn Glick Eye
Institute
Department of Ophthalmology
Indiana University School of
Medicine
Indianapolis IN
USA

Joseph Caprioli MD
David May II Professor of
Ophthalmology
Chief, Glaucoma Division
Director, Glaucoma Basic Science and
Clinical Laboratories
Jules Stein Eye Institute
University of California, Los Angeles
Los Angeles CA
USA

Roberto G Carassa MD
Associate Professor
Head, Glaucoma Service
Ophthalmology Unit
University Hospital San Raffaele
Milano
Italy

Daniel S Casper MD PhD
Associate Clinical Professor of
Ophthalmology
College of Physicians and Surgeons
Columbia University
New York NY
USA

Yara PM Catoira-Boyle MD
Assistant Professor of Clinical
Ophthalmology
Department of Ophthalmology
Indiana University School of
Medicine
Indianapolis IN
USA

Piero Ceruti MD
Eye Clinic
Department of Neurological and
Visual Sciences
University of Verona
Verona
Italy

Debasis Chakrabarti MD
Consultant
Glaucoma Services
Rotary Narayana Nethralaya
Kolkata
India

Raka (Chatterjee) Chakrabarti MD
Consultant Glaucoma Specialist
Susrut Eye Hospital and Research
Centre
Kolkata
India

Pratap Challa MD
Assistant Professor of Ophthalmology
Director of Residency Training
Programme
Department of Ophthalmology
Duke University
Durham NC
USA

Peter T Chang MD
Assistant Professor of Ophthalmology
Cullen Eye Institute
Baylor College of Medicine
Houston TX
USA

Mark Y-M Chiang MBBS
Birmingham and Midland Eye Centre
Good Hope Hospital NHS Trust
Birmingham
UK

Neil T Choplin MD
Captain (Retired)
Medical Corps, United States Navy
Adjunct Clinical Professor of Surgery
Uniformed Services University of
Health Sciences
Glaucoma Specialist
Eye Care of San Diego
San Diego CA
USA

George A Cioffi MD
Chairman of Ophthalmology
Devers Eye Institute, Legacy Health
System
Professor of Ophthalmology
Oregon Health and Sciences
University
Portland OR
USA

Anne L Coleman MD PhD
Frances and Ray Stark Professor of
Ophthalmology
Jules Stein Eye Institute
David Geffen School of Medicine
University of California, Los Angeles
Los Angeles CA
USA

Nathan G Congdon MD MPH
Professor of Ophthalmology and
Public Health
Chinese University of Hong Kong
and Professor
Joint Shantou International Eye
Center
Shantou
China

Michael A Coote MBBS FRANZCO
Centre for Eye Research Australia
University of Melbourne
Consultant, Glaucoma Investigation
and Research Unit
Royal Victoria Eye and Ear Hospital
East Melbourne
Australia

Vital P Costa MD
Director, Glaucoma Service
Associate Professor of Ophthalmology
Department of Ophthalmology
University of Campinas
São Paulo
Brazil

David P Crabb MSc PhD
Reader in Statistics and Measurement
in Vision
Department of Optometry and Visual
Science
City University
London
UK

E Randy Craven MD
Director, Glaucoma Consultants of
Colorado, PC
Denver
and Associate Clinical Professor
University of Colorado Health
Sciences Center
Aurora CO
USA

**Jonathan G Crowston PhD
FRCOphth FRANZCO**
Professor
Department of Ophthalmology
University of Melbourne
Centre for Eye Research Australia
Royal Victorian Eye & Ear Hospital
East Melbourne
Australia

Elie Dahan MD MMedOphth
Senior Lecturer
Consultant, Glaucoma and Pediatric
Ophthalmology
Eintal Eye Institute
Tel Aviv
Israel

**Annegret H Dahlmann-Noor Dr med
PhD FRCOphth FRCS(Ed) DipMedEd**
Senior Clinical Research Associate
Ocular Repair and Regeneration
Biology
Institute of Ophthalmology
London
UK

Ricardo de Lima MD
Asociacion Para Evitar La Ceguera en
Mexico
Coyoacan
Mexico City
Mexico

**Jeremy P Diamond MBBCh FRSC
FRCOphth PhD**
Consultant Ophthalmic Surgeon
Bristol Eye Hospital
Bristol
UK

Syril K Dorairaj MD
Glaucoma Associates of New York
The New York Eye and Ear Infirmary
Department of Surgery
Beth Israel Medical Center
New York NY
USA

Amish Doshi MD AB
Fellow
Department of Ophthalmology
Hamilton Glaucoma Center
University of California San Diego
La Jolla CA
USA

J Crawford Downs PhD
Associate Scientist
Director, Ocular Biomechanics
Laboratory
Devers Eye Institute
Portland OR
USA

Mohammed K El Mallah MD
Clinical Associate in Glaucoma
Department of Ophthalmology
Duke University Medical Center
Durham NC
USA

Fathi F ElSayyad FRCSEd FRCOphth
Director of ElSayyad Eye Center
Professor of Ophthalmology
Misr University for Science and
Technology
Cairo
Egypt

Douglas W Esson DVM DACVO
Ophthalmologist
Eye Care for Animals
Tustin CA
USA

Francisco Fantes MD
Professor of Clinical Ophthalmology
Bascom Palmer Eye Institute
University of Miami
Miami FL
USA

Herbert P Fechter III MD PE
Assistant Professor, Uniformed
Services University
Private Practice
Eye Physicians and Surgeons of Augusta
Augusta GA
USA

Robert D Fechtner MD
Professor of Ophthalmology
Institute of Ophthalmology and
Visual Science
New Jersey Medical School
University of Medicine and Dentistry,
New Jersey
Newark NJ
USA

Ronald L Fellman MD
Associate Clinical Professor of
Ophthalmology
University of Texas Health Science
Center
Glaucoma Associates of Texas
Dallas TX
USA

Arosha Fernando MRCOphth
Specialist Registrar
Moorfields Eye Hospital
London
UK

Ann Caroline Fisher MD
Clinical Instructor
Stanford University School of
Medicine
Pacific Eye Specialists
Daly City CA
USA

Frederick W Fitzke PhD
Professor of Visual Optics and
Psychophysics
Division of Visual Science
UCL Institute of Ophthalmology
University College London
London
UK

Josef Flammer MD
Professor
Head, Department of Ophthalmology
University Hospital Basel
Basel
Switzerland

Brad Fortune OD PhD
Associate Scientist
Discoveries in Sight Research
Laboratories
Devers Eye Institute
Portland OR
USA

**Paul J Foster BMedSci(Hons) BM
BS PhD FRCS (Ed)**
Senior Lecturer in Ophthalmic
Epidemiology
UCL Institute of Ophthalmology and
Glaucoma Service
Consultant Ophthalmologist
Moorfields Eye Hospital
London
UK

**Jeffrey Freedman MBBch PhD FCS
(SA) FRCSE**
Professor of Clinical Ophthalmology
Department of Ophthalmology
The State University of New York
Brooklyn NY
USA

Stefano A Gandolfi MD
Professor of Ophthalmology
Chairman, University Eye Clinic
Clinica Oculistica
Parma
Italy

**David (Ted) Garway-Heath MD
FRCOphth**
Honorary Visiting Professor,
City University, London
and Consultant Ophthalmologist
Moorfields Eye Hospital
London
UK

**Gus Gazzard MA MD MBBChir
FRCOphth**
Consultant Ophthalmic
Surgeon–Glaucoma
King's College Hospital
London
UK

Steven J Gedde MD
Professor of Ophthalmology
Residency Program Director
Bascom Palmer Eye Institute
University of Miami
Miller School of Medicine
Miami FL
USA

Stelios Georgoulas MD
London School of Pharmacy
Scholarship Research Fellow
The School of Pharmacy
University of London
Ocular Repair and Regeneration
Biology
Moorfields Eye Hospital and UCL
Institute of Ophthalmology
London
UK

**Ivan Goldberg MBBS (Syd)
FRANZCO FRACS**
Clinical Associate Professor
Department of Ophthalmology
University of Sydney
Head, Glaucoma Service
Sydney Eye Hospital
Sydney NSW
Australia

**Stuart L Graham MBBS MS PhD
FRANZCO**
Professor of Ophthalmology and
Visual Science
Australian School of Advanced
Medicine
Macquarie University
Sydney NSW
Australia

Alana Grajewski MD
Voluntary Associate Professor of
Ophthalmology
Bascom Palmer Eye Institute
University of Miami School of
Medicine
Miami FL
USA

David S Greenfield MD
Professor of Ophthalmology
Bascom Palmer Eye Institute
University of Miami Miller School of
Medicine
Palm Beach Gardens FL
USA

Franz Grehn MD
Professor and Chairman
Department of Ophthalmology
University Hospitals Würzburg
Würzburg
Germany

Daniel E Grigera MD
Assistant Professor of Ophthalmology
University del Salvador
Head, Glaucoma Unit
Hospital Oftalmológico Santa Lucía
Buenos Aires
Argentina

Ronald L Gross MD
Professor of Ophthalmology
The Clifton R McMichael Chair in
Ophthalmology
Cullen Eye Institute
Baylor College of Medicine
Houston TX
USA

Meenakashi Gupta MD
Glaucoma Service
Massachusetts Eye and Ear Infirmary
Harvard Medical School
Boston MA
USA

Ivan O Haefliger MD FEBO
Professor in Ophthalmology
Laboratory of Ocular Pharmacology
and Physiology
University Eye Clinic
Basel University
Basel
Switzerland

Ali S Hafez MD PhD
Assistant Clinical Professor of
Ophthalmology
University of Montreal
Montreal QC
Canada

**Matthew J Hawker BMedSci(Hons)
MBChB DM MRCOphth**
Specialist Registrar in
Ophthalmology
Department of Ophthalmology
Norfolk and Norwich University
Hospital
Norwich
Norfolk
UK

**Paul R Healey MBBS(Hons)
B(Med)Sc MMed PhD FRANZCO**
Director, Glaucoma Services
Western Sydney Eye Hospital
Clinical Senior Lecturer
Director of Glaucoma Research
University of Sydney
Centre for Vision Research
Westmead Hospital
Westmead NSW
Australia

Catherine J Heatley MRCOphth
Moorfields Eye Hospital
London
UK

Dale K Heuer MD
Professor and Chairman
Department of Ophthalmology
Medical College of Wisconsin
Director, Froedtert and the Medical
College of Wisconsin Eye Institute
Milwaukee WI
USA

Eve J Higginbotham MD
Dean and Senior Vice President for
Academic Affairs
Morehouse School of Medicine
Atlanta GA
USA

Roger A Hitchings FRCOphth
Professor of Glaucoma and Allied
Studies
Consultant Ophthalmologist
Glaucoma Unit
Moorfields Eye Hospital
London
UK

Gábor Holló MD PhD DSc
Associated Professor of
Ophthalmology
Department of Ophthalmology
Director, Glaucoma and Perimetry
Unit
Semmelweis University
Budapest
Hungary

Ann M Hoste MD
Department of Glaucoma
Goes Eye Center
Antwerp
Belgium

Camille Hylton MD
Assistant Professor
Emory University
Atlanta GA
USA

Thomas V Johnson BA
Centre for Brain Repair
University of Cambridge
Cambridge
UK

Jost B Jonas MD
Professor of Ophthalmology
Department of Ophthalmology
Medical Faculty Mannheim
Ruprecht-Karls-University
Heidelberg
Germany

Malik Y Kahook MD
Assistant Professor and Director of
Clinical Research
Department of Ophthalmology
Rocky Mountain Lions Eye Institute
University of Colorado Denver
Denver CO
USA

Michael A Kass MD
Professor and Head
Department of Ophthalmology and
Visual Sciences
Washington University School of
Medicine
St Louis MO
USA

L Jay Katz MD FACS
Professor, Jefferson Medical College
Director of Glaucoma Service and
Attending Surgeon
Wills Eye Institute
Philadelphia PA
USA

Jill E Keeffe OAM PhD
Professor, Head of Population Health
Unit
Department of Ophthalmology
University of Melbourne
Centre for Eye Research Australia
Royal Victorian Eye and Ear Hospital
Melbourne VIC
Australia

**Peng Tee Khaw PhD FRCP FRCS
FRCOphth FIBiol FRCPath FMedSci**
Director, National Institutes of
Health Research UK Biomedical
Research Centre
Ocular Repair and Regeneration
Biology Unit
Moorfields Eye Hospital and UCL
Institute of Ophthalmology
London
UK

Albert S Khouri MD
Institute of Ophthalmology and
Visual Science
New Jersey Medical School
University of Medicine and Dentistry,
New Jersey
Newark NJ
USA

Danny Kim MD
Chief Resident, Ophthalmology
Case Western Reserve University
Cleveland OH
USA

Thomas Klink Dr med.
Chief Surgeon
Eye Clinic
Würzburg University
Würzburg
Germany

Anastasios GP Konstas MD PhD
Associate Professor in Ophthalmology
Head of the Glaucoma Unit
Department of Ophthalmology
First University
AHEPA Hospital
Thessaloniki
Greece

Aachal Kotecha PhD
Lecturer, Department of Optometry
and Visual Science
City University, London
Senior Research Associate
NIHR Biomedical Research Centre
Moorfields Eye Hospital and UCL
Institute of Ophthalmology
London
UK

Theodore Krupin MD
Professor of Ophthalmology
Feinberg School of Medicine
Northwestern University
Chicago IL
USA

Avinash Kulkarni MBBS FRCSEd (Ophth)
Locum Consultant Ophthalmologist
Glaucoma Service
Moorfields Eye Hospital
London
UK

Antoine Labbé MD
Department of Ophthalmology III
Quinze-Vingts National
Ophthalmology Hospital
INSERM
Cordelier Biomedical Research Centre
University Paris V
Paris
France

Thad Labbe MD
Glaucoma Specialist
Eye Associates of Central Texas
(Private Practice)
Taylor TX
USA

Alan Lacey BSc
Department of Medical Illustration
Moorfields Eye Hospital
London
UK

Dennis SC Lam MD FRCOphth
Professor and Chairman
Department of Ophthalmology and
Visual Sciences
The Chinese University of Hong
Kong
Hong Kong Eye Hospital
Kowloon
Hong Kong SAR
China

Graham Lee MBBS (QLD) MMedSC FRANZCO
Associate Professor of Ophthalmology
University of Queensland
Visiting Surgeon, Queensland Eye
Institute
Brisbane QLD
Australia

Paul P Lee MD JD
James P Gills III, MD and Joy Gills
Professor of Ophthalmology
Department of Ophthalmology
Duke University
Durham NC
USA

Hans G Lemij MD PhD
The Rotterdam Eye Hospital
Rotterdam
Netherlands

S Fabian Lerner MD
Director, Glaucoma Section
Postgraduate Department
School of Medicine
University Favaloro
Buenos Aires
Argentina

Mark R Lesk MSc MD CM FRCS(C) DABO
Associate Professor of
Ophthalmology
University of Montreal
Director of Vision Health Research
Maisonneuve–Rosemont Hospital
Research Centre
Montreal QC
Canada

Leonard A Levin MD PhD
Canada Research Chair of
Ophthalmology and Visual Sciences
Department of Ophthalmology
University of Montreal
and Professor
Department of Ophthalmology and
Visual Sciences
University of Wisconsin
Madison WI
USA

Richard A Lewis MD
Grutzmacher and Lewis
Sacramento CA
USA

Paul R Lichter MD
F Bruce Fralick Professor of
Ophthalmology
Chair, Ophthalmology and Visual
Sciences
Director, University of Michigan
Kellog Eye Center
Ann Arbor MI
USA

Jeffrey M Liebmann MD
Clinical Professor of Ophthalmology
New York University School of
Medicine
Director, Glaucoma Services
Manhattan Eye, Ear and Throat
Hospital and
New York University Medical Center
New York NY
USA

K Sheng Lim MD
Consultant
Clinical Lead for Glaucoma Service
Department of Ophthalmology
St Thomas' Hospital
London
UK

Ridia Lim MBBS MPH FRANZCO
Ophthalmic Surgeon
Glaucoma Service
Sydney Eye Hospital
Sydney NSW
Australia

Sancy Low MBBS MRCOphth
Clinical Research Fellow
Division of Epidemiology and
Genetics
UCL Institute of Ophthalmology and
Glaucoma Service
Moorfields Eye Hospital
London
UK

Anil K Mandal MD
Director, Jasti V Ramanamma
Children's Eye Care Centre
Consultant, VST Centre for
Glaucoma Care
LV Prasad Eye Institute
LV Prasad Marg
Banjara Hills
Hyderabad AP
India

Giorgio Marchini MD
Professor of Ophthalmology
Head of the Eye Clinic
Department of Neurological and
Visual Sciences
University of Verona
Verona
Italy

Belen Martin PhD
Visiting Research Fellow
ORB Ocular Repair and Regeneration
Biology
UCL Institute of Ophthalmology and
Moorfields Eye Hospital
London
UK

**Keith R Martin DM MRCP
FRCOphth**
Senior Lecturer and Consultant in
Ophthalmology
Centre for Brain Repair
University of Cambridge
Cambridge
UK

David B Matchar MD
Professor, Department of Medicine
Director, Duke Center for Clinical
Health Policy Research
Durham NC
USA

Steven H McKinley MD
Glaucoma Section
Cullen Eye Institute
Baylor College of Medicine
Houston TX
USA

Stuart J McKinnon MD PhD
Associate Professor of Ophthalmology
and Neurobiology
Duke University Medical Center
Durham NC
USA

Felipe A Medeiros MD PhD
Associate Professor of
Ophthalmology
Hamilton Glaucoma Center
Department of Ophthalmology
University of California San Diego
La Jolla CA
USA

André Mermoud MD
Director
Glaucoma Centre
Montchoisi Clinic
Lausanne
Switzerland

Rafael V Mérula MD
Member of Glaucoma Service of São
Geraldo Hospital
Department of Ophthalmology
Federal University of Minas Gerais
Belo Horizonte
Minas Gerais
Brazil

Toni T Meyers MD
Glaucoma Consultants of Colorado
Littleton CO
USA

**Clive S Migdal MD FRCS
FRCOphth**
Senior Consultant Ophthalmologist
Glaucoma Service
Western Eye Hospital
London
UK

Dimitrios G Mikropoulos MD
Associate Specialist
Glaucoma Unit
Department of Ophthalmology
First University
AHEPA Hospital
Thessaloniki
Greece

Don Minckler MD MS
Professor of Ophthalmology and
Pathology
University of California, Irvine
Irvine CA
USA

**Anthony CB Molteno MBChB
FRCS(Ed)**
Professor of Ophthalmology
Ophthalmology Section
Department of Medical and Surgical
Sciences
University of Otago Dunedin School
of Medicine
Dunedin
New Zealand

Paolo Mora MD
Assistant Professor of Ophthalmology
Eye Imaging Unit, University Eye
Clinic
University Hospital
Parma
Italy

Javier Moreno-Montañés MD PhD
Department of Ophthalmology
Clínica Universitaria de Navarra
Pamplona
Spain

James E Morgan DPhil FRCOphth
Reader, Honorary Consultant
Department of Neurology and
Ophthalmology
University of Wales School of
Medicine
Cardiff University
Cardiff
UK

**Francisco J Muñoz-Negrete MD
PhD**
Hospital Ramón y Cajal
Glaucoma Unit
University of Alcala
Madrid
Spain

Jonathan S Myers MD
Associate Attending Surgeon
Wills Eye Institute
Philadelphia PA
USA

**Arvind Neelakantan MD
FRCOphth**
Glaucoma Associates of Texas
Assistant Clinical Professor of
Ophthalmology
University of Texas Southwestern
Medical Center
Dallas TX
USA

Anil K Negi MD FRCS FRCOphth
Consultant Ophthalmologist
Heart of England NHS Foundation
Trust
Birmingham
UK

Peter A Netland MD PhD
Siegal Professor of Ophthalmology
Director of Glaucoma, Academic
Vice-Chair
Department of Ophthalmology
Hamilton Eye Institute
University of Tennessee Health
Science Center
Memphis TN
USA

Marcelo T Nicolela MD FRCSC
Associate Professor of
Ophthalmology
Eye Care Center
Director of Fellowship Program
Department of Ophthalmology and
Visual Sciences
Dalhousie University
Halifax NS
Canada

Magdy A Nofal FRCSEd
Ophthalmic Surgeon
The Eye Surgery Unit
Torbay Hospital
Torquay
Devon
UK

Winifred Nolan MD FRCOphth
Consultant Ophthalmologist
Birmingham and Midland Eye Centre
Birmingham
UK

Baha' N Noureddin MD FACS
Professor and Chairman
Department of Ophthalmology
American University of Beirut
Beirut
Lebanon

Maria Papadopoulos MBBS FRACO
Consultant Ophthalmic Surgeon
Glaucoma Service Training Director
Moorfields Eye Hospital
London
UK

Rajul S Parikh MD
Director
Glaucoma Service
Bombay City Eye Institute
Mumbai
India

Richard K Parrish II MD
Associate Dean for Graduate Medical
Education
University of Miami Miller School of
Medicine
Anne Bates Leach Eye Hospital
Miami FL
USA

Norbert Pfeiffer MD
Professor of Medicine
Director, University Eye Clinic
Mainz University
Mainz
Germany

Jody Piltz-Seymour MD
Director
Glaucoma Care Center, PC
Philadelphia PA
USA

Harry A Quigley MD
A Edward Maumenee Professor of
Ophthalmology
Director, Dana Center for
Preventative Ophthalmology
Director, Glaucoma Service
Johns Hopkins Hospital
Baltimore MD
USA

Carolyn D Quinn MD
Assistant Professor of Clinical
Ophthalmology
Bascom Palmer Eye Institute
University of Miami Miller School of
Medicine
Palm Beach Gardens FL
USA

Pradeep Y Ramulu MD PhD
Assistant Professor of Ophthalmology
Wilmer Eye Institute
Johns Hopkins University
Baltimore MD
USA

Anthony Realini MD
Associate Professor of
Ophthalmology
West Virginia University Eye Institute
Morgantown WV
USA

Gema Rebolleda MD PhD
Professor of Ophthalmology
Alcala de Henares University
Hospital Ramon Y Cajal
Madrid
Spain

Nicolaas J Reus MD PhD
Glaucoma Service
Rotterdam Eye Hospital
Rotterdam
Netherlands

Adam C Reynolds MD
Intermountain Eye and Laser Centers
Boise ID
USA

Douglas J Rhee MD
Assistant Professor of Ophthalmology
Harvard Medical School
Massachusetts Eye and Ear Infirmary
Boston MA
USA

Robert Ritch MD
Shelley and Steven Einhorn
Distinguished Chair in
Ophthalmology
Professor of Clinical Ophthalmology
Chief, Glaucoma Services
Surgeon Director
Department of Ophthalmology
The New York Eye and Ear Infirmary
New York NY
USA

Cynthia J Roberts PhD
Professor and Martha G and
Milton Staub Chair for Research in
Ophthalmology
Departments of Ophthalmology and
Biomedical Engineering
The Ohio State University
Columbus OH
USA

Michael D Roberts PhD
Post Doctoral Research Fellow
Ocular Biomechanics Laboratory
Devers Eye Institute
Portland OR
USA

Alan L Robin MD
Professor of Ophthalmology
University of Maryland Department
of Ophthalmology
Associate Professor of Ophthalmology
Wilmer Institute, John Hopkins
University
Associate Professor of International
Health
Bloomberg School of Public Health
Baltimore MD
USA

Prin RojanaPongpun MD
Associate Professor of Ophthalmology
Department of Ophthalmology
Chulalongkorn University and
Hospital
Bangkok
Thailand

Sylvain Roy MD PhD
Senior Scientist
Glaucoma Unit
Jules Gonin Eye Hospital
University of Lausanne
Lausanne
Switzerland

Qian Ru
Dorothy Hodgkins PhD Student
ORB Ocular Repair and Regeneration
Biology
UCL Institute of Ophthalmology and
Moorfields Eye Hospital
London
UK

**John F Salmon MD FRCS
FRCOphth**
Consultant Ophthalmologist
Oxford Eye Hospital
Oxford Radcliffe NHS Trust
Honorary Senior Lecturer
Oxford University
Oxford
UK

Juan Roberto Sampaolesi MD
Professor, Department of
Ophthalmology
UCES University
Centro Oftalmológico Sampaolesi
Buenos Aires
Argentina

Chiara Sangermani MD
Glaucoma Clinic
University Eye Clinic
University Hospital
Parma
Italy

Usman A Sarodia FRCOphth
Glaucoma Service
Moorfields Eye Hospital
London
UK

Ursula Schlötzer-Schrehardt PhD
Professor
Department of Ophthalmology
Universität Erlangen-Nürnberg
Erlangen
Germany

Corinne C Schnyder MD
Adjunct Lecturer and Assistant
Professor
Resident
Department of Ophthalmology
University of Lausanne
Jules Gonin Hospital
Lausanne
Switzerland

Gregory S Schultz PhD
Professor of Obstetrics and
Gynecology, Biochemistry and
Ophthalmology
Institute for Wound Research
University of Florida
Gainesville FL
USA

Joel S Schuman MD
Eye and Ear Foundation Professor and
Chairman
Department of Ophthalmology
University of Pittsburgh School of
Medicine
Pittsburgh PA
USA

Gail F Schwartz MD
Assistant Professor
Wilmer Eye Institute
Johns Hopkins University
Glaucoma Consultants
Greater Baltimore Medical Center
Baltimore MD
USA

Tarek M Shaarawy MD MSc
Consultant Ophthalmologist and Head
Glaucoma Sector, Ophthalmology
Service
Department of Clinical Neurosciences
University Geneva
Geneva
Switzerland

Peter Shah MBChB FRCOphth
Professor of Glaucoma
Consultant Ophthalmic Surgeon
Birmingham and Midland Eye Centre
Good Hope Hospital NHS Trust
Birmingham
UK

Clinton W Sheets MD
Department of Ophthalmology
University of Florida
Gainesville FL
USA

Mark B Sherwood FRCP FRCOphth
Daniels Professor
Departments of Ophthalmology and
Cell Biology
Director of Vision Research Center
University of Florida
Gainesville FL
USA

Lineu Oto Shiroma MD
Glaucoma Service
Sadalla Amin Ghanem Eye Hospital
Joinville SC
Brazil

Lesya M Shuba MD PhD FRCSC
Assistant Professor
Department of Ophthalmology and
Visual Sciences
Dalhousie University
Halifax NS
Canada

Annapurna Singh MD
Assistant Professor of Ophthalmology
Case Western Reserve University
Cleveland OH
USA

Arun D Singh MD
Director
Department of Ophthalmic Oncology
Cole Eye Institute and Taussing
Cancer Center
Cleveland Clinic Foundation
Cleveland OH
USA

Kuldev Singh MD MPH
Professor of Ophthalmology
Director, Glaucoma Service
Stanford University School of
Medicine
Stanford CA
USA

George L Spaeth MD FACS
Louis Esposito Research Professor
Emeritus Director of the William &
Anna Goldberg Glaucoma Service
Wills Eye Institute
Jefferson Medical College
Philadelphia PA
USA

**Alexander Spratt MBBCh
MRCOphth**
Clinical Research Fellow
Glaucoma Research Unit
Moorfields Eye Hospital
London
UK

Ingeborg Stalmans MD PhD
Professor of Ophthalmology
Department of Ophthalmology
University Hospitals Leuven
Leuven
Belgium

Robert L Stamper MD
Professor and Director of Glaucoma
Service
Department of Ophthalmology
University of California, San Francisco
School of Medicine
San Francisco CA
USA

William C Stewart MD
Clinical Professor of Ophthalmology
University of South Carolina School
of Medicine
Columbia SC
USA

Remo Susanna Jr MD
Associated Professor and Chief,
Glaucoma Service
Department of Ophthalmology
University of São Paulo
São Paulo
Brazil

Ernst R Tamm MD
Professor and Chairman
Institute of Human Anatomy and
Embryology
University of Regensburg
Regensburg
Germany

Angelo P Tanna MD
Assistant Professor of Ophthalmology
Director, Glaucoma Service
Feinberg School of Medicine
Northwestern University
Chicago IL
USA

Chaiwat Teekhasaenee MD
Associate Professor of
Ophthalmology
Glaucoma Service, Department of
Ophthalmology
Ramatibodhi Hospital
Bangkok
Thailand

Celso Tello MD
Einhorn Clinical Research Center
New York Eye and Ear Infirmary
New York
Associate Professor of Ophthalmology
New York Medical College
Valhalla NY
USA

Clement CY Tham FRCS FRCOphth
Professor
Department of Ophthalmology and
Visual Science
The Chinese University of
Hong Kong
Hong Kong Eye Hospital
Kowloon
Hong Kong SAR
China

Hagen Thieme MD PhD
Senior Consultant
Assistant Professor
University Eye Clinic
Mainz
Germany

Ravi Thomas MD
Professor
Director of Glaucoma Service
Queensland Eye Institute
Brisbane QLD
Australia

**Andrew M Thompson
BPharm(Hons) MB ChB FRANZCO**
Glaucoma Fellow
Ophthalmology Section
Department of Medical and Surgical
Sciences
University of Otago
Dunedin School of Medicine
Dunedin
New Zealand

Ravilla D Thulasiraj MBA
Executive Director
LAICO – Aravind Eye Care System
Anna Nagar, Madurai
Tamilnadu
India

John Thygesen MD
Director of Glaucoma Services
Associate Professor
Department of Ophthalmology
Copenhagen
Denmark

Karim Tomey MD FACS FRCOphth
Consultant Ophthalmologist,
Glaucoma Specialist
Beirut Eye Specialist Center
Rizk Hospital
Beirut
Lebanon

Carol B Toris PhD
Professor, Director of Glaucoma
Research
Department of Ophthalmology and
Visual Sciences
University of Nebraska Medical
Center
Omaha NE
USA

Roberto Tosi MD
Eye Clinic
Department of Neurological and
Visual Sciences
University of Verona
Verona
Italy

James C Tsai MD
Robert R Young Professor and
Chairman
Department of Ophthalmology and
Visual Science
Yale University School of Medicine
Chief of Ophthalmology
Yale-New Haven Hospital
New Haven CT
USA

Sonal S Tuli MD
Program Director
Director Cornea and External
Diseases
Department of Ophthalmology
University of Florida
Gainesville FL
USA

Anja Tuulonen MD PhD
Professor of Ophthalmology
Institute of Clinical
Medicine/Ophthalmology
University of Oulu, Finland
Clinic Head (Ophthalmology)
Northern Ostrobothnian Hospital
District
Oulu, Finland
Tampere School of Public Health
University of Tampere
Tampere
Finland

Tara A Uhler MD
Director of Resident Education
Wills Eye Residency Program at
Jefferson
Assistant Professor of
Ophthalmology
Jefferson Medical College of Thomas
Jefferson University
Philadelphia PA
USA

Nicola Ungaro MD
Director
Glaucoma Clinic
University Eye Clinic
Parma
Italy

E Michael Van Buskirk MD
Clinical Professor of Ophthalmology
Devers Eye Institute, Legacy Health
System
Oregon Health and Sciences
University
Portland OR
USA

Leonieke ME van Koolwijk MD
Glaucoma Service
The Rotterdam Eye Hospital
Rotterdam
Netherlands

**Stephen A Vernon DM FRCS
FRCOphth DO**
Directorate of Ophthalmology
Queens Medical Centre
University Hospital
Nottingham
UK

Roberto M Vessani MD
Assistant Professor
Glaucoma Service
Department of Ophthalmology
University of São Paulo
São Paulo
Brazil

Ananth C Viswanathan MBBS FRCOphth MD
Consultant Surgeon, Moorfields Eye Hospital
Honorary Visiting Professor, City University
Honorary Senior Lecturer, Institute of Ophthalmology
London
UK

Robert Weinreb MD
Distinguished Professor of Ophthalmology
Department of Ophthalmology
Director, Hamilton Glaucoma Center
University of California, San Diego
La Jolla CA
USA

Anthony Wells MBChB FRANZCO
Consultant Ophthalmologist
Capital Eye Specialists
Wellington
New Zealand

Mark Werner MD
Voluntary Assistant Professor of Ophthalmology
Bascom Palmer Eye Institute
University of Miami
Miller School of Medicine
Miami FL
USA

Boateng Wiafe MD MSc
Ophthalmic Surgeon
Regional Eye Care Advisor for sub-Saharan Africa
Operation Eyesight Universal
Accra
Ghana

Jacob T Wilensky MD
Professor of Ophthalmology
Director, Glaucoma Service
University of Illinois, College of Medicine
Chicago IL
USA

Bettina K Windisch MD
Department of Ophthalmology and Visual Sciences
Dalhousie University
Halifax NS
Canada

Tina Wong FRCOphth FRCSEd PhD
Singapore National Eye Centre
Singapore Eye Research in Institute
Singapore

Darrell WuDunn MD PhD
Associate Professor of Ophthalmology
Indiana University School of Medicine
Indianapolis IN
USA

Jennifer LY Yip MRCOphth
Clinical Research Fellow
International Centre for Eye Health
London School of Hygiene and Tropical Medicine
London
UK

Linda M Zangwill MD
Professor
Hamilton Glaucoma Center
Department of Ophthalmology
University of California, San Diego
La Jolla CA
USA

Virginia E Zanutigh MD PhD
Chairman, Department of Glaucoma
Ophthalmology Center, Quilmes
Quilmes, Buenos Aires
Argentina

Thierry Zeyen MD PhD
Professor of Ophthalmology
Department of Ophthalmology
University Hospital St. Rafael
Leuven
Belgium

Thom J Zimmerman MD PhD
Chairman
Ophthalmology and Visual Sciences
University of Louisville
Louisville KY
USA

ACKNOWLEDGEMENTS

A book of this magnitude is in fact the fruit of the collective knowledge of its writers, all 234 of them, and thus carries between its pages part of their minds and souls. The editors have sought no less than the best in their fields and required nothing short of their utmost input. And we freely acknowledge that that is exactly what we got. Every contributor in this book has strived to pass along his knowledge to others and has done so diligently and patiently, and to all of them we owe loads of gratitude and appreciation.

Thanks are also due to Prof S Drance for accepting to write the Foreword. A book on glaucoma cannot ask for a better Foreword or aspire to have a more distinguished writer.

We are personally grateful to our publishing editors for making this book a reality. Geoffrey Greenwood who worked hard with us in developing the initial concept, Russell Gabbedy, our Commissioning Editor, who has steadfastly steered the book to timely completion, and to Sven Pinczewski, Senior Development Editor, whose support and thorough professionalism, made our job much easier and more enjoyable.

One of the few remaining pleasures of working in academia is the ability to share your professional life surrounded by brilliant minds from several generations. Credit is due to our colleagues, our staff members and our assistants for many years of support and encouragement.

Groucho Marx once said "outside of a dog, a book is a man's best friend. Inside of a dog it's too dark to read." We sincerely hope that in this book you will find a friend, a companion and a trustworthy ally in your professional life.

CONTRIBUTORS LOCATIONS

Glaucoma is a collaborative effort drawing on the expertise of 220 contributors in 28 countries across 6 continents.

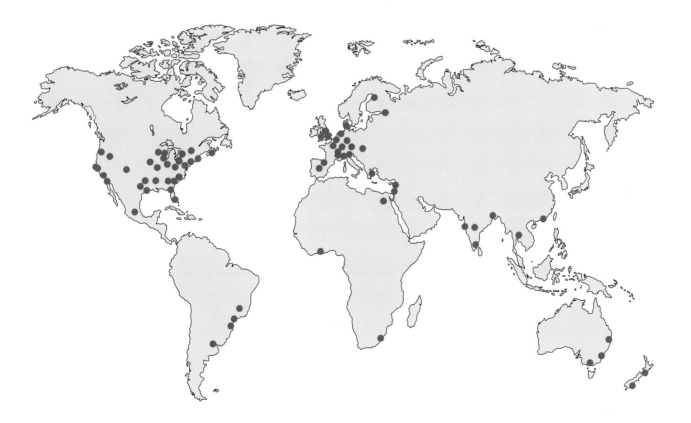

DEDICATION

This book is dedicated to a large group of people

To our Parents

*Samia Nada, Mounir Shaarawy, Gerald and Sylvia Sherwood,
Mary and Alan Hitchings, Barry and Glenda Crowston*

To our Wives

Ghada, Ruth, Virmati and Joanna

To our Children

*Hussein and Lana, Adam and Eliana, Anata and Samantha,
James and Zoe*

*Also to our mentors and teachers, colleagues and friends,
many of whom have kindly contributed to this work*

*And above all else it is dedicated to our patients who have
been a source of joy, inspiration and knowledge to all of us*

Tarek, Mark, Roger and Jonathan

THE EDITORS

TAREK M SHAARAWY

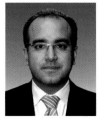

Is the Head of the Glaucoma unit, and the Glaucoma surgery research group at the University of Geneva Hospitals. He obtained both his medical bachelor and Masters Degree in ophthalmology at the University of Cairo, and his Doctorate in Medicine degree from the University of Lausanne. He trained in ophthalmology at the Cairo Research Institute of Ophthalmology and completed two glaucoma fellowships at the Universities of Lausanne and Basel. He is currently the Secretary General of the International Society of Glaucoma surgery.

His main research interests are surgical techniques of Glaucoma surgery, normal pressure glaucoma, and glaucoma patterns of practice in developed and developing countries. He is the author and editor of five text books on Glaucoma, and more than 60 book chapters and publications in peer reviewed journals.

In addition to his glaucoma practice Tarek Shaarawy is active in a number of NGOs dealing with global prevention of blindness.

ROGER HITCHINGS

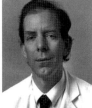

Is the IGA Professor of Ophthalmology and the senior glaucoma specialist at Moorfields Eye Hospital, London, England. He has particular interest in glaucoma surgery, imaging, Normal Tension Glaucoma and glaucoma genetics.

Roger Hitchings has authored and edited 3 books, 15 book chapters and over 240 peer-reviewed papers on glaucoma. He is currently Past President of the European Glaucoma Society. In addition to his glaucoma practice R A Hitchings is the R&D Director for Moorfields Eye Hospital, responsible for co-ordinating research between the Hospital and the Institute of Ophthalmology. He developed a national 5-year National Research Strategy for the Royal College of Ophthalmologists.

MARK B SHERWOOD

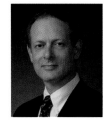

Is the Daniels Professor of Ophthalmology and Director of the Vision Research Center at the University of Florida. He trained in ophthalmology at Manchester University, St. Thomas' Hospital, London and at Moorfields Eye Hospital and completed glaucoma fellowships at Moorfields Eye Hospital, London and the Wills Eye Hospital, Philadelphia. He joined the faculty of the University of Florida in 1986 and was Chair of the Department of Ophthalmology between 1994 and 2004. He has authored and edited 4 books, 8 book chapters and more than 70 publications in peer reviewed journals.

JONATHAN CROWSTON

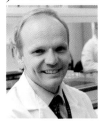

Is a clinican-scientist and Professor of Glaucoma at the Center for Eye Research Australia, University of Melbourne and Head of Glaucoma at the Royal Victorian Eye and Ear Hospital. He obtained his medical degree at the Royal Free Hospital, London and a PhD at the Institute of Ophthalmology, University College London. He trained in ophthalmology at Moorfields Eye Hospital and completed glaucoma fellowships at Westmead Hospital in Sydney and the University of California, San Diego where he was subsequently appointed to the Faculty. In 2006 he was appointed as the first Professor of Glaucoma in Australia. His research interests include neuroprotection and the modulation of wound healing after glaucoma surgery.

GLAUCOMA IN THE WORLD

CHAPTER 1

Prevalence and Geographical Variations

Winnie Nolan and Jennifer Yip

INTRODUCTION

Glaucoma is the commonest cause of irreversible blindness worldwide.[1] The World Health Organization (WHO) estimates for the number of people blind from glaucoma in 2002 were 4.4 million (12.3% of people blind worldwide). The majority of glaucoma in the world remains undiagnosed and so we rely on data collected from epidemiological surveys to estimate numbers with the disease. In recent decades there have been a number of population-based surveys investigating the prevalence of eye disease. One of the limitations of using prevalence data has been the lack of a standardized definition of glaucoma across the different surveys. The increasing use of the International Society of Geographical and Epidemiological Ophthalmology (ISGEO) definition of glaucoma[2] (Table 1.1) means it is now possible to obtain a global picture of the numbers of individuals affected by glaucoma. It also allows comparison of glaucoma prevalence and types in different regions, so highlighting populations and subgroups at increased risk of the disease.

With the accumulation of epidemiological data it is clear that glaucoma affects all populations, but that some regions and racial subgroups are more affected either due to having a higher disease prevalence or because the large population of those regions means the absolute numbers of individuals with glaucoma is very large.

In this chapter the methods of acquiring epidemiological data will be explained and the geographic and racial variations in the prevalence and types of glaucoma will be illustrated together with a discussion of contributing risk factors.

EPIDEMIOLOGICAL METHODS

PREVALENCE AND INCIDENCE

Epidemiological studies quantify and interpret frequency of disease, and factors that affect this. Two important measures that form the basis of all epidemiological studies are incidence and prevalence. *Incidence* is the number of new cases in a given population over a *specified period of time*. This can only be derived from cohort studies, trials, or disease registers. *Prevalence* is the number of all cases in a given population at *one point in time*, and this can be determined from cross-sectional studies and disease registers. Both measures alone are descriptive in nature and, when used to compare frequencies in different populations or subgroups, the analysis and search for risk factors and causal factors can begin. This will lead to new understanding and practical application in clinical care and public health.

STUDY DESIGNS: POPULATION-BASED SURVEYS

Cross-sectional surveys in glaucoma are the starting point to determine the burden of disease in a population.

TABLE 1.1 International Society of Geographical and Epidemiological Ophthalmology classification of glaucoma for use in population-based surveys[2]

GLAUCOMA

Category 1 diagnosis (structural and functional evidence)

Cup:disc ratio (CDR) or CDR symmetry ± 97.5th percentile for the normal population

Or

Neuroretinal rim width reduced to ≤0.1 CDR (between 11 to 1 o'clock or 5 to 7 o'clock)

+

A definite visual field defect consistent with glaucoma

Category 2 diagnosis (advanced structural damage with unproved field loss)

CDR or CDR asymmetry ≥99.5th percentile for the normal population

Category 3 diagnosis (optic disc not seen)

Visual acuity <3/60 and IOP >99.5th percentile

Or

Visual acuity <3/60 and evidence of glaucoma filtering surgery

---

The scientific value of a survey is dependent on its internal and external validity. Glaucoma prevalence should be determined by population-based studies, which select a representative sample. A sample is selected at random as it would be impossible to examine every person in a population, and if everyone has an equal probability of being selected, then this saves time and money without losing accuracy. The type of sampling selected should be accounted for: for example, clustered sampling requires larger sample sizes, and this inflation factor is called the design effect. It will also require a clustered analysis, as participants within the same cluster are more likely to be similar compared to those between clusters, which leads to increased variability. The sample size should be predetermined based on an expected prevalence derived from the literature or a pilot study. As glaucoma is generally a disease of the older population, most glaucoma surveys focus on people who are 40 years or older, as this decreases the required sample size and saves resources.

Internal validity is dependent on factors that can distort the results, leading to false estimates, whether this is due to chance, bias, or confounding. *Chance errors* can be minimized with adequate sample size. A low participation rate is an important source of bias in surveys, as nonparticipants may have a different experience of disease. Bias in ascertainment of disease or risk factors can result from imprecise methods and protocols. Clear criteria should be used to examine the participants and define the outcome. The ISGEO guidelines[2] described below have been adopted internationally in many surveys, and are a useful standard to allow comparisons between different studies.

Humans are prone to error, and objective measures are valued in scientific studies. The set of instruments used to assess the different parameters required in a glaucoma survey will vary. Gold standard instruments such as Goldmann applanation tonometer and Humphrey visual fields may not be feasible in some community-based projects; however, a well-designed and executed study with acceptable instruments may provide better data and more answers than a poorly thought out study with the best equipment available. If more than one set of equipment or examiners are employed in the study, then *inter-observer* assessments are required to demonstrate that both teams are comparable in performance.

Prevalence estimates include incident cases. In a fixed population with a low prevalence of disease, the prevalence is approximately equal to the incidence multiplied by average duration of disease.[3] However, as there are changes in population and prevalence with death and migration, the formula should be used as an approximation only. Incidence is not affected by differences in disease treatment and death, and is the preferable measurement when comparing disease rates in different areas. Prevalence is a useful measure of the burden of disease, especially in conditions with long duration such as glaucoma.

INTERPRETATION OF FINDINGS FROM EPIDEMIOLOGICAL STUDIES

Variation in disease frequency between difference populations is a major source of epidemiological hypotheses in the investigation of causal mechanisms. These differences can be real or artifact. The first step is to establish that a real variation exists and then look for an association between the disease and a risk factor in these groups. It is important to point out that a risk factor implies an association, and not necessarily causation, although some risk factors are causal.

Artifacts Associations between disease and risk factor can lead to the discovery of causal mechanisms, and ultimately in clinical practice, an intervention that can prevent adverse outcomes. However, observations and interpretations of inevitably inaccurate data can lead to wrong conclusions. The art of epidemiology lies in the balanced judgment of this flawed information. Artifactual associations can arise from chance, bias, changes in the population, differences in diagnosis or measurement of disease, and discrepancy in data handling and presentation.

Chance can be evaluated using statistical methods, and the effect of bias on surveys has been discussed. Changes in population can be difficult to determine. The aging of the world's population will lead to an increase in age-related diseases, such as glaucoma. Age-specific prevalence would not change, unless glaucoma itself is related to survival. Errors arising from data handling can be averted with quality assurance methods.

DEFINITIONS AND DIAGNOSTIC CRITERIA

Differences in diagnostic criteria can result in difficulties when comparing differences in glaucoma prevalence. An example of this is in comparing prevalence figures for primary angle-closure glaucoma (PACG) from different surveys. The recent ISGEO guidelines have helped to standardize definitions used in PACG studies. Previous criteria used symptoms rather than structural or functional evidence for diagnosing glaucoma. As a result, in the first publication of the Mongolia glaucoma survey, the prevalence of PACG was 1.4%,[3] but using the revised grading system, the prevalence is 0.8%. Similar problems arise when different criteria are used to evaluate glaucoma progression. Differences can occur if only disc or visual field evidence is used compared to a combination of both factors. The definitions used for perimetric progression should also be carefully assessed in each study, as this may be the true cause of an apparent variation between different areas. Care should also be taken with studies that use self-reporting as the method for case ascertainment. At least 50% of glaucoma is undiagnosed in the population, and using this method to determine association with risk factors would be biased.

DEFINITION OF GLAUCOMA FOR USE IN EPIDEMIOLOGICAL SURVEYS

In an attempt to overcome the problem of varying diagnostic criteria for glaucoma The Working Group for Defining Glaucoma of ISGEO developed a new scheme for the diagnostic classification of glaucoma.[2] This classification emphasizes the importance of visually significant end-organ (optic nerve head) damage as a requirement for the diagnosis of glaucoma.

Table 1.1 shows an abbreviated version of the ISGEO classification of glaucoma.

PRIMARY OPEN-ANGLE GLAUCOMA

According to the ISGEO classification, primary open-angle glaucoma (POAG) is defined as glaucomatous optic neuropathy in the presence of an open-angle and no other ocular abnormality to account for a secondary mechanism.

PRIMARY ANGLE-CLOSURE GLAUCOMA

The ISGEO classification of primary angle-closure glaucoma (PACG) is a revised classification which places the emphasis on evidence of glaucomatous optic neuropathy together with gonioscopic evidence.

The ISGEO classification of primary angle-closure (PAC) has three stages:

- Primary angle-closure suspect (PACS)
  Appositional contact between the peripheral iris and posterior trabecular meshwork deemed possible (i.e. occludable)
- Primary angle-closure (PAC)
  Presence of an occludable angle (as above) together with signs of trabecular meshwork obstruction, e.g. peripheral anterior synechiae, elevated IOP, excessive pigment deposition on surface of trabecular meshwork or ischemic sequelae such as glaucomflecken or iris whirling. The optic disc is healthy.
- Primary angle-closure glaucoma (PACG)
  PAC with evidence of glaucomatous optic neuropathy.

SECONDARY GLAUCOMAS

Secondary glaucoma was proposed by the ISGEO authors to be the presence of glaucomatous optic neuropathy together with signs of other pathological processes.

APPLICATIONS OF EPIDEMIOLOGICAL DATA

Obtaining glaucoma prevalence data is the starting point for prevention of blindness programs targeted at reducing the number of cases of blindness. The epidemiological data has several uses:

- Application of data to population figures to estimate the absolute numbers affected with glaucoma in different geographic regions.
- Highlighting regions or subgroups with a higher prevalence of glaucoma-related visual impairment.

- Determination of association between demographic factors, e.g. age, sex, ethnicity, and glaucoma, and ocular factors such as biometric measurements or genetic factors, which may be causal mechanisms contributing to the pathogenesis of glaucoma.
- Comparing prevalence between different regions so that prioritization in resources and research programs can be given to populations most at risk.

REGIONAL VARIATION IN GLAUCOMA PREVALENCE AND TYPE

EUROPE, NORTH AMERICA

Primary open-angle glaucoma (POAG) is the predominant glaucoma in Europe, the United States of America (USA), and in the European-derived population of Australia (Table 1.2).[4–7] Within these regions the highest prevalence of POAG is in the African and Caribbean-derived populations that live in the USA and in the Caribbean.[4,8,9]

Primary angle-closure glaucoma (PACG) is relatively uncommon compared with POAG in Blacks and Caucasians living in these geographic regions. While it is indeed likely that PACG is less frequent than POAG in these populations, unless gonioscopic assessment is included as part of the comprehensive examination of

TABLE 1.2 Recent prevalence estimates for primary open-angle glaucoma from population surveys in persons over 40 years old by region

REGION	AUTHOR	PREVALENCE (%)
Africa		
Tanzania (East Africa)	Buhrmann	3.1
Kwazulu-Natal (South Africa)	Rotchford	2.7
Temba (South Africa)	Rotchford	2.9
West Indies		
Barbados (Blacks)	Leske	7.0
United States and Europe		
Baltimore	Tielsch	
Beaver Dam	Klein	2.1
Egna-Neumarket, Italy	Bonomi	2.0
Australia		
Melbourne	Wensor	1.7
Asia (South)		
Aravind, India	Dandona	1.7
Bangladesh	Rahman	2.5
Chennai, India	Vijaya	1.62
Asia (East)		
Mongolia	Foster	0.5
Singapore	Foster	2.1
Tajimi, Japan	Iwase	3.9

glaucoma cases detected in surveys, then the true prevalence of PACG may be underestimated.

LATIN AMERICA

Two surveys have focused specifically on the Hispanic or Latino population who live in the United States. Proyecto VER (conducted in Arizona) found a POAG prevalence somewhere between that shown in White and Black people living in the North America, but increasing at a significantly more rapid rate with age compared to other ethnic groups.[10] The Los Angeles Latino Eye Study (LALES) demonstrated a high prevalence of POAG (4.74%). This is likely to be partly due to the less stringent definitions used, which required either optic disc damage *or* visual field evidence to make the diagnosis of glaucoma.[11] The population of the LALES study had mainly Mexican ancestry whereas that of Proyecto VER had a greater number of people with Native American roots. Either way, the data may or may not be applicable to Latin America as a whole, bearing in mind that the region is populated by people with Indigenous, Hispanic, and African ethnicity. There are no published figures at present for the prevalence of glaucoma in Central or South America.

ASIA

Asia is thought to harbor almost half of the glaucoma cases worldwide and the numbers affected are projected to increase considerably over the next 20 years.[12] This is due to the presence of a number of heavily populated countries including the two most populous, namely China (estimated population 1.3 billion) and India (estimated population 1.1 billion), which make up almost a third of the world's population.[13] Indonesia (245 million) is another densely and heavily populated country in the region.

Surveys carried out in Mongolia, Singapore, China, and India all show that the prevalence of primary angle-closure glaucoma (PACG) is almost equal to that of POAG (the POAG prevalence being similar to that in Caucasians).[3,14–16] But one important finding from these surveys is that a greater proportion of people affected by PACG are bilaterally blind (10% of POAG cases vs 25% with PACG).[17] Application of these prevalence and blindness figures to current and predicted population numbers indicates that glaucoma is and will be a growing public health problem in Asia.

AFRICA

The most comprehensive data available from Africa was provided by surveys conducted in East Africa (Tanzania) and South African. These reported combined primary and secondary glaucoma prevalence figures of just over 5% (see Table 1.2).[18–20] The predominant glaucoma was POAG but pseudoexfoliation (in Black South Africans), aphakic, and angle-closure mechanisms composed the remaining cases. Glaucoma prevalence among Black people living in USA is measured as being four or more times that in Caucasians.[4,8] As the ancestors of African-Americans and the Caribbean population came from West Africa, it is suspected that glaucoma prevalence in this region may be equally high. But at the present time there are no published cross-sectional data from West Africa, although surveys are under way. It is very likely that the prevalence and mechanism of glaucoma varies between heterogeneous populations of the African continent. But what has been repeatedly demonstrated is that glaucoma affects a higher proportion of African-derived people, has a younger age of onset, and that it may result in a greater visual morbidity than in other populations.[19,21]

PRIMARY OPEN-ANGLE GLAUCOMA: PREVALENCE AND NUMBERS AFFECTED

A recent meta-analysis by Rudnicka et al.[22] reviewed all POAG surveys available in the literature, and estimated pooled prevalence by race. The plotted summary of all studies reviewed is shown in Figure 1.1, which provides a useful outline of differences in prevalence estimates. The variation in prevalence estimates between different races grouped in this manner is evident, with prevalence for whites ranging from <0.5% to >10%. The overall pooled prevalence estimate was 2% (95% CI: 1.61–2.70%), which is higher than 1.69% (1.53–1.85%) presented in another meta-analysis using individual data from recent studies from the USA, Europe, and Australia.[23] There was also statistical evidence in all racial groups of heterogeneity, that is, a true variation between studies rather than variation by chance. This was attributed to differences in age groups for the different studies, survey methods, and year of publication which reflects the change in diagnostic criteria used. In this study, the prevalence is presented by different racial groups, regardless of location; therefore, glaucoma prevalence of Blacks include surveys from Africa, the West Indies, and Black populations within Europe and the USA. This would overlook potential differences in prevalence estimates caused by environmental factors, which would be another source of heterogeneity. To address these issues, Table 1.2 shows a summary of different prevalence estimates by region from more recent surveys with comparable methods in participants over 40 years old.

These and other prevalence figures have been applied to the projected global populations for 2010 to estimate the absolute numbers of individuals with glaucoma worldwide. These calculations estimate that there will be almost 45 million individuals with primary open-angle glaucoma (POAG) by 2010.[12] A breakdown for these figures by region is seen in Table 1.3.

Citation	Study (age range)

Asian
19	Hu (40+)
18	Arkell (15-70+)
22	Jacob (30-60)
21	Foster (40-89)
24	Dandona (0-102)
29	Rahman (35-85)
27	Ramakrishnan (40-90)
17	Aisbirk (40+)
23	Foster (40-81)
26	Bourne (50-70+)
11	Shiose (30-70+)
20	Rauf (30-80+)
25	Metheetrairut (60-104)
28	Iwase (40-80+)
	Subtotal

Black
30	Wallace (35-74)
35	Ekwerekwu (30-80+)
34	Rotchford (40-80+)
33	Buhrmann(40-80+)
32	Wormald (35-60+)
36	Rotchford (40-97)
2	Tielsch (40-80+)
12	Leske (40-86)
37	Ntim-Amponsah (30-100)
31	Mason (30-70+)
	Subtotal

White
4	Hollows (40-74)
12	Leske (40-86)
41	Bankes (20-80+)
6	Bengtsson (58.5-68.5)
2	Tieisch (40-80+)
10	Dielemans (55-75+)
44	Giuffre (40-99)
40	Salmon (40-70+)
49	Wensor (40-90+)
5	Coffey (50-80+)
1	Leibowitz (<65-75+)
47	Bonomi (40-80+)
39	Anton (40-79)
38	Quigley (41-90+)
3	Kiein (43-75+)
9	Mitchell (49-80+)
46	Cedrone (40-80+)
50	Kozobolis (40-80+)
48	Reidy (65-100)
7	Ringvold (65-89+)
8	Ekstrom (65-74)
42	Martinez (65-90+)
43	Gibson (76-85+)
45	Hirvela (70-95)
	Subtotal
	Overall

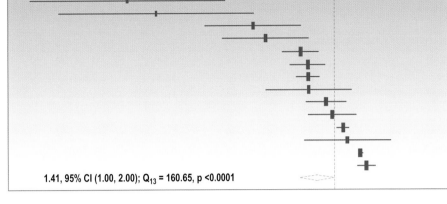
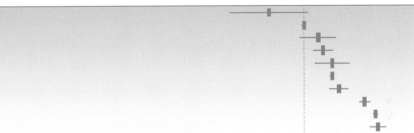
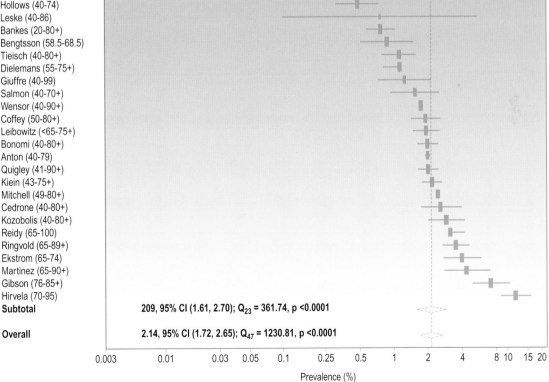

Asian Subtotal: 1.41, 95% CI (1.00, 2.00); Q_{13} = 160.65, p <0.0001

Black Subtotal: 4.23, 95% CI (3.07, 5.83); Q_9 = 173.44, p<0.0001

White Subtotal: 209, 95% CI (1.61, 2.70); Q_{23} = 361.74, p <0.0001

Overall: 2.14, 95% CI (1.72, 2.65); Q_{47} = 1230.81, p <0.0001

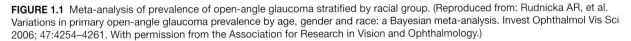

0.003   0.01   0.03   0.05   0.1   0.25   0.5   1   2   4   8   10   15   20

Prevalence (%)

FIGURE 1.1 Meta-analysis of prevalence of open-angle glaucoma stratified by racial group. (Reproduced from: Rudnicka AR, et al. Variations in primary open-angle glaucoma prevalence by age, gender and race: a Bayesian meta-analysis. Invest Ophthalmol Vis Sci 2006; 47:4254–4261. With permission from the Association for Research in Vision and Ophthalmology.)

TABLE 1.3 Estimated numbers with open-angle glaucoma (OAG) and angle-closure glaucoma (ACG) worldwide, 2010[12]

WORLD REGION	NUMBER WITH OAG	WORLD OAG %	NUMBER WITH ACG	WORLD ACG %	OAG AND ACG COMBINED
China	8 309 001	18.6	7 473 195	47.5	15 782 196
Europe (including USA, Australia)	10 693 335	23.9	1 371 405	8.7	12 064 740
India	8 211 276	18.4	3 733 620	23.7	11 944 896
Africa	6 212 179	13.9	245 844	1.6	6 458 023
Latin America	5 354 354	12	322 804	2.1	5 677 158
Japan	2 383 802	5.3	278 643	1.8	2 662 466
South East Asia	2 116 036	4.7	2 141 584	13.6	4 257 620
Middle East	1 440 849	3.2	177 869	1.1	1 618 718
World	44 720 832		15 744 965		60 465 796

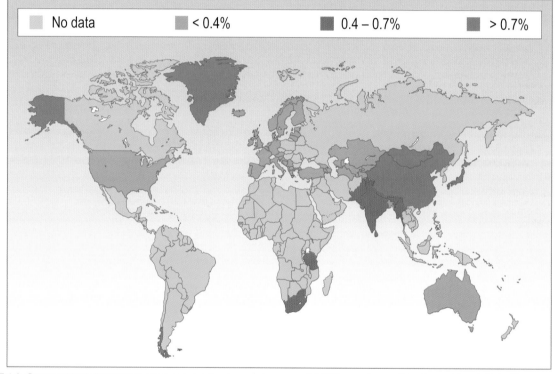

FIGURE 1.2 Geographical distribution of primary angle-closure glaucoma (PACG) prevalence. (Courtesy of Sarah Polack)

PRIMARY ANGLE-CLOSURE GLAUCOMA: PREVALENCE AND NUMBERS AFFECTED

Figure 1.2 and Table 1.4 show the global variations in prevalence of PACG. Data from Caucasian populations with European ancestry suggest relatively low numbers are affected, with figures ranging from only two cases (0.04%) in Beaver Dam to 0.6% in Egna-Neumarkt in Italy.[5,7] Again, the definitions vary and the majority of the surveys in Western countries have focused on detecting POAG. The Proyecto VER survey of Hispanic patients in the USA reported a PACG prevalence of 0.1%,[10] but there are no population-based data from Central or South America. In Africa the data available confirm that angle-closure does exist in this population, with a prevalence of 0.5% in South Africa and Tanzania.[18–20]

Recently, there has been an expansion in the number of population-based glaucoma surveys conducted in Asia. Some of the Asia-based surveys carried out in the past lacked validity due to methodological weaknesses. These included the use surrogate measures of angle width such as the oblique flashlight test, and a variation in definitions of angle-closure and glaucoma.

TABLE 1.4 Prevalence estimates for primary angle-closure glaucoma by region

REGION	AUTHOR	PREVALENCE (%)
United States, Europe, and Australia		
Baltimore whites	Personal communication	0.4
Beaver Dam	Klein	0.04
Melbourne	Wensor	0.06
Wales	Hollows	0.09
Egna-Neumarkt, Italy	Bonomi	0.6
Proyecto VER (Hispanic)	Quigley	0.1
Asia (South)		
Andra Pradesh (>30 yr)	Dandona	0.7
Aravind	Ramakrishnan	0.5
Chennai	Vijaya	0.87
Asia (East)		
Beijing, China	Hu	1.37
Guangzhou, China (>50 yr)	He	1.5
Tajimi, Japan	Yamamoto	0.6
Mongolia	Foster	0.8
Singapore	Foster	0.8
Thailand (>50 yr)	Bourne	0.9
Africa		
Tanzania	Buhrmann	0.5
Temba, South Africa	Rotchford	0.5
Cape coloreds, South Africa	Salmon	2.3

The strength of many of the more recent surveys lies in their adherence to the ISGEO glaucoma definitions, and the inclusion of gonioscopy as part of the definitive clinical examination on all subjects.

Surveys from Asia confirm that angle-closure glaucoma occurs more frequently in this region although POAG is equally if not more common. PACG prevalence figures range from 0.8% and 0.87% in Mongolia[3] and Southern India[15] to 1% in Singapore[14] and 1.5% in Guangzhou, China.[16] The higher figure for the Guangzhou study can be accounted for by the older age of the population being examined (>50 years) compared to the other study populations. When these figures are applied to the population numbers for Asia the real potential magnitude of the burden of PACG is immediately apparent (see Table 1.3). These estimates of numbers of people with PACG in 2010 predict that China will account for almost 50% angle-closure glaucoma worldwide and that 85% all individuals with PACG will be from Asia.[12] These figures are estimates but have the benefit of the reliable epidemiological data that has been collected in Asia. The increase in predicted

numbers of glaucoma-affected people is partly due to an increase in life expectancy. The higher rate of visual loss in PACG compared with POAG heightens the concern over the potential numbers with glaucoma blindness in Asia and is the stimulus for current research strategies aimed at effective methods of treatment and early detection of the disease.

SECONDARY GLAUCOMAS

Secondary glaucomas are defined by the presence of a primary ophthalmic or systemic disease causing raised intraocular pressure, which if sustained then leads to glaucomatous optic neuropathy.[14] Although it is relatively uncommon when compared with POAG, these cases have a greater risk of blindness. This is partly as a result of the underlying disease, but also due to the higher levels of IOP seen in these cases and the fact that they are often refractory to conventional glaucoma treatment. The geographical distribution of these types of glaucoma will follow that of the causal ocular pathology. For example, in countries where intracapsular cataract surgery is still practiced there is a higher prevalence of aphakic glaucoma.[19,24] However, with the increasing use of extracapsular cataract surgery and intraocular lens (IOL) implantation in most parts of the world, the incidence of this type of glaucoma should be on the decrease.

GEOGRAPHICAL VARIATION IN RISK FACTORS

RACE AND ETHNICITY

There is much debate about the role and use of race in epidemiological research. The biological concept of race is outdated. There is less genetic variation between races or groups separated geographically compared to individuals from the same ethnic group.[25] Ethnicity refers to a group with shared cultural and geographical origins, and is being increasingly used as a euphemism for race, although they are distinct but overlapping entities. Ethnicity is difficult to measure accurately, and at present, is dependent on self-assessment. However, in studies that use ethnicity or race as a source of variation, the implication is that it encompasses genetic, environmental, and cultural differences. The variation in glaucoma prevalence found in different races, ethnicities, and geographical locations will be due to multiple causes. Previous surveys have suggested that people of African Caribbean descent have higher prevalence of POAG and lower prevalence of PACG,[4,8] while the trend is reversed in East Asians.[3,15] A meta-analysis of POAG surveys (see Fig. 1.1) calculated the pooled prevalence estimates for each Asian, Black, and white populations, and these were 1.4%, 4.2%, and 2.1%, respectively.[22]

INTRAOCULAR PRESSURE

The evidence for a causal association between intraocular pressure (IOP) and glaucoma is robust. Randomized, controlled trials have shown that removal of the risk factor (higher IOP) can reduce disease.[26,27] A 'high' IOP is arbitrary based on the distribution of IOP in the population. In Western populations, 21 mmHg is traditionally used as the cut-off point, as this represents the mean (16 mmHg) plus 2 standard deviations. The distribution of IOP is Asian populations is shifted to the left, that is, they have lower IOPs with a lower mean, and the cutoff point is approximately 1–2 mmHg lower. In Mongolia and Singapore, the mean and cutoff were 13 mmHg and 19 mmHg, respectively.[3,28] A higher prevalence of normal tension glaucoma (NTG) has been observed in the Japanese population.[29] The distribution of IOP in this population presents a cutoff point of 20 mmHg with a mean of 14.5 mmHg. Prevalence estimates for NTG used 21 mmHg as the boundary; however, authors from the Tajimi study suggested that there were very few patients that would have been recategorized as a result of this. There is a suggestion that Blacks have higher IOP. The Barbados Eye Study (BES) showed that the distribution of IOP in Blacks have a mean of 18.7 mmHg and standard deviation of 5.2 mmHg, which was higher than the Mixed and White participants in the study.[8]

Central corneal thickness (CCT) has been shown to vary in different populations. It has also associated with variations in IOP. The gold standard for IOP measurement is currently the Goldmann applanation tonometer, which assumes a standard CCT. Thicker corneas are associated with higher IOP and thinner corneas with lower IOP. This could result from a measurement artifact. An ancillary cross-sectional study to The Ocular Hypertension Treatment Study (OHTS) concluded that thinner CCT was associated with progression from ocular hypertension (OHT) to glaucoma.[30] However, OHTS followed a population with ocular hypertension and higher CCT than normal populations, and their results could be interpreted as a protective effect of thicker corneas. Clinic-based studies have demonstrated that thinner corneas are associated with glaucoma progression;[31] however, it is unclear whether this is due to a mechanism independent of IOP measurement. Results from BES and other hospital-based studies have shown that Blacks have a thinner CCT compared to Whites.[32] Variations between different population studies should also take into account the type of instruments used, as this can also have an effect on the absolute figure for CCT.

SYSTEMIC FACTORS

There is some evidence of an association between patients with POAG and systemic cardiovascular disease.[33] Glaucoma patients are more likely to have arteriosclerotic changes in the ocular[34] and systemic vasculature. Both arterial hypertension and hypotension have been linked with POAG. It is likely that these apparently contradictory associations are due to heterogeneous populations with differences in risk mediated through perfusion pressure (blood pressure, intraocular pressure) and autonomic function of the optic nerve head. There is also evidence to suggest that POAG is associated with vasospasm. This is defined as inappropriate constriction in the microcirculation in response to stimuli. The eye can be more sensitive to alterations in perfusion pressure as vasospasm can obstruct autoregulation of the ocular vasculature. This also relates to the association between migraine and glaucoma.

There are varied reports from large surveys on the association between diabetes and POAG. The Rotterdam Study,[35] Beaver Dam Eye Study,[36] and the Blue Mountains Eye Study[37] all showed an increased prevalence of glaucoma in diabetic patients, whereas the Framingham Study[38] and the Baltimore Eye Survey[39] failed to demonstrate an association. However, diabetes was associated with higher IOP in the Baltimore Eye Survey. There is also no evidence on the association between higher body mass index (BMI) and obesity, a strong risk factor for diabetes, and glaucoma. An association between BMI and IOP has been demonstrated in a Japanese population in a cross-sectional and longitudinal study.[40] It is difficult to unravel the complex associations and mechanisms between these diseases. There are difficulties in comparison between studies, as different diagnostic criteria for both diseases were used. If the association is mediated through IOP, then adjusting for IOP in multivariate models will remove the effect of BMI or diabetes as an independent risk factor.

PSEUDOEXFOLIATION

The finding of pseudoexfoliative (PXF) material on the lens surface is strongly associated with glaucoma and raised intraocular pressure.[41] Glaucoma patients with PXF have higher IOPs than POAG patients without PXF[42] and it is a risk factor for blindness due to cataract or glaucoma.[43] One of the problems in establishing the epidemiological distribution of PXF is that to be sure of its presence or absence on the lens surface requires pupil dilation, otherwise it may be missed. PXF is a frequent finding in the Scandinavian countries of Northern Europe such as Iceland (31% glaucoma cases)[44] but other regions where it is prevalent include southern India,[43] Mongolia,[3] and in the Mediterranean countries such as Turkey and Greece. It is rare in the Chinese and is so far unreported in African-American/Caribbean people, West Africans,[45] and in Tanzania,[18] but has high prevalence in Black South Africans (16% all glaucoma cases)[19,20] and Ethiopians.[46] The clustering of PXF in families and populations gives support to the theory of a genetic basis for the condition although nongenetic factors have also been put forward as potential contributors.[47] The epidemiology and etiology of PXF is an area that merits further research as it is the commonest identifiable cause of open-angle glaucoma worldwide.

PRIMARY ANGLE-CLOSURE GLAUCOMA: RISK FACTORS AND MECHANISMS

A more detailed description of the factors predisposing individuals to angle-closure is set out in another chapter but it is worth touching on some of them in this section. It was established by Ron Lowe that there is an association between certain biometric characteristics and an increased risk of developing angle closure, these being a smaller eye, shallower central anterior chamber, and steep corneal curvature and relatively anterior positioned lens. These risk factors for angle-closure were also reported by Danish ophthalmologists working with the Greenland Inuit people.[48–50] The values for age-specific mean central anterior chamber depth (ACD) measured in Mongolians were shown by Foster et al. to lie between those found in Caucasian populations (which have deeper chambers) and those of the Greenland Inuit (with shallower chambers) demonstrating the inverse relationship between mean population central ACD and the prevalence of PACG.[51]

The other main risk factors for angle-closure are directly related to the latter factors. With age, enlargement of the lens shallows the chamber and narrows the angle, and women tend to have smaller eyes and anterior segments than men, putting these groups at greater risk.

The strong link between these anatomical characteristics and PACG has been the basis for studies looking at the use of ACD measurement as a simple method of detecting cases of angle-closure in high-risk populations.

MECHANISMS OF ANGLE CLOSURE

As well as the number of people with established PACG, there is a much greater number of individuals who have narrow angles alone (primary angle-closure suspects). A proportion of these (between one-fifth to one-third) will progress to angle-closure and an even smaller number develop PACG, but the rest remain healthy.[52,53] So there must be other as yet unknown factors apart from crowding of the anterior segment which contribute to the pathogenesis of the angle-closure process to result in glaucoma. The traditional thinking is that angle-closure presents as acute symptomatic episodes in Caucasians and in a more chronic asymptomatic form in Asian people. While studies confirm that the majority of angle-closure in Asia is asymptomatic there are insufficient data from European studies to allow us to draw conclusions on the natural history of the disease

TABLE 1.5 Proportion of people with glaucoma cases detected in population-based surveys that were previously undiagnosed

POPULATION STUDIED	PERCENTAGE OF CASES PREVIOUSLY UNDIAGNOSED
South Africa (Temba)[19]	87% (POAG)
Chennai – Southern India[55]	98.5% (POAG)
Los Angeles Latinos (LALES)[11]	75% (POAG)
Australia – Blue Mountains Eye Study[56]	51% (POAG)
Melbourne (Visual impairment project)[6]	50% (POAG)
Rotterdam[57]	53% (POAG)

and underlying mechanisms in this group. What is becoming more apparent to angle-closure researchers, both in Asia and the West, is that while pupil block is a significant mechanism in the pathogenesis of angle-closure, it is not the only one.[54] It may be that there are regional variations both globally and within Asia in the causal mechanisms of angle closure. This has major implications for treatment, as laser iridotomy only acts to relieve pupil block and so may not be effective in all people with the disease.

PREVALENCE OF UNDETECTED GLAUCOMA

The proportion of glaucoma cases detected in population-based surveys that were previously undiagnosed is high in all regions of the world. The figure for the high-income areas such as Europe and Australia is fairly consistent at about 50% (Table 1.5). In the middle- and low-income regions of Asia and Africa the percentage is much higher, approaching 90% and above, and can be linked with late presentation of glaucoma cases and the higher risk of glaucoma blindness in these populations. Contributing factors to the late presentation of glaucoma patients in developing countries include poor public knowledge about glaucoma and limited access to healthcare services. In developed countries with better access to optometry and eye care services the principal reason for the poor glaucoma detection rate is the lack of a good screening test for a largely asymptomatic disease. However, within populations such as the UK, demographic factors including ethnicity (African Caribbean and Asian), older age, and lower socioeconomic status have been associated with a higher risk of late presentation with glaucoma.[58,59]

Late presentation is more likely to lead to visual morbidity. These issues indicate that global and national health inequalities could contribute to glaucoma blindness.

PREVALENCE AND GEOGRAPHICAL VARIATIONS

Harry A Quigley

Dramatic change is not too drastic a term to describe what has happened during the last decade in glaucoma research. The definition of glaucoma, in all its primary forms, was literally in chaos until the last 10 years. Open-angle glaucoma (OAG) was typically defined by what is unflatteringly called the 'three guys in a room' method – namely, anything that self-anointed experts called OAG, was OAG. Fortunately, we are now in possession of structural and functional measures of glaucoma damage that allow the definition of disease in concrete terms that may be applied to every study of the disease and permit standardization. Clearly, such new definitional systems will evolve as both logic and technology dictate. Their validity is dependent upon their usefulness. But, the era of 'expert' definition is over.

Even more arcane was the definition (or lack thereof) of angle-closure glaucoma. Terms such as creeping, subacute, intermittent, and chronic were applied in various studies, without any documentation. No clarity to the natural history of disease is possible until we can agree on what is being studied, and can compare it among reports. Fortunately, initial attempts at consensus are being developed.

Just as prehistoric is the use of the term 'low tension glaucoma.' Intraocular pressure (IOP) is a major risk factor for both OAG and angle-closure glaucoma (ACG), but we are now aware that more than half of those with OAG have IOP levels that are within the range of the non-OAG population. And, their phenotypic change in the disc and field are minimally different, if at all, from those with OAG at higher IOP. We should be studying risk factors that lead to OAG among both those with normal and those with higher IOP, but artificial divisions at magic numbers are clearly no longer justified by any scientific data.

In many discussions in developed countries, when one says 'glaucoma' it is assumed to be OAG that is being considered. Yet, recent evaluations of worldwide data make it clear that one-third of those with glaucoma have ACG and half of world glaucoma blindness is due to ACG. Emphasis on the mechanisms and treatment of ACG is merited not only because of its frequency, but because it is likely that its therapy is probably more relevant to immediate public health intervention in many Asian settings. The theory of why ACG is more common in Chinese persons deserves more attention, particularly because past emphasis on anatomic features of eye size cannot explain its prevalence. We must focus on physiological responses that lead to ACG.

The fact that most glaucoma worldwide is not diagnosed is an embarrassment for ophthalmology, but 'screening' for the glaucomas is not yet practical or useful. Methods must be developed that separate those at significant risk for these disorders from the population, and we must develop algorithms that deserve consideration to segregate glaucoma patients from adults who have no eye disease. The problem is not easily solved, but lies at the heart of attacking the second leading cause of world blindness.

Therapy for glaucoma has been proven to slow the progression of disease in developed country settings where complex diagnostic evaluation and expensive treatment are considered feasible. For the majority of the world, we have not yet determined at what stage of disease treatment is better than natural history, and how to train those who would deliver such treatment or how to implement a program for glaucoma within the other priorities of national healthcare schemes. We seem to have a situation in which too many are probably being treated in developed countries and few if any are receiving sight-saving care in the developing world.

SPOTLIGHT: CLINICAL EPIDEMIOLOGY: STIMULATING AND APPLYING GLAUCOMA RESEARCH TO THE PATIENT

R Thomas and R Parikh

While population-based studies have vastly increased our knowledge of glaucoma, the epidemiological principles used in such investigations are also applicable to clinical care and research. We all know excellent clinicians, who intuitively make correct diagnoses, assign prognoses, and tailor therapy for the individual patient. They practice the 'art' of clinical medicine; there is, in fact, a science behind this 'art.' Epidemiological concepts form the foundation of this science of clinical epidemiology, the mother of evidence-based or, for those who abhor the term, best data-based medicine.

Number needed to treat and number needed to harm (derived from absolute risk difference) allow assessment of clinical significance as apposed to statistical significance; their logical extension, 'likelihood of help versus harm,' facilitates individualized therapy, especially in difficult cases. Similarly, an understanding of relative risk as well as the jargon of its manipulations (relative risk reduction; excess risk) permit us to correctly interpret (and apply) statements like '10% reduction per mmHg.' These principles are detailed in the chapter on risk versus benefit.

Concepts such as sensitivity, specificity, and predictive values are not limited to research. They play a crucial clinical role in 'ruling in' or 'ruling out' diagnoses. If a highly specific test (around 95%), is positive, it 'rules in' (confirms) the diagnosis. For example, any three abnormal points on a 20-1 frequency-doubling test have a specificity of 99%. This finding confirms (rules in) a field defect. The rule can be remembered as SpPIN (*Sp*ecific test if *P*ositive, rules *IN*). Similarly, a highly sensitive test (95% or so), if negative, rules out a diagnosis. As illustration, absence of venous pulsations has a sensitivity of 99% for papilledema. If this sign is absent, that is venous pulsations are present, one can literally 'rule out' papilledema; at least at that point in time. This rule can be remembered as SnNOUT (*Sn*ensitive test if *N*egative rules *OUT*).

Furthermore, the formula: $1 - (1 - \text{specificity test 1})$ $(1 - \text{specificity test 2})$, allows tests to be combined to establish a diagnosis. Consider a glaucoma suspect with an intraocular pressure (IOP) of 25 mmHg (specificity 90%) AND a van Herrick test less than one-fourth the corneal thickness (85% specificity for angle closure). The formula provides a combined test specificity of 98.5%: one is almost sure that the patient has angle closure. The same formula can also combine sensitivities to 'rule out' a diagnosis. Clinical signs can be combined with investigations to establish (or exclude) a diagnosis. And multilevel likelihood ratios calculated from sensitivity and specificity for individual test results are probably the best way to use investigations, including imaging.

The concept of positive predictive value explains why many patients with field defects on SWAP do not convert on follow-up with conventional perimetry. The specificity of

SWAP is high, but as only 1–2% of cases actually progress, false positives will be higher. This principle also explains the limitation of follow-up using imaging techniques. It is not that the technology is bad; unless the specificity is >99%, there will be more false positives compared to true positives.

Knowledge of these and other epidemiological principles (such as causality) encourage valid questions and are also pertinent in the 'how to' of clinical practice research. All these principles are detailed in our clinical bibles.[1–3]

References
1. Sackett DL, Haynes RB, Guyatt GH, et al. Clinical epidemiology. A basic science for clinical medicine. 2nd edn. New York: Little, Brown; 1991.
2. Haynes RB, Sactett DL, Guyatt GH, et al. Clinical epidemiology: how to do clinical practice research. 3rd edn. London: Lippincott Williams & Wilkins; 2006.
3. Straus SE, Richardson WS, Glasziou P, et al. Evidence-based medicine: how to practice and teach EBM. 3rd edn. Edinburgh: Churchill Livingstone; 2005.

Summary
Glaucoma is the commonest cause of irreversible visual morbidity worldwide. The covert nature of the disease requires representative surveys to determine the true burden of glaucoma. Good-quality surveys with standardized definitions and methods are the starting point with which to tackle this global public health problem and in recent decades the number of well-conducted prevalence surveys has increased considerably. However, data from areas such as Latin America and Africa are needed to further quantify this problem. Global and regional strategies can then be developed to address the challenge of glaucoma blindness in the Vision 2020 agenda.

REFERENCES

1. Resnikoff S, et al. Global data on visual impairment in the year 2002. Bull World Health Organization 2004; 82:844–851.
2. Foster PJ, Burhmann R, Quigley HA, et al. The definition and classification of glaucoma in prevalence surveys. Br J Ophthalmol 2002; 86:238–242.
3. Foster PJ, Baasanhu J, Alsbirk PH, et al. Glaucoma in Mongolia. A population-based survey in Hovsgol province, northern Mongolia. Arch Ophthalmol 1996; 114:1235–1241.
4. Tielsch J, Sommer A, Katz J, et al. Racial variations in the prevalence of primary open-angle glaucoma: the Baltimore Eye Survey. JAMA 1991; 266:369–374.
5. Bonomi L, Marchini G, Marraffa M, et al. Epidemiology of angle-closure glaucoma. Prevalence, clinical types, and association with peripheral anterior chamber depth in the Egna-Neumarkt glaucoma study. Ophthalmology 2000; 107:998–1003.
6. Wensor MD, McCarty CA, Stanislavsky YL, et al. The prevalence of glaucoma in the Melbourne Visual Impairment Project. Ophthalmology 1998; 105:733–739.
7. Klein BE, Klein R, Sponsel WE, et al. Prevalence of glaucoma. The Beaver Dam Eye Study. Ophthalmology 1992; 99:1499–1504.
8. Leske C, Connell A, Schahat A, et al. The Barbados Eye Study: prevalence of open-angle glaucoma. Arch Ophthalmol 1994; 112:821–829.
9. Mason RE, Kosoko O, Wilson MR, et al. National survey of the prevalence and risk factors of glaucoma in St Lucia, West Indies I: prevalence findings. Ophthalmology 1989; 96:1363–1368.
10. Quigley HA, West SK, Rodriguez J, et al. The prevalence of glaucoma in a population-based study of Hispanic subjects: Proyecto VER. Arch Ophthalmol 2001; 119:1819–1826.
11. Varma R, Ying-Lai M, Francis BA, et al. Prevalence of open-angle glaucoma and ocular hypertension in Latinos: the Los Angeles Latino Eye Study. Ophthalmology 2004; 111:1434–1439.
12. Quigley HA, Broman AT. The number of people with glaucoma worldwide in 2010 and 2020. Br J Ophthalmol 2006; 90:262–267.
13. www.globalhealthfacts.org.
14. Foster PJ, Oen FT, Machin D, et al. The prevalence of glaucoma in Chinese residents of Singapore: a cross-sectional population survey of the Tanjong Pagar district. Arch Ophthalmol 2000; 118:1105–1111.
15. Vijaya L, George R, Arvind H, et al. Prevalence of angle-closure disease in a rural southern Indian population. Arch Ophthalmol 2006; 124:403–409.
16. He M, Foster PJ, Ge J, et al. Prevalence of clinical characteristics of glaucoma in adult Chinese: a population-based study in Liwan district, Guangzhou. Invest Ophthalmol Vis Sci 2006; 47:2782–2788.
17. Foster PJ, Johnson GJ. Glaucoma in China: how big is the problem? Br J Ophthalmol 2001; 85:1277–1282.
18. Buhrmann RR, Quigley HA, Barron Y, et al. Prevalence of glaucoma in a rural East African population. Invest Ophthalmol Vis Sci 2000; 41:40–48.
19. Rotchford AP, Kirwan JF, Muller MA, et al. Temba glaucoma study: a population-based cross-sectional survey in urban South Africa. Ophthalmology 2003; 110:376–382.
20. Rotchford AP, Johnson GJ. Glaucoma in Zulus: a population-based cross-sectional survey in a rural district in South Africa. Arch Ophthalmol 2002; 120:471–478.
21. Sommer A, Tielsch JM, Katz J, et al. Racial differences in cause-specific prevalence of blindness in east Baltimore. N Engl J Med 1991; 325:1412–1417.
22. Rudnicka AR, Mt-Isa S, Owen CG, et al. Variations in primary open-angle glaucoma prevalence by age, gender, and race: a Bayesian meta-analysis. Invest Ophthalmol Vis Sci 2006; 47(10):4254–4261.
23. Friedman DS, Wolfs RC, O'Colmain BJ, et al. Prevalence of open-angle glaucoma among adults in the United States. Arch Ophthalmol 2004; 122(4):532–538.
24. Arvind H, George R, Raju P, et al. Glaucoma in aphakia and pseudophakia in the Chennai glaucoma study. Br J Ophthalmol 2005; 89:699–703.
25. Rose S, Kamin L, Lewontin R. Not in our genes: biology, ideology and human nature. New York: Penguin; 1984.
26. The AGIS Investigators. The Advanced Glaucoma Intervention Study (AGIS): 7. The relationship between control of

intraocular pressure and visual field deterioration. Am J Ophthalmol 2000; 130(4):429–440.

27. Heijl A, Leske MC, Bengtsson B, et al. Reduction of intraocular pressure and glaucoma progression: results from the Early Manifest Glaucoma Trial. Arch Ophthalmol 2002; 120(10):1268–1279.

28. Foster PJ, Machin D, Wong TY, et al. Determinants of intraocular pressure and its association with glaucomatous optic neuropathy in Chinese Singaporeans: the Tanjong Pagar Study. Invest Ophthalmol Vis Sci 2003; 44(9):3885–3891.

29. Iwase A, Suzuki Y, Araie M, et al. The prevalence of primary open-angle glaucoma in Japanese: the Tajimi Study. Ophthalmology 2004; 111(9):1641–1648.

30. Brandt JD, Beiser JA, Kass MA, et al. Central corneal thickness in the Ocular Hypertension Treatment Study (OHTS). Ophthalmology 2001; 108(10):1779–1788.

31. Medeiros FA, Sample PA, Zangwill LM, et al. Corneal thickness as a risk factor for visual field loss in patients with preperimetric glaucomatous optic neuropathy. Am J Ophthalmol 2003; 136(5):805–813.

32. Nemesure B, Wu SY, Hennis A, et al. Corneal thickness and intraocular pressure in the Barbados eye studies. Arch Ophthalmol 2003; 121(2):240–244.

33. Pache M, Flammer J. A sick eye in a sick body? Systemic findings in patients with primary open-angle glaucoma. Surv Ophthalmol 2006; 51(3):179–212.

34. Hayreh SS. Retinal and optic nerve head ischemic disorders and atherosclerosis: role of serotonin. Prog Retin Eye Res 1999; 18(2):191–221.

35. Dielemans I, de Jong PT, Stolk R, et al. Primary open-angle glaucoma, intraocular pressure, and diabetes mellitus in the general elderly population. The Rotterdam Study. Ophthalmology 1996; 103(8):1271–1275.

36. Klein BE, Klein R, Jensen SC. Open-angle glaucoma and older-onset diabetes. The Beaver Dam Eye Study. Ophthalmology 1994; 101(7):1173–1177.

37. Mitchell P, Smith W, Chey T, et al. Open-angle glaucoma and diabetes: the Blue Mountains eye study, Australia. Ophthalmology 1997; 104(4):712–718.

38. Kahn HA, Leibowitz HM, Ganley JP, et al. The Framingham Eye Study. I. Outline and major prevalence findings. Am J Epidemiol 1977; 106(1):17–32.

39. Tielsch JM, Katz J, Quigley HA, et al. Diabetes. intraocular pressure, and primary open-angle glaucoma in the Baltimore Eye Survey. Ophthalmology 1995; 102(1):48–53.

40. Mori K, Ando F, Nomura H, et al. Relationship between intraocular pressure and obesity in Japan. Int J Epidemiol 2000; 29(4):661–666.

41. Grodum K, Heijl A, Bengtsson B. Risk of glaucoma in ocular hypertension with and without pseudoexfoliation. Ophthalmology 2005; 112(3):386–390.

42. Thomas R, Nirmalan PK. S. Skishnaiah. Pseudoexfoliation in southern India. The Andra Pradesh Eye Disease Study,. Invest Ophthalmol Vis Sci 2005; 46:1170–1176.

43. Arvind H, Raju P, Paul PG, et al. Pseudoexfoliation in south India. Br J Ophthalmol 2003; 87(11):1321–1323.

44. Jonasson F, Damji KF, Arnarsson A, et al. Prevalence of open-angle glaucoma in Iceland: Reykjavik Eye Study. Eye 2003; 17(6):747–753.

45. Herndon LW, Chalia P, Ababio-Danso B, et al. Survey of glaucoma in an eye clinic in Ghana, West Africa. J Glaucoma 2002; 11:421–425.

46. Teshome T, Regassa K. Prevalence of pseudoexfoliation syndrome in Ethiopian patients scheduled for cataract surgery. Acta Ophthalmol Scand 2004; 82(3 Pt 1):254–258.

47. Damji KF, Bains HS, Stefansson E, et al. Is pseudoexfoliation syndrome inherited? A review of genetic and nongenetic factors and a new observation. Ophthalmic Genet 1998; 19:175–185.

48. Lowe RF. Primary angle-closure glaucoma: a review of ocular biometry. Aust J Ophthalmol 1977; 5:9–17.

49. Alsbirk PH. Anterior chamber depth and primary angle-closure glaucoma. I. An epidemiologic study in Greenland Eskimos. Acta Ophthalmol 1975; 53:89–104.

50. Clemmesen V, Alsbirk PH. Primary angle-closure glaucoma in Greenland. Acta Ophthalmol 1971; 49:47–58.

51. Foster PJ, Alsbirk PH, Baasanhu J, et al. Anterior chamber depth in Mongolians: variation with age, sex, and method of measurement. Am J Ophthalmol 1997; 124:53–60.

52. Thomas R, George R, Parikh R, et al. Five-year risk of progression of primary angle-closuresuspects to primary angle closure: a population-based study. Br J Ophthalmol 2003; 87:450–454.

53. Thomas R, Parikh R, Muliyil J, et al. Five-year risk of progression of primary angle-closure to primary angle-closure glaucoma: a population-based study. Acta Ophthalmol Scand 2003; 81:480–485.

54. He M, Foster PJ, Johnson GJ, et al. Angle-closure glaucoma in Asian and European people. Different diseases? Eye 2006; 20:3–12.

55. Vijaya L, George R, Paul PG, et al. Prevalence of open-angle glaucoma in a rural south Indian population. Invest Ophthalmol Vis Sci 2005; 46:4461–4467.

56. Mitchell P, Smith W, Attebo K, et al. Prevalence of open-angle glaucoma in Australia. The Blue Mountains Eye Study. Ophthalmology 1996; 103:1661–1669.

57. Dielemans I, VIngerling JR, Wolfs RCW, et al. The prevalence of primary open-angle glaucoma in a population-based study in The Netherlands. Ophthalmology 1994; 11:1851–1855.

58. Fraser S, Bunce C, Wormald R. Risk factors for late presentation in chronic glaucoma. Invest Ophthalmol Vis Sci 1999; 40:2251–2257.

59. Fraser S, Bunce C, Wormald R, et al. Deprivation and late presentation of glaucoma: case-control study. Br Med J 2001; 322:639–643.

CHAPTER 2

Screening for Glaucoma

Paul R Healey

INTRODUCTION

The basis for healthcare in most countries is for individuals to seek care for symptomatic conditions. This approach depends on a number of requirements:

- Individuals must know what symptoms require health assessment and when to seek it.
- Individuals must be able to access healthcare assessment and treatment.
- The healthcare system must be able to diagnose disease and/or treat the symptoms satisfactorily.

No society can satisfy all factors for every member. The effectiveness of a symptom-based healthcare system is dependent on the outcome of the disease and its treatment, at both individual and societal levels. For certain highly prevalent or contagious diseases with significant morbidity or cost, primary prevention in the form of treatment of unaffected individuals is practised. In many countries, primary prevention includes vaccination against infectious diseases, water fluoridation to prevent dental caries, and food supplementation (e.g. iodine) to prevent diseases of nutrient deficiency.

In contrast to treating unaffected individuals, secondary prevention aims to improve outcomes of prevalent disease by its earlier detection and treatment. But where it has a long presymptomatic phase, symptom-based healthcare is unable to detect and therefore treat such a disease. The detection of disease in individuals without symptoms is known as disease screening. Successful screening shortens the time between onset of disease and diagnosis. It can occur at an individual level within a doctor–patient relationship or at a public health level as part of a defined program to improve health outcomes.

Disease screening is usually considered within the context of the detection and treatment of a disease or disability within the entire healthcare system. Test accuracy and cost constrain the screening population and type of screening tests used. However, follow-on costs of treating and following positive screenees must also be considered. Therefore, for some screening programs, the aim of the screening test is not to diagnose disease but to provide a smaller population enriched with disease that requires further testing to make a definitive diagnosis. This includes screening tests for breast and prostate cancer. For other conditions, such as systemic or ocular hypertension, the screening test may be definitive.

For public health screening to be effective there must be a way of implementing the screening program in the group of interest. The terms 'mass screening' or 'community-based screening' are usually used to refer to a public health program where a group of at-risk individuals are targeted for screening. It is usually expensive, as the target group needs to be contacted and a healthcare service episode created specifically for the screening test.

In contrast, 'opportunistic screening' or 'case detection' offers screening to those who are already attending the health service for other reasons. As such, direct program-to-target population contact is not required and the cost of screening is marginal to the preexisting healthcare episode.

Some screening guidelines have suggested opportunistic screening should be considered when evidence is poor or lacking for the utility of a mass screening program.[1] In this sense, it is used to justify clinical activity in the absence of good evidence. In reality, opportunistic screening can provide the same service as mass screening, but only to that proportion of the target population who attend the health service intercurrently. Therefore, as a screening methodology, its efficacy is dependent on the proportion of the target population that could be reached.

CRITERIA FOR SCREENING

The question of whether screening is worthwhile is complex. Forty years ago, Wilson and Junger[2] proposed six prerequisites for screening (Table 2.1).

If glaucoma is assessed against these criteria, it has a number features which make it a good candidate for screening.

1. **The condition sought should be an important health problem.**

TABLE 2.1 Wilson and Junger's prerequisites for disease screening
The condition sought should be an important health problem.
There must be an accepted and effective treatment for patients with the disease that must be more effective at preventing morbidity when initiated in the early, asymptomatic stage than when begun in the later, symptomatic stages.
Facilities for diagnosis and treatment should be available.
There must be an appropriate, acceptable, and reasonably accurate screening test.
The natural history of the condition, including development from latent to manifest disease, should be adequately understood.
The cost of case-finding (including diagnosis and treatment of patients diagnosed) should be economically balanced in relation to possible expenditure on medical care as a whole.

Epidemiologic studies have shown glaucoma to be an important public health problem. Projections from some of these studies estimate that 60.5 million people will be affected by open-angle and angle-closure glaucoma in 2010, rising to 79.6 million by 2020. Bilateral glaucoma blindness will affect 8.4 million people in 2010 and 11.2 million in 2020.[3] Visual loss from glaucoma can not be reversed.

2. **There must be an accepted and effective treatment for patients with the disease that must be more effective at preventing morbidity when initiated in the early, asymptomatic stage than when begun in the later, symptomatic stages.**
   Glaucoma is irreversible but presymptomatic throughout much of its course. A severe symptomatic stage of glaucoma usually occurs when visual acuity decreases at the end stage of the disease. Lowering intraocular pressure (IOP) with medicines, laser, or surgery is an accepted and effective treatment for glaucoma. A number of studies have suggested that the onset[4] and progression[5–7] of open-angle glaucoma is delayed by these methods. Earlier disease state at commencement of treatment also appears to reduce the risk of progression.[5]

3. **Facilities for diagnosis and treatment should be available.**
   Almost all nations have resident or visiting medically trained ophthalmologists. In some countries, optometrists also provide primary eye care. The saturation of diagnostic and treatment facilities for eye disease varies greatly, usually in proportion to GDP and health spending as a whole. Access to health services also varies greatly between and within countries, related to geographic, cultural, and financial factors.

4. **There must be an appropriate, acceptable, and reasonably accurate screening test.**
   The development of screening tests for glaucoma has principally focused on open-angle glaucoma using risk factor assessment, in particular IOP measurement.[8–10] Screening algorithms based on functional criteria such as visual field defects[11–13] and to a lesser extent structural (optic disc and nerve fiber layer) criteria have also been developed.[14–17] For angle-closure glaucoma, the focus has been on detection of narrow angles or angle closure. The accuracy of individual and to some extent multiple screening tests has been generally thought to be disappointing for early glaucoma. However, diagnostic test characteristics are generally more favorable for more advanced disease.

5. **The natural history of the condition, including development from latent to manifest disease, should be adequately understood.**
   The natural history of open-angle glaucoma is reasonably well understood. The Early Manifest Glaucoma Trial reported a 62% rate of progression over 6 years among controls.[18] Estimates of 10-year progression in a cohort study ranged from 50% to 70% depending on the visual field criteria.[19] The same study reported the cumulative risk of blindness due to advanced field loss as 16%. A long-term cohort study reported a 27% risk of blindness over 20 years.[20] A number of reports suggest that the risk of blindness is greater in those who first present with visual field loss, particularly moderate to advanced loss.[21,22] This is consistent with other data suggesting that the rate of visual field loss on standard automated perimetry increases with greater field loss on initial examination.[23,24]

6. **The cost of case-finding (including diagnosis and treatment of patients diagnosed) should be economically balanced in relation to possible expenditure on medical care as a whole.**
   The cost of case-finding depends on the mode of screening and the diagnostic algorithm used. The least expensive form of screening would focus on short, simple examination methods such as history taking and physical examination (of the eye) in people already presenting to eye care services for other reasons. Treatment and monitoring of glaucoma are major potential costs of screening. There are few estimates of these costs in comparison to health spending as a whole. An important problem is the lack of high-quality data in this area. Two recent papers have reported models for open-angle glaucoma screening in Europe.[25,26] The first[25] compared an organized mass screening program at 5-year intervals between 50 and 79 years to opportunistic screening (case-detection). The authors reported a cost of €9023 per quality-adjusted life year (QALY) gained from the screening program with an overall prevention of 930 years of visual disability. The model was particularly sensitive to screening cost and specificity of diagnostic tests. The other report[26] also modeled an organized mass-screening program, in comparison to opportunistic screening, using a somewhat different methodology. A 10-year interval mass-screening program in a 50-year-old cohort with a 4% glaucoma prevalence was considered likely to be cost-effective. The model was highly sensitive to perspective on costs and test specificity.

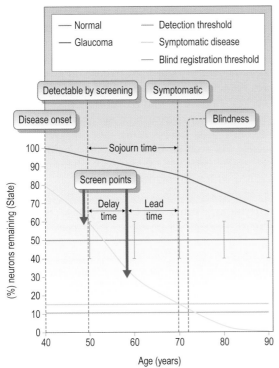

FIGURE. 2.1 The State/Rate/Risk Factor graph as it relates to open-angle glaucoma screening. (From Spaeth GL. Visual loss in a glaucoma clinic. I. Sociological considerations. Invest ophthalmol 1970; 9: 73–82.)[27]

SCREENING CONCEPTS

Because the aim of screening is to steal a march on time, temporal relationships are critical to the understanding of when and who to screen. Figure 2.1 shows glaucoma expressed in terms of its State, Rate, and Risk Factors. In this figure, *time* is shown along the abscissa and the *state* of glaucomatous damage on the ordinate. The instantaneous slope of the line represents the *rate* of progression. The determinants of that rate of progression are the known and unknown *risk factors* for that patient's disease.

While the aim of screening is to detect disease earlier than the symptomatic period, the earliest state of the disease may not be detectable. A theoretical threshold of detection is shown as a light-blue line. For visual field loss on standard automated perimetry, it has been proposed that 40% neuronal loss is required for detection.[28] The error bars around the blue line represent the uncertainty of diagnosis. The orange line represents the average state at which the vision loss might become sufficiently symptomatic for eye care to be sought. This level has not been reported. However, it can be estimated as between 80% and 90%.[28] The red line represents a theoretical level at which vision loss meets the criteria for blind registration (less then 10° of intact visual field).[28]

The time between positive screening and onset of symptoms is the time gained by screening. It is known as the 'lead time.' However, if the time of positive

screening occurs after the disease state crosses the detection threshold then some potential lead time is lost. This is known as the 'delay time.' The lead time and delay time together make up the 'sojourn time.'

The yellow line represents an imaginary person with open-angle glaucoma (OAG) to illustrate the features of the figure. In this case, the glaucomatous neural loss commenced some time before age 40. At age 49, the person screens negative because of the insensitivity of the tests used. From age 50, the test would be able to detect the OAG, but the person does not return for screening until age 60, by which time almost two-thirds of the optic nerve neurons have been lost. At this stage, disc and field changes are so great that screening is positive. Although 10 years and 25% of neurons have been lost by the delay (delay time), the positive diagnosis at age 60 has gained 10 years and 25% of neurons from the time the person would have presented with reduced vision (lead time). If aggressive risk factor reduction (in the absence of being able to directly arrest the cellular processes) changed the rate of loss (slope of the yellow line) to approximate the green 'normal' rate, the subject may retain useful vision until death in his eighties. This 10-year lead time would prevent 10 years of blindness if the same improvement of rate was initiated at the time of symptomatic presentation.

Both lead and delay time vary with sojourn time, which is a function of the sensitivity of the test and the rate of progression. Sojourn time can vary with disease subtype and age. In breast cancer, sojourn time was estimated as 2 years in women aged 40–49 years regardless of histological type. In women aged 50–69 years, sojourn time varied strongly with histological type (between 1.2 and 7.7 years).[29] This has lead to increased screening frequency in younger women.[30]

There are few data in the glaucoma literature concerning estimates and risk factors for sojourn time. Given that glaucoma is symptomatic only at an advanced stage, it might be reasonable to use advanced visual field loss or blindness as a surrogate for symptomatic presentation and use cohort data (most of whom would be treated) to gauge a rough idea of the lead time of cases detected by current screening methods. Jay and Murdoch used ages at presentation for patients with early and advanced field loss to estimate rates of progression for untreated open-angle glaucoma.[31] They reported that IOP had an important influence, with lead times of 14.4 years for IOPs of 21–25 mmHg, 6.5 years for IOPs 25–30 mmHg, and 2.9 years for IOPs over 30 mmHg. A number of studies have confirmed IOP as a risk factor for progression,[5,32,33] and some have also found older age at diagnosis to be a risk factor as well.[5,33] It is not known whether sojourn or lead times vary with glaucoma subtype. Primary angle-closure glaucoma causes disproportionately more blindness for its prevalence, suggesting it is a more aggressive disease.[34–36] However, this may be an IOP effect, as a stronger correlation between IOP and visual field loss has been reported in angle-closure glaucoma compared with open-angle glaucoma.[37]

While increasing lead time diagnoses cases with less disease burden and increases the opportunity for treatment, the trade-off is less reliable screening because screening points lie closer to the limit of detection. The magnitude will depend on the characteristics of the screening test. This effect was seen in the Ocular Hypertension Treatment Trial, which followed 1636 subjects with ocular hypertension and no detectable OAG for 5 years, with one half randomized to receive IOP-lowering treatment. Of 703 reliable visual field tests that showed the first development of glaucomatous field loss, 604 (85.9%) did not show the field loss on repeated testing.[38] In addition to confirmed glaucomatous field loss, study end points also included loss of neural rim tissue observed by trained graders of stereo-optic disc photographs. Of confirmed OAG cases, initial end points were found on optic disc grading in 50% of treated and 57% of control subjects. This contrasts with 42% of treated and 33% of control subjects for whom visual field testing provided the first OAG end point.[4]

The reliability of testing for glaucoma will have an important impact on not only sensitivity, but also health resources due to false-positive screening. The ideal region within the sojourn time to screen would be one where a simple, inexpensive screening test would be quite reliable, yet still giving patients enough lead time for treatment to be effective.

IMPORTANT QUESTIONS IN GLAUCOMA SCREENING

Discussion of glaucoma at a public health or governmental level is based on concepts supplied by the ophthalmic community. A misunderstanding of fundamental concepts in glaucoma or screening can lead to erroneous conclusions about the utility of screening for glaucoma. The questions below address some of these misconceptions.

WHAT CONSTITUTES EARLY DIAGNOSIS?

An important misconception concerns what constitutes early glaucoma diagnosis. Frequently, it is thought to mean diagnosis at either an extremely early stage of the disease, or even diagnosis *before* any damage has occurred. Studies of early diagnosis have examined ocular hypertension or the use of sophisticated and sensitive technologies for detecting the earliest evidence of structural or functional damage. Focusing on this stage of the disease is not only unnecessary, it causes a multitude of problems related to the uncertainty of diagnosis and dilutes the effectiveness of intervention. From a public health perspective, early diagnosis means diagnosis at an earlier stage than would have presented symptomatically. Given that symptomatic presentation of glaucoma occurs at its end stage, almost any stage of glaucoma is early disease from the point of view of screening. If we ask a screening strategy to deliver a complete cohort of at-risk patients with the earliest

signs of disease, it will fail. But if we focus later in the sojourn period, our diagnostic accuracy will be much improved, the group detected will be closer to symptomatic disease and the time to blindness, and therefore, the time-benefit of treatment will be, in general, much greater. An additional problem with trying to screen for the earliest disease is that screening cycles need to be very short, greatly increasing cost. Moving further into the sojourn time allows more cost-effective screening frequency. As seen in Figure 2.1, decades of lead time can be gained from early detection without being overly concerned with minimizing delay time.

SCREENING FOR DISEASE VERSUS SCREENING FOR RISK FACTORS

Focusing on screening for the earliest stages of glaucoma naturally leads to the idea of screening for and treating ocular hypertension in order to prevent glaucoma. This is perhaps the primary fault with current screening strategies. The Ocular Hypertension Treatment Study[4] (OHTS) demonstrated a reduction in the development of glaucoma if people with ocular hypertension are treated with pressure-lowering medications. Indeed, only 4.4% of those treated developed glaucoma. This contrasts with the results of the Early Manifest Glaucoma Trial[5] (EMGT) which treated people discovered to have glaucoma after screening for the disease. In this study, the rate of glaucoma progression in the treatment group was 45% over a similar time period. At face value, it would seem that there is a much better chance to prevent glaucoma if we detect and treat ocular hypertension rather than wait for glaucoma to develop. However, the reason for conducting randomized, controlled trials is to compare the treatment group to the control group, and this analysis paints quite a different picture. In the OHTS, only 9.5% of the untreated control group developed glaucoma compared with 62% of the control group of the EMGT. The reduction in risk that treatment confers is the difference in rate between treatment and control. The Early Manifest Glaucoma Trial showed a 17% absolute reduction in risk of progression compared to 5.1% in the OHTS (or 6.6% for the comparative [white] group of OHTS subjects).

The reason for this is that there are known and unknown risk and protective factors which alter the effect of a particular risk factor on the onset of a disease. For some people, ocular hypertension leads to a rapid progression to glaucoma. For this group, treatment is certainly worthwhile as would be finding them through IOP screening. However, for others with ocular hypertension, glaucoma may not develop for many decades, or may never develop at all. For this latter group, there is a benefit in not screening, as it would save the individuals from anxiety, cost, and treatment of side effects. For the former group, any benefit of IOP screening will depend on whether there is gain in starting treatment immediately compared to waiting until the disease became detectable. We do not yet know the answer to this question and trial evidence would

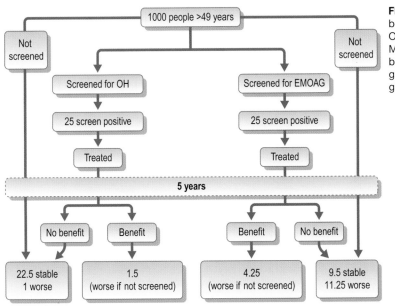

FIGURE 2.2 The effect of screening on treatment benefit. Data from Blue Mountains Eye Study, Ocular Hypertension Treatment Study, and Early Manifest Glaucoma Trial. OH, Ocular hypertension between 24 and 32 mmHg without evidence of glaucoma; EMOAG, Early Manifest open-angle glaucoma.

be helpful. While protective factors may also occur in someone with glaucoma, the fact that the disease has already occurred shows that the risk factors outweigh the protective factors and make *further* progression of the disease much more likely. To explore the benefit of screening on outcome, we can examine the number of people we would need to screen to prevent one case of progressing glaucoma (Fig. 2.2). This is called the number needed to screen.

THE NUMBER NEEDED TO SCREEN

Using the Blue Mountains Eye Study as an older screening population, for every 1000 people we screen with IOP measurement using OHTS criteria, we will find about 25 with ocular hypertension between 24 mmHg and 32 mmHg (Healey PR; unpublished data). Data from the OHTS non-African-American population tells us that of these 25, about 2.5 will develop glaucoma over 5 years if untreated. If everyone who screened positive was treated successfully 1 person would develop glaucoma, sparing 1.5 people who would have otherwise developed the disease over the 5-year period.

If we screened another 1000 people for manifest glaucoma with a matching optic disc and visual field examination, about 30 cases of glaucoma would be found.[39] Excluding advanced disease[40] leaves us with 25 people. The EMGT tells us that over 5 years, glaucoma will progress in 15.5 of these if untreated and 11.25 if treated, leaving 4.25 people whose glaucoma progression was prevented.

If we optimistically regard progression in both ocular hypertension and manifest glaucoma to be equally bad and compliance with treatment to be equally good, there would still be almost threefold more people who benefit from glaucoma rather than ocular hypertension screening. Under these ideal conditions, the number

needed to screen for ocular hypertension screening to prevent one case of glaucoma in 5 years is 670 (1000/1.5). If, instead, we screen for glaucoma, we only need to screen 235 people (1000/4.25) to prevent one case of progression over the same time period.

An alternative approach is to look at what benefit we can confer by screening (see Fig. 2.2). For every 1000 people screened for ocular hypertension (OH), after 5 years 1.5 would benefit from the screening (if they were all treated), one would progress despite treatment, and 22.5 would just be inconvenienced by treatment (as they would not have progressed even without treatment). In contrast, if the same 1000 were screened for OAG, after 5 years 4.25 would benefit against 9.5 who would not benefit from treatment (because their disease would not progress even if untreated). Eleven and one-quarter would progress despite treatment. Whether any of those in the 'no treatment benefit' groups would be better off if not screened depends on how the negative aspects of diagnosis and treatment compare to benefits not related to treatment at that time or whether there may be some later benefit (after 5 years) from screening positive. Given that those with glaucoma already have a disease, the case for a delayed or nontreatment benefit will be stronger for the OAG group compared with the OH group. The ratios of people benefiting to not benefiting from screening and treatment are 1:15 for OH and 1:2.2 for OAG.

The above examples necessarily make many assumptions about disease rates and do not take into account finding previously diagnosed glaucoma when screening for glaucoma or finding glaucoma when screening for ocular hypertension. However, population studies suggest that, in developed countries, most glaucoma with raised IOP is already diagnosed and conversely most undiagnosed glaucoma is not associated with high IOP,[39] making the difference between screening strategies even greater.

Another important consideration is the effect of false-positive and false-negative outcomes from the screening program and the impacts of screening frequency. The effect of false positives is to increase the number who do not benefit from screening. False negatives can be 'caught' in later screening cycles. The benefit they receive depends on the screening frequency. Frequent screening will pick up previous false negatives before their disease has progressed very much. But frequent screening is more costly. Screening benefit will also depend on life expectancy. From Figure 2.1, it can be seen that someone with a longer life expectancy will have more time to gain a benefit from screening. Someone screening positive close to death may not have sufficient time to benefit from treatment.

These analyses demonstrate a finding that has been previously reported for other diseases,[41] namely that there will always be less benefit if we screen for risk factors rather than the disease itself. That is not to say that intraocular pressure is not important. We know that, along with increasing age, increasing intraocular pressure is the strongest risk factor for the prevalence, incidence, and progression of glaucoma. As part of a strategy to screen for glaucoma, IOP measurement, along with other risk factor assessment, may well be helpful. However, the screening outcome should be glaucoma and not ocular hypertension.

SCREENING FOR ANGLE CLOSURE

If a very great proportion of people with a disease risk factor develop the disease, then it may indeed be worthwhile using it in screening. This is particularly true if the time from the appearance of the risk factor to the occurrence of the disease is short in relation to the sojourn time. Although less common than open-angle glaucoma, primary angle closure glaucoma causes more blindness[3] and most probably has a shorter sojourn time.

Angle closure is the primary risk factor for angle-closure glaucoma, its effect being mediated through increasing intraocular pressure.[37] Given this relationship, it may be feasible to screen for angle closure (with or without intraocular pressure) in order to detect angle-closure glaucoma.

There have been very few reports of screening for angle closure or even the risk of glaucoma in people with angle closure. The Liwan Eye Study reported the prevalence of narrow iridocorneal angles, angle closure, and angle-closure glaucoma in a well-defined older Southern Chinese population. Ten percent of the population had gonioscopically narrow angles and, of these, one in five had primary (synechial) angle closure (2.4% of the population).[34,42] Angle-closure glaucoma was found in 1.5% of the entire population,[34] suggesting an ideal positive predictive value of angle closure for angle-closure glaucoma of 64% with 100% sensitivity in this higher-risk general population. If the incidence of angle-closure glaucoma was high in those with angle closure, the case for screening for angle closure would be even stronger. But this risk has not been well reported. One

TABLE 2.2 **Key questions from the OTA report on open-angle glaucoma screening**
KQ 1: Is there new evidence that screening for open-angle glaucoma reduces severe visual impairment?
KQ 3: Is there new evidence that feasible screening tests are accurate and reliable in detecting increased intraocular pressure or open-angle glaucoma?
KQ 4: Is there new evidence that treating increased intraocular pressure reduces the incidence of primary open-angle glaucoma?
KQ 5: Is there new evidence that treating increased intraocular pressure reduces severe visual impairments?
KQ 6: Is there new evidence that treating open-angle glaucoma with drugs, laser, and/or surgery reduces severe visual impairment?
KQ 7: Is there new evidence that screening results in adverse effects? Is screening acceptable to patients?
KQ 8: Is there new evidence that treatment of increased intraocular pressure and/or open-angle glaucoma results in adverse effects?
Note: there was no KQ 2 in the list.

cohort study in Indian eyes suggested a 5-year incidence of angle-closure glaucoma of 28.5% among subjects with angle closure.[43] The alternative strategy would be to screen for the glaucomatous optic neuropathy itself. But there are no studies comparing the efficacy and outcomes of these two approaches. As this disease is a major cause of glaucoma blindness, well-designed and conducted studies are urgently needed.

CURRENT STATUS SCREENING FOR GLAUCOMA

There have been a number of public health analyses of open-angle glaucoma screening.[44–47] The first addressed by government in North America occurred almost 20 years ago and has been reviewed several times since. The most recent review was by the United States Preventive Services Task Force (USPSTF) in 2005.[45,47] It was based on an initial report in 1988[45] and a review in 1996.[46]

For the 2005 review, a Medline-based literature review was undertaken to answer seven key questions (Table 2.2). The only evidence found were trials of IOP-lowering treatment which were rated good to poor as an evidence source (KQ 5, KQ 8). The report made some specific and important statements concerning inadequacy of evidence for glaucoma screening. They included:

- no studies assessing the screening and treatment of open-angle glaucoma in a population setting
- no population-based studies demonstrating that screening is feasible, accurate, or reliable for detecting early glaucoma
- no studies that directly assess the sensitivity and specificity of the adult medical eye examination for the diagnosis of glaucoma

- no studies that assessed the treatment of ocular hypertension using delay of progression to severe visual impairment as an end point
- no new studies (since the last review in 1996) addressing the harms or acceptability of screening for ocular hypertension or primary open-angle glaucoma

Lastly, the task force reported that there was no clear way to quantitatively relate specific degrees of visual field loss to impairment of vision-specific quality of life (QOL), and studies examining these associations had not established a relationship between changes in vision-specific QOL and specific treatment approaches. The recommendation statement was therefore that: 'There is insufficient evidence to recommend for or against routine screening for intraocular hypertension or glaucoma by primary care clinicians.' This was the same conclusion reached in previous assessments and underscored a relatively negative attitude to glaucoma screening in a contemporary editorial by a task force member.[48]

The irony in the negative reports concerning glaucoma screening is that, in the developed world at least, most diagnosed glaucoma is discovered by routine opportunistic screening either for the disease or its risk factors. This may take the form of a comprehensive eye examination by an ophthalmologist during a visit for another reason or noncontact tonometry performed by an optometrist during the prescription of glasses. We can therefore reasonably attribute the vast majority of any treatment benefit to screening. In developing regions where screeing is sparse, rates of undiagnosed glaucoma are extremely high and disease morbidity correspondingly higher.[50]

However, in developed regions, the large number of people with glaucoma who remain undiagnosed[39,49] despite frequent screening opportunities[51,52] tells us that screening strategies are far from ideal and reinforces the need to improve our screening algorithms.

The comments by the task force offer challenges to the ophthalmic and public health communities. Given the results of treatment studies such as EMGT and OHTS, with appropriate data on the performance of glaucoma screening tests,[53] it may not be necessary to conduct randomized, controlled trials of screening for glaucoma. With a better understanding of what constitutes early glaucoma and the difference between screening for disease and risk factors, it may also be unnecessary to conduct a trial to show that treating ocular hypertension prevents blindness. Nevertheless, there is a clear need for further research into glaucoma screening. We know very little about the determinants of sojourn time in glaucoma or the relationship between disease state and disability.

Since the time of Wilson and Junger,[2] a number of alternative models have evolved for assessing screening for a disease. The international Evidence-Based Medicine Working Group has published a number of users' guides, including one for evaluating screening guidelines and recommendations.[54] They suggest asking two simple sets of questions:

1. Validity
   A. Is there randomized, controlled trial evidence that earlier intervention works?
   B. Were the data identified, collected, and combined in an unbiased fashion?
2. Impact
   A. What are the benefits compared to the harms?
   B. How do these compare in different target groups and with different screening strategies?
   C. What are the impacts of screenees' values and preferences?
   D. What is the impact of uncertainty?
   E. What is the cost-effectiveness?

The evidence for the first set is now good. Answering the second set of questions may facilitate the development of accurate, cost-effective glaucoma screening strategies. The broad implementation of such strategies may have the single biggest impact on the prevention of blindness and disability from glaucoma.

ACKNOWLEDGEMENTS

I would like to thank Les Irwig, Professor of Epidemiology, School of Public Health, University of Sydney, NSW, Australia, for his assistance in the preparation of this manuscript. I would also like to acknowledge George Spaeth, Louis J Esposito Glaucoma Research Professor, Wills Eye Institute, Philadelphia, USA as the originator of the graph[27] on which Figure 2.1 is based.

REFERENCES

1. The American Cancer Society: guidelines for the cancer-related checkup. Recommendations and rationale. CA Cancer J Clin 1992; 30:4–50.

2. Wilson JMG, Junger F. Principles and practice of screening for disease. [34]. Public Health Papers. Geneva: World Health Organization; 1968.

3. Quigley HA, Broman AT. The number of people with glaucoma worldwide in 2010 and 2020. Br J Ophthalmol 2006; 90: 262–267.

4. Kass MA, Heuer DK, Higginbotham EJ, et al. The Ocular Hypertension Treatment Study: a randomized trial determines that topical ocular hypotensive medication delays or prevents the onset of primary open-angle glaucoma. Arch Ophthalmol 2002; 120:701–713.

5. Heijl A, Leske MC, Bengtsson B, et al. Reduction of intraocular pressure and glaucoma progression: results from the Early Manifest Glaucoma Trial. Arch Ophthalmol 2002; 120: 1268–1279.

6. Collaborative Normal-Tension Glaucoma Study Group. The effectiveness of intraocular pressure reduction in the treatment of normal-tension glaucoma. Collaborative Normal-Tension Glaucoma Study Group. Am J Ophthalmol 1998; 126:498–505.

7. Collaborative Normal-Tension Glaucoma Study Group. Comparison of glaucomatous progression between untreated patients with normal-tension glaucoma and patients with therapeutically reduced intraocular pressures. Collaborative Normal-Tension Glaucoma Study Group. Am J Ophthalmol 1998; 126:487–497.

8. Le Blanc R. Value of intraocular pressure measurement as a screening tool for glaucoma. Surv Ophthalmol 1989; 33(Suppl):445–446.

9. Vernon SA, Jones SJ, Henry DJ. Maximising the sensitivity and specificity of non-contact tonometry in glaucoma screening. Eye 1991; 5(Pt 4):491–493.

10. Katz J, Tielsch JM, Quigley HA, et al. Automated suprathreshold screening for glaucoma: the Baltimore Eye Survey. Invest Ophthalmol Vis Sci 1993; 34:3271–3277.

11. Heijl A. Automatic perimetry in glaucoma visual field screening. A clinical study. Graefe's Arch Clin Exp Ophthalmol 1976; 200:21–37.

12. Henson DB. An optimized visual field screening method. Surv Ophthalmol 1989; 33(Suppl):443–444.

13. Johnson CA, Samuels SJ. Screening for glaucomatous visual field loss with frequency-doubling perimetry. Invest Ophthalmol Vis Sci 1997; 38:413–425.

14. Sommer A, Pollack I, Maumenee AE. Optic disc parameters and onset of glaucomatous field loss. II. Static screening criteria. Arch Ophthalmol 1979; 97:1449–1454.

15. Hitchings RA, Brown DB, Anderton SA. Glaucoma screening by means of an optic disc grid. Br J Ophthalmol 1983; 67: 352–355.

16. Cooper RL, Grose GC, Constable IJ. Mass screening of the optic disc for glaucoma: a follow-up study. Aust NZ J Ophthalmol 1986; 14:35–39.

17. Harper R, Reeves B. The sensitivity and specificity of direct ophthalmoscopic optic disc assessment in screening for glaucoma: a multivariate analysis. Graefe's Arch Clin Exp Ophthalmol 2000; 238:949–955.

18. Heijl A, Leske MC, Bengtsson B, et al. Reduction of intraocular pressure and glaucoma progression: results from the Early Manifest Glaucoma Trial. Arch Ophthalmol 2002; 120:1268–1279.

19. Wilson MR, Kosoko O, Cowan CL Jr, et al. Progression of visual field loss in untreated glaucoma patients and glaucoma suspects in St. Lucia, West Indies. Am J Ophthalmol 2002; 134:399–405.

20. Hattenhauer MG, Johnson DH, Ing HH, et al. The probability of blindness from open-angle glaucoma. Ophthalmology 1998; 105:2099–2104.

21. Oliver JE, Hattenhauer MG, Herman D, et al. Blindness and glaucoma: a comparison of patients progressing to blindness from glaucoma with patients maintaining vision. Am J Ophthalmol 2002; 133:764–772.

22. Grant WM, Burke JF Jr. Why do some people go blind from glaucoma? Ophthalmology 1982; 89:991–998.

23. Wilson R, Walker AM, Dueker DK, et al. Risk factors for rate of progression of glaucomatous visual field loss: a computer-based analysis. Arch Ophthalmol 1982; 100:737–741.

24. Mikelberg FS, Schulzer M, Drance SM, et al. The rate of progression of scotomas in glaucoma. Am J Ophthalmol 1986; 101:1–6.

25. Vaahtoranta-Lehtonen H, Tuulonen A, Aronen P, et al. Cost effectiveness and cost utility of an organized screening programme for glaucoma. Acta Ophthalmol Scand 2007; 85:508–518.

26. Burr JM, Mowatt G, Hernandez R, et al. The clinical effectiveness and cost-effectiveness of screening for open-angle glaucoma: a systematic review and economic evaluation. Health Technology Assessment 2007; 11:41.

27. Spaeth GL. Visual loss in a glaucoma clinic. I. Sociological considerations. Invest Ophthalmol 1970; 9:73–82.

28. Bartz-Schmidt KU, Thumann G, Jonescu-Cuypers CP, et al. Quantitative morphologic and functional evaluation of the optic nerve head in chronic open-angle glaucoma. Surv Ophthalmol 1999; 44(Suppl 1):S41–S53.

29. Tabar L, Fagerberg G, Chen HH, et al. Tumour development, histology and grade of breast cancers: prognosis and progression. Int J Cancer 1996; 66:413–419.

30. Tabar L, Fagerberg G, Chen HH, et al. Efficacy of breast cancer screening by age. New results from the Swedish Two-County Trial. Cancer 1995; 75:2507–2517.

31. Jay JL, Murdoch JR. The rate of visual field loss in untreated primary open angle glaucoma. Br J Ophthalmol 1993; 77: 176–178.

32. The Advanced Glaucoma Intervention Study (AGIS): 7. The relationship between control of intraocular pressure and visual field deterioration. The AGIS Investigators. Am J Ophthalmol 2000; 130:429–440.

33. Gordon MO, Beiser JA, Brandt JD, et al. The Ocular Hypertension Treatment Study: baseline factors that predict the onset of primary open-angle glaucoma. Arch Ophthalmol 2002; 120:714–720.

34. He M, Foster PJ, Ge J, et al. Prevalence and clinical characteristics of glaucoma in adult Chinese: a population-based study in Liwan District, Guangzhou. Invest Ophthalmol Vis Sci 2006; 47:2782–2788.

35. Foster PJ, Oen FT, Machin D, et al. The prevalence of glaucoma in Chinese residents of Singapore: a cross-sectional population survey of the Tanjong Pagar district. Arch Ophthalmol 2000; 118:1105–1111.

36. Foster PJ, Baasanhu J, Alsbirk PH, et al. Glaucoma in Mongolia. A population-based survey in Hovsgol province, northern Mongolia [see comments]. Arch Ophthalmol 1996; 114: 1235–1241.

37. Gazzard G, Foster PJ, Devereux JG, et al. Intraocular pressure and visual field loss in primary angle closure and primary open angle glaucomas. Br J Ophthalmol 2003; 87:720–725.

38. Keltner JL, Johnson CA, Quigg JM, et al. Confirmation of visual field abnormalities in the Ocular Hypertension Treatment Study. Ocular Hypertension Treatment Study Group. Arch Ophthalmol 2000; 118:1187–1194.

39. Mitchell P, Smith W, Attebo K, et al. Prevalence of open-angle glaucoma in Australia. The Blue Mountains Eye Study. Ophthalmology 1996; 103:1661–1669.

40. Lee AJ, Wang JJ, Rochtchina E, et al. Patterns of glaucomatous visual field defects in an older population: the Blue Mountains Eye Study. Clin Exp Ophthalmol 2003; 31:331–335.

41. Khaw KT, Rose G. Cholesterol screening programmes: how much potential benefit? Br Med J 1989; 299:606–607.

42. He M, Foster PJ, Ge J, et al. Gonioscopy in adult Chinese: the Liwan Eye Study. Invest Ophthalmol Vis Sci 2006; 47: 4772–4779.

43. Thomas R, Parikh R, Muliyil J, et al. Five-year risk of progression of primary angle closure to primary angle closure glaucoma: a population-based study. Acta Ophthalmol Scand 2003; 81:480–485.

44. Periodic health examination, 1995 update: 3. Screening for visual problems among elderly patients. Canadian Task Force on the Periodic Health Examination. CMAJ 1995; 152: 1211–1222.

45. Office of Technology Assessment. Screening for Open-Angle Glaucoma in the Elderly. Preventive Health Services Under Medicare. Washington, DC: Congress of the United States; 1988.

46. Guide to Clinical Preventive Services. 2nd edn. Washington, DC: US Preventive Services Task Force, 1996.

47. Fleming C, Whitlock EP, Beil T, et al. Screening for primary open-angle glaucoma in the primary care setting: an update for the US Preventive Services Task Force. Ann Fam Med 2005; 3:167–170.

48. Harris R. Screening for glaucoma. Br Med J 2005; 331: E376–E377.

49. Dielemans I, Vingerling JR, Wolfs RC, et al. The prevalence of primary open-angle glaucoma in a population-based study in The Netherlands. The Rotterdam Study. Ophthalmology 1994; 101:1851–1855.

50. Vijaya R, George L, Paul PG, et al. Prevalence of open-angle glaucoma in a rural south Indian population. Invest Ophthalmol Vis Sci 2005; 46:4461–4467.

51. Grodum K, Heijl A, Bengtsson B. A comparison of glaucoma patients identified through mass screening and in routine clinical practice. Acta Ophthalmol Scand 2002; 80:627–631.

52. Wong EY, Keeffe JE, Rait JL, et al. Detection of undiagnosed glaucoma by eye health professionals. Ophthalmology 2004; 111:1508–1514.

53. Lord SJ, Irwig L, Simes RJ. When is measuring sensitivity and specificity sufficient to evaluate a diagnostic test, and when do we need randomized trials? Ann Intern Med 2006; 144: 850–855.

54. Barratt A, Irwig L, Glasziou P, et al. Users' guides to the medical literature: XVII. How to use guidelines and recommendations about screening. Evidence-Based Medicine Working Group. JAMA 1999; 281:2029–2034.

CHAPTER 3

Economics of Glaucoma Care

Paul Lee and David B. Matchar

INTRODUCTION

Glaucoma, both closed/narrow (NAG) and open-angle (OAG), constitutes one of the world's leading causes of blindness and vision loss according to the World Health Organization.[1] It is the second specific cause of blindness in the world and the leading cause of irreversible blindness.[1] The associated economic impact of glaucoma is likely to increase over the next 20 years as the numbers of those most likely to develop OAG – those over age 65 – increase throughout the world. Indeed, the number of people with OAG is projected to exceed those with NAG, even in countries that have traditionally had high rates of NAG.[2] As noted elsewhere in this text, the global population is aging relentlessly, with expansion being especially notable for those over age 65 and particularly among the oldest old (80 years and older). In addition, as the incidence of diabetes mellitus (DM) continues to rise rapidly in nearly all populations,[3] not just those of the developed societies such as the United States and Western Europe, vision loss due to the complications associated with DM (including neovascular glaucoma) will surely rise as well.

The rapid rise in prevalence of OAG affects not only the individuals with the condition, but also the societies in which these people live. As OAG becomes more evident, so will the chronic nature of the economic burden, due to both the long-term treatment and the costs of reduced vision. With the increase in the number of persons with glaucoma and growing societal needs for resources for other health and broader social conditions, a better understanding of the economics of glaucoma, its treatment, and its sequelae will be important not only to patients and their doctors but to policymakers as well. The increasing importance of economic analyses is highlighted by the work of agencies such as National Institute for Clinical Excellence (NICE) in the United Kingdom and similar bodies in Australia, New Zealand, and Canada, all of which provide evaluations of not only the safety and effectiveness of treatments but also of their economic impact, including cost-effectiveness studies. Indeed, in these countries such analyses are required prior to governmental approval of new therapies.[4,5]

METHODS AND COMPONENTS OF ECONOMIC ANALYSES OF GLAUCOMA

TYPES OF ECONOMIC ANALYSES

Economic analyses come in a variety of forms. Most simply, an economic analysis can consist of an assessment of the *costs* of the condition (so-called 'cost of illness' studies, which assess both the natural history/untreated impact of the disease on productivity, morbidity overall, and mortality as well as the costs of interventions). More sophisticated analyses aim to assist decision-makers in allocating research, clinical, or public health resources by assessing the *value* of treatments – costs relative to benefits.[6,7] As seen in Table 3.1, many studies have been published that provide information about almost all aspects of the economics of glaucoma, although they may be limited in scope, study population, or country of origin.

Costs of illness analyses Costs of illness analyses measure the costs of the disease or the interventions (generally both together, since very few populations exist in developed economies with untreated glaucoma over a long term). Such analyses typically include a range of costs associated with the disease and/or its treatments. The *disease-related costs*[8–12] include: (1) the time lost from work; (2), the associated economic value of disability for loss of productivity even if at work; (3) the costs of care in alternate (non-home) living facilities due to disease impacts; (4) the costs of care for in-home living assistance due to the disease; (5) the direct costs of family members and social support persons to assist an individual with a disease; (6) the costs to those family and social support members from taking time off from work (loss of productivity) to provide care and support for those with a condition; (7) government support payments to those with disabilities from a given condition; (8) loss of government tax revenue from loss of economic productivity of those with the disease and those who support them; and (9) years of life lost due to having the disease, and associated financial impacts. In assessing costs analyses, particular care must be taken not to

TABLE 3.1 Overview of types (and examples) of economic analyses in open-angle glaucoma[6,7]

	SOCIETY	GROUP	INDIVIDUAL
Costs analyses – condition/disease			
Direct medical costs (intervention)	Taylor Rein	Taylor Traverso Lee	Taylor numerous
Other direct costs (intervention)	Taylor Rein, Frick	Taylor Traverso Lee	Taylor numerous
Social support costs (disease + intervention)	Taylor Rein, Frick	Taylor	Taylor
Productivity losses (disease + intervention)	Taylor Rein, Frick	Taylor	Taylor
Budgetary impact (disease)	Taylor Rein, Frick	Taylor	Taylor
Value analyses – interventions		—	—
Cost-minimization	numerous		
Cost-benefit ($)	Taylor	n/a	n/a
Cost-effectiveness	Kymes	—	—
Cost-utility	Kymes	—	—

'double count' or otherwise count costs more than once among these categories, since there can be significant overlap in some of these elements. For example, lost government tax revenue is often already included as part of the overall productivity loss, since tax revenue is based on work productivity. Similarly, costs associated with any disease-associated increase in mortality need to be carefully separated from lost work productivity in general, and such work productivity losses also need to be adjusted downward for the shorter life spans.

The *costs of treatment interventions* then add additional costs, including: (1) costs of provider care (outpatient and inpatient); (2) costs of medications; (3) costs of devices and aids; (4) additional productivity losses of the patient due to the time and side effects of treatment; (5) incremental productivity losses of family members and those unpaid support members to assist in treatment-related activities (e.g. to take the patient to physicians' offices; (6) marginal costs of additional home health and other healthcare facility costs due to treatments and their side effects; and (7) costs of care due to the need to treat side effects of treatment. By including the costs attributed to the condition but not overall total medical costs, cost of illness studies provide a means of comparing the costs burdens of different diseases and even different groups of conditions. Such studies, however, do not provide direct guidance on allocation of resources, such as research or clinical funds.[13]

Assessment of the value of treatments Assessment of the value of treatments are generally conducted in one of four ways, based on how the overall benefit of treatment is measured relative to the costs.[6,7] While these have traditionally been labeled 'cost-effectiveness' analyses, true *cost-effectiveness analysis* (CEA) technically refers to a comparison of the costs relative to a single natural unit of outcome of interest, in the form of an incremental cost effectiveness ratio. This ratio is calculated for pairs of interventions and consists of the additional cost of the more expensive option compared to the less expensive, divided by the additional effectiveness of the more expensive option compared to the less expensive. The effectiveness measure in the denominator can consist of any clinically important outcome. For glaucoma, this could be a measure of visual disability. For example, the Ocular Hypertension Study provides data on visual field progression which have been incorporated into a calculation of an incremental cost-effectiveness ratio – the extra cost of treatment per extra case of visual field progression avoided.[14,15]

Cost-utility analysis (CUA) is similar to CEA in that it includes both costs and the impact of the intervention. However, in CUA the outcome is assessed specifically in terms of a metric termed 'utility.' Utility incorporates both impacts on quality of life and on life span. Currently, the standard way to assess utility for policy-relevant analysis is a 'quality-adjusted life year' (QALY) – life expectancy weighted by disease-related quality of life. The weightings used to calculate QALYs are based on empirical studies of patients' preferences regarding vision. Such studies have been relatively sparse in the literature,[16–19] hindering the use of this important methodology for glaucoma.[14]

Cost-minimization analysis (CMA) is used to compare the cost of two or more interventions when it is assumed that each provides comparable health outcomes. For example, CMA could be used to compare the costs of surgery to medications over a stated time period, where both achieve a comparable annual rate of visual field worsening. Many studies have been performed comparing different drug therapies for their impact on the intermediate outcome of intraocular pressure (IOP) lowering to a certain level or for a given level of effectiveness.[20,21] While similar analyses are uncommon for

TABLE 3.2 Different perspectives on outcomes of interest by perspective			
PERSPECTIVE	ORGAN	SYSTEM	PERSON
MD	IOP / RNFL	Va / VF	Vision-related quality of life
Person	Symptoms	Task ability	General quality of life
Payor	Cost of care	Cost-effective	Satisfaction
Society	Surveillance	Utilities	Disability

With permission from Lee PP. Outcomes and endpoints in glaucoma. J Glaucoma 1996; 5:295–297.

surgical versus medical interventions for structural or visual field end points, such an analysis might be possible using data from a study such as the Collaborative Initial Glaucoma Treatment Study (CIGTS).[22]

Cost-benefit analysis (CBA) measures both the costs and outcomes of alternative treatments in terms of common monetary units such as dollars. For example, a CBA of cataract surgery versus no cataract surgery would evaluate the net cost of having surgery and the net benefits of the intervention in monetary units (i.e. including the monetary value of any improvement in quality or length of life). The Melbourne Center for Eye Research Analysis study for Australia demonstrates, for example, that many interventions for vision care are actually cost savings for society, in that each dollar spent on vision care yields more than one dollar in net savings.[11,12] The work performed is a model for CBA assessment in vision in general and could readily be applied to glaucoma care in societies with developed market economies.

WHOSE PERSPECTIVE IS USED IN ANALYSIS

In assessing these different potential methods of expressing the 'economics of glaucoma,' one also needs to bear in mind whose perspective is incorporated in measuring the costs and, particularly, the end points or 'outcomes' of interest (as noted in Table 3.2). On the cost side, patients are concerned about how much they personally have to pay, in monetary terms, time lost, and opportunities foregone. Payors are concerned about balancing the revenue to support care with the outgoing expenditures to the entities that provide care. Societies are more concerned about the economic value of the healthcare that is provided, but the political leadership is also focused on the political ramifications of the level of care that is accessible and available to their citizens.

From a benefits perspective, patients, providers, payors, and society as a whole likewise have very different interests in assessing the benefits of detecting and treating various health conditions, including glaucoma. Thus, having a clear explication of the interests in question is particularly relevant in any discussion, particularly those that extend beyond costs to some measure of benefit of intervention. For example, physicians have a strong interest in analyzing the value of services relative to the costs of preventing worsening of the optic nerve or visual field, while patients may be more interested in the value of treatments relative to their ability to drive, cook, or enjoy a sporting activity (things which have a strong but not exclusively visual component).

Based on theoretical considerations, it has been proposed that all economic analyses be performed from the 'societal perspective.' However, practically speaking, a key concern is whether the analysis is perceived to be relevant to a particular decision-maker. The nature of the analysis should take the audience into account – for example, whether the analysis is developed for ophthalmologists eager to present the societal case treatments aimed at preventing visual field loss, or employers interested in productivity of the worker related to their visual impairment.

CURRENT STATE OF ECONOMIC ASSESSMENT IN GLAUCOMA

Currently, very few studies have directly assessed the resource impacts of detecting and treating NAG, whether in a modern market economy or, particularly, a less developed economy. In an analysis of the direct costs of treating acute primary angle-closure glaucoma, Singapore estimated that individuals would spend between US$879 and US$2577 over 5 years for their treatment after an initial angle-closure episode.[23] While reliable estimates for the costs of screening for NAG are unavailable due to the lack of an affordable, reliable screening system for NAG, it has been estimated that five to six higher-risk individuals suspected of being susceptible to angle-closure glaucoma would have to be treated to avoid one case of acute NAG over 5 years.[24] As such, for the purposes of this chapter, the authors will focus on the resource use issues associated with OAG, understanding that NAG remains an important and underexplored area for subsequent analyses, particularly for the developing economies.[2,24]

Yet, even concentrating on OAG, one sees that little work has been done on the economics of OAG care in developing and less developed economies, often because the resources to provide care for OAG are often unavailable for a large majority of those societies. In many countries, even basic epidemiological data on the prevalence and incidence of disease are lacking. For example, in Ghana[25] the best estimates come from clinic-based studies as opposed to population-based censuses. Further, even among these patients, most did not know they had glaucoma until diagnosed with visual impairment. In contrast, in the USA and Australia, while almost 50% do not know they have glaucoma,[26,27] nearly half of these individuals in Australia had actually seen an eye care provider in the prior year.[28] Thus, for the purposes of this chapter, the authors will also limit the discussion of OAG to the analyses available in developed countries and await additional information for less developed economies. As data are developed for India, China, and other countries with the assistance of the World Health Organization, the National Eye Institute, and other organizations, there will be more data to further the understanding in these contexts.

COSTS OF ILLNESS: GLAUCOMA AND ITS TREATMENT[8,10,12,29–37]

Studies in the USA and Australia have assessed the total cost burden imposed on society from glaucoma and other causes of visual impairment.[8–12] Figures 3.1 through 3.3 from the analysis of costs in Australia illustrate the nature of the analyses and the proportion due to glaucoma. As can be seen, for glaucoma (1) physician costs are only a small component of direct medical costs (Fig. 3.1); (2); the disease represents only a small proportion of overall direct costs associated with vision loss and visual disorders (Fig. 3.2); and (3), perhaps even more importantly, is associated with greater indirect (i.e. productivity) costs than direct costs of medical care (Fig. 3.3). Indeed, glaucoma care constitutes less than 15% of overall healthcare costs for an individual patient with glaucoma in the United States.[38] It is not surprising that the per capita direct costs of glaucoma care in the USA exceed that of Australia given the relative costs of medications and healthcare in general in the two countries and the nature of the financing systems in each country.

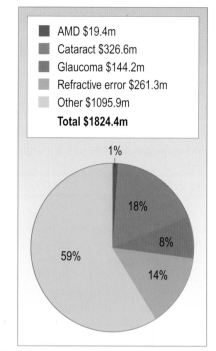

FIGURE 3.2 Direct costs for eye condition care in Australia in 2004. (From Taylor HR, Pezzullo ML, Keeffe JE. The economic impact and cost of visual impairment in Australia. Br J Ophthalmol 2006; 90:272–275.)

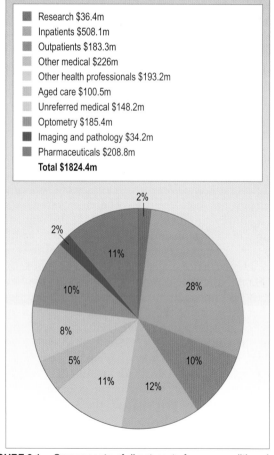

FIGURE 3.1 Components of direct costs for eye conditions in Australia in 2004. (From Taylor HR, Pezzullo ML, Keeffe JE. The economic impact and cost of visual impairment in Australia. Br J Ophthalmol 2006; 90:272–275.)

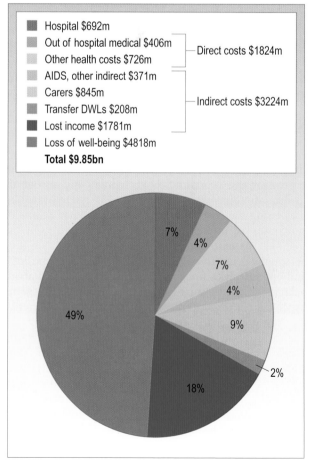

FIGURE 3.3 Total costs, including indirect costs, for eye care in Australia in 2004. (From Taylor HR, Pezzullo ML, Keeffe JE. The economic impact and cost of visual impairment in Australia. Br J Ophthalmol 2006; 90:272–275.)

Specifically, if the USA had the same direct costs of glaucoma care as Australia (Australian$144 million), expenditures in the USA would be US$1.9 billion. However, current estimates of actual direct medical costs for the comparable period is at least US$2.9 billion, suggesting that direct costs for glaucoma care in the USA is greater than Australia by about one-third.

The estimates above relate to aggregate estimates from administrative sources. Several studies in the last decade provide estimates of the direct costs of medical care in developed countries for *individual patients* with OAG, generally based on empirical data alone or combined with modeling.[29–39] A consistent finding is that pharmaceuticals constituted the single largest component of costs, ranging from 25% to 50% generally of total costs. Compared to European countries and Canada, the USA has the highest per patient costs (e.g. US mean cost of care per year at glaucoma specialty centers of US$1581 vs 540 to 960 in Italy and Germany, respectively).[28,29] Figures 3.4A and 3.4B provide illustrations of the total direct medical costs per patient and how they are allocated in the USA and Europe (see also Fig. 44.6).

In addition, these studies consistently show that certain factors are associated with higher costs of treatment for glaucoma. Individuals with OAG have higher costs than those who are only suspected of having OAG or who only have ocular hypertension. Treatment costs are higher in the first year of diagnosis, due to additional testing and treatment initiation. Costs are also greater for individuals with more severe disease, measured by visual field, optic nerve head structure, or by IOP. Also, costs are increased if side effects or resistance develops to IOP lowering.

For practical reasons, no data have been published on the *costs associated with the untreated natural history of glaucoma* in order to isolate the costs of the disease separate from its treatment. While data are available on the natural history of untreated glaucoma leading to severe visual loss or blindness in certain populations (notably those of African descent in the Barbados study),[40] this information has not been converted into cost analyses. As such, the only costs estimates are those for either treated groups or those with mixed treated and untreated groups (i.e. based on real world usage of medications).[29]

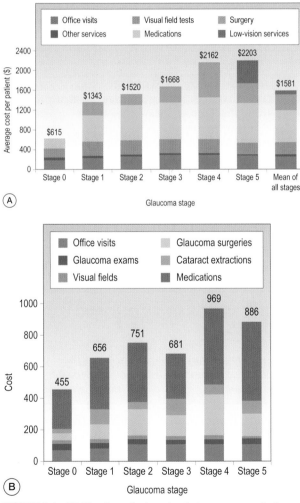

FIGURE 3.4 **(A)** Direct medical costs of glaucoma care in the United States by stage of disease. Costs adjusted for national Medicare allowable rates and for realistic adherence and persistence in use of medications. (From Lee PP, Walt JG, Doyle JJ, et al. A multicenter, retrospective pilot study of resource use and costs associated with severity of disease in glaucoma. Arch Ophthalmol 2006; 124:12–19.) **(B)** Direct medical costs of glaucoma care in Europe by stage of disease. (From Traverso CE, Walt JG, Kelly SP, et al. Direct costs of glaucoma and severity of the disease: a multinational long term study of resource utilisation in Europe. Br J Ophthalmol 2005; 89:1245–1249.)

COSTS ASSOCIATED WITH BLINDNESS AND VISUAL IMPAIRMENT[8–12]

The costs of blindness and visual impairment are critical in assessing the economics of glaucoma and are a key to the assessment of the analysis of 'value' associated with treatments. If there was no disability or harm to be ameliorated, there would be no 'benefit' to be gained from treatment either preventing or retarding loss of functioning. Relatively good data are available on rates of blindness associated with treated glaucoma. From a study in Olmsted County, 3% of individuals presenting with glaucoma will be blind in at least one eye; at 20 years 9% will develop bilateral blindness and 27% unilateral blindness.[41] Since most of the cases of blindness occur later in the course of disease and the life expectancy of patients with glaucoma is less than 20 years (12.8 years in whites and 16.3 years in blacks[38]), the overall rate of blindness from glaucoma is likely lower than the 20-year rates in Olmsted County.

Fewer population data are available about visual impairment short of blindness. Data from the Baltimore Eye Study demonstrate substantial heterogeneity in disease severity,[42] with many patients having advanced field loss short of legal blindness. The impact of visual impairment in visual acuity and contrast sensitivity short of blindness has been shown to be linear, based on results from the Salisbury Eye Evaluation.[43] Recent data confirm that early visual field loss may be associated with significant decrements on vision-related function, even with one normal eye, suggesting that visual field effects may also be linear to at least some degree.[44,45]

VALUE OF CARE/BENEFITS OF GLAUCOMA CARE

While studies now demonstrate that visual functioning and quality of life vary with the degree of visual field loss (as well as visual acuity and contrast sensitivity),[43–47] there is less information about how individual patients value their vision when impaired by glaucoma. Unlike the several CUAs of various retinal treatments and cataract surgery,[7] there are few such analyses of glaucoma treatment. However, many studies comparing the annual costs of treatment of different medications or therapies have been published,[48] while a smaller number have sought to conduct, in effect, *cost-minimization studies*, comparing the costs of achieving similar degrees of IOP lowering.[20,21]

Cost-utility analyses in glaucoma are limited thus far to one publication based on the results of the Ocular Hypertension Treatment Study (OHTS).[14] In this study, investigators determined that treating all patients similar to the OHTS population who had a 5% or greater risk of progressing to glaucoma per year would have an incremental cost-effectiveness ratio of US$3670 per QALY compared to US$42 430 per QALY if all patients with a 2% or greater annual risk were treated.

An important insight in this CUA is that the value of treatment is particularly sensitive to the quality-of-life weightings assigned to visual impairment provided by respondents. Several methods are available for expressing preference weights, including: (1) the time tradeoff (TTO) technique, where respondents are asked to trade-off a certain number of years of life to have perfect health (or vision in some studies) for the remaining years; (2) standard gamble, where respondents are asked to provide the 'threshold probability' at which a gamble between the worst possible outcome and a perfect outcome (say a gamble between death and well-being with normal vision) is equivalent in value to the certainty of an intermediate undesirable outcome such as visual impairment; (3) a 'feeling thermometer' approach, where they are asked to value a specific health state on a scale of 0 to 100; or (4) a questionnaire approach using specific instruments such as the EQ-5D that have been cross-referenced to a TTO or standard gamble approach.[7,16–19]

While only a few studies have assessed utility weights for the vision-related impact of glaucoma,[16–19] several insights are evident. First, individuals with relatively early glaucoma do not perceive a major loss of quality of life in terms of willingness to make tradeoffs. The vast majority of subjects (up to 87%) would not trade any remaining life span or risk blindness (compared to their current visual state) to make their vision perfect again.[16–19] An example can be found in Fig. 3.5, adapted from the work by Jampel and colleagues[16] Second, though there is some discrepancy in the relative effects of visual loss independent of acuity, utility weights are strongly related to visual acuity loss.[17,18]

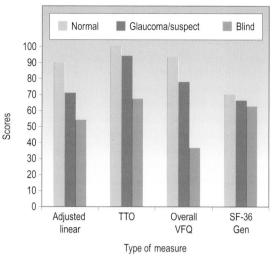

FIGURE 3.5 Quality of life and utility values in glaucoma. TTO, time tradeoff values (mean); Overall VFQ, mean total NEI-Visual Functioning Questionnaire score; SF-36, Short-form 36 general health subscale. (From Egge K, Zahl PH. Survival of glaucoma patients. Acta Ophthalmol Scand 1999; 77:397–401.)

To date, the best example of a true *cost-benefit analysis* (CBA) that has been published in glaucoma has come from the University of Melbourne in assessing vision programmatic areas overall in Australia.[11,12] Their analysis of programs for the detection, early treatment, or prevention of glaucoma damage indicates that such programs would actually be cost-saving for Australian society. In other words, more than one dollar would be saved for every dollar that is spent in glaucoma programs. Clearly, additional studies, particularly of CUA and CBA, are needed to better understand the impact and nature of glaucoma from an economic perspective, not only in developed economies but also those in developing economies.

FUTURE NEEDS IN ECONOMIC ANALYSES

Significant opportunity exists to better utilize economic analyses in glaucoma to help guide decision-making and resource allocation.[49] First, having a standardized set of definitions and factors to consider in constructing various analytical models would help both diffuse such analyses to more societies and increase the comparability of different models across different societies. Coincident with this, identifying where data are available and where they are lacking – and how to impute data from other sources and societies – will help identify priority areas for fundamental research for different societies. A critical area in this endeavor is to develop and more widely implement innovative methods of capturing the indirect costs of glaucoma or any other health condition.[50,51] In addition, defining standard (and thus routine) use of sensitivity analysis methods and techniques for incorporating uncertainty into model outputs will help make all such work more robust and thus more useful to policymakers.

Second, significant work is needed, as noted above, in creating more representative and larger samples from which to derive patient preferences and utility values. Indeed, there may be a need for a fundamentally new approach to capturing patient preferences and values across all health conditions, not just glaucoma or other ocular disorders. In glaucoma, available data suggest that there is not a normal distribution of utilities or preferences, particularly relative to the large majority of patients with nonend-stage glaucoma who have relatively normal visual acuities (or at least unaffected by glaucoma) but abnormal visual fields. Better characterizing and modeling this situation is critical to making CUA accurate and useful.

Third, once more data are available about how to better characterize both costs and utilities or preference states, performing additional CEAs and CUAs will be critical to placing glaucoma care in context to other pressing ocular and nonocular diseases and conditions. Further, once such data are available, we can better understand the value and desirability of having screening programs to detect glaucoma and other ocular conditions. In particular, this will help to place studies describing costs for detecting each case of glaucoma in context.[52–54]

Finally, these studies, which are already routine in the European Union (EU) and the Commonwealth countries, may well become standard assessments in the United States. Whether they will be used in the same way as they are in the EU and the Commonwealth is uncertain, due to unique legal traditions and legislative rules in the United States. As health systems around the world adapt and change to pressing future demands, economic analyses will likely become ever more important tools in deciding how to allocate resources within a society. Such uses, however, will ultimately be dependent upon the philosophy used in determining a society's healthcare financing system. For systems where individuals are empowered with their own decision-making and control over financing for routine healthcare, the operation of a structured 'marketplace' and individual consumer decisions will increase the sensitivity of healthcare decisions to the true value placed by each individual patient and thus decrease the need for society to determine if a particular intervention is sufficiently 'valuable' to be covered for each individual.

REFERENCES

1. World Health Organization. Magnitude and causes of visual impairment. Fact Sheet 282. November 2004. Online. Available: http://www.who.int/mediacentre/factsheets/fs282/en (accessed July 18, 2007).

2. Quigley HA, Broman AT. The number of people with glaucoma worldwide in 2010 and 2020. Br J Ophthalmol 2006; 90:262–267.

3. World Health Organization. Prevention of blindness from diabetes mellitus: report of a WHO consultation in Geneva, Switzerland. November 2005. On line. Available: http://www.who.int/blindness/en/ (accessed July 24, 2007).

4. Raftery J. NICE: faster access to modern treatments? Analysis of guidance on health technologies. Br Med J 2001; 323:1300–1303.

5. Morgan SG, McMahon M, Mitton C, et al. Centralized drug review processes in Australia, Canada, New Zealand, and the United Kingdom. Health Aff 2006; 25:337–347.

6. Lee PP. Economic analysis in eye disease. Arch Ophthalmol 2007; 121:115–116.

7. Brown MM, Brown GC, Sharma S, et al. Health care economic analyses and value-based medicine. Surv Ophthalmol 2003; 48:204–223.

8. Rein DB, Zhang P, Wirth KE, et al. The economic burden of major adult visual disorders in the United States. Arch Ophthalmol 2006; 124:1754–1760.

9. Lee PP. Economic impact of visual impairment and blindness in the United States. Arch Ophthalmol 2007; 135:544–550.

10. Taylor HR, Pezzullo ML, Keeffe JE. The economic impact and cost of visual impairment in Australia. Br J Ophthalmol 2006; 90:272–275.

11. Taylor HR, Pezzullo ML, Nesbitt SJ, et al. Costs of interventions for visual impairment. Am J Ophthalmol 2007; 143:561–565.

12. Centre for Eye Research Australia. Clear insight: the economic impact and cost of vision loss in Australia. Melbourne: Centre for Eye Research Australia; 2004.

13. Shiell A, Gerard K, Donaldson C. Cost of illness studies: an aid to decision-making. Health Policy 1987; 8:317–323.

14. Kymes SM, Kass MA, Anderson DR, et al. Ocular Hypertension Treatment Study Group (OHTS). Management of ocular hypertension: a cost-effectiveness approach from the Ocular Hypertension Treatment Study. Am J Ophthalmol 2006; 141:997–1008.

15. Weinreb RN, Friedman DS, Fechtner RD, et al. Risk assessment in the management of patients with ocular hypertension. Am J Ophthalmol 2004; 138:458–467.

16. Jampel HD, Schwartz A, Pollack I, et al. Glaucoma patients' assessment of their visual function and quality of life. J Glaucoma 2002; 11:154–163.

17. Kobelt G, Jonsson B, Bergstrom A, et al. Cost-effectiveness analysis in glaucoma: what drives utility? Results from a pilot study in Sweden. Acta Ophthalmol Scand 2006; 84:363–371.

18. Gupta V, Srinivasan G, Mei SS, et al. Utility values among glaucoma patients: an impact on the quality of life. Br J Ophthalmol 2005; 89:1241–1244.

19. Saw SM, Gazzard G, Au Eong KG, et al. Utility values in Singapore Chinese adults with primary open-angle and primary angle-closure glaucoma. J Glaucoma 2005; 14(6):455–462.

20. Goldberg LD, Walt J. Cost considerations in the medical management of glaucoma in the US: estimated yearly costs and cost effectiveness of bimatoprost compared with other medications. Pharmacoeconomics 2006; 24:251–264.

21. Fiscella R, Walt J. Estimated comparative costs of achieving a 20% reduction in intraocular pressure with bimatoprost or latanoprost in patients with glaucoma or ocular hypertension. Drugs Aging 2006; 23:39–47.

22. Lichter PR, Musch DC, Gillespie BW, et al. CIGTS Study Group. Interim clinical outcomes in the Collaborative Initial Glaucoma Treatment Study comparing initial treatment randomized to medications or surgery. Ophthalmology 2001; 108:1943–1953.

23. Wang JC, Chew PT. What is the direct cost of treatment of acute primary angle closure glaucoma? The Singapore model. Clin Exp Ophthalmol 2004; 32:578–583.

24. Thomas R, Sekhar GC, Parikh R. Primary angle closure glaucoma: a developing world perspective. Clin Exp Ophthalmol 2007; 35:374–378.

25. Herndon LW, Challa P, Ababio-Danso B, et al. Survey of glaucoma in an eye clinic in Ghana, West Africa. J Glaucoma 2002; 11:421–425.

26. Wong EY, Keeffe JE, Rait JL, et al. Detection of undiagnosed glaucoma by eye health professionals. Ophthalmology 2004; 111:1508–1514.

27. Friedman DS, Wolfs RC, O'Colmain BJ, et al. Eye Diseases Prevalence Research Group. Prevalence of open-angle glaucoma among adults in the United States. Arch Ophthalmol 2004; 122:532–538.

28. Traverso CE, Walt JG, Kelly SP, et al. Direct costs of glaucoma and severity of the disease: a multinational long term study of resource utilisation in Europe. Br J Ophthalmol 2005; 89:1245–1249.

29. Lee PP, Walt JG, Doyle JJ, et al. A multicenter, retrospective pilot study of resource use and costs associated with severity of disease in glaucoma. Arch Ophthalmol 2006; 124:12–19.

30. Lindblom B, Nordmann JP, Sellem E, et al. A multicentre, retrospective study of resource utilization and costs associated with glaucoma management in France and Sweden. Acta Ophthalmol Scand 2006; 84:74–83.

31. Iskedjian M, Walker J, Vicente C, et al. Cost of glaucoma in Canada: analyses based on visual field and physician's assessment. J Glaucoma 2003; 12:456–462.

32. Oostenbrink JB, Rutten-van Molken MP, Sluyter-Opdenoordt TS. Resource use and costs of patients with glaucoma or ocular hypertension: a one-year study based on retrospective chart review in the Netherlands. J Glaucoma 2001; 10:184–191.

33. Kobelt G, Jonsson L, Gerdtham U, et al. Direct costs of glaucoma management following initiation of medical therapy. A simulation model based on an observational study of glaucoma treatment in Germany. Graefe's Arch Clin Exp Ophthalmol 1998; 236:811–821.

34. Kobelt-Nguyen G, Gerdtham UG, Alm A. Costs of treating primary open-angle glaucoma and ocular hypertension: a retrospective, observational two-year chart review of newly diagnosed patients in Sweden and the United States. J Glaucoma 1998; 7:95–104.

35. Vicente C, Walker J, Buys Y, et al. Association between mean intraocular pressure, disease stability and cost of treating glaucoma in Canada. Curr Med Res Opin 2004; 20:1245–1251.

36. Denis P, Lafuma A, Berdeaux G. Medical outcomes of glaucoma therapy from a nationwide representative survey. Clin Drug Investig 2004; 24:343–352.

37. Rouland JF, Berdeaux G, Lafuma A. The economic burden of glaucoma and ocular hypertension: implications for patient management: a review. Drugs Aging 2005; 22:315–321.

38. Quigley HA, Vitale S. Models of open-angle glaucoma prevalence and incidence in the United States. Invest Ophthalmol Vis Sci 1997; 38:83–91.

39. Lee PP, Levin LA, Walt JG, et al. Cost of patients with primary open-angle glaucoma: a retrospective study of commercial insurance claims data. Ophthalmology 2007; 114:1241–1247.

40. Hyman L, Wu SY, Connell AM, et al. Prevalence and causes of visual impairment in The Barbados Eye Study. Ophthalmology 2001; 108:1751–1756.

41. Hattenhauer MG, Johnson DH, Ing HH, et al. The probability of blindness from open-angle glaucoma. Ophthalmology 1998; 105:2099–2104.

42. Quigley HA, Tielsch JM, Katz J, et al. Rate of progression in open-angle glaucoma estimated from cross-sectional prevalence of visual field damage. Am J Ophthalmol 1996; 122:355–363.

43. West SK, Rubin GS, Broman AT, et al. How does visual impairment affect performance on tasks of everyday life? The SEE Project. Salisbury Eye Evaluation. Arch Ophthalmol 2002; 120:774–780.

44. McKean-Cowdin R, Varma R, Wu J, et al. Los Angeles Latino Eye Study Group. Severity of visual field loss and health-related quality of life. Am J Ophthalmol 2007; 143:1013–1023.

45. Ringsdorf L, Owsley G, McGwin C. Visual field defects and vision-specific health-related quality of life in African Americans and whites with glaucoma. J Glaucoma 2006; 15:414–418.

46. Parrish RK. Visual impairment, visual functioning, and quality of life assessments in patients with glaucoma. Trans Am Ophthalmol Soc 1996; 94:919–1028.

47. Gutierrez P, Wilson MR, Johnson C, et al. Influence of glaucomatous visual field loss on health-related quality of life. Arch Ophthalmol 1997; 115:777–784.

48. Schmier JK, Halpern MT, Jones ML. The economic implications of glaucoma: a literature review. Pharmacoeconomics 2007; 25:287–308.

49. Taylor HR. Eye care: dollars and sense. Am J Ophthalmol 2007; 143:1–8.

50. Melese M, Alemayehu W, Friedlander E, et al. Indirect costs associated with accessing eye care services as a barrier to service use in Ethiopia. Trop Med Int Health 2004; 9:426–431.

51. Chou SL, Misajon R, Gallo J, et al. Measurement of indirect costs for people with vision impairment. Clin Exp Ophthalmol 2003; 31:336–340.

52. Hitzl W, Ortner C, Hornykewycz K, et al. Resource use and costs for a glaucoma screening program in Austria: an 8-year review: a cost-consequence analysis based on the Salzburg-Moorfields Collaborative Glaucoma Study. Eur J Ophthalmol 2006; 16:92–99.

53. Peeters A, Schouten JS, Webers CA, et al. Cost-effectiveness of early detection and treatment of ocular hypertension and primary open-angle glaucoma by the ophthalmologist. Eye 2008; 22:354–362.

54. Lee PP. Outcomes and endpoints in glaucoma. J Glaucoma 1996; 5(4):295–297.

CHAPTER 4

Practical Application of Glaucoma Care in Different Societies

Alan L Robin, Donald L Budenz, Nathan Congdon, and Ravilla D Thulasiraj

INTRODUCTION

Glaucoma therapy in less developed countries is challenging and requires a different set of thought processes and skills than are currently used in more developed nations. Problems faced in developing nations are appreciably magnified and reach a greater level of significance because of generalized poorer training, later diagnosis, less access to care, poorer utilization of care, folklore, and beliefs. In essence, there are more extremes. In this chapter, the authors will discuss these issues and look at some potential tools needed to solve them.

Even in situations where there is the best of care, the detection of glaucoma in a prosperous population is relatively poor. In a more developed society, one would expect that with a high number of physicians and optometrists per capita, and with a financial incentive to capture each new patient, hardly anyone with a disease would go undetected. Glaucoma, however, because it is generally an asymptomatic disease, is often not detected. Even within a 5–mile radius of the Wilmer Institute (Johns Hopkins University, Baltimore, Maryland, USA) almost 50% of subjects were unaware of the disease.[1] Similar patterns of subjects being unaware that they are glaucomatous have been seen in other parts of the United States[2] as well as through Western Europe and Australia.[3–7]

The prevalence of the disease and the lack of therapy may be different in the elderly (those over 73 years). In a recent study in Salisbury, Maryland, USA, almost 20% of subjects had a best corrected presenting vision of less than 6/12 and the rate of blindness varied between 1.3% and 5.3%.[8] Additionally, one-third of who were diagnosed with glaucoma were never told previously that they had the disease. In developing nations, this problem becomes more extreme. In south India, the authors found that 21% of subjects in a population-based survey (mean age 60 years) were blind in either eye at presentation and that 93% had not been previously diagnosed with the disease.[9] There are many possible reasons for this discrepancy between the developed and less developed nations. One common reason is that many in less developed nations accept visual impairment as a natural consequence of aging. The concept of 'white hair and white eyes' as a normal occurrence is not uncommon. That is, as one accepts the natural aging and whitening of hair, blindness is also an accepted consequence of maturation. Concepts of public health and preventive care are foreign to most, even in more developed nations. Individuals are unaware of diseases such as glaucoma or diabetic retinopathy, so they do not routinely access care. Visual impairment is as much an accepted part of daily life as is poor mobility from arthritis.

When individuals do come in for care, as their vision is dimming, doctors and paramedical personnel are usually geared towards cataract blindness and often do not measure the intraocular pressure, do not perform perimetry, and do not examine the fundus. Part of this is due to lack of adequate training.[10] This may be a question of priorities, skill levels, or inadequate time. The issue of staffing is not only that the absolute number of ophthalmologists per capita is far less. This situation is compounded by the fact that the proportion of ophthalmologists who are well trained in glaucoma is even less.[11] In many places, applanation tonometry is not commonly done and physicians rely upon digital intraocular pressure (IOP) measurements. Slit lamps may be a luxury in areas of China and Africa. Likewise, diseases such as normal-tension glaucoma are impossible to diagnose in eyes with cataract in which the lens opacity makes it quite difficult to either view the fundus or perform perimetry.

Cataract and refraction have become major hurdles in themselves.[12] The mere diagnosis of and surgery for visually disabling cataract is often a significant problem in and of itself. The skillful performance of cataract surgery with intraocular lens insertion is now becoming commonplace.[8] Following surgery, subjects are often sent back to their homes and villages without a thorough fundus examination. Little counseling outside of postoperative cataract care is given. Later, subjects may become visually disabled from posterior capsule opacification. If that occurs, they may return to the clinic and receive a capsulotomy. Following the capsulotomy, time and material restraints often dictate that the fundus is not viewed. Minimal postoperative instructions are given to the patient outside of those necessary for a capsulotomy. The actions associated with this type of care teach the patient an incorrect lesson. They have twice seen that blindness may occur, but that blindness can be easily cured by either surgery or laser. The implication is, of course, is that there is no need for yearly or every-other-yearly preventive visits. If the patient then develops glaucoma or diabetic retinopathy, he will not return until he has become blind as, of course, he has learned that this blindness can be reversed. However, as people age, the prevalence of blinding diseases such as glaucoma markedly increases, especially over the age of 73. It may also be that the prevalence of glaucoma may be increased in both aphakic and pseudophakic eyes[13] and blindness due to glaucoma is seen in 22% in either one or both eyes.

Detecting glaucoma is often difficult. Modern equipment such as computerized perimetry and scanning laser ophthalmoscopy is not commonly available in many urban and most rural centers. Intraocular pressure measurements (often tactile or Schiotz) and monocular fundus examinations are the rule, if they occur at all. Gonioscopy is not often done even in developing countries like the United States.[14] In the majority of more developed nations, the primary angle-closure glaucomas are relatively infrequent whereas in developing nations they can account for one-half of primary glaucomas.[15] The accurate diagnosis of angle-closure disease is imperative for prompt and appropriate care, and these cases need to be discovered early to prevent permanent synechial closure and the need for more involved surgery. In many areas lasers are not available, but surgical iridectomy is relatively easy to perform. It may be more difficult to perforate a thick brown iris with a laser in a narrow anterior chamber and if iridotomy closure occurs, the patient may not have returned for follow-up care and may be totally unaware of this problem. Additionally, care has to be taken to train surgeons to also convince patients to have surgery on fellow eyes.

Early diagnosis must be emphasized. In developing countries, most individuals with glaucoma have visual disability or blindness upon entry into the healthcare system. In the Aravind Comprehensive Eye Care Study in southern India, 21% of those with glaucoma were blind in either eye (one-third of these were bilaterally blind with an additional 14% blind in one eye alone). Ninety-three percent of these had never been previously diagnosed with glaucoma.[16] Screening for glaucoma alone is not often cost-effective because of the relatively low prevalence of the disease and problems with both sensitivity and specificity of most screening tests. However, if screening for glaucoma is coupled with other disease screening, such as screening for diabetic retinopathy, it may become much more cost-effective as both diseases require disc and fundus photography. Simple perimetry testing such as frequency doubling technology (FDT) can be cost-effective when coupled with fundus examinations or either dilated or undilated fundus photography. This type of screening can make a large impact as telemedicine becomes more widely utilized. Currently, telemedicine is being performed at two separate institutions in both Chennai and Madurai, India. Telemedicine has the ability to bring eye care screening to the people, rather than having patients come to specific centers. This is more convenient for patients and frees them to get expert opinions without being subject to long-distant travel and allows them potentially freer access to better-quality eye care.

Since subjects with glaucoma typically present with more advanced disease, the presence of so many visually disabled individuals and monocular patients makes it necessary to be appropriately aggressive when treating these individuals and much more so than one might be with either high-risk ocular hypertensives or early glaucoma subjects in more developed countries. Once the diagnosis of open-angle glaucoma is made, the main question is how to proceed with therapy. Although the American Academy of Ophthalmology states that all newly diagnosed glaucoma patients should be given the option of either medical, surgical, or laser therapy, in the USA medical therapy is predominantly the first choice. Medical therapy is problematic from many perspectives in the developing countries. These potential problems include not only cost, adherence, and the ability of a patient with an eye of low visual function to successfully get a drop into the eye, but also quality and accessibility of pharmaceutical agents. In more developed nations cost can be prohibitive in patients taking glaucoma medications, especially those on fixed and lower incomes. The quality of a generic product may also be questionable.[17] Adherence is a problem that has been well discussed, and is not limited to those with chronic asymptomatic eye diseases. However, in developed nations, one rarely worries about the quality of medications or a patient's ability to procure a specific medication.

Adherence with medical therapy is most likely far poorer in less developed countries. No formal compliance studies in glaucoma have been published relating to developing nations with medical glaucoma therapies, but some have suggested that compliance may be much poorer. Within 5 years of diagnosis, fewer than 10% of patients still continue follow-up care or return for therapy (unpublished data, Aravind Hospital System, Coimbatore India). The cost of locally produced drugs is often affordable with medications such as pilocarpine hydrochloride, timolol maleate, and brimonidine tartrate relatively inexpensive, often costing less than €1 per bottle. There is, however, a distribution problem. In cities, it is usually possible to get any type of medications. In rural areas, it may be difficult to get anything more than pilocarpine or timolol, making it useless to prescribe other IOP-lowering medications. This definitely limits the options available to more rural patients before surgical interventions. Also, as urban dwellers may earn more than rural patients, the influence of cost may unduly hamper those who are more rural.

Cost issues are paramount. Costs of therapy are, of course, as important in the developing world as they are in the more developed world. In the United States, the cost of therapy can cause patients to use their medications less often than prescribed (taking a twice-daily medication once daily, or using a once-daily medication less often than prescribed to help save on the cost of the prescription).

In developing nations, medications are far cheaper in terms of US dollars compared with their prices in the USA or even Europe. However, they are expensive in terms of an individual's daily income. The National Bureau of Statistics in China in 2004[18] found that in 2004 the average income per person in rural China was US$0.97/day and US$3.11/day in urban China. That needs to cover the average cost of food per day (US$0.34/day and US$0.90/day in rural and urban China, respectively), and housing (US$0.11/day and US$0.24/day, rural and urban China, respectively). China has some basic medical insurance which means that the government will pay 80% of the cost of further medical treatment for a person after the person has paid the first US$241.00. This, however, does not apply to some urban and most rural citizens. In most cities, basic medical insurance does not seem to cover the newer glaucoma medications such as prostaglandins and topical carbonic anhydrase inhibitors.

In some parts of China, especially rural China, traditional treatments, such as acupuncture, are still considered costless therapy.[19] In some parts of China, even the medications with the lowest costs are not available.

What are the costs of glaucoma care in China?[20] The cost of a laser trabeculoplasty ranges from US$36.19 to US$72.39, while the cost of filtration surgery was US$72.39. The average costs of medications (assuming full compliance and no wasting) is US$0.71/day in China.

The quality of many generics is often suspect. The authors have seen this with ophthalmic antibiotics[21] and have seen that generic glaucoma medications do not lower IOP as well as nongeneric brand names.[22] This, however may, lead to a quandary. Does one use a potentially inferior but inexpensive generic medication or instead ask a patient to pay a significant part of his or her salary for a slightly more consistent and more efficacious medication? Often, this decision is made on the basis of cost. In addition, generic medications such as timolol and pilocarpine are widely available and can be sourced almost anywhere Also, if gonioscopy is not accurately performed, angle-closure disease may be inappropriately treated with medications rather than laser or surgical intervention, causing needless blindness. The diagnosis of all forms of angle closure requires an adequate skill set, including gonioscopy and proficiency with a slit lamp, which is most often not acquired in residency.[23] Should laser trabeculoplasty be used in developing nations? Some reports have found it potentially effective in a limited number of subjects for a relatively short time period.[24] However, long-term studies are needed. Additionally, in many areas power

and maintenance may be limiting factors. For a laser to be effective, it must be durable, often it should be portable, and self-contained battery power is needed because of fluctuations in power.[25] Additionally, lasers are relatively expensive and may not be cost-effective in other than teaching institutions and major hospital centers with a higher ratio of paying patients. Often, they may be as effective as a single medication, but over half of individuals with open-angle glaucomas may require more than one type of IOP-lowering medication.

Some have considered diode laser ciliary body ablation as an initial therapy. This machine is sturdy, which is a major advantage in that it is unlikely to need costly repairs. This has the potential advantage of minimal training, quick therapy, and minimal intraoperative and postoperative care. However, there is a risk of sympathetic ophthalmia[26] which could make the relative risks far outweigh the benefits of simplicity and cost.

Superficially, surgery seems like a good option, but if one considers a filtering procedure, should one just perform a trabeculectomy? Cataract is one of the primary complications of filtering surgery.[27] An asymptomatic subject with 6/6 visual acuity could go in for glaucoma surgery, seeing well, and after filtration surgery, have poorer vision from subsequent cataract. This 'poor vision' would obviously be blamed on the glaucoma surgery and this could be a horrible situation, especially in someone who was asymptomatic. In the best of situations, this takes someone temporarily out of the workforce and requires a second trip to the operating theater. This increases the risk not only of endophthalmitis, but also bleb failure, leaving the patient back where he or she started, but two surgeries later. This could be compounded by poor cataract surgical techniques in some regions. Also, one poor result, through social marketing, could destroy the relationship between the eye care providers and the community. Therefore, should one consider a combined cataract and glaucoma operation so the patient might have a sense of positive social marketing and feel better than one might after a trabeculectomy alone where dysesthesia is a major side effect.[28] In a disease where no discomfort is experienced, adding discomfort to a potentially blinding condition might cause the person and the people associated with him to lose faith in the healthcare provider. Regrettably, most individuals who come in complaining about glaucoma do not have visually significant cataracts and the IOP-lowering that results from combined procedures appears worse than glaucoma surgery alone. A low dose of an antimetabolite might best be used. If not filtering surgery, perhaps a shunt? Shunt surgery is technically easier than a trabeculectomy, involves minimal intraocular intervention, and requires minimal postoperative care. Although in some studies the results appear comparable between filters and shunts, the initial cost of a shunt (hundreds of US dollars) is definitely prohibitive for most. Soon, relatively expensive versions of glaucoma drainage devices will be available through Aurolab in Madurai, India, and will hopefully be less than US$10.00.

Various skill levels are required for filtering surgery. As an example of the variability of training and surgical skills, the authors first will examine cataract surgery, the bread and butter of ophthalmic surgery. In Madurai, India,[29] fewer than 1.9% of patients had final visual acuities less than 6/18, whereas in Hyderabad[30] 41.6% had visual disability or blindness following cataract surgery. This suggests that if the skill level needed for cataract surgery can vary so much in a developing nation where cataract is a frequently performed procedure, the outcomes for filtering surgery might vary even more considerably since this is not as routine a surgical procedure.

Ideally, surgery could be the best option, as it could be a one-time procedure that would obviate compliance issues, be cost-effective, and be socially acceptable. Work is currently going on in various centers to help develop easy, universal surgical techniques. However, as of now, this is not the case nor does it appear to be the case for the near future.

PRACTICAL CONSIDERATIONS IN THE MANAGEMENT OF GLAUCOMA IN SUB-SAHARAN AFRICA

Sub-Saharan Africa, because of its paucity of trained healthcare providers, rural settings, and lack of infrastructure, may require additional consideration compared to other areas of the world. The following description of the management of glaucoma in Africa is based solely on personal experience in Ghana, West Africa, and may not be generalizable to the entire continent but is likely to relate to many developing sub-Saharan African countries.

Several factors contribute to the unique management of glaucoma in sub-Saharan Africa. First, the prevalence of primary open-angle glaucoma in black Africans is estimate at 3% of people 40 years and older in glaucoma surveys done in Tanzania[31] and South Africa.[32–34] In studies conducted in Nigeria, glaucoma accounts for 16% to 24% of blindness, falling just behind cataract and trachoma.[35] Second, glaucoma in blacks may have an earlier age of onset[36–41] and take a more aggressive course,[42,43] leading to visual disability and blindness at an earlier age. And third, the extremely limited resources in the developing countries of sub-Saharan Africa make diagnosis and management difficult.[44]

The diagnosis of glaucoma in West Africa is most often based on intraocular pressure and disc appearance alone. There appears to be little or no emphasis placed on gonioscopy. Manual kinetic perimetry requires relatively expensive equipment, skilled perimetrists, and considerable time to perform. Automated visual field equipment would be ideal, but equipment is expensive and difficult to both obtain and maintain in developing countries. Portable, inexpensive, and less technology- and personnel-dependent perimetry have not gained popularity in West Africa. Relying on IOP and optic disc visualization alone to diagnose and follow glaucoma is problematic. First, the cup-to-disc ratio is known to be larger and more variable in blacks with a mean of 0.4 compared to 0.3 in Caucasians.[45–47] Due to the high cost of fundus photographic instrumentation, following optic discs for evidence of increased cupping is not feasible in developing parts of the world. Further complicating IOP monitoring is the fact that blacks have thinner corneas than non-blacks. Thus, many cases of glaucoma are missed because of 'normal' IOPs on screening examinations that do not include optic disc visualization. Not uncommonly, the diagnosis of glaucoma in developing Africa is made after unilateral blindness is discovered by the patient. Ideally, diagnosis would be based on a combination of optic disc and visual field information where skilled observers and perimetry are available. Following known glaucoma patients for evidence of progression is also hindered by the same lack of technology as mentioned above. Specifically, baseline photographs of the optic disc would be useful in follow-up but are rarely available, and serial visual fields analysis is uncommon as well. Generally, IOP is the only parameter followed. Ideally, if the IOP has been lowered 30–50% from baseline, the patient is considered 'stable,' although it is known that a subset of these patients will, in fact, progress.

Practically speaking, medical management of glaucoma is rarely successful in sub-Saharan Africa due to the cost of the medications and difficulty in obtaining them. Verrey and colleagues[48] reviewed the records of 397 patients with chronic glaucoma in rural Ghana and found that only 17% of patients receiving medical treatment had IOPs lower than 22 mmHg. In contrast, 84% of patients treated surgically had IOPs lower than 22 mmHg. As in India and China, even generic β-blockers and miotics may cost more per day than basic necessities such as food. Medications are also not practical, even for those with money. The hot climate and periods without electricity sometimes lasting weeks make unstable and other relatively unstable compounds ineffective.

Given the problems with medical and laser therapy of glaucoma in sub-Saharan Africa, primary surgical treatment might appear to be a reasonable first-line therapy for people with sight-threatening glaucoma in this part of the world. However, in interactions and discussions with ophthalmologists in West Africa, the authors have discovered reluctance to treat glaucoma with surgery. Since cataract extraction remains the most commonly performed ocular surgical procedure in West Africa, patient expectations, based upon outcomes after cataract surgery, are generally high after any type of eye surgery. Patients often cannot distinguish between blindness caused by cataract and glaucoma. They therefore may expect 'cataract surgery-like success' after glaucoma surgery. With glaucoma surgery, the best visual outcome to be expected is retention of preoperative vision. Patients who have lost central vision from glaucoma are disappointed when their visual acuity does not improve following trabeculectomy as with acquaintances who have had cataract surgery. Despite the best efforts of ophthalmologists to temper expectations, such outcomes are not 'practice builders.' Social marketing of services is very important. Good results after cataract surgery build trust and inspire other members of the community to have their cataracts operated upon. This, in turn, inspires still others to have surgery. Glaucoma surgery, despite warnings, provides negative social marketing. This is, in fact, a good way to alienate a community from ophthalmic care. Rather than bringing sight to a village, performing glaucoma surgery does not allow many to see better but causes some to lose vision and have discomfort. Communities may quickly lose faith even in the best of surgeons performing procedures that do not offer visual improvement.

Standard trabeculectomy is known to have a higher risk for failure in blacks compared to Caucasians,[49–51] presumably due to a more vigorous wound healing response in the former.[52] Several investigators have reported success and safety when using antifibrotic agents in black Africans.[53–55] A prospective, randomized trial by Egbert et al.[53] showed a clear advantage to using a single intraoperative application of 5–fluorouracil (5–FU) (50 mg/mL on a soaked surgical sponge applied for 5 minutes) compared to no antifibrotic agent in glaucoma patients undergoing trabeculectomy in Ghana. Mermoud et al.[54] compared a series of black South African patients treated with low-dose mitomycin C (0.2 mg/mL on a soaked surgical sponge for 5 minutes) to historical controls who received no antifibrotic agents. These investigators found an 83% success rate in the mitomycin C group compared to 37% in the control group, after an average follow-up of 9 months. Singh et al.,[55] in a prospective, randomized trial comparing intraoperative 5–FU (50 mg/mL for 5 minutes) versus high-dose mitomycin C (0.5 mg/mL on a soaked surgical sponge for 3.5 minutes) in glaucoma patients undergoing trabeculectomy in Ghana, found that the success rate in the mitomycin C group was 93% compared to 73% in the 5-FU group after an average follow-up of 10 months. Practically speaking, it makes little sense to perform trabeculectomy without mitomycin C, even as a primary procedure, in this population. The value of glaucoma drainage tube implant (GDI) surgery has yet to be evaluated in this population. Currently, GDIs are not practical in developing countries primarily due to the high cost of implants and the lack of tissue banking needed for patch grafts to cover the tube.

In summary, glaucoma management in sub-Saharan Africa is difficult, as it is in other parts of the developing world, due to scarce resources and lack of infrastructure. Add to this is the fact that the prevalence of glaucoma is very high in this population, glaucoma takes on an apparently more aggressive form, and failure of trabeculectomy is higher in this racial group, and the problems are compounded. Practically speaking, if one is sure a patient has glaucoma, primary trabeculectomy with mitomycin C is currently the best option. Yet a marked lack of skilled surgeons makes this impractical to some extent as well. Hopefully, a simpler and more successful operation will be developed that would help the treatment of glaucoma in this part of the world.

GLAUCOMA CARE: THE NONGOVERNMENTAL ORGANIZATION PERSPECTIVE

In many nations, there is reliance upon nongovernmental organizations (NGOs) for staffing, supplies, and education. The following section provides an NGO perspective of care.

CURRENT SITUATION

Glaucoma is the second leading cause of blindness in the world,[56] but is rarely engaged by blindness prevention NGOs. Glaucoma is not mentioned on the websites of Christoffel Blindenmission (CBM)[57] and Helen Keller International,[58] and is described on the webpage of Sightsavers International as 'not one of the core conditions that we work with.'[59] Orbis has limited glaucoma programs, for example in Northern China in the Shenyang Region.[60]

The following areas are often mentioned as barriers to wider glaucoma programming on the part of blindness prevention NGOs. First, there is a competition between glaucoma and other ophthalmic diseases, such as cataract. Cataract remains the leading cause of blindness in the world;[61] studies have demonstrated excellent potential for return to normal vision with extraction of the cataractous lens in both the developed[62] and developing[63] world. The production of low-cost intraocular lenses, sutures, and medications, together with high-volume surgical approaches, has generally brought the cost per case into the range of US$25–40 in efficient programs. Primarily for these reasons, most blindness prevention NGOs focus on cataract as their primary target.[64–66]

Studies have also demonstrated treatment of vitamin A deficiency (VAD) to be a highly effective and inexpensive way to avoid blindness,[67] and programs to alleviate VAD are an important part of the portfolio of NGOs such as Helen Keller International.[68] Childhood refractive error, childhood cataract, trachoma, and onchocerciasis are other diseases affecting vision for which proven treatments exist and in which one or more blindness prevention NGOs have invested significant resources. Given the limited resources of most blindness prevention NGOs, new programs to combat glaucoma blindness would be in direct competition with programs for these other diseases, all of which still remain important causes of blindness.

Another reason glaucoma rarely figures as a primary objective for NGOs is that glaucoma screening is difficult to perform. Screening usually involves assessment of the optic nerve and/or testing for typical changes in the visual field. Existing technologies and/or combinations of technologies have not been demonstrated to produce good sensitivity and specificity in screening for glaucoma.[69] Evaluation of the optic nerve even among experienced observers may be subject to significant variation.[70] Machines which might replace or supplement human evaluation of the optic nerve are expensive and ill-suited for use in the rural areas of the developing world where many blindness prevention NGOs operate (and where 90% of world blindness exists). Important questions remain about the accuracy of visual field testing in a developing world setting, particularly with regards to sensitivity.[71] Gonioscopy remains the standard modality to screen for the presence of narrow anterior chamber angles, but is often poorly taught, subjective, and requires significant training and the presence of a slit lamp. Newer modalities to evaluate the angle[72] are expensive and not appropriate to the rural developing world setting.

Additionally, there are many problems with our current modalities. In general, medical therapy for glaucoma requires lifetime treatment. Though low-cost eyedrop medications (as little as US$1 per bottle or less in India and China) are sold in many countries, rural availability is limited and the follow-up involved in chronic drop therapy impractical in rural areas, where 60% of Asia's population, for example, resides.[73] The quality, safety, and efficacy of inexpensive, locally available drop preparations is often not known. Surgical therapy is known to be limited because of the risks of infection after incisional glaucoma. This is especially true in the presence of the antimetabolite agents that have become common in modern glaucoma surgery.[74–78] As glaucoma drainage surgery results in the deliberate creation of a fistula into the eye, it appears likely that the prevalence of endophthalmitis after glaucoma surgery is higher than for cataract surgery. The risk of endophthalmitis after glaucoma surgery, particularly in rural areas where treatment may not be delivered in a timely fashion, is a significant concern for many NGO program planners considering large-scale glaucoma interventions.

Elevation of IOP can be observed after laser peripheral iridotomy,[79,80] and pretreatment with pressure-lowering medication is usually recommended to prevent this. Focal[81,82] or generalized[83] corneal decompensation after laser peripheral iridotomy (LPI) may also be observed. This is often due to improper aiming and energy application. Various visual symptoms have been reported after LPI, including monocular blurring, shadows, ghost images, and glare.[84,85] Large prospective studies will be needed to accurately quantify the risks and benefits associated with laser peripheral iridotomy.

All of the common treatments for glaucoma (any therapy lowering IOP) have been linked with increased risk of lens opacification and cataract. Evidence from a number of trials in both the developed[86–88] and developing[89] world indicates that there is an increased incidence of lens opacity in persons undergoing trabeculectomy surgery. Though the evidence is less clear, some studies suggest an elevated risk of lens opacification with medical glaucoma therapy as well.[90] Similarly, limited evidence suggests that LPI may also increase the rate of cataract progression.[91] The possibility of increasing cataract prevalence is of concern to blindness prevention NGOs, most of whom have adopted the prevention of cataract blindness as a central mission.

Well-performed cataract surgery has been reported to have a high potential for patient satisfaction in both the developed[92] and developing world.[93] Blindness prevention NGOs and others attempting to create sustainable cataract surgical programs often depend in their financial planning on the word-of-mouth advertising provided by satisfied patients. This is in distinction to glaucoma treatment: negative impact on quality of life has been demonstrated with both medical and surgical glaucoma therapies.[94] There is concern on the part of program planners that 'negative social marketing' as a result of glaucoma treatments, particularly surgery, might undercut the success of cataract programs.

WHAT ARE THE ACTUAL REQUIREMENTS FOR BLINDNESS PREVENTION NONGOVERNMENTAL ORGANIZATIONS TO TAKE A MORE ACTIVE ROLE IN GLAUCOMA PROGRAMMING?

This section assesses the arguments made above against NGO programming for glaucoma, and attempts to determine what is actually needed before NGOs begin widespread programs targeting glaucoma.

Competition from other diseases In fact, there is a growing consensus in the NGO community that vertical, disease-targeted programs are not an efficient way to deliver eye care. Potential areas of synergy and program overlap are most obvious for glaucoma with adult cataract:

- Both diseases affect principally older age groups.
- The preoperative examination for cataract surgery may be the only opportunity to detect glaucoma in a rural resident with little access to healthcare.
- The setting of cataract surgery may provide an appropriate venue to intervene surgically for glaucoma at the same time.

Though research in this area is badly needed, it seems unlikely that carrying out a basic examination for advanced glaucoma and combined cataract/trabeculectomy surgery where indicated would significantly reduce the efficiency of cataract programs. *The 'competition' argument does not represent a significant impediment to NGOs beginning to support clinic-based programs to detect and operate on advanced glaucoma at this time.*

Detection of early glaucoma is a challenge even for specialists in the area. However, in a setting of limited resources and restricted access to eye care, the appropriate focus is likely to be on patients with advanced disease, who can be detected by simple disc examination, and without the need for visual field testing. The presence of dense cataracts mandates that some patients will not be identified until the early postoperative period. The ability to detect even moderately advanced glaucoma by examination of the disc presupposes familiarity with stereo examination of the optic nerve and the presence of simple equipment (e.g. 90 D lens) which may not exist in many settings.

With regard to angle closure, there exists growing evidence that LPI may not be sufficient to control IOP without surgery once an acute attack[95] and/or optic nerve damage[96] have occurred. It is thus desirable to identify patients with narrow angles requiring treatment before they progress to this stage. In a hospital-based program, this would imply routine gonioscopic screening of all patients with laser treatment as needed on eyes not scheduled for cataract surgery. This presupposes the ready availability of a goniolens and the knowledge to use it, which may not exist in many settings.

Screening for glaucoma and narrow angles requiring treatment in a clinic-based, developing world setting is not complex and does not pose an impediment to NGOs undertaking such programs at this time. Training of clinical staff in basic disc examination and gonioscopy will be a key feature of such programs.

Trabeculectomy is no more inherently expensive or difficult to perform than cataract surgery, but follow-up requirements are comparatively burdensome and the risk of sight-threatening complications (cataract, endophthalmitis) is probably higher. Medicines are unlikely to be appropriate for use in the rural developing world. While the current state of information regarding the safety and efficacy of LPI is not sufficient to warrant population-based screening programs, the technique is sufficiently well understood for routine hospital-based use. The current state of glaucoma surgery is not an absolute impediment to the involvement of NGOs in hospital-based glaucoma screening and treatment programs, but for such programs to become widespread, new, safer, longer lasting procedures are needed. Research in the area of patient satisfaction with glaucoma surgery and the ability of educational messaging to mediate satisfaction levels is an important prerequisite for large-scale NGO involvement in glaucoma programming. NGOs themselves are well positioned to take a role in such research.

The following are suggested roles for NGOs in the area of glaucoma programming in the near future:

1. Support hospital-based identification and surgical treatment of advanced glaucoma as a part of comprehensive ophthalmic care provided in NGO cataract programs.
2. Support educational initiatives to improve the skills of medical practitioners in three key areas: slit lamp use, stereoscopic examination of the optic nerve, and (indentation) gonioscopy.
3. Support simple studies on patient satisfaction with glaucoma surgery, and the impact on satisfaction of simple educational messages.

GLAUCOMA SERVICES IN DEVELOPING COUNTRY SETTING

It is important to understand the context in which eye care in general is provided in developing countries.

In these countries, the ratio of population to ophthalmologist varies from 100 000 to one million plus per ophthalmologist. In the African countries, the population density is also very low. The population in these countries lives largely in rural areas; in many countries over 80% of the population lives in rural areas. On the other hand, the ophthalmologists and eye hospitals are usually located in urban centers, with most of them being in the capital or bigger cities in the country. All these factors make access to even very basic eye care service a major challenge. Studies have shown that even in an outreach eye camp only about 7% of the people in need of eye care are able to access it.[97] Not only this, but there are also issues relating to affordability.

It is in this context that one has to view the treatment of glaucoma. In most places, eye care is largely synonymous with cataract surgery and correction for refractive errors. Even when patients present themselves at a hospital or an eye camp, examination for glaucoma is not done routinely. In most hospitals, measurement of intraocular pressure using Schiotz tonometers and fundus examination are the only means of detecting glaucoma. In many areas, especially the smaller African countries, such facilities may not be available anywhere in the country. Apart from the lack of infrastructure, the diagnostic and clinical management skills among ophthalmologists are also wanting. In many of the residency programs either the required equipment or skills and sometimes both are not in place, resulting in inadequately trained ophthalmologists. As a consequence of the challenges in the community and the inadequacy among the providers, the discipline of glaucoma treatment is quite underdeveloped in most of the developing countries.

Several population-based studies estimate the prevalence of glaucoma to be roughly 1% in the Indian population. In these studies[16] it is also shown that most of those diagnosed as having glaucoma were newly diagnosed, demonstrating the poor penetration of glaucoma services into the community.

Looking ahead, this is a challenge that needs to be addressed, especially in view of the commitment to eliminate avoidable blindness by the year 2020. Some initiatives are already in place to address this. To bridge the skills gap among the ophthalmologists, a short-term skills development course of 8 weeks' duration is being offered to train them in diagnostic, laser, and surgical procedures. Guidelines are being formulated for routine examination for glaucoma as they enter the eye care system through eye camps or an eye hospital. In order to enhance community access, rural primary eye care centers called Vision Centers are being established at a density of one for every 50 000 population. In these centers, slit lamp examination, fundus examination, and applanation tonometry are being recommended with reference to screening for glaucoma. As these developments are falling in place, the ophthalmologist and the other eye care providers have to develop other innovative methods for reaching those at risk and scale up the other initiatives described above.

REFERENCES

1. Tielsch JM, Sommer A, Katz J, et al. Racial variations in the prevalence of primary open-angle glaucoma. The Baltimore Eye Survey. JAMA 1991; 266:369–374.

2. Quigley HA, West SK, Rodriguez MD, et al. The prevalence of glaucoma in a population-based study of Hispanic subjects. Arch Ophthalmol 2001; 119:1819–1826.

3. Dielemans I, Vingerling JR, Wolfs RCW, et al. The prevalence of primary open-angle glaucoma in a polpulation-based study in The Netherlands: The Rotterdam Study. Ophthalmology 1994; 101:1851–1855.

4. Mitchell P, Smith W, Attebo K, et al. Prevalence of open-angle glaucoma in Australia: The Blue Mountains Eye Study. Ophthalmology 1996; 103:1661–1669.

5. Leske MC, Connell AMS, Schachat AP, et al. The Barbados Eye Study: prevalence of open angle glaucoma. Arch Ophthalmol 1994; 112:821–829.

6. Klein BEK, Klein R, Sponsel WE, et al. Prevalence of glaucoma: the Beaver Dam Eye Study. Ophthalmology 1992; 99:1499–2504.

7. Wensor MD, McCarty CA, Stanislavsky YL, et al. The prevalence of glaucoma in the Melbourne Visual Impairment Project. Ophthalmology 1998; 105:733–739.

8. Friedman DS, Jampel HD, Munoz B, et al. The prevalence of open-angle glaucoma among blacks and whites 73 years and older: the Salisbury Eye Evaluation Glaucoma Study. Arch Ophthalmol 2006; 124:1625–1630.

9. Ramakrishnan R, Nirmalan PK, Krishnadas R, et al. Glaucoma in a rural population of southern India: the Aravind Comprehensive Eye Survey. Ophthalmology 2003; 110:1484–1490.

10. Thomas R, Dogra M. An evaluation of medical college departments of ophthalmology in India and change following provision of modern instrumentation and training. Ind J Ophthalmol 2008; 56:9–16.

11. Grover AK. Postgraduate education in India: are we on the right track? Ind J Ophthalmol 2008; 56:3–4.

12. Resnikoff S, Pascolini D, Mariotti SP, et al. Global magnitude of visual impairment caused by uncorrected refractive errors in 2004. Bull World Health Organ 2008; 86:63–70.

13. Arvind H, George R, Raju P, et al. Glaucoma in aphakia and pseudophakia in the Chennai Glaucoma Study. Br J Ophthalmol 2005; 89:699–703.

14. Freemont AM, Lee PP, Mangione CM, et al. Patterns of care for open-angle glaucoma in managed care. Arch Ophthalmol 2003; 121:777–783.

15. Quigley HA, Broman AT. The number of people with glaucoma worldwide in 2010 and 2020. Br J Ophthalmol 2006; 90: 262–267.

16. Ramakrishnan R, Praveen K, Nirmalan MPH, et al. Glaucoma in a rural population of southern India: the Aravind Comprehensive Eye Survey. Ophthalmology 2003; 110:1484–1490.

17. Cantor LB. Ophthalmic generic drug approval process: implications for safety and efficacy. J Glaucoma 1997; 6:344–349.

18. China Statistical Yearbook 2005. National Bureau of Statistics of China. 2005.

19. Xujing LU, Aiqin L, Pinzheng L. A review of literature on present situation of glaucoma for research and treatment with Acupuncture. Chinese Traditional Ophthalmology 2003; 13(2):119–121.

20. Ying G, Lingling W, Jijun L. Daily cost of glaucoma medications in China. J Glaucoma. In press.

21. Weir RE, Zaidi FH, Charteris DG, et al. Variability of the content of Indian generic ciprofloxacin eye drops. Br J Ophthalmol 2005; 89:1094–1096.

22. Narayanaswamy A, Neog A, Baskaran M, et al. A randomized, crossover, open label pilot study to evaluate the efficacy and safety of Xalatan in comparison with generic Latanoprost (Latoprost) in subjects with primary open angle glaucoma or ocular hypertension. Ind J Ophthalmol 2007; 55(2):127–131.

23. Thomas R, Mangat T. An evaluation of medical college departments of ophthalmology in India and change following provision of modern instrumentation and training. Ind J Ophthalmol 2007; 56:9–16.

24. Thomas JV, El-Mofty A, Hamdy EE, et al. Argon laser trabeculoplasty as initial therapy for glaucoma. Arch Ophthalmol 1984; 102(5):702–703.

25. Robin AL, Arkell S, Gilbert SM, et al. Q-switched neodymium: YAG laser iridotomy. A field trial with a portable laser system. Arch Ophthalmol 1986; 104:526–530.

26. Lam S, Tessler HH, Lam BL, et al. High incidence of sympathetic ophthalmia after contact and noncontact neodymium:YAG cyclotherapy. Ophthalmology 1993; 100(6):798–799.

27. Robin AL, Ramakrishnan R, Krishnadas R, et al. A long-term dose response study of mitomycin C in glaucoma filtration surgery. Arch Ophthalmol 1997; 115:969–974.

28. Budenz DL, Hoffman K, Zacchei A. Glaucoma filtering bleb dysesthesia. Am J Ophthalmol 2001; 131:626–630.

29. Natchiar GN, Thulasiraj RD, Negrel AD, et al. The Madurai Intraocular Lens Study. I: A randomized clinical trial comparing complications and vision outcomes of intracapsular cataract extraction and extracapsular cataract extraction with posterior chamber intraocular lens. Am J Ophthalmol 1998; 125:1–35.

30. Dandona L, Dandona R, Naduvilath TJ, et al. Population-based assessment of the outcome of cataract surgery in an urban population in southern India. Am J Ophthalmol 1999; 127:650–658.

31. Buhrmann RR, Quigley HA, Barron Y, et al. Prevalence of glaucoma in a rural East African population. Invest Ophthalmol Vis Sci 2000; 41:40–48.

32. Rotchford AP, Kirwan JF, Muller MA, et al. Temba Glaucoma Study: a population-based cross-sectional survey in urban South Africa. Ophthalmology 2003; 110:376–382.

33. Ayanryo JO. Blindness in the Midwestern state of Nigeria. Tropical Geogr Med 1974; 26:325–332.

34. Schwab L, Steinkuller PG. Surgical treatment of open angle glaucoma is preferable to medical management in Africa. Soc Sci Med 1983; 17:1723–1727.

35. Nwosu SNN. Blindness and visual impairment in Anambra State, Nigeria. Trop Geogr Med 1994; 46:346–349.

36. Tielsch JM, Sommer A, Witt K, et al. Blindness and visual impairment in an American urban population: the Baltimore Eye Survey. Arch Ophthalmol 1990; 108:286–290.

37. Mason RP, Kosoko O, Wilson MR, et al. National survey of the prevalence and risk factors of glaucoma in St. Lucia, West Indies. Part I. Prevalence findings. Ophthalmology 1989; 96:1363–1368.

38. Olurin O, Ghandi N, Pan T. Primary glaucoma in Nigeria. E African Med J 1972; 49:725–734.

39. Wallace J, Lovell H. Glaucoma and intra-ocular pressure in Jamaica. Am J Ophthalmol 1969; 67:93–100.

40. Wilensky JT, Gandhi N, Pan T. Racial influences in open angle glaucoma. Ann Ophthalmol 1978; 10:1398–1402.

41. Quigley HA. Number of people with glaucoma worldwide. Br J Ophthalmol 1996; 80:389–393.

42. Grant WM, Burke JF. Why do some people go blind from glaucoma? Ophthalmology 1982; 89:991–998.

43. Hiller R, Khan H. Blindness from glaucoma. Am J Ophthalmol 1975; 80:62–69.

44. Budenz DL, Singh K. Glaucoma care in West Africa. J Glaucoma 2001; 10:348–353.

45. Beck RW, Messner DK, Musch DC, et al. Is there a racial difference in physiologic cup size? Ophthalmology 1985; 92:873–876.

46. Chi T, Beck RW, Messner DK, et al. Racial differences in optic nerve head parameters. Arch Ophthalmol 1989; 107:836–839.

47. Varma R, Tielsch JM, Quigley HA, et al. Race-, age-, gender-, and refractive error-related differences in the normal optic disc. Arch Ophthalmol 1994; 112:1068–1076.

48. Verrey JD, Foster A, Wormald R, et al. Chronic glaucoma in northern Ghana – a retrospective study of 397 patients. Eye 1990; 4:115–120.

49. Welsh NH. Trabeculectomy with fistula formation in the African. Br J Ophthalmol 1972; 56:32–36.

50. Freedman J, Shen E, Ahrens M. Trabeculectomy in a black American glaucoma population. Br J Ophthalmol 1976; 60:573–574.

51. Merrit JC. Filtering procedures in American blacks. Ophthalmic Surg 1980; 11:91–94.

52. Skuta GL, Parrish RK. Wound healing in glaucoma filtering surgery. Surv Ophthalmol 1987; 32:149–170.

53. Egbert PR, Williams AS, Singh KS, et al. A prospective trial of intraoperative fluorouracil during trabeculectomy in a black population. Am J Ophthalmol 1993; 116:612–616.

54. Mermoud A, Salmon JF, Murray AND. Trabeculectomy with mitomycin C for refractory glaucoma in Blacks. Am J Ophthalmol 1993; 116:72–78.

55. Singh KS, Egbert PR, Byrd S, et al. Trabeculectomy with intraoperative 5-fluorouracil vs. mitomycin C. Am J Ophthalmol 1997; 123:48–53.

56. Quigley HA, Broman AT. The number of people with glaucoma worldwide in 2010 and 2020. Br J Ophthalmol 2006; 90(3):262–267.

57. Online. Available: http://www.cbmuk.org.uk/what/blindness.html (accessed 20 February 2007).

58. Online. Available: http://www.hki.org/ (accessed 20 February 2007).

59. Online. Available: http://www.sightsavers.org/what%20we%20do/eye%20conditions/glaucoma/world1222.html (accessed 20 February 2007).

60. Online. Available: http://www.orbis.org/bins/content_page.asp?cid = 589-598-694-1166&langπ = 9 (accessed 20 February 2007).

61. Resnikoff S, Pascolini D, Etya'ale D, et al. Global data on visual impairment in the year 2002. Bull World Health Organ 2004; 82(11):844–851.

62. Powe NR, Schein OD, Gieser SC, et al. Synthesis of the literature on visual acuity and complications following cataract extraction with intraocular lens implantation. Cataract Patient Outcome Research Team. Arch Ophthalmol 1994:239–252.

63. Prajna NV, Chandrakanth KS, Kim R, et al. The Madurai Intraocular Lens Study. II: clinical outcomes. Am J Ophthalmol 1998; 125(1):14–25.

64. Online. Available: http://www.cbmuk.org.uk/what/cataracts.html (accessed 20 February 2007).

65. Online. Available: http://www.sightsavers.org/What%20We%20Do/Eye%20Conditions/Cataract/World1414.html (accessed 20 February 2007).

66. Online. Available: http://www.orbis.org/bins/content_page.asp?cid = 589-598-693-1444&lang = 9 (accessed 20 February 2007).

67. Loevinsohn BP, Sutter RW, Costales MO. Using cost-effectiveness analysis to evaluate targeting strategies: the case of vitamin A supplementation. Health Policy Plan 1997; 12(1):29–37.

68. Online. Available: http://www.hki.org/programs/vitamina.htm (accessed 20 February 2007).

69. Tielsch JM, Katz J, Singh K, et al. A population-based evaluation of glaucoma screening: the Baltimore Eye Survey. Am J Epidemiol 1991; 134(10):1102–1110.

70. Hanson S, Krishnan SK, Phillips S. Observer experience and cup:disc ratio assessment. Optom Vis Sci 2001; 78(10):701–705.

71. Mansberger SL, Johnson CA, Cioffi GA, et al. Predictive value of frequency doubling technology perimetry for detecting glaucoma in a developing country. J Glaucoma 2005; 14(2):128–134.

72. Radhakrishnan S, Goldsmith J, Huang D, et al. Comparison of optical coherence tomography and ultrasound biomicroscopy for detection of narrow anterior chamber angles. Arch Ophthalmol 2005; 123(8):1053–1059.

73. Online. Available: http://www.un.org/esa/population/publications/wup1999/WUP99ANNEXTABLES.pdf (accessed 12 January 2007).

74. Wolner B, Liebmann JM, Sassani JW, et al. Late bleb-related endophthalmitis after trabeculectomy with adjunctive 5-fluorouracil. Ophthalmology 1991; 98:1053–1060.

75. Higginbotham EJ, Stevens RK, Musch DC, et al. Bleb-related endophthalmitis after trabeculectomy with mitomycin C. Ophthalmology 1996; 103:650–656.

76. Greenfield DS, Suner IJ, Miller MP, et al. Endophthalmitis after filtering surgery with mitomycin. Arch Ophthalmol 1996; 114:943–949.

77. Mills KB. Trabeculectomy: a retrospective long-term follow-up of 444 cases. Br J Ophthalmol 1981; 65:790–795.

78. The Fluorouracil Filtering Surgery Study Group. Five-year follow-up of the Fluorouracil Filtering Surgery Study. Am J Ophthalmol 1996; 121:349–366.

79. Stilma JS, Boen-Tan TN. Timolol and intra-ocular pressure elevation following neodymium:YAG laser surgery. Doc Ophthalmol 1986; 61:2339.

80. Kumar N, Feyi-Waboso A. Intractable secondary glaucoma from hyphema following YAG iridotomy. Can J Ophthalmol 2005; 40:85–86.

81. Wishart PK, Sherrard ES, Nagasubramanian S, et al. Corneal endothelial changes following short pulsed laser iridotomy and surgical iridectomy. Trans Ophthalmol Soc UK 1986; 105:541–548.

82. Lim LS, Ho CL, Ang LP, et al. Inferior corneal decompensation following laser peripheral iridotomy in the superior iris. Am J Ophthalmol 2006; 142:166–168.

83. Schwartz AL, Martin NF, Weber PA. Corneal decompensation after argon laser iridectomy. Arch Ophthalmol 1988; 106:1572–1574.

84. Murphy PH, Trope GE. Monocular blurring. A complication of YAG laser iridotomy. Ophthalmology 1991; 98:1539–15342.

85. Spaeth GL, Idowu O, Seligsohn A, et al. The effects of iridotomy size and position on symptoms following laser peripheral iridotomy. J Glaucoma 2005; 14:364–367.

86. Collaborative Normal-Tension Glaucoma Study Group. Comparison of glaucomatous progression between untreated patients with normal-tension glaucoma and patients with therapeutically reduced intraocular pressures. Am J Ophthalmol 1998; 126:487–497.

87. The AGIS Investigators. The Advanced Glaucoma Intervention Study, 6: effect of cataract on visual field and visual acuity. Arch Ophthalmol 2000; 118:1639–1652.

88. Musch DC, Gillespie BW, Niziol LM, et al. Collaborative Initial Glaucoma Treatment Study Group. Cataract extraction in the collaborative initial glaucoma treatment study: incidence, risk factors, and the effect of cataract progression and extraction on clinical and quality-of-life outcomes. Arch Ophthalmol 2006; 124(12):1694–1700.

89. Robin AL, Ramakrishnan R, Krishnadas R, et al. A long-term dose response study of mitomycin in glaucoma filtration surgery. Arch Ophthalmol 1997; 115:969–974.

90. Chandrasekaran S, Cumming RG, Rochtchina E, et al. Associations between elevated intraocular pressure and glaucoma, use of glaucoma medications, and 5-year incident cataract: the Blue Mountains Eye Study. Ophthalmology 2006; 113(3):417–424.

91. Lim LS, Husain R, Gazzard G, et al. Cataract progression after prophylactic laser peripheral iridotomy: potential implications

for the prevention of glaucoma blindness. Ophthalmology 2005; 112:1355–1359.

92. Lundstrom M, Stenevi U, Thorburn W, et al. Catquest questionnaire for use in cataract surgery care: assessment of surgical outcomes. J Cataract Refract Surg 1998; 24(7): 968–974.

93. Fletcher A, Vijaykumar V, Selvaraj S, et al. The Madurai Intraocular Lens Study. III: visual functioning and quality of life outcomes. Am J Ophthalmol 1998; 125(1):26–35.

94. Janz NK, Wren PA, Lichter PR, et al. CIGTS Study Group. The Collaborative Initial Glaucoma Treatment Study: interim quality of life findings after initial medical or surgical treatment of glaucoma. Ophthalmology 2001; 108(11):1954–1965.

95. Aung T, Ang LP, Chan SP, et al. Acute primary angle-closure: long-term intraocular pressure outcome in Asian eyes. Am J Ophthalmol 2001; 131:7–12.

96. Rosman M, Aung T, Ang LP, et al. Chronic angle-closure with glaucomatous damage: long-term clinical course in a North American population and comparison with an Asian population. Ophthalmology 2002; 109:2227–2231.

97. Fletcher AE, Donoghue M, Devavaram J, et al. Low uptake of eye services in rural India: a challenge for programs of blindness prevention. Arch Ophthalmol 1999; 117(10):1393–1399.

PATHOGENESIS

CHAPTER 5

Pathogenesis of Glaucomatous Optic Neuropathy

James Morgan

BACKGROUND

The loss of retinal ganglion cells (RGCs) is a signature event in glaucoma. The loss of visual field usually occurs in arcuate fashion which matches the location of damage within the retinal nerve fiber and the optic nerve head. These clinical observations provide compelling evidence that the pathophysiological events initiating RGC loss occur at the optic nerve head. Secondary changes such as hemorrhages in the peripapillary retinal nerve fiber layer, posterior deviation of the lamina cribrosa, or loss of cribrosal tissue with the development of optic nerve head pits are all associated with the exacerbation of vision loss.

Our knowledge of the clinical risk factors for the development of glaucoma has been important in shaping our views of the events that occur in the optic nerve head in this disease. Advancing age remains the single most important (but untreatable) risk factor. Of the treatable risk factors, elevated intraocular pressure is the most easily identified, though it is clear that refractive error and optic disc size also play a role. In addition, there is strong evidence that the blood supply of the optic nerve head influences retinal ganglion cell survival. It is now clear that these risk factors do not act in isolation; the challenge has been the development of a framework in which they can interact to generate vision loss.

In the past, the pathophysiological processes that result in axon loss have been considered separately as either mechanical or vascular factors in the initiation and propagation of retinal ganglion cell death. A more contemporary view is that they can be treated as a continuum in which each factor contributes to the damage of retinal ganglion cell axons. Therefore, rather than being mutually exclusive it now seems likely that that vascular and mechanical factors combine to cause axon loss. Our understanding of the way in which these forces can result in neural damage has advanced considerably in the last decade. It has highlighted the importance of determining not just the gross organization of the optic nerve head and lamina cribrosa, but also the behaviors of its various cellular elements under stress.

NORMAL ORGANIZATION OF THE LAMINA CRIBROSA: RELEVANCE TO THE PATHOGENESIS OF GLAUCOMATOUS OPTIC NEUROPATHY

The human optic disc represents an elliptical opening in the sclera through which optic nerves pass to leave the eye and enter the retrobulbar optic nerve. For the million or so axons that comprise the optic nerve this is a zone of transition and vulnerability. Axons have to rotate through 90° to exit the eye and, in doing this, to rearrange so that they come to lie in the appropriate topographic organization within the optic nerve. The posterior part of the optic nerve also sees the myelination of the axons as each is invested in an oligodendrocyte-derived sheath to facilitate saltatory conduction. Retinal ganglion cells are unique in the retina in that they are the only cells to generate action potentials. This is an energy intensive process; analysis of retinal nerve fiber layer anatomy has shown that the mitochondria tend to concentrate in varicosities along the retinal ganglion cell axons.[1] It is perhaps not surprising that RGCs are particularly vulnerable to the diseases where mitochondrial function is compromised. Studies of the distribution of mitochondrial enzymes such as cytochrome-c oxidase have shown that these are concentrated at the optic nerve head (Figs 5.1 and 5.2).[2]

Axons are supported in this passage by a complex arrangement of glial supportive tissue in the anterior part of the optic nerve head which lies in continuity with pores that run through the lamina cribrosa. These glial processes are effectively contiguous with those lying within the retinal nerve fiber layer. The optic nerve head is divided into an anterior glial prelamina region that lies anterior to the collagenous lamina cribrosa. At the part of the optic nerve that is clinically apparent as the lamina cribrosa, the lamina is comprised of the collagenous cribrosal plates, approximately 10 layers thick, that lie at the level of the scleral opening.[3] Each plate is perforated to provide room for the axons to pass in bundles approximately 100 μm wide. When viewed in cross-section, the plates appear to be discrete and separated. Digest studies in which the cellular components (and the glial prelamina are removed by enzymatic or chemical digestion) have revealed that the plates have abundant connections between each other and form a compact three-dimensional array of pores through which the axon bundles run (Fig. 5.3).[4]

The scleral lamina can therefore be regarded as a meshlike structure in which any forces that result in distortion of one part will be transmitted throughout the lamina cribrosa.

AXON ORGANIZATION IN THE OPTIC NERVE HEAD: A ROLE FOR MECHANICAL FACTORS

The detailed organization of axons as they pass through the optic nerve remains a source of continued debate.[5] At a coarse level, axon bundles are arranged so that those arising from peripheral parts of the retina come to lie in the periphery of the optic nerve.[6] Analysis of the movement of the cribrosal plates in glaucoma has shown that these rotate around the margin of the scleral opening (Elschnig's rim) in a way that is likely to induce the greatest compressive force on axons lying in the peripheral part of the optic nerve. This pattern of events fits with clinical observations that peripheral loss of visual field is a characteristic feature in glaucoma. Electron microscopic studies of retinal ganglion cell axons in experimental glaucoma provides confirmatory evidence that axons may be damaged as the cribrosal structures are distorted and collapse (Fig. 5.4).[7]

While these events are likely to occur in the end stages of disease, the extent to which this occurs with early axon damage is unclear. Detailed analysis of the trajectories taken by individual axons through the optic nerve head suggests that even minor displacement of the lamina cribrosa could have an adverse effect on axonal function. When the paths taken by individual axons are traced it is apparent that they can deviate from the expected path observed when the population is considered as a whole.[5,8] This topographic 'noise' can give rise to populations of axons in which some pass between the cribrosal plates, which might render them more vulnerable to the pressure on the optic nerve

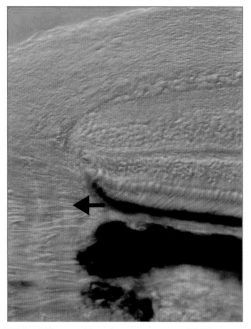

FIGURE 5.1 Differential interference contrast (DIC) image of a primate optic nerve head showing the relationship between the retinal nerve fiber layer and lamina cribrosa. The arrow indicates the demarcation between the anteriorly located glial prelamina and the scleral lamina cribrosa. (Reproduced with permission from British Journal of Ophthalmology 1998; 82:6.)

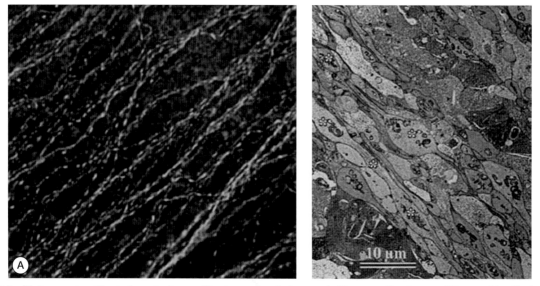

FIGURE 5.2 (A) Axon varicosities in the retinal nerve fiber layer of a whole mounted human retina from an 85-year-old patient. The varicosities coincide with regions in the axon where mitochondria and other organelles are concentrated. (From Wang L, Dong J, Cull G, et al. Varicosities of intraretinal ganglion cell axons in human and nonhuman primates. Invest Ophthalmol Vis Sci 2003; 44:2–9.)

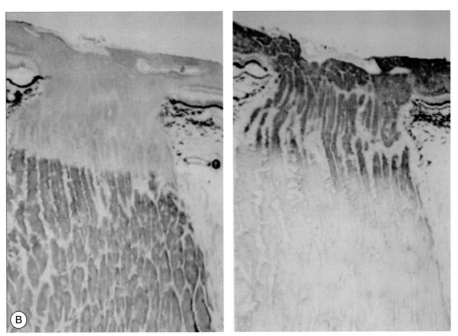

FIGURE 5.2 **(Continued)**: (B) Distribution of cytochrome oxidase activity in the human optic nerve head. (From Andrews RM, Griffiths PG, Johnson MA, Turnbull DM. Histochemical localisation of mitochondrial enzyme activity in human optic nerve and retina. Br J Ophthalmol 1999; 83:231–235.)

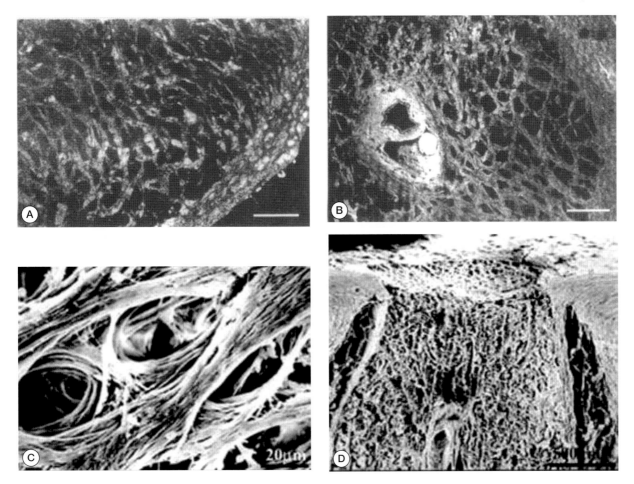

FIGURE 5.3 (A, B) Immunofluorescent staining of cross-section through the human lamina cribrosa stained with antibodies against collagens I and III. Scale, 100 μm. (From Albon J, Karwatowski WS, Avery N, et al. Changes in the collagenous matrix of the aging human lamina cribrosa. Br J Ophthalmol 1995; 79:368–375.) (C, D) Scanning electron micrographs of human optic nerve head following partial enzymatic digestion. (From Albon J, Farrant S, Akhtar S, et al. Connective tissue structure of the tree shrew optic nerve and associated ageing changes. Invest Ophthalmol Vis Sci 2007; 48:2134–2144.)

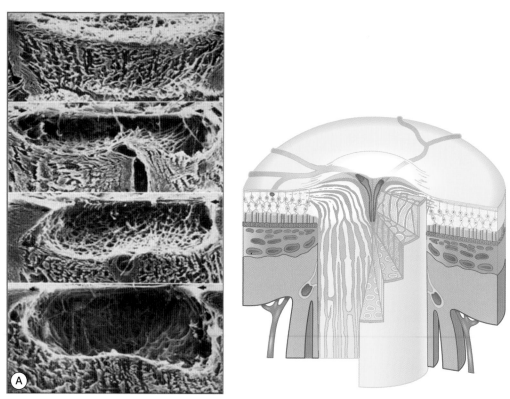

FIGURE 5.4 (A) Scanning electron micrographs of human optic nerve head in glaucoma showing characteristic rotation of the plates of the lamina cribrosa at the edge of the optic nerve. (From Quigley HA, Addicks EM. Regional differences in the structure of the lamina cribrosa and their relation to glaucomatous optic nerve damage. Arch Ophthalmol 1981; 99:137–143.) (B) Diagrammatic representation of the orientation of the glial columns in the prelamina part of the human optic nerve head, based on staining for GFAP, a marker of astrocytes. (From Triviño A, Ramírez JM, Salazar JJ, et al. Immunohistochemical study of human optic nerve head astroglia. Vis Res 1996; 36:2015–2028.)

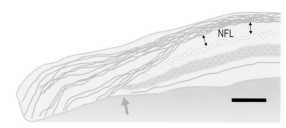

FIGURE 5.5 Path taken by axons within the primate (macaque) retinal nerve fiber layer. Note that axons from the superficial layers of the retinal nerve fiber layer are distributed throughout the optic nerve at the level of the scleral canal. (Redrawn from Ogden TE. Nerve fiber layer of the macaque retina: retinotopic organization. Invest Ophthalmol Vis Sci 1983; 24:85–98.)

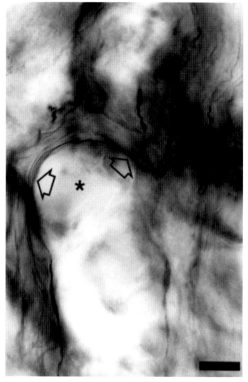

head. A degree of axon deviation is to be expected when the difference in the dimensions of the anterior and posterior parts of the scleral lamina are considered. The anterior part of the scleral lamina receives unmyelinated axons, whereas the posterior part interfaces with the junction at which axons become myelinated. As a result, the number of pores increases with depth in the lamina cribrosa such that there are more pores in the deeper part of the lamina, than in the superficial part (Figs 5.5 and 5.6).[3]

FIGURE 5.6 Axon deviation in the human lamina cribrosa. A single axon is indicated (*open arrows*) that passes between the plates of the lamina cribrosa (*the middle of a plate is shown by the asterisk*). (From Morgan JE, Jeffery G, Foss AJ. Axon deviation in the human lamina cribrosa. Br J Ophthalmol 1998; 82:680–683.)

ASTROGLIAL INTERACTIONS WITHIN THE LAMINA CRIBROSA: TRANSLATING THE EFFECTS OF STRESS AND STRAIN

In the early stages of glaucoma, it is unlikely that the cribrosal plates are grossly distorted in ways that will result in axonal constriction. A simple mechanical model of axon damage therefore seems unlikely in the early stages of the disease. Studies indicating local axon enlargement with accumulation of mitochondria at the level of the lamina cribrosa now seem more likely to reflect axonal metabolic demands[2] rather than gross axon compression. Clinical evaluation of the optic nerve head suggests little distortion of the lamina cribrosa and this has been confirmed by digital imaging studies of the optic nerve head. Yet even at this stage in glaucoma, axons are lost and the challenge has been to determine the mechanisms by which this can occur.

Several key studies have recently been undertaken which have analyzed the interaction between the shape of the optic nerve and the stress and strain that might be built up in the optic nerve head. These have been based on meticulous high-resolution reconstructions of the optic nerve head which have allowed the generation of three-dimensional computer models of the nerve head.[9-11] These models can then be subject to finite element analysis in which the forces that lie within the beams of the lamina cribrosa are modeled to develop three-dimensional stress and strain maps of the lamina cribrosa. An important finding from this work is that it has highlighted the stresses that can build up in the lamina cribrosa, and that these changes can occur shortly after experimental elevation in intraocular pressure (IOP) (Fig. 5.7).[10]

Forces acting within the optic nerve head are dynamic and reflect pulsation in the central retinal artery and its interaction with the intraocular pressure. The degree to which the lamina cribrosa can be distorted varies with age. In younger eyes it shows considerable elasticity and can, after increased pressure has been removed, return to its normal configuration. With older eyes, the elasticity of the tissue is reduced and there is less of a tendency for the deformation to resolve with resolution of the imposed pressure.[12] These observations all point to the lamina cribrosa as playing a key role in mediating axon damage.

Recent evidence that the lamina cribrosa thickness increases following short-term elevation of IOP in the primate is consistent with the idea that changes in the optic nerve are dynamic.[13] The increase could arise from axonal swelling or from remodeling of the cribrosa itself with the deposition of new connective tissue. It is important to note that these data are derived from observations on young eyes. Further work is required to determine the extent to which these changes occur in older eyes.

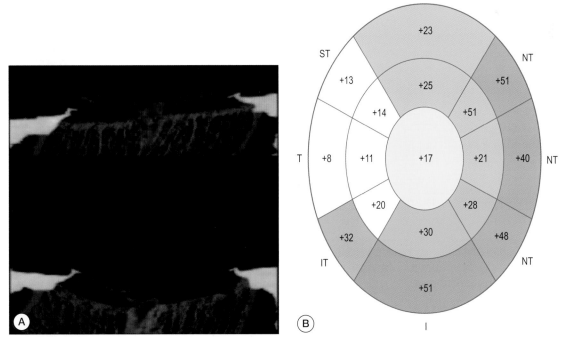

FIGURE 5.7 (A) Digital reconstruction of a primate optic nerve showing the effects of experimental elevation of intraocular pressure on the scleral lamina. Note the posterior bowing of the lamina with preservation of the pore alignment. The rotation of the laminar plates is greatest at the periphery of the nerve. (From Burgoyne CF, Downs JC, Bellezza AJ, Hart RT. Three-dimensional reconstruction of normal and early glaucoma monkey optic nerve head connective tissues. Invest Ophthalmol Vis Sci 2004 Dec; 45(12):4388–4399.) (B) Image shows the thickening in the lamina cribrosa that occurs with a short-term increase in IOP in the primate. (Redrawn from Yang H, Downs JC, Girkin C, et al. 3-D histomorphometry of the normal and early glaucomatous monkey optic nerve head: lamina cribrosa and peripapillary scleral position and thickness. Invest Ophthalmol Vis Sci 2007 Oct; 48(10):4597–4607.)

OPTIC NERVE HEAD ASTROCYTES: TRANSLATING OPTIC NERVE STRESS INTO AXON DAMAGE

Astrocytes are the predominant glial support cell in the optic nerve head.[14] They surround the beams of the lamina cribrosa and are connected and communicate via a network of gap junctions to form, effectively, a syncytium to provide an environment to support the retinal ganglion cell axons. The astrocyte population can be distinguished on the basis of the expression of the adhesion molecule (NCAM) into those that line the glial tubes that guide the axons to the scleral lamina and those that line the plates of the lamina cribrosa (NCAM−). Other astrocytes (IB) show a wider distribution throughout the optic nerve.[14] The close association of these cells and the beams of the lamina cribrosa where they are effectively interposed between the cribrosa and the axons, makes them ideally placed to mediate the effects of changes in the cribrosal beams to the axon population. As axons conduct action potentials, it is critical that the appropriate extracellular environment is maintained to support the associated ionic changes. The astrocytes are also important for the maintenance of cribrosal structure, where they are involved in the production of collagens and elastins that contribute to the structural integrity of the cribrosal beams.[14]

Numerous experiments have indicated how astrocytes may go from exerting a supportive effect on axons to a mode in which they can inflict damage. If the ability of astrocytes to support axons is compromised, this will result in axonal stress and loss. For example, astrocytes can also generate harmful agents such as nitrous oxide (NO) by upregulating the expression of NOS-2, which can result in direct axonal damage (Fig. 5.8). There is some evidence that agents limiting the generation of NO can reduce the loss of retinal ganglion cells in a model of experimental glaucoma.[15]

In addition to astrocytes, a significant population of lamina cribrosal cells has been isolated.[16] These are classed as glial cells but differ in that they do not express glial fibrillary acid protein (GFAP).[17] These cells are star-shaped and lie within the cribriform plates; they are likely to be important in maintaining their integrity but are localized to the scleral lamina. The relation of these cells to RGC axons requires clarification. In experiments where the cells are subject to the stresses and strains that might be seen in glaucoma, these cells can upregulate the expression of genes such as TGF-β_2 that may be important in regulating the remodeling of the lamina cribrosa.[18]

BLOOD SUPPLY: NORMAL AND GLAUCOMA

BLOOD SUPPLY OF THE OPTIC NERVE HEAD

Clinical studies suggest that deficits in the blood supply of the optic nerve head may be important in generating

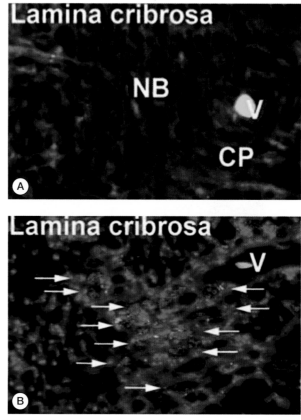

FIGURE 5.8 Immunohistochemistry for NOS-2 (*red*) and GFAP (*green*) in the normal (A) and glaucomatous (B) optic nerve head. NB, nerve bundle; CP, cribriform plate; V, blood vessel. *Arrows* colocalize GFAP abd NOS-2. (From Liu B, Neufeld AH. Expression of nitric oxide synthase-2 (NOS-2) in reactive astrocytes of the human glaucomatous optic nerve head. Glia 2000; 30:78–86. Reprinted with permission of Wiley-Liss, Inc., a subsidiary of John Wiley & Sons, Inc.)

RGC loss. Glaucoma-like cupping of the optic nerve head has been observed in patients in whom the systemic blood supply has been compromised (by systemic hypotension).[19] The blood supply of the optic nerve is complicated and unusual in that the central retinal artery does not contribution to the supply of the optic nerve head. Instead, the blood supply comes from a series of 15–20 short posterior ciliary arteries which in turn come off the long posterior ciliary arteries (off the ophthalmic artery). These arteries form an incomplete anastomosis around the optic nerve at the level of the scleral lamina (as such, they run in the sclera). The precise anatomy of these vessels has been characterized by resin cast studies of postmortem tissue in which the vasculature is filled with a resin and, following tissue digestion, the anatomy of the vasculature revealed.[20] The short posterior ciliary arteries lie within the sclera and form an incomplete anastomosis around the optic nerve, the so-called circle of Zinn Haller. Small, end-arterial branches are sent from this circle into the optic nerve head to supply it with oxygen (Fig. 5.9).

These end-stage arteries expose the optic nerve head to the risk that it will be compromised when the systemic

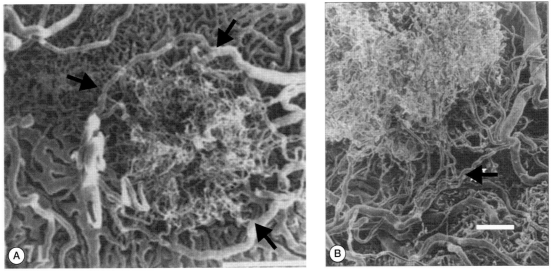

FIGURE 5.9 Scanning electron micrograph of a corrosion cast of human optic nerve head vasculature. (A) Anastomosis of Zinn Haler indicated (arrows) sending short posterior ciliary vessels into the optic nerve head at the level of the lamina cribrosa. (B) *Arrow* indicates area where the anastomosis is narrowed. (From Olver JM, Spalton DJ, McCartney AC. Quantitative morphology of human retrolaminar optic nerve vasculature. Invest Ophthalmol Vis Sci 1994 Oct; 35(11):3858–3866.)

blood supply is affected; this agrees with clinical observations that low systemic blood pressure can be associated with an increased risk of glaucoma progression. Patients with conditions such as Raynaud's syndrome also appear to be at slightly increased risk of developing glaucoma. There is evidence that patients with low-tension glaucoma may demonstrate abnormalities in the peripheral circulation in response to changes in temperature.[20]

These observations do not, in themselves, prove that deficits in the blood supply are important factors, but they are persuasive. In the clinical setting some patients have been reported with elevated systemic levels of endothelin-1, a potent vasoconstrictor. In the rodent and primate models of glaucoma, chronic delivery of endothelin, which results in vasoconstriction of the short poasterior ciliary arteries (SPCAs), can result in the loss of axons in a distribution, similar to that seen in glaucoma associated with elevated intraocular pressure.[21]

WHAT IS THE ROLE OF INTRAOCULAR PRESSURE IN INITIATING AXON LOSS?

The relationship between IOP and axon loss is complex. The IOP level remains a key influence on the health of the axon population; even small differences in IOP between the eyes in a single patient correlate with differences in glaucoma severity.[22] Recent evidence suggests that long-term IOP fluctuation may play a significant role in determining the degree of visual field loss,[23,24] in that eyes with greater variation in IOP have an increased risk of progressive visual field loss. These observations fit nicely with the idea that stress and strain in the lamina cribrosa, acting through cellular elements, will promote the loss of retinal ganglion cell

axons. It now seems likely that the non-neuronal glial cell population plays a major role in integrating the effects of IOP elevation and fluctuation with exacerbating factors such as a compromised optic nerve head circulation. For any given case, the relative importance of all these factors may vary but the phenotypic outcome is similar.

HOW DOES AXONS DAMAGE RESULT IN RETINAL GANGLION CELL LOSS?

Early studies of the effects of elevated intraocular pressure on axonal anatomy revealed ballooning of axons at the sites of compression of the plates of the lamina cribrosa.[25] This provided an attractive hypothesis for the way in which axons were affected and how this might result in the loss of retinal ganglion cells. Axons are important in regulating the activity and survival of the cell soma by the retrograde transport of neurotrophins from the target regions contacted by the axons. They terminate in both the lateral geniculate nucleus (LGN) and the superior colliculus, and these are sites which produce neurotrophins that are then retrogradely transported to the retinal ganglion cells. Compromised transport of neurotrophins from these target locations to the retinal ganglion cells would predispose to cell death. Histological studies demonstrating the building of tyrosine kinase B (TRKB) receptor in the optic nerve head of rodent and primate glaucomatous optic nerves[26] supports this hypothesis. However, it is not yet clear the extent to which other cells in the retina (and optic nerve) can compensate by local production of neurotrophins. Upregulation of brain-derived neurotrophic factor (BDNF) levels in experimental glaucoma are associated with reduced loss of retinal ganglion

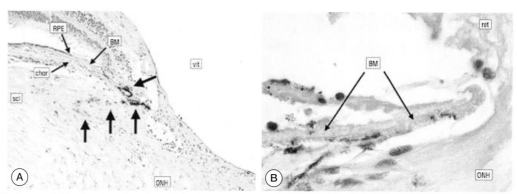

FIGURE 5.10   Immunohistochemistry for microglia in the human optic nerve head. (A) Clusters of HLA-DR labeled cells. (B) Cells positive for CD45. The cells are clustered along Bruch's membrane, which extends beyond the termination of the retinal pigment epithelium. (From Neufeld AH. Microglia in the optic nerve head and the region of parapapillary chorioretinal atrophy in glaucoma. Arch Ophthalmol 1999; 117:1050–1056.)

cells,[27] but further work is required to see if this is a persistent effect.

RETINAL FACTORS IN THE INITIATION OF RETINAL GANGLION CELL DEATH

It is possible that retinal ganglion cell loss in itself will influence the viability of surviving cells. Of most interest in this respect has been the suggestion that the release of glutamate from dying cells is directly toxic to surrounding RGCs. Measurement of glutamate levels from the vitreous of patients with glaucoma suggested a selective rise in glutamate which can cause neural damage.[28] However, subsequent studies have not confirmed this elevation[29,30] and the consensus is now that an elevated glutamate concentration in the vitreous is unlikely to be a prime factor in the initiation of retinal ganglion cell death. It is likely that glutamate uptake mechanisms, in particular glutamate transporters, are important for clearing glutamate from the inner retina, limiting the effects of its toxicity. At a local level, the possibility remains that glutamate release may exacerbate retinal ganglion cell death though there is no evidence as yet that glutamate uptake mechanisms are compromised in experimental glaucoma.[31] Even so, work in the rodent suggests that the loss of one group of RGCs, following optic nerve transection, can result in greater loss of surrounding cells.[32] Further work is required to see whether this is the case in glaucoma.

IMMUNOLOGICAL FACTORS IN GLAUCOMATOUS OPTIC NEUROPATHY

Clinical investigations have revealed that immunological factors are likely to be important in influencing the degree of retinal ganglion cell death in glaucoma. Systemic investigations are consistent with activation of the immune system in initiating retinal ganglion cell

loss, for example with elevation of autoantibodies to both retinal and optic nerve antigens.[33] Whether these changes are secondary to the loss of retinal ganglion cells remains unclear. Treatments based on immuno-modulation by boosting the protective effects of T cells within the central nervous system (CNS) have shown some benefit in limiting retinal ganglion cell death in a rodent glaucoma model.[34] The protective effect also extends to acute increases in IOP[35] but not to the prevention of secondary retinal ganglion cell loss in models of more severe optic nerve damage (e.g. by partial optic nerve transection).[36]

Histological studies of the human optic nerve head have suggested that microglial cells, which can be resident or recruited from the systemic circulation, might be important in the initiation of retinal ganglion cell death.[37] Microglia are important in the CNS and can act in both a protective and a destructive role; there is good evidence for their role in retinal conditions such as uveitis and photoreceptor degeneration.[38] They usually act as scavengers to clear the debris of dead or dying neurons, but can also act to harm cells by the release of cytokines such as tumor necrosis factor (TNF)-α (Fig. 5.10).

In experimental models of glaucoma there is evidence that microglia are activated as a result of the elevation in intraocular pressure.[39] The activity of these cells can be reduced by the application of agents such as minocycline, and it is possible that this can be beneficial in reducing the degree of retinal ganglion cell loss.[40] Although the protective effect is partial, this is an important novel avenue for treatment, given the safety of agents such as minocycline.

More recently, attention has turned to the role of the complement pathway in initiating retinal ganglion cell death. Evidence from the rodent model of glaucoma has indicated the deposition of C1q, C3, and membrane attack complex (MAC) within the retinal ganglion cell layer following the induction of experimental glaucoma.[41] Labeling for the membrane attack complex, the

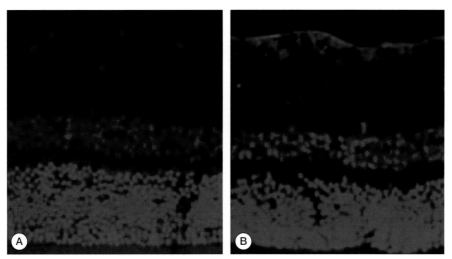

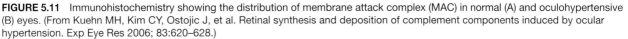

FIGURE 5.11 Immunohistochemistry showing the distribution of membrane attack complex (MAC) in normal (A) and oculohypertensive (B) eyes. (From Kuehn MH, Kim CY, Ostojic J, et al. Retinal synthesis and deposition of complement components induced by ocular hypertension. Exp Eye Res 2006; 83:620–628.)

outcome from activation of the complement pathway, also shows increased labeling in glaucomatous eyes (Fig. 5.11).

Summary

Considerable progress has been made in our understanding of the factors that influence axon loss in glaucoma. There is a broad consensus that the lamina cribrosa and its cellular elements play a key role in initiating axonal damage, which then precipitates retinal ganglion cell death. The relationship between the beams of the lamina cribrosa and surrounding astrocytes provides a pivotal point for the generation of cytokines and agents that would damage passing axons. More recently attention has also turned to the role played by other factors such as the immune system and the possibility that dying retinal ganglion cells may also contribute to the death of adjacent cells.

Key Points

- The optic nerve is the focal point for the loss of retinal ganglion cells.
- Both focal and diffuse damage in the optic nerve head can generate the characteristic patterns of retinal ganglion cell death.
- The shape and structure of any given optic nerve may increase its vulnerability to damage.
- Stress/strain and mechanical factors at the level of the lamina cribrosa will influence the initiation of retinal ganglion cell death.
- Vascular factors such as systemic hypotension or vasospasm may exacerbate RGC death.
- Other elements within the retina may influence the pattern of RGC death, for example the presence of immune cells in the optical nerve head and retina (microglia) and the possible involvement of the immune system in glaucoma.

REFERENCES

1. Wang L, Dong J, Cull G, et al. Varicosities of intraretinal ganglion cell axons in human and nonhuman primates. Invest Ophthalmol Vis Sci 2003; 44:2–9.

2. Bristow EA, Griffiths PG, Andrews RM, et al. The distribution of mitochondrial activity in relation to optic nerve structure. Arch Ophthalmol 2002; 120:791–796.

3. Ogden T, Duggan J, Danley K, et al. Morphometry of nerve bundle pores in the optic nerve head of the human. Exp Eye Res 1988; 46:559–568.

4. Quigley HA, Hohman RM, Addicks EM, et al. Morphologic changes in the lamina cribrosa correlated with neural loss in open-angle glaucoma. Am J Ophthalmol 1983; 95:673–691.

5. Fitzgibbon T, Taylor S. Retinotopy of the human retinal nerve fibre layer and optic nerve head. J Comp Neurol 1996; 375:238–251.

6. Radius RL, Anderson DR. The course of axons through the retina and optic nerve head. Arch Ophthalmol 1979; 97:1154–1158.

7. Quigley H, Addicks E. Regional differences in the structure of the lamina cribrosa and their relation to glaucomatous optic nerve damage. Arch Ophthalmol 1981; 99:137–143.

8. Morgan J, Jeffery G, Foss A. Axon deviation in the human lamina cribrosa. Br J Ophthalmol 1998; 82:680–683.

9. Bellezza AJ, Rintalan CJ, Thompson HW, et al. Deformation of the lamina cribrosa and anterior scleral canal wall in early experimental glaucoma. Invest Ophthalmol Vis Sci 2003; 44:623–637.

10. Burgoyne CF, Downs JC, Bellezza AJ, et al. Three-dimensional reconstruction of normal and early glaucoma monkey optic nerve head connective tissues. Invest Ophthalmol Vis Sci 2004; 45:4388–4399.

11. Burgoyne CF, Downs JC, Bellezza AJ, et al. The optic nerve head as a biomechanical structure: a new paradigm for understanding the role of IOP-related stress and strain in the pathophysiology of glaucomatous optic nerve head damage. Prog Retin Eye Res 2005; 24:39–73.

12. Albon J, Purslow PP, Karwatowski WS, et al. Age related compliance of the lamina cribrosa in human eyes. Br J Ophthalmol 2000; 84:318–323.

13. Yang H, Downs JC, Girkin C, et al. 3-D histomorphometry of the normal and early glaucomatous monkey optic nerve head: lamina

cribrosa and peripapillary scleral position and thickness. Invest Ophthalmol Vis Sci 2007; 48:4597–4607.

14. Hernandez MR. The optic nerve head in glaucoma: role of astrocytes in tissue remodeling. Prog Retin Eye Res 2000; 19:297–321.

15. Neufeld AH, Sawada A, Becker B. Inhibition of nitric-oxide synthase 2 by aminoguanidine provides neuroprotection of retinal ganglion cells in a rat model of chronic glaucoma. Proc Natl Acad Sci USA 1999; 96:9944–9948.

16. Lambert W, Agarwal R, Howe W, et al. Neurotrophin and neurotrophin receptor expression by cells of the human lamina cribrosa. Invest Ophthalmol Vis Sci 2001; 42:2315–2323.

17. Kirwan RP, Leonard MO, Murphy M, et al. Transforming growth factor-beta-regulated gene transcription and protein expression in human GFAP-negative lamina cribrosa cells. Glia 2005; 52:309–324.

18. Kirwan RP, Fenerty CH, Crean J, et al. Influence of cyclical mechanical strain on extracellular matrix gene expression in human lamina cribrosa cells in vitro. Mol Vis 2005; 11: 798–810.

19. Drance SM, Morgan RW, Sweeney VP. Shock-induced optic neuropathy: a cause of nonprogressive glaucoma. N Engl J Med 1973; 288:392–395.

20. Drance S, Douglas G, Wijsman K, et al. Response of blood flow to warm and cold in normal and low tension glaucoma patients. Am J Ophthalmol 1988; 105:35–39.

21. Cioffi GA. Ischemic model of optic nerve injury. Trans Am Ophthalmol Soc 2005; 103:592–613.

22. Cartwright M, Anderson D. Correlation of asymmetric damage with asymmetric intraocular pressure in normal-tension glaucoma (low-tension glaucoma). Arch Ophthalmol 1988; 106:898–900.

23. Nouri-Mahdavi K, Hoffman D, Coleman AL, et al. Predictive factors for glaucomatous visual field progression in the Advanced Glaucoma Intervention Study. Ophthalmology 2004; 111:1627–1635.

24. Asrani S, Zeimer R, Wilensky J, et al. Large diurnal fluctuations in intraocular pressure are an independent risk factor in patients with glaucoma. J Glaucoma 2000; 9:134–142.

25. Quigley H, Addicks E. Chronic experimental glaucoma in primates. II. Effect of extended intraocular pressure on optic nerve head and axonal transport. Invest Ophthalmol Vis Sci 1980; 19:137–152.

26. Pease ME, McKinnon SJ, Quigley HA, et al. Obstructed axonal transport of BDNF and its receptor TrkB in experimental glaucoma. Invest Ophthalmol Vis Sci 2000; 41:764–774.

27. Martin KR, Quigley HA, Zack DJ, et al. Gene therapy with brain-derived neurotrophic factor as a protection: retinal ganglion cells in a rat glaucoma model. Invest Ophthalmol Vis Sci 2003; 44:4357–4365.

28. Dreyer E, Zurakowski D, Schumer R, et al. Elevated glutamate levels in the vitreous body of humans and monkeys with glaucoma. Arch Ophthalmol 1996; 114:299–305.

29. Honkanen RA, Baruah S, Zimmerman MB, et al. Vitreous amino acid concentrations in patients with glaucoma undergoing vitrectomy. Arch Ophthalmol 2003; 121:183–188.

30. Wamsley S, Gabelt BT, Dahl DB, et al. Vitreous glutamate concentration and axon loss in monkeys with experimental glaucoma. Arch Ophthalmol 2005; 123:64–70.

31. Hartwick AT, Zhang X, Chauhan BC, et al. Functional assessment of glutamate clearance mechanisms in a chronic rat glaucoma model using retinal ganglion cell calcium imaging. J Neurochem 2005; 94:794–807.

32. Levkovitch-Verbin H, Quigley HA, Kerrigan-Baumrind LA, et al. Optic nerve transection in monkeys may result in secondary degeneration of retinal ganglion cells. Invest Ophthalmol Vis Sci 2001; 42:975–982.

33. Tezel G, Wax MB. The immune system and glaucoma. Curr Opin Ophthalmol 2004; 15:80–84.

34. Bakalash S, Kessler A, Mizrahi T, et al. Antigenic specificity of immunoprotective therapeutic vaccination for glaucoma. Invest Ophthalmol Vis Sci 2003; 44:3374–3381.

35. Ben Simon GJ, Bakalash S, Aloni E, et al. A rat model for acute rise in intraocular pressure: immune modulation as a therapeutic strategy. Am J Ophthalmol 2006; 141:1105–1111.

36. Blair M, Pease ME, Hammond J, et al. Effect of glatiramer acetate on primary and secondary degeneration of retinal ganglion cells in the rat. Invest Ophthalmol Vis Sci 2005; 46:884–890.

37. Neufeld AH. Microglia in the optic nerve head and the region of parapapillary chorioretinal atrophy in glaucoma. Arch Ophthalmol 1999; 117:1050–1056.

38. Hughes EH, Schlichtenbrede FC, Murphy CC, et al. Minocycline delays photoreceptor death in the rds mouse through a microglia-independent mechanism. Exp Eye Res 2004; 78:1077–1084.

39. Ju KR, Kim HS, Kim JH, et al. Retinal glial cell responses and Fas/FasL activation in rats with chronic ocular hypertension. Brain Res 2006; 1122:209–221.

40. Levkovitch-Verbin H, Kalev-Landoy M, Habot-Wilner Z, et al. Minocycline delays death of retinal ganglion cells in experimental glaucoma and after optic nerve transection. Arch Ophthalmol 2006; 124:520–526.

41. Kuehn MH, Kim CY, Ostojic J, et al. Retinal synthesis and deposition of complement components induced by ocular hypertension. Exp Eye Res 2006; 83:620–628.

CHAPTER 6

Aqueous Humor Dynamics and Intraocular Pressure Elevation

Carol B Toris

INTRODUCTION

A fine balance between the production, circulation, and drainage of ocular aqueous humor from the posterior chamber (aqueous humor dynamics) is essential to maintain intraocular pressure (IOP) at a steady-state level, provide nutritive support to avascular ocular tissues, and keep the shape of the globe constant. Parameters of aqueous humor dynamics include the rate of aqueous humor production, the facility of trabecular outflow, the rate of fluid drainage through the uveoscleral outflow pathway, and the pressure in the episcleral veins (Fig. 6.1). When one or more of these parameters is altered and the balance between inflow and outflow is disturbed, various pathological conditions affecting IOP can result. Elevated IOP is usually attributed to an increase in resistance to outflow but other factors may be involved. Understanding the complex mechanisms that regulate aqueous humor circulation is essential

for better management of glaucoma. To that end, this chapter explores aqueous humor dynamics in healthy eyes and in various syndromes affecting IOP.

AQUEOUS HUMOR DYNAMICS IN THE HEALTHY HUMAN EYE

AQUEOUS FLOW

Ocular aqueous humor is produced continuously by the ciliary processes of the ciliary body to supply nutrients to the lens, cornea, and avascular tissues of the anterior chamber angle and to flush away their metabolic waste products. Other functions include transport of neurotransmitters, stabilization of the ocular structure, and regulation of the homeostasis of ocular tissues. The circulation of aqueous humor also provides the mechanism for removal of inflammatory cells and mediators under

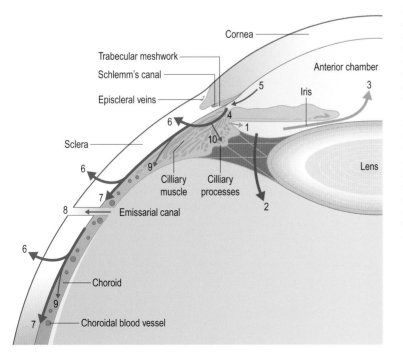

FIGURE 6.1 Aqueous humor dynamics. Aqueous humor that is secreted into the posterior chamber (1) flows across the vitreous cavity (2) or through the pupil into the anterior chamber (3). Fluid circulates around the anterior chamber and eventually drains into the anterior chamber angle (4). Aqueous humor drains from the anterior chamber angle via two routes, the trabecular meshwork, Schlemm's canal, and episcleral veins (5), or the uveoscleral outflow route. The latter route starts with the ciliary muscl e. From there, fluid may flow in many directions, including: across the sclera (6), within the supraciliary and suprachoroidal spaces (7), through emissarial canals (8), into uveal vessels (9) and vortex veins (not drawn), and possibly into ciliary processes (10) where it could be secreted again. (Redrawn, with permission, from Figures 1 and 3 of Toris CB. Aqueous humor dynamics I, measurement methods and animal studies. The eye's aqueous humor. In: Mortimer M. Civan, ed. Current topics in membranes. Elsevier: San Diego; 2008, in press.)

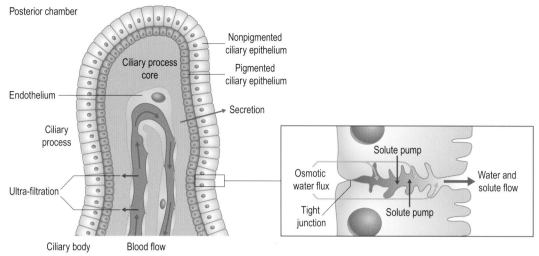

FIGURE 6.2   Aqueous humor production. Aqueous humor is produced in a series of steps. An ultrafiltrate of blood that flows through the ciliary process moves across the leaky capillaries into the core of the process (*Ultrafiltration*). Solute and fluid from the core are actively transported via solute pumps into the intercellular spaces of the nonpigmented epithelium (*Secretion*). An osmotic gradient draws water into the intercellular space. Water and solute diffuse in the direction opposite the tight junction at the apical end, and into the posterior chamber. The figure on the right is an enlargement of the intercellular spaces between two nonpigmented ciliary epithelial cells.

some pathological conditions, and it enables drugs to be distributed to the different ocular structures.

Aqueous humor is produced in a series of steps (Fig. 6.2), starting with a copious amount of blood flowing through the core of the ciliary processes. Plasma from the blood moves by ultrafiltration into the tissue spaces of the ciliary process stroma, a process involving the flow of water and water-soluble substances across the capillary endothelium in response to a hydrostatic pressure gradient.[1] Next, anions, cations, and other substances are actively transported across the nonpigmented ciliary epithelial cells and deposited into the clefts between cells. The ions create a hyperosmotic environment and subsequent diffusion of water into the intercellular spaces. The intercellular spaces are closed by tight junctions at the apical end and opened to the posterior chamber at the basal end, a design that directs the flow of fluid into the posterior chamber. Nutrients and other substances necessary for the survival of the avascular ocular tissues are added by diffusion to this fluid as it courses through the anterior chamber. Additionally, some solutes such as iodopyracet, *p*-aminohippurate, and prostaglandins are removed from the aqueous humor by the ciliary epithelium itself.[2,3]

The rate of aqueous flow is relatively constant, with little physiological need for variation. A true regulatory mechanism to control the flow rate has not been found. There is a predictable rhythm of aqueous flow throughout a 24-hour day (Table 6.1). In healthy humans, aqueous flow is highest in the late morning and lowest in the middle of the night. The flow rate at night during sleep is only 43% of the rate in the morning after awakening.[4] Daytime aqueous flow averages about 2.9 μL/min in young healthy humans and 2.2 μL/min in those over 80 years of age.[5] During one's lifetime, the rate of aqueous flow slows at a rate of about 2.4% per decade.[5]

The mechanisms regulating the circadian rhythm of aqueous flow have been elusive. A series of clinical studies[6] has found that aqueous flow is stimulated by β-adrenergic agonists including epinephrine, norepinephrine, terbutaline, and isoproterenol. Corticosteroids appear to augment the catecholamine effect.[7] Melatonin might be involved in the nocturnal nadir of aqueous flow.[8] Inconsistent with these findings are other studies reporting that subjects treated with topical epinephrine had reduced rather than increased aqueous flow[9] and patients with surgical adrenalectomy who completely lacked circulating epinephrine had normal rhythms of aqueous flow.[10] A mixture of various hormonal factors of varying concentrations may be only a part of the complex formula needed to regulate the circadian rhythm of aqueous flow.

The rate of aqueous production by the ciliary processes cannot be measured in the living eye but it can be estimated by monitoring the movement of fluid through the anterior chamber (aqueous flow). In a clinical research setting, aqueous flow is measured by the method known as fluorophotometry (Fig. 6.3).[11] First, multiple drops of fluorescein are applied topically to the cornea to establish a corneal depot. Over a period of several hours, fluorescein from the cornea diffuses into the anterior chamber, mixes with aqueous humor, and begins to drain through the anterior chamber angle. With a fluorophotometer, the fluorescein concentrations in the cornea and anterior chamber are measured periodically for several hours. The log of the fluorescein concentrations are plotted over time. The total fluorescein mass in the anterior segment is the product of the fluorescein concentrations in the cornea and anterior chamber and their respective volumes. The aqueous flow rate is calculated by the mass of fluorescein lost from the cornea and anterior chamber over time, divided by the average concentration in the anterior chamber during the time interval.[6]

TABLE 6.1 Average values of aqueous humor dynamics in healthy humans

PARAMETER	MEAN VALUE	COMMENTS	METHOD OF MEASUREMENT	SELECT REFERENCES
IOP (mmHg)	18.7 ± 0.7 (OD day) 16.6 ± 0.6 (OD night)	Lower at night (supine)	Tonometry	Perlman et al. 2007[84]
	15.7 ± 0.5 (day) 17.4 ± 0.6 (night)	Higher at night (seated) Higher at night (supine)	Tonometry	Liu et al. 2003[85]
	20.0 ± 0.3 (day) 21.3 ± 0.4 (night) 13.9 ± 0.3 (day) 13.2 ± 0.4 (night) 19.3 ± 0.4 (day) 18.1 ± 0.3 (night)	No change at night (seated) Lower at night (supine)	Tonometry	Sit et al. 2007[86]
Aqueous flow (μL/min)	3.0 ± 0.8 (morning) 2.7 ± 0.6 (afternoon) 1.3 ± 0.4 (night)	Slower at night	Fluorophotometry	Brubaker 1998[5,6]
	2.9 ± 0.9 (young) 2.4 ± 0.6 (old)	Slower with aging	Fluorophotometry	Toris et al. 1999[20]
Outflow facility (μL/min/mmHg)	0.28 ± 0.01 (young) 0.19 ± 0.01 (old)	Lower with aging	Tonography	Gaasterland et al. 1978[24]
	0.21 ± 0.10 (young) 0.25 ± 0.10 (old)	No change with aging	Fluorophotometry	Toris et al. 1999[20]
	0.29 ± 0.02 (day) 0.25 ± 0.01 (night)	Lower at night	Tonography	Sit et al. 2007[86]
Episcleral venous pressure (mmHg)	10.1 ± 1.3 8.8 ± 2.0 (seated) 9.5 ± 1.9 (supine)	No change with aging Higher in the supine Position	Various methods Venomanometry	Zeimer 1989[26] Sultan et al. 2003[87]
Uveoscleral outflow (μl/min)	1.52 ± 0.81 (young) 1.10 ± 0.81 (old)	Slower with aging	Calculation	Toris et al. 1999[20]

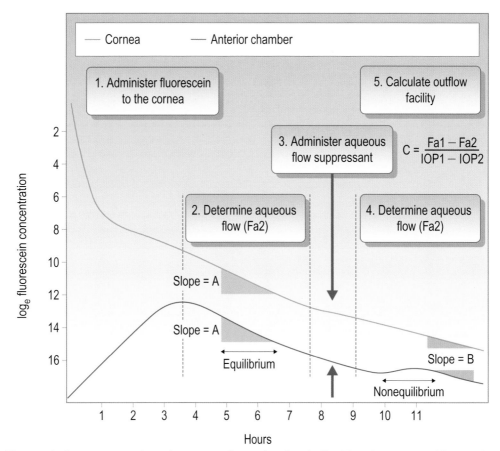

FIGURE 6.3 Fluorescein decay curves to determine aqueous flow and outflow facility. Plotted are curves of fluorescein concentration in the cornea and anterior chamber over time. Steps 1 and 2 are used to measure aqueous flow. Steps 1–5 are needed to determine outflow facility. (1) Fluorescein drops are applied to the eye. (2) Starting 4-to-8 hours later, the cornea and anterior chamber fluorescein concentrations are measured at 45–60 minute intervals for several hours using a fluorophotometer. The disappearance rates of fluorescein from the cornea and anterior chamber are the decay *slopes A*. Aqueous flow is calculated from the equilibrium data when the cornea and anterior chamber decay curves are parallel and the volumes of the cornea and anterior chamber remain constant (*Fa1*). (3) If one wishes to determine outflow facility, the experiment continues by administering an aqueous flow suppressant, such as a β-blocker or carbonic anhydrase inhibitor, immediately after measuring intraocular pressure (*IOP1*). (4) Aqueous flow suppressants will change the slope of the curve, after a period of nonequilibrium, to a new slope, *slope B*. The post-treatment aqueous flow rate (*Fa2*) is determined by fluorophotometry and IOP is measured again (*IOP2*). (5) Outflow facility (C) is calculated as the ratio of the change in flow (Fa1 − Fa2) to change in IOP (IOP1 − IOP2).

Fluorophotometry is a very well-established method with good reproducibility[12] but four important limitations and assumptions associated with this technique require consideration:

1. Diffusion of fluorescein into the iris, limbal vessels, and tear film is assumed.[6,13] It also is assumed that the diffusion rate remains undisturbed during an experimental manipulation. It is difficult to measure aqueous flow in eyes with uveitis because of the increased permeability of the blood–aqueous barrier and the change in diffusion rate of fluorescein.[14]

2. The distribution of fluorescein throughout the anterior chamber and cornea is uniform. Nonuniformity of fluorescein may occur in some conditions such as keratoconus. In these eyes, measurements of fluorescein concentration over time could be more variable, and consequently the accuracy of the aqueous flow determination would be poor.

3. The back flow of tracer from the anterior chamber into the posterior chamber is blocked by the lens–iris barrier.[15] The accuracy of fluorophotometry is diminished if the lens–iris barrier is missing or compromised such as in pseudophakia, a dilated pupil, or a previous iridotomy or iridectomy.

4. Several hours of fluorophotometric scans taken at intervals of at least 30 minutes are required to determine a reasonably accurate aqueous flow rate in humans.[6] Rapid and brief changes in aqueous flow cannot be detected by fluorophotometry.

TRABECULAR OUTFLOW

Once in the anterior chamber, aqueous humor drains through the anterior chamber angle by passive flow via one of two pathways (see Fig. 6.1). The trabecular outflow pathway is illustrated in Figure 6.4. The uveal meshwork is a forward extension of the ciliary muscle

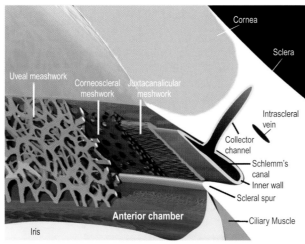

FIGURE 6.4 Trabecular outflow route. In the anterior chamber angle, aqueous humor percolates through the uveal and corneoscleral meshwork, juxtacanalicular connective tissue, and endothelial lining of Schlemm's canal (inner wall) before reaching the lumen of the canal. Fluid in Schlemm's canal is drained by 25–35 collector channels into aqueous veins and episcleral veins before entering the systemic circulation (veins not drawn). (From Figure 2 of Toris CB. Aqueous humor dynamics I, measurement methods and animal studies. The eye's aqueous humor. In: Mortimer M. Civan, ed. Current topics in membranes. Elsevier: San Diego; 2008, in press.)

consisting of large overlapping holes and flattened sheets which branch and interconnect in multiple planes. The middle layer, the corneoscleral meshwork, includes several perforated sheets of connective tissue extending between the scleral spur and Schwalbe's line. The openings in these sheets are small and do not overlap. The sheets are interconnected by tissue strands and endothelial cells. The juxtacanalicular meshwork, lying adjacent to the inner wall of Schlemm's canal, contains collagen, glycosaminoglycans, glycoproteins, fibroblasts, and endothelial-like cells. Elastic fibers also are present that may provide support for the inner wall of Schlemm's canal. This meshwork contains very narrow, irregular openings. Experimental evidence and theoretical predictions indicate that normal aqueous humor outflow resistance resides in the inner wall region of Schlemm's canal.[16,17] This region is composed of an endothelial layer, its basement membrane, and the adjacent juxtacanalicular (cribriform, subendothelial) connective tissue. The presence of micron-size pores in the inner wall endothelium explains why this endothelium has one of the highest hydraulic conductivities in the body, comparable only to that of fenestrated endothelia. The endothelium allows passage of microparticles 200–500 nm in size. Some outflow resistance is generated by the funneling of aqueous humor into the pores of the inner wall endothelium.[17] Another pathway, composed of the open spaces in the juxtacanalicular connective tissue creates an insignificant fraction of outflow resistance, unless extracellular matrix material fills the spaces. Interestingly, the amount of extracellular matrix material in the juxtacanalicular tissue increases with aging, thus providing an explanation for the apparent reduction in outflow facility in older subjects.[18]

Other factors affecting trabecular outflow resistance are ciliary muscle tone and trabecular cell function. The ciliary muscle is connected to the juxtacanalicular region and inner wall endothelium of the trabecular meshwork. When the ciliary muscle contracts, this region is mechanically deformed in such a way as to open up the spaces in the trabecular meshwork and dilate Schlemm's canal, thus decreasing the resistance to fluid flow. Trabecular cells actively change shape, altering the geometry of the open spaces in the meshwork, and they modulate extracellular matrix turnover which fills or empties the spaces in the juxtacanalicular connective tissue.[19]

Outflow facility in healthy human eyes ranges between 0.1 and 0.4 μL/min/mmHg.[20–24] By tonography or perfusion of enucleated human cadaver eyes, trabecular outflow resistance increased with aging.[18] However, when measured by fluorophotometry in healthy humans on no known prescription drugs, no age-related changes in outflow facility were observed.[20]

Critical evaluation of published studies of outflow facility requires an understanding of the methods by which this parameter is accessed. Tonography and fluorophotometry are the two methods used in clinical studies. Two or four minutes of tonography measures a reduction in IOP from application of a weight placed on the eye of a supine subject. A corresponding change in aqueous flow, to account for the IOP change, is obtained from the Friedenwald Tables.[25] Outflow facility is the ratio of the change in flow to change in IOP. Tonographic outflow facility includes trabecular outflow facility, uveoscleral outflow facility (considered to be small), and pseudofacility (also considered to be small) in the measurement. Another factor, ocular rigidity (a measure of the stiffness of the eye), affects the measurement of IOP during tonography. A fluorophotometric method (see Fig. 6.3) measures rather than assumes an aqueous flow change with an IOP change. The changes in IOP and aqueous flow are induced by administering an aqueous flow suppressant such as acetazolamide, dorzolamide, or timolol. The fluorophotometric method avoids pseudofacility and ocular rigidity but the measurement takes several hours to complete and is more variable than tonography. Neither method works well in ocular normotensive volunteers who do not have much change in IOP during the assessment.

EPISCLERAL VENOUS PRESSURE

Aqueous humor traversing the trabecular meshwork eventually drains into the episcleral veins. In healthy humans the pressure in the episcleral veins ranges from 7 to 14 mmHg,[26] with values between 9 and 10 mmHg being reported most often (see Table 6.1). There does not appear to be a correlation between episcleral venous pressure and age.[27] Episcleral venous pressure increases from 1 to 9 mmHg by changing body position from seated to supine and this in turn increases IOP directly. When body position does not change, episcleral venous pressure is relatively stable. A change in episcleral venous pressure of 0.8 mmHg corresponds to a change in IOP

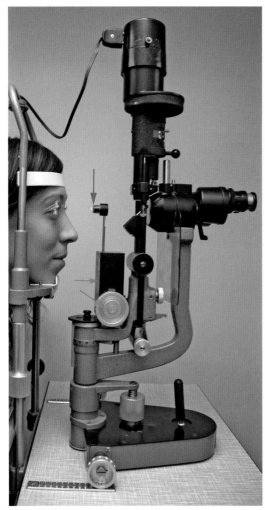

FIGURE 6.5 Venomanometry. An episcleral venomanometer (*blue arrow*) is mounted on a simple Haag Streit slit lamp. With the aid of the binoculars on the slit lamp, the lighted membrane (*red arrow*) is positioned on a vessel near the limbus. The silver dial (*green arrow*) is used to increase the pressure behind the membrane until the vessel collapses. The reading on the dial is considered episcleral venous pressure (mmHg).

of 1 mmHg. The circadian variations in IOP parallel the circadian variations in episcleral venous pressure.[28] In addition to postural changes, other factors affect episcleral venous pressure including inhalation of O_2,[29] application of cold temperature,[30] and vasoactive drugs.[31]

Measurement of episcleral venous pressure in human subjects is usually made with a commercially available venomanometer (Eyetech, Morton Grove, IL) attached to a slit lamp (Fig. 6.5). The membrane at the tip of the device is placed on the conjunctiva near the limbus. Episcleral veins underlying the conjunctiva are identified with the aid of the slit lamp biomicroscope. By turning the dial on the side of the device, the pressure within the membrane tip is raised until the appropriate vessel collapses. This pressure is considered episcleral venous pressure. The procedure requires a cooperative, unmoving subject and a clear conjunctiva to allow an unobstructed view of an appropriate vessel. Identification and visualization of an appropriate vessel can be difficult.

UVEOSCLERAL OUTFLOW

Drainage of aqueous humor from the anterior chamber other than through the trabecular meshwork is called uveoscleral outflow. Unlike the trabecular outflow pathway, the uveoscleral outflow pathway does not contain recognizable channels and vessels. Instead, fluid seeps through the anterior face of the ciliary muscle and other tissues in and around the uvea. In 1965, Anders Bill[32] observed that large tracers, as markers of bulk flow, exited the anterior chamber through the ciliary muscle and out through the sclera into the extraocular tissues and ultimately into the lymphatic system. Normally, most constituents of aqueous flow probably do not traverse the sclera but instead are absorbed into the suprachoroidal space and choroidal vessels.

Drainage of fluid through the uvea is sometimes described as 'unconventional outflow' because it seeps through tissue rather than flows through channels, or 'pressure-independent outflow' because it does not depend on IOP to the same extent as trabecular outflow. It should be clarified that some pressure dependence is required of all flow. Although very small, there is a pressure gradient for flow from the anterior chamber into the supraciliary and suprachoroidal spaces. Studies of monkeys have shown that uveoscleral outflow changes little at IOPs in the normal to high range (11–35 mmHg).[33] A change in IOP apparently has little effect on the pressure gradient between the anterior chamber and the suprachoroidal space. When IOP is well below normal (4 mmHg), uveoscleral outflow does become pressure dependent.[34]

Uveoscleral outflow in healthy subjects 20–30 years of age is reported to be in the range of 25–57% of total aqueous flow.[20,35,36] As one ages, uveoscleral outflow gradually slows.[20] One study of 104 healthy subjects divided into two age groups found that the group 20–30 years of age had uveoscleral outflow rates that were 54% of total aqueous flow whereas the group over 60 years of age had significantly slower uveoscleral outflow rates that were 45% of total aqueous flow. Even in the older subjects, uveoscleral outflow was substantially greater than what was first reported in the original pivotal human study.[37] In that classic study, uveoscleral outflow was measured using a radioactive tracer just prior to enucleation. Several hours later, the enucleated eyes were analyzed for radioactivity. In the two nonglaucomatous eyes that had received no ocular drug for 48 hours prior to the study, uveoscleral outflow was 4% and 14% of total drainage. Three decades later we have learned that uveoscleral outflow in humans is substantially greater than once thought.

Of all the parameters of aqueous humor dynamics, uveoscleral outflow is the most difficult to determine in a clinical setting. It cannot be measured directly but it is calculated from the modified Goldmann equation:

$$F_u = F_a - C(IOP - P_{ev})$$

Aqueous flow (F_a), outflow facility (C), IOP, and episcleral venous pressure (P_{ev}) are measured and uveoscleral outflow (F_u) is calculated mathematically. Inherent variability with this method is great and reproducibility is fair. Improved techniques are sorely needed to advance our understanding of uveoscleral outflow in the healthy and diseased human eye.

AQUEOUS HUMOR DYNAMICS IN CLINICAL SYNDROMES AFFECTING INTRAOCULAR PRESSURE

Clinical syndromes associated with IOP elevations may not lead to glaucoma but glaucomatous damage is often the result. The pressure elevations are usually attributed to an imbalance in aqueous humor dynamics. The source of the problem is attributed to changes often in trabecular outflow, occasionally in uveoscleral outflow, and rarely in aqueous flow. Following is a summary of the syndromes causing an elevation in IOP for which aqueous humor dynamics have been measured. Related conditions with ocular normotension are included for comparison.

OCULAR HYPERTENSION

Ocular hypertension is the condition in which the IOP is elevated above what is considered normal but the eye remains healthy with no pathologic optic nerve cupping and visual field defects. The IOP is considered abnormal when it is at least 21 mmHg which is two standard deviations above the mean in several population-based studies.[38] When patients with ocular hypertension are compared with age-matched healthy ocular normotensive volunteers, aqueous flow is within the normal range[5,21,39] but both outflow facility[21,22,39] and uveoscleral outflow[21] are significantly reduced. The elevated IOP in ocular hypertension can be explained by pathologic changes in both outflow pathways (Table 6.2).

PRIMARY OPEN-ANGLE GLAUCOMA

Primary open-angle glaucoma (POAG) is a disease involving disturbance of the structural or functional integrity of the eye leading to elevated IOP accompanied by progressive damage to the optic nerve and visual field loss. The glaucomatous damage often can be arrested or diminished by adequate lowering of IOP. When compared with healthy age-matched subjects, aqueous flow in patients with primary open-angle glaucoma was found to be normal during the day but significantly elevated at night.[40] The nocturnal aqueous flow effect is small and not sufficient to explain the elevated IOP. The major contributing factor for the elevated IOP in primary open-angle glaucoma, and most other glaucomas accompanied by ocular hypertension for that matter, appears to be increased resistance to fluid flow through the trabecular meshwork. This was reported in 1951,[22] 1961,[41] and again in 1995[40] using tonography as the method of measurement. There is little known about uveoscleral outflow in patients with primary open-angle glaucoma other than a small study[42] of 14 patients with IOPs uncontrolled on maximally tolerated medical therapy. In that study, it was found that uveoscleral outflow was substantially elevated as much as 80% of total outflow in severely glaucomatous eyes, compared to 37% in contralateral eyes with less severe glaucoma. Outflow facility when measured by the fluorophotometric method was very low in these patients on multiple medications (0.02 µL/min/mmHg)[42] compared to a separate study[20] of healthy subjects (0.25 µL/min/mmHg) on no known prescription drug. A summary of aqueous humor dynamics in patients with primary open-angle glaucoma is found in Table 6.2.

Systemic and ocular medications may have contributed to this large difference in uveoscleral outflow between studies but another possibility exists. The aqueous humor may have been redirected from the trabecular meshwork, an area of abnormally high resistance, to the uvea, a region where flow is less dependent on IOP. In support of this idea is a study[43] of untreated monkeys with experimentally-induced unilateral glaucoma from laser burns to the trabecular meshwork to establish a stable chronic elevation in IOP.[44] Outflow facility was significantly reduced in the hypertensive eyes (0.06 µL/min/mmHg) when compared with the contralateral healthy eyes (0.16 µL/min/mmHg). In the absence of drugs that might alter uveoscleral drainage, the hypertensive eyes also demonstrated elevated uveoscleral outflow (2.25 µL/min) when compared to the contralateral control eyes (1.05 µL/min).[43] These clinical and animal studies suggest that, in ocular hypertension[21] and the initial stages of glaucoma, uveoscleral outflow and outflow facility are below normal. As the disease progresses, trabecular outflow facility continues to decline while the facility of uveoscleral outflow remains constant (pressure independent). When trabecular outflow facility is reduced to a critical level, aqueous humor is redirected from the trabecular to the uveal pathway.

Morphological and biochemical changes in the tissues of the drainage pathways help to explain the increased resistance in the trabecular outflow pathway in patients with glaucoma. Within the trabecular meshwork of glaucomatous specimens, endothelial cell numbers are decreased[45] yet basement membrane is thickened, suggesting increased cellular activity. Plaques consisting of clusters of material appear in the corneoscleral beams and juxtacanalicular meshwork. These plaques appear to be derived from elastic-like fibers that make up a subendothelial tendon sheath. The increased thickness of the sheath of the elastic fibers and connecting fibrils reduces the intertrabecular spaces and narrows the flow pathways to the inner wall endothelium. The presence of plaques also increases with aging but the total amount of this material is greater in eyes with POAG.[46] Alteration of the extracellular matrix components that are produced and maintained by trabecular meshwork cells have been found. Collagen abnormalities in POAG include fragmentation, altered orientation, and abnormal spacing. Fibronectin[47] is deposited in the subendothelial region of Schlemm's canal. Expression of myocilin and the amount of αB-crystalline, a small stress protein, is increased in the trabecular meshwork

TABLE 6.2 Aqueous humor dynamics in syndromes associated with ocular hypertension and related conditions associated with ocular normotension

SYNDROME	IOP	F_a	C	P_{ev}	F_u
Ocular hypertension	↑	↔[5,21,39]	↓[21,22,39]	↔↑[21]	↓[21]
Glaucoma					
Primary open-angle glaucoma	↑	↔ day and night[40] (↑ night[40])	↓[22,40,42]		↑[42] (on maximally tolerated medical therapy)
Normal-tension glaucoma	↔	↔[55]	↔[55]		
Pigment dispersion syndrome (PDS)					
PDS with normal IOP	↔	↔[57,58]	↔[57,58]	↔[58]	↔[58]
PDS with ocular hypertension	↑	↔[57,58]	↓[57,58]	↔[58]	↔[58]
Exfoliation syndrome (XFS)					
XFS with normal IOP	↔	↔[62,64]	↔[62,64]	↔[64]	→[64]
XFS with ocular hypertension	↑	↔[64]	↓[64]	↔[64]	→[64]
Diabetes					
Type 1, with complications	→↓	↓[66,67]	↔[67]		
Type 1, without complications	↔	↔[68]			
Inflammatory conditions					
Glaucomatocyclitic crisis	↑	↑[73,81,83] ↔[22,72,82]	↓[22,70-74]		
Fuch's heterochromic iridocyclitis	↔	↔[14]	↔[14]		

Superscripted numbers indicate key citations. Reference 58 is an ARVO abstract. Arrows indicate values greater than (↑), or less than (↓) healthy age-matched subjects. C, outflow facility; F_a, aqueous flow; F_u, uveoscleral outflow; IOP, intraocular pressure; P_{ev}, episcleral venous pressure.

of some glaucomatous eyes.[48] The interaction of the extracellular matrix components with proteins such as cochlin[49] may lead to the formation of deposits that obstruct the outflow pathway. Clearly many complex changes within the trabecular meshwork contribute to increased outflow resistance in glaucomatous eyes.

It should be mentioned that factors other than aqueous humor drainage may be involved in the elevated IOP and optic neuropathy in primary open-angle glaucoma. It has been reported that blood pressure decreases[50] and IOP increases at night,[51–54] both factors reported to increase the risk of glaucomatous damage to the retina.

NORMAL-TENSION GLAUCOMA

Normal-tension glaucoma is defined as cupping and visual field loss characteristic of glaucoma despite IOPs within the 'normal' range. Ten patients with normal-tension glaucoma had no change in daytime IOP, aqueous flow or outflow facility, or nighttime aqueous flow when compared to 10 age-matched healthy controls (see Table 6.2).[55] The primary difference in patients with normal-tension glaucoma is increased variability of nighttime blood pressure[56] and nocturnal hypotension that may reduce the optic nerve head blood flow to an unhealthy level.[50] Fluctuations in ocular perfusion pressure cause episodes of ischemia during which time the optic nerve head is at great risk of permanent damage. These events are not detectable on routine clinical examination and are independent of aqueous humor dynamics.

PIGMENT DISPERSION SYNDROME

Pigment dispersion syndrome is a condition in which friction between the posterior surface of the iris making contact with the anterior zonules of the lens releases pigment and cells from the iris, debris that is flushed into the anterior chamber and the trabecular meshwork where it may become trapped in the drainage pathway. Patients with pigment dispersion syndrome have deeper anterior chambers than normal which predisposes them to the condition.[57] When pigment dispersion syndrome is not accompanied by ocular hypertension, aqueous humor inflow and outflow are normal. When pigment dispersion is accompanied by ocular hypertension, outflow facility is reduced[57] but uveoscleral outflow remains normal (data presented at the 2003 ARVO annual meeting).[58] This is distinctly different from ocular hypertension without pigment dispersion syndrome, in that both uveoscleral outflow and outflow facility are reduced (see Table 6.2).[21]

EXFOLIATION SYNDROME

Exfoliation syndrome is characterized by white deposits on the anterior capsule of the lens and tissues of the ciliary body, iris, cornea, and trabecular meshwork.[59] Exfoliation syndrome tends to convert into exfoliation glaucoma mainly in elderly patients. This is because there is age-related narrowing of the outflow pathways to the inner wall of Schlemm's canal[60] and build-up of

extracellular material and other debris. This material is easily flushed from the trabecular meshwork in young persons, but becomes trapped in the trabecular meshwork of older persons. When exfoliative material becomes trapped in sufficient quantity near the endothelial cells of the trabecular meshwork and Schlemm's canal, it causes degradation of the tissues and further obstruction of the aqueous humor outflow pathways. The amount of trapped material has been positively correlated with increasing IOP and the presence of glaucoma.[61]

Distinct changes in aqueous humor dynamics have been found in exfoliation syndrome. When comparing the affected eye of 18 untreated patients with unilateral exfoliation syndrome and ocular normotension with its contralateral unaffected eye,[62] there was no difference in IOPs (14 mmHg and 12 mmHg, respectively), aqueous flow rates (2.4 μL/min in both eyes) and outflow facilities (0.15 μL/min/mmHg and 0.19 μL/min/mmHg, respectively). When exfoliation syndrome was accompanied by ocular hypertension[63] (mean IOP of 32 mmHg in the affected eye and 18 mmHg in the unaffected eye, $n = 10$), aqueous flow and outflow facility were significantly lower in the affected eye (2.02 μL/min and 0.07 μL/min/mmHg, respectively) than the unaffected eye (2.38 μL/min and 0.15 μL/min/mmHg, respectively). The lower rate of aqueous flow was originally thought to be due to damage to the ciliary epithelia from the disease process.[63] However, later it was thought that the lower aqueous flow was the result of insufficient time for washout of the timolol that had been used to treat the affected eye.[6] In a recent study (data presented at the 2006 ARVO annual meeting)[64] aqueous humor dynamics in 40 patients with exfoliation syndrome with and without ocular hypertension were compared to a group of 40 age- and IOP-matched patients without exfoliation syndrome. Aqueous flow was not different between groups (2.05 ± 0.73 in the exfoliation group and 2.23 ± 0.61 μL/min in the control group) but uveo-scleral outflow was significantly ($p < 0.0001$) lower in the group with exfoliation syndrome (0.11 ± 0.69 versus 0.78 ± 0.81 μL/min, respectively). When these subjects were divided by IOP and not exfoliation syndrome, the patients with ocular hypertension had reduced outflow facility compared to the ocular normotensive controls. It was concluded that the reduced outflow facility was IOP-dependent and unrelated to the exfoliation syndrome. The reduced uveoscleral outflow was dependent on the presence of exfoliation syndrome and unrelated to IOP. These effects on aqueous humor dynamics are distinctly different from those found in ocular hypertension and in pigment dispersion syndrome (see Table 6.2).

DIABETES MELLITUS

Diabetes mellitus is associated with abnormalities of the general circulation including decreased tissue oxygenation, vascular leakiness, increased blood viscosity, capillary shunting, and capillary nonperfusion. Ocular effects include changes in aqueous humor dynamics, increases or decreases in IOP, presence of aqueous flare, increased permeability of the blood–ocular barriers, and abnormalities in the retinal vasculature. Diabetes has been listed as a risk factor for glaucoma, but in some studies IOP in diabetes mellitus has been reported to be below normal with reduced risk of glaucoma. Consensus among studies is lacking.[65] Aqueous humor dynamics have been studied in patients with diabetes and reduced IOP. The cause of the lower IOP is a reduction in the rate of aqueous flow.[66,67] IOP and aqueous flow were correlated with severity of diabetic retinopathy, age of onset, duration of diabetes, and age of the patient. There was a significant negative correlation between the degree of retinopathy and aqueous flow rate, i.e. as the severity of retinopathy increased, aqueous flow decreased.[67]

Patients with type 1 diabetes are prescribed insulin to control circulating glucose levels. Insulin is a hormone with vasoactive properties that could directly affect the production rate of aqueous humor. It has been proposed that the insulin treatment and not the disease might account for the reduction in aqueous flow in diabetes. A study[68] designed to control for the insulin treatment during the time of aqueous flow assessment maintained insulin at one of two fixed levels by a hyperinsulin-emic-euglycemic glucose clamp. During each clamp, aqueous flow was measured in 11 patients with type 1 diabetes and 17 age-matched healthy control subjects. At the higher insulin level, aqueous flow was slightly greater than at the lower insulin level but this did not reach statistical significant ($p = 0.09$). A more important finding was that despite the normal IOPs and the absence of microvascular complications (retinopathy and microalbuminurea), a significant reduction in aqueous flow was found. For IOP to be normal in the presence of reduced aqueous flow, other parameters of aqueous humor dynamics must change. When measured by tonography, patients with type 1 diabetes had normal outflow facilities (see Table 6.2).[67,68] Uveoscleral outflow and episcleral venous pressure have yet to be investigated in diabetes.

FUCHS' HETEROCHROMIC IRIDOCYCLITIS

Chronic, unilateral iridocyclitis characterized by iris heterochromia are hallmarks of Fuchs' uveitis syndrome or Fuchs' heterochromic iridocyclitis. Abnormal uveal pigment is associated with chronic low-grade inflammation that is believed to cause iris atrophy and secondary glaucoma in some patients. In the affected eyes of 10 patients with unilateral Fuchs' uveitis syndrome and normal IOP (17 mmHg) no change was found in outflow facility but the permeability of the blood–aqueous barrier was increased when compared with the unaffected contralateral eye.[14] When fluorescein was applied to both eyes to measure aqueous flow, there was 7% greater clearance of fluorescein in the affected eye, which may have been caused by increased diffusion of fluorescein. Differences in the diffusion of fluorescein may be interpreted as differences in aqueous flow that may not be real. Nevertheless, the authors suggested that aqueous flow could be lower in eyes with Fuchs'

uveitis syndrome (see Table 6.2). In agreement with this, a study[34] in monkeys with experimental iridocyclitis found hypotony associated with a reduction in aqueous flow and an increase in uveoscleral outflow.

GLAUCOMATOCYCLITIC CRISIS (POSNER-SCHLOSSMAN SYNDROME)

A condition with recurrent episodes of markedly elevated IOP usually ranging between 40 and 60 mmHg accompanied by anterior chamber inflammation is called glaucomatocyclitic crisis or Posner-Schlossman syndrome.[69] It appears that the cause of the elevated IOP is a reduction of outflow facility (see Table 6.2).[70] During the interval between attacks, outflow facility returns to normal or slightly increases compared to the contralateral healthy eye.[22,71–73] One study[74] found reduced outflow facility in both the affected and healthy eye in 6 of 11 patients. It has been proposed that the inflammation is mediated by prostaglandins. Prostaglandin E has been found in higher concentration in the aqueous humor of patients during but not between attacks.[75] Evidence against this theory is found in studies[39,76–80] reporting topical prostaglandins increase, rather than decrease outflow facility, which would contribute to a reduction, not an increase, in IOP.

Two studies[73,81] have reported that an increase in aqueous production contributed to the elevated IOP in glaucomatocyclitic crisis. To complicate matters, three studies[22,72,82] that evaluated this parameter did not find an aqueous flow increase. All of these studies were conducted decades ago when fluorophotometry was not available and aqueous flow was determined in an indirect manner using the Goldmann equation. Uveoscleral outflow was not considered in the calculation and episcleral venous pressure was assumed to be normal. Later, when fluorophotometry was used to measure aqueous flow,[83] the clearance rate of fluorescein was found to be reduced, suggesting that aqueous flow was increased during an attack. However, measurement of intracameral fluorescein may have been fraught with errors from the presence of proteins and flare in the anterior chamber.[12] Taking this into consideration, it is unlikely that hypersecretion contributes to the elevated IOP in glaucomatocyclitic crisis.[70]

Summary

A primary function of the production and circulation of aqueous humor is the maintenance of IOP at a healthy and stable level. When IOP becomes elevated, as seen in ocular hypertension, primary open-angle glaucoma, and various syndromes described in this chapter, it is always accompanied by a reduction in outflow facility. Changes in uveoscleral outflow are not consistent among the various syndromes. Uveoscleral outflow is reduced with aging, ocular hypertension, and exfoliation syndrome, unchanged in pigment dispersion syndrome accompanied by elevated IOP, and may be increased in severe glaucoma. Aqueous flow is increased in glaucomatocyclitic crisis, and unchanged in all other conditions in which IOP is increased. It is clear that each of these conditions associated with elevated IOP produces distinctive changes in aqueous humor dynamics. Tailoring a treatment to target the specific abnormality is a logical approach in the management of ocular hypertension and glaucoma.

REFERENCES

1. Civan MM, Macknight ADC. The ins and outs of aqueous humour secretion. Exp Eye Res 2004; 78:625–631.

2. Bill A. Blood circulation and fluid dynamics in the eye. Physiol Rev 1975; 55:383–417.

3. Bito LZ, Wallenstein MC. Transport of prostaglandins across the blood–brain and blood–aqueous barriers and the physiological significance of these absorptive transport processes. Exp Eye Res 1977; 25:229–243.

4. Reiss GR, Lee DA, Topper JE, et al. Aqueous humor flow during sleep. Invest Ophthalmol Vis Sci 1984; 25:776–778.

5. Brubaker RF. Flow of aqueous humor in humans. Invest Ophthalmol Vis Sci 1991; 32:3145–3166.

6. Brubaker RF. Clinical measurements of aqueous dynamics: implications for addressing glaucoma. In: Civan MM, ed. The eye's aqueous humor. From secretion to glaucoma. San Diego: Academic Press; 1998:233–284.

7. Jacob E, FitzSimon JS, Brubaker RF. Combined corticosteroid and catecholamine stimulation of aqueous humor flow. Ophthalmology 1996; 103:1303–1308.

8. Viggiano SR, Koskela TK, Klee GG, et al. The effect of melatonin on aqueous humor flow in humans during the day. Ophthalmology 1994; 101:326–331.

9. Wang Y-L, Hayashi M, Yablonski ME, et al. Effects of multiple dosing of epinephrine on aqueous humor dynamics in human eyes. J Ocul Pharmacol Ther 2002; 18:53–63.

10. Maus TL, Young WF Jr, Brubaker RF. Aqueous flow in humans after adrenalectomy. Invest Ophthalmol Vis Sci 1994; 35:3325–3331.

11. Jones RF, Maurice DM. New methods of measuring the rate of aqueous flow in man with fluorescein. Exp Eye Res 1966; 5:208–220.

12. Brubaker RF. Clinical evaluation of the circulation of aqueous humor. In: Tasman W, Jaeger EA, eds. Duane's clinical ophthalmology. Philadelphia: Lippincott-Raven; 1997:1–11.

13. McLaren JW, Niloofar Z, Brubaker RF. A simple three-compartment model of anterior segment kinetics. Exp Eye Res 1993; 56:355–366.

14. Johnson D, Liesegang TJ, Brubaker RF. Aqueous humor dynamics in Fuchs' uveitis syndrome. Am J Ophthalmol 1983; 95:783–787.

15. Maus TL, Brubaker RF. Measurement of aqueous humor flow by fluorophotometry in the presence of a dilated pupil. Invest Ophthalmol Vis Sci 1999; 40:542–546.

16. Ethier CR. The inner wall of Schlemm's canal. Exp Eye Res 2002; 74:161–172.

17. Johnson M. 'What controls aqueous humour outflow resistance?'. Exp Eye Res 2006; 82:545–557.

18. Gabelt BT, Kaufman PL. Changes in aqueous humor dynamics with age and glaucoma. Prog Retin Eye Res 2005; 24:612–637.

19. Soto D, Comes N, Ferrer E, et al. Modulation of aqueous humor outflow by ionic mechanisms involved in trabecular meshwork cell volume regulation. Invest Ophthalmol Vis Sci 2004; 45:3650–3661.

20. Toris CB, Yablonski ME, Wang Y-L, et al. Aqueous humor dynamics in the aging human eye. Am J Ophthalmol 1999; 127:407–412.

21. Toris CB, Koepsell SA, Yablonski ME, et al. Aqueous humor dynamics in ocular hypertensive patients. J Glaucoma 2002; 11:253–258.

22. Grant WM. Clinical measurements of aqueous outflow. AMA Arch Ophthalmol 1951; 46:113–131.

23. Becker B. The decline in aqueous secretion and outflow facility with age. Am J Ophthalmol 1958; 46:731–736.

24. Gaasterland D, Kupfer C, Milton R, et al. Studies of aqueous humour dynamics in man. VI. Effect of age upon parameters of intraocular pressure in normal human eyes. Exp Eye Res 1978; 26:651–656.

25. Friedenwald JS. Some problems with the calibration of tonometers. Am J Ophthalmol 1948; 31:935–944.

26. Zeimer RC. Episcleral venous pressure. In: Ritch R, Shields MB, Krupin T, eds. The glaucomas. St. Louis: The CV Mosby; 1989:249–255.

27. Zeimer RC, Gieser DK, Wilensky JT, et al. A practical venomanometer. Measurement of episcleral venous pressure and assessment of the normal range. Arch Ophthalmol 1983; 101:1447–1449.

28. Blondeau P, Tétrault JP, Papamarkakis C. Diurnal variation of episcleral venous pressure in healthy patients: a pilot study. J Glaucoma 2001; 10:18–24.

29. Yablonski ME, Gallin P, Shapiro D. Effect of oxygen on aqueous humor dynamics in rabbits. Invest Ophthalmol Vis Sci 1985; 26:1781–1784.

30. Ortiz GJ, Cook DJ, Yablonski ME, et al. Effect of cold air on aqueous humor dynamics in humans. Invest Ophthalmol Vis Sci 1988; 29:138–140.

31. Toris CB, Tafoya ME, Camras CB, et al. Effects of apraclonidine on aqueous humor dynamics in human eyes. Ophthalmology 1995; 102:456–461.

32. Bill A. The aqueous humor drainage mechanism in the cynomolgus monkey (*Macaca irus*) with evidence for unconventional routes. Invest Ophthalmol 1965; 4:911–919.

33. Bill A. Conventional and uveo-scleral drainage of aqueous humour in the cynomolgus monkey (*Macaca irus*) at normal and high intraocular pressures. Exp Eye Res 1966; 5:45–54.

34. Toris CB, Pederson JE. Effect of intraocular pressure on uveoscleral outflow following cyclodialysis in the monkey eye. Invest Ophthalmol Vis Sci 1985; 26:1745–1749.

35. Townsend DJ, Brubaker RF. Immediate effect of epinephrine on aqueous formation in the normal human eye as measured by fluorophotometry. Invest Ophthalmol Vis Sci 1980; 19:256–266.

36. Mishima HK, Kiuchi Y, Takamatsu M, et al. Circadian intraocular pressure management with latanoprost: diurnal and nocturnal intraocular pressure reduction and increased uveoscleral outflow. Surv Ophthalmol 1997; 41:S139–sS144.

37. Bill A, Phillips CI. Uveoscleral drainage of aqueous humour in human eyes. Exp Eye Res 1971; 12:275–281.

38. Coleman AL. Epidemiology of glaucoma. In: Morrison JC, Pollack IP, eds. Glaucoma: science and practice. New York: Thieme Medical; 2003:2–11.

39. Ziai N, Dolan JW, Kacere RD, et al. The effects on aqueous dynamics of PhXA41, a new prostaglandin $F_{2\alpha}$ analogue, after topical application in normal and ocular hypertensive human eyes. Arch Ophthalmol 1993; 111:1351–1358.

40. Larsson L-I, Rettig ES, Brubaker RF. Aqueous flow in open-angle glaucoma. Arch Ophthalmol 1995; 113:283–286.

41. Becker B. Tonography in the diagnosis of simple (open angle) glaucoma. Trans Am Acad Ophthalmol Otolaryngol 1961; 65:156–162.

42. Yablonski ME, Cook DJ, Gray J. A fluorophotometric study of the effect of argon laser trabeculoplasty on aqueous humor dynamics. Am J Ophthalmol 1985; 99:579–582.

43. Toris CB, Zhan G-L, Wang Y-L, et al. Aqueous humor dynamics in monkeys with laser-induced glaucoma. J Ocul Pharmacol Ther 2000; 16:19–27.

44. Quigley HA, Hohman RM. Laser energy levels for trabecular meshwork damage in the primate eye. Invest Ophthalmol Vis Sci 1983; 24:1305–1307.

45. Alvarado J, Murphy C, Juster R. Trabecular meshwork cellularity in primary open-angle glaucoma and nonglaucomatous normals. Ophthalmology 1984; 91:564–579.

46. Lütjen-Drecoll E, Shimizu T, Rohrbach M, et al. Quantitative analysis of 'plaque material' in the inner and outer wall of Schlemm's canal in normal and glaucomatous eyes. Exp Eye Res 1986; 42:443–455.

47. Babizhayev MA, Brodskaya MW. Fibronectin detection in drainage outflow system of human eyes in ageing and progression of open-angle glaucoma. Mech Ageing Dev 1989; 47:145–157.

48. Lütjen-Drecoll E, May CA, Polansky JR, et al. Localization of the stress proteins aB-crystalline and trabecular meshwork inducible glucocorticoid response protein in normal and glaucomatous trabecular meshwork. Invest Ophthalmol Vis Sci 1998; 39:517–525.

49. Bhattacharya SK, Rockwood EJ, Smith SD, et al. Proteomics reveal Cochlin deposits associated with glaucomatous trabecular meshwork. J Biol Chem 2005; 280:6080–6084.

50. Hayreh SS, Zimmerman MB, Podhajsky P, et al. Nocturnal arterial hypotension and its role in optic nerve head and ocular ischemic disorders. Am J Ophthalmol 1994; 117:603–624.

51. Liu JHK, Kripke DF, Hoffman RE, et al. Nocturnal elevation of intraocular pressure in young adults. Invest Ophthalmol Vis Sci 1998; 39:2707–2712.

52. Liu JHK, Kripke DF, Hoffman RE, et al. Elevation of human intraocular pressure at night under moderate illumination. Invest Ophthalmol Vis Sci 1999; 40:2439–2442.

53. Liu JHK, Kripke DF, Twa MD, et al. Twenty-four-hour pattern of intraocular pressure in the aging population. Invest Ophthalmol Vis Sci 1999; 40:2912–2917.

54. Liu JHK, Zhang X, Kripke DF, et al. Twenty-four-hour intraocular pressure pattern associated with early glaucomatous changes. Invest Ophthalmol Vis Sci 2003; 44:1586–1590.

55. Larsson L-I, Rettig ES, Sheridan PT, et al. Aqueous humor dynamics in low-tension glaucoma. Am J Ophthalmol 1993; 116:590–593.

56. Plange N, Kaup M, Daneljan L, et al. 24-h blood pressure monitoring in normal tension glaucoma: night-time blood pressure variability. J Hum Hypertens 2006; 20:137–142.

57. Brown JD, Brubaker RF. A study of the relation between intraocular pressure and aqueous humor flow in the pigment dispersion syndrome. Ophthalmology 1989; 96:1468–1470.

58. Camras CB, Haecker NR, Zhan G, et al. Aqueous humor dynamics in patients with pigment dispersion syndrome. Invest Ophthalmol Vis Sci 2003; 44:2207 (ARVO E-Abstract).

59. Hammer T, Schlötzer-Schrehardt U, Naumann GOH. Unilateral or asymmetric pseudoexfoliation syndrome? An ultrastructural study. Arch Ophthalmol 2001; 119:1023–1031.

60. Lütjen-Drecoll E. Morphological changes in glaucomatous eyes and the role of TGFβ₂ for the pathogenesis of the disease. Exp Eye Res 2005; 81:1–4.

61. Schlötzer-Schrehardt U, Naumann GOH. Trabecular meshwork in pseudoexfoliation syndrome with and without open-angle glaucoma. A morphometric, ultrastructural study. Invest Ophthalmol Vis Sci 1995; 36:1750–1764.

62. Gharagozloo NZ, Baker RH, Brubaker RF. Aqueous dynamics in exfoliation syndrome. Am J Ophthalmol 1992; 114:473–478.

63. Johnson DH, Brubaker RF. Dynamics of aqueous humor in the syndrome of exfoliation with glaucoma. Am J Ophthalmol 1982; 93:629–634.

64. Johnson T, Fan S, Toris CB, et al. Uveoscleral outflow is reduced in exfoliation syndrome. Invest Ophthalmol Vis Sci 2006; 47:2943 (ARVO E-Abstract).

65. Oh SW, Lee S, Park C, et al. Elevated intraocular pressure is associated with insulin resistance and metabolic syndrome. Diabetes Metab Res Rev 2005; 21:434–440.

66. Hayashi M, Yablonski ME, Boxrud C, et al. Decreased formation of aqueous humour in insulin-dependent diabetic patients. Br J Ophthalmol 1989; 73:621–623.

67. Larsson L-I, Pach JM, Brubaker RF. Aqueous humor dynamics in patients with diabetes mellitus. Am J Ophthalmol 1995; 120:362–367.

68. Lane JT, Toris CB, Nakhle SN, et al. Acute effects of insulin on aqueous humor flow in patients with type 1 diabetes. Am J Ophthalmol 2001; 132:321–327.

69. Posner A, Schlossman A. Syndrome of unilateral recurrent attacks of glaucoma with cyclitic symptoms. Arch Ophthalmol 1948; 39:517–535.

70. Camras CB, Chacko DM, Schlossman A, et al. Posner-Schlossman syndrome. In: Prepose JS, Holland GN, Wilhelmus KR, eds. Ocular infection & immunity. St. Louis: Mosby-Year Book; 1996:529–537.

71. Higgitt AC. Secondary glaucoma. Trans Ophthal Soc UK 1956; 76:73–82.

72. Mansheim BJ. Aqueous outflow measurements by continuous tonometry in some unusual forms of glaucoma. AMA Arch Ophthalmol 1953; 50:580–587.

73. Spivey BE, Armaly MF. Tonographic findings in glaucomatocyclic crises. Am J Ophthalmol 1963; 55:47–51.

74. Kass MA, Becker B, Kolker AE. Glaucomatocyclic crisis and primary open-angle glaucoma. Am J Ophthalmol 1973; 75:668–673.

75. Masuda K, Izawa Y, Mishima S. Prostaglandins and glaucomato-cyclitic crisis. Jpn J Ophthalmol 1975; 19:368–375.

76. Brubaker RF, Schoff EO, Nau CB, et al. Effects of AGN 192024, a new ocular hypotensive agent, on aqueous dynamics. Am J Ophthalmol 2001; 131:19–24.

77. Christiansen GA, Nau CB, McLaren JW, et al. Mechanism of ocular hypotensive action of bimatoprost (Lumigan) in patients with ocular hypertension or glaucoma. Ophthalmology 2004; 111:1658–1662.

78. Dinslage S, Hueber A, Diestelhorst M, et al. The influence of Latanoprost 0.005% on aqueous humor flow and outflow facility in glaucoma patients: a double-masked placebo-controlled clinical study. Graefe's Arch Clin Exp Ophthalmol 2004; 242:654–660.

79. Toris CB, Zhan G, Fan S, et al. Effects of travoprost on aqueous humor dynamics in patients with elevated intraocular pressure. J Glaucoma 2007; 16:189–195.

80. Toris CB, Zhan G, Camras CB. Increase in outflow facility with unoprostone treatment in ocular hypertensive patients. Arch Ophthalmol 2004; 122:1782–1787.

81. Sugar HS. Heterochromia iridis with special consideration of its relation to cyclitic disease. Am J Ophthalmol 1965; 60:1–18.

82. Hart CT, Weatherill JR. Gonioscopy and tonography in glaucomatocyclic crises. Br J Ophthalmol 1968; 52:682–687.

83. Nagataki S, Mishima S. Aqueous humor dynamics in glaucomato-cyclitic crisis. Invest Ophthalmol Vis Sci 1976; 15:365–370.

84. Perlman JI, Delany CM, Sothern RB, et al. Relationships between 24h observations in intraocular pressure vs blood pressure, heart rate, nitric oxide and age in the medical chronobiology aging project. Clin Ter 2007; 158:31–47.

85. Liu JHK, Bouligny RP, Kripke DF, et al. Nocturnal elevation of intraocular pressure is detectable in the sitting position. Invest Ophthalmol Vis Sci 2003; 44:4439–4442.

86. Sit AJ, Nau CB, McLaren JW, et al. Circadian variation of aqueous dynamics in young, healthy adults. Invest Ophthalmol Vis Sci 2008; 49:1473–1479.

87. Sultan M, Blondeau P. Episcleral venous pressure in younger and older subjects in the sitting and supine positions. J Glaucoma 2003; 12:370–373.

CHAPTER 7

Mechanical Strain and Restructuring of the Optic Nerve Head

J Crawford Downs, Michael D Roberts, and Claude F Burgoyne

THE OPTIC NERVE HEAD AS A BIOMECHANICAL STRUCTURE

The optic nerve head (ONH) is of particular interest from a biomechanical perspective because it is a weak spot within an otherwise strong corneoscleral envelope. While there are likely to be important pathophysiologies within the lateral geniculate and visual cortex[1] as well as evidence both for[2] and against[3] direct, intraocular pressure (IOP)-induced damage to the retinal photoreceptors, most evidence suggests that the lamina cribrosa is the principal site of retinal ganglion cell (RGC) axonal insult in glaucoma.[4]

The lamina cribrosa provides structural and functional support to the RGC axons as they pass from the relatively high-pressure environment in the eye to a low-pressure region in the retrobulbar cerebrospinal space. To protect the RGCs in this unique anatomic region, the lamina cribrosa in higher primates has developed into a complex structure composed of a three-dimensional (3D) network of flexible beams of connective tissue (Fig. 7.1). The ONH is nourished by the short posterior ciliary arteries, which penetrate the immediate peripapillary sclera to feed capillaries contained within the laminar beams. This intrascleral and intralaminar vasculature is unique in that it is encased in load-bearing connective tissue, either within the scleral wall adjacent to the lamina cribrosa, or within the laminar beams themselves (see Fig. 7.1). Glaucoma is a multifactorial disease, and the authors believe that biomechanics not only determines the mechanical environment in the ONH but also mediates IOP-related reductions in blood flow and cellular responses through various pathways (Fig. 7.2).

Consideration of the anatomy of the lamina cribrosa and peripapillary sclera suggests that the classic 'mechanical' and 'vascular' mechanisms of glaucomatous injury are inseparably intertwined (see Figs 7.1 and 7.2).

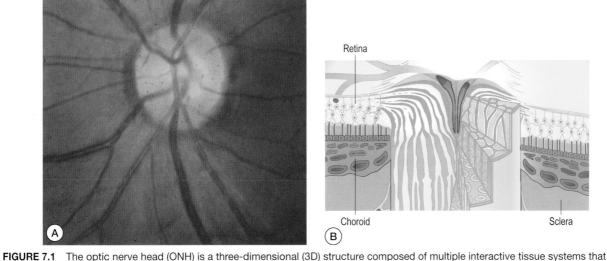

FIGURE 7.1 The optic nerve head (ONH) is a three-dimensional (3D) structure composed of multiple interactive tissue systems that exist on different scales. This complexity has been a formidable deterrent to characterizing its mechanical environment. **(A)** While clinicians are familiar with the clinically visible surface of the optic nerve head (referred to as the optic disc), in fact the ONH **(B)** is a dynamic, 3D structure (seen here in an illustrated sectional view) in which the retinal ganglion cell (RGC) axons in bundles (*white*) surrounded by glial columns (*red*), pass through the connective tissue beams of the lamina cribrosa (*light blue*), isolated following trypsin digestion in a scanning electron micrograph (SEM) of the scleral canal in **(C)**.

(continued)

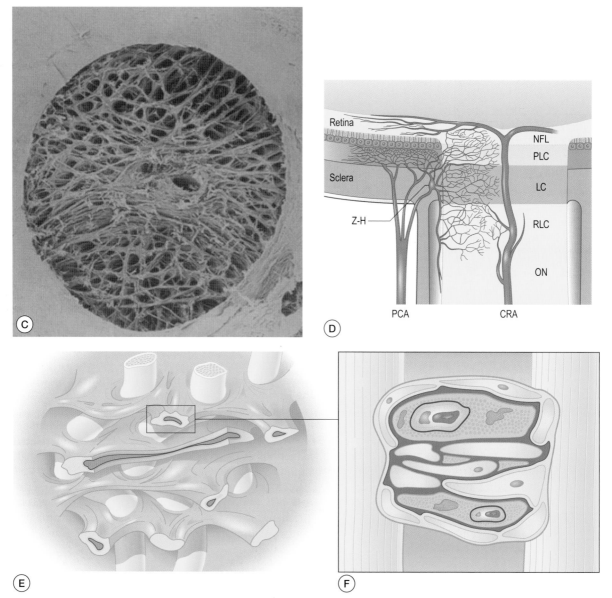

FIGURE 7.1 (Continued) The blood supply for the connective tissues of the lamina cribrosa **(D)** derives from the posterior ciliary arteries and the circle of Zinn-Haller (Z-H). **(E,F)** The relationship of the laminar beams to the axon bundles is shown in schematic form in **(E)**. **(F)** Individual beams of the lamina cribrosa are lined by astrocytes. Together, they provide structural and metabolic support for the adjacent axon bundles. Within the lamina, the retinal ganglion cell (RGC) axons have no direct blood supply. Axonal nutrition requires diffusion of nutrients from the laminar capillaries (*solid red*), across the endothelial and pericyte basement membranes, through the extracellular matrix (ECM) of the laminar beam (*stippled*), across the basement membranes of the astrocytes (*thick black*), into the astrocytes (*yellow*), and across their processes (not shown) to the adjacent axons (*vertical lines*). Chronic age-related changes in the endothelial cell and astrocyte basement membranes, as well as intraocular pressure (IOP)-induced changes in the laminar ECM and astrocyte basement membranes, may diminish nutrient diffusion to the axons in the presence of a stable level of laminar capillary volume flow. In advanced glaucoma, the connective tissues of the normal lamina cribrosa (sagittal view of the center of the optic nerve head (ONH); vitreous above, orbital optic nerve below). (A, Reproduced with permission of J Glaucoma. Burgoyne CF, Downs JC. Premise and prediction – how optic nerve head biomechanics underlies the susceptibility and clinical behavior of the aged optic nerve head. J Glaucoma 2008;17:318-328.)

For example, prior to structural damage, purely IOP-related stress could detrimentally affect the blood supply to the laminar segments of the axons through deformation of the capillary-containing connective tissue structures. Also, IOP-related remodeling of the extracellular matrix (ECM) of the laminar beams could limit the diffusion of nutrients to RGC axons in the ONH. Reciprocally, primary insufficiency in the blood supply to the laminar region could induce cell-mediated connective tissue changes that would serve to weaken the laminar beams, making them more prone to failure under previously 'safe' levels of IOP-related mechanical stress.

To incorporate these concepts into a global conceptual framework, the authors have previously proposed that the ONH is a biomechanical structure.[5] This paradigm assumes that IOP-related stress (force/cross-sectional area) and strain (local deformation of the tissues) are central determinants of both the physiology

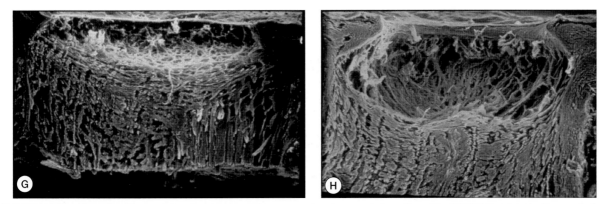

FIGURE 7.1 (Continued)   G) remodel and restructure into a cupped and excavated configuration (H). ((B) Reprinted with permission from Anderson DR. Ultrastructure of human and monkey lamina cribrosa and optic nerve head. Arch Ophthalmol 1969; 82:800–814;[61] (C) reprinted with permission from Quigley HA, Brown AE, Morrison JD, et al. The size and shape of the optic disc in normal human eyes. Arch Ophthalmol 1990; 108:51–57;[62] (D) reprinted with permission from Cioffi GA, Van Buskirk EM. Vasculature of the anterior optic nerve and peripapillary choroid. In: Ritch R, Shields MB, Krupin T, eds. The glaucomas. St. Louis: Mosby; 1996:177–197;[63] (E) reprinted with permission from Quigley HA. Overview and introduction to session on connective tissue of the optic nerve in glaucoma. In: Drance SM, Anderson DR, eds. Optic nerve in glaucoma. Amsterdam/New York: Kugler Publications; 1995:15–36;[64] (F) reprinted with permission from Morrison JC, L'Hernault NL, Jerdan JA, et al. Ultrastructural location of extracellular matrix components in the optic nerve head. Arch Ophthalmol 1989; 107:123–129;[65] (G, H) Courtesy of Harry A Quigley, MD.)

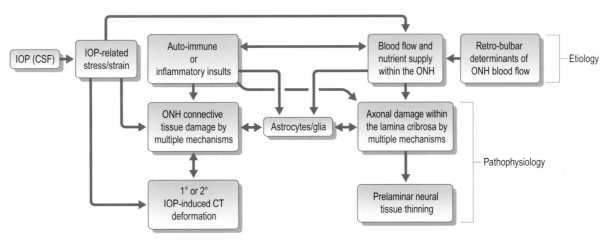

FIGURE 7.2   Intraocular pressure (IOP)-related stress and strain are a constant presence within the optic nerve head (ONH) at all levels of IOP. In a biomechanical paradigm, IOP-related strain influences the ONH connective tissues and the volume flow of blood (primarily), and the delivery of nutrients (secondarily) through chronic alterations in connective tissue stiffness and diffusion properties (explained in Fig. 7.1). Non-IOP-related effects such as autoimmune or inflammatory insults and retrobulbar determinants of ocular blood flow can primarily damage the ONH connective tissues and/or axons, leaving them vulnerable to secondary damage by IOP-related mechanisms at normal or elevated levels of IOP. (Adapted from Burgoyne CF and Downs, JC. Premise and prediction–how optic nerve head biomechanics underlies the susceptibility and clinical behavior of the aged optic nerve head. Invited original article, J Glaucoma 2008;17:318–328.)

and pathophysiology of the ONH tissues and their blood supply (see Fig. 7.2) at all levels of IOP. These changes include not only alterations to the load-bearing connective tissues of the lamina cribrosa and the peripapillary sclera but also to the cellular components of these tissues, including astrocytes, glial cells, endothelial cells, and pericytes, along with their basement membranes and the RGC axons in the ONH. Experienced over a lifetime at physiologic levels, they underlie 'normal' ONH aging. However, acute or chronic exposure to pathophysiologic levels results in glaucomatous damage.

Although clinical IOP lowering remains the only proven method of preventing the onset and progression of glaucoma, the role of IOP in the development and progression of the disease remains controversial. This largely arises from the clinical observation that significant numbers of patients with normal IOPs develop glaucoma (normotensive glaucoma), while other individuals with elevated IOP show no signs of the disease. While there is a wide spectrum of individual susceptibility to IOP-related glaucomatous vision loss, the biomechanical effects of IOP on the tissues of the optic nerve head likely play a central role in the development and progression of the disease at all IOPs. The individual susceptibility of a particular patient's ONH to IOP insult is likely a function of the biomechanical response of the constituent tissues and the resulting mechanical, ischemic, and cellular events driven by that response.

Hence, eyes with a particular combination of tissue geometry and stiffness may be susceptible to damage at normal IOP, while others may have a combination of ONH tissue geometry and stiffness that can withstand even high levels of IOP.

In this chapter, the authors focus on ocular biomechanics along two main themes: what is known about how mechanical forces and the resulting deformations are distributed in the posterior pole and ONH (biomechanics), and what is known about how the living system responds to those deformations (mechanobiology).

MECHANICAL ENVIRONMENT OF THE OPTIC NERVE HEAD AND PERIPAPILLARY SCLERA

BASIC ENGINEERING CONCEPTS

The following are fundamental terms and concepts from engineering mechanics that may not be familiar to clinicians and nonengineering scientists. The interested reader may pursue these ideas in greater depth by referring to appropriate textbooks on engineering science, mechanics of materials, and biomechanics.[6,7]

Stress is a measure of the load applied to, transmitted through, or carried by a material or tissue. Stress can be defined as the amount of force applied to a tissue divided by the cross-sectional area over which it acts (e.g. pressure is a stress and can be expressed in pounds per square inch [psi]). Stress may be decomposed into components that act in perpendicular (tension or compression) and tangential directions (Fig. 7.3). The perpendicular components are called *normal* stresses and act to elongate or compress the tissue. The tangential components are called *shear* stresses and act to distort the shape of the tissue (see Fig. 7.3).

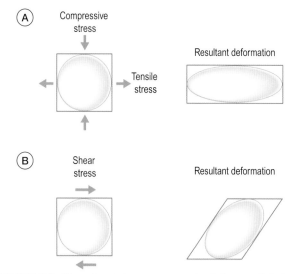

FIGURE 7.3 *Normal* and *shear* components of stress and strain. **(A)** The normal tensile and compressive stresses acting on a small square in the manner shown will act to elongate the region in one direction and compress it in the other. **(B)** The shear stresses acting on a similar region will act to distort the shape of the region.

Because tissues generally exhibit spatial variations in shape and cross-sectional area and the points of load application can be nonuniform, the stress within a biologic structure can vary considerably from region to region. Some regions may bear very little stress while other regions experience very high stresses due to their proximity to a particular loading point or geometric feature. It is important to note that stress is a mathematical quantity that can be calculated, but cannot be measured, felt, or observed. Furthermore, the notion of stress as a mathematical description of mechanical load-bearing is distinct from and not synonymous with notions of stress typically used in physiologic or metabolic contexts (e.g. *ischemic* or *oxidative* stress).

Strain is a measure of the local deformation in a material or tissue induced by an applied stress, and is usually expressed as the percentage change in length of the original geometry (e.g. a wire that was originally 10 mm long that has been stretched an additional 1 mm exhibits 10% strain). Like stress, strain may also be decomposed into normal (tensile or compressive) and shear (distortional) components (see Fig. 7.3). It is important to recognize that strain, unlike stress, may be observed and measured. It is also important to appreciate the distinction between the deformation of a structure and strain within its constituent parts. While a structure may exhibit an overall, global deformation in response to an applied load, the localized relative displacement described by the strain provides a measurable indicator of the level of microdeformation (stretch, compression, or shearing) experienced by the tissue. In the ONH, an increase in IOP may induce a net posterior displacement of the lamina cribrosa, but it will also stretch (strain) the constituent laminar beams themselves. The concept of strain has important consequences in biomechanics at all levels, because it is strain, not stress, which causes damage to tissues. Furthermore, mechanosensation by cells is likely dependent on the local deformations associated with tissue strain and may play a role in tissue remodeling.

The *material properties* of a tissue describe its ability to resist deformation under an applied load and therefore relate *stress* to *strain* (*i.e.* load to deformation). Material properties can be thought of as the stiffness or compliance of a particular tissue or material that is intrinsic to the material itself. Hence, a stiff tissue such as sclera can have high stress, but low strain, while an equal volume of compliant tissue like retina might have high strain even at low levels of stress. Material properties are generally determined through rigorous experimental testing of the material in tension, compression, and shear.

Material properties are often described in terms of their material symmetry (isotropic or anisotropic), the nature of the relationship between load and deformation (linear or nonlinear), and the time-dependence of their response to loading (elastic or viscoelastic). Isotropic materials exhibit identical resistance to load in all directions while anisotropic materials can exhibit higher or lower stiffness properties along different directions. For instance, concrete may be isotropic by itself, but the introduction of rebar during fabrication would produce an anisotropic material with higher resistance to tension along the direction of the rebar. The load–deformation, or stress–strain relationship which characterizes a material can also be described in terms of whether it is linear or nonlinear. In linear materials, stress is directly proportional to strain, by a constant factor known as the Young's modulus. Nonlinear materials, on the other hand, have a nonconstant proportionality between stress and strain, and hence do not have a unique or

constant Young's modulus. Figure 7.4 illustrates the behavior of a nonlinear anisotropic material.

In some materials, the load–deformation response is time-dependent. Viscoelastic materials, for instance, exhibit higher resistance when loaded quickly than when loaded slowly (similar to the behavior of a hydraulic shock absorber). Viscoelastic materials also exhibit the phenomena of *creep* and *stress relaxation*. Creep refers to the tendency of a material to deform over time under a constant load. Similarly, stress relaxation refers

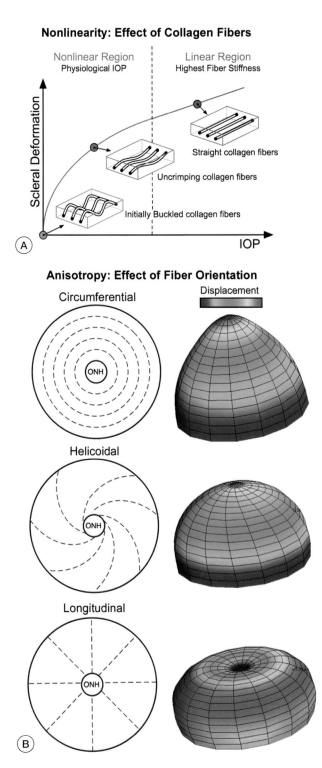

FIGURE 7.4 The material properties of the peripapillary sclera are influenced by nonlinearity and collagen fiber orientation (anisotropy). Separate from its thickness, the behavior of the sclera is governed by its material properties, which in turn are influenced by nonlinearity and fiber orientation. **(A)** Nonlinearity is an engineering term for tissues or structures whose material properties are altered by loading. This figure demonstrates that the sclera becomes stiffer as it is loaded uniaxially (in one direction). In the case of the sclera, this is likely due to the fact collagen fibers embedded within the surrounding ground matrix start out crimped and progressively straighten as the load is increased. This conformational change in the fibrils accounts for the transition from an initially compliant, nonlinear response to a stiffened linear response as intraocular pressure (IOP) increases. **(B)** Apart from nonlinearity, collagen fiber orientation (anisotropy) within the sclera strongly influences its mechanical behavior. Fiber orientation can be totally random (isotropic; not shown) or have a principal direction (anisotropic; three idealized cases shown). Finite element (FE) models of an idealized posterior pole with principal collagen fiber orientation in the circumferential, helicoidal, and longitudinal directions are shown. As the displacement plots show, the underlying fiber orientation can have profound effects on the deformation that occurs for a given IOP. Note that the displacement scale is exaggerated for illustrative purposes. (Courtesy of Michael Girard.)

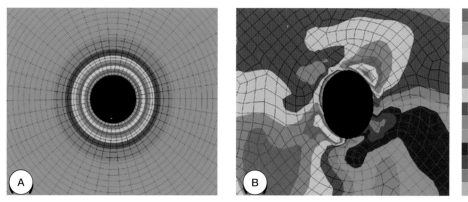

FIGURE 7.5 The thickness of the peripapillary sclera, and the size and shape of the scleral canal influence the magnitude and distribution of intraocular pressure (IOP)-related stress within the peripapillary sclera. Stress plots within 3D biomechanical models of the posterior sclera and optic nerve head (ONH) demonstrate that stress concentrates around a defect (scleral canal) in a pressure vessel (eye) and varies according to the geometry of the peripapillary sclera and scleral canal. The idealized model in **(A)** shows the stress concentration around a circular canal in a perfectly spherical pressure vessel with uniform wall thickness (the ONH has been removed from these images for visualization purposes). The model in **(B)** shows the IOP-related stress concentration around an anatomically shaped scleral canal with realistic variation in peripapillary scleral thickness. In this case, the highest stresses (*red*) occur where the sclera is thinnest and the lowest stresses (*blue*) occur where the sclera is thickest, and also tend to concentrate around areas of the scleral canal with the smallest radius of curvature. The response of the sclera to this load is determined by its structural stiffness, which is the combination of geometry (how much tissue is bearing the load) and material properties (how rigid or compliant is the tissue).

to the phenomenon wherein the mechanical stress borne by a material diminishes with time following an imposed constant displacement. It is important to note that viscoelastic material responses are not necessarily indicative of mechanical yield or failure (see below). Materials which exhibit no time-dependent behavior are termed elastic materials.

The simplest material property description is that of an isotropic, linearly elastic material (e.g. steel). Biologic soft tissues (e.g. sclera or tendon) are usually nonlinear, anisotropic, viscoelastic materials and so exhibit increased resistance to strain at higher load levels, are stiffer when loaded in a particular direction, and respond to load in a rate- and time-dependent manner. Characterization of the material properties of biologic soft tissues is a formidable undertaking and requires extensive experimental effort. Once established, material descriptions for tissues may be used in conjunction with descriptions of geometry and loading conditions to model the stress and strain fields borne throughout a structure.

Another useful concept in biomechanics is *structural stiffness*, which incorporates both the material properties and geometry of a complex load-bearing structure into a composite measure of the structure's resistance to deformation. In the cornea, both the geometry (thickness) and the material properties contribute to its structural stiffness and hence influence the accuracy of IOP measurements that rely on deformation. In the posterior pole, both the geometry and material properties of the sclera and lamina cribrosa contribute to structural stiffness, and hence determine the ability of the ONH and peripapillary sclera to withstand strain when exposed to IOP. As such, individual ONH biomechanics is governed by the geometry (size and shape of the scleral canal, scleral thickness, and regional laminar density and beam orientation) and the material properties

(stiffness) of the lamina cribrosa and sclera. Hence, two eyes exposed to identical IOPs may exhibit very different strain fields due to differences in their structural stiffness (Fig. 7.5).

Mechanical yield occurs when a material is strained beyond its elastic limit, and is therefore unable to return to its undeformed shape. A material or tissue that has yielded in response to high strains is permanently damaged and deformed and is usually less resistant to further loading (hypercompliance). *Mechanical failure* occurs at even higher strain, typically follows yield, and generally manifests in soft tissues as catastrophic rupture or pulling apart. For any individual ONH there will likely be an IOP that induces widespread yield in the laminar beams, but does not result in visible failure of individual trabeculae. At even higher IOPs, some catastrophic failure of individual laminar beams will be evident, while a new population of beams may now demonstrate yield. Yield and failure are short-term mechanical processes that likely induce a long-term cellular remodeling response that serves to restructure the ONH to alter its future load-bearing capacity.

OVERVIEW OF THE MECHANICAL ENVIRONMENT OF THE OPTIC NERVE HEAD AND PERIPAPILLARY SCLERA

From an engineering perspective, the eye is a vessel with inflow and outflow facilities that regulate its internal pressure. IOP imposes a pressure load normal to the inner surface of the eye wall, generating an in-wall circumferential stress known as the hoop stress (Fig. 7.6). This IOP-generated stress is primarily borne by the stiff, collagenous sclera, while the more compliant retina and nerve fiber tissues bear little of the in-wall stress load and are therefore exposed primarily to the compressive

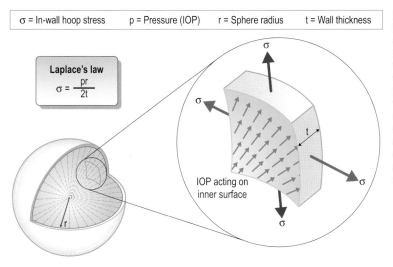

σ = In-wall hoop stress   p = Pressure (IOP)   r = Sphere radius   t = Wall thickness

Laplace's law

$$\sigma = \frac{pr}{2t}$$

IOP acting on inner surface

FIGURE 7.6 In-wall stress engendered by intraocular pressure (IOP) loading. In an idealized spherical shell, the majority of the stress generated by IOP is transferred into a hoop stress borne within the thickness of the wall. Laplace's Law, which relates the in-wall hoop stress to the internal pressure, is only applicable to spherical pressure vessels with isotropic material properties and uniform wall thickness, and can only be used to calculate very rough estimates of hoop stress in actual eyes. In pressure vessel geometries like the eye, with variable wall thickness, aspherical shape, and anisotropic material properties, the hoop stress may vary substantially by location.

stress of IOP. IOP is borne in the ONH by the fenestrated connective tissues of the lamina cribrosa, which span the scleral canal opening and tether into the stiff outer ring of circumferential collagen and elastin fibers in the peripapillary sclera (like a trampoline). While Laplace's Law[7] is useful to describe the pressure–deformation relationship in a spherical vessel of uniform thickness, it is inadequate for describing the eye's response to variations in IOP (Fig. 7.7). There are several characteristics of the ocular load-bearing tissues that complicate the study of the mechanical environment to which the ONH and its resident cell populations are exposed.

First, the three-dimensional connective tissue geometry of the eye is complex and difficult to measure. For instance, the thickness of monkey sclera can vary as much as fourfold from the equator to the peripapillary region,[8,9] and the 3D morphology of lamina cribrosa is more regionally complex and individualized than is generally appreciated.[10–12] Secondly, the cornea, sclera, and lamina cribrosa have extremely complex ECM microstructures with highly anisotropic collagen and elastin fibril orientations. As a result, the *experimental* characterization and *theoretical/mathematical* description of their constituent material properties are complex and difficult to obtain. Thirdly, the cells that maintain the ocular connective tissues are biologically active. As such, the geometry and material properties of the sclera and lamina cribrosa change in response to both physiologic (age) and pathologic (IOP-related damage) factors. Fourthly, the eye is exposed to ever changing loading conditions because IOP undergoes acute, short-term and long-term fluctuations ranging from blinks and eye rubs to circadian rhythms.

Finally, IOP-related stress generates strain patterns in the ONH and peripapillary sclera that are not only dependent on differing connective tissue geometries and material properties but also are influenced by complex loading conditions. The important factors contributing to this biomechanical component include the alignment and density of collagen fibrils in each tissue (stiffness and anisotropy), the rate of change in IOP (via tissue viscoelasticity), and the level of IOP-related strain at the time of altered loading (via tissue nonlinearity). In broad terms, the ONH connective tissues should be stiffer when there is already considerable strain present and/or if the IOP load is applied quickly. Conversely, the ONH should be more compliant in response to slow changes in IOP and/or at low levels of strain.

MECHANICAL RESPONSE OF THE OPTIC NERVE HEAD TO ACUTELY ELEVATED INTRAOCULAR PRESSURE

It is important to note that the ONH responds to IOP elevations as a structural system, so the acute mechanical response of the lamina cribrosa is confounded with

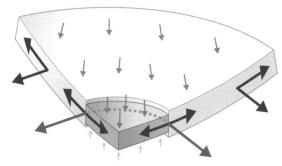

FIGURE 7.7 Stress, relative to intraocular pressure (IOP) (*red arrows*) in the lamina cribrosa (*light green*) and peripapillary sclera (*gray*) engendered by IOP loading. Cutaway diagram of IOP-induced stress in an idealized spherical scleral shell with a circular scleral canal spanned by a more compliant lamina cribrosa. In this case, the majority of the stress generated by IOP (*red arrows*) is transferred into a hoop stress borne within the thickness of the sclera and lamina (*blue arrows*) that is concentrated circumferentially around the scleral canal (*green arrows*). Note that the difference between IOP (*red arrows*) and the retrolaminar cerebrospinal fluid pressure (*pink arrows*) is the translaminar pressure gradient that generates both a net posterior force on the surface of the lamina and a hydrostatic pressure gradient within the neural and connective tissues of the prelaminar and laminar regions. *Most importantly, note that the in-plane hoop stress transferred to the lamina from the sclera is much larger than stress induced by the translaminar pressure gradient.*

the responses of the peripapillary sclera, prelaminar neural tissues, and retrolaminar optic nerve. Also, because the lamina lies buried underneath the prelaminar neural tissues and the acute structural responses of these two tissues to acute IOP elevations are quite different, acute laminar deformation cannot be directly measured from imaging the surface topography of the ONH.[13] A final confounding effect is the cerebrospinal fluid pressure which, along with IOP, determines the translaminar pressure gradient that must be borne by the lamina cribrosa.

Intuitively, it may seem that for a given acute increase in IOP, the lamina cribrosa should deform posteriorly, and there have been several experimental studies designed to measure acute IOP-related laminar deformation. Yan and co-workers found that increasing IOP from 5 to 50 mmHg for 24 hours produced an average posterior deformation of the central lamina of 79 µm in human donor eyes.[14] Crapps and Levy reported a 12 µm average posterior movement of the central lamina with acute IOP elevations of 10–25 mmHg for shorter time periods in human eyes.[15] More recently, Bellezza and colleagues reported a small but significant posterior laminar deformation of 10–23 µm (95% confidence interval [CI]) in a histologic evaluation of monkey eyes perfusion fixed

with one eye at 10 mmHg and the contralateral eye at 30 or 45 mmHg for 15 minutes prior to death.[16] However, these deformations, while statistically significant, did not substantially exceed the 95% CI for intra-animal physiologic differences (1–17 µm) between normal eyes bilaterally immersion fixed at an IOP of 0 mmHg.

The previous studies were performed using two-dimensional (2D) measurements of laminar compliance within actual histologic sections. Angled sectioning, section warping, and the lack of a stable measurement reference plane can influence the accuracy of this technique. To overcome these problems, Downs, Yang, and co-workers developed a technique for 3D delineation and measurement of ONH structures within high-resolution, digital 3D reconstructions (Fig. 7.8).[17–20] While the authors' initial reports have concentrated on monkeys with early experimental glaucoma in one eye, preliminary data from a larger group of bilaterally normal monkeys perfusion fixed with both eyes at an IOP of 10 mmHg (n = 5), one eye at 10 mmHg and the other at 30 mmHg (n = 3), and one eye at 10 mmHg and the other at IOP 45 mmHg (n = 3) suggest that while acute IOP elevation causes expansion of the scleral canal, in most monkey eyes there is no net posterior laminar deformation from the

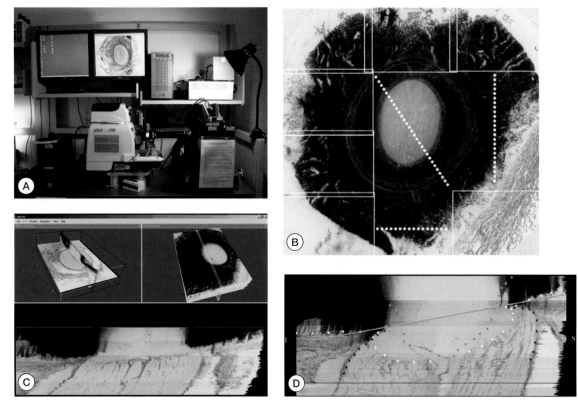

FIGURE 7.8 Three-dimensional (3D) delineation of optic nerve head (ONH) and peripapillary scleral landmark points within digital 3D ONH reconstructions.[17,18] **(A)** Photograph of the authors' microtome-based 3D reconstruction device allows for serial sectioning and high-resolution image capture of the stained block face of embedded ONH specimens. **(B)** Images are acquired in a mosaic, then stitched into a composite of the entire 6-mm-diameter specimen, and stacked into a digital 3D reconstruction of the connective tissues of the ONH with 1.5 × 1.5 × 1.5 µm voxel resolution **(C)**. Once loaded into custom software, the reconstruction can be digitally sectioned and landmarks delineated. In this view **(D)** the measurement reference plane, Bruch's membrane opening (BMO), is marked and shown with a *light blue line*.

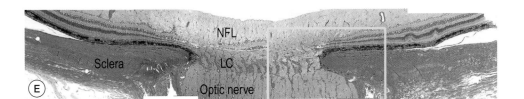

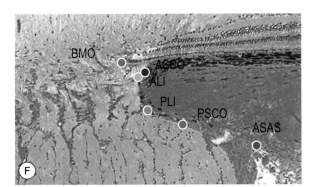

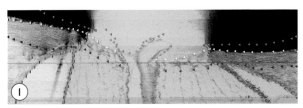

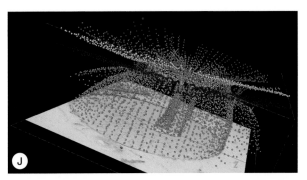

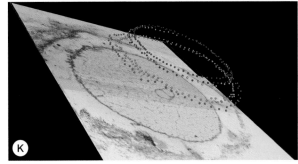

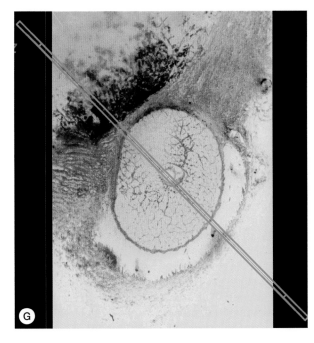

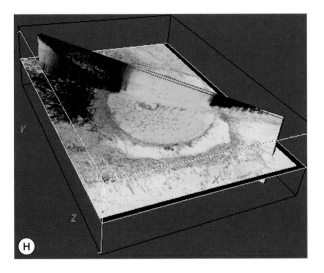

FIGURE 7.8 (Continued) **(E)** Central horizontal histologic section through a representative normal monkey eye showing the ONH anatomy. **(F)** Magnified view of the nasal side of the neural canal showing the following landmark points: BMO (*red*), the anterior scleral canal opening (ASCO, *dark blue*), the anterior laminar insertion point (ALI, *yellow*), the posterior laminar insertion point (PLI, *green*), the posterior scleral canal opening (PSCO, *pink*), the anterior-most aspect of the subarachnoid space (ASAS, *light blue*). **(G, H)** With the 3D digital ONH reconstruction, a total of 40 radial, sagittal slices (each 7 voxels thick) are served to the delineator at 4.5° intervals. **(I)** A representative digital sagittal slice, showing the marks for 7 landmark surfaces and 6 landmark point pairs. These features are interactively delineated within the 3D volume by viewing the position of a marking cursor displayed simultaneously within the sagittal **(G)** and transverse section images **(H)**. **(J)** Representative 3D point cloud showing all delineated points for a normal monkey ONH in relation to the last section image of the reconstruction. **(K)** A subset of the 3D point cloud showing the neural canal landmarks depicted in **(F)**. (D, F, G, H, I, J and K, Reproduced with permission of Invest Ophthalmol Vis Sci. Downs JC, Yang H, Girkin C, et al. Three-dimensional histomorphometry of the normal and early glaucomatous monkey optic nerve head: neural canal and subarachnoid space architecture. Invest. Ophthalmol Vis Sci. 2007;48:3195–3208.)

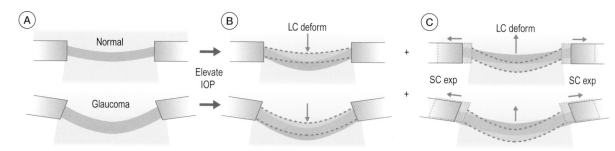

FIGURE 7.9 There are two components of acute intraocular pressure (IOP)-induced optic nerve head (ONH) deformation in normal and early-glaucoma eyes. **(A)** Sagittal section diagram of the ONH, showing the peripapillary sclera (*gray*) and the lamina cribrosa (LC) for normal (*upper*) and early-glaucoma (*lower*) eyes. Note that the early-glaucoma eye has undergone permanent changes in ONH geometry including thickening of the lamina, posterior deformation of the lamina and peripapillary sclera, and posterior scleral canal expansion (SC exp). Upon acute IOP elevation, the authors believe two phenomena occur simultaneously and with interaction: the lamina displaces posteriorly due to the direct action of IOP **(B)**, but much of this posterior laminar displacement is counteracted as the lamina is pulled taut by simultaneous SC exp **(C)**. It is important to note that even though the net result of these IOP-related deformations is a small amount of posterior displacement of the lamina, substantial levels of IOP-related strain are induced in both the peripapillary sclera and lamina in this scenario. (Reproduced with permission from Yang H, Downs JC, Bellezza AJ, et al. 3-D histomorphometry of the normal and early glaucomatous monkey optic nerve head: prelaminar neural tissues and cupping. Invest Ophthalmol Vis Sci. 2007;48:5068–5084.)

plane of the sclera. Thus, the authors' current understanding of the aggregate response of the young adult monkey ONH to acute IOP elevation is that expansion of the scleral canal pulls the lamina taut within the plane of the sclera, making it more resistant to posterior deformation out of that plane (Fig. 7.9). These data are preliminary and their interpretation may change with further study.

It is important to note that the lack of laminar deformation in these eyes does not mean that the lamina is not strained. In this scenario, the expansion of the canal stretches the lamina cribrosa within the plane of the sclera, generating substantial strain within the laminar beams. Estimation of laminar beam strain within these same 3D reconstructions is one of the outputs of finite element (FE) modeling, an engineering technique that is discussed below.

THE CONTRIBUTION OF THE SCLERA TO OPTIC NERVE HEAD BIOMECHANICS

The data described above, as well as the closed-form analyses and computational models described in the next section, suggest that the sclera plays an important role in ONH biomechanics. The peripapillary sclera provides the boundary conditions for the ONH, i.e. the peripapillary sclera is the tissue through which load and deformation are transmitted to the ONH, and that the structural stiffness of the peripapillary sclera therefore influences how the lamina deforms (see Fig. 7.9). This can be understood from the discussion above in which a compliant sclera allows the scleral canal to expand following an acute IOP elevation, pulling the laminar beams taut within the canal and thereby increasing laminar resistance to posterior deformation. In contrast, a rigid sclera allows less expansion of the canal or none at all, forcing the structural stiffness of the lamina alone to bear the IOP-related stress. Hence, characterization of both components of scleral structural stiffness (geometry and material properties) is essential to understanding the effects of IOP on the ONH.

Characterization of scleral geometry Maps of the thickness variation for the posterior pole of human[21] and monkey eyes[8,9] show extreme spatial variation in scleral thickness, with very thin regions near the equator (as low as 300 μm in the human and 111 μm in the monkey). In both species the peripapillary sclera is notably thicker (1000 μm in the human and 415 μm in the monkey). Interestingly, this thick ring of peripapillary sclera is absent in the nasal quadrant of monkey eyes due to the oblique nasal insertion of the optic nerve through the scleral canal. Variations in peripapillary scleral thickness that occur naturally or in pathologic conditions such as myopia may be important in assessing individual susceptibility to glaucomatous damage.

Characterization of scleral material properties Several researchers have characterized scleral material properties in various species.[22,23] Most recently, Downs and co-workers used a strain-rate controlled, servo-hydraulic materials testing system to determine the viscoelastic material properties of normal rabbit and monkey peripapillary sclera. They found that the material properties of peripapillary sclera are highly time-dependent (viscoelastic), but reported no significant differences in material properties by quadrant.[24,25]

However, uniaxial testing of scleral strips is limited in its ability to describe the nonlinear and anisotropic responses of the sclera (see Fig. 7.5), leading Girard and colleagues to develop a new 3D approach. Using a customized scleral shell pressurization apparatus, precise IOP control, and laser-based electronic speckle pattern interferometry, they measure the 3D deformation of the entire posterior scleral shell in response to small, stepped increases in IOP (5–45 mmHg). Preliminary results suggest that the monkey posterior sclera is highly nonlinear (it gets stiffer as IOP increases) and anisotropic (the underlying collagen fibril distribution is nonuniform and changes throughout the scleral shell, which affects directional stiffness) (Fig. 7.10).[26] By using an FE model (see below) backfitting method, they

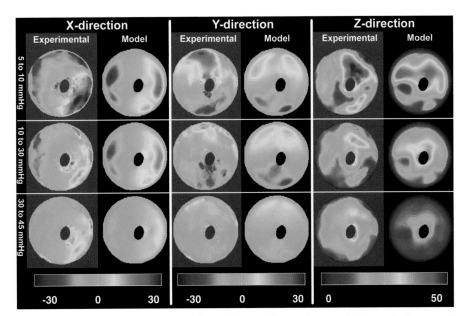

FIGURE 7.10 Experimental results and finite element model predictions of the nonlinear, anisotropic displacement behavior of an individual monkey posterior scleral shell as intraocular pressure (IOP) increases from 5 to 10 mmHg (*top row*), 10 to 30 mmHg (*middle row*), and 30 to 45 mmHg (*bottom row*). Experimental (*gray background*) and predicted (Model, *black background*) displacements for the X direction (left-to-right) , Y direction (top-to-bottom), and Z direction (in-and-out) directions are mapped onto the outer surface of the scleral shell of a right eye (for each map superior top, inferior bottom, temporal left and nasal right). The inhomogeneity of the experimental displacement patterns are indicative of underlying tissue anisotropy, and the much greater displacements seen in the 5 to 10 mmHg IOP elevation as compared to the 30 to 45 mmHg IOP elevation reflect the highly nonlinear behavior (i.e. the sclera is stiffer and therefore more resistant to deformation at higher levels of strain). (Courtesy of Michael Girard.) (Reproduced with permission of Invest Ophthalmol Vis Sci. Girard M, Downs JC, Burgoyne CF, et al. IOVS 2007;48:ARVO E-Abstract 3304.)

have calculated the nonlinear, hyperelastic, anisotropic material properties for the entire posterior scleral shell of normal monkeys, and work is ongoing to characterize changes in these properties due to age and stage of glaucomatous damage.

ENGINEERING MODELS OF STRESS AND STRAIN IN THE OPTIC NERVE HEAD AND PERIPAPILLARY SCLERA

Closed-form solutions Attempts to mathematically model the mechanical environment of the ONH generally fall into two broad categories: closed-form solutions and numerical solutions. In closed-form solutions, engineering principles are used to derive equations that can be analyzed to understand the effects of selected biological parameters. Examples of closed-form approaches include work by Dongqi and Zeqin,[27] Edwards and Good,[28] and a hybrid cellular solid approach by Sander et al.[29] The appeal of closed-form solutions is that general conclusions may be drawn from a model cast in terms of a limited number of geometric and material parameters that are felt to be of interest or might be clinically measurable. However, closed-form solutions may be of limited utility because of the complexity of the ONH and peripapillary scleral tissues (e.g., the nonuniform and asymmetric geometry and material properties). The most sophisticated of these studies suggest that the structural stiffness of the sclera is the most important determinant of macrolevel ONH biomechanics.[29]

Numerical solutions: finite element analysis To overcome the inherent limitations of closed-form solutions, researchers often utilize numerical methods to study more complex biological systems. One of the most powerful of these is finite element (FE) analysis. In FE analysis, complex load-bearing structures are broken into small, regularly shaped elements (see Fig. 7.4). Stress and strain within each element is calculated and then superposed to predict the mechanical response of the entire structure.

The power of FE analysis lies in its ability to model structures with highly complex geometries using material properties with varying levels of complexity as warranted (e.g. inhomogeneous, anisotropic, nonlinear, or viscoelastic material descriptions). The three components necessary as inputs for FE models are the 3D geometry of the tissue structure to be modeled, the material properties of the different tissues in the model, and appropriate loading and boundary conditions. These requirements have spurred the development of methodologies to isolate and describe the 3D geometry of the ONH and peripapillary sclera (see Fig. 7.8) and experimentally characterize their constituent material properties (see Fig. 7.10).

There are two basic approaches to FE modeling of the ONH: parametric and individual-specific. Parametric modeling involves computing stress and strain in average, idealized geometries that do not conform to any individual's particular anatomy. Within these models, parameters such as peripapillary scleral thickness and laminar stiffness can be varied independently to gauge that parameter's effects on ONH biomechanics as a whole. This is a similar approach to analytical modeling, but the analyzed geometries are much more fidelic and the results more relevant and intuitive. Although parametric FE models are by nature simplified in their geometries and there are limited cases that can be modeled, these investigations yield interesting insight into the contributions of individual anatomical elements and tissue material properties to overall ONH biomechanics.

Bellezza et al. used parametric FE modeling to study the mechanical environment of an idealized 3D model of the posterior pole.[30] In this study, the effects of the size and shape (aspect ratio) of an elliptical scleral canal within a spherical scleral shell of uniform thickness were studied. Idealized beamlike structures spanning the ONH were also incorporated into the model to simulate the lamina cribrosa. This study illustrated that IOP-related stress concentration within the load-bearing connective tissues of the ONH is substantial, even at low levels of IOP. Specifically, models with larger scleral canal diameters, more elliptical canals, and thinner sclera all showed increased stresses in the ONH and peripapillary sclera for a given level of IOP. In the peripapillary sclera and ONH, stresses were as much as one and two orders of magnitude greater than IOP, respectively. While the model used in this study was idealized in terms of its material properties and geometry, it served to reinforce the concept of the peripapillary sclera and ONH as a high-stress environment even at normal levels of IOP.

Sigal and co-workers used idealized axisymmetric FE models to pursue a more complex parametric analysis of the factors that influence the biomechanical environment within the ONH (Fig. 7.11).[31,32] In these studies, various geometric and material details of a generic model were parameterized and independently varied to assess their impact on a host of outcome measures such as strain in the lamina cribrosa and prelaminar neural tissue (see Fig. 7.11). This work identified the five most important determinants of ONH biomechanics (in rank order) as: the stiffness of the sclera, the size of the eye, IOP, the stiffness of the lamina cribrosa, and the thickness of the sclera. The finding that scleral stiffness plays a key role in ONH biomechanics is especially interesting, and was also found to be important in the analytical models of Sander and co-workers.[29] Parametric studies such as these are important because they can be used to identify important biomechanical factors that warrant more in-depth study, thus narrowing and focusing future experimental and modeling efforts.

To address the limitations of idealized geometric and material property descriptions inherent in parametric FE models, individual-specific FE models can be created from the reconstructed geometries of particular eyes.[12,33] At present, individual-specific modeling is based on high-resolution 3D reconstructions of monkey and human cadaver eyes (see Fig. 7.8), with a long-term goal to build models based on clinical imaging of living eyes to use them in the assignment of target IOP. This is especially important given that the 3D geometry of the scleral canal and peripapillary sclera largely determine the stress and strain transmitted to the contained ONH. (Figure 7.7 notes specifically how the 3D geometry of the scleral canal and peripapillary sclera alter the stress environment.) Anatomically accurate 3D models are necessary to capture the biomechanics of anisotropic scleral material properties (varying collagen fibril orientation) and scleral canals that are noncircular and have varying optic nerve insertion angles (i.e. the optic nerve inserts from the nasal side resulting in a thinner peripapillary sclera in that quadrant). When modeling an ONH with anatomic fidelity, the tissue geometries

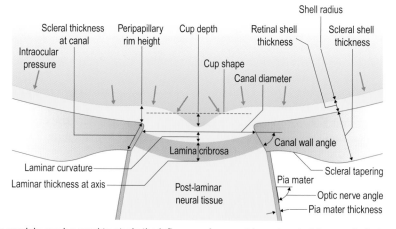

FIGURE 7.11 Parametric models can be used to study the influence of geometric and material property factors. To model the optic nerve head (ONH), Sigal et al.[32] created an idealized, axisymmetric (symmetric about the anterior-to-posterior axis) reference geometry and varied geometric and material property factors to assess their influence on various outcome measures of stress and strain within the model. This type of parametric sensitivity analysis is useful for identifying the tissues and anatomic structures that may be most important in the mechanical response of the ONH. Such information can serve to focus future biomechanics research and clinical device development efforts on the tissues and structures determined to be most important in ONH biomechanics. (Courtesy of Ian Sigal.) (Reproduced with permission from Sigal IA, Roberts MD, Girard M, et al. Biomechanical changes of the optic disc. In: Levin LA, Albert DM (eds), Ocular disease: mechanisms and management. New York: Elsevier; 2009 [Forthcoming].)

can be constructed either by serial histologic methods or 3D imaging, and material properties are generally determined through direct mechanical testing (see Fig. 7.10). Unfortunately, imaging of the lamina in vivo is not yet possible at the resolutions required for modeling, and no technology exists for experimental biomechanical testing of laminar beams. As a result, ONH FE models are typically constructed from eyes that are perfusion or immersion fixed at a selected IOP, and then undergo ex vivo 3D reconstruction of their connective tissues.

Bellezza developed a histologic technique to 3D reconstruct the trabeculated structure of the lamina cribrosa from individual monkey eyes that have been perfusion fixed at varying levels of IOP (see Fig. 7.8).[17] The resulting 3D data sets form the geometries[18–20] of individual-specific FE models of the ONH at macro- and microscale. Roberts, Downs, and co-workers have developed macroscale continuum FE models of the posterior pole and ONH connective tissues from individual monkey eyes (Fig. 7.12).[12] In these models, the laminar microarchitecture is modeled using a continuum approach, with anisotropic material properties assigned to each finite element in the ONH based on the connective tissue volume fraction and the predominant beam orientation of the contained laminar microarchitecture (Fig. 7.13). Regional variations in connective tissue volume fraction and predominant orientation are translated into variations in local oriented stiffness so that regions of higher and lower porosity reflect greater and lesser compliance, respectively. The inclusion of regional laminar material properties (connective tissue volume fraction and beam orientation) into FE models has a pronounced effect on the ONH's response to IOP (Fig. 7.14). This indicates that the regional variations in laminar geometry and structural stiffness must be represented in models to fully capture the biomechanical behavior of the ONH and suggests that the lamina is biologically optimized to withstand IOP-induced deformation.

Downs and colleagues have also used the 3D reconstruction and continuum modeling approaches to characterize and explore laminar beam biomechanics.[34] This microscale modeling approach utilizes a substructuring technique based on parent macroscale FE models to calculate the IOP-related stress and strain fields in laminar beams (Fig. 7.15). This technique reveals a complexity of IOP-related strains and stresses within the lamina cribrosa microarchitecture that is not available through macroscale FE modeling. There have been several interesting preliminary results from this work. First, stress and strain in the laminar microarchitecture are likely higher than predicted by macroscale models of the ONH. Secondly, even at normal levels of IOP, the micro-FE models predict that while the majority of laminar beams are within physiologic strain ranges, there are individual laminar beams with levels of IOP-related strain that are likely pathologic. Thirdly, mean strain within the laminar beams of different monkeys varies greatly, and is generally dependent on the 3D geometry of each eye's ONH connective tissues. Finally, strain is not equally distributed through the ONH, and is concentrated in regions with less dense laminar beams.

This work, while still in its early stages, holds the possibility of testing hypotheses about failure mechanisms and cellular responses at the level of the laminar beams.

OTHER ACUTE, INTRAOCULAR PRESSURE-RELATED CHANGES IN THE OPTIC NERVE HEAD

Optic nerve head, retinal, and choroidal blood flow are all affected in different ways by acute IOP elevations.[35,36] Previous studies using microspheres have suggested that volume flow within the prelaminar and anterior laminar capillary beds is preferentially diminished once ocular perfusion pressure (defined as the systolic arterial blood pressure plus one-third of the difference between systolic and diastolic pressures minus IOP) is less than 30 mmHg.[35,36]

While a direct link to mechanical strain has not been established, axonal transport is compromised in the lamina cribrosa at physiologic levels of IOP[37,38] and is further impaired following acute IOP elevations.[4,39,40] Several hypotheses regarding this behavior emerge when considering ONH biomechanics. First, as the pores in the lamina cribrosa change conformation due to IOP-related mechanical strain, the path of the axons through those pores may be disrupted, thereby directly impeding axoplasmic transport. Secondly, it may be that the IOP-related reduction in blood flow in the laminar region impairs the mitochondrial metabolism that drives axoplasmic transport. Finally, axoplasmic transport could be sensitive to the magnitude of the translaminar pressure gradient, and as that hydrostatic pressure gradient gets larger with increasing IOP (or lower cerebrospinal fluid pressure), the mechanisms driving that transport are unable to overcome the resistance of the pressure gradient (see Fig. 7.7).

In summary, while connective tissue dynamics should, by themselves, directly and indirectly influence astrocyte and glial metabolism and axonal transport, glaucomatous damage within the ONH may not necessarily occur at locations with the highest levels of IOP-related connective tissue strain, but rather at those locations where the translaminar tissue pressure gradient is greatest and/or where the axons, blood supply, and astrocytes and glia have been made most vulnerable. Further studies are necessary to elucidate the link(s) between IOP, mechanical strain, blood flow, astrocyte and glial cell homeostasis, and axoplasmic transport in the ONH, in both the physiologic and diseased states.

RESTRUCTURING AND REMODELING OF THE OPTIC NERVE HEAD

NORMAL AGING

The ONH connective tissues are exposed to substantial levels of IOP-related stress and strain at normal levels of IOP (see Fig. 7.7). The authors believe that physiologic levels of stress and strain experienced over a lifetime induce a broad spectrum of changes in both the connective tissues and vasculature that are central to

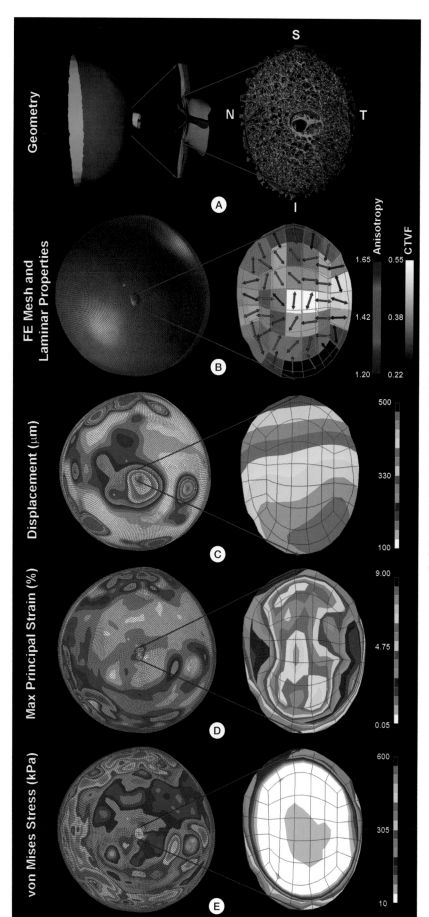

FIGURE 7.12 Construction and results from a macroscale continuum finite element (FE) model of the posterior scleral shell and optic nerve head (ONH) of a normal monkey eye. **(A)** To construct the model geometry, the 3D-delineated lamina cribrosa and surrounding peripapillary sclera (see Fig. 7.8) of an individual eye are incorporated into a generic anatomic scleral shell with regional thickness variations mapped from previous histologic measurements.[15,16] The segmented 3D reconstruction of the laminar connective tissue (shown) is represented in each model. **(B)** A continuum FE mesh of the posterior pole is generated from the geometry. The sclera in this model is assigned uniform isotropic material properties based on previous experimental testing.[35] The continuum elements representing the porous load-bearing laminar architecture are assigned anisotropic material properties that reflect the microstructure of the lamina enclosed by each laminar FE. This material property description is defined using a combination of the connective tissue volume fraction (CTVF) and the predominant laminar beam orientation. A visualization of the CTVF and predominant beam orientation are presented. Note that in this visualization an anisotropy value of 1 would represent an isotropic material with no predominant orientation, while larger values imply oriented laminar beams that impart higher stiffness in the direction of the plotted arrow. **(C–E)** FE results showing predicted displacement, strain, and stress distributions due to an increase in intraocular pressure (IOP) from 10 to 45 mmHg. Note that in this eye, the model predicts that the ONH tilts inferiorly, the strains are highest along the superior-inferior axis of the ONH, and that the sclera bears most of the IOP-related stress.

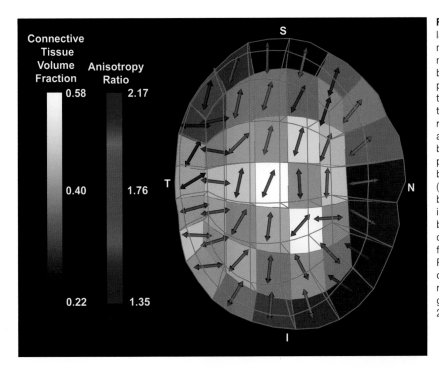

FIGURE 7.13 Regional differences in laminar microarchitecture in a normal monkey eye. Characterization of the laminar microarchitecture utilizes the element boundaries of a continuum finite mesh to partition the lamina cribrosa connective tissue into 45 subregions. The connective tissue volume fraction (CTVF) for each region is expressed as a percentage and mapped to a gray-scale value in the background. The arrows indicate the predominant orientation of the laminar beams in each region, with higher values (color coded) indicating regions in which the beams are more highly oriented. Note that in the peripheral regions of the lamina, the beams are tethered radially into the scleral canal wall. (Reproduced with permission from Yang H, Downs JC, Burgoyne CF. Physiologic intereye differences in monkey optic nerve head architecture and their relation to changes in early experimental glaucoma. Invest Ophthalmol Vis Sci 2009;50:224–234.)

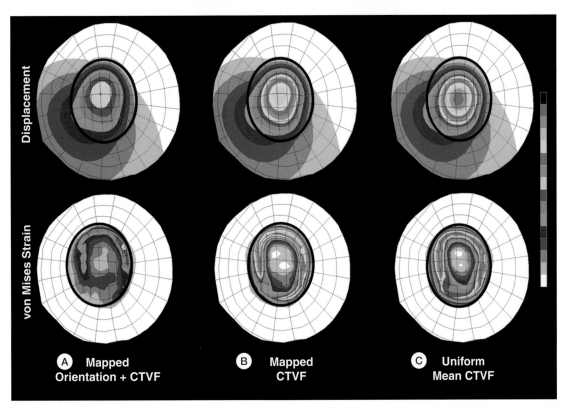

FIGURE 7.14 Incorporation of laminar beam orientation and connective tissue volume fraction (CTVF) into the material description of the lamina cribrosa affects the predictions of finite element (FE) models. Internal (vitreous) surface views of the displacement and strain in the optic nerve head (ONH) (*within the heavy black outline*) and peripapillary sclera in continuum models of the same eye following acute intraocular pressure (IOP) elevation. In column (**A**), the stiffness of each laminar element is determined from both the predominant laminar beam orientation and CTVF of the contained lamina. In column (**B**) the orientation information (i.e. using an isotropic material stiffness), but retaining mapped CTVF, produces a substantial increase in the displacement of the lamina with markedly higher strains. In column (**C**) all elements in the lamina are assigned the same isotropic material stiffness based on an average CTVF (with no beam orientation information). This model has slightly more central laminar displacement than case (**B**), but actually has lower strain in the superior lamina cribrosa owing to the fact that the superior elements in case (**B**) had lower CTVFs in that region (i.e. below the mean CTVF). These results suggest that representing regional laminar microarchitecture in FE models is essential to accurately predict ONH biomechanical behavior.

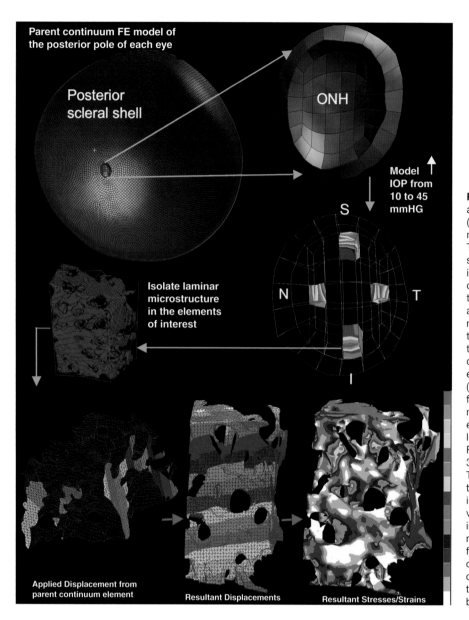

FIGURE 7.15 Construction and analysis of micro-finite element (FE) models of the laminar microarchitecture of a monkey eye. The complexity of the stresses and strains at the laminar beam level is not captured in the macroscale continuum FE models because the details of the microstructure are homogenized into a bulk material description. To address this limitation, a substructuring technique has been developed to characterize the beam-level strain environment within optic nerve head (ONH) models. The displacement field calculated from a continuum model is used along with individual element boundaries to define input loading conditions for microscale FE models of subregions of the 3D reconstructed lamina cribrosa. These micro-FE models illustrate that the stress and strain borne by the individual laminar beams are highly variable and complex. Modeling of individual beam mechanics will be necessary to predict the yield and failure of individual beams, model changes in blood flow in the laminar capillaries, and determine the strains to which the laminar astrocyte basement membrane are subjected.

normal aging. Thus, the restructuring and remodeling of glaucomatous damage (described in the following sections) should be understood to occur in the setting of the physiologic restructuring and remodeling inherent in normal aging.

Age-related alterations of the laminar ECM have been reported to include increased collagen deposition, thickening of astrocyte basement membranes, and increased rigidity of the lamina and sclera.[41-43] The aged ONH is thus more likely to have stiff connective tissues. Age-related hardening of the laminar ECM not only stiffens the connective tissues but also it should diminish nutrient diffusion from the laminar capillaries through the laminar ECM, across the astrocyte basement membranes, and into the adjacent axons (see Fig. 7.1). Thus, in addition to the effects of age-related decreases in the volume flow within the laminar capillaries, axonal nutrition in the aged eye may be further impaired as a result of diminished nutrient diffusion from the laminar capillaries to the center of the axon bundles.

ALTERATIONS IN CONNECTIVE TISSUE ARCHITECTURE, CELLULAR ACTIVITY, AXOPLASMIC TRANSPORT, AND BLOOD FLOW IN EARLY GLAUCOMA

Pathophysiologic stress and strain induce pathologic changes in cell synthesis and tissue microarchitecture that exceed the effects of aging and underlie the two governing pathophysiologies in glaucoma: (1) mechanical yield and/or failure of the load-bearing connective tissues of the ONH (Fig. 7.16; see also Fig. 7.2), and (2) progressive damage to the adjacent axons by a variety of mechanisms (see Fig. 7.2).

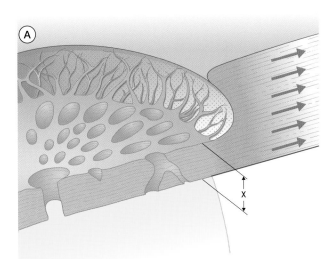

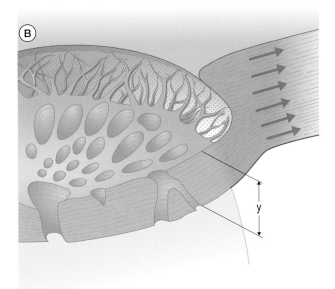

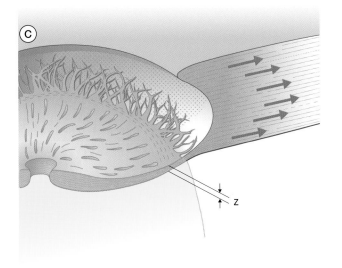

FIGURE 7.16 Progression of connective tissue morphology from normal health to early glaucoma to end-stage glaucoma. **(A)** Diagram of normal optic nerve head (ONH) connective tissue showing the thickness of the lamina cribrosa (x) and the in-wall hoop stress generated by intraocular pressure (IOP) in the peripapillary sclera. **(B)** In early experimental glaucoma, the authors' data to date suggest that rather than catastrophic failure of the laminar beams, there is permanent posterior deformation and thickening (y) of the lamina which occurs in the setting of permanent expansion of the posterior scleral canal. These changes indicate that a combination of mechanical yield and subsequent remodeling of the connective tissues occur very early in glaucoma that is not yet accompanied by physical disruption of the beams or frank excavation. **(C)** As the disease progresses to end-stage damage, the authors believe that the anterior laminar beams eventually fail, the lamina compresses (z) and scars, the laminar insertion into the sclera displaces posteriorly, and the scleral canal enlarges to the typical cupped and excavated morphology. Very little is known about the biomechanics, cellular processes, and remodeling that drives the morphological progression from the earliest detectable stage of glaucoma to end-stage damage, but it is likely that these processes continue to be driven by the distribution of IOP-related stress and strain within the connective tissues either primarily or through their effects on the capillaries contained within the laminar beams and the adjacent astrocytes. (Modified from Burgoyne CF, Downs JC, Bellezza AJ, et al. The optic nerve head as a biomechanical structure: a new paradigm for understanding the role of IOP-related stress and strain in the pathophysiology of glaucomatous optic nerve head damage. Prog Retin Eye Res 2005; 24:39–73.[5])

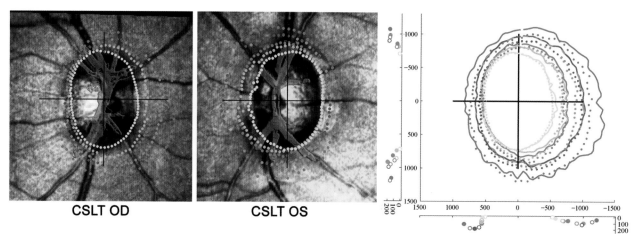

CSLT OD   CSLT OS

FIGURE 7.17 (**Left** and **Middle**) the authors' method of 3D reconstruction and delineation (see Fig. 7.8) includes the central retinal vessels, which allows clinical alignment of the delineated point clouds to clinical images and demonstrates the anatomic expansion of the neural canal under the clinically visible disc margin.[18] Here, just the neural canal landmark points are three-dimensionally overlaid onto Heidelberg retinal tomograph images of the normal (*OD*, **Left**) and early experimental glaucoma (*OS*, **Middle**) eye of a monkey. Note that the clinically visible disk margin in these eyes has been histomorphometrically determined to be Bruch's membrane opening (*yellow dots*) in both eyes. Note also that the neural canal is not the size of the clinical visible disc margin, but rather it enlarges dramatically as it passes through the sclera. Because the data are digital, the left eye data can be converted to right eye orientation and overlaid onto the right eye data as shown (**Right**). Here the early glaucoma (*solid line*) and normal (*dotted line*) eye data can be directly compared. Note that expansion of the neural canal is present at the onset of early glaucomatous damage in the monkey eye and is greatest in the posterior aspects of the canal. (Reproduced with permission from Downs JC, Yang H, Girkin C, et al. Three dimensional histomorphometry of the normal and early glaucomatous monkey optic nerve head: neural canal and subarachnoid space architecture. Invest Ophthalmol Vis Sci. 2007;48:3195–3208.)

Early glaucomatous damage has not been rigorously studied in humans because human cadaver eyes with well-characterized early damage are rare. In monkeys, following moderate experimental IOP elevations, the authors have described the following changes in ONH and peripapillary scleral connective tissue architecture and material properties at the onset of confocal scanning laser tomography-detected ONH surface change (clinical cupping): (1) enlargement and elongation of the neural canal (Fig. 7.17); (2) posterior deformation and thickening of the lamina cribrosa accompanied by mild posterior deformation of the scleral flange and peripapillary sclera (Fig. 7.18); (3) hypercompliance of the lamina in some cases; and (4) alteration in the viscoelastic material properties of the peripapillary sclera.[24] These findings are accompanied by prelaminar neural tissue thickening and are summarized in Figure 7.19.[18,20,44]

The increase in laminar thickness in these early-glaucoma monkey eyes is likely a combination of axonal swelling, tissue edema, gliosis, connective tissue remodeling, and new connective tissue synthesis. Preliminary quantification of the amount of connective tissue within the authors' 3D reconstructions of the lamina suggests an increase in connective tissue volume of 50–100% in early glaucoma (Fig. 7.20). These data strongly support the notion that connective tissue remodeling, and new connective tissue synthesis, are present at this early stage of the neuropathy.

Alterations in cellular activity, axoplasmic transport, and blood flow in early glaucoma have not been rigorously studied. However, in a recent study in rat eyes (which has a very minimal lamina cribrosa) Johnson et al. used genomic techniques to characterize the alterations in the genome of ONH tissues following 5 weeks' exposure to elevated IOP.[45] Within the large group of animals studied, a subset of eyes had an early 'focal' stage of orbital optic nerve axon loss. Within these animals, expression of genes governing initiation of cell division was maximally elevated (compared to later stages of damage) as well as the genes for several ECM components, including fibulin 2, tenascin C, and the matrix metalloproteinase inhibitor TIMP-1. While gene expression for TGF-β_1 increased linearly with severity of damage in all studied eyes, gene expression for transforming growth factor (TGF)-β_2 was lowest in the focally damaged eyes, suggesting differential expression of TGF-β isoforms at this early stage of the neuropathy. Similar to TGF-β_2, gene expression for the principal water channel protein in astrocytes, aquaporin-4, demonstrated the largest degree of downregulation in focal damage. Most importantly, Johnson and co-workers characterized gene expression patterns in a group of eyes 2-weeks after optic nerve transection eyes and found a pattern of expression similar to the most severely damaged high IOP eyes, suggesting that the changes in gene expression in the focal group were likely IOP-related, not simply a reflection of early axonal loss.

ALTERATIONS IN CONNECTIVE TISSUE ARCHITECTURE, CELLULAR ACTIVITY, AXOPLASMIC TRANSPORT, AND BLOOD FLOW IN LATER STAGES OF GLAUCOMATOUS DAMAGE

The classic descriptions of profound laminar deformation, excavation of the scleral canal beneath the optic disc margin, compression, and increased rigidity of the lamina are largely based upon human and monkey

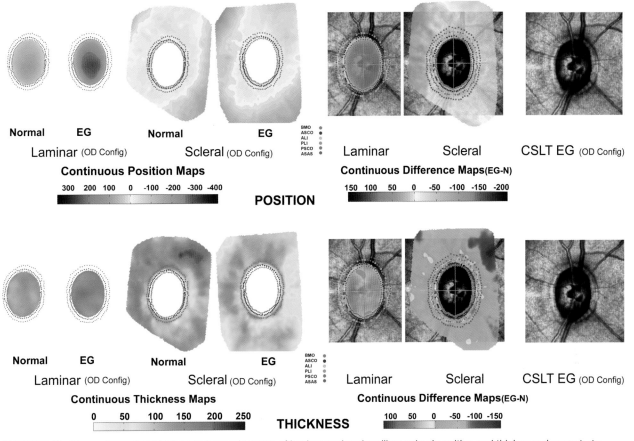

FIGURE 7.18 Three-dimensional histomorphometric maps of laminar and peripapillary scleral position and thickness demonstrate profound permanent posterior deformation of the lamina cribrosa and peripapillary sclera and thickening of the lamina cribrosa in the early-glaucoma eye of one monkey.[19] Laminar and peripapillary scleral position (*above*) and thickness (*below*) are co-localized with the neural canal landmark points for both the normal and early-glaucoma eyes of one monkey (*left four columns*). Early-glaucoma eye difference maps for each parameter are shown in the first two columns to the right, followed by a confocal scanning laser tomograph (CSLT) image of the early glaucoma (EG) eye prior to sacrifice for orientation. These maps are typical for early glaucomatous changes in the monkey eye and demonstrate the permanent posterior deformation of the lamina and immediate peripapillary sclera, as well as the marked thickening of the lamina in the glaucoma eye compared to its contralateral control. (Reproduced with permission from Yang H, Downs JC, Girkin C, et al.. 3-D histomorphometry of the normal and early glaucomatous monkey optic nerve head: lamina cribrosa and peripapillary scleral position and thickness. Invest Ophthalmol Vis Sci. 2007;48:4597–4607.)

eyes with moderate, severe, and end-stage glaucomatous damage.[46–48] Because these studies describe a broad range of damage that has occurred in response to an IOP insult that is uncharacterized in magnitude and duration, a common description of events has yet to emerge. However, astrocyte basement membrane disruption and thickening as well as damage to elastin, physical disruption of the laminar beams, and remodeling of the ECM are consistent phenomenon within these reports.[47,49,50] It is assumed that IOP-induced alterations in the synthetic activities of the cells associated with these tissues underlie these changes.[51–53]

Within the more severely damaged eyes in Johnson's study, expression of genes governing initiation of cell division were also elevated (compared to normals) but to a lesser degree than in eyes with focal damage. Genes associated with activation of microglia, immune response, ribosomes, and lysosomes were all linearly elevated in the more severely damaged eyes. Genes for the ECM components including fibulin 2, tenascin C, and the matrix metalloproteinase inhibitor TIMP-1

were elevated nonlinearly (most elevated in early damage, less elevated in more severe) while genes for periostin, collagen IV, and collagen VI were elevated linearly. Differential gene expression for TGF-β_1 and TGF-β_2, as well as nonlinear expression of aquaporin, are described above.

Axoplasmic transport alterations at the lamina cribrosa[54] and a complicated array of ONH, retinal, and choroidal blood flow alterations[55,56] have been described following chronic IOP elevation in monkey and human eyes. However, direct observation of ONH blood flow at the level of the peripapillary sclera and lamina cribrosa capillaries is not yet possible either experimentally or clinically. Thus, it is not possible to study primary interactions between IOP and non-IOP-induced alterations in ONH blood flow, ONH connective tissue integrity, ONH glial cell activity, and RGC axonal transport within individual human and animal eyes.

Integrins are mechanotransduction proteins that span the laminar astrocyte and capillary endothelial cell basement membranes to bind to ligands in the

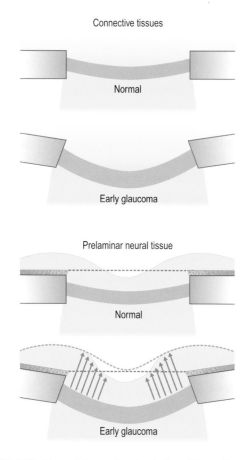

FIGURE 7.19 Remodeling and restructuring of the optic nerve head (ONH) in early experimental glaucoma. Sagittal section diagrams of the ONH, showing the peripapillary sclera (*gray*) and the lamina cribrosa for normal and early glaucoma eyes. **(Top)** The early glaucoma eye has undergone permanent changes in ONH geometry, including thickening of the lamina, posterior deformation of the lamina and peripapillary sclera, and posterior scleral canal expansion. **(Bottom)** Recent work has also shown[20] that although the cup deepens relative to Bruch's membrane opening (*dotted pink line*) as can be detected by longitudinal confocal scanning laser tomography imaging (*pink line*) in early glaucoma, the prelaminar neural tissues (*yellow*) are actually thickened rather than thinned. (Yang H, Downs JC, Bellezza AJ, et al. 3D histomorphometry of the normal and early glaucomatous monkey optic nerve head: prelaminar neural tissues and cupping. Invest Ophthalmol Vis Sci 2007; 48:5068–5084.[20])

ECM and interact with the cell cytoskeleton. Morrison has described the location and alteration of integrin subunits in normal and glaucomatous human and monkey eyes,[57] and proposed them as an important link between laminar deformation and damage, laminar connective tissue remodeling, and laminar astrocyte-mediated axonal insult in glaucoma.

BIOMECHANICAL MANIPULATION OF OPTIC NERVE HEAD AND PERIPAPILLARY SCLERAL CELLS IN CULTURE

Laminar astrocytes have been shown to respond to changes in hydrostatic or barometric pressure.[58]

However, the uncertain role of hypoxia and lack of astrocyte basement membrane deformation in the barometric pressure model has led to genomic and biochemical characterization of ONH astrocytes exposed to controlled levels of strain.[59,60] At present, these strain-based techniques are in their infancy and a consistent stimulation cycle and pattern of gene and protein expression has yet to emerge. Eventually, strain predictions from FE models and data on IOP fluctuation from telemetric IOP monitoring studies will allow these experiments to more closely model physiologic/pathophysiologic conditions in the normal and glaucomatous human and animal eye.

FUTURE DIRECTIONS

CLINICAL IMPLICATIONS

There are currently no science-based tools to predict at what level of IOP an individual ONH will be damaged. As described herein, FE modeling is a computational tool for predicting how a biological tissue of complicated geometry and material properties will behave under varying levels of load. The goal of basic research FE modeling in monkey and human cadaver eyes is to learn what aspects of ONH neural, vascular, and connective tissue architecture are most important to the ability of a given ONH to maintain structural integrity, nutritional and oxygen supply, and axoplasmic transport at physiologic and nonphysiologic levels of IOP. In the future, clinical imaging of the ONH will seek to capture the architecture of these structures so as to allow clinically derived biomechanical models of individual patient ONHs to make predictions regarding physiologic and pathophysiologic levels of IOP. Eventually, knowing the relationship between IOP, mechanical strain, systemic blood pressure, and the resultant astrocyte and axonal mitochondrial oxygen levels will drive the clinical assessment of safe target IOP. Clinical characterization of the actual IOP insult through telemetric IOP monitoring will eventually allow better-controlled studies of ONH-directed neuroprotection. Finally, these FE modeling-driven targets for deep (subsurface) ONH imaging will likely allow early detection of lamina cribrosa deformation and thickening. Once clinically detectable, early stabilization, and perhaps reversal, of these laminar changes will become a new end point for target IOP lowering in most ocular hypertensive and all progressing eyes.

BASIC RESEARCH DIRECTIONS

From an engineering standpoint, large challenges remain to achieve basic and clinical knowledge regarding: (1) the mechanisms and distributions of IOP-related yield and failure in the laminar beams and peripapillary sclera; (2) the mechanobiology of the astrocytes, scleral fibroblasts, and lamina cribrosa and

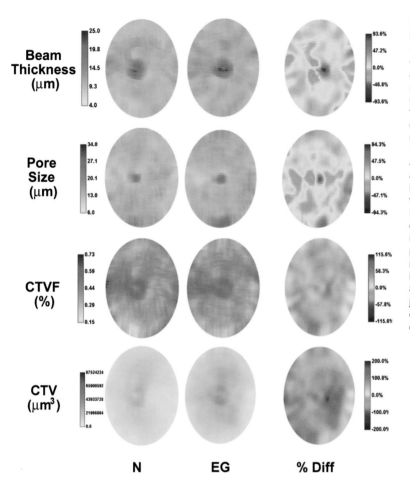

N   **EG**   **% Diff**

FIGURE 7.20 Three-dimensional (3D) histomorphometric maps of laminar microarchitecture in paired normal (N) and early-glaucoma (EG) eyes for three monkeys. **(Left and Center)** Maps of laminar beam thickness, pore size, connective tissue volume fraction (CTVF), and connective tissue volume (CTV) for contralateral normal and early-glaucoma eyes of a monkey derived from the same 3D reconstruction technique described in Figure 7.8. **(Right)** The differences between the normal and early glaucoma eyes for each parameter are mapped as a percentage. Note that CTVF is a ratio of laminar connective tissue volume to total tissue volume in each regional sample. In early glaucoma, the CTVF and total laminar connective tissue volume increase significantly in all regions, and laminar beam thickness and pore size increase in most regions but decrease in others. These results together indicate that the increase in laminar thickness described in Figure 8.18 in early experimental glaucoma is due not just to axonal swelling or tissue edema but also contains a very substantial component of laminar connective tissue synthesis.

glial cells; (3) the mechanobiology of axoplasmic flow and within the lamina cribrosa; (4) the fluid dynamics governing the volume flow of blood within the laminar capillaries and scleral and laminar branches of the posterior ciliary arteries; and (5) nutrient diffusion to the astrocytes in young and aged eyes. The authors predict that knowledge gained from these studies will importantly contribute to new therapeutic interventions aimed at the ONH and peripapillary sclera of glaucomatous eyes.

REFERENCES

1. Yucel YH, Zhang Q, Weinreb RN, et al. Effects of retinal ganglion cell loss on magno-, parvo-, koniocellular pathways in the lateral geniculate nucleus and visual cortex in glaucoma. Prog Retin Eye Res 2003; 22:465–481.

2. Kendell KR, Quigley HA, Kerrigan LA, et al. Primary open-angle glaucoma is not associated with photoreceptor loss. Invest Ophthalmol Vis Sci 1995; 36:200–205.

3. Panda S, Jonas JB. Decreased photoreceptor count in human eyes with secondary angle-closure glaucoma. Invest Ophthalmol Vis Sci 1992; 33:2532–2536.

4. Minckler DS, Bunt AH, Johanson GW. Orthograde and retrograde axoplasmic transport during acute ocular hypertension in the monkey. Invest Ophthalmol Vis Sci 1977; 16:426–441.

5. Burgoyne CF, Downs JC, Bellezza AJ, et al. The optic nerve head as a biomechanical structure: a new paradigm for understanding the role of IOP-related stress and strain in the pathophysiology of glaucomatous optic nerve head damage. Prog Retin Eye Res 2005; 24:39–73.

6. Ethier CR, Simmons CA. Introductory biomechanics: from cells to organisms. 1st edn. New York: Cambridge University Press; 2007.

7. Timoshenko SP. Theory of elasticity. 3rd edn. New York: McGraw-Hill; 1970.

8. Downs JC, Ensor ME, Bellezza AJ, et al. Posterior scleral thickness in perfusion-fixed normal and early-glaucoma monkey eyes. Invest Ophthalmol Vis Sci 2001; 42:3202–3208.

9. Downs JC, Blidner RA, Bellezza AJ, et al. Peripapillary scleral thickness in perfusion-fixed normal monkey eyes. Invest Ophthalmol Vis Sci 2002; 43:2229–2235.

10. Quigley HA, Addicks EM. Regional differences in the structure of the lamina cribrosa and their relation to glaucomatous optic nerve damage. Arch Ophthalmol 1981; 99:137–143.

11. Radius RL. Regional specificity in anatomy at the lamina cribrosa. Arch Ophthalmol 1981; 99:478–480.

12. Roberts MD, Hart RT, Liang Y, et al. Continuum-level finite element modeling of the optic nerve head using a fabric tensor based description of the lamina cribrosa. ASME Summer Bioengineering Conference. Keystone, CO: American Society of Mechanical Engineers; 2007.

13. Morgan WH, Chauhan BC, Yu D-Y, et al. Optic disc movement with variations in intraocular and cerebrospinal fluid pressure. Invest Ophthalmol Vis Sci 2002; 43:3236–3242.

14. Yan DB, Coloma FM, Metheetrairut A, et al. Deformation of the lamina cribrosa by elevated intraocular pressure. Br J Ophthalmol 1994; 78:643–648.

15. Crapps EE, Levy NS. Displacement of the lamina scleralis with pressure elevation. Invest Ophthalmol Vis Sci 1981; 20:82.

16. Bellezza AJ, Rintalan CJ, Thompson HW, et al. Deformation of the lamina cribrosa and anterior scleral canal wall in early experimental glaucoma. Invest Ophthalmol Vis Sci 2003; 44:623–637.

17. Burgoyne CF, Downs JC, Bellezza AJ, et al. Three-dimensional reconstruction of normal and early glaucoma monkey optic nerve head connective tissues. Invest Ophthalmol Vis Sci 2004; 45:4388–4399.

18. Downs JC, Yang H, Girkin C, et al. Three dimensional histomorphometry of the normal and early glaucomatous monkey optic nerve head: neural canal and subarachnoid space architecture. Invest Ophthalmol Vis Sci 2007; 48:3195–3208.

19. Yang H, Downs JC, Girkin C, et al. 3D histomorphometry of the normal and early glaucomatous monkey optic nerve head: lamina cribrosa and peripapillary scleral position and thickness. Invest Ophthalmol Vis Sci 2007; 48:4597–4607.

20. Yang H, Downs JC, Bellezza AJ, et al. 3D Histomorphometry of the normal and early glaucomatous monkey optic nerve head: prelaminar neural tissues and cupping. Invest Ophthalmol Vis Sci 2007; 48:5068–5084.

21. Olsen TW, Aaberg SY, Geroski DH, et al. Human sclera: thickness and surface area. Am J Ophthalmol 1998; 125: 237–241.

22. Phillips JR, Khalaj M, McBrien NA. Induced myopia associated with increased scleral creep in chick and tree shrew eyes. Invest Ophthalmol Vis Sci 2000; 41:2028–2034.

23. Woo SL, Kobayashi AS, Schlegel WA, et al. Nonlinear material properties of intact cornea and sclera. Exp Eye Res 1972; 14: 29–39.

24. Downs JC, Suh JK, Thomas KA, et al. Viscoelastic characterization of peripapillary sclera: material properties by quadrant in rabbit and monkey eyes. J Biomech Eng 2003; 125:124–131.

25. Downs JC, Suh JK, Thomas KA, et al. Viscoelastic material properties of the peripapillary sclera in normal and early-glaucoma monkey eyes. Invest Ophthalmol Vis Sci 2005; 46:540–546.

26. Girard M, Downs JC, Burgoyne CF, et al. Nonlinear finite element modeling of monkey posterior sclera under intraocular pressure. ASME Summer Bioengineering Conference. Keystone, CO: American Society of Mechanical Engineers; 2007.

27. Dongqi H, Zeqin R. A biomathematical model for pressure-dependent lamina cribrosa behavior. J Biomech 1999; 32: 579–584.

28. Edwards ME, Good TA. Use of a mathematical model to estimate stress and strain during elevated pressure induced lamina cribrosa deformation. Curr Eye Res 2001; 23:215–225.

29. Sander EA, Downs JC, Hart RT, et al. A cellular solid model of the lamina cribrosa: mechanical dependence on morphology. J Biomech Eng 2006; 128:879–889.

30. Bellezza AJ, Hart RT, Burgoyne CF. The optic nerve head as a biomechanical structure: initial finite element modeling. Invest Ophthalmol Vis Sci 2000; 41:2991–3000.

31. Sigal IA, Flanagan JG, Ethier CR. Factors influencing optic nerve head biomechanics. Invest Ophthalmol Vis Sci 2005; 46:4189–4199.

32. Sigal IA, Flanagan JG, Tertinegg I, et al. Finite element modeling of optic nerve head biomechanics. Invest Ophthalmol Vis Sci 2004; 45:4378–4387.

33. Sigal IA, Flanagan JG, Tertinegg I, et al. Predicted extension, compression and shearing of optic nerve head tissues. Exp Eye Res 2007; 85:312–322.

34. Downs JC, Roberts MD, Burgoyne CF, et al. Finite element modeling of the lamina cribrosa microarchitecture in the normal and early glaucoma monkey optic nerve head. ASME Summer Bioengineering Conference. Keystone, CO: American Society of Mechanical Engineers; 2007.

35. Geijer C, Bill A. Effects of raised intraocular pressure on retinal, prelaminar, laminar, and retrolaminar optic nerve blood flow in monkeys. Invest Ophthalmol Vis Sci 1979; 18:1030–1042.

36. Alm A, Bill A. Ocular and optic nerve blood flow at normal and increased intraocular pressures in monkeys (Macaca irus): a study with radioactively labelled microspheres including flow determinations in brain and some other tissues. Exp Eye Res 1973; 15:15–29.

37. Ernest JT, Potts AM. Pathophysiology of the distal portion of the optic nerve. I. Tissue pressure relationships. Am J Ophthalmol 1968; 66:373–380.

38. Minckler D. Correlations between anatomic features and axonal transport in primate optic nerve head. Trans Am Ophthalmol Soc 1986; 84:429–451.

39. Quigley H, Anderson DR. The dynamics and location of axonal transport blockade by acute intraocular pressure elevation in primate optic nerve. Invest Ophthalmol Vis Sci 1976; 15: 606–616.

40. Quigley HA, Anderson DR. Distribution of axonal transport blockade by acute intraocular pressure elevation in the primate optic nerve head. Invest Ophthalmol Vis Sci 1977; 16:640–644.

41. Albon J, Purslow PP, Karwatowski WS, et al. Age related compliance of the lamina cribrosa in human eyes. Br J Ophthalmol 2000; 84:318–323.

42. Morrison JC, Jerdan JA, Dorman ME, et al. Structural proteins of the neonatal and adult lamina cribrosa. Arch Ophthalmol 1989; 107:1220–1224.

43. Albon J, Karwatowski WS, Avery N, et al. Changes in the collagenous matrix of the aging human lamina cribrosa. Br J Ophthalmol 1995; 79:368–375.

44. Yang H, Downs JC, Girkin C, et al. 3D histomorphometry of the normal and early glaucomatous monkey optic nerve head: lamina cribrosa and peripapillary scleral position and thickness. Invest Ophthalmol Vis Sci 2007; 48:4597–4607.

45. Johnson EC, Jia L, Cepurna WO, et al. Global changes in optic nerve head gene expression after exposure to elevated intraocular pressure in a rat glaucoma model. Invest Ophthalmol Vis Sci 2007; 48:3161–3177.

46. Emery JM, Landis D, Paton D, et al. The lamina cribrosa in normal and glaucomatous human eyes. Trans Am Acad Ophthalmol Otolaryngol 1974; 78:OP290–OP297.

47. Quigley HA, Addicks EM, Green WR, et al. Optic nerve damage in human glaucoma. II. The site of injury and susceptibility to damage. Arch Ophthalmol 1981; 99:635–649.

48. Quigley HA, Hohman RM, Addicks EM, et al. Morphologic changes in the lamina cribrosa correlated with neural loss in open-angle glaucoma. Am J Ophthalmol 1983; 95: 673–691.

49. Quigley HA, Dorman-Pease ME, Brown AE. Quantitative study of collagen and elastin of the optic nerve head and sclera in human and experimental monkey glaucoma. Curr Eye Res 1991; 10:877–888.

50. Hernandez MR, Andrzejewska WM, Neufeld AH. Changes in the extracellular matrix of the human optic nerve head in primary open-angle glaucoma. Am J Ophthalmol 1990; 109:180–188.

51. Hernandez MR, Yang J, Ye H. Activation of elastin mRNA expression in human optic nerve heads with primary open-angle glaucoma. Glaucoma 1994; 3:214–225.

52. Hernandez MR, Ye H, Roy S. Collagen type IV gene expression in human optic nerve heads with primary open angle glaucoma. Exp Eye Res 1994; 59:41–51.

53. Clark AF, Browder SL, Steely HT, et al. Cell biology of the human lamina cribrosa. In: Drance SM, Anderson DR, eds. Optic nerve in glaucoma. Amsterdam/New York: Kugler Publications; 1995:79–105.

54. Quigley HA, Addicks EM. Chronic experimental glaucoma in primates. II. Effect of extended intraocular pressure elevation on optic nerve head and axonal transport. Invest Ophthalmol Vis Sci 1980; 19:137–152.

55. Grunwald JE, Riva CE, Stone RA, et al. Retinal autoregulation in open-angle glaucoma. Ophthalmology 1984; 91:1690–1694.

56. Ulrich WD, Ulrich C, Bohne BD. Deficient autoregulation and lengthening of the diffusion distance in the anterior optic nerve circulation in glaucoma: an electro-encephalo-dynamographic investigation. Ophthalmic Res 1986; 18:253–259.

57. Morrison JC. Integrins in the optic nerve head: potential roles in glaucomatous optic neuropathy (an American Ophthalmological Society thesis). Trans Am Ophthalmol Soc 2006; 104:453–477.

58. Yang JL, Neufeld AH, Zorn MB, et al. Collagen type I mRNA levels in cultured human lamina cribrosa cells: effects of elevated hydrostatic pressure. Exp Eye Res 1993; 56:567–574.

59. Kirwan RP, Fenerty CH, Crean J, et al. Influence of cyclical mechanical strain on extracellular matrix gene expression in human lamina cribrosa cells in vitro. Mol Vis 2005; 11: 798–810.

60. Yamaoka A, Matsuo T, Shiraga F, et al. TIMP-1 production by human scleral fibroblast decreases in response to cyclic mechanical stretching. Ophthalmic Res 2001; 33:98–101.

61. Anderson DR. Ultrastructure of human and monkey lamina cribrosa and optic nerve head. Arch Ophthalmol 1969; 82:800–814.

62. Quigley HA, Brown AE, Morrison JD, et al. The size and shape of the optic disc in normal human eyes. Arch Ophthalmol 1990; 108:51–57.

63. Cioffi GA, Van Buskirk EM. Vasculature of the anterior optic nerve and peripapillary choroid. In: Ritch R, Shields MB, Krupin T, eds. The glaucomas. St. Louis: Mosby; 1996:177–197.

64. Quigley HA. Overview and introduction to session on connective tissue of the optic nerve in glaucoma. In: Drance SM, Anderson DR, eds. Optic nerve in glaucoma. Amsterdam/New York: Kugler Publications; 1995:15–36.

65. Morrison JC, L'Hernault NL, Jerdan JA, et al. Ultrastructural location of extracellular matrix components in the optic nerve head. Arch Ophthalmol 1989; 107:123–129.

Role of Ocular Blood Flow in the Pathogenesis of Glaucoma

Ali S Hafez and Mark R Lesk

INTRODUCTION

Although the clinical picture of glaucoma is well described, the exact mechanism leading to this specific type of damage to the optic nerve head (ONH) is not yet clear. It is generally accepted that the mechanism of damage in glaucoma is almost certainly multifactorial.[1] But while elevated intraocular pressure (IOP) remains the risk factor most commonly associated with glaucomatous optic neuropathy (GON), numerous other variables involved in the development and progression of glaucoma have been identified.[2] Vascular risk factors in particular have been extensively studied. These include systemic blood pressure alterations,[3–5] diabetes[6,7] reduced ocular blood flow (OBF),[8–10] and vasospasm.[11–13]

Conventionally, two theories have been presented for the pathogenesis of glaucoma, pressure and vascular:

- *Pressure theory*, introduced by Muller, supposes that GON is a direct consequence of elevated IOP, damaging the lamina cribrosa and neural axons.
- *Vascular theory*, suggested by von Jaeger, considers GON as a consequence of insufficient blood supply to the ONH due to either elevated IOP or to other risk factors reducing OBF.

Both theories have been vigorously studied and defended by various research groups for over a century.

The role of axoplasmic transport blockage in GON was later introduced by Anderson and Hendrickson in 1974.[14] Retrograde axoplasmic transport is essential for the delivery of many substances necessary for the survival of the retinal ganglion cell (RGC) bodies. Interruption of this process could trigger pathways that lead to RGC death via apoptosis.[15] Obstruction of axoplasmic transport at the level of the lamina cribrosa in response to elevated IOP has been demonstrated in the primate glaucoma model using radioactive tracers.[16,17] It is not yet known to what degree obstruction of axoplasmic flow might be influenced by IOP-dependent blood flow changes in the optic nerve.

Both experimental and clinical studies have proven the role of IOP and the benefits of IOP-lowering therapy in glaucoma. Yet therapeutic IOP reduction was shown to improve the prognosis of glaucoma patients but does not stop progression of the disease. The existence of normal-tension glaucoma (NTG) on the one hand and ocular hypertension (OHT) on the other indicates that other factors might be involved in the pathogenesis of GON either directly or by rendering the eye more sensitive to IOP changes.

FINDINGS OF OCULAR BLOOD FLOW STUDIES IN GLAUCOMA AND THEIR INTERPRETATION

Investigations using epidemiological, histological, and noninvasive clinical techniques point to defective ocular blood flow as an important risk factor in glaucoma. Among the vascular theories, hypoperfusion of the ONH was reported to be caused by atherosclerosis, vasospasm, and systemic blood pressure alterations.[4,12]

Other proposed mechanisms involve abnormal scleral and lamina cribrosa structure,[18–21] abnormal cerebrospinal fluid pressure,[22] and autoimmune mechanisms.[23]

In general, studies have reported slower ocular blood flow velocities in glaucoma patients compared to normals. Blood flow velocities have been found to be lower in the retina, ONH, and choroid as well as in the retro-ocular vessels and in the peripheral circulation. Normal-tension glaucoma patients were shown to have lower blood flow velocities than those with high-tension glaucoma.

The facts that the reduction of OBF has often been observed to precede the damage and that blood flow was shown to be reduced in other parts of the body of glaucoma patients suggest that the hemodynamic alterations may at least partially be primary.[24] Also, given the probable variability in the vascular mechanisms, the observed variability in blood flow reduction is expected.

Studies have also shown that glaucoma patients are more likely to demonstrate ocular as well as systemic vascular changes compared to normal subjects. Such

TABLE 8.1 Ocular vascular findings in glaucoma
Impaired perfusion of the optic nerve head
Impaired circulation in peripapillary retinal arteries
Optic disc hemorrhages
Localized constriction of retinal arteries

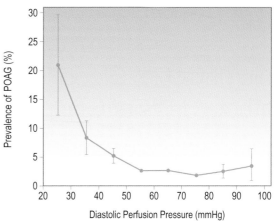

FIGURE 8.1 Systemic vascular findings in glaucoma showing correlation between glaucoma and OPP. There is an epidemiologic link between ocular perfusion pressure and glaucoma. The risk of glaucoma is sixfold for those with the lowest ocular perfusion pressure. (Redrawn from Tielsch JM, Katz J, Sommer A, et al. Hypertension, perfusion pressure and primary open-angle glaucoma. A population-based assessment. Arch Ophthalmol 1995; 113:216–221.)

observations could well point to an underlying vascular mechanism for glaucomatous optic neuropathy.

OCULAR VASCULAR CHANGES IN GLAUCOMA

A number of ocular signs point indirectly to the fact that at least in some glaucoma patients, blood flow plays an important role (Table 8.1). Changes in conjunctival capillaries (e.g. perilimbal aneurysms), localized constriction of peripapillary retinal arteries,[25] increased prevalence of disc hemorrhages,[26] preservation of nerve fibers around retinal vessels,[27] and the possible significance of cilioretinal arteries[28] have all been described in glaucoma patients.

Studies have also shown that glaucoma patients are twice as likely to have crescent-shaped RPE and/or choroidal atrophic changes at the disc margin which might be attributed to ischemia.[29]

SYSTEMIC VASCULAR FINDINGS IN GLAUCOMA

Epidemiologic links have been reported between ocular perfusion pressure (OPP) and glaucoma (Baltimore Eye Survey,[3] Rotterdam Eye Study,[30] Egna-Neumarkt Eye Study,[31] Barbados Eye Study[32]). In the Baltimore Eye Survey, there was a sixfold risk of glaucoma for those with the lowest ocular perfusion pressure (Fig. 8.1).

The Collaborative Normal Tension Glaucoma Study[33] demonstrated a highly significant association between the rate of progression and the presence of migraines in normal-tension glaucoma patients. Studies have also reported exaggerated nocturnal blood pressure dips in open-angle glaucoma (OAG) and NTG patients with progressive field loss. It was hypothesized that such dips might compromise perfusion of the ONH.[5,34]

INTERPRETATION OF OCULAR BLOOD FLOW STUDIES

Findings of ocular blood flow studies in glaucoma are difficult to interpret for various reasons:[24] authors use different techniques and therefore measure different aspects of ocular circulation; they include glaucoma patients at different stages, e.g. early versus late; different types of glaucoma are studied, e.g. normal-tension glaucoma versus high-tension glaucoma; and some studies include provocation tests while others do not. Consequently, the interpretation of the available data is difficult and blood flow reduction may, at least partly, be secondary to a reduced demand. Furthermore, blood flow alterations have been described in various parts of

the ocular circulation and it remains unclear how circulatory disorders in parts of the eye other than the anterior optic nerve may affect survival of axons and retinal ganglion cells. Finally, the influence of additional factors such as systemic blood pressure, vasospasm, vascular dysregulation, and plasma levels of vasoactive agents such as endothelin-1 remain to be clarified.

POTENTIAL MECHANISMS OF OCULAR BLOOD FLOW REDUCTION IN GLAUCOMA PATIENTS

Theoretically, there are three components contributing to ocular blood flow reduction in glaucoma patients: (1) increased local resistance to flow, (2) decreased ocular perfusion pressure (OPP), and (3) increased blood viscosity.

Several indications point to the role of both increased local resistance to flow and decreased ocular perfusion pressure in the development and progression of glaucoma:

LOCAL RESISTANCE TO BLOOD FLOW

Increased resistance to blood flow is manifested as reduced vascular diameter and is affected by either structural changes due to anatomic variations in the vessels, vasculitis, or mechanical obstruction of the lumen (via thrombosis or arteriosclerosis) or functional changes such as abnormal or defective autoregulation of blood flow. Reduced vascular diameter can also be due to reversible spasm of the smooth muscle cells in the vessel wall.

OCULAR PERFUSION PRESSURE

Ocular perfusion pressure equals mean arterial blood pressure minus venous blood pressure in a specific vascular bed. Normally, venous pressure is slightly higher than

IOP and for practical purposes IOP is a good indicator of the venous pressure. Therefore, OPP can be considered as the difference between mean arterial blood pressure and IOP (where mean arterial blood pressure = diastolic blood pressure + {1/3} [systolic blood pressure − diastolic blood pressure]). Reduced ocular perfusion pressure might be attributed to either increased IOP or decreased systemic blood pressure or to both.

During the past four decades an increasing amount of evidence was found to support each of the above theories hypothesized to play a crucial role in the pathogenesis of glaucomatous optic neuropathy.

Studies by Hayreh[35–37] have shown a close association between glaucomatous optic neuropathy and systemic vascular disorders such as hypertension, hypercholesterolemia, cardiovascular diseases, and diabetes. Hayreh[38] hypothesized that serotonin released from carotid, ophthalmic, and posterior cerebral arteries in atherosclerotic patients produces transient vasospasms of the ONH and thus contributes to the development and progression of glaucomatous optic neuropathy and in particular NTG. In their analysis of optic nerve blood flow abnormalities in glaucoma, Flammer and Orgul[24] considered arteriosclerosis as a less important factor for increased local resistance to blood flow which contributes to defective optic nerve perfusion. Although experimental studies by Hayreh et al.[39] indicated that arteriosclerosis might increase the sensitivity to IOP elevations, and although some arteriosclerotic patients were shown to present with a sclerotic type of glaucoma,[38] Flammer and Orgul[24] believed there was currently very little evidence linking glaucomatous optic neuropathy to arteriosclerosis or its risk factors (gender, obesity, hypercholesterolemia, smoking, diabetes, hypertension, carotid stenosis). They attributed increased local resistance to blood flow to a functional rather than a structural change, namely to abnormal or defective autoregulation of blood flow.

Autoregulation refers to the capacity of an organ or tissue to regulate its blood supply in accordance with its functional or metabolic needs. With intact autoregulation, changes in ocular perfusion pressure or metabolic demands are associated with local constriction or dilatation of the terminal arterioles, which causes vascular resistance to increase or decrease, thereby maintaining a constant supply of oxygen and nutrients to the tissues. Conversely, abnormal autoregulation could be expressed not only as an excessive arterial constriction (vasospasm) but also as an inadequate arterial dilatation.[40] Observations by Drance and co-workers[13] have confirmed an increased prevalence of vasospasm in patients with NTG.

Optic nerve blood flow was also reported to be influenced by systemic blood pressure.

NTG patients were reported to have a clearly increased prevalence of systemic hypotension. Lower systemic blood pressure, both systolic and diastolic, was also found, particularly during the night, in patients with progressive glaucoma compared to stable patients (Fig. 8.2).[34] This association between glaucomatous damage and low blood pressure has been confirmed by

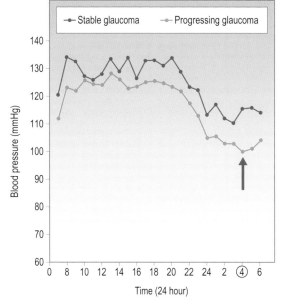

FIGURE 8.2 Nocturnal hypertension in progressive visual field loss. Lower levels of blood pressure were found, particularly during the night, in patients with progressive glaucoma (*arrow*) compared to stable patients. (Redrawn from Graham SL, Drance SM, Wijsman K, et al. Ambulatory blood pressure monitoring in glaucoma. The nocturnal dip. Ophthalmology 1995; 102:61–69.)

several authors.[41–43] Consequently, there is little doubt that low blood pressure is an essential risk factor as is increased IOP.

Increased systemic blood pressure, on the other hand, was reported to shift the autoregulatory plateau to a higher level compared to normals. This adaptation improves the person's tolerance to hypertension but at the same time makes the individual less tolerant to low systemic blood pressure and more susceptible to an immediate and permanent damage from ischemia. Consequently, patients with chronic hypertension are considered to be at greater risk for cerebral or coronary ischemia as well as for GON when subjected to reduced OPP.[4] In general, epidemiologic studies suggest that systemic hypertension is protective against glaucoma in younger patients (presumably through improved OPP) but deleterious in older patients (presumably through atherosclerosis or loss of autoregulation).[3]

INCREASED BLOOD VISCOSITY

Finally, the contribution of hypercoagulability states to GON has been investigated by several authors. Drance et al.[1] found a relative hyperviscosity in NTG patients, though this was not confirmed by subsequent publications.[44,45] A study by O'Brien et al.[46] reported activation of coagulation cascades and fibrinolysis pathways in untreated OAG compared with controls. Hamard et al.,[47] using a laser Doppler velocimeter, found decreased blood flow in NTG and also increased red cell aggregability. It can be concluded that although as yet there is no consistent evidence as to the presence of an abnormal rheology in NTG, the presence of abnormalities should be considered in each NTG patient.

TABLE 8.2 Summary of ocular blood flow assessment techniques and the respective perfusion parameters measured

TECHNIQUE	MEASURED PERFUSION PARAMETER
Color Doppler imaging	Blood velocities used to calculate resistive index in retrobulbar vessels
Pulsatile ocular blood flow	Change in ocular volume used to calculate the pulsatile component of ocular blood flow mostly from the choroid
Fluorescein/ICG angiography	Parameters from both retinal and choroidal vasculature (AVP times, capillary velocities)
Laser Doppler velocimetry	Velocity at the center of a single major vessel of the ONH and retina
Laser Doppler flowmetry	Blood flow in capillary beds of the rim, cup, and choroid in relative units
Scanning laser Doppler flowmetry	Blood flow in capillary beds of neuroretinal rim and peripapillary retina in relative units
Laser speckle technique	Retinal and superficial ONH blood velocities used for the quantification of flow
Retinal vessel analyzer	Continuous on-line measurement of the diameter of a segment of a retinal vessel in relative units
Canon laser blood flowmeter	Blood column diameter, blood velocity, and blood flow in a major retinal vessel in μL/min

CURRENT EVIDENCE OF ABNORMAL OCULAR BLOOD FLOW IN GLAUCOMA

Evidence that defective perfusion of the ONH plays an important role in the pathogenesis of glaucomatous optic neuropathy has been accumulating over the past four decades. Studies have reported strong associations between GON and systemic blood pressure alterations, diabetes, cardiovascular and cerebrovascular disorders, vasospastic responses, age, hypercoagulability states, and increased local resistance to flow.

Recent technical advances have made possible the quantification of blood flow in different intraocular tissues as well as of retrobulbar and peripheral blood flow (Table 8.2). A description of the currently available OBF assessment techniques, their advantages, and limitations has been detailed in Chapter 21.

The following section reviews briefly the current evidence of the role of defective perfusion of the ONH, retina, and choroid as well as the various vascular factors involved in the pathogenesis of GON.

IMPAIRED OPTIC NERVE HEAD, RETINAL, AND CHOROIDAL BLOOD FLOW IN GLAUCOMA

Some of the main evidence implicating blood flow deficits in glaucoma is derived from fluorescein angiography.[48,49] These studies have shown delayed retinal circulation as well as impaired perfusion of the ONH, peripapillary retina, and choroid in glaucoma patients. The severity of perfusion defects progresses with the severity of glaucoma and the defects correlate well with visual field loss and nerve fiber layer dropouts.[49]

Techniques using color Doppler imaging[50,51] and pulsatile ocular blood flow[52,53] have demonstrated that both retrobulbar blood flow and bulk choroidal blood flow are reduced in glaucoma patients in contrast to normal subjects. Using single-point laser Doppler flowmetry, several authors reported decreased blood flow in the ONH of OAG when compared to control subjects[54] and to glaucoma suspects.[55]

Scanning laser Doppler flowmetry (SLDF) was also used for several comparisons between flow measurements in OAG patients and normal subjects. Michelson and associates[56] reported that both neuroretinal rim blood flow and peripapillary retinal blood flow were significantly decreased in OAG patients compared to controls. Neuroretinal rim blood flow was less by 71% while peripapillary retinal flow was less by 49%. Findl and associates[10] reported reduced blood flow in both the disc cup (−46%) and the neuroretinal rim (−18%) in patients with OAG when compared to control subjects. Nicolela et al.[57] reported a significant decrease in blood flow in the lamina cribrosa in OAG patients compared to control subjects.

SLDF has also been used to compare ONH and retinal perfusion between OAG patients and ocular hypertensives. Kerr and associates[58] reported reduced blood flow in the lamina cribrosa and the temporal neuroretinal rim of glaucoma patients in comparison to ocular hypertensives. Using full-field perfusion image analysis, Hafez et al.[59] reported a significantly lower neuroretinal rim blood flow in OAG patients when compared to both OHT patients and normal subjects, with no significant difference between ocular hypertensives and normals.

IMPROVEMENTS IN OCULAR BLOOD FLOW FOLLOWING THERAPEUTIC INTRAOCULAR PRESSURE REDUCTION

Ocular perfusion has been evaluated in both glaucoma patients and ocular hypertensives in response to sustained therapeutic IOP reduction.

The ability of topical antiglaucoma medications to alter perfusion has been reported by different authors using different methods to assess different aspects of ocular circulation.[60–63] Investigators have also reported improved ocular perfusion following sustained IOP reduction in glaucoma patients following surgery. Color Doppler imaging demonstrated significant improvements

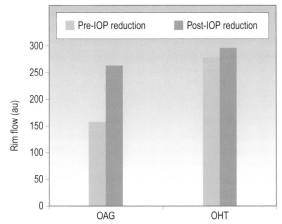

FIGURE 8.3 Scanning laser Doppler flowmetry measurements for the parameter flow in OAG and OHT groups before and after therapeutic IOP reduction. (From Hafez AS, Bizzarro RLG, Rivard M, Lesk MR. Changes in optic nerve head blood flow after therapeutic intraocular pressure reduction in glaucoma patients and ocular hypertensives. Ophthalmology 2003; 110(1):201–210.)

in retrobulbar hemodynamics following trabeculectomy in patients with glaucoma.[64] Pulsatile ocular blood flow measurements similarly demonstrated a significant increase (+29%) in ocular blood flow following reduction of IOP post-trabeculectomy.[65]

Changes in ONH and retinal blood flow were also examined by Hafez et al. using SLDF.[66] The study was performed on OAG patients who required therapeutic IOP reductions and using ocular hypertensives as a control group. Following a similar percentage of therapeutic IOP reduction, rim blood flow did not change in the OHT group while in the OAG group it demonstrated a significant increase of 67% (Fig. 8.3).

The reported changes suggest evidence consistent with the hypothesis concerning defective autoregulation of the ONH blood flow in glaucoma patients. They also demonstrate the close relationship between neuroretinal rim blood flow and IOP in glaucoma patients. A similar close relationship between neuroretinal rim blood flow and the mechanical properties of the ONH has been explored.[67]

BLOOD FLOW RESPONSES TO AN INDUCED CHANGE IN INTRAOCULAR PRESSURE USING SUCTION CUP

The ability of the eye to adjust to a sudden increase in IOP was thoroughly investigated both in experimental animals and in humans. Blood flow responses to an induced change in IOP using a suction cup have been studied using single-point laser Doppler flowmetry,[68] color Doppler imaging,[69] and scanning laser Doppler flowmetry.[70] In general, suction-induced IOP elevations reduced retrobulbar, retinal, and ONH perfusion parameters in both normal and glaucomatous eyes. Such hemodynamic changes were reversed following normalization of IOP.

Induced changes in IOP using a suction cup have also demonstrated the highly dependent relationship between the hemodynamics of the central retinal artery and short posterior ciliary arteries, on the one hand, and acute changes in IOP, on the other.[69] Acute incremental elevation of IOP in healthy humans resulted in a progressive drop in both central retinal artery and short posterior ciliary arteries flow velocities, implying a close link between mechanical and hemodynamic properties of the ONH. In contrast, ophthalmic artery flow velocities were found to be unaffected by such changes.

CORRELATION BETWEEN REDUCED NEURORETINAL RIM BLOOD FLOW VALUES AND LARGE CUP-TO-DISC RATIO

An inverse correlation has been proposed between neuroretinal rim flow values and cup-to-disc ratio which could be suggestive of a link between defective ONH perfusion and the severity of glaucomatous disc changes.[59]

The reported correlation with the cup-to-disc ratio was across a mixed population of OAG and OHT patients and, in contrast, there was no similar correlation between rim flow and visual field mean defect. Ocular hypertensives with larger cup-to-disc ratios were found to have significantly lower neuroretinal rim blood flow compared to OHT patients with smaller cup-to-disc ratios, suggesting that the defect in rim blood flow takes place early in the development of glaucomatous optic neuropathy.

A similar significant inverse correlation has been reported between neuroretinal rim blood flow and cup-to-disc ratio in both glaucoma suspects[55] and glaucoma patients.[56]

DEFECTIVE AUTOREGULATION OF THE OPTIC NERVE HEAD BLOOD FLOW IN GLAUCOMA

As previously mentioned, autoregulation maintains a relatively constant blood flow in spite of changes in OPP, which in turn depends on systemic blood pressure and IOP. In the absence of autoregulation, there is an inverse relationship between IOP and OPP. The higher the IOP, the lower the OPP and, consequently, the lower is the blood flow to the ONH. On the other hand, reduction of IOP would be expected to improve OPP and consequently increase ONH blood flow.

Changes in OPP occur routinely in daily life as mediated by stress and exercise-induced elevations in systemic blood pressure, by nocturnal reductions in systemic blood pressure, and by diurnal variations in IOP.[3] When such OPP changes occur with intact autoregulation, local constriction or dilatation in the terminal retinal arterioles causes vascular resistance to increase or decrease respectively, thereby maintaining constant blood flow and nutrient supply to the ocular tissues.[24]

The existence of intact autoregulation in the normal ONH has been demonstrated in a large number of experimental[71–73] and clinical[74,75] studies. Autoregulation has been reported to operate only within a critical range of OPP and becomes ineffective when the OPP goes below or above this critical range. This range of OPP has been investigated in different species using various methodologies.[71–73,76] In healthy monkeys, Geijer and Bill[71] reported ONH autoregulation to be normal at an OPP of >30 mmHg. Ernest[76] reported similar findings with pressures >50 mmHg.

Breakdown of the autoregulatory mechanism that normally keeps blood flow at levels adequate for tissue requirements was reported to take place at an OPP of <30 mmHg by Sperber and Bill,[73] at <25 mmHg by Sossi and Andersen,[72] and at 30–35 mmHg OPP by Hayreh and co-workers.[39] It was speculated to be caused by systemic diseases[76] or acquired with age.[72]

Substantial evidence in the literature suggests that glaucomatous optic neuropathy may be due to a breakdown in autoregulation. Pillunat et al.[77] and Hafez et al.[66] presented evidence of defective autoregulation in the ONH of NTG and OAG, respectively, whereas Grunwald et al.[78] reported evidence suggestive of abnormal autoregulation of macular blood flow in OAG. In a recent study, Riva et al.[79] reported an increase in ONH blood flow, as measured by laser Doppler flowmetry, of 39.0% in normals versus only 17.5% in ocular hypertensives and 10.4% in early glaucoma patients when the fundus was stimulated with a 15 Hz monochromatic green light flicker. Flicker stimulation was reported to increase metabolic demands and consequently induce an increase in blood flow via vasodilatation mediated by nitric oxide release.

It has been generally assumed that the choroid does not possess the capacity to autoregulate. However, recent studies provide evidence that the choroid has some autoregulatory capacity in response to changes in OPP in healthy subjects. In OAG patients, such autoregulation was reported to be considerably impaired while in OHT patients the autoregulation was found to be normal, increased, or slightly decreased.[80]

EFFECT OF INHALED CARBON DIOXIDE ON RETROBULBAR CIRCULATION IN GLAUCOMA

Earlier studies on the response of retinal circulation to changes in arterial oxygen and carbon dioxide were limited to measurements of vessel diameter. The studies reported that hyperoxia decreased retinal vessel diameter whereas hypoxemia increased it.[81] Later, Riva et al.,[82] using laser Doppler velocimetry, measured changes in retinal blood velocity in normal subjects following induced hyperoxia. After 5 minutes of oxygen breathing, blood velocity was reduced by 53%, vessel diameter by 12%, and calculated flux by 60%. Studies using blue-field entoptic stimulation also found decreased velocities of perimacular leukocytes associated with hyperoxia and increased velocities with hypoxemia.[83]

Induced gas perturbations were also used to test the hypothesis that glaucoma patients show preexisting and reversible vasoconstriction of retrobulbar vasculature and thus differ from normals in their response to vasoactive stimuli. In a study by Harris et al.,[51] color Doppler imaging was performed on the eyes of NTG patients and control subjects, before and after breathing of CO_2. Baseline values for end-diastolic velocities were found to be lower in the ophthalmic arteries of NTG patients compared to those of healthy subjects and the resistivity index was found to be higher. When PCO_2 was increased, controls remained unchanged whereas end-diastolic velocity increased in NTG. Similar findings were recently reported by Hosking et al.[84]

These studies suggest the presence of a relative vasoconstriction in some orbital vessels of glaucoma patients, which might be the result of vasospasm, and which could be partially reversed by hypercapnia.

ROLE OF VASOSPASM IN THE DEVELOPMENT AND PROGRESSION OF GLAUCOMA

A high prevalence of peripheral vasospasticity (Fig. 8.4) has been reported in glaucoma patients. This vasospasticity has been consistently linked to abnormal ocular blood flow. Phelps and Corbett, in 1985,[85] were the first to suggest the possible role of vasospastic phenomena in the development and progression of glaucomatous optic neuropathy. They found that 47% of their patients with normal-tension glaucoma also suffered from migraine. Gasser and Flammer, in 1987,[86] described ocular vasospasm in which patients with unexplained scotomas had abnormal capillaroscopic response to cold in the nailfold of the fingers. These scotomas were aggravated by the immersion of a hand in cold water. They assumed that patients with tendency to vasospasm exhibit ocular vascular reactions similar to those that occur in the capillaries of the fingers. In 1988, Guthauser et al.[11] demonstrated a statistically significant relationship between patient's history of cold hands and the outcome of both the visual field cold water test and the nailfold capillaroscopic test. The visual field results were also found to correlate significantly with the capillaroscopic results.

Strong associations have been also established between NTG, migrainous headaches, and vasospasm. Drance et al., in 1988,[13] using Doppler blood flow measurements in the finger and a cold test, showed that in nonglaucomatous subjects, 26% without migraine had a positive vasospastic response while 64% with classic migraine showed such a response. Of the patients with low-tension glaucoma, 65% showed a positive vasospastic response.

These findings were later supported by results from the Collaborative Normal Tension Glaucoma Study[33] that demonstrated a 2.58-fold increased risk of progression in glaucoma patients suffering from migraines.

Studies have also suggested a possible role for systemic vasodilators in patients with progressive NTG and an underlying vasospastic disorder. Improvements in visual fields were demonstrated following treatment

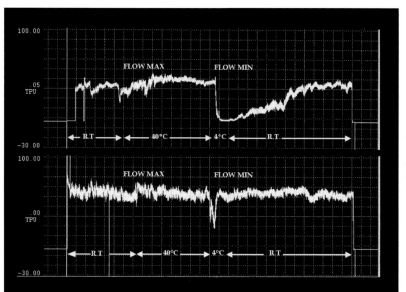

FIGURE 8.4 (*Top*) Tracing of peripheral blood flow in a vasospastic patient showing a low baseline flow at room temperature and a marked decrease in flow after immersion of the hand in cold water (4°C) with a delayed recovery to baseline. (*Bottom*) Tracing of peripheral blood flow in a nonvasospastic patient showing a normal baseline flow at room temperature and a rapid decrease after immersion of the hand in cold water (4°C) with a rapid recovery to baseline. (Hafez AS, Bizzarro R, Descovich D, Lesk MR. Correlation between finger blood flow and changes in ocular blood flow following therapeutic intraocular pressure reduction. J Glaucoma 2005; 14:448–454.)

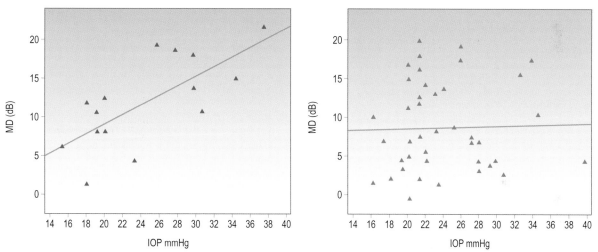

FIGURE 8.5 Correlations between IOP and visual field mean defect (*MD*) in two distinct OAG populations: vasospastic and atherosclerotic. (Redrawn from Schulzer M, Drance SM, Carter CJ, et al. Biostatistical evidence for two distinct chronic open angle glaucoma populations. Br J Ophthalmol 1990; 74:196–200.)

by calcium channel blocker (nifedipine) for 6 months.[87] Netland et al.[88] looked retrospectively at NTG patients on calcium channel blockers and found that they were less likely to progress, whereas Pillunat et al.[89] reported that NTG patients showed an increase in ocular pulse amplitude and an improvement in central visual fields during rebreathing of carbon dioxide, a known systemic vasodilator.

Evidence of two distinct OAG populations was presented by Schulzer et al. (Fig. 8.5). Vasospastic OAG patients had visual field damage that was proportional to their level of IOP while the degree of visual field damage in atherosclerotic OAG patients was independent of IOP level. Subsequently, Hafez et al.[91] demonstrated that ONH blood flow was more sensitive to changes in IOP in vasospastic than in nonvasospastic OAG and OHT patients. An interaction between IOP and ONH blood flow in vasospastic subjects was thus hypothesized.

Summary

In summary, clinical, epidemiological, and experimental data consistently link abnormal ocular perfusion to open-angle glaucoma. The vast majority of published studies on ocular blood flow report reduced ocular perfusion in glaucoma patients. Blood flow decreases with increase in glaucoma damage, and this reduction occurs both in early and later stages of glaucoma. The reduction in blood flow involves different parts of the eye, including the ONH, choroid, and retinal circulation, as well as in retrobulbar and even peripheral blood flow. Blood flow alterations are more pronounced in normal-pressure glaucoma than in high-pressure glaucoma, and in progressive than in nonprogressive eyes. In studies applying provocation tests, differences between OAG patients and normal subjects were more pronounced under provocation.

Current evidence also suggests that abnormalities in ocular blood flow can be explained partly by low OPP, and partly by vasospasm and abnormal autoregulation of blood flow, which can manifest as an inability to adapt to increased or fluctuating IOP or to decreased systemic blood pressure or to both.

REFERENCES

1. Drance SM, Sweeny VP, Morgan RW, et al. Studies of factors involved in the production of low-tension glaucoma. Arch Ophthalmol 1973; 89:457–465.

2. Quigley HA, Enger C, Katz J, et al. Risk factors for the development of glaucomatous field loss in ocular hypertension. Arch Ophthalmol 1994; 112:644–649.

3. Tielsch JM, Katz J, Sommer A, et al. Hypertension, perfusion pressure and primary open-angle glaucoma. A population-based assessment. Arch Ophthalmol 1995; 113:216–221.

4. Hayreh SS, Zimmerman MB, Podhajsky P, et al. Nocturnal arterial hypotension and its role in optic nerve head and ocular ischemic disorders. Am J Ophthalmol 1994; 117:603–624.

5. Graham SL, Drance SM, Wijsman K, et al. Ambulatory blood pressure monitoring in glaucoma. The nocturnal dip. Ophthalmology 1995; 102:61–69.

6. Becker B. Diabetes mellitus and primary open-angle glaucoma. The XXVII Edward Jackson Memorial Lecture. Am J Ophthalmol 1971; 71:1–16.

7. Corbett JJ, Phelps CD, Eslinger P, et al. The neurologic evaluation of patients with low-tension glaucoma. Invest Ophthalmol Vis Sci 1985; 26:1105–1108.

8. Nicolela MT, Drance SM, Rankin SJ, et al. Color Doppler imaging in patients with asymmetric glaucoma and unilateral visual field loss. Am J Ophthalmol 1996; 121:502–510.

9. Schumann J, Gugleta K, Dubler B, et al. Interocular difference in progression of glaucoma correlates with interocular differences in retrobulbar circulation. Am J Ophthalmol 2000; 129:728–733.

10. Findl O, Rainer G, Dallinger S, et al. Assessment of optic disk blood flow in patients with open-angle glaucoma. Am J Ophthalmol 2000; 130:589–596.

11. Guthauser U, Flammer J, Mahler G. The relationship between digital and ocular vasospasm. Graefe's Arch Clin Exp Ophthalmol 1988; 226:224–226.

12. Gasser P. Ocular vasospasm: a risk factor in the pathogenesis of low-tension glaucoma. Int Ophthalmol 1989; 13(4):281–290.

13. Drance SM, Douglas GD, Wijsman K, et al. Response of blood flow to warm and cold in normal and low tension glaucoma patients. Am J Ophthalmol 1988; 105:35–39.

14. Anderson DR, Hendrickson A. Effect of intraocular pressure on rapid axoplasmic transport in monkey optic nerve. Invest Ophthalmol 1974; 13:771–783.

15. Quigley HA. Ganglion cell death in glaucoma: pathology recapitulates ontogeny. Aust NZ J Ophthalmol 1995; 23:85–91.

16. Quigley H, Anderson D. The dynamics and location of axonal transport blockade by acute intraocular pressure elevation in primate optic nerve. Invest Ophthalmol Vis Sci 1976; 15: 505–515.

17. Quigley H, Flower R, Addicks E, et al. The mechanism of optic nerve damage in experimental acute intraocular pressure elevation. Invest Ophthalmol Vis Sci 1980; 19:505–517.

18. Yan DB, Coloma FM, Metheetrairut A, et al. Deformation of the lamina cribrosa by elevated intraocular pressure. Br J Ophthalmol 1994; 78:643–648.

19. Burgoyne CF, Quigley HA, Thomson HW, et al. Early changes in optic disc compliance and surface position in experimental glaucoma. Ophthalmology 1995; 102:1800–1809.

20. Levy NS, Crapps EE. Displacement of optic nerve head in response to short-term intraocular pressure elevation in enucleated human eyes. Arch Ophthalmol 1984; 102:782–786.

21. Jonas JB, Gareis O, Naumann GOH. Optic disc topography and short-term increase in intra-ocular pressure. Graefe's Arch Clin Exp Ophthalmol 1990; 228:524–527.

22. Minckler DS, Spaeth GL. Optic nerve damage in glaucoma. Surv Ophthalmol 1981; 26:128–148.

23. Bill A. Vascular physiology of the optic nerve. In: Varma R, Spaeth GL, Parker K, eds. The optic nerve in glaucoma. Philadelphia: Lippincott; 1993; 47:37–50.

24. Flammer J, Orgul S. Optic nerve blood flow abnormalities in glaucoma. Prog Retin Eye Res 1998; 17:267–289.

25. Rankin SJ, Drance SM. Peripapillary focal retinal arteriolar narrowing in open angle glaucoma. J Glaucoma 1996; 5:22–28.

26. Drance SM. Disc hemorrhages in the glaucomas. Surv Ophthalmol 1989; 33:331–337.

27. Chihara E, Honda Y. Preservation of nerve fiber layer by retinal vessels in glaucoma. Ophthalmology 1992; 99:208–214.

28. Shihab ZM, Beebe WE, Wentlandt T. Possible significance of cilioretinal arteries in open angle glaucoma. Ophthalmology 1985; 92:880–883.

29. Jonas JB. Clinical implications of peripapillary atrophy in glaucoma. Curr Opin Ophthalmol 2005; 16:84–88.

30. Ikram MK, de Voogd S, Wolfs RC, et al. Retinal vessel diameters and incident open-angle glaucoma and optic disc changes: the Rotterdam study. Invest Ophthalmol Vis Sci 2005; 46:1182–1187.

31. Bonomi L, Marchini G, Marraffa M, et al. Vascular risk factors for primary open angle glaucoma: the Egna-Neumarkt Study. Ophthalmology 2000; 107:1287–1293.

32. Leske MC, Connell AM, Wu SY, et al. Risk factors for open-angle glaucoma. The Barbados Eye Study. Arch Ophthalmol 1995; 113:918–924.

33. Drance SM, Anderson DR, Schulzer M. Risk factors for progression of visual field abnormalities in normal tension glaucoma. Am J Ophthalmol 2001; 131:699–708.

34. Graham SL, Drance SM. Nocturnal hypotension: role in glaucoma progression. Surv Ophthalmol 1999; 43:10–16.

35. Hayreh SS. Factors influencing blood flow in the optic nerve head. Glaucoma 1997; 6:412–425.

36. Hayreh SS. Evaluation of optic nerve head circulation: review of the methods used. J Glaucoma 1997; 6:319–330.

37. Hayreh SS. Progress in the understanding of the vascular etiology of glaucoma. Curr Opin Ophthalmol 1994; 5:26–35.

38. Hayreh SS. Retinal and optic nerve head ischemic disorders and atherosclerosis: role of serotonin. Prog Retin Eye Res 1999; 18:191–221.

39. Hayreh SS, Bill A, Sperber GO. Effects of high intraocular pressure on the glucose metabolism in the retina and optic nerve in old atherosclerotic monkeys. Graefe's Arch Clin Exp Ophthalmol 1994; 232:745–752.

40. Flammer J. The vascular concept in glaucoma. Surv Ophthalmol 1994; 38(Suppl):3–6.

41. Hayreh SS, Podhajsky P, Zimmerman MB. Role of nocturnal arterial hypotension in optic nerve head ischemic disorders. Ophthalmologica 1999; 213:76–96.

42. Kaiser HJ, Flammer J. Systemic hypotension: a risk factor for glaucomatous damage? Ophthalmologica 1991; 203:105–108.

43. Choi J, Kim KH, Jeong J, et al. Circadian fluctuation of mean ocular perfusion pressure is a consistent risk factor for normal-tension glaucoma. Invest Ophthalmol Vis Sci 2007; 48:104–111.

44. Carter CJ, Brooks DE, Doyle DL, et al. Investigations into a vascular etiology for low-tension glaucoma. Ophthalmology 1990; 97:49–55.

45. Goldberg I, Hollows FC, Kass MA, et al. Systemic factors in patients with low-tension glaucoma. Br J Ophthalmol 1981; 65:56–62.

46. O'Brien C, Butt Z, Ludlam C, et al. Activation of the coagulation cascade in untreated primary open-angle glaucoma. Ophthalmology 1997; 104:725–730.

47. Hamard P, Hamard H, Dufaux J, et al. Optic nerve head blood flow using a laser Doppler velocimeter and haemorrheology in primary open angle glaucoma and normal pressure glaucoma. Br J Ophthalmol 1994; 78:449–453.

48. Spaeth GL. Fluorescein angiography: its contributions towards understanding the mechanisms of visual loss in glaucoma. Trans Am Ophthalmol Soc 1975; 73:491–553.

49. Plange N, Kaup M, Huber K, et al. Fluorescein filling defects of the optic nerve head in normal tension glaucoma, primary open angle glaucoma, ocular hypertension and healthy controls. Ophthalmic Physiol Opt 2006; 26:26–32.

50. Galassi F, Nuzzaci G, Sodi A, et al. Color Doppler imaging in evaluation of optic nerve blood supply in normal and glaucomatous subjects. Int Ophthalmol 1992; 16:273–276.

51. Harris A, Sergott RC, Spaeth GL, et al. Color Doppler analysis of ocular vessel blood velocity in normal-tension glaucoma. Am J Ophthalmol 1994; 118:642–649.

52. Langham ME, Farrell RA, O'Brien V, et al. Non-invasive measurement of pulsatile blood flow in the human eye. In: Lambrou GN, Greve EL, eds. Ocular blood flow in glaucoma. Amsterdam: Kugler & Ghedini; 1989:93–99.

53. James CB, Smith SE. Pulsatile ocular blood flow in patients with low tension glaucoma. Br J Ophthalmol 1991; 75:466–470.

54. Grunwald JE, Piltz-Seymour JR, Hariprasad SM, et al. Optic nerve and choroidal circulation in glaucoma. Invest Ophthalmol Vis Sci 1998; 39:2329–2336.

55. Piltz-Seymour JR, Grunwald JE, Hariprasad SM, et al. Optic nerve blood flow is diminished in eyes of primary open-angle glaucoma suspects. Am J Ophthalmol 2001; 132:63–69.

56. Michelson G, Langhans MJ, Groh MJM. Perfusion of the juxtapapillary retina and the neuroretinal rim area in primary open angle glaucoma. J Glaucoma 1996; 5:91–98.

57. Nicolela MT, Hnik P, Drance SM. Scanning laser Doppler flowmeter study of retinal and optic disk blood flow in glaucomatous patients. Am J Ophthalmol 1996; 122:775–783.

58. Kerr J, Nelson P, O'Brien C. A comparison of ocular blood flow in untreated primary open-angle glaucoma and ocular hypertension. Am J Ophthalmol 1998; 126:42–51.

59. Hafez AS, Bizzaro RLG, Lesk MR. Optic nerve head blood flow in glaucoma patients, ocular hypertensives and normal subjects measured by scanning laser Doppler flowmetry. Am J Ophthalmol 2003; 136:1022–1031.

60. Harris A, Arend O, Kagemann L, et al. Dozolamide, visual function and ocular hemodynamics in normal-tension glaucoma. J Ocul Pharmacol Ther 1999; 15:189–197.

61. Araie M, Tamaki Y, Muta K. Effect of long-term topical beta blocker on optic nerve head circulation. In: Drance SM, ed. Vascular risk factors and neuroprotection in glaucoma. New York: Kugler; 1996:209–216.

62. Drance SM, Crichton A, Mills RP. Comparison of the effect of latanoprost 0.005% and timolol 0.5% on the calculated ocular perfusion pressure in patients with normal tension glaucoma. Am J Ophthalmol 1998; 125:585–592.

63. Carlsson AM, Chauhan BC, Lee A, et al. The effect of brimonidine tartrate on retinal blood flow in patients with ocular hypertension. Am J Ophthalmol 2000; 129:297–301.

64. Trible JR, Sergott RC, Spaeth GL, et al. Trabeculectomy is associated with retrobulbar hemodynamic changes: a color Doppler analysis. Ophthalmology 1994; 101:340–351.

65. James CB. Effect of trabeculectomy on pulsatile ocular blood flow. Br J Ophthalmol 1994; 78:818–822.

66. Hafez AS, Bizzaro RLG, Rivard M, et al. Changes in optic nerve head blood flow after therapeutic intraocular pressure reduction in glaucoma patients and ocular hypertensives. Ophthalmology 2003; 110:201–210.

67. Lesk MR, Hafez AS, Descovich D. Relationship between central corneal thickness and changes of optic nerve head topography and blood flow after intraocular pressure reduction in open-angle glaucoma and ocular hypertension. Arch Ophthalmol 2006; 124:1568–1572.

68. Riva CE, Hero M, Titze P, et al. Autoregulation of human optic nerve blood flow in response to acute changes in ocular perfusion pressure. Graefe's Arch Clin Exp Ophthalmol 1997; 235:618–626.

69. Harris A, Joos K, Kay M, et al. Acute IOP elevation with scleral suction: effects on retrobulbar haemodynamics. Br J Ophthalmol 1996; 80:1055–1059.

70. Michelson G, Groh MJ, Langhans M. Perfusion of the juxtapapillary retina and optic nerve head in acute ocular hypertension. Ger J Ophthalmol 1996; 5:315–321.

71. Geijer C, Bill A. Effects of raised intraocular pressure on retinal, prelaminar, laminar, and retrolaminar optic nerve blood flow in monkeys. Invest Ophthalmol Vis Sci 1979; 18:1030–1042.

72. Sossi N, Anderson DR. Effect of elevated intraocular pressure on blood flow. Occurrence in cat optic nerve head studied with iodoantipyrine I 125. Arch Ophthalmol 1983; 101:98–101.

73. Sperber GO, Bill A. Blood flow and glucose consumption in the optic nerve, retina and brain: effects of high intraocular pressure. Exp Eye Res 1985; 41:639–653.

74. Pillunat LE, Stodtmeister R, Wilmanns I, et al. Autoregulation of ocular blood flow during changes in intraocular pressure. Graefe's Arch Clin Exp Ophthalmol 1985; 223:219–223.

75. Pillunat LE, Anderson DR, Knighton RW, et al. Autoregulation of human optic nerve head circulation in response to increased intraocular pressure. Exp Eye Res 1997; 64:737–744.

76. Ernest JT. Optic disc blood flow. Trans Ophthalmol Soc UK 1976; 96:348–351.

77. Pillunat LE, Stodtmeister R, Wilmanns I. Pressure compliance of the optic nerve head in low tension glaucoma. Br J Ophthalmol 1987; 71:181–187.

78. Grunwald JE, Riva CE, Stone RA, et al. Retinal autoregulation in open-angle glaucoma. Ophthalmology 1984; 91:1690–1694.

79. Riva CE, Salgarello T, Logean E, et al. Flicker-evoked response measured at the optic disc rim is reduced in ocular hypertension and early glaucoma. Invest Ophthalmol Vis Sci 2004; 45:3662–3668.

80. Ulrich A, Ulrich C, Barth T, et al. Detection of disturbed autoregulation of the peripapillary choroid in primary open angle glaucoma. Ophthalmic Surg Lasers 1996; 27:746–757.

81. Hickam JB, Frayser R. Studies of the retinal circulation in man: observation on vessel diameter, arteriovenous oxygen difference and mean circulation time. Circulation 1966; 33:302–316.

82. Riva CE, Grunwald JE, Sinclair SH. Laser Doppler velocimetry of the effect of pure oxygen breathing on retinal blood flow. Invest Ophthalmol Vis Sci 1983; 24:47–51.

83. Fallon TJ, Maxwell D, Kohner EM. Retinal vascular autoregulation in conditions of hyperoxia and hypoxia using blue field entoptic phenomenon. Ophthalmology 1985; 92:701–705.

84. Hosking SL, Harris A, Chung HS, et al. Ocular haemodynamic responses to induced hypercapnia and hyperoxia in glaucoma. Br J Ophthalmol 2004; 88:406–411.

85. Phelps CD, Corbett JJ. Migraine and low-tension glaucoma. A case control study. Invest Ophthalmol Vis Sci 1985; 26:1105.

86. Gasser P, Flammer J. Influence of vasospasm on visual function. Doc Ophthalmol 1987; 66:3–18.

87. Kitazawa Y, Shirai H, Go FJ. The effect of Ca^{2+}-antagonists on visual field in low-tension glaucoma. Graefe's Arch Clin Exp Ophthalmol 1989; 227:408–412.

88. Netland PA, Chaturvedi N, Dreyer EB. Calcium channel blockers in the management of low-tension and open-angle glaucoma. Am J Ophthalmol 1993; 115:608–613.

89. Pillunat LE, Lang GK, Harris A. The visual response to increased ocular blood flow in normal pressure glaucoma. Surv Ophthalmol 1994; 38:139–148.

90. Schulzer M, Drance SM, Carter CJ, et al. Biostatistical evidence for two distinct chronic open angle glaucoma populations. Br J Ophthalmol 1990; 74:196–200.

91. Hafez AS, Bizzaro R, Descovich D, et al. Correlation between finger blood flow and changes in ocular blood flow following therapeutic intraocular pressure reduction. J Glaucoma 2005; 14:448–454.

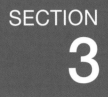

DIAGNOSIS OF GLAUCOMA

CHAPTER 9

Tonometry and Intraocular Pressure Fluctuation

Aachal Kotecha, Sheng Lim, and David Garway-Heath

INTRODUCTION

Raised intraocular pressure (IOP) is the most important modifiable risk factor for the development and progression of glaucomatous optic neuropathy. The accurate and precise measurement of IOP is, therefore, of great clinical importance. Several tonometers are in common usage, and an understanding of the principles of IOP measurement and sources of measurement error for each of the tonometers facilitates the correct interpretation of clinical IOP readings. The 'accuracy' of a measurement refers to how close the measurement is to the true value; the 'precision' of a measurement refers to how reproducible it is. All current forms of clinical tonometry measure the IOP through the cornea and the accuracy of their measurements are, therefore, subject to the biomechanical properties of the cornea. This topic is considered in detail in Chapter 16. Measurement precision may be quantified for repeat observations by the same observer (the repeatability coefficient) or by different observers (95% limits of agreement). The repeatability coefficient gives the value within which two readings by the same observer will fall for 95% of subjects/patients. Recently, it has been suggested that IOP fluctuation, in addition to raised IOP, may be a risk factor for glaucoma progression. Variation in IOP measurements may arise from measurement error or from true IOP fluctuation. This chapter considers the operating principles of the tonometers in common use, and the sources and clinical significance of IOP measurement variation.

GOLDMANN APPLANATION TONOMETRY

TONOMETER PRINCIPLE

Hans Goldmann and Theo Schmidt introduced the Goldmann applanation tonometer (GAT) in 1957. The IOP is estimated by measuring the force required to flatten a fixed area of the cornea ('applanation' tonometry). The optimal applanation area was derived from empirical experimentation and the Imbert–Fick principle.

The Imbert–Fick principle states that the pressure *(P)* of a body of fluid encapsulated within a sphere is directly proportional to the force *(W)* required to applanate an area *(A)* of the sphere:

$$W = PA \qquad (9.1)$$

The principle holds provided that the surface encapsulating the fluid is infinitely thin, perfectly elastic, dry, and perfectly flexible and that the only force being exerted upon it is from the applanating surface. However, with respect to the cornea, none of these assumptions is true. Goldmann recognized that the equation would need to be modified to account for certain corneal characteristics (a finite thickness, measurable rigidity, and the capillary attraction forces of the precorneal tear film). An assumption was made that, in the absence of corneal pathology, the central corneal thickness (CCT) did not vary much around $500\,\mu m$. The modified equation included factors to account for the resistance of the cornea to applanation and the action of surface tension from the tear meniscus on the tonometer prism:

$$W + s = PA + b \qquad (9.2)$$

where W = tonometer force, s = surface tension of precorneal tear film, P = intraocular pressure, A = area of applanation, and b = corneal rigidity/ resistance to bending (Fig. 9.1).

The effects of corneal rigidity and tear film surface tension forces (see Fig. 9.1) approximately cancel when the area applanated is $7.35\,mm^2$. When applanating this area, a force of $0.1\,g$ corresponds to an IOP of $1\,mmHg$.

GAT is the reference standard for tonometry.

The GAT is slit lamp mounted and is available in a modified hand-held form (the Perkins tonometer). When viewed through the slit lamp, the tonometer biprism splits the image of the fluorescent tear meniscus into two semicircular rings. A dial on the side of the tonometer is adjusted to vary the force applied to the eye, causing a movement of the rings either together or

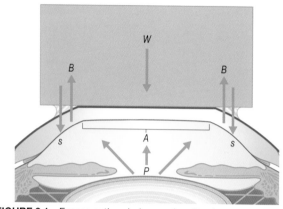

FIGURE 9.1 Forces acting during applanation tonometry. *W*, tonometer force; *s*, surface tension of precorneal tear film; *P*, intraocular pressure; *A*, area of applanation; *b*, corneal rigidity/resistance to bending.

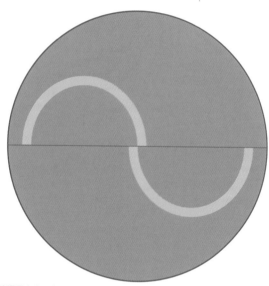

FIGURE 9.2 Correct mire alignment in GAT.

apart. The end point is achieved when the inner edges of the semicircles touch (Fig. 9.2).

ACCURACY OF INTRAOCULAR PRESSURE MEASUREMENTS AND PRECISION OF TECHNIQUE

Sources of IOP measurement error[1] using this technique are summarized in Table 9.1.

Other sources of error include: 'digit preference' – a subconscious bias towards certain digits, such as a preference for figures that end in 0, 5, or even numbers; eyelid squeezing (attempted eyelid closure during tonometry); patient obesity (may give high readings); and a tight necktie.

Typical repeatability coefficients are 2.2–5.5 mmHg for GAT.[2] For different observers measuring IOP in the same subjects, the 95% limits of agreement have been reported to be ±2.2–3.8 mmHg for GAT.[2,3]

NONCONTACT TONOMETRY

TONOMETER PRINCIPLE

Developed in the early 1970s, the noncontact tonometer (NCT) uses a jet of air to applanate the cornea. As corneal anesthesia is not required to perform the test, it remains the most commonly used device in optometric practice.

The system consists of a central air plenum flanked either side by an infrared light emitter and detector. In the resting state, the convex cornea scatters light and no signal is picked up by the detector (Fig. 9.3A). The pressure of the air pulse is gradually increased to deform the cornea. At corneal applanation, the corneal surface behaves like a plane mirror reflecting light to the detector (Fig. 9.3B). This signal is the trigger to switch off the air pressure pulse.

In early NCTs, IOP was determined from the time taken for the air jet to applanate the cornea. With the introduction of the pressure transducer in the late 1980s, IOP was measured from the actual air jet pressure required to applanate the cornea. The NCT is simple to use and requires minimal training to master.

ACCURACY AND PRECISION OF INTRAOCULAR PRESSURE MEASUREMENTS

Most studies assessing the accuracy of the NCT have compared the device to GAT IOP measurements. At the time of writing, no data from manometric studies assessing IOP accuracy have been published.

The NCT measurement is made in 1–3 milliseconds. IOP variation caused by the cardiac cycle can, therefore, be a significant source of NCT IOP measurement variability. Studies assessing the repeatability of NCT have found repeatability coefficients of between 3.0 mmHg and 4.0 mmHg,[2] although measurements with hand-held NCTs may be less repeatable.

Studies assessing the agreement between IOP measurements made by the table-mounted NCT and GAT have for the most part shown good agreement between the devices, with little systematic relative over- or underestimation in normotensive and glaucomatous subjects.[2] However, there may be a greater disparity at higher IOP levels with hand-held NCTs.

THE OCULAR RESPONSE ANALYZER

The Ocular Response Analyzer (ORA; Reichert Corporation; New York, USA) is an NCT that measures dynamic aspects of corneal deformation by an air pulse. A metered airpulse is directed at the cornea until applanation is achieved. This acts as a trigger to switch off the airpulse. A small time delay results in a further increase in air pressure which causes a degree of corneal indentation. After reaching a peak, the air pressure steadily reduces until it is completely removed. The instrument makes two measurements: the force

TABLE 9.1 Common sources of error with Goldmann applanation tonometry[1]

SOURCE OF ERROR	EFFECT ON MIRES	EFFECT ON IOP MEASUREMENT
Excessive tears	Wide/broad fluorescein rings	Overestimation
Insufficient tears	Narrow fluorescein rings	Underestimation
Absence of fluorescein		Underestimation
Corneal astigmatism (>3 dioptres)	Changes area of applanation from circle to ellipse	Underestimation in with-the-rule astigmatism
		Overestimation in against-the-rule astigmatism
Corneal curvature		Steeper corneas require more force to produce correct area of applanation – overestimation of IOP
Corneal epithelial edema		Underestimation
Corneal stromal edema		Underestimation
Breath-holding/increased venous pressure from tight clothing around neck		Increase in IOP
Sustained accommodation		Decrease in IOP
Deviation of gaze from primary position		Increase in IOP, especially with upgaze

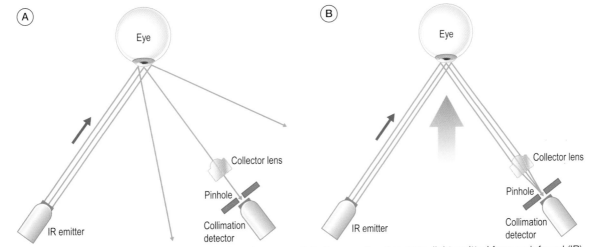

FIGURE 9.3 Noncontact tonometer principle. (**A**) When the cornea is in its normal resting state, light emitted from an infrared (IR) source is scattered by the convex corneal surface. (**B**) When the cornea is applanated by the pressure of the air jet, it acts as a plane reflecting surface causing the light to be reflected into the light detector.

required to flatten the cornea as the air pressure rises ('force-in' applanation, P1) and the force at which the cornea flattens again as the air pressure falls ('force-out' applanation, P2). The 'force-out' applanation occurs at a lower pressure than the 'force-in' applanation, and this has been attributed to the viscoelastic dampening effects of the cornea. The pressure difference between the two applanation events is termed *corneal hysteresis* (Fig. 9.4). Corneal hysteresis is a direct measure of the corneal biomechanical properties and may more completely describe the contribution of corneal resistance to IOP measurements than CCT alone.[4]

Two measurements of corneal biomechanical properties are made, corneal hysteresis (CH) and the corneal response factor (CRF). While CH represents the absolute difference between the applanation pressures P1 and P2,

the CRF is derived from the formula (P1 − kP2), where k is a constant. It has been suggested that CH predominantly reflects the viscous properties of the cornea, while CRF better reflects the elastic properties (also see Ch. 16).

THE TONOPEN

TONOMETER PRINCIPLE

Introduced in the late 1980s, the Tonopen is based on the Mackay Marg tonometer. The system comprises a central, moveable plunger of diameter 1.02 mm that is surrounded by a larger footplate. Pressing the instrument tip against the cornea activates a strain gauge that senses the force generated by the plunger to applanate the central cornea.

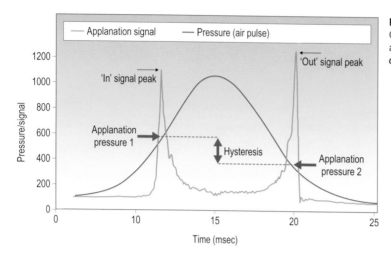

FIGURE 9.4 Signal/applanation plot from Reichert ORA. The difference between the 'force-in' applanation and 'force-out' applanation is termed *corneal hysteresis*. (Copyright © 2004 Reichert Inc.)

As the rest of the tonometer comes into contact with the cornea, the force exerted on the plunger reduces until the plunger is flush with the footplate. The effect of corneal rigidity is transferred to the surrounding footplate and at that point the force exerted on the plunger is considered to be only the IOP. This change in force generates a waveform tracing which is analyzed by a microprocessor.

ACCURACY AND PRECISION OF INTRAOCULAR PRESSURE MEASUREMENTS

In an ex vivo manometric study, the Tonopen exhibited high concordance with transducer pressures at IOP levels up to 40 mmHg, showing an underestimation of IOP when the transducer set IOP at levels >40 mmHg. In an in vivo manometric study of adult Chinese eyes, the Tonopen underestimated true IOP by an average 2 mmHg, with a range of error between −8 mmHg and 4 mmHg. The variation of IOP readings and disagreement between true IOP and Tonopen-measured IOP increased at higher levels of true IOP.

Studies assessing the repeatability of the Tonopen find repeatability coefficients up to 4.3 mmHg.[2] In clinical studies, the Tonopen has been shown to relatively underestimate GAT, particularly at higher levels of IOP whilst other studies find good agreement between the devices with minimal systematic bias.[2]

THE PASCAL® DYNAMIC CONTOUR TONOMETER

The Pascal® Dynamic Contour Tonometer (DCT; Swiss Microtechnology® AG, Port, Switzerland) was introduced in 2002. The tonometer is a non-applanating, slit lamp mounted, contact tonometer (Fig. 9.5).

TONOMETER PRINCIPLE

Applanation tonometers measure the force required to flatten a defined area of the cornea. The force required is proportional to the IOP, but readings may be affected

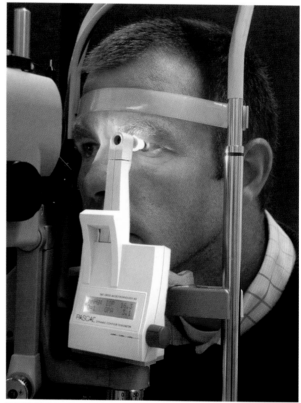

FIGURE 9.5 Pascal DCT.

by complex corneal biomechanical properties leading to measurement error (see Ch. 16 for further details).

The design purpose of the DCT was to develop a noninvasive and direct method for IOP measurement that would be relatively unaffected by the inter-individual variations of corneal biomechanics. The DCT measurement principle is based on contour matching, which assumes that if the eye were enclosed by a contoured, tight-fitting shell, the forces generated by IOP would act on the shell wall. Replacing part of the shell wall with a pressure sensor would enable measurement of these forces and therefore the IOP.[5]

The DCT has a contoured tonometer tip surface that is designed to match the contour of the cornea. The

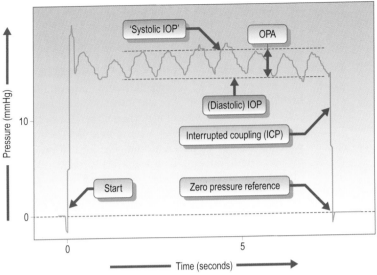

FIGURE 9.6 Pressure curve from DCT recording. The instrument displays the diastolic IOP and ocular pulse amplitude (OPA).

radius of curvature of the tip is 10.5 mm with a contact surface approximately 7 mm in diameter. A piezoresistive pressure sensor of diameter ≈ 1.2 mm is integrated flush within the contour surface, enabling transcorneal measurements of the anterior chamber fluid pressure. The tip is mounted into housing similar to that used for GAT, which provides a constant appositional force of 1 g.

An electric signal is generated by the pressure sensor and IOP readings are sampled at 100 Hz with measurements being recorded to a resolution of 0.1 mmHg.

Diastolic IOP is displayed on a LCD screen within the housing. The dynamic sampling of IOP yields pressure curves from which the ocular pulse amplitude (OPA) is determined (Fig. 9.6). The OPA value displayed on the LCD screen is a peak-to-peak difference of the average systolic and average diastolic IOP, in units of mmHg. The DCT provides an audible signal, the pitch of which modulates regularly, indicating pulse oscillations.

For IOP measurement, a disposable silicone tip is placed on the tonometer head and is changed between patients to prevent cross-contamination of tear fluid. As the tonometer is a contact tonometer, topical corneal anesthesia is required. A minimum of five cardiac cycles need to be recorded, although it is recommended that five to eight cycles are recorded to allow for a pulse curve of sufficient quality to be generated. This can be determined from the audible signal provided by the instrument. Once adequate measurements are obtained, the LCD display will generate an IOP and OPA value (in mmHg), and a 'quality score,' which relates to the quality of pulse curve obtained. Readings of value 1 and 2 only should be accepted, although readings of quality 3 may be acceptable. Readings of 4 or 5 should be discarded.

ACCURACY AND PRECISION OF INTRAOCULAR PRESSURE MEASUREMENTS

At the time of writing, the only published study assessing the accuracy of the DCT has been by Kniestedt

et al.[6] comparing the performance of DCT, pneumatonometry and GAT on 16 freshly enucleated cadaver eyes with the corneal epithelium removed. The IOP was altered from 5 mmHg to 58 mmHg in incremental steps using a closed-stopcock system and the study found that for all manometrically set IOP values, the DCT was more accurate compared with pneumatonometry and GAT. The DCT readings also showed the least variability, quantified by the standard deviation of IOP measurements. However, although this is a carefully performed study, the behavior of eyes postmortem may differ to that of the living eye. The authors acknowledge that de-epithelialization may affect the accuracy of GAT.

A clinical study has shown a prototype DCT to have good to moderate intraobserver variability, with a repeatability coefficients of 3.2 mmHg.[3] DCT IOP measurements are on average higher than those of GAT, which has been attributed to calibration differences. It has been suggested that since manometric studies have shown that GAT IOP measurements are 1.2–2 mmHg lower than intracameral measurements, the DCT values may be more accurate.[7] The limits of agreement between DCT and GAT are quite wide, ranging from +3.0 mmHg to +5.5 mmHg.[3,8]

PNEUMATONOMETRY

TONOMETER PRINCIPLE

Pneumatonometry is a form of applanation tonometry, the principle of the technique first being described by Durham and co-workers in 1964, with modifications developed by Langham in 1969.

The tonometer probe consists of a hollow central tube flanked by side exhausts. The probe tip is covered by a flexible Silastic diaphragm. Air flows under pressure through the central tube, forcing a small gap between the diaphragm and probe edge. When placed against cornea, the force of air eventually results in applanation

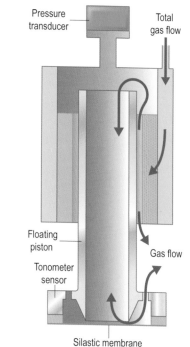

FIGURE 9.7 Principle of pneumatonometer probe.

of the cornea and closure of the diaphragm gap. Pressure within the central tube rises until it balances the IOP (Fig. 9.7). The instrument records the fluctuations in IOP caused by the cardiac cycle, a manifestation of ocular blood flow (OBF), which is recorded as the ocular pulse amplitude (OPA). A minimum of seven cycles are required for an adequate reading of OBF.

ACCURACY AND PRECISION OF INTRAOCULAR PRESSURE MEASUREMENTS

The accuracy of OBF tonometry has been determined relative to GAT. Bhan et al. assessed OBF IOP measurement repeatability in a group of normal eyes. OBF readings were more variable than those made with GAT, with repeatability coefficients of 7.7 mmHg (95% confidence intervals 6.6–8.8 mmHg) for OBF compared with 4.8 mmHg for GAT.[9] There was a consistent positive bias, with the pneumatonometer reading up to 3 mmHg greater than GAT, a finding confirmed by other studies.[10] Lower repeatability coefficients have been reported (3.7 mmHg for the OBF and 2.2–5.5 mmHg for GAT[2]).

REBOUND TONOMETRY

TONOMETER PRINCIPLE

A more recent introduction to the tonometry family is rebound tonometry, which uses a dynamic electromechanical method for measuring IOP. The device consists of a solenoid propelling coil and a sensing coil positioned around a central shaft containing a lightweight magnetized probe. The application of a transient electrical current to the solenoid coil propels the probe to the cornea. The movement of the magnetized probe induces a voltage within the system which is monitored by the sensor. As the probe impacts cornea, it decelerates and rebounds from the surface; deceleration is less at low, compared with high, IOP and consequently the higher the IOP the shorter the duration of impact.

A commercial rebound tonometer, the ICare, became available in 2003. This is a hand-held device and corneal anesthesia is not required. On activation of the measurement button, it automatically takes six readings of IOP, and discards the highest and lowest reading before presenting a digital readout of the average IOP. Studies have shown that it is relatively easy to use and is useful in inexperienced hands.

ACCURACY AND PRECISION OF INTRAOCULAR PRESSURE MEASUREMENTS

To date, no intracameral studies assessing rebound tonometer accuracy have been reported; most studies have assessed agreement with GAT. In normal eyes, the ICare shows a relative positive bias ranging from 0.50 mmHg to 1.50 mmHg over GAT and up to 3.35 mmHg over the Perkins tonometer.[11] A similar bias has been found in ocular hypertensive and glaucomatous eyes.

Studies assessing the effects of learning on the use of the rebound tonometer found no effect. Repeatability coefficients have yet to be published.

HOME TONOMETRY

Attempts have been made to produce tonometric devices that can be administered by the patient at home in order to give the clinician a record of IOP measurements between clinic visits. Zeimer and co-workers developed the first home tonometry device in 1983.[12] The system monitored the amount of light reflected by a flexible membrane that was brought into contact with the patient's cornea by a stream of air, the pressure of which was controlled by the patient depressing a small 'bulb' at the back of the device. The profile of reflected light changed as the cornea was flattened by the membrane, and at the point of applanation the system produced an audible signal for the patient to release the bulb. The air pressure required to applanate the cornea with the membrane was proportional to the patient's IOP. The device required the patient to self-administer corneal anesthesia and, as a result, did not enter widespread use.

The Proview phosphene tonometer, developed in the late 1990s, utilizes the entoptic phenomenon of pressure phosphenes that become visible when pressure is applied to the globe.[13] The device consists of a spring compression probe that is applied through a closed eyelid in the superior nasal area. The amount of force required to induce a pressure phosphene is proportional to the IOP.

ACCURACY AND PRECISION OF INTRAOCULAR PRESSURE MEASUREMENTS

In a study by Fresco evaluating the phosphene tonometer and comparing it to GAT, the mean IOP difference between GAT and the phosphene tonometer was -0.34 mmHg (95% limits of agreement -5.1 mmHg to 4.8 mmHg).[13] However, other authors have found the agreement between GAT and the phosphene tonometer to be poor and it still remains uncertain whether pressure-induced phosphene generation correlates with IOP, or whether the effects of individual eyelid resistance, scleral rigidity, or phosphene threshold limit the usefulness of the device.

INTRAOCULAR PRESSURE FLUCTUATION

Sidler-Huguenin first reported the concept of diurnal IOP variation in 1898 and this was refined by Maslenikow in 1904. The factors affecting IOP fluctuation are still not fully understood. However, a good knowledge of IOP variation characteristics is essential in the management of patients with glaucoma.

There is currently no clinical tool for continuous monitoring of normal variations and spontaneous fluctuations of IOP. In studies, subjects either undergo repeated IOP measurement during office (clinic) hours, or are admitted for regular IOP measurement over a 24-hour period. There have also been studies in which patients performed 'self-tonometry,' using the device developed by Zeimer and colleagues, during their waking hours.[14] The main advantage of this paradigm is that patients are in their natural environment, although the tonometer may not be as accurate and precise as the Goldmann tonometer.

In all studies, IOP is usually measured in patients after a brief period of rest in order to minimize the influence of spontaneous changes in physiological and environmental factors on IOP.

Although many aspects of IOP fluctuation have been reported, the peak, mean, and range and are probably the most important parameters of IOP fluctuation.

GOLDMANN'S AND FRIEDENWALD'S EQUATIONS

There are three categories of IOP fluctuation: ultra-short-term fluctuation (those occurring within seconds and minutes), short-term fluctuation (those occurring over hours and days), and long-term fluctuation (those occurring over months and years).

IOP fluctuation is best understood in the context of aqueous dynamics and the relationship between intraocular volume and IOP, described by the modified Goldmann (9.3) and Friedenwald (9.4) equations, respectively.

$$F_f = (P_i - P_e)\,C\ + F_u \qquad (9.3)$$

where F_f is aqueous humor flow rate, P_i is the intraocular pressure, P_e is the episcleral venous pressure, C is trabecular facility, and F_u is uveoscleral outflow.

$$K = dP/dV \qquad (9.4)$$

where, K is the rigidity coefficient ($=0.021$ mmHg/μL), dP is the change in pressure (mmHg), and dV is the change in volume (μL).

In a nonsteady state, the Friedenwald equation explains ultra-short-term IOP fluctuation. Such circumstances include: increased choroidal blood volume during the systolic cardiac cycle, external ocular pressure, and the Valsalva maneuver. These all lead to sudden IOP spikes due to the scleral rigidity.

However, during a steady state, the IOP is explained by the Goldmann equation. The formula may be rearranged:

$$P_i = F_f/C - F_u/C + P_e \qquad (9.5)$$

or

$$P_i = (F_f - F_u + P_e)/C \qquad (9.6)$$

The steady state IOP is therefore dependent on aqueous humor flow rate, episcleral venous pressure, trabecular outflow, and uveoscleral outflow. Any change in these parameters will result in an IOP change.

What is the evidence for fluctuations in each of these parameters?

1. Aqueous humor flow rate

Aqueous flow averages about $2.9\,\mu$L/min in young healthy humans. Drinking a large amount of water over a short time, as in the classic water drinking test, can induce hypotonicity of the plasma and increase the aqueous production rate over an ultra-short time period. It is possible that IOP variation itself may affect the aqueous production rate in the ultra-short term. This is conceptualized as 'pseudofacility' – the effect of increased IOP during tonography measurement causing a reduction in aqueous production rate. This effect is probably fairly small and has not been shown to be significant in a fluorophotometry study.

There is a slight reduction of aqueous flow rate with age, with an estimated reduction of 2.4% per decade, reaching a mean level of only $2.2\,\mu$L/min in octogenarians.[15]

Aqueous flow also has a distinctive circadian rhythm. The flow rate at night, during sleep, is only 43% of the rate in the morning after awakening. If all other parameters were stable, the highest IOP would be first thing in the morning on waking, while the lowest would be when one is sleeping.[16]

2. Episcleral venous pressure

Episcleral venous pressure in healthy humans is in the range of 7 to 14 mmHg.[17] This parameter is liable to ultra-short-term and short-term fluctuation as this is the only component of aqueous humor dynamics that is affected by body position. Episcleral venous pressure increases by 3.6 mmHg by changing body position from seated to supine. Otherwise, when body position does not change, episcleral pressure appears to be relatively stable. A change in episcleral venous pressure of 0.8 mmHg corresponds to a change in IOP of 1 mmHg. Long-term fluctuation of episcleral venous pressure remains unknown.

3. Trabecular outflow

Outflow facility in healthy human eyes is in the range of 0.1–0.4 μL/min/mmHg.[18] There is some evidence of diurnal variation in outflow facility. In addition, trabecular outflow resistance increases with age, demonstrated by tonography or perfusion of enucleated human cadaver eyes.[19] Outflow facility is reduced in primary open-angle glaucoma, ocular hypertension, and exfoliation and pigment dispersion syndromes with secondary ocular hypertension.

4. Uveoscleral outflow

Calculated uveoscleral outflow is 25–57% of total aqueous flow in young healthy subjects 20–30 years of age and decreases with age.[18] Uveoscleral outflow is reduced in ocular hypertension with and without pseudoexfoliation syndrome, and is increased in uveitis. There are no data on diurnal variation of uveoscleral outflow pathway.

ULTRA-SHORT-TERM FLUCTUATION OF INTRAOCULAR PRESSURE

Ultra-short-term IOP fluctuation can be caused by the systolic cardiac cycle, changing external ocular pressure, episcleral venous pressure, and aqueous flow, and by other (unknown) factors. One of the most important factors determining the IOP spike height in the ultra-short term is scleral rigidity.[20] Experimental data suggest scleral rigidity increases significantly with age, and this leads to greater spikes in IOP, other parameters being equal.[21] However, the clinical significance of ultra-short-term fluctuation of IOP is unclear.

SHORT-TERM FLUCTUATION OF INTRAOCULAR PRESSURE

Short-term IOP fluctuation is variation occurring over hours or days. Twenty-four-hour IOP variation can be further subdivided into: diurnal (daytime), nocturnal (nighttime), and circadian (24-hour). This fluctuation is likely to be caused by changes in aqueous flow rate, episcleral venous pressure, trabecular outflow, and other factors (Table 9.2). Of these, the most important variables are aqueous flow rate and episcleral venous pressure. The circadian pattern of aqueous flow rate has been known for many years and has a marked effect on the IOP, if all other parameters remained unchanged. For example, IOP would be lowest during sleep and

TABLE 9.2 Aqueous dynamics parameters: the evidence of fluctuation and its effect on intraocular pressure

	ULTRA-SHORT TERM	SHORT TERM	LONG TERM
Aqueous flow	Yes	Yes	Yes
Trabecular outflow	?	?Yes	Yes
Uveoscleral outflow	?	?	?
EVP	Yes	Yes	?
IOP	Yes	Yes	Yes

EVP, episcleral venous pressure; IOP, intraocular pressure.

TABLE 9.3 Mean range of circadian IOP fluctuation in normal eyes

AUTHORS	NUMBER OF EYES	TIME	MEAN RANGE (mmHg)	SD	MAXIMUM RANGE
Drance[22]	404	6:00 – 22:00	3.7	1.8	10
De Venecia[23]	230	05:00 – 24:00	5.0	2.4	N/A
Katavisto[24]	50	04:00 – 24:00	3.17	1.2	6

highest on waking, with a difference of around 43% (Equation 9.6), but this has not always been borne out in clinical studies. Body position has a clear effect on episcleral venous pressure and this affects the IOP accordingly; for example, IOP is 4–5 mmHg higher in subject lying down compared to the sitting position.

In glaucomatous eyes, the IOP fluctuation response to challenges such as the water drinking test probably differs from normal eyes; the abnormally low (pressure sensitive) trabecular outflow facility may result in both the peak and the duration of IOP elevation being prolonged.

The pattern of diurnal (day time) and circadian (24-hour) IOP fluctuation varies widely between individuals (glaucomatous and healthy).

Circadian fluctuation and peak intraocular pressure in normal subjects The circadian fluctuation and time of IOP peaks in normal eyes from published studies are summarized in Table 9.3 and Table 9.4. The mean range of IOP circadian fluctuation is between 3 mmHg and 6.5 mmHg, with a maximum reported range of 11 mmHg. Normal eyes, on average, are likely to have low pressure (recorded in the sitting position) in the night and have the highest pressures early in the morning, before decreasing gradually through out the day. There is a nearly 70% chance of capturing the peak IOP between 08:00 and 16:00 (see Table 9.4).

Circadian fluctuation and peaks of intraocular pressure in glaucoma subjects The most obvious

TABLE 9.4 Probability of peak IOP at different time points of the day in normal eyes

AUTHORS	NUMBER OF EYES	4:00	8:00	12:00	16:00	20:00	24:00
Drance[22]	306		42%	11%	27%	2%	18%
De Venecia[23]	230		38%	17%	10%	9%	26%
Katavisto[24]	100	19%	25%	25%	14%	5%	11%
Newell[25]	60		44%	35%		24%	0%
Kitazawa[26]	24	6%	16%	28%	26%	16%	6%
Average probability		11%	30%	21%	17%	10%	11%

TABLE 9.5 Mean range of circadian IOP fluctuation in untreated glaucomatous eyes

AUTHORS	NUMBER OF EYES	TIME	MEAN RANGE (mmHg)	SD	MAXIMUM RANGE
Drance[22]	138		7.5	3.1	16
David[27]	280	08:00–18:00	5.8	2.9	
Yamagami[28]	228	04:00–24:00	4.8	1.8	
Smith[29]	800		5.8	3.0	
Katavisto[24]	329		11	5.7	

TABLE 9.6 Probability of peak IOP at different time points of the day in glaucoma eyes

AUTHORS	NUMBER OF EYES	4:00	8:00	12:00	16:00	20:00	24:00
Drance[22]	140		46%	11%	21%	7%	14%
Drance[30]	133		25%	38%	4%	11%	22%
Katavisto[24]	507	19%	27%	21%	12%	9%	12%
Kitazawa[26]	27	21%	10%	3%	0%	21%	45%
Yamagami[28]	228	19%	22%	18%	19%	11%	11%
Average probability		16%	24%	22%	9%	14%	15%

TABLE 9.7 Mean range of circadian IOP fluctuation in ocular hypertensive eyes

AUTHORS	NUMBER OF EYES	TIME	MEAN RANGE (mmHg)	SD	MAXIMUM RANGE
Kitazawa[26]	28	00:00 – 24:00	8.1	2.6	16

TABLE 9.8 Probability of peak IOP at different time points of the day in ocular hypertensive eyes

AUTHORS	NUMBER OF EYES	4:00	8:00	12:00	16:00	20:00	24:00
Kitazawa[26]	28	39%	22%	10%	3%	7%	19%
Smith[29]	400		44%	43%	13%		

difference in diurnal IOP fluctuation between untreated glaucomatous eyes (Table 9.5) and eyes of normal subjects (see Table 9.3) is the greater mean IOP range in the glaucomatous eyes. Once again, the trend is for IOP to be highest early in the morning and gradually decreasing throughout the day. IOP monitoring between 08:00 and 16:00 has a nearly 60% chance of capturing the peak pressure (Table 9.6).

Circadian fluctuation and peaks of intraocular pressure in ocular hypertensive subjects There have been relatively few studies of diurnal IOP fluctuation in ocular hypertensive subjects. It is thus difficult to draw any conclusion about the trends. The study by Kitazawa and Horie[26] seemed to suggest that the mean range of IOP fluctuation is more in keeping with that of glaucomatous eyes (Table 9.7 and Table 9.8).

LONG-TERM VARIATION OF INTRAOCULAR PRESSURE

There are two means of assessing 'true' long-term IOP fluctuation: performing repeated diurnal IOP curves over a period of few years or by measuring IOP at the same time of the day over a few years. However, studies have tended to use the standard deviation of IOP measured at different time points during multiple office visits as a surrogate for long-term IOP fluctuation, but this method is probably affected more by the inherent diurnal fluctuation than long-term fluctuation of IOP.

The other two parameters of long-term IOP variations which are thought to be important in the management of glaucoma are mean and peak IOP.

Intraocular pressure variability and clinical management of glaucoma There is conflicting evidence as to whether long-term IOP variation is a risk factor for conversion of ocular hypertension (OHT) to glaucoma, or for progression of established primary open-angle glaucoma (POAG).

Drance[30] was one of the first to suggest that diurnal IOP variation may be a risk factor for progression of POAG. Retrospective analyses of diurnal IOP measurements generated by home tonometry[31] and during clinic hours[32] suggest a significant association between the range and peak of IOP measurements and progression of visual field damage. In a study of predominantly pseudoexfoliative glaucoma patients, Bergea and colleagues prospectively measured the daytime IOP curve at 2 monthly intervals for 2 years and found IOP fluctuation to be associated with disease progression.[33] However, this appears to be the only prospective study in which multiple diurnal IOP curves have been measured. Many studies have assessed the variation of single IOP measurements between office visits.

The European Glaucoma Prevention Study (EGPS) assessed the role of IOP fluctuation, defined as the standard deviation (SD) of inter-visit IOP over the study period, on the conversion of OHT to POAG. In a multiple variable analysis of risk factors, mean IOP was significantly associated with conversion (adjusted hazard ratio [HR] = 1.12 per 1 mmHg, 95% confidence intervals [CI], 1.03–1.22, $p < 0.01$), while IOP fluctuation was not a significant risk.[34] Other studies have also found mean IOP level to be a significant risk factor for conversion of OHT to POAG, with no effect of IOP fluctuation.[35]

In a post hoc analysis of IOP data from the Advanced Glaucoma Intervention Study (AGIS), Nouri-Mahdavi and colleagues found that long-term IOP fluctuation

was a significant risk factor for visual field progression. As for the EGPS, fluctuation was defined as the SD of inter-visit IOP measurements.[36] Eyes that had an SD <3 mmHg over the follow-up period showed no signs of progression, while eyes exhibiting an SD >3 mmHg had significant disease progression. In a multiple variable analysis it was found that every 1 mmHg IOP fluctuation was associated with 31% higher odds for developing progression. Conversely, assessment of IOP fluctuation in the Early Manifest Glaucoma Trial (EMGT) found no association between IOP fluctuation and visual field progression.[37] Both these studies included mean IOP over the follow-up period in the multiple variable analyses. In the EMGT analysis, IOP fluctuation was also defined as the SD of inter-visit IOP measurements, but only measurements up to the point where progression was first detected (or, in the case of nonprogressors, up to and including the final follow-up visit) were included. IOP fluctuation was found to be 2.02 mmHg and 1.78 mmHg, respectively, in patients who did and did not show progression. A multiple variable analysis showed that mean IOP and not IOP fluctuation was a significant factor for progression, with every 1 mmHg higher mean IOP associated with an 11% increase in risk (IOP fluctuation increases with the level of IOP).

Differences between the two studies may be explained by the differences in study design and population investigated. Unlike the EMGT analysis, the AGIS analysis included IOP measurements following identification of progression. In addition, the goal of patient treatment in the AGIS was to maintain IOP below 18 mmHg and, as such, clinicians could add supplementary topical hypotensive therapy when deemed necessary.[38] These two points introduce bias into the data analysis, as treatment is usually intensified once progression is detected, thus artificially increasing IOP fluctuation. Indeed, when IOP measurements following progression were included, the EMGT authors found IOP fluctuation to be a significant risk factor for progression (HR 1.66, 95% CI 1.44–1.93, $p < 0.001$), and mean IOP was no longer important (HR 0.97, 95% CI 0.92–1.02, $p = 0.26$).

Inter-visit IOP fluctuation has been found to be a risk factor for the progression of pseudoexfoliative glaucoma,[39] and in a retrospective analysis of IOP and progression of primary angle-closure glaucoma and POAG patients undergoing a combined phacoemulsification and trabeculectomy procedure, inter-visit IOP fluctuation was a significant risk factor even in the presence of low postoperative IOP.[40]

The role of IOP fluctuation in progression of disease remains to be clarified. It has been suggested that IOP fluctuation has a greater impact on progression in eyes with low IOP, while IOP level has greater importance in eyes with higher IOP.[41] However, further prospective studies investigating longer-term diurnal IOP variation are needed to confirm whether or not it plays an important role in glaucomatous progression.

REFERENCES

1. Whitacre MM, Stein R. Sources of error with use of Goldmann-type tonometers. Surv Ophthalmol 1993; 38(1):1–30.

2. Tonnu PA, Ho T, Sharma K, et al. A comparison of four methods of tonometry: method agreement and interobserver variability. Br J Ophthalmol 2005; 89(7):847–850.

3. Kotecha A, White ET, Shewry JM, et al. The relative effects of corneal thickness and age on Goldmann applanation tonometry and dynamic contour tonometry. Br J Ophthalmol 2005; 89(12):1572–1575.

4. Kotecha A, Elsheikh A, Roberts CR, et al. Corneal thickness-and age-related biomechanical properties of the cornea measured with the ocular response analyzer. Invest Ophthalmol Vis Sci 2006; 47(12):5337–5347.

5. Kanngiesser HE, Kniestedt C, Robert YC. Dynamic contour tonometry: presentation of a new tonometer. J Glaucoma 2005; 14(5):344–350.

6. Kniestedt C, Nee M, Stamper RL. Accuracy of dynamic contour tonometry compared with applanation tonometry in human cadaver eyes of different hydration states. Graefe's Arch Clin Exp Ophthalmol 2005; 243(4):359–366.

7. Kaufmann C, Bachmann LM, Thiel MA. Comparison of dynamic contour tonometry with Goldmann applanation tonometry. Invest Ophthalmol Vis Sci 2004; 45(9):3118–3121.

8. Doyle A, Lachkar Y. Comparison of dynamic contour tonometry with Goldmann applanation tonometry over a wide range of central corneal thickness. J Glaucoma 2005; 14(4):288–292.

9. Bhan A, Bhargava J, Vernon SA, et al. Repeatability of ocular blood flow pneumatonometry. Ophthalmology 2003; 110(8):1551–1554.

10. Spraul CW, Lang GE, Ronzani M, et al. Reproducibility of measurements with a new slit lamp-mounted ocular blood flow tonograph. Graefe's Arch Clin Exp Ophthalmol 1998; 236(4):274–279.

11. Garcia-Resua C, Gonzalez-Meijome JM, Gilino J, et al. Accuracy of the new ICare rebound tonometer vs. other portable tonometers in healthy eyes. Optom Vis Sci 2006; 83(2):102–107.

12. Zeimer RC, Wilensky JT, Gieser DK, et al. Evaluation of a self tonometer for home use. Arch Ophthalmol 1983; 101(11):1791–1793.

13. Fresco BB. A new tonometer – the pressure phosphene tonometer: clinical comparison with Goldman tonometry. Ophthalmology 1998; 105(11):2123–2126.

14. Zeimer RC, Wilensky JT, Gieser DK, et al. Application of a self-tonometer to home tonometry. Arch Ophthalmol 1986; 104(1):49–53.

15. Brubaker RF, Nagataki S, Townsend DJ, et al. The effect of age on aqueous humor formation in man. Ophthalmology 1981; 88(3):283–288.

16. Reiss GR, Lee DA, Topper JE, et al. Aqueous humor flow during sleep. Invest Ophthalmol Vis Sci 1984; 25(6):776–778.

17. Zeimer RC, Gieser DK, Wilensky JT, et al. A practical venomanometer. Measurement of episcleral venous pressure and assessment of the normal range,. Arch Ophthalmol 1983; 101(9):1447–1449.

18. Toris CB, Yablonski ME, Wang YL, et al. Aqueous humor dynamics in the aging human eye. Am J Ophthalmol 1999; 127(4):407–412.

19. Gabelt BT, Kaufman PL. Changes in aqueous humor dynamics with age and glaucoma. Prog Retin Eye Res 2005; 24(5): 612–637.

20. Friedenwald JS. Contribution to the theory and practice of tonometry. Am J Ophthalmol 1937; 20:985–1024.

21. Pallikaris IG, Kymionis GD, Ginis HS, et al. Ocular rigidity in living human eyes. Invest Ophthalmol Vis Sci 2005; 46(2): 409–414.

22. Drance SM. The significance of the diurnal tension variations in normal and glaucomatous eyes. Arch Ophthalmol 1960; 64:494–501.

23. De Venecia G, Davis MD. Diurnal variation of intraocular pressure in the normal eye. Arch Ophthalmol 1963; 69:752–757.

24. Katavisto M. The diurnal variations of ocular tension in glaucoma. Acta Ophthalmol 1964(Suppl 78):1–130.

25. Newell FW, Krill AE. Diurnal tonography in normal and glaucomatous eyes. Am J Ophthalmol 1965; 59:840–853.

26. Kitazawa Y, Horie T. Diurnal variation of intraocular pressure in primary open-angle glaucoma. Am J Ophthalmol 1975; 79(4):557–566.

27. David R, Zangwill L, Briscoe D, et al. Diurnal intraocular pressure variations: an analysis of 690 diurnal curves. Br J Ophthalmol 1992; 76(5):280–283.

28. Yamagami J, Araie M, Aihara M, et al. Diurnal variation in intraocular pressure of normal-tension glaucoma eyes. Ophthalmology 1993; 100(5):643–650.

29. Smith J. Diurnal intraocular pressure. Correlation to automated perimetry. Ophthalmology 1985; 92(7):858–861.

30. Drance SM. Diurnal variation in intraocular pressure in treated glaucoma. Arch Ophthalmol 1963; 70:302–311.

31. Asrani S, Zeimer R, Wilensky J, et al. Large diurnal fluctuations in intraocular pressure are an independent risk factor in patients with glaucoma. J Glaucoma 2000; 9(2):134–142.

32. Collaer N, Zeyen T, Caprioli J. Sequential office pressure measurements in the management of glaucoma. J Glaucoma 2005; 14(3):196–200.

33. Bergea B, Bodin L, Svedbergh B. Impact of intraocular pressure regulation on visual fields in open-angle glaucoma. Ophthalmology 1999; 106(5):997–1004; discussion 1004–1005.

34. Miglior S, Torri V, Zeyen T, et al. Intercurrent factors associated with the development of open-angle glaucoma in the European glaucoma prevention study. Am J Ophthalmol 2007; 144(2):266–275.

35. Bengtsson B, Heijl A. Diurnal IOP fluctuation: not an independent risk factor for glaucomatous visual field loss in high-risk ocular hypertension. Graefe's Arch Clin Exp Ophthalmol 2005; 243(6):513–518.

36. Nouri-Mahdavi K, Hoffman D, Coleman AL, et al. Predictive factors for glaucomatous visual field progression in the Advanced Glaucoma Intervention Study. Ophthalmology 2004; 111(9):1627–1635.

37. Bengtsson B, Leske MC, Hyman L, et al. Fluctuation of intraocular pressure and glaucoma progression in the Early Manifest Glaucoma Trial. Ophthalmology 2007; 114(2): 205–209.

38. The Advanced Glaucoma Intervention Study (AGIS): 7. The relationship between control of intraocular pressure and visual field deterioration. The AGIS Investigators. Am J Ophthalmol 2000; 130(4):429–440.

39. Konstas AG, Hollo G, Astakhov YS, et al. Factors associated with long-term progression or stability in exfoliation glaucoma. Arch Ophthalmol 2004; 122(1):29–33.

40. Hong S, Seong GJ, Hong YJ. Long-term intraocular pressure fluctuation and progressive visual field deterioration in patients with glaucoma and low intraocular pressures after a triple procedure. Arch Ophthalmol 2007; 125(8):1010–1013.

41. Caprioli J. Intraocular pressure fluctuation: an independent risk factor for glaucoma? Arch Ophthalmol 2007; 125(8):1124–1125.

CHAPTER 10

Visual Fields

David P Crabb

INTRODUCTION

This chapter summarizes the use of standard visual field measures that are most likely used in modern glaucoma detection and management. For the interested reader there are some excellent complete texts on the subject, notably Henson,[1] Cubbidge,[2] and also chapters in Edgar and Rudnicka.[3]

The visual field is simply the portion of space from which light can enter the eye, reach the retina, stimulate the photoreceptors, and evoke a sensation of light. Perimetry is a diagnostic examination technique for recognizing disturbances in the visual field. It is of basic importance for ophthalmologists and optometrists, and extends to other medical specialties, notably neurology and neurosurgery. In current clinical practice perimetry remains central to the detection and monitoring of visual function in glaucoma.

Perimetry normally tests the light-difference sensitivity across the visual field. This sensitivity reflects the capability of the eye to perceive a brightness difference between a test target and its background. Light-difference sensitivity depends upon the tested location on the retina and upon the parameters of the measurement technique, such as intensity of background luminance and target size. The normal visual field extends further away from fixation temporally and inferiorly than superiorly and nasally. The physiological blind spot corresponds to the location where the optic nerve enters the eye and its center is located about 15° temporal from fixation. From the center of the retina this sensitivity decreases towards the periphery, evoking the classically defined 'hill of vision:' a three-dimensional representation of retinal light sensitivity. In this analogy there is a peak at the center of the hill of vision which represents the increasing sensitivity to light from the retinal periphery to the fovea. A visual field defect is any departure from the normal topography of the hill of vision (Fig. 10.1).

The history of the recognition of visual field defects is a fascinating one and the interested reader is directed towards a short review by Atchison.[4] The first true

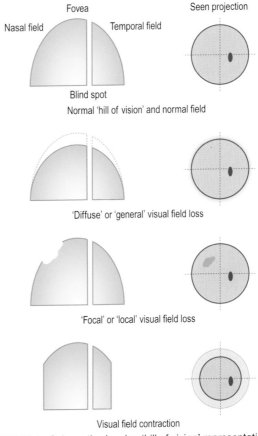

FIGURE 10.1 Schematic showing 'hill of vision' representation and 'projected' form of the visual field. Early glaucomatous defects are typically diffuse or focal (scotomas).

clinical description of a perimetric technique to examine and quantify the visual field was by von Graefe in the mid-nineteenth century. A chalk board with a central fixation point was used in conjunction with a large, moving illuminated object. Marks were recorded on the board as the object moved from seen to unseen areas. One of von Graefe's early figures crudely illustrated a peripheral field defect in a patient with glaucoma. In 1857, Aubert and Foerster introduced a perimetric technique where a test stimulus was presented on an arc. Several directions or meridians could be examined by rotating the arc. In the late 1800s, Landesberg used similar methods to define as scotomas visual field defects that are surrounded by areas with more normal sensitivity and Bjerrum developed a tangent screen examination whereby a subject fixates the center of a flat observation surface: this was used to establish the characteristic arcuate distribution of glaucomatous visual field loss that still bears his name. In the early twentieth century, Rönne used this type of perimetry to define the glaucomatous nasal step, relating it to the anatomical arrangement of the retinal nerve fiber layer.

MANUAL VISUAL FIELD TESTING

Perimetry, using stimuli moving across a background surface, was advanced significantly by Goldmann in the 1930s with the development of standardized kinetic perimetry: this elegantly designed device allowed control of the luminance of both the background and stimuli with the latter projected onto a hemispheric bowl, being moved from 'not seen' areas to sites where it was first perceived. The stimuli devised at that time have become standards: the smallest being Goldmann size 0, with a diameter of 0.43° and area of {1/16} mm². On the Goldmann scale the diameter size doubles each time; the standard used in both manual and automated perimetry is Goldmann III (0.05° and area of 4 mm²). In Goldmann perimetry, lines called isopters are drawn to connect points which exhibit the same sensitivity to differences between stimulus and background luminance. These isopters generate a type of contour map of the sensitivity of the visual field. The direct mechanical

link between the stimulus control and a plotting pen provided the first visual field measurement with a degree of reproducibility and accuracy.

Goldmann perimetry is still widely used today, including in some centers in glaucoma diagnosis and management (Fig. 10.2). The high-resolution shape information obtained by the 'improvisation' of kinetic testing in real time allows for detailed delineation of visual field defects that can be invaluable for neuro-ophthalmologic diagnosis. However, kinetic or manual perimetry is subjective, being heavily reliant on training and experience, and colloquially bears resemblance more to an 'art' rather than a standardized scientific measurement. There are serious technical limitations, especially with regards to the psychophysical response to the moving target and spatial summation effects, along with subject's response time to the examiner. More simply, the examiner may simply overlook areas of the field which are not thought to be important and the configuration of field defects may be biased to fulfill preconceived ideas. Moreover, kinetic testing gives poorly reproducible results in the central field and at the edges of gradually deepening scotomas such as those found in glaucoma. Therefore, when quantifiable, reproducible results are required, automated perimetry is preferred.

AUTOMATED VISUAL FIELD TESTING

The modern benchmark used for measuring the visual field in glaucoma is standard automated perimetry (SAP) (Fig. 10.3) Considerable research evidence has established that glaucomatous loss is detected and managed much more reliably with automated perimetry

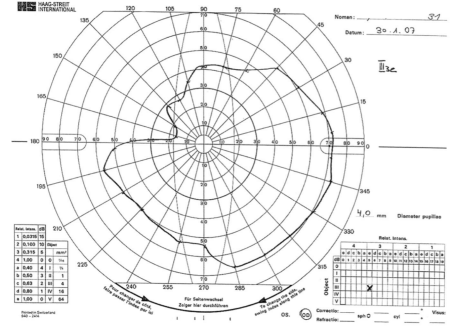

FIGURE 10.2 Example printout from Goldmann perimetry for a glaucomatous patient (right eye) with a significant defect using a Goldmann size III stimulus. The area within the contour line is the 'seeing' part of the field.

as compared to Goldmann perimetry.[5] In contrast to the kinetic strategy used in manual Goldmann perimetry these automated devices are examples of static perimetry: the stimuli presented to the subject do not move. Luminance sensitivity is established at a fixed matrix of test points by varying the stimulus intensity until each test location is just seen: this point is known as the threshold. A light stimulus presented below the threshold will not be detected by the subject, whereas a stimulus above the threshold will be detected by the subject. The threshold sensitivity at each test location, which is the reciprocal of the threshold, is typically presented in decibels (dB) indicating the logarithmic nature of light intensity on a linear scale where, for example, 0 dB would represent the brightest stimulus intensity on the perimeter, with, very approximately, values around 30 dB being 'normal' values. These values are a relative scale and are not directly comparable across different makes of perimeter.

SAP is the modern clinical standard for measuring glaucomatous visual field defects: it is mainly operator independent and yields clinically measurable numerical data relating to the measured threshold at a grid of points in the visual field. SAP can be divided into suprathreshold strategies, typically used in glaucoma detection and screening, and full-threshold strategies, mainly used for more detailed testing and monitoring disease worsening or glaucomatous progression.

Suprathreshold techniques are relatively quick to administer: they simply record whether a location is normal (stimulus seen) or abnormal (stimulus not

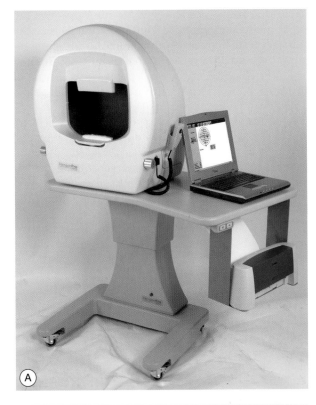

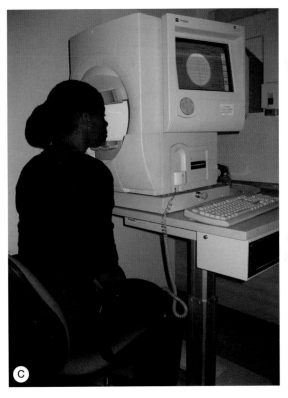

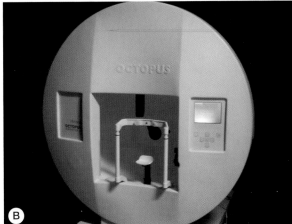

FIGURE 10.3 Examples of modern automated perimeters. **(A)** Henson (Tinsley Medical Instruments, UK), **(B)** Octopus (Haag-Streit AG, Switzerland), **(C)** Humphrey Field Analyzer (Zeiss-Humphrey Instruments, Dublin, CA, USA).

seen). This is done by presenting a stimulus calculated to be slightly more intense than the subject's threshold (suprathreshold increment), normally set between 4 dB and 6 dB higher. Most suprathreshold tests take account of the fact that sensitivity declines with age and also varies by location with, for example, relatively reduced sensitivity of the peripheral visual field compared to the central field. These suprathreshold tests therefore use a list of values held as a database from which the testing threshold is determined.

Some suprathreshold tests attempt to determine the subject's unique overall threshold, usually by means of a full-threshold examination using a few selected test points and then use this information. The Henson perimeter is an exemplar of suprathreshold instruments: these have recently incorporated other improved types of suprathreshold testing including the HEART algorithm[6] and multisampling techniques.[7]

Full-threshold techniques provide more detailed information than suprathreshold strategies since they indicate the depth of scotomas rather than merely their presence or absence. However, full-threshold testing is much more protracted, which has important implications in the clinical setting and in terms of the demand on the patient. In full-threshold testing each location is examined using a staircase or bracketing technique. An example of this is the widely employed 4–2 staircase strategy used, for example, in Octopus (Haag-Streit AG, Switzerland) and Humphrey (Zeiss-Humphrey Instruments, US) perimetry (Fig. 10.4). The intensity of the initial stimulus depends on age-matched normal values: if this is seen, the next presentation at that location is 4 dB less intense. If this is also seen, the following stimulus at that location is

reduced by a further 4 dB in intensity, and so on until the subject fails to see a stimulus presentation: this is the 'first reversal.' The stimuli following this are increased in intensity by 2 dB each time until the subject now reports a stimulus as seen: this is the 'second reversal.' The threshold is typically estimated as the mean of the final and the penultimate presentation intensities, but this final calculation varies between instruments with, for example, the Octopus applying a final correction. If the initial presentation is not seen, intensities of subsequent presentations are increased by 4 dB until one is seen ('first reversal') then decreased by 2 dB until one is missed ('second reversal').

Thresholds are initially estimated in this manner at four locations in the visual field, one in each quadrant at approximately 9° from the fovea. Although each of the four 'seed' locations is measured in turn, the perimeter does this in random order so that the position on the staircase is different for each location and the observer is not preconditioned to the location of the next stimulus presentation. Points adjacent to the seed points are tested next: the initial stimulus presentation is set at the brightness determined from the threshold previously obtained at the seed point. This testing of contiguous points 'spirals' outwards such that all points in the grid are eventually measured.

The threshold is a peculiar measurement: it isn't measured directly, and is based on a probability of 'yes' and 'no' sequences. Moreover, the physiological nature of the threshold varies during a test (short-term fluctuation) and between tests (long-term fluctuation). In psychophysics, staircase testing is often designed so that the threshold is crossed many times, so that the threshold can be estimated with acceptable precision but at the cost of lengthy examination. This time luxury cannot be afforded in the clinic. Over the years much research has been aimed at developing clinically useful perimetric testing strategies that reduce the test time; some of these, for example FASTPAC and TOP,[8] reduce test time, but at the cost of poorer measurement accuracy. However, in the mid-1990s, the Swedish Interactive Testing Algorithm (SITA) developed by Heijl and colleagues[9] accomplished the task of reducing time while maintaining the standard of accuracy observed in 4–2 full-threshold testing.

SITA reduces the actual number of stimulus exposures required by measuring closer to the patient's true seeing threshold using a principle of Bayesian probability: this can be explained with a simple analogy. In horseracing, certain animals have a higher probability of winning than others and this is reflected in the different odds offered by a bookmaker covering the 'favorite' to 'outsiders' or 'long shots:' these probabilities are adjusted before the race commences to account for previous winning form, quality of the jockey, and other factors. Similarly, at the start of SITA testing (before the subject presses the response button!) not all thresholds are assumed to have an equal probability of occurring; they are adjusted based on the

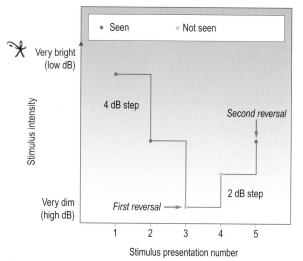

FIGURE 10.4 Schematic illustrating the staircase algorithm for standard full-threshold perimetry. The stimulus intensity is varied in 'steps' of 4 dB until the first reversal occurs and subsequently in steps of 2 dB. With the Humphrey, intensity of the last seen presentation is taken as the final threshold estimate, after a second response reversal has occurred.

expected response (using factors such as the patient's age, location in the field, and previous normal reference data). Moreover, like a fluctuating betting market, the probability of establishing the final response varies as the test progresses: as the patient responds to seeing different thresholds with 'yes' and 'no' answers, the underlying probability of a particular measured threshold being the final outcome is adjusted during the test. The range of possible outcomes is summarized by likelihood functions which can be thought of as graphs of all the likely final thresholds with the

final position and shape of the graphs giving the estimated threshold (Fig. 10.5). Moreover, SITA uses prior information about sensitivity values at neighboring locations using a physiological map of the expected relationship between the sensitivity at points in the field that adjusts the testing sequence at points and quickens the examination.

SITA testing takes approximately half the time (about 7 minutes per eye) to complete than examination with the standard 4–2 algorithm. Very noteworthy is the main reduction in test time is a result of novel features for monitoring patient attention and reliability during the visual field examination, reviewed later. These techniques tailor the pacing of the test to the individual and save as much testing time as the clever mathematics of the testing strategy.

One problem with SITA is that the technicalities are far from explicit; the interested reader can find more detail in Olsson and Rootzén.[10] There are other caveats in the use SITA: it has been designed for glaucoma and use with other clinical conditions should only be considered with caution. In addition, interchanging SITA and full-threshold testing is not recommended in longitudinal follow-up of patients.[11,12] Nevertheless, SITA is rightly becoming the new clinical gold standard for threshold perimetry in glaucoma because quicker tests are naturally appealing to the patient and clinician. Sound research evidence reassuringly suggests measurements from SITA are in close agreement with those from FT,[13] albeit defects from SITA appear slightly shallower.[14] However, there is no evidence to suggest that SITA provides more accurate measurement or better test-retest variability than FT; in fact, the test-retest variability may have a different 'profile', which may be important in terms of developing methods for detecting progression.[15] Research continues in this area, especially with function-specific perimetry, and other fast but reliable testing strategies, especially when used in follow-up, may soon become available.

It is worth pointing out that 'SITA Fast' is a different algorithm to 'SITA standard:' the former deliberately uses larger step sizes in stimulus presentation and is, therefore, quicker still. SITA Fast may have a role in testing subjects that find longer tests impossible to complete, but SITA Fast does manifest significantly greater measurement variability than both SITA and 4–2 full-threshold testing and should not be used in follow-up. Other fast strategies, notably FASTPAC and TOP, with the latter being used on Octopus instrumentation, also have prohibitive levels of measurement variability associated with them and again should only be used clinically when patients find the standard tests beyond them.

Sometimes, binocular visual field testing is required for the assessment of true functional disability or for sociolegal reasons. For example, in the UK, the binocular Esterman Test is currently used for assessing the visual fields component in terms of legal fitness

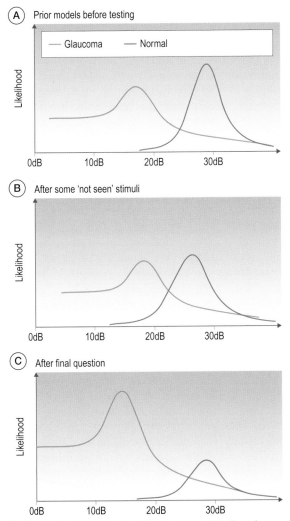

FIGURE 10.5 Schematic illustrating the use of likelihood functions for efficiently estimating thresholds in SITA. Each point in the visual field has two starting likelihood functions as illustrated in panel **(A)**. (In full threshold testing the 'curves' would simply be rectangles with all responses equally likely). The curve for the normal response has the higher peak to start with but the shape of both functions alters as a patient responds to the stimulus at different intensities. For example, **(B)** illustrates what the curves look like after a series of stimuli are not seen, thus indicating that the patient's response is more likely to fall within the curve for glaucoma. After more unseen responses the glaucoma likelihood function 'dominates' and the threshold is estimated from some location on the curve, normally the peak of the curve, but this can be further adjusted when compared to neighboring locations.

to drive. The Esterman is a suprathreshold test where patients simply have both eyes open and is available on automated perimeters. Recent work has suggested that equivalent information can be gleaned by merging monocular results.[16] At this stage, it is worth emphasizing the difficulty that some patients have with perceiving their visual field defects and the importance of binocular assessment. Although it is critical to assess the function of each eye individually to determine the presence, severity, and progression status of glaucoma, the visual world is determined by the input from both eyes to the brain. Patients' perception of the severity of their visual field loss is often difficult because an unaffected eye essentially fills in for the other. The interested reader is directed towards the results from Viswanathan et al.[17] on the role and importance of binocular testing, and for a wider discussion on the visual field and functional correlates by Spaeth et al.[18]

PATTERNS OF VISUAL FIELD LOSS IN GLAUCOMA

There is no simple blueprint for the pattern of visual field loss in glaucoma. However, typical loss is directed by the arrangement of the retinal nerve fiber layers as they congregate on entry into the optic disc, with those fibers from the temporal retina usually most susceptible to damage resulting in defects occurring more frequently in the superior hemifield. The damaged nerve fiber layers typically give isolated damage in the paracentral areas (10–20°), eventually forming arcuate scotomas. Another important configuration of early loss can be the 'nasal step,' resulting in asymmetry in retinal sensitivity either side of the temporal horizontal midline. As the disease advances, both hemifields may become involved (Fig. 10.6). Other patterns of loss are thought to occur, including baring or enlargement of the blind spot and generalized depression of the sensitivity of the field, but these are more typically non-specific signs of glaucomatous loss. For example, diffuse loss can occur in many diseases affecting visual function, such as opacification of the lens and cataract, with the latter sometimes causing difficulty when trying to establish if a visual field defect is worsening on follow-up.

Various spatial grids are available in automated static perimetry to detect these patterns of loss. A common testing pattern used for general visual field testing involves a 'square' grid of 6° separated points tested out to 30° on the Humphrey instrument (called the 30–2), or the slightly more constricted 24–2 pattern shown in Fig. 10.6A. (This only tests to 30° in the region of the nasal defect.) Various different configurations are used for screening algorithms on suprathreshold perimetry, where it is important to assess the spatial extent of the defect and Henson[1] provides a good discussion of this. The Octopus perimeters use regular spatial grids similar to the Humphrey, but the stimulus separation varies a little. In end-stage glaucoma the 10–2 spatial grid is sometimes used on the Humphrey perimeters covering the macular area to 10° with points separated by 2°. The main point here is that defect detection is determined by the size of the scotomas and the resolution of the visual field examination; certain testing patterns have become fixed standards for testing in glaucoma because fewer test points mean shorter tests, but the 24–2 pattern can only probably detect and monitor about 90% of glaucomatous defects.

MEASUREMENT VARIABILITY

Visual field testing examines the impact of a defect on visual function and is therefore the cornerstone of glaucoma assessment. However, despite the advances in automated perimetry the subjective nature of the test remains; after all, it is completely reliant on a subject reliably answering questions and pressing a button! The variability in response or measurement noise is overwhelmingly multifactorial. To start with there is variability within a single examination (short-term fluctuation): this is influenced by physiological factors, such as the magnitude of visual sensitivity itself, with lower thresholds manifesting greater fluctuation. In short, patients with defects are considerably more variable than subjects with normal fields. Short-term fluctuation also appears to vary in different parts of the field with, for example, noise increasing with eccentricity. Moreover, the fatigue effect, which tends

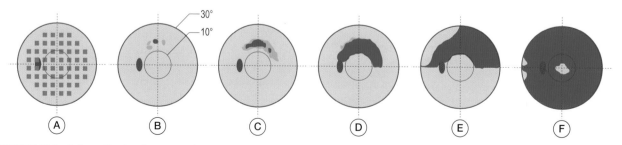

FIGURE 10.6 Schematic showing worsening patterns of visual field loss in open-angle glaucoma. **(A)** Location of testing points of the 24–2, Humphrey visual field. **(B)** Isolated defects in paracentral area. **(C)** Small isolated defects combine to form a larger defect. **(D,E)** Arcuate defect forms and worsens and eventually breaks through to the periphery. **(F)** End-stage defect, with only small functional macular area remaining.

to increase variability in response with examination duration is a widely accepted contributor to short-term fluctuation and is difficult to control or measure. Other factors that influence measurement variability, including refractive error, lens artifacts, pupil size, and even droopy eyelids, are, to a certain extent, controllable with diligent testing. Media opacity also affects measurements but a tweak in the analysis of results attempts to correct for this. Unsurprisingly, short-term fluctuation also varies with the reliability of the subject's response: inattentiveness (false-negative errors); 'trigger happy' reactions (false-positive errors); loss of fixation – for these the automated perimeter attempts (sometimes quite cleverly) to measure patient reliability. To cap it all, there is the problem of long-term fluctuation encountered when tests are performed on separate occasions; this in turn is influenced by the learning effect, where subjects simply get better at the examination and more reliable with experience, yielding an improvement in sensitivity, with defects falsely appearing to get better! A number of investigators believe most of the learning to be complete after the performance of the first two fields, whilst some published studies indicate that improvements in performance remain beyond this, especially when baseline sensitivity is very low. In general, it is good practice to allow at least one training visual field test per eye to account for most of the learning effect, especially if establishing a baseline measurement for follow-up.

INTERPRETATION OF VISUAL FIELD RESULTS

Results for automated perimetry are typically presented as printouts which vary from instrument to instrument but almost all automated perimeters have some features in common. (Fig. 10.7) A grid of numbers representing the 'raw' thresholds measured at all the test locations are typically displayed as a grid of values. The gray scale of the visual field provides an image which is

FIGURE 10.7 Humphrey Field Analyzer output showing a single field analysis of results from a normal subject **(A)** and a glaucomatous patient.

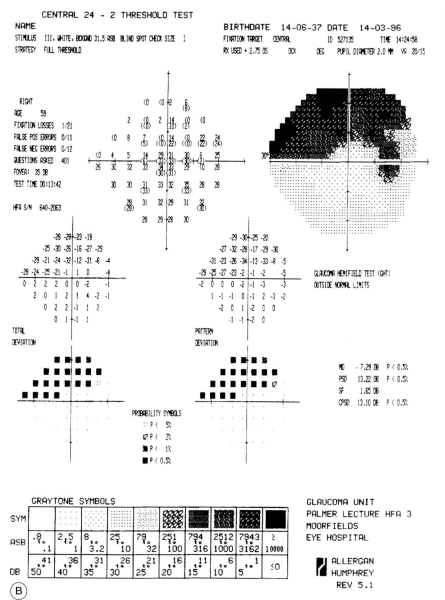

FIGURE 10.7 (Continued) (B) using the full-threshold 24–2 program.

more readily interpreted, with darker areas representing defects. For suprathreshold tests there is normally only one of two categories being represented by a symbol indicating whether the stimulus at that location was seen or not (Fig. 10.8).

Since automated perimetry generates numerical results, a vast array of statistical analyses has been applied to visual fields. Quantification procedures applied to visual field results can be put into three main categories: single field analysis, analysis of patient response reliability, and series of visual field results (analysis of progression).

SINGLE FIELD ANALYSIS

Analyses based on a single field test typically compare a visual field with results from a normal population or by using within-eye comparisons. This section briefly summarizes single visual field analysis with the emphasis on results from automated perimetry, specifically the Humphrey. Reviews of the single field analysis of results from other types of perimetry and other automated instruments, including the widely-used Octopus, can be found in Henson.[1]

The difficulty of interpreting the stand-alone raw values and gray scale is compounded by the existence of sensitivity threshold values that decrease with increasing age and eccentricity in the normal field. Hence, to further aid the interpretation of the raw data, age-corrected normal values have been established and are stored in the Humphrey (Fig. 10.9). These can be subtracted from the recorded sensitivity threshold at each test location to give a defect depth representation, usefully displayed as a total deviation plot. This is expressed in decibels, and charted as symbols representing the different levels of probability with which

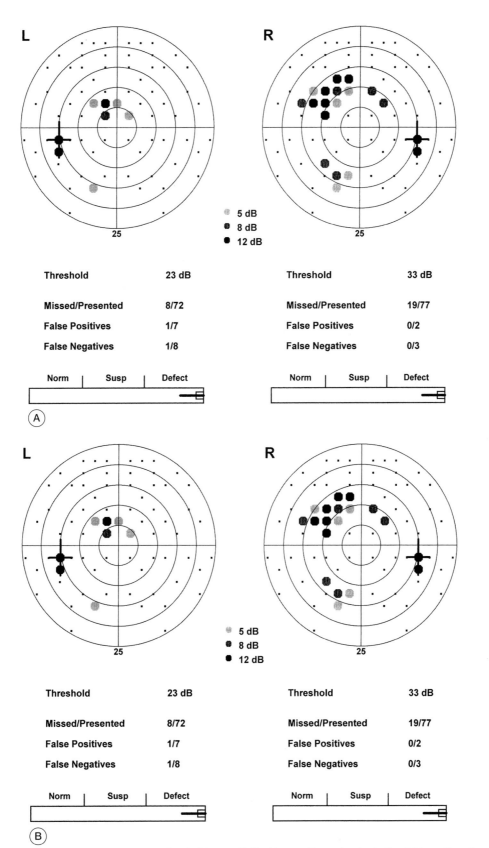

FIGURE 10.8 Results from a single stimulus suprathreshold test with the Henson Pro perimeter. In the right eye there is a superior arcuate defect and an inferior paracentral defect, while in the left eye there is a paracentral defect that is close to fixation. Each visual field is quantified, based upon the number of missed stimuli, their depth, and clustering properties. The results of this analysis are given on the scales at the bottom of the chart. The box represents the value and the horizontal line the confidence limits.

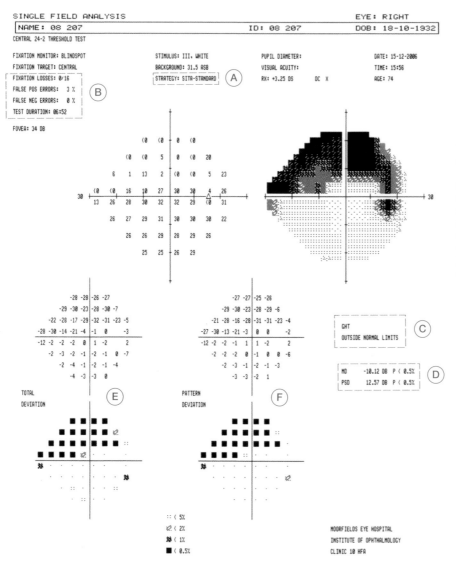

FIGURE 10.9 Humphrey Field Analyzer output showing a single field analysis of results from a glaucomatous patient using the SITA standard program **(A)**. Reliability indices and test duration is shown in the top left-hand corner **(B)**. The results for the GHT **(C)** and global indices **(D)** are shown below the main gray scale. For this subject there is little difference in the appearance of the total deviation plot **(E)** and the pattern deviation plot **(F)**. Nevertheless, the latter is the most important defect plot on the chart for assessing glaucomatous defects because this attempts to correct for any general loss of sensitivity that may be present because of media opacity or cataract.

the particular value would occur in a normal population. The symbols beneath indicate probability statements about the measured threshold at each test location when compared with a normal database.[19] For example, a black symbol indicates that the deviation from normal at that point occurs in less than 0.5% of normal subjects and, therefore, must be regarded as highly suspect. The pattern deviation grids are similar to the total deviation plots, but a possible shift in the direction of a general reduction in retinal sensitivity is mathematically removed. This essentially makes this representation more sensitive to localized defects. It is worth emphasizing that in glaucoma detection the pattern deviation plot is by far the most useful graphical display on the entire printout.

Information relating to the amount of visual field loss, and whether the loss is generalized or focal, is summarized in a set of summary measures known as global indices. For the Octopus perimeter the main indices are mean defect and loss variance. The corresponding measures for the Humphrey perimeter are now described in

more detail. The mean deviation (MD) is simply the average deviation from the age-corrected normal reference field. It is an estimate of the total field loss, both general and localized. Pattern standard deviation (PSD) is the standard deviation of the differences between the measured thresholds and the normal reference values at individual test locations. PSD estimates the nonuniform part of the deviation. A small value for PSD indicates close agreement in shape between the subject's field and the normal reference field. Conversely, a high value of PSD indicates an irregular hill of vision and a field with localized defects. Limits for normal subjects have been evaluated for all the indices and if a calculated value falls outside these limits a probability statement is given. These levels of probability are associated with the distribution of the value of the particular index in a normal population. Therefore, in this instance $p < 5\%$ simply means that less than 5% of the normal population demonstrate a larger value for the calculated index. It does not equate to a 5% chance that the result is normal. Like all summary measures, global indices

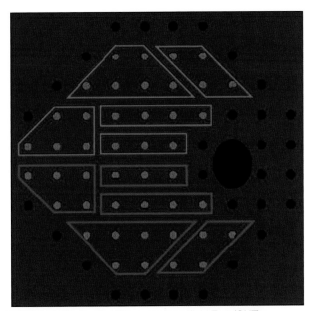

FIGURE 10.10 For the Glaucoma Hemifield Test (GHT) five anatomical sectors (*red*) in the superior visual field are superimposed on the Humphrey test pattern selected according to the normal arrangement of the retinal nerve fiber layers. Within each sector, the sum of the probability scores is calculated and the difference compared with the mirror image sector (*green*) in the inferior hemifield. If there are significant differences between the sectors then the GHT is 'outside normal limits.' GHT is a reasonably precise diagnostic procedure for early glaucomatous loss.

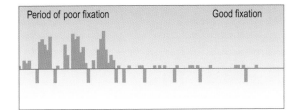

FIGURE 10.11 An example of a graph indicating eye movements, with upward spikes indicating eye movements and downward spikes indicating blinking during stimulus presentation. This is typically given as a trace on the bottom of the results printout that can be reviewed at the end of the examination.

are a form of data reduction and, while useful in giving an overall numerical value to the field, should always be considered secondary to the deviation plots, especially in the early detection of glaucomatous defects.

Additionally, the Humphrey printout gives the results of the Glaucoma Hemifield Test (GHT) used to determine whether a single field is normal or has a suspected glaucomatous defect (Fig. 10.10).[20] It was devised to detect field loss that is asymmetric about the horizontal meridian, a characteristic of glaucomatous loss. Analysis is performed in five corresponding pairs of sectors that are based on the normal anatomy of the retinal nerve fiber layer. Deviations from the age-corrected normal threshold in the most sensitive areas of the field are used to detect overall glaucomatous loss. Fields are classified as outside or within normal limits, borderline, or as having a general reduction in retinal sensitivity. This automated algorithm has been proven to give good levels of sensitivity and specificity for separating glaucomatous from normal fields,[21] especially if a repeated GHT was considered. In Octopus perimetry, the Bebie curve is a cumulative distribution of the defect depth at each location and, like the GHT, is designed to separate normal visual fields from those with early diffuse loss.

RELIABILITY INDICES

In practice, consideration of the reliability measures should be the first step when examining the printout from automated perimetry. The full-threshold program on the Humphrey is typical of modern automated perimeters in performing 'catch trials' throughout the test to determine subject reliability. These are known as false-positive (FP) trials, false-negative (FN) trials, and fixation losses (FL).

The movement of the stimulus projection system used by the Humphrey is audible to the subject. Periodically during each test, the projector moves as if to present a stimulus but does not do so. If the subject responds, an FP error is recorded. At other times, a stimulus which is much brighter than threshold is presented at a site where sensitivity has already been determined. If the patient does not respond, an FN error is recorded. Hence, a large number of FP errors may denote a 'trigger happy' subject, while a large proportion of FN errors may indicate an inattentive or fatigued subject. Fixation is monitored throughout the test by the Heijl-Krakau method: this presents stimuli at the site of the predetermined blind spot. If seen, there is an indication that fixation has been lost, and an FL error is recorded. Visual fields which have a large proportion of fixation losses, false negatives, or especially false positives are likely to be unreliable. Automated perimeters may alert the examiner to this; for example, the Humphrey displays a 'low patient reliability' message.

An additional indicator for patient response reliability or measurement variability is assessed by the short-term fluctuation (SF) index in full-threshold testing programs in the Humphrey and the Octopus. On the Humphrey, SF is calculated as a weighted mean of the standard deviations at 10 predetermined test points where the threshold is measured twice during the examination. This procedure is costly in terms of test time, offers limited precision, and may not be useful because of the nature of the points being preselected: for example, they may be in defect areas where the response variability is known to be greater.

In Humphrey SITA testing the reliability measures are estimated differently and are completed without the need for extra catch trials, thus significantly reducing test time.[22] For example, FP rates are estimated by use of the patient's reaction time, with overly quick responses disregarded and retested. This procedure does more than estimate FP responses but tailors the pacing of the test

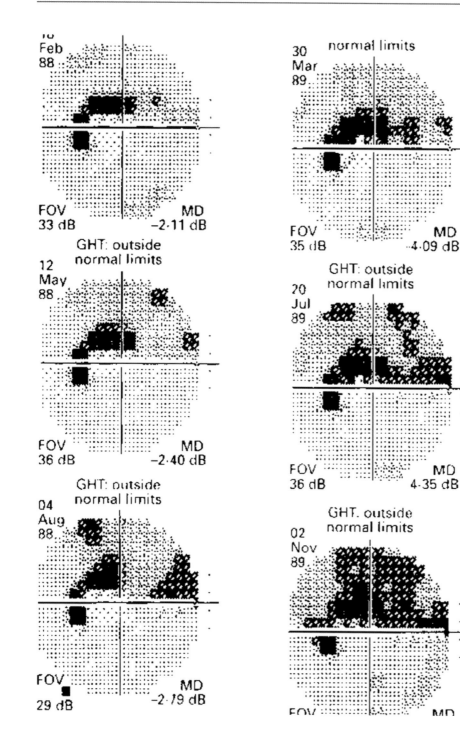

FIGURE 10.12 Series of Humphrey visual fields (*gray scales*) of the same eye showing clear and obvious progression of a superior hemifield defect.

to the individual's reaction time and makes a significant contribution towards the quicker test times in SITA. Furthermore, FN is estimated in SITA by examining the subject's sequence of responses and, again, no extra testing is required. It is recognized that the Heijl-Krakau method is limited by correct initial mapping of the blindspot area and the fact that the stimuli is relatively small in comparison to the area that it is projected on the optic disc, meaning that patient's fixation will have to move a long way for the stimulus to fall outside the blind spot. For these reasons, newer instruments have abandoned this method and provide gaze tracking to monitor eye movements using an infrared camera projected onto the

cornea. This provides a trace or gaze graph that can be assessed by the examiner at the end of the test (Fig. 10.11). In the Octopus version the test is automatically interrupted if fixation is lost during examination. In summary, the reliability indices are important, but often the examiners qualitative judgment is as useful in determining if a subject has preformed the test well.

VISUAL FIELD PROGRESSION

The accurate detection of glaucomatous change in a series of visual field results is important in the clinical management of a patient, and in the evaluation of

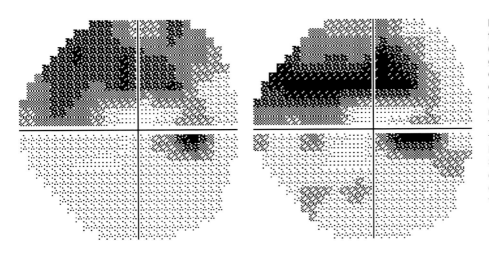

FIGURE 10.13 Baseline and follow-up Humphrey visual fields (*gray scales*) for a patient with glaucoma. Has the visual field defect worsened and progression occurred? No! Both visual fields were measured on the same morning in a very reliable patient! The difference between the two fields illustrates the typical level of between-test variability. Separating true physiological change from this noise is a challenging task in detecting visual field progression.

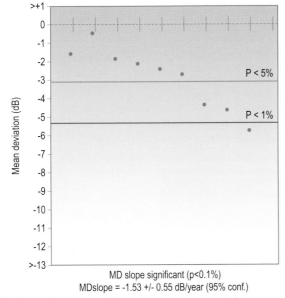

FIGURE 10.14 A plot of MD against time extracted from a Humphrey printout of serial analysis. Each symbol represents the MD at a different visit in follow-up. Worsening of MD can be assessed as the point falls below population reference values or a trend analysis such as linear regression of MD against time of follow-up. In this case, there is clear evidence that the patient's overall visual field sensitivity is deteriorating.

which treatments are most effective in arresting progression. The slow, often equivocal rate of sensitivity loss, and the variability that exists between field results, makes this a difficult task. Sometimes, with sufficient follow-up, it is easy to determine even though it might be difficult to exactly quantify (Fig. 10.12). Often, however, it is normally much more difficult: take a quick look at the gray-scale representation of a baseline field and follow-up for the glaucomatous patient shown in Fig. 10.13 and make a judgment about whether the field defect has worsened without looking at the details in the legend! Separating any physiological change (signal) from the between-test measurement variability (noise) is a real challenge.

There is certainly no gold-standard method for determining visual field progression.[23] Moreover, there is no direct or external measure of disease progression in glaucoma that can be used to validate visual field changes: current clinical devices for measuring structural deficits using optical imaging techniques still only provide a surrogate measure of the biological variables of real interest, namely retinal ganglion cell count and function. In practice, visual field progression is often determined by clinical 'judgment' and 'experience' in looking at series of visual field charts. For research purposes, a 'panel' of such expertise is often used as a surrogate gold standard. However, agreement between experts has been shown to be spectacularly poor,[24] and this approach provides only qualitative information rather than a numerical value for change or the probability of change.

One set of methods relies on estimates of change in the global indices of the field such as the mean defect value (Fig. 10.14). However, summary measures largely or completely ignore detailed spatial information contained within a visual field and are insensitive to early localized change. They do, however, provide a very specific method for determining change, meaning that if a patient is showing change with the global indices then the patient is almost certainly progressing, with the caveat that overall depression in the visual field may also simply be a sign of the onset or worsening of concomitant cataract. Other methods for 'scoring' visual fields (for example AGIS criteria[25]) have been used in clinical trials but these 'scores' share similar attributes to analysis of the global indices.

Methods that consider the change in sensitivity at individual test locations have been suggested as a means of more accurately estimating visual field progression in glaucoma. These point-wise methods are becoming more readily used because of available software and are generally thought to be sensitive to change. A good example of these methods is the glaucoma progression analysis (GPA) which was recently used to quantify progression in the first large, controlled, randomized clinical trial to evaluate the effect of lowering the intraocular pressure on changes in defects in newly detected, open-angle glaucoma.[26] GPA is designed to evaluate change in sensitivity from baseline data, and

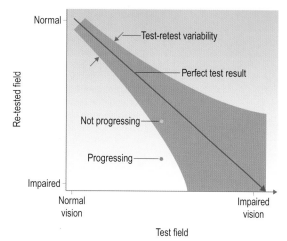

FIGURE 10.15 GPA quantifies change in relation to the between-visual-field test measurement error. On retest the 'perfect' test result would be on the diagonal; the shaded areas around the line represents the variably in 'stable' glaucoma. A point is only declared progressing if it falls beyond this expected error. The shaded area increases as the sensitivity of the visual field declines: a greater magnitude of change is required in a field with low sensitivity, whereas more subtle differences between baseline and follow-up are flagged as change in fields with higher overall sensitivity. These limits are derived from a population data set and do not account for the patient's own level of measurement variability.

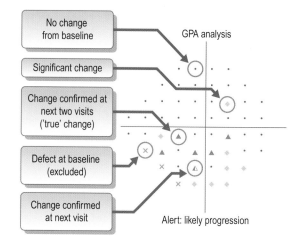

FIGURE 10.16 Interpretation of the GPA symbols. A significant change from baseline in the same three or more locations in three consecutive follow-up tests generates a 'likely progression' alert (three filled black triangles).

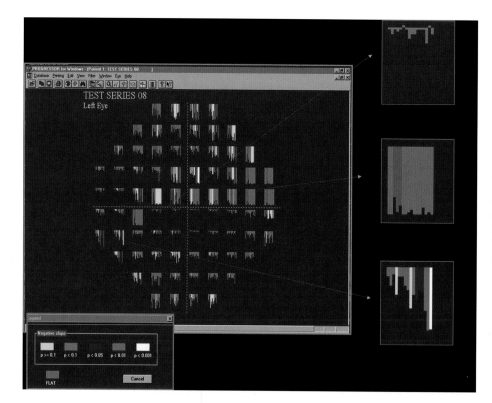

FIGURE 10.17 PROGRESSOR software showing an analysis of a series of 16 visual fields from the left eye of a patient with progressive field loss. Each location is represented by a bar graph with each bar representing, from left to right, a visual field in the series. Longer bars are defects and shorter bars are nearer to normal sensitivity. The 'hotter' colors indicate that the rate of loss at that point is statistically significant. There is considerable evidence of widespread progression mainly in the superior hemifield and at inferior points close to the blind spot location.

evaluates the amount of change with respect to empirical results of repeated tests derived from a population of patients with stable glaucomatous field loss (Fig. 10.15). Two of the first three fields in a series are automatically selected and averaged to give a merged baseline field.

The change from baseline (dB) is evaluated and displayed at each test location. The objective is to highlight locations where sensitivity changes by more than is typically observed in the stable glaucoma patient database. The analysis takes into consideration the location of the test

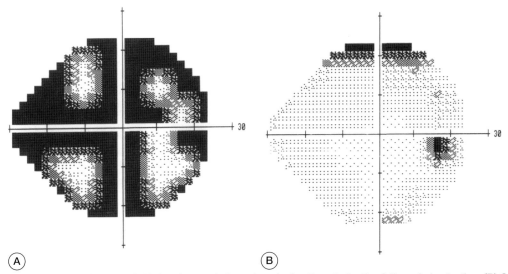

FIGURE 10.18 **(A)** Gray scale of a visual field showing an obvious cloverleaf pattern, indicating fatigue during testing. **(B)** Gray scale of a visual field where the subject has a superior lid artifact.

point within the field, the initial amount of sensitivity loss, and the MD of the field as a whole. These results are given as symbols on GPA plot with a triangle indicating a degree of deterioration found less than 5% of the time at that location in the group of stable glaucoma patients. Other symbols indicate confirmed change in subsequent follow-up, and an overall statement of change is also provided (Fig. 10.16). GPA is an 'event-type' analysis with each individual follow-up field compared with baseline, and intermediate tests are not used. It is also dependent on the population-based reference data it uses to adequately describe the variability that needs to be exceeded to flag change.

A potentially better approach is afforded by using linear regression of sensitivity values at each location.[27,28] This provides a clinically useful rate of loss at each point which is estimated by how well the sensitivity values follow the trend over time. This method is solely based on the subject's own data, with more variable patients requiring a greater rate of loss before significance can be assumed; equally, points which are slowly deteriorating with little noise are likely to be flagged earlier. The PROGRESSOR visual field analysis software (developed at Moorfields and the Institute of Ophthalmology, London) uses this method and additionally presents the results in a useful and easily interpretable way (Fig. 10.17). Each test location is represented as a small bar graph, with one bar for each test. The length of each bar corresponds to the sensitivity of the location at that test: the longer the bar, the lower the sensitivity. The color of the bar relates to the significance of the slope of the regression line at that test. Thus, undamaged locations are seen as series of short gray bars, damaged but stable locations are seen as long series of long gray bars, and progressing locations are seen as series of progressively lengthening bars

which change color as the regression slope becomes more significant. Another promising adjunct to this method is the use of a technique widely used in digital image processing which further improves diagnostic precision of the analysis.[29]

Point-wise methods are certainly more sensitive than using global measures but are not so specific; there is no evidence of consensus on what level of point-wise change constitutes 'real' progression, or whether there should be a requirement for contiguous points to show this behavior and whether it should be maintained in subsequent fields. The latter is important because no decision should be made on progression at the very first signs of it. Developing better methods for quantifying progression will continue to occupy the researchers in the field, with the hope that these will be blended with structural measures to improve the clinically useful data management tools available.

TECHNICAL TIPS FOR USERS

Automated visual field examination is an easy procedure, but the examiner should be aware of a number of factors when setting up the subject for testing. These are briefly summarized here.

Patients should be set up comfortably and be instructed to keep the occluded eye open. Importantly, subjects should be encouraged to blink normally: too often subjects will unnaturally stare without blinking, and this inhibits good test performance. One should remember that although the test is automated, good results are achieved if the patients is counseled carefully and the test is carefully explained, especially the importance of fixation. An important message is that is better to stop the test and re-instruct rather than wait for obvious flags appearing on the reliability indices on the printout after the test has been done. Other aspects to testing that have a real bearing on the quality of the results are rims of frames if subjects use their own correction and correct refraction. Good practical advice is offered on the latter in Henson[1] and Cubbidge.[2]

Patient fatigue is a big problem with visual field testing. The classic presentation of the fatigue effect on visual field outcome is the cloverleaf pattern, where patients have tired after the four primary points have been tested at the beginning of the test (Fig. 10.18A). For this reason, the second eye examined will generally perform slightly worse than the first eye. It is therefore useful to remember, when carrying out series of visual fields during follow-up, that the eye testing order remains constant. In elderly patients, lid ptosis (Fig. 10.18B) may be present and this often manifests an artifact in the final field; precautions in these cases using comfortable taping should be instituted before testing.

The most important technical tip in terms of interpreting visual field results is never to make a clinical decision based on one test result! Repeated fields and follow-up fields must be done to confirm or verify any kind of clinical decision. Remember, for glaucoma, the pattern deviation plot is by far the most useful graphical tool on the printout and that all statistical analysis should be interpreted in conjunction with the subject's reliability indices and the examiner's overall feel for how well the subject has performed the test.

Summary

Modern automated perimetry is the current standard for assessing visual field defects in glaucoma. Despite the problem with measurement variability, they should remain the benchmark by which we interpret glaucoma because they directly assess what the patient can see, as opposed to indirect measures such as imaging or intraocular pressure measurements. Their role as the most important outcome measure in clinical trials of different new treatments for glaucoma should be established. Systematically and correctly examining the statistical analysis accompanying visual field plots assists in deciding whether physiological field loss is present or worsening. However, the wealth of statistical information on the visual field chart is no substitute for careful clinical interpretation.

REFERENCES

1. Henson DB. Visual fields. 2nd edn. Oxford: Butterworth-Heinemann; 2000.

2. Cubbidge RP. Visual fields. Edinburgh: Elsevier; 2005.

3. Edgar DF, Rudnicka AR. Glaucoma identification and co-management. Oxford: Butterworth-Heinemann; 2006.

4. Atchinson DA. History of visual field measurement. Aust J Optom 1979; 62:345–354.

5. Katz J, Tielsch JM, Quigley HA, et al. Automated perimetry detects visual field loss before manual Goldmann perimetry. Ophthalmology 1995; 102:21–26.

6. Henson DB, Artes PH. New developments in suprathreshold perimetry. Ophthalm Physiol Opt 2002; 22:463–468.

7. Artes PH, Henson DB, Harper R, et al. Multisampling suprathreshold perimetry: a comparison with conventional suprathreshold and full-threshold strategies by computer simulation. Invest Ophthalmol Vis Sci 2003; 44: 2582–2587.

8. Morales J, Weitzman ML, de la Rosa MG. Comparison between Tendency-Oriented-Perimetry (TOP) and Octopus threshold perimetry. Ophthalmology 2000; 107:137–142.

9. Bengtsson B, Olsson J, Heijl A, et al. A new generation of algorithms for computerized threshold perimetry, SITA. Acta Ophthalmol Scand 1997; 75:368–375.

10. Olsson J, Rootzén H. An image model for quantal response analysis in perimetry. Scand J Statist 1994; 21:373–387.

11. Heijl A, Bengtsson B, Patella VM. Glaucoma follow-up when converting from long to short perimetric threshold tests. Arch Ophthalmol 2000; 118:489–493.

12. Musch DC, Gillespie BW, Motyka BM, et al. Converting to SITA-standard from full-threshold visual field testing in the follow-up phase of a clinical trial. Invest Ophthalmol Vis Sci 2005; 46:2755–2759.

13. Wild JM, Pacey IM, Hancock SA, et al. The SITA perimetric threshold algorithms in glaucoma. Invest Ophthalmol Vis Sci 1999; 40:1998–2009.

14. Budenz DL, Rhee P, Feuer WJ, et al. Comparison of glaucomatous visual field defects using standard full threshold and Swedish Interactive Threshold Algorithms. Arch Ophthalmol 2002; 120:1136–1141.

15. Artes PH, Iwase A, Ohno Y, et al. Properties of perimetric threshold estimates from full threshold, SITA standard and SITA Fast strategies. Invest Ophthalmol Vis Sci 2002; 43:2654–2659.

16. Crabb DP, Fitzke FW, Hitchings RA, et al. A practical approach to measuring the visual field component of fitness to drive. Br J Ophthalmol 2004; 88:1191–1196.

17. Viswanathan AC, McNaught AI, Poinoosawmy D, et al. Severity and stability of glaucoma: patient perception compared with objective measurement. Arch Ophthalmol 1999; 117: 450–454.

18. Spaeth G, Walt J, Keener J. Evaluation of quality of life for patients with glaucoma. Am J Ophthalmol 2006; 141:S3–S14.

19. Heijl A, Lindgren G, Olsson J, et al. Visual field interpretation with empiric probability maps. Arch Ophthalmol 1989; 107:204–208.

20. Åsman P, A Heijl. Glaucoma Hemifield Test: automated visual field evaluation, Arch Ophthalmol 1992; 110:812–819.

21. Katz J, Quigley HA, Sommer A. Repeatability of the Glaucoma Hemifield Test in automated perimetry. Invest Ophthalmol Vis Sci 1995; 36:1658–1664.

22. Olsson J, Bengtsson B, Heijl A, et al. An improved method to estimate frequency of false positive answers in computerised perimetry. Acta Ophthalmol Scand 1997; 75:36181–36183.

23. Spry PGD, Johnson CA. Identification of progressive glaucomatous visual field loss. Surv Ophthalmol 2002; 47:158–173.

24. Viswanathan AC, Crabb DP, McNaught AI, et al. Interobserver agreement on visual field progression in glaucoma: a comparison of methods. Br J Ophthalmol 2003; 87:726–730.

25. The AGIS Investigators. The Advanced Glaucoma Intervention Study (AGIS): 2.Visual field test scoring. Ophthalmology 1994; 101:1445–1455.

26. Heijl A, Leske MC, Bengtsson B, et al., for the EMGT Group. Reduction of intraocular pressure and glaucoma progression: results from the Early Manifest Glaucoma Trial. Arch Ophthalmol 2002; 120:1268–1279.

27. Fitzke FW, Hitchings RA, Poinoosawmy D, et al. Analysis of visual field progression in glaucoma. Br J Ophthalmol 1996; 80:40–48.

28. Gardiner SK, Crabb DP. Examination of different pointwise linear regression methods for determining visual field progression. Invest Ophthalmol Vis Sci 2002; 43:1400–1407.

29. Strouthidis NG, Scott A, Viswanathan AC, et al. Monitoring glaucomatous visual field progression: the effect of a novel spatial filter. Invest Ophthalmol Vis Sci 2007; 48:251–257.

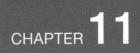

Function-Specific Perimetry

Felipe A Medeiros and Luciana M Alencar

INTRODUCTION

Irreversible visual field defects are the final common feature of glaucomatous damage to the retinal ganglion cells (RGCs). For many years, functional evaluation of the RGCs relied solely on standard achromatic automated perimetry (SAP), also known as white-on-white perimetry. However, although SAP remains the most commonly performed method of visual field assessment in glaucoma, histological and clinical studies have shown that in many cases visual field defects on SAP are detectable only when a substantial number of ganglion cells have been lost.[1–3] These findings suggest that SAP is relatively insensitive to early structural damage from glaucoma, and have prompted investigation into psychophysical tests capable of detecting earlier functional losses.

Several factors seem to be related to the relative insensitivity of SAP to early RGC damage, including the variability of the test and the considerable redundancy of the human visual system. Whereas light detection can be perceived by almost all RGCs, more specific features, such as contrast sensitivity, movement perception, and color vision, are encoded by specific subsets of the RGCs. The knowledge that different features of the visual information are transmitted by specific RGCs has been used to develop function-specific perimetric tests for visual field assessment in glaucoma, by using stimuli that target specific subgroups of cells.

A BRIEF OVERVIEW OF THE HUMAN VISUAL SYSTEM

After reaching the retina, light is detected by photoreceptors (cones and rods) which transmit electric signals to bipolar cells. The bipolar cells, in turn, connect to the retinal ganglion cells whose function is to send electric signals to the cerebral centers associated with vision. The axons of the RGCs project through the optic nerve and visual pathways to make synaptic connections with neurons at the dorsal lateral geniculate nucleus (LGN) of the thalamus.

The human retina has three different groups of cone photoreceptors. Each variety of cones has a maximal sensitivity to a specific region of the color spectrum: the blue cones are most sensitive to short-wavelength stimulus (440 nm, blue band), the green cones to medium wavelengths (530–540 nm), and the red cones to long wavelengths (560–580 nm). Yellow light is perceived as the stimulation of both red and green cones, but not blue ones, whereas the visual perception of the white color is the result of proportional stimulation of cones of all types. Functional overlap exists because even though a photoreceptor of a particular type is more sensitive to a certain color, it still has some sensitivity to other wavelengths throughout the visual spectrum. The proportion of stimulation of the three different types of cones for a determined wavelength is what results in the notion of a specific color.[4,5] After information is sent to the RGCs, it is processed using two chromatic mechanisms of opponency (blue-yellow and red-green) and one achromatic mechanism (light-dark).[6] While red-green opponency occurs between red and green cones, blue-yellow opponency occurs between the blue cones and the combination of red-green cones.

The retinal ganglion cells are primarily classified based on their projection to the lateral geniculate nucleus. There are several subpopulations of RGCs, which are both morphologically and physiologically distinct (Table 11.1). The parasol ganglion cells are located throughout the retina and account for 10% of all RGCs. They project to the magnocellular visual pathway and are also called M cells. They have large bodies, large axons, and large dendritic fields (Fig. 11.1). These cells subserve motion perception, high temporal, and low spatial resolution with high-contrast sensitivity, and stereopsis.[7] The small midget ganglion cells represent the most numerous group, and account for 80% of all ganglion cells in the retina and project to the parvocellular layers in the LGN (thus also called P cells). They outnumber parasol ganglion cells by about 7 to 1 and this ratio may increase to as much as 30 to 1 in the central retina.[8] They subserve central visual acuity, low temporal, and high spatial resolution with low-contrast sensitivity, static stereopsis, and pattern recognition.

M cells respond to broadband light of different wavelengths, whereas P cells convey color information (red-green) and shape.[9] A third system has also been isolated, corresponding to the small bistratified blue-on ganglion cells, formerly considered as a subset of the parvocellular system (Type 2 P cells, and now K cells) and which comprise 10% of all RGC.[10] These neurons are located within and between the principal layers of the LGN, and make up the koniocellular system. These K cells mediate almost exclusively the blue-yellow signal.[10–12] Details of most other RGC types are still unknown.

As mentioned above, each system conveys different features of visual information, but because SAP uses a static achromatic stimulus, it is thought to nonselectively invoke all systems. Since there is considerable functional overlap between the RGCs, and also redundancy in the coverage of a given retinal location, many neighbor cells are stimulated simultaneously by the type of stimulus used in SAP. Thus, even with death of a significant number of ganglion cells, the signal is still transmitted, and early loss may not be detected.[13] In contrast, function-specific perimetric tests attempt to isolate subpopulations of ganglion cells by evaluating a specific visual function characteristically processed by that cell subtype. When a single system is isolated by function-specific perimetric tests, relatively fewer cells are being tested at the same time. As a result, there is less redundancy in the coverage of a given retinal location and less overlap in the responses that could potentially 'mask' ganglion cell losses. Therefore, early glaucomatous damage becomes easier to detect when specific subpopulations of RGCs are being evaluated by these tests.

Several function-specific perimetric tests have been developed to target specific subgroups of RGCs, including frequency doubling technology (FDT) perimetry, short-wavelength automated perimetry (SWAP), and high-pass resolution perimetry (HPRP). SWAP requires detection by the short-wavelength cones from the koniocellular pathway, and is only processed through the blue-yellow ganglion cells. FDT and various forms of motion perimetry target the parasol ganglion cells of the magnocellular pathway. HPRP is thought to selectively target the midget ganglion cells of the parvocellular system.[14] Each one of these tests is discussed in detail below.

TABLE 11.1 Characteristics of the M, P, and K cell pathways

	M	P	K
Subset of RGC	Parasol	Midget	Bistratified (blue-on)
Percentage of all RGC	10%	80%	9%
Projection to LGN	Magnocellular layers	Parvocellular layers	Interlaminar
Most sensitive to	Motion perception, contrast sensitivity, broadband light perception	Central visual acuity, red-green opponency	Blue-yellow opponency

RGC, retinal ganglion cells; LGN, lateral geniculate nucleus.

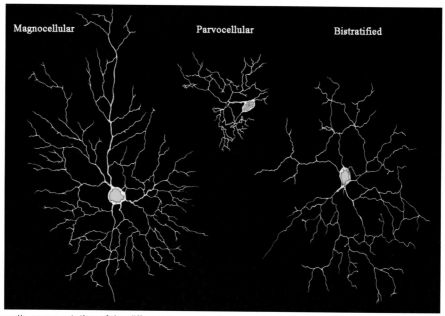

FIGURE 11.1 Schematic representation of the different types of retinal ganglion cells. Note the different sizes for body, axons, and field coverage.

SHORT-WAVELENGTH AUTOMATED PERIMETRY

Short-wavelength automated perimetry (SWAP) is a visual field test designed to assess the short-wavelength-sensitive color system. SWAP isolates the short-wavelength-sensitive pathway throughout the retino-geniculo-cortical route. The motivation for the development of SWAP as a visual field test was based on original reports showing the existence of color vision defects in glaucomatous patients.[15–17]

The short-wavelength-sensitive color system originates at the receptor level in the retina with the short-wavelength (blue) cones. These cones send projections to the blue-cone bipolar cells, which then project to the small bistratified retinal ganglion cells. The small bistratified retinal ganglion cells project to the interlaminar (koniocellular) layers of the lateral geniculate nucleus. They are responsible for encoding and transmission of information related to the blue-yellow opponency, where blue activates and yellow suppresses the system. The short-wavelength cones and the koniocellular pathway have only recently been separated from the parvocellular 'color system,' as evidence showed that these cells are larger than P cells and project their axons to the interlaminar layers of the LGN, and not to the parvocellular layers.[10–12] The small bistratified retinal ganglion cells make up approximately 9% of the population of retinal ganglion cells and are sparsely distributed across the retina.

It is believed that SWAP is able to detect early functional loss not because the small bistratified cells are affected first in glaucoma, but because it specifically tests only one type of ganglion cell, reducing the redundancy of the system. When the short-wavelength-sensitive pathway is isolated, a deficit may be manifest even when a small proportion of cells are affected, because even if other cell types are still functioning in a given retinal area, they are unable to detect the specific stimulus until it becomes much brighter than normal.

MODE OF ACTION

Short-wavelength automated perimetry (SWAP) was initially developed from modifications in SAP, and it can be performed both with the Humphrey Field Analyzer (HFA; Carl-Zeiss Meditec, Dublin, CA) and the Octopus 1-2-3 (Haag-Streit, Interzeag AC, Schlieren, Switzerland) perimeters. It differs from conventional perimetry for its narrow-band blue-light stimulus and the yellow background illumination (Table 11.2). The large blue stimulus presented has a peak wavelength of 440 nm, which approximates the peak response of the S cones, and has a Goldmann size V. These cones send their signals via the bipolar cells to the blue-yellow retinal ganglion cells. Before the actual testing procedure, the patient should initially undergo an adaptation period of at least 3 minutes under a bright yellow background (100 cd/m²) in order to fatigue the medium-wavelength (green) and long-wavelength (red) cones,

and suppress rod activity.[18] The target used in SWAP needs to be larger mainly due to its lesser brightness and to the necessity of larger stimulus to test this system. These fibers are slower to respond and the potential visual acuity of this system is only 20/200. The results are reported in log units relative to a threshold of 0 dB (10 000 apostilbs). All other aspects of testing are identical to conventional SAP.

SWAP (or blue-yellow perimetry) is run on the same equipment as conventional SAP, with the same general procedures. It is commercially available on the HFAII in 30–2, 24–2, and 10–2 patterns, and Macula threshold (central 5°). Used strategies are also similar to SAP, viz full-threshold, FASTPAC, and the latest SITA-SWAP. Both Octopus 101 and 300 series (default on 311 but optional on 301) also provide blue-yellow perimetry, available on G1, G2, 32, and M2 programs for the normal, dynamic, and tendency-oriented perimetry (TOP) strategies.

CLINICAL INTERPRETATION OF SHORT-WAVELENGTH AUTOMATED PERIMETRY

Figure 11.2 shows a printout of a SWAP examination obtained with the Humphrey HFAII perimeter. Similarly to SAP, a statistical package (Statpac II) compares the results with age-related normal subjects and provides numerical and probability plots. During the examination, fixation is monitored in the same way as conventional perimetry, providing an index of fixation losses (FL). However, even with steady central fixation, some patients will present increased FL with SWAP. As FL is monitored using repeated stimulation over the blind spot, and the stimulus used for SWAP is larger, subjects with small blind spots may still detect the target. This situation can be managed either by turning off the fixation monitor, or by reducing the size of the stimulus used. Blinking and eye movement are also displayed on a gaze-tracking plot on the bottom of the printout. Catch trials are used to test reliability of the responses, providing false-positive (FP) and

TABLE 11.2 Comparison of parameters for standard achromatic perimetry (SAP) and short-wavelength automated perimetry (SWAP)

	SAP	SWAP
Stimulus size (Goldmann/degree)	III/0.47°	V/1.8°
Stimulus color	White	Blue
Stimulus duration (msec)	200	200
Maximum stimulus brightness (cd/m²)	10 000	65
Background color	White	Yellow
Background brightness [cd/m² (asb)]	10 (31.5)	100 (315)

false-negative (FN) indexes, which refer respectively to responses in the absence of a target and targets missed on suprathreshold brightness.

Sensitivity values are provided for each location tested and a corresponding gray-scale map is shown next to it. The gray-scale pattern on SWAP printouts, however, can be misleading. This scale uses the same conversion factor as SAP. However, because of the reduced visual perception of blue cones, sensitivity thresholds are usually 1.5–2.5 dB lower with SWAP than with SAP. This results in a darker gray-scale map in SWAP when compared to SAP even for normal subjects, as illustrated in Fig. 11.2. Although gray-scale maps on SWAP may appear to show a diffuse loss of sensitivity, the probability maps, which display significant deviations from age-corrected thresholds, will appear more similar to SAP.

The total and pattern deviation plots, and the global indices (MD, mean deviation; PSD, pattern standard deviation; SF, short fluctuation; CPSD, corrected PSD) follow the same principles as SAP. The printout also shows the results of the Glaucoma Hemifield Test (GHT), which compares and evaluates asymmetries between superior and inferior hemispheres. It is important to note, however, that normal subjects tested on SWAP tend to show asymmetries that are more pronounced than those shown on SAP. More frequently, the inferior hemisphere will show higher sensitivity thresholds than the superior hemisphere, with differences increasing with eccentricity.[19] The reasons for these findings are not clear.

Overall, the interpretation of the results of SWAP testing should follow the same principles as for conventional achromatic perimetry. However, because of the pronounced affect that lens opacities may have on SWAP results, causing diffuse loss of sensitivity (see below), more emphasis should be given to the evaluation of the pattern deviation plot and indices that

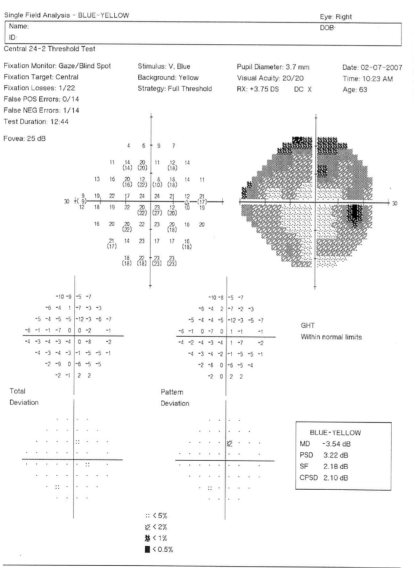

FIGURE 11.2 Printout of a SWAP examination from a healthy subject obtained with the full-threshold strategy on a Humphrey HFAII perimeter. Note the darker gray-scale plot. However, analyses from the total deviation and pattern deviation plot are normal, as well as the global indices.

measure localized loss or asymmetries such as PSD and GHT.

STRENGTHS AND LIMITATIONS

Early detection of functional damage Of all new psychophysical procedures, SWAP is the one that has had the most extensive validation. There is mounting evidence that indicates that SWAP is more sensitive than SAP for detection of early functional deficits due to glaucoma. Longitudinal studies performed by two independent laboratories showed that SWAP defects may occur 3 to 5 years before abnormalities are seen on SAP, and that they were predictive of both the onset and location of future SAP defects.[20–22] Johnson et al.[22] followed a group of 38 ocular hypertensive patients for 5 years. At the beginning of the study, all patients had normal achromatic visual fields, and nine patients had abnormal SWAP. From the nine patients with initial SWAP defects, five later developed defects on SAP, all of which were on the same locations as the defects previously seen on SWAP. During follow-up, none of the patients with normal SWAP tests at the beginning of the study showed changes with SAP. Although these results suggested earlier detection of functional damage with SWAP than with SAP, it is important to note that subjects were initially recruited based on the presence of normal SAP results. This could have potentially favored SWAP sensitivity, as any subject showing abnormal SAP but normal SWAP would have been excluded from the investigation.

Because of its potential ability to detect early functional damage in glaucoma, SWAP has traditionally been indicated as a test to evaluate visual function in glaucoma suspects. Published studies have reported that from 8% to 30% of ocular hypertensive patients with normal SAP results already have visual field defects when tested with SWAP, depending on the criteria used and the specific characteristics of the population being evaluated. Also, ocular hypertensive patients at higher risk for developing glaucoma tend to show a greater prevalence of SWAP defects than those considered to be at a lower risk for developing the disease. Figure 11.3 shows a high-risk ocular hypertensive patient, with defects on SWAP, but not on SAP. A study by Medeiros et al.[23] showed that patients with thin corneas, a known risk factor for developing glaucoma,[24] had a significantly greater prevalence of SWAP defects compared to patients with thick corneas. In another investigation, Sample et al.[21] stratified a population of glaucoma suspects with normal SAP into risk groups based on cup-to-disc ratio and intraocular pressure (IOP) levels. They observed that both the high-risk group and the glaucoma group had more damage on SWAP than the medium- and low-risk groups. Interestingly, even though the prevalence of field defects in populations of ocular hypertensive patients is higher when

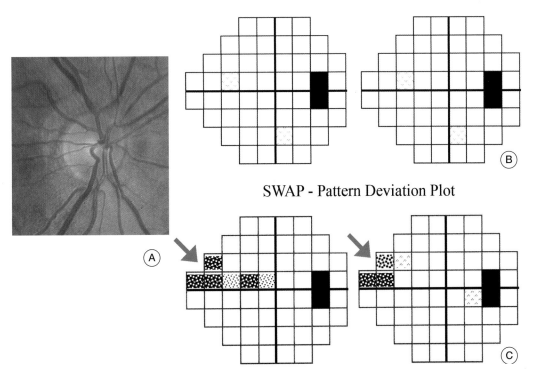

SAP - Pattern Deviation Plot

SWAP - Pattern Deviation Plot

FIGURE 11.3 High-risk ocular hypertensive patient tested with both SWAP and SAP. The patient had intraocular pressure of 28 mmHg and a thin cornea of 496 μm. The neuroretinal rim and retinal nerve fiber layer **(A)** do not show any clear evidence of damage. Although SAP visual fields were still within normal limits, a superior nasal defect could be demonstrated on the SWAP pattern deviation plot **(C)**, which was confirmed in a subsequent test.

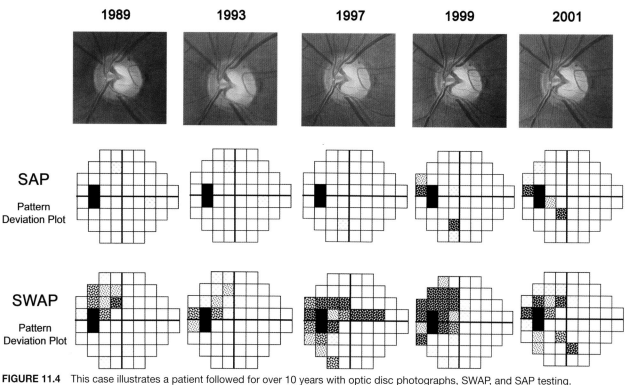

FIGURE 11.4 This case illustrates a patient followed for over 10 years with optic disc photographs, SWAP, and SAP testing. Progressive neuroretinal rim thinning in the nasal, superior temporal, and inferior temporal sectors of the optic nerve are seen on the photographs over time. Corresponding and reproducible visual field defects were apparent on SWAP testing 10 years before their detection by SAP.

assessed with SWAP than with SAP, the incidence rates of new defects have been found to be similar with the two tests.[25] This supports the concept that both tests are identifying the same underlying damage, but SWAP is catching it at an earlier stage. Figure 11.4 shows an example of a glaucomatous patient who had visual field defects identified by SWAP several years earlier than by SAP.

In glaucomatous patients already presenting with visual field loss, the defect is usually larger and deeper with SWAP than with SAP.[20,21,26] One study observed that among subjects who showed progression, the SWAP defects were three to four times larger than the ones detected with SAP.[20] SWAP has also been shown to have a higher correlation with structural tests of glaucomatous damage than SAP in some studies. Patients with structural evidence of glaucomatous optic neuropathy tend to have a greater prevalence of SWAP defects than those without evidence of optic nerve damage.[27] In addition, correlations between SWAP and retinal nerve fiber layer or optic disc imaging technologies have been found to be stronger than those found for SAP.[28,29]

Detection of progressive damage Short-wavelength automated perimetry has also been evaluated for its ability to detect progression. Some studies have shown it detects progression 1 to 3 years in advance compared to SAP.[20,26] Further, in eyes already presenting a glaucomatous visual field defect, the rate of progression has

been shown to be faster with SWAP than with SAP.[20] SWAP defects also seem to correspond closely to structural changes seen on the optic nerve head in glaucomatous patients.[27,30] In addition, when compared to SAP, SWAP has been demonstrated to have a greater sensitivity to assess progressive functional damage in subjects who developed progressive changes on the appearance of the optic nerve over time.[31]

Limitations An important limitation of the SWAP full-threshold strategy is the longer duration of the test, which is around 15% longer than full-threshold SAP, taking approximately 10 to 15 minutes per eye. Although this limitation has largely been overcome with the recent introduction of the SITA-SWAP testing, the yellow background and the blue spot target of SWAP are still relatively more difficult to recognize than the white-on-white test, which could potentially increase patient fatigue and discomfort during the test. The presence of a possible learning effect must also be considered when initiating follow-up with SWAP. Even for subjects with previous experience with SAP, a learning effect for SWAP novices can still be demonstrated.

The variability of measurements of sensitivity threshold is an important consideration when evaluating a perimetric test. Variability can usually be divided into short-term and long-term components. Short-term variability refers to the variation of threshold values for the same point on the visual field, when repetitive measurements are performed during the same examination.

On the other hand, long-term variability refers to the test-retest variation occurring among examinations performed over time, in the absence of clinically detectable pathologic changes. The short-term variability (or short-term fluctuation) for SWAP has been shown to be 25% to 30% higher than SAP. For long-term variability, studies with normal subjects and stable glaucoma patients have shown that the full-threshold SWAP strategy has a variability that is higher than SAP by about 0.55 dB, on average.[32,33] The greater variability could potentially make it more difficult to differentiate random variations of visual function from true progression of glaucomatous damage. However, this greater variability needs to be considered in light of the significant increase in sensitivity found with the test. In fact, despite this increased variability, one study suggested that when a defect appears on SWAP, it is more likely to persist in follow-up tests than when a defect appears on SAP.[25] As with conventional perimetry, any evidence of progression seen on SWAP testing should always be confirmed by additional examinations.

Another limitation of the SWAP assessment of visual function is the known influence of the aging crystalline lens on the results of the test. The aging lens may acquire a yellow tone as a result of initial nuclear cataract development, which acts as a blue filter and may account for as much as 63% of the variability in threshold measurements for SWAP.[34] The effect of cataract usually presents itself as a diffuse depression of sensitivity. Therefore, any diffuse depression of sensitivity seen on SWAP testing should be interpreted with caution. As glaucomatous defects generally present a localized component, it is important to evaluate maps and indices that are designed to detect the presence of localized defects on SWAP testing, such as the pattern standard deviation and pattern deviation plots.[20,22,26,35–38]

Another drawback of SWAP testing is that in more advanced cases, especially those with cataracts, the test is limited by the perimeter's dynamic range. Even after adjusting for the lens effect, as on the pattern deviation plot, there is still a lower range of perceived luminance of the target when compared to SAP. In advanced cases, the patient may not recognize even the brightest target, and because of this narrow dynamic range, the test may not be sensitive enough to accurately monitor progression in more advanced cases of glaucoma. Therefore, for subjects with advanced visual field defects, follow-up should generally be pursued with conventional SAP.

SWEDISH INTERACTIVE THRESHOLDING ALGORITHM-SHORT-WAVELENGTH AUTOMATED PERIMETRY

Swedish Interactive Thresholding Algorithm-Short-Wavelength Automated Perimetry (SITA-SWAP) is a combination of short-wavelength automated perimetry and the Swedish Interactive Thresholding Algorithm. It has been developed in an attempt to reduce some of the disadvantages of the full-threshold SWAP. The full-threshold strategy tests each point in the visual field using a staircase strategy, progressively decreasing the values of stimulus brightness until the patient is not able to see them anymore. Although generally accurate, this procedure can be very time consuming. In SITA strategy, 'guesses' are made as to the value of the threshold at a determined location on the visual field and the stimulus brightness is varied around the initial estimate until the actual threshold is obtained. These values are based on the probable hill of vision height derived from the foveal threshold values (measured before the test starts), the patient's age, and the results obtained in adjacent points in the visual field. SITA-SWAP 24–2 threshold fields can often be obtained in an average of 3.6 minutes, reducing by 30–50% the time of traditional SWAP full-threshold testing.[38] Figure 11.5 shows a printout of a SITA-SWAP test performed on a glaucomatous patient.

Correlation of results of SITA-SWAP to traditional full-threshold SWAP testing has been good, but further refinement seems necessary. When compared to full-threshold SWAP, the SITA-SWAP strategy presented significantly higher normal thresholds of sensitivity. This results in a larger dynamic range, potentially increasing the number of subjects that can be tested with SWAP. SITA-SWAP presents also a smaller intersubject variance.[39,40] Even though the consequent narrower normal limits could lead to more sensitive probability maps, studies are still necessary to confirm this hypothesis.

On a recent comparison with full-threshold SWAP and SAP-SITA, the SITA-SWAP strategy identified a similar number of abnormal points to the other two, with the advantage of a reduced testing time when compared to full-threshold SWAP. In contrast, another study reported that the SITA-SWAP was not significantly more sensitive than the SAP-SITA to detect abnormalities on visual fields of glaucoma suspects and early glaucoma subjects.[39] Longitudinal studies are still necessary to evaluate the ability of SITA-SWAP strategy to detect early functional damage and progression in glaucomatous patients.

FREQUENCY DOUBLING PERIMETRY

As the name suggests, frequency doubling technology (FDT) perimetry determines the contrast sensitivity for detecting the frequency doubling stimulus. This phenomenon is thought to be mediated by a subset of the magnocellular retinal ganglion cells with nonlinear response properties called My. Because the My cells are a small group that represents 15–25% of all M cells and only 3–5% of all RGCs, a deficit would be manifest even when a small proportion of cells is affected, due to the reduced redundancy in coverage of a given location in the retina.[41,42] Indeed, several independent studies have shown that FDT has high sensitivity and specificity to discriminate glaucomatous patients from normal subjects, and that its results are predictive of future onset and location of functional loss assessed by SAP in glaucoma suspects.[43–50]

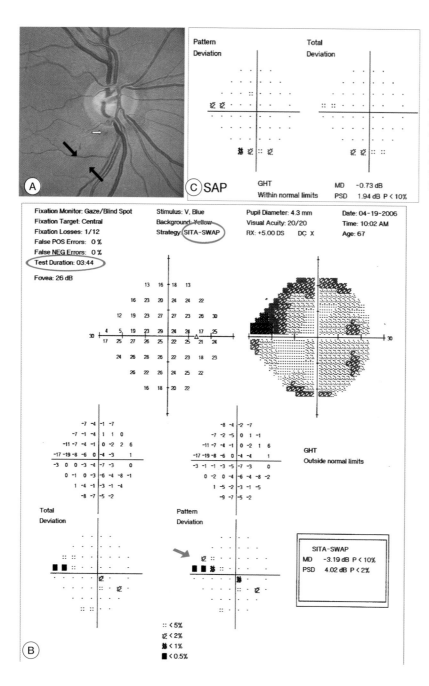

FIGURE 11.5 Printout of an abnormal SITA-SWAP examination from a glaucomatous patient. **(A)** The optic nerve shows inferior neuroretinal rim thinning with a corresponding localized retinal nerve fiber layer defect (*black arrows*) and a small hemorrhage (*white arrow*). **(B)** The SITA-SWAP printout shows a well-defined superior nasal defect, corresponding to the inferior temporal optic nerve damage. **(C)** Although the SAP examination shows a cluster of two suspicious abnormal points on the superior nasal region, all the other test indices were still within the normal limits.

MODE OF ACTION

The FDT stimulus is a large 10° × 10° square consisting of black and white bars, undergoing a rapid counterphase flicker at a frequency of 25 Hz. The spatial frequency doubling illusion occurs as a result of this rapidly flickering of low spatial sinusoidal gratings (0.25 cycle/degree). Alternating the black and the white bands in rapid sequence makes the eye perceive the stimulus as having twice as many bars (Fig. 11.6). In the normal eye it will happen at a certain level of contrast, which is related to the My cells functional status.[41,43] However, some authors believe that at this contrast threshold all magnocellular cells are likely to respond to this type of stimulus, and others believe that it is the result of a combination of retinal and cortical mechanisms.[51]

The FDT perimeter (perimeter from Humphrey-Zeiss Systems, Dublin, CA with frequency doubling technology from Welch Allyn, Skaneateles Falls, NY) can use both suprathreshold (C-20–5 and C-20–1, covering the central 20°) and threshold strategies (N-20 for the central 20° and N-30 extending to the nasal sector). Seventeen points are tested with the C-20 and N-20 strategies, four in each 10° quadrant and an extra central 5° circular target. For the N-30, two additional points are tested on the nasal field, totaling 19 points. Threshold strategies take up to 4–5 minutes, whereas suprathreshold modes require less than 1 minute per eye and have mostly been used for glaucoma screening.[46,52] The device is portable and easy to use for both the technician and the patient. Subjects can use their own distance spectacles, and must press the response

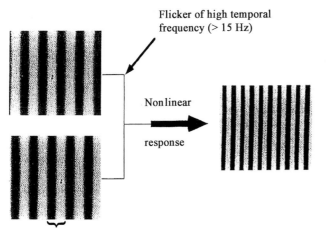

Flicker of high temporal
frequency (> 15 Hz)

Nonlinear

response

< 1 cycle/°

FIGURE 11.6 Schematic representation of the frequency doubling illusion phenomenon. Alternating the black and the white bands in rapid sequence makes the eye perceive the stimulus as having twice as many bars. This phenomenon seems to be perceived by nonlinear visual mechanisms from the magnocellular pathway.

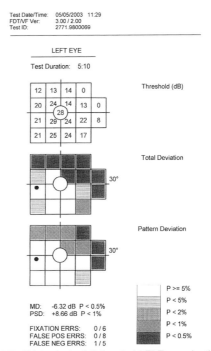

FULL THRESHOLD N-30

Test Date/Time: 05/05/2003 11:29
FDT/VF Ver: 3.00 / 2.00
Test ID: 2771.9800069

LEFT EYE

Test Duration: 5:10

Threshold (dB)

12	13	14	0	
20	24	14	13	0
21	29	24	22	8
21	25	24	17	

(28)

Total Deviation

30°

Pattern Deviation

30°

P >= 5%
P < 5%
P < 2%
P < 1%
P < 0.5%

MD: -6.32 dB P < 0.5%
PSD: +8.66 dB P < 1%

FIXATION ERRS: 0 / 6
FALSE POS ERRS: 0 / 8
FALSE NEG ERRS: 1 / 5

FIGURE 11.7 Printout of a full-threshold FDT examination obtained in a patient with glaucoma. Similarly to conventional perimetry, the full-threshold FDT gives the raw sensitivity values, the total deviation plot, and the pattern deviation plot. The global indices mean deviation (MD) and pattern standard deviation (PSD), and the reliability indices, are shown on the bottom of the printout.

button whenever they are able to see the bars. It has been suggested that the test is resistant to blurring effects of up to 6 diopters.

For the threshold strategies, the instrument uses a modified binary search staircase threshold procedure, presenting the stimulus for a maximum of 720 msec and varying the contrast in order to assess the minimum contrast perceived. During the first 160 msec, stimulus contrast is increased gradually from zero to the contrast selected for that presentation. If the stimulus is not seen, it remains at this contrast for up to 400 msec and then is gradually decreased to zero during the final 160 msec. The interstimulus interval varies randomly up to 500 msec.

The screening procedure C-20–5 presents the stimulus at the contrast level expected based on estimates of normal age-adjusted 5% probability level. If the stimulus is detected, the device moves on to the next location; if the stimulus is missed, it repeats the presentation at the 5% probability level, then on the 2% and 1% probability levels. The results are presented in terms of $p = 5\%$ (stimulus seen on initial or repeated presentation at the 5% probability level), $p < 5\%$ (stimulus missed both times at the 5% level), $p < 2\%$ (stimulus missed at the 2% level), and $p < 1\%$ (stimulus missed at the 1% level, which 99% of normal subjects are supposed to detect). The C-20–1 is more specific but less sensitive than the C-20–5 as it starts with probability levels of 1%. Better values for sensitivity and specificity can be obtained using the threshold modes.

CLINICAL INTERPRETATION OF FREQUENCY DOUBLING TECHNOLOGY

Figure 11.7 shows a printout of a full-threshold FDT examination obtained in a patient with glaucoma.

Similarly to conventional perimetry, the full-threshold FDT gives both the raw sensitivity values and probability plots. After comparing the results with age-matched normal individuals from the internal database, a statistical analysis package provides the total and pattern deviation plots, and the global indices mean deviation (MD) and pattern standard deviation (PSD). Reliability is also measured and shown with similar indices as conventional SAP perimetry: fixation losses, false positives, and false negatives.

The criteria for abnormality on FDT perimetry are not well established, and several different criteria have been proposed.[53] Using the screening protocol, Quigley[46] found that the criterion with best performance to discriminate between glaucoma and normal eyes was the presence of two or more abnormal locations, regardless of the severity of the defect. This criterion resulted in a sensitivity of 91% with specificity of 94%. In his study, he also found that the severity of abnormal points with FDT was not as well correlated with glaucoma damage as the total number of abnormal points. Several authors have also proposed that an FDT examination should be considered abnormal in the presence of at least one abnormal point. This criterion, however, may result in lower specificity values. Therefore, other investigators have suggested the use of scores including all contrast levels presented in

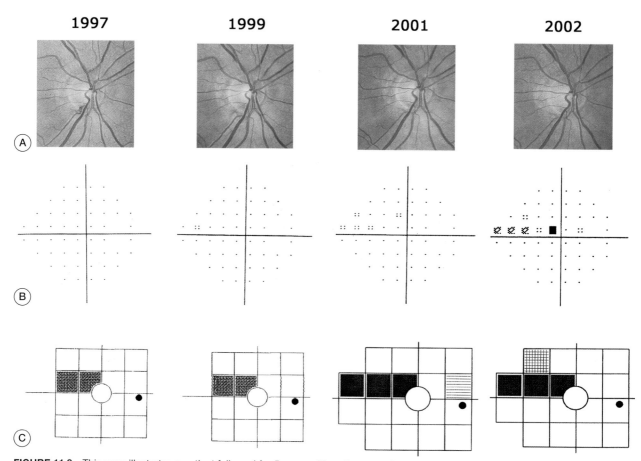

FIGURE 11.8 This case illustrates a patient followed for 5 years with optic nerve photographs, SAP, and FDT testing. The neuroretinal rim showed progressive thinning on the inferior temporal sector **(A)**, but SAP visual fields remained normal until 2002 **(B)**. A superior nasal defect could be demonstrated with FDT several years before SAP **(C)**.

test locations.[44,49,52,54] Using such scores, Patel et al.[54] found a strong correlation between the score result in the FDT and the losses defined by SAP. In contrast, another study has reported that the difference of validity between a score system and a simple one-missed-point criterion was marginal.[55] It is important to emphasize that, whichever the criteria used, it is always necessary to confirm that the defect is repeatable on subsequent tests.

STRENGTHS AND LIMITATIONS

Early detection of functional damage Previous investigations have found high sensitivity and specificity values for FDT perimetry in the detection of patients with confirmed glaucomatous damage.[43–46,48,52,54,56–58] Most of these studies, however, have included only patients with glaucomatous visual field loss as identified by SAP. In studies evaluating and comparing functional tests, it is important to have a reference standard for disease diagnosis that is independent of the tests being evaluated. In a study comparing several tests for glaucoma diagnosis, but using optic nerve appearance as the reference standard for diagnosing the disease, Sample et al.[57] reported that FDT parameters had

higher diagnostic accuracy when compared to other functional tests such as SAP and SWAP.

In patients suspected of having glaucoma, FDT has also been shown to be able to detect functional loss before SAP.[59–61] Figure 11.8 shows an example of a patient whose FDT detected a visual field loss several years before SAP. In a prospective longitudinal study by Medeiros et al.,[50] 105 glaucoma suspect patients were followed for approximately 3.5 years. All patients had normal visual fields at the beginning of the study as assessed by SAP, and suspicion was based on optic disc appearance and IOP levels. At baseline, 24% of the 105 patients had repeatable abnormal FDT tests. During follow-up, 16% developed repeatable SAP visual field abnormalities. An abnormal FDT examination at baseline was able to predict the onset and location of future SAP visual field defects. After adjustment for other risk factors, a patient with an abnormal FDT test at baseline was threefold more likely to develop a confirmed abnormal SAP visual field during follow-up than a patient with a normal FDT (Fig. 11.9). These findings have also been confirmed by prospective studies conducted by Landers and colleagues.[62,63] These studies suggest that FDT could potentially be used as a tool for providing earlier diagnosis and risk assessment in glaucoma.

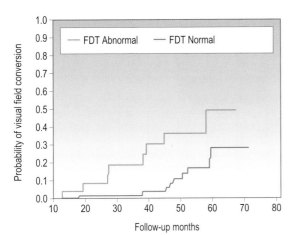

FIGURE 11.9 Cumulative probability of development of visual field abnormality in patients with abnormal FDT examination at baseline, and in patients with normal FDT examination at baseline. (Modified from Medeiros et al. Frequency doubling technology perimetry abnormalities as predictors of glaucomatous visual field loss. Am J Ophthalmol 2004; 137(5):863–871.)

Glaucoma screening with frequency doubling technology Because of its portability, ease of use, short testing time, and high sensitivity and specificity values, FDT has been suggested as a potential screening tool for glaucoma.[43,64] FDT also seems to have reduced variability when compared to both SAP and SWAP and, therefore, fewer examinations would be required to confirm an abnormal result with this technology.[65,66] The reduced variability may be explained by the smaller influence of media opacities, pupil diameter, and refractive errors on perimetric testing.[65]

Recently, a large population-based study has evaluated the performance of the FDT for glaucoma screening.[67] In this study, definite glaucoma diagnosis was determined by SITA-SAP and optic disc stereophotographs. Over 5000 eyes of patients older than 40 years were evaluated in the study. Using FDT, the sensitivity and specificity for detecting definite glaucoma were 55.6% and 92.7%, respectively. The reported sensitivity was lower than that from previous hospital-based studies.[46,52,60] However, most of the 107 patients who were diagnosed with glaucoma in this population-based study had earlier stages of disease when compared to previous studies reported in the literature.

Detection of progressive damage There is evidence that FDT may detect progressive visual field loss earlier than SAP. In a prospective clinical study, Bayer and Erb[59] found that FDT identified future progression of existing SAP visual field defects in 74% of eyes with glaucoma. FDT was able to detect progression on average 12 to 24 months before SAP. In another prospective longitudinal study, Haymes et al.[68] followed 65 patients with glaucoma tested every 6 months with both SAP and FDT. Using different criteria to assess progression, FDT detected 31–49% of patients as progressing.

SAP was able to detect 35–49% of progressions. Only 15–25% were detected at the same time by both FDT and SAP. Criteria for progression included several different scores using glaucoma change probability analysis and linear regression analysis. Even though progression rates varied with the method of analysis for both tests, FDT was able to detect progression in more patients than SAP for most of the criteria used. Further, when patients progressed in both tests, abnormalities were seen with FDT before SAP in most cases.

Limitations One of the main limitations of previous versions of FDT perimetry was the relatively large size of the stimulus and the low number of targets presented, resulting in suboptimal spatial resolution and reduced ability to detect localized defects.[69,70] Also, the low number of targets made difficult the evaluation of progressive damage over time, which may limit the use of this instrument for glaucoma follow-up. This limitation has been addressed by the recently released FDT Matrix perimeter (see below).

Threshold sensitivity values obtained by FDT also seem to be affected by cataract, although probably at a lower degree than other function-specific perimetric tests such as SWAP. An improvement in sensitivity values is seen both in glaucomatous as well as in normal patients after cataract surgery.[71] Therefore, the effects of cataract need to be taken into account in the evaluation of FDT examinations.

FREQUENCY DOUBLING TECHNOLOGY MATRIX

The FDT Matrix (Carl-Zeiss Meditc, Dublin, CA) is the latest commercially available version of the FDT. It offers a new additional testing program along with the same tests provided by the previous versions of this technology. In the new testing pattern, the FDT Matrix utilizes grating targets smaller than the original FDT to enable standard 24–2 and 30–2 test patterns, which look identical to those in SAP. The stimulus is a 5° × 5° square (half of the original) with a spatial frequency of 0.5 cycles/degree and temporal frequency of 18 Hz. The first-generation FDT was able to evaluate contrast sensitivity for only 17 or 19 test locations, whereas the FDT Matrix can evaluate 54 (24–2) or 69 (30–2) locations. Figure 11.10 shows a glaucomatous eye tested with the standard FDT and the 24–2 FDT.

The FDT Matrix uses a maximum likelihood threshold Bayesian strategy called zippy estimation of sequential testing (ZEST). In brief, the intensity of the first stimulus presented is based on the mean of a population's probability density function (PDF). For each location, the subsequent stimulus is based on the modified PDF after the patient's previous response, which determines the likelihood that this patient will see the stimulus, given the internal variability in response. This strategy of testing has been shown to have reduced test-retest variability and to reduce the testing time by 40–50%.[72–74] In FDT Matrix, the Bayesian strategy has a

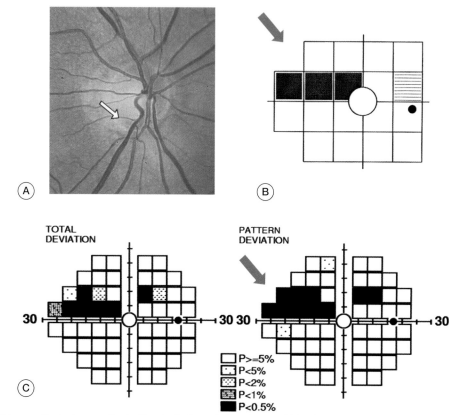

FIGURE 11.10 This case illustrates a patient with a typical nasal step shown with both conventional FDT **(B)** and FDT Matrix 24–2 **(C)**. Note the correspondence of the visual field defect and the inferior thinning of the optic disc rim **(A)**. When compared to the conventional FDT, the defect shown on the FDT Matrix **(C)** delimits better the superior nasal arcuate pattern.

fixed number of presentations at each test location and a flat previous probability density function that reduces duration of the test while keeping similar accuracy and reliability.[72,73,75] Test duration with FDT Matrix is slightly shorter than with SAP-SITA, with average testing times ranging from 5 to 6 minutes.

Due to its relatively recent introduction in the market, only a few studies have evaluated the diagnostic ability of the FDT Matrix.[76–79] In a recent investigation by Sakata and colleagues,[79] FDT Matrix enabled detection of abnormal visual function in more eyes with glaucomatous neuropathy than did SAP-SITA, although the difference between the two tests was not statistically significant. Another study by Burgansky-Eliash et al.[80] did not find differences in the performance of these tests for detection of patients with evidence of glaucomatous structural damage by optic disc photographs or optical coherence tomography. It is important to emphasize, however, that studies comparing diagnostic instruments should take into account the influence of disease severity on the performance of the tests. It is possible that the comparison of the diagnostic abilities of different tests will be influenced by the severity of glaucomatous damage. For example, a particular test may be more sensitive at early stages of the disease, whereas another test may be more sensitive for moderate or advanced stages. Therefore, it is important to characterize the relationship between the performance

of the diagnostic test and the severity of disease and to evaluate how this relationship affects the comparison between different tests. Disregarding the effect of disease severity in the comparison of the tests may mask significant differences in performance. In a recent study, Medeiros et al.[76] compared the abilities of FDT Matrix and SAP-SITA to diagnose glaucoma, taking into account the influence of disease severity on the evaluation of the performance of the tests. The study included 370 eyes of 211 participants. One hundred and seventy-four eyes of 110 patients had glaucomatous optic neuropathy, whereas 196 eyes of 101 subjects were normal. All patients underwent visual function testing with FDT 24–2 Humphrey Matrix and SAP-SITA within 6 months. The authors found that FDT Matrix performed significantly better than SAP-SITA for detection of early glaucomatous damage. That is, for patients with smaller values of neuroretinal rim loss (as assessed by confocal scanning laser ophthalmoscopy), FDT Matrix performed significantly better than SITA-SAP (Fig. 11.11). In patients with more severe disease, however, the performance of FDT Matrix was no different from SAP.

The FDT Matrix is a promising instrument for providing early diagnosis of glaucomatous functional loss. However, further studies are necessary in order to investigate the ability of this instrument for longitudinal assessment of progressive glaucomatous damage.

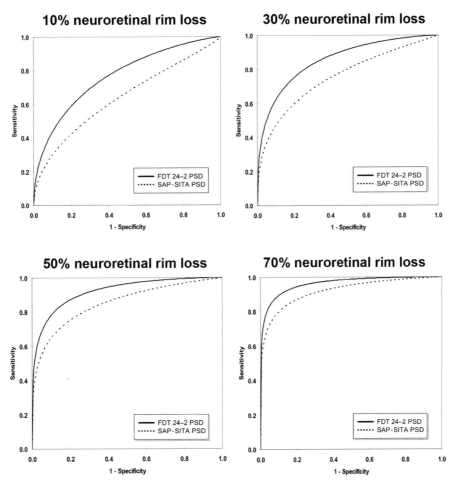

FIGURE 11.11 Receiver operating characteristic (ROC) curves for SAP-SITA PSD and FDT Matrix 24–2 PSD for discriminating patients with glaucomatous optic neuropathy from healthy subjects. ROC curves are presented for different values of percentage neuroretinal rim loss. Larger areas under ROC curves indicate better diagnostic performance. Note that the areas under the ROC curves are larger for FDT Matrix 24–2 than SAP-SITA, with the differences between the two tests being more pronounced at earlier stages of the disease (smaller values of neuroretinal rim area loss). (Reproduced from Medeiros et al. Invest Ophthalmol Vis Sci 2006; 47(6):2520–2527.)

HIGH-PASS RESOLUTION PERIMETRY

High-pass resolution perimetry (HPRP) was designed originally as a method to estimate retinal ganglion cell density, more specifically small parvocellular cells sensitive to high spatial and low temporal frequency stimulus. It uses ring-shaped targets of different sizes to determine resolution over the central 30 degrees of the visual field (Fig. 11.12). The luminances are 25 cd/m² for the ring cores, 15 cd/m² for the ring border, and 20 cd/m² for the background. Thus, the average luminance of the target and the background are equal, what gives it the property of 'vanishing optotype.' The targets are of 14 different sizes with a step factor of 1.26, with dark borders surrounding a brighter core. Instead of a change in contrast or brightness of the target, the perimeter determines resolution thresholds based on the size of the stimulus seen for each one of the 50 locations.[81,82] Each step size is defined as 1 dB and the smallest is set to zero. At each point location, the score is the smallest size identified, so that the better the resolution, the lower the score. It is believed that the thresholds of

HPRP are related to the spatial density of the functional receptive fields, with good anatomic correlation.

Currently, HPRP is commercially available on the Ophthimus system (Visumetrics and High Tech Vision, Goteberg, Sweden). It is a rapid test, lasting about 5 minutes, and is well tolerated by the patients. The test uses a staircase strategy to determine the smallest stimulus the individual is able to discern at each location.[82] Catch trials and blank trials are also presented. In addition, the instrument provides statistical analyses, which include a mean score, global deviation values, local deviation values, and an estimate of functional channels, i.e. an estimate of the number of ganglion cells. However, it is controversial if this latter estimate truly correlates with number of ganglion cells.[83]

Some authors have reported that the HPRP is useful in the detection of glaucomatous visual field loss, with relatively high sensitivity and specificity.[83–87] In addition, it has been suggested that the HPRP could potentially be used to assess early functional damage in glaucoma, before SAP defects would become apparent. Unlike SAP, the variability of HPRP thresholds does not increase

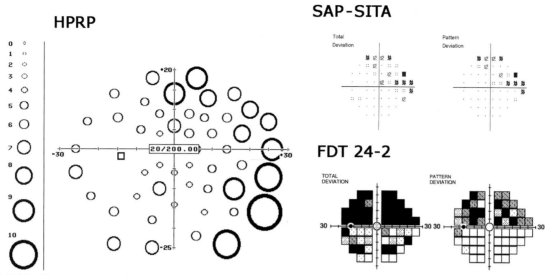

FIGURE 11.12 Glaucomatous patient tested with SAP-SITA, HPRP, and FDT 24–2. The SAP printout shows a superior arcuate defect. The FDT similarly shows a defect superiorly, more extensive and deeper than the one seen on SAP. In agreement with FDT and SAP, the HPRP shows reduced sensitivity on the superior nasal area. However, in contrast to the other two, HPRP also shows reduced sensitivity on the inferior nasal quadrant.

with eccentricity, ensuing a lower test-retest variability, which may translate into earlier detection of visual field changes.[82] In a longitudinal study, Chauhan et al.[86] followed 113 glaucoma patients and 119 control subjects for a median time of 4.5 years, performing both full-threshold SAP and HPRP every 6 months. Among the patients showing progressive visual field loss over time, HPRP detected progression earlier than full-threshold SAP in 54% of the cases, whereas full-threshold SAP detected progression earlier than HPRP in 19% of the cases. Concomitant progression was seen with both tests in 27% of the cases. The average time difference between detection of progression with these two tests was 12 months.

Despite some positive results obtained with HPRP by a few researchers, this test has not been widely used in clinical practice. The benefit of HPRP over SAP seems to have disappeared with the incorporation of the SITA strategy on SAP testing. In fact, in a recent comparison of HPRP with other tests of visual function (FDT, SWAP, and SAP-SITA), Sample et al.[88] found that HPRP generally performed worse than the other tests in identifying patients with glaucomatous optic neuropathy.

COMPARISON AMONG INSTRUMENTS

Only a few studies have compared the performance of the different visual function-specific tests in the same population. In a recent study, Sample et al.[88] evaluated a large group of 246 individuals with SAP-SITA, full-threshold SWAP, FDT, and HPRP. These subjects were classified as normal, ocular hypertensive, or glaucomatous, based on the appearance of the optic nerve and levels of intraocular pressure. Visual fields were not used for classification. From the glaucoma group, 54% of the eyes were normal on SAP-SITA, and 90% were identified by at least one of the function-specific visual field tests. In general, FDT showed higher sensitivity

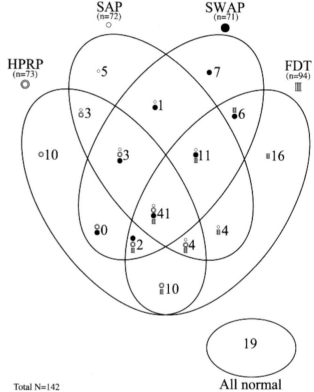

FIGURE 11.13 Venn diagram showing the overall agreement among SAP-SITA, full-threshold SWAP, FDT, and HPRP in the diagnosis of functional loss in a group of patients with glaucomatous optic neuropathy. Abnormality was based on the PSD index and all tests were matched for specificity at 80%. (Reproduced from Sample et al. Invest Ophthalmol Vis Sci 2006; 47(8): 3381–3389.)

values than the other tests for detection of patients with glaucomatous optic neuropathy, at the same levels of specificity. It is interesting to note, however, that each test identified a different subset of eyes with glaucomatous optic neuropathy as abnormal (Fig. 11.13),

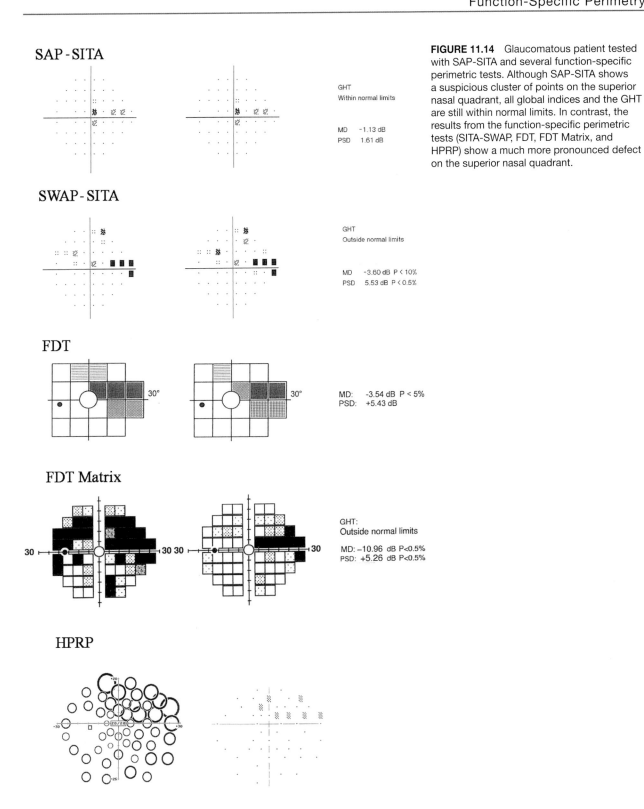

SAP-SITA

GHT
Within normal limits

MD   −1.13 dB
PSD   1.61 dB

SWAP-SITA

GHT
Outside normal limits

MD   −3.60 dB P < 10%
PSD   5.53 dB P < 0.5%

FDT

MD: −3.54 dB P < 5%
PSD: +5.43 dB

FDT Matrix

GHT:
Outside normal limits

MD: −10.96 dB P<0.5%
PSD: +5.26 dB P<0.5%

HPRP

FIGURE 11.14 Glaucomatous patient tested with SAP-SITA and several function-specific perimetric tests. Although SAP-SITA shows a suspicious cluster of points on the superior nasal quadrant, all global indices and the GHT are still within normal limits. In contrast, the results from the function-specific perimetric tests (SITA-SWAP, FDT, FDT Matrix, and HPRP) show a much more pronounced defect on the superior nasal quadrant.

and that combining the tests improved sensitivity with only a slight reduction in specificity.[88] Further, when more than one test was abnormal, the location of the defect was the same in all tests. Since these methods stimulate different types of ganglion cells, this evidence seems to support the existence of nonselective ganglion cell loss in glaucoma. Figure 11.14 shows an example of a glaucomatous patient evaluated by all previously discussed tests of visual function.

Although SAP is still considered the gold standard for functional evaluation in glaucoma, function-specific perimetric tests may offer several advantages for early diagnosis of functional loss. Hardware and software upgrades have overcome several limitations of the first generations of these instruments, but prospective longitudinal studies are still necessary in order to provide guidelines for clinicians on how to best incorporate the results from these new instruments into clinical practice.

REFERENCES

1. Harwerth RS, Carter-Dawson L, Shen F, et al. Ganglion cell losses underlying visual field defects from experimental glaucoma. Invest Ophthalmol Vis Sci 1999; 40(10):2242–2250.

2. Kerrigan-Baumrind LA, Quigley HA, Pease ME, et al. Number of ganglion cells in glaucoma eyes compared with threshold visual field tests in the same persons. Invest Ophthalmol Vis Sci 2000; 41(3):741–748.

3. Harwerth RS, Quigley HA. Visual field defects and retinal ganglion cell losses in patients with glaucoma. Arch Ophthalmol 2006; 124(6):853–859.

4. Brown PK, Wald G. Visual pigments in human and monkey retinas. Nature 1963; 200:37–43.

5. Smith VC, Pokorny J. Spectral sensitivity of the foveal cone photopigments between 400 and 500 nm. Vision Res 1975; 15(2):161–171.

6. Hering E. Outlines of a theory of the light sense. MA: Cambridge: Harvard University Press; 1964. xxvii, 317.

7. Ogden TE. Nerve fiber layer of the primate retina: morphometric analysis. Invest Ophthalmol Vis Sci 1984; 25(1):19–29.

8. Dacey DM, Petersen MR. Dendritic field size and morphology of midget and parasol ganglion cells of the human retina. Proc Natl Acad Sci USA 1992; 89(20):9666–9670.

9. Schiller PH, Malpeli JG. Functional specificity of lateral geniculate nucleus laminae of the rhesus monkey. J Neurophysiol 1978; 41(3):788–797.

10. Martin PR, White AJ, Goodchild AK, et al. Evidence that blue-on cells are part of the third geniculocortical pathway in primates. Eur J Neurosci 1997; 9(7):1536–1541.

11. Dacey DM, Lee BB. The 'blue-on' opponent pathway in primate retina originates from a distinct bistratified ganglion cell type. Nature 1994; 367(6465):731–735.

12. Dacey DM. Morphology of a small-field bistratified ganglion cell type in the macaque and human retina. Vis Neurosci 1993; 10(6):1081–1098.

13. Johnson CA. Selective versus nonselective losses in glaucoma. J Glaucoma 1994; 3:S32–S44.

14. Frisen L. High-pass resolution perimetry: central-field neuroretinal correlates. Vision Res 1995; 35(2):293–301.

15. Adams AJ, Rodic R, Husted R, et al. Spectral sensitivity and color discrimination changes in glaucoma and glaucoma-suspect patients. Invest Ophthalmol Vis Sci 1982; 23(4):516–524.

16. Flammer J, Drance SM. Correlation between color vision scores and quantitative perimetry in suspected glaucoma. Arch Ophthalmol 1984; 102(1):38–39.

17. Hamill TR, Post RB, Johnson CA, et al. Correlation of color vision deficits and observable changes in the optic disc in a population of ocular hypertensives. Arch Ophthalmol 1984; 102(11):1637–1639.

18. Wild JM. Short wavelength automated perimetry. Acta Ophthalmol Scand 2001; 79(6):546–559.

19. Sample PA, Irak I, Martinez GA, et al. Asymmetries in the normal short-wavelength visual field: implications for short-wavelength automated perimetry. Am J Ophthalmol 1997; 124(1):46–52.

20. Johnson CA, Adams AJ, Casson EJ, et al. Progression of early glaucomatous visual field loss as detected by blue-on-yellow and standard white-on-white automated perimetry. Arch Ophthalmol 1993; 111(5):651–656.

21. Sample PA, Taylor JD, Martinez GA, et al. Short-wavelength color visual fields in glaucoma suspects at risk. Am J Ophthalmol 1993; 115(2):225–233.

22. Johnson CA, Adams AJ, Casson EJ, et al. Blue-on-yellow perimetry can predict the development of glaucomatous visual field loss. Arch Ophthalmol 1993; 111(5):645–650.

23. Medeiros FA, Sample PA, Weinreb RN. Corneal thickness measurements and visual function abnormalities in ocular hypertensive patients. Am J Ophthalmol 2003; 135(2):131–137.

24. Gordon MO, Beiser JA, Brandt JD, et al. The Ocular Hypertension Treatment Study: baseline factors that predict the onset of primary open-angle glaucoma. Arch Ophthalmol 2002; 120(6):714–720; discussion 729–730.

25. Demirel S, Johnson CA. Incidence and prevalence of short wavelength automated perimetry deficits in ocular hypertensive patients. Am J Ophthalmol 2001; 131(6):709–715

26. Sample PA, Weinreb RN. Progressive color visual field loss in glaucoma. Invest Ophthalmol Vis Sci 1992; 33(6): 2068–2071.

27. Johnson CA, Sample PA, Zangwill LM, et al. Structure and function evaluation (SAFE): II. Comparison of optic disk and visual field characteristics. Am J Ophthalmol 2003; 135(2):148–154.

28. Teesalu P, Vihanninjoki K, Airaksinen PJ, et al. Correlation of blue-on-yellow visual fields with scanning confocal laser optic disc measurements. Invest Ophthalmol Vis Sci 1997; 38(12):2452–2459.

29. Ferreras A, Polo V, Larrosa JM, et al. Can frequency-doubling technology and short-wavelength automated perimetries detect visual field defects before standard automated perimetry in patients with preperimetric glaucoma? J Glaucoma 2007; 16(4):372–383.

30. Sanchez-Galeana CA, Bowd C, Zangwill LM, et al. Short-wavelength automated perimetry results are correlated with optical coherence tomography retinal nerve fiber layer thickness measurements in glaucomatous eyes. Ophthalmology 2004; 111(10):1866–1872.

31. Girkin CA, Emdadi A, Sample PA, et al. Short-wavelength automated perimetry and standard perimetry in the detection of progressive optic disc cupping. Arch Ophthalmol 2000; 118(9):1231–1236.

32. Blumenthal EZ, Sample PA, Zangwill L, et al. Comparison of long-term variability for standard and short-wavelength automated perimetry in stable glaucoma patients. Am J Ophthalmol 2000; 129(3):309–313.

33. Kwon YH, Park HJ, Jap A, et al. Test-retest variability of blue-on-yellow perimetry is greater than white-on-white perimetry in normal subjects. Am J Ophthalmol 1998; 126(1):29–36.

34. Sample PA, Martinez GA, Weinreb RN. Short-wavelength automated perimetry without lens density testing. Am J Ophthalmol 1994; 118(5):632–641.

35. Sample PA, Weinreb RN. Color perimetry for assessment of primary open-angle glaucoma. Invest Ophthalmol Vis Sci 1990; 31(9):1869–1875.

36. Chauhan BC, LeBlanc RP, Shaw AM, et al. Repeatable diffuse visual field loss in open-angle glaucoma. Ophthalmology 1997; 104(3):532–538.

37. Moss ID, Wild JM, Whitaker DJ. The influence of age-related cataract on blue-on-yellow perimetry. Invest Ophthalmol Vis Sci 1995; 36(5):764–773.

38. Bengtsson B. A new rapid threshold algorithm for short-wavelength automated perimetry. Invest Ophthalmol Vis Sci 2003; 44(3):1388–1394.

39. Bengtsson B, Heijl A. Diagnostic sensitivity of fast blue-yellow and standard automated perimetry in early glaucoma: a comparison between different test programs. Ophthalmology 2006; 113(7):1092–1097.

40. Bengtsson B, Heijl A. Normal intersubject threshold variability and normal limits of the SITA SWAP and full threshold SWAP perimetric programs. Invest Ophthalmol Vis Sci 2003; 44(11):5029–5034.

41. Kelly DH. Nonlinear visual responses to flickering sinusoidal gratings. J Opt Soc Am 1981; 71(9):1051–1055.

42. Ansari EA, Morgan JE, Snowden RJ. Psychophysical characterisation of early functional loss in glaucoma and ocular hypertension. Br J Ophthalmol 2002; 86(10):1131–1135.

43. Johnson CA, Samuels SJ. Screening for glaucomatous visual field loss with frequency-doubling perimetry. Invest Ophthalmol Vis Sci 1997; 38(2):413–425.

44. Cello KE, Nelson-Quigg JM, Johnson CA. Frequency doubling technology perimetry for detection of glaucomatous visual field loss. Am J Ophthalmol 2000; 129(3):314–322.

45. Horn FK, Wakili N, Junemann AM, et al. Testing for glaucoma with frequency-doubling perimetry in normals, ocular hypertensives, and glaucoma patients. Graefe's Arch Clin Exp Ophthalmol 2002; 240(8):658–665.

46. Quigley HA. Identification of glaucoma-related visual field abnormality with the screening protocol of frequency doubling technology. Am J Ophthalmol 1998; 125(6):819–829.

47. Sponsel WE, Arango S, Trigo Y, et al. Clinical classification of glaucomatous visual field loss by frequency doubling perimetry. Am J Ophthalmol 1998; 125(6):830–836.

48. Thomas R, Bhat S, Muliyil JP, et al. Frequency doubling perimetry in glaucoma. J Glaucoma 2002; 11(1):46–50.

49. Burnstein Y, Ellish NJ, Magbalon M, et al. Comparison of frequency doubling perimetry with Humphrey visual field analysis in a glaucoma practice. Am J Ophthalmol 2000; 129(3):328–333.

50. Medeiros FA, Sample PA, Weinreb RN. Frequency doubling technology perimetry abnormalities as predictors of glaucomatous visual field loss. Am J Ophthalmol 2004; 137(5):863–871.

51. Anderson AJ, Johnson CA. Mechanisms isolated by frequency-doubling technology perimetry. Invest Ophthalmol Vis Sci 2002; 43(2):398–401.

52. Wadood AC, Azuara-Blanco A, Aspinall P, et al. Sensitivity and specificity of frequency-doubling technology, tendency-oriented perimetry, and Humphrey Swedish Interactive Threshold Algorithm-fast perimetry in a glaucoma practice. Am J Ophthalmol 2002; 133(3):327–332.

53. Gardiner SK, Anderson DR, Fingeret M, et al. Evaluation of decision rules for frequency-doubling technology screening tests. Optom Vis Sci 2006; 83(7):432–437.

54. Patel SC, Friedman DS, Varadkar P, et al. Algorithm for interpreting the results of frequency doubling perimetry. Am J Ophthalmol 2000; 129(3):323–327.

55. Casson R, James B, Rubinstein A, et al. Clinical comparison of frequency doubling technology perimetry and Humphrey perimetry. Br J Ophthalmol 2001; 85(3):360–362.

56. Yamada N, Chen PP, Mills RP, et al. Screening for glaucoma with frequency-doubling technology and Damato campimetry. Arch Ophthalmol 1999; 117(11):1479–1484.

57. Sample PA, Bosworth CF, Blumenthal EZ, et al. Visual function-specific perimetry for indirect comparison of different ganglion cell populations in glaucoma. Invest Ophthalmol Vis Sci 2000; 41(7):1783–1790.

58. Bowd C, Zangwill LM, Berry CC, et al. Detecting early glaucoma by assessment of retinal nerve fiber layer thickness and visual function. Invest Ophthalmol Vis Sci 2001; 42(9):1993–2003.

59. Bayer AU, Erb C. Short wavelength automated perimetry, frequency doubling technology perimetry, and pattern electroretinography for prediction of progressive glaucomatous standard visual field defects. Ophthalmology 2002; 109(5):1009–1017.

60. Paczka JA, Friedman DS, Quigley HA, et al. Diagnostic capabilities of frequency-doubling technology, scanning laser polarimetry, and nerve fiber layer photographs to distinguish glaucomatous damage. Am J Ophthalmol 2001; 131(2):188–197.

61. Wu LL, Suzuki Y, Kunimatsu S, et al. Frequency doubling technology and confocal scanning ophthalmoscopic optic disc analysis in open-angle glaucoma with hemifield defects. J Glaucoma 2001; 10(4):256–260.

62. Landers JA, Goldberg I, Graham SL. Detection of early visual field loss in glaucoma using frequency-doubling perimetry and short-wavelength automated perimetry. Arch Ophthalmol 2003; 121(12):1705–1710.

63. Landers J, Sharma A, Goldberg I, et al. A comparison of diagnostic protocols for interpretation of frequency doubling perimetry visual fields in glaucoma. J Glaucoma 2006; 15(4):310–314.

64. Harasymowycz PJ, Papamatheakis DG, Fansi AK, et al. Validity of screening for glaucomatous optic nerve damage using confocal scanning laser ophthalmoscopy (Heidelberg Retina Tomograph II) in high-risk populations: a pilot study. Ophthalmology 2005; 112(12):2164–2171.

65. Chauhan BC, Johnson CA. Test-retest variability of frequency-doubling perimetry and conventional perimetry in glaucoma patients and normal subjects. Invest Ophthalmol Vis Sci 1999; 40(3):648–656.

66. Spry PG, Johnson CA, McKendrick AM, et al. Variability components of standard automated perimetry and frequency-doubling technology perimetry. Invest Ophthalmol Vis Sci 2001; 42(6):1404–1410.

67. Iwase A, Tomidokoro A, Araie M, et al. Performance of frequency-doubling technology perimetry in a population-based prevalence survey of glaucoma: the Tajimi study. Ophthalmology 2007; 114(1):27–32.

68. Haymes SA, Hutchison DM, McCormick TA, et al. Glaucomatous visual field progression with frequency-doubling technology and standard automated perimetry in a longitudinal prospective study. Invest Ophthalmol Vis Sci 2005; 46(2):547–554.

69. Johnson CA, Cioffi GA, Van Buskirk EM. Frequency doubling technology perimetry using a 24–2 stimulus presentation pattern. Optom Vis Sci 1999; 76(8):571–581.

70. Anderson AJ, Johnson CA. Frequency-doubling technology perimetry. Ophthalmol Clin North Am 2003; 16(2):213–225.

71. Siddiqui MA, Azuara-Blanco A, Neville S. Effect of cataract extraction on frequency doubling technology perimetry in patients with glaucoma. Br J Ophthalmol 2005; 89(12):1569–1571.

72. Turpin A, McKendrick AM, Johnson CA, et al. Performance of efficient test procedures for frequency-doubling technology perimetry in normal and glaucomatous eyes. Invest Ophthalmol Vis Sci 2002; 43(3):709–715.

73. Turpin A, McKendrick AM, Johnson CA, et al. Development of efficient threshold strategies for frequency doubling technology perimetry using computer simulation. Invest Ophthalmol Vis Sci 2002; 43(2):322–331.

74. Turpin A, McKendrick AM, Johnson CA, et al. Properties of perimetric threshold estimates from full threshold, ZEST, and SITA-like strategies, as determined by computer simulation. Invest Ophthalmol Vis Sci 2003; 44(11):4787–4795.

75. Artes PH, Hutchison DM, Nicolela MT, et al. Threshold and variability properties of matrix frequency-doubling technology and standard automated perimetry in glaucoma. Invest Ophthalmol Vis Sci 2005; 46(7):2451–2457.

76. Medeiros FA, Sample PA, Zangwill LM, et al. A statistical approach to the evaluation of covariate effects on the receiver operating characteristic curves of diagnostic tests in glaucoma. Invest Ophthalmol Vis Sci 2006; 47(6):2520–2527.

77. Patel A, Wollstein G, Ishikawa H, et al. Comparison of visual field defects using matrix perimetry and standard achromatic perimetry. Ophthalmology 2007; 114(3):480–487.

78. Spry PG, Hussin HM, Sparrow JM. Clinical evaluation of frequency doubling technology perimetry using the Humphrey Matrix 24–2 threshold strategy. Br J Ophthalmol 2005; 89(8):1031–1035.

79. Sakata LM, Deleon-Ortega J, Arthur SN, et al. Detecting visual function abnormalities using the Swedish Interactive Threshold Algorithm and matrix perimetry in eyes with glaucomatous appearance of the optic disc. Arch Ophthalmol 2007; 125(3):340–345.

80. Burgansky-Eliash Z, Wollstein G, Patel A, et al. Glaucoma detection with matrix and standard achromatic perimetry. Br J Ophthalmol 2007; 91(7):933–938.

81. Frisen L. High-pass resolution perimetry. A clinical review. Doc Ophthalmol 1993; 83(1):1–25.

82. Wall M, Chauhan B, Frisen L, et al. Visual field of high-pass resolution perimetry in normal subjects. J Glaucoma 2004; 13(1):15–21.

83. Sample PA, Ahn DS, Lee PC, et al. High-pass resolution perimetry in eyes with ocular hypertension and primary open-angle glaucoma. Am J Ophthalmol 1992; 13(3):309–316.

84. Birt CM, Shin DH, McCarty B, et al. Comparison between high-pass resolution perimetry and differential light sensitivity perimetry in patients with glaucoma. J Glaucoma 1998; 7(2):111–116.

85. Kono Y, Chi QM, Tomita G, et al. High-pass resolution perimetry and a Humphrey Field Analyzer as indicators of glaucomatous optic disc abnormalities. A comparative study. Ophthalmology 1997; 104(9):1496–1502.

86. Chauhan BC, House PH, McCormick TA, et al. Comparison of conventional and high-pass resolution perimetry in a prospective study of patients with glaucoma and healthy controls. Arch Ophthalmol 1999; 117(1):24–33.

87. Iester M, Altieri M, Vittone P, et al. Detection of glaucomatous visual field defect by nonconventional perimetry. Am J Ophthalmol 2003; 135(1):35–39.

88. Sample PA, Medeiros FA, Racette L, et al. Identifying glaucomatous vision loss with visual-function-specific perimetry in the diagnostic innovations in glaucoma study. Invest Ophthalmol Vis Sci 2006; 47(8):3381–3389.

CHAPTER 12

Electrophysiology in Glaucoma Assessment

Stuart Graham and Brad Fortune

INTRODUCTION

ELECTROPHYSIOLOGICAL MEASURES IN GLAUCOMA

The two most common electrophysiological measures of vision function are the electroretinogram (ERG) and visual evoked cortical potential (VECP). Specific variations of these two general test types have been applied to glaucoma both as clinical diagnostic tools and for research purposes. The ERG is typically recorded from the surface of the eye by placing some conductive fiber or thin wire 'electrode' on the cornea or bulbar conjunctiva. The VECP (often abbreviated as visual evoked potential or simply VEP) is recorded using one or more surface electrodes, such as small gold-plated discs, held in contact with the occipital scalp by some conductive paste or gel. Both the ERG and VEP represent compound electrical 'field' potentials recorded in response to a visual stimulus, such as a flash of light or a counter-reversing checkerboard pattern. Thus, both of these signal types are event-related potentials and therefore require specialized equipment for synchronization between stimulus events and recorded responses. Most state-of-the-art recording systems enable the user to perform this and other necessary functions seamlessly, including data storage, data analyses, and generation of reports. The following sections provide an overview of the most common types of clinical ERG and VEP techniques in practice, each with a specific focus on potential usefulness in glaucoma diagnosis. Detailed reviews of ERG and VEP signal origins, analyses, recording techniques, and equipment can be found in more general textbooks about electrophysiology of the visual system.[1,2]

The full-field flash electroretinogram The full-field or standard flash ERG has the longest history and widest range of clinical applications. In response to a single diffuse flash of light, its form will depend on the state of retinal adaptation (dark or light adapted) as well as the intensity (and less critically, the chromaticity) of the stimulus flash. In the dark-adapted (scotopic) state, dim flashes (those within ≈ 2 log units of the human psychophysical threshold) produce a monophasic positive response like the blue trace shown at the bottom of Figure 12.1. This broad, smooth peak, known as the scotopic b-wave, reflects currents produced by rod bipolar cells. As the flash intensity increases, a faster negative potential known as the a-wave emerges, creating a more biphasic-shaped ERG. The scotopic a-wave predominantly reflects the response of the rod photoreceptors. As the flash intensity becomes even brighter, the a-wave becomes larger and faster (steeper) and the oscillatory potentials (OPs) become quite prominent along the leading edge and peak of the b-wave (e.g. orange trace). When a sufficiently strong background light is introduced to create a photopic adaptation state, these same bright flashes produce a much smaller ERG (e.g. red trace at top of Fig. 12.1), whose a-wave reflects the less numerous cone photoreceptors, as well as hyperpolarizing (or 'off') bipolar cells, and to a lesser extent, third-order retinal neurons. The photopic b-wave is shaped predominantly by the activity of depolarizing (or 'on') and off bipolar cells, but also reveals OPs, which are thought, like the scotopic OPs, to depend on feedback circuitry within the inner plexiform layer. None of these major features of the full-field ERG response is thought to depend significantly on intact retinal ganglion cell (RGC) function. Therefore, it is not surprising that they contribute little to glaucoma diagnosis.

Most reports show that the full-field ERG is unhelpful in glaucoma diagnosis,[3–5] with only mild amplitude reductions and/or latency delays found for the glaucoma population average compared with healthy controls, substantial overlap of population distributions, and most individual cases remaining well within the normal range.[6–8] The full-field ERG showed poor sensitivity in identifying glaucoma patients compared to the

---

At the time of publication, the AccuMap® system is not in production, however, the principles used in the AccuMap® can be applied to the other recording systems.

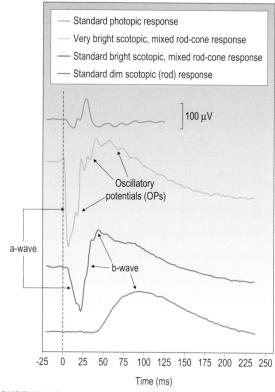

FIGURE 12.1 Representative examples of normal full-field flash electroretinogram (ERG) responses. The *blue trace* at the bottom is a response to a dim flash from a dark-adapted eye; the intensity of the flash is 24 dB below the 'standard' flash intensity (recommended by the International Society for Clinical Electrophysiology of Vision, ISCEV) and is thus used as a diagnostic of rod pathway (scotopic) function. The *green trace* is the dark-adapted response to the standard flash intensity, while the *orange trace* is the response to a flash 20 dB more intense than the standard. Both are considered 'mixed' responses, reflecting activity of both rod and cone dark-adapted pathways. The *red trace* at the top shows a response to the standard flash intensity after the eye has been light-adapted; the rod-suppressing background adaptation light serves to isolate cone-system response activity; thus, this response is used as a diagnostic of photopic retinal function.

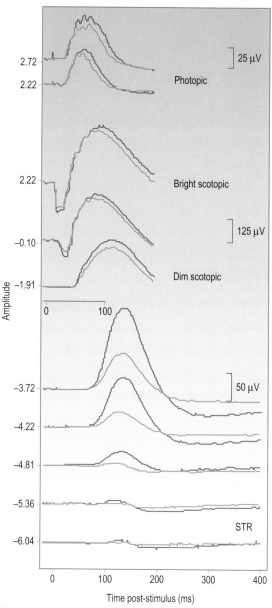

FIGURE 12.2 Full-field flash ERG responses to increasing intensity from a rat eye with experimental glaucoma (5 weeks' unilateral chronic IOP elevation), *red traces*, and from the fellow control eye, *blue traces*. In this rat model of glaucoma, there was selective loss of STR amplitude (*red traces*, dim flash responses, bottom), while responses to brighter flashes and photopic ERG responses were more similar between the control eye and the eye with experimental chronic IOP elevation (compare traces labeled dim scotopic, bright scotopic, and photopic). (Modified from Fortune et al.[25])

pattern ERG (PERG).[9] Again, considering that the ERG has predominantly an outer retinal signal origin, this is not surprising.

Most studies have found that OPs are normal after optic nerve damage[10] and that OP amplitudes have a poor sensitivity for glaucoma detection.[9] Wanger and Persson[11] found the OPs were normal while the PERG was reduced in unilateral glaucoma. However, other studies have reported OP reductions in human or experimental glaucoma.[12,13]

The scotopic threshold response Careful investigations of the dark-adapted, full-field ERG have shown that the response to a very dim stimulus, near the psychophysical scotopic threshold, is a reflection of inner retinal activity in cats,[14,15] mice,[16] rats,[17,18] monkeys,[19,20] and humans.[21,22] Accordingly, this ERG response has been called the scotopic threshold response (STR).[14] Although it is technically demanding to record, it has been shown to have exquisite

sensitivity for detection of retinal functional abnormalities in experimental models of RGC disease such as optic nerve transection,[18] acutely elevated IOP,[23,24] and experimental glaucoma;[20,25] Figure 12.2 shows selective loss of STR amplitude (red traces, bottom) in a rat model of experimental glaucoma;[25] responses to brighter flashes and photopic ERG responses were more similar between the control eye (blue traces), and the eye with experimental chronic IOP elevation (red traces).

Elevated scotopic thresholds have been measured psychophysically in early human glaucoma.[26] However,

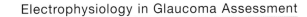

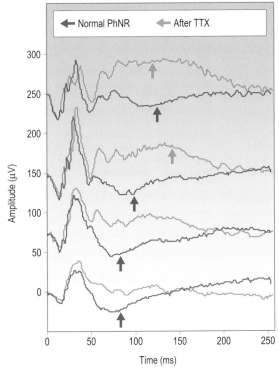

FIGURE 12.3 Photopic ERG of monkey before and after intravitreal injection of tetrodotoxin (TTX). (Traces are modified from Fortune et al.[38])

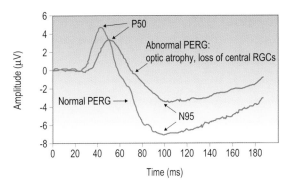

FIGURE 12.4 Representative example of a normal 'transient' PERG response (*blue trace*) from a normal rhesus monkey eye. The normal transient PERG is characterized by the initial positive peak around 50 ms (the 'P50') and a larger negative component at about 95 ms (the 'N95'). In monkeys with bilateral optic atrophy and loss of central RGCs (*green trace*), the PERG, particularly the N95 component, is substantially reduced while the full-field flash ERG remains normal. (Modified from Fortune et al.[61])

selective STR abnormalities have not yet been reported in human glaucoma.[27] Indeed, the human STR may not be as sensitive to RGC loss[28] compared with the STR of monkeys[20] or rats.[18,25] Further studies are needed.

The photopic negative response A more recently characterized component of the full-field ERG, called the photopic negative response (PhNR) because it is a slower negative component following the b-wave peak, may be more promising than other ERG components described above.[29] The PhNR is much easier to record than the STR, for both patient and clinician. Evidence suggests that the PhNR depends on intact RGC function, especially on spiking activity dominated in the retina by RGCs, and is thus more likely to be affected by glaucoma.[29–32] Figure 12.3 shows an example of how the photopic ERG changes in a monkey eye after intravitreal injection of tetrodotoxin (TTX) to block spiking activity. There is substantial reduction in the slower negative component (50–150 ms) known as the PhNR following the relatively unaffected a- and b-waves. Further evidence supporting the utility of the PhNR derives from studies showing much larger effects on the PhNR, relative to other ERG components, in other optic nerve diseases, including compressive, traumatic, ischemic, and inflammatory optic neuropathies.[33,34]

Other investigators have also evaluated the PhNR in glaucoma. In a small sample of 11 glaucoma patients, the PhNR was reported to correlate with PERG reductions.[35] A further study with 18 glaucoma subjects found the s-cone PhNR to be more sensitive in glaucoma detection than the PERG.[36] However, one report suggested that the late negative ERG component of either scotopic or photopic ERGs was unable to distinguish between human controls and glaucoma.[37,38]

The pattern electroretinogram The pattern electroretinogram (PERG, Fig. 12.4) is a small biphasic electrical signal thought to originate in the inner retinal layers in response to patterned stimuli (for reviews see references 39–44). The PERG response is generated by the macula and shows spatial frequency selectivity, an indication of postreceptoral origins.

More specific evidence that the PERG response originates from elements within the inner retina came from studies showing that responses to patterned stimuli were abolished after optic nerve transection in cat,[45] monkey,[46] and human,[47] while responses to uniform field stimulation remained normal. Current source density analyses have also indicated that ERG responses to patterned stimuli are generated by currents within the innermost layers of the retina (peak at ≈20–30% depth), between the middle of the inner plexiform layer and retinal nerve fiber layer.[48,49] The fundamental response to uniform field stimulation, in contrast, was shown to derive from a source-sink pair in the distal half of the retina.[49] Structure–function correlations have also suggested a proximal retinal origin to the pattern ERG response.[50,51]

Consistent with this background, altered PERG responses have been detected after experimental RGC lesions,[52,53] in experimental glaucoma,[31,50,54] human glaucoma,[11,55–57] ocular hypertension,[58,59] and other diseases of the optic nerve[60,61] in the presence of normal flash ERGs. Given the vast body of supporting literature, the PERG is considered to be one of the best electrophysiological tools for assessment of RGC function in clinical and laboratory settings.[40,42,43]

Figure 12.4 shows an example of a normal 'transient' PERG response (blue trace) from a normal monkey eye. For faster rates of pattern reversal, a 'steady

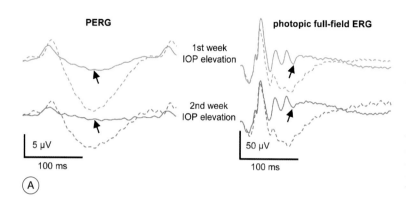

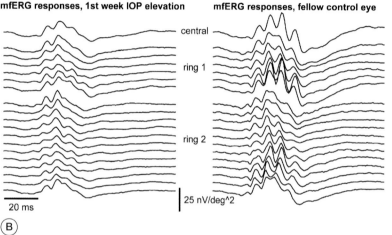

FIGURE 12.5 Examples of transient PERG and PhNR changes (A) and multifocal ERG (mfERG) changes (B) detected in a non-human primate experimental model of glaucoma during the first and second week of detectable IOP elevation. The dashed traces in experimental glaucoma during the first week (top row) and second week (bottom row) of left column and to the reduced PhNR in the right column. Panel B shows the reduction in the mfERG high frequency components in the experimental eye (left column) as compared with the fellow control eye (right column) in the same subject during the first week of IOP elevation.

state' response takes a form similar to a sine wave. The normal transient PERG is characterized by the initial positive peak around 50 ms (the 'P50') and a larger negative component at about 95 ms (the 'N95'). In monkeys with bilateral optic atrophy and loss of central RGCs (green trace, Fig. 12.4), the PERG, particularly the N95 component, is substantially reduced while the full-field flash ERG remains normal.[61]

Many studies dating back to the 1980s have described abnormal PERGs in patients with glaucoma.[56,57,62–69] Changes have been observed in the amplitudes and latencies of the P50, N95, their sum (P50 + N95) and their relative reductions. It appears that both components are affected in glaucoma[9,42] but that the N95 may be the most reduced (see review by Holder[43]). In ocular hypertension the results have been less consistent, with some studies reporting no changes, while others confirm a delay with or without a reduction in amplitude. One study reported abnormal PERGs in 40% of 206 OHT eyes.[70] Parisi et al. recently reported a very high abnormality rate in OHT eyes with 85% delayed P50 latency, and 69% showing reduced P50–N95 amplitude.[71]

Topographic localization of pattern ERG changes has been attempted with some success, for example using a ring stimulu [68] or hemifield PERGs.[72] A PERG stimulus has also been linked to an SLO to project the stimulus into quadrants, which gave a sensitivity of 82%, and a specificity of 80%, based on 34 glaucomas. A PERG recorded to frequency-doubled (FD) stimuli has been described, with nine test stimulus regions within the field. This multiregion FD PERG was able to detect 100% of moderate to severe glaucoma, and found abnormalities in 67% of high-risk suspects.[73]

In a recent prospective, longitudinal study of ocular hypertensive patients,[59] the PERG (ratio of small versus large check response amplitudes) was able to predict conversion to manifest glaucoma (defined by reliable new visual field defects) with a sensitivity of 80% and specificity of 71% 1 year prior to conversion. The predictive value of PERG measurements acquired at longer durations before conversion was poorer. Nonetheless, these results provide further evidence that the PERG becomes abnormal prior to standard automated perimetry, as has been suggested by many prior cross-sectional studies. It should be noted, however, that the predictive value of PERG was not substantially better even at the time of conversion, still misclassifying more than 20% of eyes. Variability of control and glaucoma populations,[74,75] as well as confounding effects of other sources from more distal retinal generators,[75] ultimately constrain the diagnostic performance of PERG in glaucoma. Yet any eye with a markedly reduced PERG should still warrant close attention and follow-up.

The pattern visual evoked potential The conventional flash or pattern VEP is generally agreed to be abnormal in glaucoma,[76–78] but many cases are not successfully detected by VEP and the sensitivity of

VEP, especially early in the disease, is not high. It is recognized that the pattern VEP is predominantly generated in the visual cortex by areas receiving projections from the central retina.[79–82] A small, unified check size, which is commonly used for stimulation, is another factor that tends to bias the central response.[83,84] This limits application of the method in detection of peripheral field changes in glaucoma.

Due to the large interindividual variability in VEP amplitude, most studies have concentrated on VEP latency. In an early study with an age-corrected cohort of patients with OAG and OHT, the central field pattern VEP showed about 50% and 25% of patients, respectively, to have a delay in latency compared to normals. The VEP latency was correlated with severity of field defects and the degree of cupping and pallor of the optic disc.[85] Other groups have also reported delayed VEPs, such that glaucoma suspects with OHT were found to have 15 to 20 ms delay in P100 latency compared with controls.[86] Parisi et al. reported 100% sensitivity using VEP latency for glaucoma detection.[71]

Flicker VEPs in POAG and suspects were studied retrospectively in 428 patients; visual fields and amplitude was found to be reduced, correlating with optic cup size and visual field grade, but not with peak time IOP.[87] In monkeys with monocular laser-induced glaucoma there was a reduction in amplitude, but no phase shift seen in the pattern VEP.[50]

Flash VEP P1 amplitudes have been found to correlate with the size of optic disc cupping and field loss[88] and to be reduced in glaucomatous eyes compared with normal or OHT eyes.[89] However, the luminance-contrast pattern VEP, corrected for age in patients with glaucoma (mean deviation of 8.9 ± 5.3), showed little change in amplitude or latency, whereas abnormalities were detected with color-contrast pattern VEP.[90]

Therefore, while the conventional VEP to either flash or pattern stimulation is reflecting the disease process in glaucoma, results are variable across different studies, and the conventional VEP still does not perform as well as required for accurate, reliable diagnosis and monitoring of disease, particularly early-stage glaucoma.

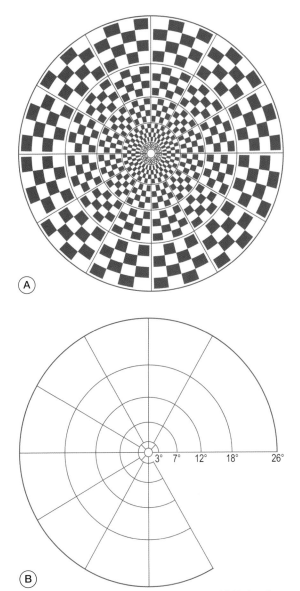

FIGURE 12.6 (A) Stimulus for multifocal pattern VEP showing dartboard array or cortically scaled checks with 60 test zones each with 16 checks. **(B)** Eccentricity of stimulus.

MULTIFOCAL RECORDING TECHNIQUES FOR ELECTRORETINOGRAM/PATTERN VISUAL EVOKED POTENTIAL

A significant advancement in stimulus and recording technology was introduced by Sutter and Tran[91] which enables the presentation of a multifocal stimulus with efficient calculation of the corresponding local response. This is now available commercially in several different electrophysiological systems. Visual stimuli typically consist of preset numbers of hexagons in arrays (or segments in a dart board) with the possibility of flash or pattern stimuli within each hexagon or dartboard segment. The stimulus areas can be retinally or cortically scaled. This means that the area of each hexagon or dartboard segment increases with eccentricity, in proportion to cone density for retinal stimulation, or to a cortical magnification factor (M-scale) for VEP recording (Fig. 12.6). For the pattern stimulus it utilizes a pseudorandom binary exchange of two opposite checkerboard pattern conditions at each of the test sites of the visual field. According to this sequence, there is a 50% probability for the checkerboard pattern to reverse its polarity with every frame of the stimulating display (e.g. every 15 ms).

Each input (stimulation site) is modulated in time according to the same pseudorandom binary m-sequence, but shifted in time (by an integer number of stimulus frames). This allows computation of cross-correlation kernels with very low-level 'contamination' by adjacent stimulus sectors, as well as characterization of nonlinear interactions between sequential visual events.[91,92] The first-order 'kernel' is similar to a conventional impulse response. Second-order kernels, however, show the difference between the anticipated summation response in a linear system when consecutive flashes (or polarity reversals) are presented, and the response that is actually recorded. In other words, it is a measure of the temporal nonlinearity of the visual system. The 'slices' of the second-order kernel represent nonlinearities observed when the consecutive stimulus event occurs in subsequent frames (e.g. at 15 ms, 30 ms, 45 ms, etc.). This technique of nonlinear analysis is important since the human visual system exhibits temporal nonlinearities. Thus, this technique enables characterization of these effects.

Alternatively, different pseudorandom sequences can be used to drive the temporal sequence at each individual stimulus element[93] using families of different binary or ternary sequences, and subsequent cross-correlations performed to extract the local responses. The latter technique does not allow for examination of higher-order kernels.

The great advantage of multifocal recording is that one can record a detailed multifocal photopic flash ERG that shows a topographic distribution of signal amplitudes (Fig. 12.7), instead of just a mass response reflecting the average response across the entire retina. The mfERG amplitudes are very useful in delineating areas of outer retinal damage in many diseases (for reviews, see Hood[94] and Lai et al.[95]). By changing the stimulus design to an alternating pattern of black and white triangular checks, which reverse according to the pseudorandom sequence, it becomes possible to record the responses of a *pattern mfERG*.

In addition to mfERGs, the technique also makes possible recordings of multifocal cortical responses to flash and pattern stimuli, producing a multifocal VEP (mfVEP). Responses to pattern stimuli are superior to flash mfVEP, being more uniform throughout the field. Figure 12.8 shows a *pattern mfVEP* recorded to a cortically scaled stimulus pattern of checks.

While several anatomical and perimetric studies have demonstrated a diffuse component of damage in glaucoma, the most characteristic visual field defects are spatially localized within the midperiphery.[96] Given the localized nature of glaucomatous damage, the development of multifocal techniques stirred great interest because it offered a significant advantage over other ERG and VEP types, that is, topographical assessment of localized function.

MULTIFOCAL TECHNIQUES IN GLAUCOMA

Multifocal flash electroretinogram It has become clear that the multifocal electroretinogram (mfERG) technique,[91,97] can detect pathological changes within

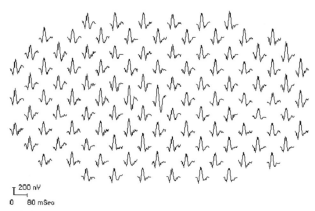

FIGURE 12.7 Normal multifocal ERG trace. Note larger signal at fovea (VERIS).

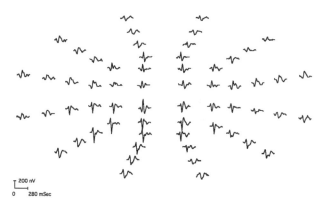

FIGURE 12.8 Normal combined multichannel mfVEP using bipolar electrodes (VERIS).

the outer retina with relatively high spatial resolution and sensitivity.[94,95,98] The clinical utility of the mfERG for evaluation of local outer retinal function has been validated by basic studies showing mfERG responses are similar to scaled-down versions of photopic ganzfeld ERGs.[99–101] The underlying mechanisms which generate the dominant features of each ERG type, namely cone photoreceptor and cone bipolar cell currents, are also similar.[100,102,103]

Compelling evidence suggests that mfERG responses also contain significant contributions from inner retinal neurons and circuitry, including RGCs and their action potentials.[32,53,61,100,101,104–108] In addition to local inner retinal contributions, mfERG responses may also reflect electrical events arising at the optic nerve head. For example, the optic nerve head component (ONHC), first proposed by Sutter and Bearse,[109] is believed to represent activity of RGC axons and to be generated in the vicinity of the optic nerve head.[107,109] The ONHC theory provides the most parsimonious explanation for the nasal–temporal asymmetries prominent in every normal mfERG response array.

Initial studies in both human glaucoma[104,110–115] and experimental glaucoma in nonhuman primates[106,108] showed that mfERG responses are indeed abnormal. However, the abnormalities, at least those determined by conventional measurements such as peak-to-trough amplitude, implicit time, and scalar-product amplitude density, generally do not show spatial correspondence with local sensitivity losses measured perimetrically.[112,115,116] One possible explanation is that RGC losses lead to reduction of the ONHC, whose latency varies according to response location, while remaining local mfERG components maintain a more constant latency throughout the retina. Thus, the effect of a missing or diminished ONHC on the shape and features of any local composite response might be location dependent. Furthermore, the fast luminance flicker stimulus common to most of the above-mentioned studies typically elicits only a relatively small ONHC in normal eyes.[117,118] Therefore, only subtle differences are revealed by the common mfERG flicker stimulus for eyes with early or moderately advanced glaucoma.[104,110,112–115] Surprisingly, even use of multifocal *pattern-reversal* ERG stimuli did not improve diagnostic capability greatly: although moderate loss has been demonstrated for glaucoma population averages, there is substantial overlap with control populations and no relationship to disease severity measured perimetrically.[116,119,120]

Sutter and colleagues have developed alternative modes of mfERG stimulation, which are thought to elicit a relatively larger ONHC in normal eyes.[117,121,122] Glaucomatous abnormalities of the ONHC should become more apparent using this type of mfERG stimulus. Initial studies of human[118,121,123] and experimental glaucoma[118,124] supported this hypothesis. However, other clinical applications of this stimulus type have demonstrated that response variability hinders diagnostic performance.[125]

While the application of the mfERG technique to human glaucoma has thus far met with limited success,[112–116,123,125] several studies have demonstrated powerful utility in nonhuman primate models of glaucoma[32,106,108,126] and other forms of RGC damage.[53,61] It remains unknown why the monkey mfERG appears to contain a relatively greater RGC contribution and/or ONHC than the human mfERG.

Multifocal pattern visual evoked potential The multifocal pattern VEP (mfVEP) was the first electrophysiological test described that appeared capable of topographically mapping visual field defects in detail.[127] It showed definite focal reductions in signal that corresponded to areas of visual field loss. By employing a cortically scaled pattern stimuli and appropriate electrode positions it was possible to record VEP responses from as far as 20–26° eccentricity.[127] Several groups have now verified this using different recording systems and techniques.[128–132]

The mfVEP technique has been refined with addition of multiple channels, together with adjusted filter settings, electrode positions, and analysis of resulting waveforms to maximize signals and improve interpretation. Bipolar electrodes, placed near or straddling the inion, allow a larger response to be recorded than the conventional fronto-occipital electrode placements (where the upper hemifield responses are consistently smaller). Adding at least one additional pair of electrodes oriented at 90° (i.e. horizontally) from the first pair allows detection of additional signals that are otherwise very small for the vertically oriented set (Klistorner; Fig. 12.9). This is most likely a consequence of the cortical representation of the visual field, with the upper hemifield

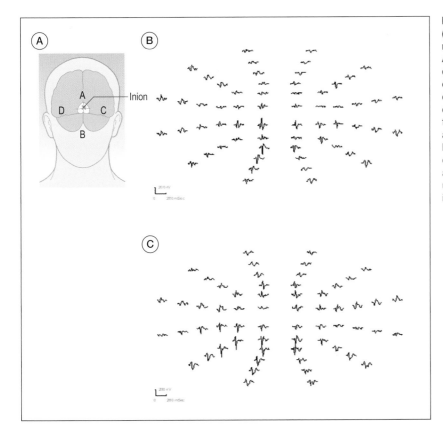

FIGURE 12.9 (A) Electrode positions (Klistorner and Graham[133]) for multichannel mfVEP recording surrounding striate cortex. AB locations linked for vertical bipolar channel, CD for horizontal channel. Oblique channels can be created by linking other combinations. **(B)** A recording from vertical channel and **(C)** a horizontal channel. Note that signals in certain areas, especially along the horizontal meridian, are often better detected in either one of the two orthogonal channels. Combining data from all channels provides better coverage of all underlying signals and produces traces as in Figure 12.8.

representation being on the inferior bank of the calcarine sulcus, further away from the recording electrode on the occiput, and whose cells are oriented differently from those of the lower visual field. This may explain why using a full-field stimulus to record the VEP has previously shown variable results in glaucoma patients, depending on the distribution of the field loss relative to the surface electrodes. An upper field defect, for example, may not produce a significant change in the signal on a conventional VEP (Fig. 12.10).

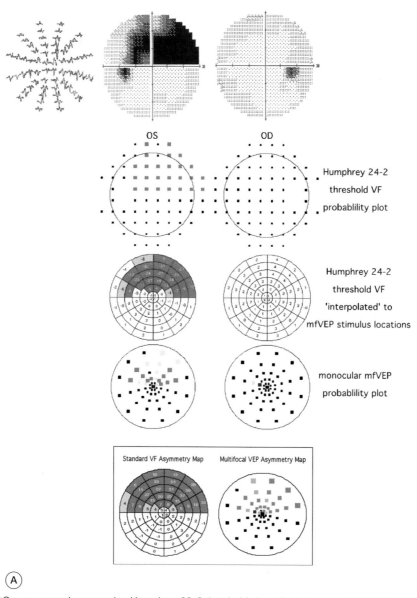

FIGURE 12.10 (A) POAG case example comparing Humphrey 30–2 threshold visual fields (*gray-scale plots, top row*) with mfVEP (*to left of visual field gray-scale plots, right eye traces are blue, left eye traces are red*), as well as with the CVEP (ISCEV standard VEP responses for full-field checkerboard stimulation shown by *blue traces, third pair from bottom,* as well as for lower hemifield stimulation, *red pair of traces,* and upper hemifield stimulation, *green pair of traces at bottom*). The patient has a moderately severe superior arcuate scotoma, with dense nasal step in the left eye and a normal visual field in the right eye (shown by *gray-scale plots top row* and visual field total deviation probability plots in the *second row*). The *third row* shows the visual field total deviation map interpolated to the mfVEP stimulus pattern for comparison with the mfVEP.[134] The *fourth row* displays the monocular probability maps for the mfVEP signal-to-noise ratio (SNR),[134] which show a very clear mfVEP defect superiorly in the left eye and a small paracentral cluster of two abnormal points in the superior hemifield of the right eye mfVEP. The interocular comparison[134] (*fifth row*) shows a clear superior hemifield defect in the left eye (*red color indicates left eye*) for both standard visual field (*left panel*) and mfVEP (*right panel*). **(B)** The ISCEV standard CVEP (*blue pair of traces in sixth row*) shows a normal response in both eyes (*bold trace right eye and thinner trace left eye*), with little or no asymmetry between eyes. As expected, based on visual field results, when stimulation was limited to the lower hemifield (*red pair of traces in seventh row*), the CVEP responses had equal amplitude, morphology, and timing, which were all within normal limits. However, when stimulation was limited to the upper hemifield, the CVEP responses were also equal, despite the dramatic difference in upper hemifield sensitivity between the two eyes. Upper hemifield CVEP responses from both eyes were within normal limits.[135] This case serves to underscore how the CVEP will frequently miss even severe damage, especially when limited to the upper hemifield. (Fortune et al. Invest Ophthalmol Vis Sci 2002; 43:E-Abstract 2126.)

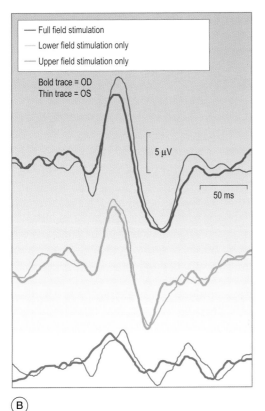

Full field stimulation
Lower field stimulation only
Upper field stimulation only

Bold trace = OD
Thin trace = OS

5 μV

50 ms

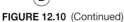

FIGURE 12.10 (Continued)

MODE OF ACTION

Since the PERG and mfVEP are the principal tests shown to be able to consistently identify glaucoma, only these two will be described in more detail in the sections below.

PERG TECHNIQUE

The PERG is typically recorded in response to a slowly reversing uniform checkerboard pattern (or grating) with the subject centrally fixating a stimulus that is usually 10–20° in width. The PERG response to slower temporal stimulation is 'transient,' consisting of a biphasic potential that is much smaller in amplitude than the ERG (4 μV compared to 400 μV, compare Figs 12.4 and 12.1 above). PERGs can also be recorded to chromatic patterns (e.g. red/green or blue/yellow) but they are even smaller in amplitude.[136] International recording standards have been published (ISCEV Standard, see http://www.iscev.org/standards/index. html). The PERG is sensitive to optical blur and retinal illuminance, so refractive error, media opacities, or pupil size will affect the response.

The transient PERG (see Fig. 12.4 above) has an initial small negative component with an implicit time of about 25 ms (N1) followed by a large positive component peaking at about 50 ms (P1 or P50). This is followed by a further negative wave at around 95 ms implicit time (N2 or N95). If the pattern reversal frequency is fast, with >10 reversals per second, the N95

becomes obscured by the subsequent P50, producing a steady-state periodic response.

MULTIFOCAL VEP TECHNIQUE

Stimulation and recording The electrophysiological method used is similar in most studies, but no international standards are yet defined. Investigators have either used the VERIS Scientific™ system (Electro-Diagnostic Imaging, Inc., Redwood City, CA), the AccuMap (ObjectiVision, Sydney, Australia), or the Retiscan system (Roland Instruments, Wiesbaden, Germany).

The visual stimulus is usually generated on a CRT screen (e.g. 22″-high resolution display). With faster refresh rates, flat screens (LCD and plasma) can now be used (author's unpublished data, SLG). The most commonly used stimulus consists of 60 close-packed segments see (Fig. 12.6 above), the sizes of which are cortically scaled with eccentricity to stimulate approximately equal areas of cortical (striate) surface.[82,137] The scaling would therefore be expected to produce a signal of similar order of amplitude from each stimulating segment. The insert in Figure 12.6 demonstrates the relationship between size of the stimulus segments and visual field. Each segment includes a checkerboard pattern (16 checks) with the size of individual checks being proportional to the size of the segment and therefore also dependent on eccentricity. Checks are alternated in pseudorandom sequences from which local responses are calculated using cross-correlation of the digitized output signal with the binary input sequences.

Subjects are comfortably seated in a chair and asked to fixate on a point at the center of the dartboard pattern, or in the case of the AccuMap a randomly changing central fixation symbol is presented, to which the patient is asked to respond. This task serves both as a test of fixation accuracy and to aid patient concentration. The distance to the screen is usually 30 cm, corresponding to a total angular subtense 52° for stimulus diameter. All subjects need to be appropriately refracted for near. Pupils are not dilated and recordings are collected using monocular stimulation.

The signal is amplified 100 000 times and band-pass filtered between 1 and 100 Hz. More recent studies have used tighter filter settings with digital filters down to 1–30 Hz, or even 1–20 Hz. With the VERIS system the full m-sequence has to be run before data can be analyzed, using either 8- or 16-minute total recordings broken up into short 30-second presentations. With the AccuMap system, results are updated after each 55-second run, and runs continue until an acceptably stable signal is achieved (usually 6–10 runs). Runs can be rejected on both systems if too noisy or artifacts are recognized.

Data from at least two orthogonally oriented channels are collected and the maximal response chosen from each segment of the visual field. The results are then presented in a combined trace array. For example, the two channels shown in Figure 12.9 are combined with at least two oblique channels to produce a trace array similar to that seen in Figure 12.8. The amplitude and peak time (latency) of the signal can be calculated for each point and compared to a normal database. Inter-eye asymmetries for both parameters are also calculated.

STRENGTHS AND LIMITATIONS

Both the PERG and mfVEP have the significant advantage of providing objective information on visual function. The limitations of subjective tests are well known. Elderly patients find subjective tests difficult to understand and perform, and many report the experience as stressful. In a recent study of the performance of the gold standard (Humphrey SITA full-threshold visual field testing),[138] the specificity of SITA in normals was only 38% at first test and 73.7% after two tests. Clinical trials have shown large fluctuations in subjective defects from test to test and patients may be repeatedly poor performers. There is also a learning curve associated with subjective perimetry that complicates interpretation in new patients, such that 2–3 field tests need to be done before a reliable result is achieved. Therefore, any objective functional information is useful for the clinician, particularly in those who are poor perimetry performers.

The only other form of objective perimetry (pupil perimetry) is dependant on having both an intact afferent and efferent pathway. Any condition that affects pupil function such as diabetes, PXF, previous iritis, trauma, and medications will therefore influence results.

PERG

The PERG technique is relatively easy for an electrophysiological test in that it does not require pupil dilation or dark/light adaptation and is easy for the patient to perform. It does require electrodes in contact with the eye (or lower eye lid) so it is minimally invasive.

The clinical utility of the PERG is limited by the intersubject and intrasubject variability of the response.[139] However, through the use of standardized recording procedures, this variability can be minimized.[140,141] A differential loss of N95 signal over P50 may have clinical relevance suggesting optic nerve rather than retinal disease.[43]

Limitations are that the PERG only provides a summed signal from the central visual field, so it cannot localize abnormalities (unless modifications are made to the method of presentation, see above). Also, since it is acuity dependent, any cause of retinal image blurring from tear film problems to cornea, lens, and vitreous opacities will confound its interpretation.

Abnormal PERGs have been reported in diabetes, retinopathies, age-related macular degeneration, optic neuropathies, amblyopia, and Alzheimer's disease. Pathologic processes in the outer retina also produce significant PERG deficits, meaning that if retinal cells distal to the ganglion cells are disordered then the PERG is also reduced.

mfVEP

With the use of multiple recording channels for the mfVEP, signals from all areas of the visual field can be combined to provide an objective map of visual function.[128,129,131,133,134,142] Signal amplitudes are compared to normal population values and probability plots can be created. Using this technique, sensitivity has been reported to be >90%, depending on the criteria used to define abnormality and the degree of glaucoma severity.[129,131,133,134,142–145] However, in contrast to signal amplitude, mfVEP latency does not demonstrate good correlation with visual field loss (Fig. 12.11).[146,147]

Inter-eye asymmetry analysis has been described as a useful technique for detecting early changes.[143,148] The close proximity in the striate cortex of the signal generators for the right and left eye visual fields means that the signals are normally close to identical for the two eyes, assuming no other pathology or amblyopia. However, interocular asymmetry analysis will not be reliable in cases where symmetric field loss occurs between both eyes, or for detecting damage in the less affected eye when one eye has more advanced loss. It is therefore necessary to examine both the monocular amplitude deviation and the interocular asymmetry in combination.

The mfVEP is noninvasive with only scalp electrodes required. No pupil dilation, light adaptation, or shielding is required. Test time is longer than the newer subjective test algorithms (e.g. SITA), being around 8 minutes per eye, with additional set-up time for the electrode application. With VERIS, an m-sequence run of 8 minutes is performed and this is often repeated. The mfVEP can also be useful in other optic neuropathies such as optic neuritis[148–151] or ischemic optic neuropathy.[128] Studies have described mfVEP in subjects with cortical lesions[152–154] and for assessment of the visual field in children.[155]

Limitations that need to be addressed include standardizing electrode positioning, accounting for interindividual variability in signal amplitude, minimizing noise artifacts, controlling fixation, and consensus on how to analyze data. Currently, the between-test amplitude variability of the mfVEP is 10–16%, and is greatest in the zones with smaller signals. This limits the application of the data to progression analysis. Improved signal-to-noise ratios (SNRs) are needed to enable better reproducibility and potential for serial analysis (see below).

One study showed very little effect of pupil size on the signal amplitude.[156] There was a slight latency change (decrease) with pupil dilation, which would need to be considered if investigating conditions where latency is important (e.g. optic neuritis).

Cataract and visual blur can reduce central amplitudes,[157] while the more peripheral points remain unaffected. It is still possible to record an mfVEP in subjects

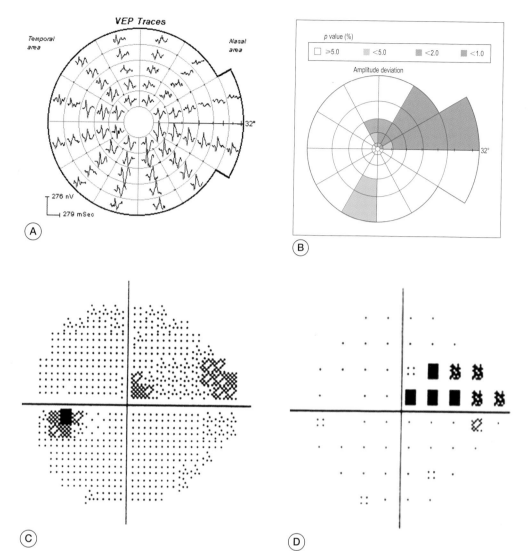

FIGURE 12.11 Superior arcuate scotoma identified by mfVEP trace array and probability plot (**A** and **B**, AccuMap) and Humphrey VF gray-scale and total deviation plot (**C** and **D**).

with poor central vision but maintaining accurate fixation can be difficult and results need to be interpreted with caution. As for the PERG, the resultant VEP signal can be affected by other pathology in the retina, so is not a specific test for glaucoma.

The possibility of simultaneous binocular recording of mfVEPs has recently been established using virtual reality goggles.[158] The advantage of this technique is that inter-eye comparisons should be even more valuable due to the identical recording conditions for each eye. Limitations will exist, however, with patients who have underlying strabismus or other disparity in the fixation angle between the two eyes.

REFERENCE POPULATION

For the PERG, individual labs are required to collect their own databases, and these need to be age stratified since the PERG does show age-related amplitude decline and latency changes.

For the mfVEP the approach varies depending on the system used. The AccuMap has an internal normative database of 200 controls and a defined recording protocol with electrode positions set in a recording electrode cross. Due to the scaling of signals using underlying EEG amplitudes with alpha rhythm removed,[93] age matching is not required for adults. In children the mfVEP evolves significantly through to early teen years, so a normative database is required.[155]

For VERIS, individual users develop their own protocol for testing and reference populations need to be recorded. Age matching is not as important if SNRs are used rather than absolute amplitudes.[159]

COMPARISON WITH OTHER TESTS

PERG

The PERG shows reductions in glaucoma, but the PERG sensitivity varies between studies. In a study where 43 glaucoma patients and 43 age-matched normal subjects underwent extensive psychophysical testing and an ERG/PERG protocol, the PERG performed much better than any other ERG parameter.[9] Using ROC analysis, the N95 amplitude of the PERG had an Az score of 0.89, with sensitivity of 85.4% and specificity of 87.8%. This was also greater than high-pass resolution perimetry, contrast sensitivity, motion detection, and an early version of short-wavelength automated perimetry (SWAP).

However, in a large multivariate analysis of psychophysical and electrophysiological techniques in 203 glaucoma patients, where glaucoma was assessed according to disc and nerve fiber layer changes rather than visual fields or IOP, psychophysical tests performed better than PERG or blue/yellow VEP.[160]

Bach et al. have attempted to improve PERG detection rates in glaucoma by introducing a ratio (the Freiburg PERG paradigm) for steady-state PERGs recorded in response to 0.8- and 16-degree check sizes.[42,59] The use of a ratio helps overcome interindividual differences in PERG amplitudes. The PERG recorded to the smaller check size tends to be differentially reduced in glaucoma. However, reduced visual acuity such as cataract can also affect the response. They report abnormalities in OHT patients subsequently converting to glaucoma, although only four eyes of 67 patients converted to manifest glaucoma during the study, which limited the conclusions that could be drawn. The ROC analysis specificity for the test was 85%. A recent report by Parisi et al. found a very high sensitivity for the PERG in glaucoma detection at 100%, and a high abnormality rate among OHT subjects.[71]

mfVEP

A retrospective case series examined 436 consecutive subjects referred for glaucoma investigation who were tested with the AccuMap™ V1.3 system within a defined 12-month period.[132] Sensitivity was determined compared to SAP and in a subgroup using masked stereo-optic disc photos as an alternative reference standard. The mfVEP changes were correlated with both stage of disease and with Humphrey MD (r = 0.78). The overall sensitivity for detecting glaucoma with established subjective field loss was 97.5% (early glaucoma 95%, defined as HFA MD <6 dB) while 92.2% of low-risk suspects had normal mfVEPs. When masked disc assessment alone was used for diagnosis of abnormality, sensitivities for both mfVEP (80.6%) and HVF (81.9%) were similar, but mfVEP specificity was greater (89.2% vs 79.5%). The mfVEP was particularly useful in assessing excessive subjective field loss (45 eyes), showing a much closer correlation with the clinical picture.

Hood et al. have demonstrated that mfVEP amplitude correlates with subjective visual field sensitivity.[128,161] In a study of 50 patients with early glaucoma (MD <8 dB) they found agreement between automated perimetry and mfVEP in 74% of hemifields as defined by a cluster of points affected. More cases were abnormal on the mfVEP. The same group examined 50 normals, 25 OHT, and 25 glaucoma suspects all with normal subjective fields. The mfVEP was abnormal in 4% of normals, 16% of OHT, and 20% of glaucoma suspects.[162] These proportions were similar to those found in the study by Graham et al. discussed above.[132]

In another recent study[145] of 185 individuals with high-risk ocular hypertension or early glaucoma (average SAP MD was +0.3 ± 2.1 dB; average PSD was 2.3 ± 1.9 dB), the diagnostic performance of mfVEP was similar to that of SAP. This was true whether the diagnostic standard was masked evaluation of stereo-optic disc photographs or the HRT Moorfields Regression Analysis. However, SAP and mfVEP agreed in only ≈80% of eyes, suggesting that they may detect slightly different functional deficits. Further, there was less agreement between the diagnoses based on function versus those based on optic disc structure, indicating that structural and functional abnormalities are not highly coincident during early-stage glaucoma (Fig. 12.12).

A comparison study of mfVEP with objective imaging using the HRT[163] showed that there was some limited correlation between structural measures assessed by the HRT and changes on the mfVEP. There was also a similar correlation found for Humphrey and HRT. There were some cases of glaucoma missed by either HRT or mfVEP; however, all cases were abnormal on one of the tests, suggesting that it may now be possible to detect most glaucoma cases using these two objective tests: mfVEP for functional deficits and HRT for structural change.

Newer stimulus techniques such as sparse stimulation or blue/yellow patterns have the potential to provide better signal-to-noise ratios, at least in the central field, and possibly greater sensitivity to early glaucoma. Further work needs to be done on the effects of age and cataract.

The dynamic range of the mfVEP signal is narrower than that of subjective perimetry, particularly in the superior visual field, which means that there is a limitation to the number of changes that could be detected over time.[164]

There are several studies looking at repeatability and these have implications for the ability of the technique to be used in some form of progression analysis.[164–166] Since there is still significant variability between tests, a larger degree of change is needed to reach statistical significance. It is interesting to note that the intersession variability of the mfVEP was reported to be less than that for SAP.[164] However, when intersession variability is expressed relative to dynamic range, it is not clear which test will allow detection of the greater number of progressive step changes. Further study in this area is required.

STORAGE AND RETRIEVAL OF DATA

For PERGs, data are stored on a computer, and after signal averaging for a few minutes of recording, an acceptable trace is normally achieved. It is common practice

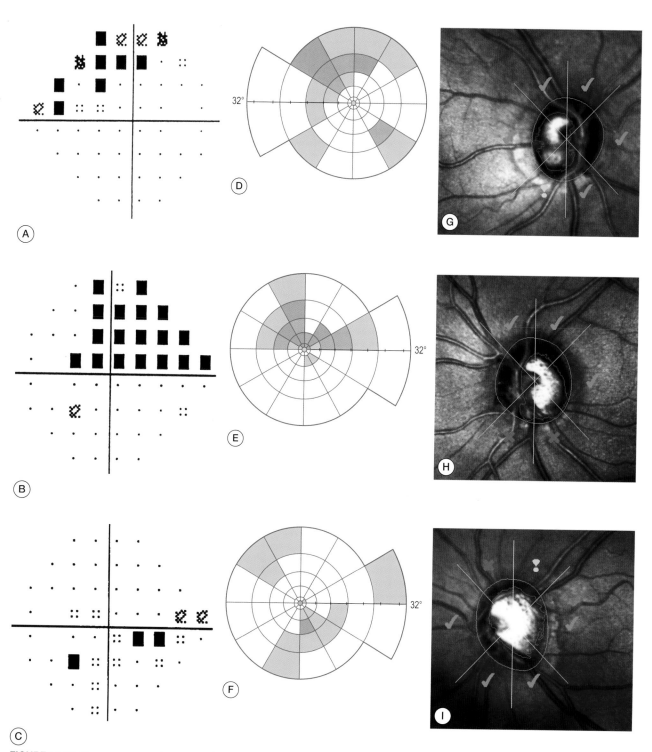

FIGURE 12.12 Glaucoma examples comparing results of subjective perimetry (Humphrey visual field-HVF), objective perimetry mfVEP (AccuMap), and disc imaging (Heidelberg HRT), showing a variable correlation between the two functional tests and the structural changes seen on imaging.

to repeat the test to gain two similar recordings, which can then be compared and averaged off line.

For mfVEP, data are stored on a computer with individual files and raw signals from each channel retrievable for export to external analysis programs such as Excel or MATLAB. In AccuMap, individual channels are still accessible for post hoc quality analysis, but are combined to form the multichannel trace array that is used for the result printout. In VERIS, it is necessary to manually export the data since the software does not yet automatically combine channels.[134]

INSTRUMENT PRINTOUTS AND INTERPRETATION OF DATA

Pattern ERG printouts vary depending on the electrophysiology system used, but usually present the recorded on-line averaged run(s) as a standard waveform

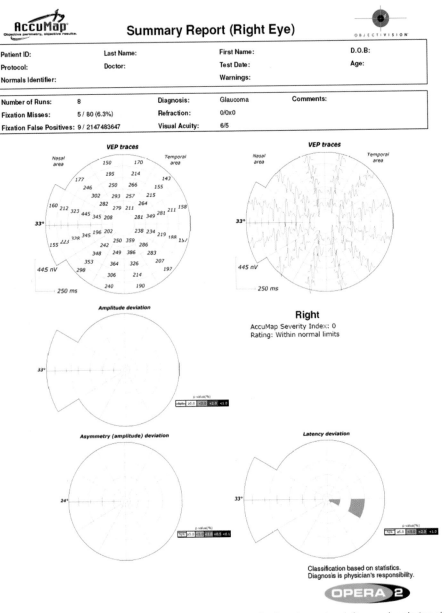

FIGURE 12.13 AccuMap summary printout for a normal subject. Actual amplitudes shown *top left*, raw signals *top right*. Monocular Amplitude deviation, asymmetry deviation, and latency deviation plots are compared to normal database.

marked with a P50 peak and N95 trough. The operator can usually adjust these markers, and corresponding amplitudes and latencies can be read from them. For a steady-state PERG, a sinusoidal-like trace is produced, and peak-to-trough amplitudes can be determined, often using Fourier analysis techniques.

For the mfVEP, VERIS produces printouts of individual channel trace arrays (see Fig. 12.9). If multichannel data is collected, then the raw data need to be exported to Excel, MATLAB, or other similar program to combine channels, as in Figure 12.8.[134] It is also possible to average signals over operator-defined areas or rings. However, the latter needs to be done with caution since, unlike the mfERG, the mfVEP waveforms change configuration depending on underlying cortex, and cancellation of opposite signals can occur. Averaging along radial sectors usually combines signals of similar waveform shape, polarity, and timing.

The AccuMap has a standard printout (Figs 12.13 and 12.14) with combined channel data already processed, and probability plots for amplitude deviation, amplitude inter-eye asymmetry, and latency deviation. Separate printouts can be obtained for inter-eye latency values, and sectoral analysis of waveforms. Individual raw channel data can also be examined post recording. The AccuMap severity index gives a rating within normal limits, borderline, or outside normal limits. This is based on scoring of clusters of abnormal points on the amplitude and asymmetry plots.

ARTIFACTS AND HOW TO PREVENT THEM

For all electrophysiological recording the subject needs to be relaxed, sitting comfortably in a chair, and in a

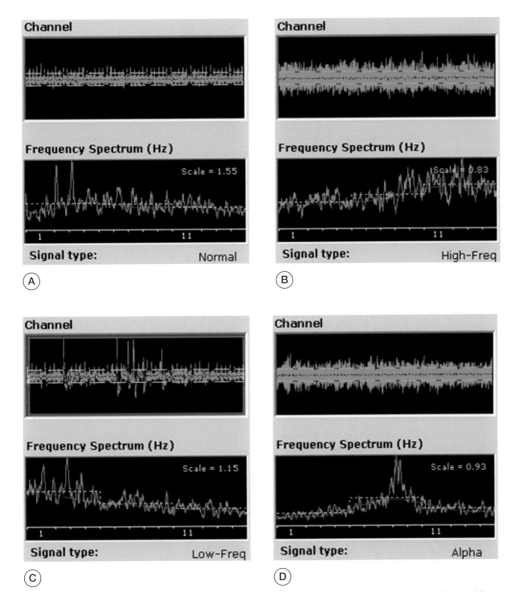

FIGURE 12.14 Noise artifacts identified by Fourier analysis (AccuMap). **(A)** Normal frequency distribution with roughly even contribution across frequencies, but ECG rhythm identified as regular-pulsed signal throughout recording, and seen as two spikes of low frequency on Fourier. **(B)** High-frequency noise, e.g. faulty contacts or electrode cables. **(C)** Low-frequency noise, eye or muscle movement. **(D)** Alpha rhythm, peaks at 8–12 Hz.

room without significant distractions or other sources of noise or extraneous light. For the mfVEP, the authors have found there is less noise from the neck muscles if the subject has the chin slightly elevated, with the back straighter rather than in a hunched position.

In recording the PERG, noise from electrodes and eye movements are the main problem encountered. Careful attention needs to be paid to the electrode position, particularly with the gold foil types. The latter are supposed to be for single use (disposable) but are frequently used for multiple tests leading to eventual loss of quality. Electrodes/cables should be checked for impedance levels prior to recording. Monitoring the recording closely and rejecting noisy traces is important. The subject should be allowed to blink frequently between recording runs, but minimize blinks during the run. Topical lubricants may help the subject tolerate the electrode and improve the resulting recording.

In the mfVEP, alpha rhythm, which is found to increase when subjects lose concentration or become sleepy, can contaminate recordings and reduce reliability, producing a false-positive result. Unfortunately, it can occur in a small proportion of young normal healthy subjects, so its recognition is critical when interpreting results. A study on fixation tasks[167] showed the importance of designing a task which keeps the patient concentrating to reduce alpha rhythm. The more difficult tasks enhanced the signal amplitude from the paracentral rings and reduced alpha rhythm.

Other problems can include high- and low-frequency noise, and contamination by electrocardiogram ECG signals (Fig. 12.15A). The latter does not significantly affect the final trace results but it can reduce the signal-to-noise ratio. The AccuMap provides an analysis of noise levels after the recording, warning if noise levels are excessive enough to influence interpretation.

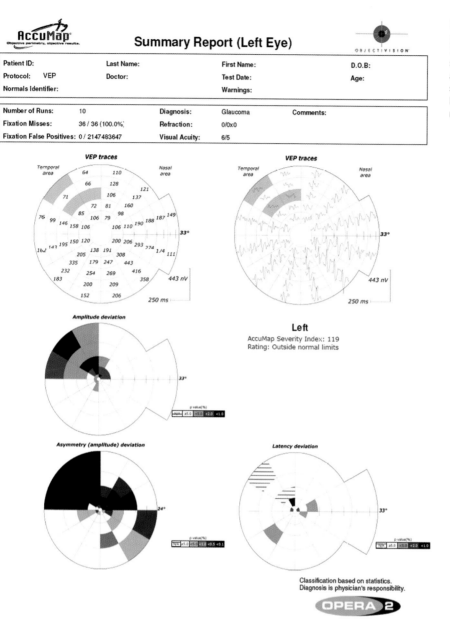

FIGURE 12.15 AccuMap summary printout for a glaucoma subject. Monocular Amplitude deviation shows superior arcuate defect, asymmetry deviation is more significant with early inferior field loss as well. Latency changes are minimal.

Large subject variations in amplitude within the population can be reduced by applying a method of scaling based on underlying EEG levels[93] or by using signal-to-noise ratios rather than peak-to-trough amplitudes.[134] This also reduces sex differences between males and females, and seems to remove any age-related change as well.[159] Without scaling, normal variability is too great to show statistically significant changes in some cases of mild loss.

The main limitation of the mfVEP as a form of objective perimetry remains intraindividual reproducibility and noisy recordings, which can lead to false positives. There is still a level of patient cooperation required together with technician experience to recognize noise and intervene during the recording. The latest versions of software (e.g. AccuMap 2) have included noise warnings and a noise index to flag alpha rhythm (patient losing concentration) and low-frequency and high-frequency noise. Hood et al. have reported a post-recording analysis to detect noise and alpha rhythm when using the VERIS system.

TECHNICAL TIPS FOR USERS

These are covered in the artifacts section above. At present, the mfVEP technique is in evolution, and different systems and authors have advocated slightly different approaches. It is important to realize that results will differ substantially based on the number and position of electrodes, number of channels used, and how the data is combined. Filter settings may differ and potentially affect noise levels and latencies. Without accounting for these differences, the various recording systems will appear to produce signals of quite different character, whereby amplitudes and latencies are not comparable. As the technique evolves, it is likely that standards may be agreed upon, allowing convergence of different approaches.

Summary

Electrophysiological testing provides a valuable adjunct for assessment of function in glaucoma, providing an objective measure of visual function. While the conventional ERG is predominantly outer retinal, and thus has not been helpful in assessing glaucomatous loss, the PhNR is a promising inner retinal ERG component, which deserves further study. The PERG has long been known to reflect glaucomatous damage, and appears to be largely ganglion cell driven, although the conventional PERG does not provide any topographic information. The mfVEP, using a multichannel bipolar recording technique, does shows a strong relationship between the locally recorded cortical response and subjective visual field loss at corresponding locations. The mfVEP can objectively demonstrate glaucomatous field defects. The mfERG has application to animal models of glaucoma but as yet has not been able to demonstrate topographical correlations with other damage measures such as visual field sensitivity in human patients.

In the clinical setting, electrophysiological testing with PERG and/or mfVEP either supports the diagnosis or helps to rule out subjective field loss. In some early or high-risk glaucoma cases it may detect functional damage earlier than other measures, enabling commencement of treatment at an earlier stage. Electrophysiological testing reassures the clinician and patient when perimetry results are inconsistent, variable, or when unexpectedly excessive changes are seen, and may thus help prevent overtreatment. The latter situations are frequently encountered in clinical practice due to the large number of patients who have trouble with perimetry. Cases with excessive field loss might otherwise be sent for diagnostic imaging with CT scan or MRI, since the clinician is uncomfortable accepting the disparity between structural and functional loss. Less commonly, when both subjective and objective tests are out of proportion to disc changes, further pathology should be suspected (e.g. intracranial tumor) and CT/MRI should be considered.

The mfVEP provides a new alternative approach for visual field assessment. It is very easy for patients to perform, even when it is their first time, and has a high level of patient acceptance.[165] It is likely that this form of testing will continue to develop in the future as an objective means of monitoring glaucoma patients. With improved signal detection, greater reproducibility, and shortened test times, it will provide the clinician with a valuable adjunct for assessing function in glaucoma.

REFERENCES

1. Heckenlively JR, Arden GB. Principles and practice of clinical electrophysiology of vision. 2nd edn. Cambridge, MA: The MIT Press; 2006.

2. Fishman GA, Birch DG, Holder GE, et al. Electrophysiological testing in disorders of the retina, optic nerve, and visual pathway. 2nd edn. San Francisco: American Academy of Ophthalmology; 2001.

3. Leydhecker G. The electroretinogram in glaucomatous eyes. Br J Ophthalmol 1950; 34:550–554.

4. Henkes HE. The electroretinogram in glaucoma. Ophthalmologica 1951; 121:44.

5. Alvis DL. Electroretinographic changes in controlled chronic open-angle glaucoma. Am J Ophthalmol 1966; 61:121–131.

6. Fazio DT, Heckenlively JR, Martin DA, et al. The electroretinogram in advanced open angle glaucoma. Doc Ophthalmol 1986; 63:45–54.

7. Holopigian K, Seiple W, Mayron C, et al. Electrophysiological and psychophysical flicker sensitivity in patients with primary open angle glaucoma and ocular hypertension. Invest Ophthalmol Vis Sci 1990; 31:1863–1868.

8. Velten IM, Horn FK, Korth M, et al. The b-wave of the dark adapted flash electroretinogram in patients with advanced asymmetrical glaucoma and normal subjects. Br J Ophthalmol 2001; 85:403–409.

9. Graham SL, Drance SM, Chauhan BC, et al. Comparison of psychophysical and electrophysiological testing in early glaucoma. Invest Ophthalmol Vis Sci 1996; 37:2651–2662.

10. Wachtmeister L, el Azazi M. Oscillatory potentials of the electroretinogram in patients with unilateral optic atrophy. Ophthalmologica 1985; 191:39–50.

11. Wanger P, Persson HE. Pattern-reversal electroretinograms in unilateral glaucoma. Invest Ophthalmol Vis Sci 1983; 24:749–753.

12. Gur M, Zeevi YY, Bielik M, et al. Changes in the oscillatory potentials of the electroretinogram in glaucoma. Curr Eye Res 1987; 6:457–466.

13. Bayer AU, Danias J, Brodie S, et al. Electroretinographic abnormalities in a rat glaucoma model with chronic elevated intraocular pressure. Experiment Eye Res 2001; 72:667–677.

14. Sieving PA, Frishman LJ, Steinberg RH. Scotopic threshold response of proximal retina in cat. J Neurophysiol 1986; 56:1049–1061.

15. Frishman LJ, Steinberg RH. Intraretinal analysis of the threshold dark-adapted ERG of cat retina. J Neurophysiol 1989; 61:1221–1232.

16. Saszik SM, Robson JG, Frishman LJ. The scotopic threshold response of the dark-adapted electroretinogram of the mouse. J Physiol 2002; 543:899–916.

17. Naarendorp F, Sato Y, Cajdric A, et al. Absolute and relative sensitivity of the scotopic system of rat: electroretinography and behavior. Vis Neurosci 2001; 18:641–656.

18. Bui BV, Fortune B. Ganglion cell contributions to the rat full-field electroretinogram. J Physiol 2004; 555:153–173.

19. Frishman LJ, Sieving PA. Evidence for two sites of adaptation affecting the dark-adapted ERG of cats and primates. Vision Res 1995; 35:435–442.

20. Frishman LJ, Shen FF, Du L, et al. The scotopic electroretinogram of macaque after retinal ganglion cell loss from experimental glaucoma. Invest Ophthalmol Vis Sci 1996; 37:125–141.

21. Sieving PA, Nino C. Scotopic threshold response (STR) of the human electroretinogram. Invest Ophthalmol Vis Sci 1988; 29:1608–1614.

22. Frishman LJ, Reddy MG, Robson JG. Effects of background light on the human dark-adapted electroretinogram and psychophysical threshold. J Opt Soc Am A 1996; 13:601–612.

23. Bui BV, Edmunds B, Cioffi GA, et al. The gradient of retinal functional changes during acute intraocular pressure elevation. Invest Ophthalmol Vis Sci 2005; 46:202–213.

24. He Z, Bui BV, Vingrys AJ. The rate of functional recovery from acute IOP elevation. Invest Ophthalmol Vis Sci 2006; 47:4872–4880.

25. Fortune B, Bui BV, Morrison JC, et al. Selective ganglion cell functional loss in rats with experimental glaucoma. Invest Ophthalmol Vis Sci 2004; 45:1854–1862.

26. Glovinsky Y, Quigley HA, Drum B, et al. A whole-field scotopic retinal sensitivity test for the detection of early glaucoma damage. Arch Ophthalmol 1992; 110:486–490.

27. Korth M, Nguyen NX, Horn F, et al. Scotopic threshold response and scotopic PII in glaucoma. Invest Ophthalmol Vis Sci 1994; 35:619–625.

28. Sieving PA. Retinal ganglion cell loss does not abolish the scotopic threshold response (STR) of the cat and human ERG. Clin Vision Sci 1991; 6:149–158.

29. Viswanathan S, Frishman LJ, Robson JG, et al. The photopic negative response of the flash electroretinogram in primary open angle glaucoma. Invest Ophthalmol Vis Sci 2001; 42:514–522.

30. Viswanathan S, Frishman LJ, Robson JG, et al. The photopic negative response of the macaque electroretinogram: reduction by experimental glaucoma. Invest Ophthalmol Vis Sci 1999; 40:1124–1136.

31. Viswanathan S, Frishman LJ, Robson JG. The uniform field and pattern ERG in macaques with experimental glaucoma: removal of spiking activity. Invest Ophthalmol Vis Sci 2000; 41:2797–2810.

32. Rangaswamy NV, Zhou W, Harwerth RS, et al. Effect of experimental glaucoma in primates on oscillatory potentials of the slow-sequence mfERG. Invest Ophthalmol Vis Sci 2006; 47:753–767.

33. Rangaswamy NV, Frishman LJ, Dorotheo EU, et al. Photopic ERGs in patients with optic neuropathies: comparison with primate ERGs after pharmacologic blockade of inner retina. Invest Ophthalmol Vis Sci 2004; 45:3827–3837.

34. Gotoh Y, Machida S, Tazawa Y. Selective loss of the photopic negative response in patients with optic nerve atrophy. Arch Ophthalmol 2004; 122:341–346.

35. Colotto A, Falsini B, Salgarello T, et al. Photopic negative response of the human ERG: losses associated with glaucomatous damage. Invest Ophthalmol Vis Sci 2000; 41:2205–2211.

36. Drasdo N, Aldebasi YH, Chiti Z, et al. The s-cone PHNR and pattern ERG in primary open angle glaucoma. Invest Ophthalmol Vis Sci 2001; 42:1266–1272.

37. Cursiefen C, Korth M, Horn FK. The negative response of the flash electroretinogram in glaucoma. Doc Ophthalmol 2001; 103:1–12.

38. Fortune B, Bui BV, Cull G, et al. Inter-ocular and inter-session reliability of the electroretinogram photopic negative response (PhNR) in non-human primates. Exp Eye Res 2004; 78(1):83–93.

39. Berninger TA, Arden GB. The pattern electroretinogram. Eye 1988; 2(Suppl):S257–S283.

40. Korth M. The value of electrophysiological testing in glaucomatous diseases. J Glaucoma 1997; 6:331–343.

41. Graham SL, Klistorner A. Electrophysiology: a review of signal origins and applications to investigating glaucoma. Aust NZ J Ophthalmol 1998; 26:71–85.

42. Bach M. Electrophysiological approaches for early detection of glaucoma. Eur J Ophthalmol 2001; 11:S41–S49.

43. Holder GE. Pattern electroretinography (PERG) and an integrated approach to visual pathway diagnosis. Prog Retin Eye Res 2001; 20:531–561.

44. Bui BV, Fortune B, Cull G, et al. Baseline characteristics of the transient pattern electroretinogram in non-human primates: inter-ocular and inter-session variability. Exp Eye Res 2003; 77:555–566.

45. Maffei L, Fiorentini A. Electroretinographic responses to alternating gratings before and after section of the optic nerve. Science 1981; 211:953–955.

46. Maffei L, Fiorentini A, Bisti S, et al. Pattern ERG in the monkey after section of the optic nerve. Exp Brain Res 1985; 59:423–425.

47. Dawson WW, Maida TM, Rubin ML. Human pattern-evoked retinal responses are altered by optic atrophy. Invest Ophthalmol Vis Sci 1982; 22:796–803.

48. Sieving PA, Steinberg RH. Contribution from proximal retina to intraretinal pattern ERG: the M-wave. Invest Ophthalmol Vis Sci 1985; 26:1642–1647.

49. Baker CL Jr, Hess RR, Olsen BT, et al. Current source density analysis of linear and non-linear components of the primate electroretinogram. J Physiol 1988; 407:155–176.

50. Johnson MA, Drum BA, Quigley HA, et al. Pattern-evoked potentials and optic nerve fiber loss in monocular laser induced glaucoma. Invest Ophthalmol Vis Sci 1989; 30:897–907.

51. Drasdo N, Thompson DA, Arden GB. A comparison of pattern ERG amplitudes and nuclear layer thickness in different zones of the retina. Clin Vis Sci 1990; 5:415–420.

52. Dawson WW, Stratton RD, Hope GM, et al. Tissue responses of the monkey retina: tuning and dependence on inner layer integrity. Invest Ophthalmol Vis Sci 1986; 27:734–745.

53. Fortune B, Wang L, Bui BV, et al. Local ganglion cell contributions to the macaque electroretinogram revealed by experimental nerve fiber layer bundle defect. Invest Ophthalmol Vis Sci 2003; 44:4567–4579.

54. Marx MS, Podos SM, Bodis-Wollner I, et al. Signs of early damage in glaucomatous monkey eyes: low spatial frequency losses in the pattern ERG and VEP. Exp Eye Res 1988; 46:173–184.

55. Trick GL. Retinal potentials in patients with primary open-angle glaucoma: physiological evidence for temporal frequency tuning deficits. Invest Ophthalmol Vis Sci 1985; 26:1750–1758.

56. Bach M, Hiss P, Rover J. Check-size specific changes of pattern electroretinogram in patients with early open-angle glaucoma. Doc Ophthalmol 1988; 69:315–322.

57. O'Donaghue E, Arden GB, O'Sullivan F, et al. The pattern electroretinogram in glaucoma and ocular hypertension. Br J Ophthalmol 1992; 76:387–394.

58. Trick GL. PRRP abnormalities in glaucoma and ocular hypertension. Invest Ophthalmol Vis Sci 1986; 27:1730–1736.

59. Bach M, Unsoeld AS, Philippin H, et al. Pattern ERG as an early glaucoma indicator in ocular hypertension: a long-term prospective study. Invest Ophthalmol Vis Sci 2006; 47:4881–4887.

60. Fiorentini A, Maffei L, Pirchio M, et al. The ERG in response to alternating gratings in patients with diseases of the peripheral visual pathway. Invest Ophthalmol Vis Sci 1981; 21:490–493.

61. Fortune B, Wang L, Bui BV, et al. Idiopathic bilateral optic atrophy in the rhesus macaque. Invest Ophthalmol Vis Sci 2005; 46:3943–3956.

62. Holder GE. Significance of abnormal pattern electroretinography in anterior visual pathway dysfunction. Br J Ophthalmol 1987; 71:166–171.

63. Korth M, Horn F, Storck B, et al. The pattern-evoked electroretinogram (PERG): age-related alterations and changes in glaucoma. Graefe's Arch Clin Exp Ophthalmol 1989; 227:123–130.

64. Weinstein G, Arden G, Hitchings R, et al. The pattern electroretinogram in ocular hypertension and glaucoma. Arch Ophthalmol 1988; 106:923–928.

65. Wanger P, Persson HE. Pattern-reversal electroretinograms and high-pass resolution perimetry in suspected or early glaucoma. Ophthalmology 1987; 94:1098–1103.

66. Trick G. Pattern reversal retinal potentials in ocular hypertensives at high and low risk of developing glaucoma. Doc Ophthalmol 1987; 65:79–85.

67. Pfeiffer N, Tillmon B, Bach M. Predictive value of the pattern electroretinogram in high-risk ocular hypertension. Invest Ophthalmol Vis Sci 1993; 34:1710–1715.

68. Watanabe I, Iijima H, Tsukahara S. The pattern electroretinogram in glaucoma: an evaluation by relative amplitude from the Bjerrum area. Br J Ophthalmol 1989; 73:131–135.

69. Van den Berg TJTP, Riemslag FCC, de Vos GWGA, et al. Pattern ERG and glaucomatous visual field defects. Doc Ophthalmol 1986; 61:335–341.

70. Ruben ST, Arden GB, O'Sullivan F, et al. Pattern electroretinogram and peripheral colour contrast thresholds in ocular hypertension and glaucoma: comparison and correlation of results. Br J Ophthalmol 1995; 79:326–331.

71. Parisi V, Miglior S, Manni GL, et al. Clinical ability of pattern electroretinograms and visual evoked potentials in detecting visual dysfunction in ocular hypertension and glaucoma. Ophthalmology 2006; 113:216–228.

72. Graham SL, Wong VA, Drance SM, et al. Pattern electroretinograms from hemifields in normal and glaucoma patients. Invest Ophthalmol Vis Sci 1994; 35:3347–3356.

73. Maddess T, James AC, Goldberg I, et al. A spatial frequency-doubling illusion-based pattern electroretinogram for glaucoma. Invest Ophthalmol Vis Sci 2000; 41:3818–3826.

74. Ventura LM, Porciatti V, Ishida K, et al. Pattern electroretinogram abnormality and glaucoma. Ophthalmology 2005; 112:10–19.

75. Hood DC, Xu L, Thienprasiddhi P, et al. The pattern electroretinogram in glaucoma patients with confirmed visual field deficits. Invest Ophthalmol Vis Sci 2005; 46:2411–2418.

76. Howe JW, Mitchell KW. Visual evoked potential changes in chronic glaucoma and ocular hypertension. Trans Ophthalmol Soc UK 1986; 105:457–462.

77. Motolko M, Drance SM, Douglas GR. The early psychophysical disturbances in chronic open-angle glaucoma. A study of visual functions with asymmetric disc cupping. Arch Ophthalmol 1982; 100:1632–1634.

78. Sokol S. The visually evoked cortical potential in optic nerve and visual pathway disorders. In: Fishman GA, ed. Electrophysiological testing in disorders of the retina, optic nerve and visual pathway. San Fransisco: American Academy of Ophthalmology; 1990:105–141.

79. Regan D. Evoked potentials in psychology, sensory physiology and clinical medicine. London: Chapman & Hall; 1972.

80. Weinstein GW, Odom JV, Cavender S. Visually evoked potentials and electroretinography in neurologic evaluation [Review]. Neurol Clin 1991; 9:225–242.

81. Gray LG, Galetta SL, Siegal T, et al. The central visual field in homonymous hemianopia. Evidence for unilateral foveal representation. Arch Neurol 1997; 54:312–317.

82. Horton JC, Hoyt F. The representation of the visual field in the human striate cortex. Arch Ophthalmol 1991; 109:816–824.

83. Harter MR. Evoked cortical responses to checkerboard patterns: effect of check-size as a function of retinal eccentricity. Vision Res 1970; 10:1365–1376.

84. Yiannikas C, Walsh JC. The variation of the pattern shift visual evoked response with the size of the stimulus field. Electroencephalogr Clin Neurophysiol 1983; 55: 427–435.

85. Towle VL, Moskowitz A, Sokol S, et al. The visual evoked potential in glaucoma and ocular hypertension: effects of check size field size and stimulation rate. Invest Ophthalmol Vis Sci 1983; 24:175–183.

86. Accornero N, Gregori B, Galie E, et al. A new color VEP procedure discloses asymptomatic visual impairments in optic neuritis and glaucoma suspects. Acta Neurol Scand 2000; 102:258–263.

87. Schmeisser ET, Smith TJ. Flicker visual evoked potential differentiation of glaucoma. Optom Vis Sci 1992; 69: 458–462.

88. Watts MT, Good PA, O'Neill EC. The flash stimulated VEP in the diagnosis of glaucoma. Eye 1989; 3:732–737.

89. Nykänen H, Raitta C. The correlation of visual evoked potentials (VEP) and visual field indices (Octopus G1) in glaucoma and ocular hypertension. Acta Ophthalmol (Copenh) 1989; 67:393–395.

90. Horn FK, Bergua A, Junemann A, et al. Visual evoked potentials under luminance contrast and color contrast stimulation in glaucoma diagnosis. J Glaucoma 2000; 9:428–437.

91. Sutter EE, Tran D. The field topography of ERG components in man – 1. The photopic luminance response. Vision Res 1992; 32:443–446.

92. Sutter EE. Imaging visual function with the multifocal m-sequence technique. Vision Res 2001; 41:1241–1255.

93. Klistorner A, Graham SL. Electroencephalogram-based scaling of multifocal visual evoked potentials: effect on intersubject amplitude variability. Invest Ophthalmol Vis Sci 2001; 42:2145–2152.

94. Hood DC. Assessing retinal function with the multifocal technique. Prog Retinal Eye Res 2000; 19:607–646.

95. Lai TY, Chan WM, Lai RY, et al. The clinical applications of multifocal electroretinography: a systematic review. Surv Ophthalmol 2007; 52:61–96.

96. Heijl A, Patella VM. Essential perimetry. 3rd edn. Dublin, CA: Carl Zeiss Meditec Inc; 2002.

97. Sutter EE. The fast m-transform: a fast computation of cross-correlations with binary m-sequences. SIAM J Computing 1991; 20:686–694.

98. Kretschmann U, Bock M, Gockeln R, et al. Clinical applications of multifocal electroretinography. Doc Ophthalmol 2000; 100:99–113.

99. Hood DC, Seiple W, Holopigian K, et al. A comparison of the components of the multifocal and full-field ERGs. Vis Neurosci 1997; 14:533–544.

100. Hood DC, Frishman LJ, Saszik S, et al. Retinal origins of the primate multifocal ERG: implications for the human response. Invest Ophthalmol Vis Sci 2002; 43:1673–1685.

101. Rangaswamy NV, Hood DC, Frishman LJ. Regional variations in local contributions to the primate photopic flash ERG: revealed using the slow-sequence mfERG. Invest Ophthalmol Vis Sci 2003; 44:3233–3247.

102. Horiguchi M, Suzuki S, Kondo M, et al. Effect of glutamate analogues and inhibitory neurotransmitters on the electroretinograms elicited by random sequence stimuli in rabbits. Invest Ophthalmol Vis Sci 1998; 39:2171–2176.

103. Hare WA, Ton H. Effects of APB PDA and TTX on ERG responses recorded using both multifocal and conventional methods in monkey. Effects of APB PDA and TTX on monkey ERG responses. Doc Ophthalmol, 2002; 105:189–222.

104. Hood DC, Greenstein V, Frishman L, et al. Identifying inner retinal contributions to the human multifocal ERG. Vis Res 1999; 39:2285–2291.

105. Hood DC, Frishman LJ, Viswanathan S, et al. Evidence for a ganglion cell contribution to the primate electroretinogram (ERG): effects of TTX on the multifocal ERG in macaque. Vis Neurosci 1999; 16:411–416.

106. Frishman LJ, Saszik S, Harwerth RS, et al. Effects of experimental glaucoma in macaques on the multifocal ERG. Multifocal ERG in laster-induced glaucoma. Doc Ophthalmol 2000; 100:231–251.

107. Hood DC, Bearse MA Jr, Sutter EE, et al. The optic nerve head component of the monkey's (Macaca mulatta) multifocal electroretinogram (mERG). Vision Res 2001; 41:2029–2041.

108. Hare WA, Ton H, Ruiz G, et al. Characterization of retinal injury using ERG measures obtained with both conventional and multifocal methods in chronic ocular hypertensive primates. Invest Ophthalmol Vis Sci 2001; 42:127–136.

109. Sutter EE, Bearse MA. The optic nerve head component of the human ERG. Vis Res 1999; 39:419–436.

110. Bearse MA Jr, Sutter EE, Sim D, et al. Glaucomatous dysfunction revealed in higher order components of the electroretinogram. In: Vision science and its applications, OSA Technical Digest Series, Vol. 1. Washington, DC: Optical Society of America; 1996:104–107.

111. Chan HL, Brown B. Multifocal ERG changes in glaucoma. Ophthalmic Physiol Opt 1999; 19:306–316.

112. Hood DC, Greenstein VC, Holopigian K, et al. An attempt to detect glaucomatous damage to the inner retina with the multifocal ERG. Invest Ophthalmol Vis Sci 2000; 41:1570–1579.

113. Hasegawa S, Takagi M, Usui T, et al. Waveform changes of the first-order multifocal electroretinogram in patients with glaucoma. Invest Ophthalmol Vis Sci 2000; 41:1597–1603.

114. Palmowski AM, Allgayer R, Heinemann-Vemaleken B. The multifocal ERG in open angle glaucoma – a comparison of high and low contrast recordings in high- and low-tension open angle glaucoma. Doc Ophthalmol 2000; 101:35–49.

115. Fortune B, Johnson. CA, Cioffi GA. The topographic relationship between multifocal electroretinographic and behavioural perimetric measures of function in glaucoma. Optom Vision Sci 2001; 78:206–214.

116. Klistorner AI, Graham SL, Martins A. Multifocal pattern electroretinogram does not demonstrate localised field defects in glaucoma. Doc Ophthalmol 2000; 100:155–165.

117. Sutter EE, Shimada Y, Bearse MA Jr. Mapping inner retinal function through enhancement of adaptive components in the M-ERG. In: Vision science and its applications, OSA Technical Digest Series, Vol. 1. Washington, DC: Optical Society of America; 1999:52–55.

118. Sutter EE, Bearse MA Jr, Stamper RL, et al. Monitoring retinal ganglion cell function with the mERG: recent advances. In: Vision science and its applications, OSA Technical Digest Series, Vol. 1. Washington, DC: Optical Society of America; 2001:10–13.

119. Stiefelmeyer S, Neubauer AS, Berninger T, et al. The multifocal pattern electroretinogram in glaucoma. Vision Res 2004; 44:103–112.

120. Harrison WW, Viswanathan S, Malinovsky VE. Multifocal pattern electroretinogram: cellular origins and clinical implications. Optom Vis Sci 2006; 83:473–485.

121. Bearse MA Jr, Sutter EE, Stamper RL. Detection of glaucomatous dysfunction using a global flash multifocal electroretinogram (mERG) paradigm. In: Vision science and its applications, OSA Technical Digest Series, Vol.1. Washington, DC: Optical Society of America; 2001:14–17.

122. Shimada Y, Li Y, Bearse MA, et al. Assessment of early retinal changes in diabetes using a new multifocal ERG protocol. Br J Ophthalmol 2001; 85:414–419.

123. Fortune B, Bearse MA, Cioffi GA, et al. Selective loss of an oscillatory component from temporal retinal multifocal ERG responses in glaucoma. Invest Ophthalmol Vis Sci 2002; 43:2638–2647.

124. Fortune B, Cull G, Wang L, et al. Factors affecting the use of multifocal electroretinography to monitor function in a primate model of glaucoma. Doc Ophthalmol 2002; 105:151–178.

125. Palmowski AM, Allgayer R, Heinemann-Vernaleken B, et al. Multifocal electroretinogram with a multiflash stimulation technique in open-angle glaucoma. Ophthalmic Res 2002; 34:83–89.

126. Raz D, Seeliger MW, Geva AB, et al. The effect of contrast and luminance on mfERG responses in a monkey model of glaucoma. Invest Ophthalmol Vis Sci 2002; 43:2027–2035.

127. Klistorner AI, Graham SL, Grigg JR, et al. Multifocal topographic visual evoked potential: improving objective detection of local visual field defects. Invest Ophthalmol Vis Sci 1998; 39:937–950.

128. Hood DC, Greenstein VC, Odel JG, et al. Visual field defects and multifocal visual evoked potentials. Arch Ophthalmol 2002; 120:1672–1681.

129. Thienprasidhi P, Greenstein VC, Chen C, et al. Multifocal visual evoked potential responses in glaucoma patients with unilateral hemifield defect. Am J Ophthalmol 2003; 136:34–40.

130. Lindenberg T, Peters A, Horn FK, et al. Diagnostic value of multifocal VEP using cross-validation and noise reduction in glaucoma research. Graefe's Arch Clin Exp Ophthalmol 2004; 242:361–367.

131. Fortune B, Goh K, Demirel S, et al. Detection of glaucomatous field loss using multifocal VEP. In: IPS Proceedings 2002/2003 The Hague: Kugler Publications; 2004:251–260.

132. Graham SL, Klistorner AI, Goldberg I. Clinical application of objective perimetry using multifocal visual evoked potentials in glaucoma practice. Arch Ophthalmol 2005; 123:729–739.

133. Klistorner A, Graham SL. Objective perimetry in glaucoma. Ophthalmology 2000; 107:2283–2299.

134. Hood DC, Greenstein VC. Multifocal VEP and ganglion cell damage: applications and limitations for the study of glaucoma. Prog Retinal Eye Res 2001; 22:201–251.

135. Fortune B, Hood DC. Conventional pattern-reversal VEPs are not equivalent to summed multifocal VEPs. Invest Ophthalmol Vis Sci 2003; 44:1364–1375.

136. Berninger TA, Arden GB, Hogg CR, et al. Separable evoked retinal and cortical potentials from each major visual pathway: preliminary results. Br J Ophthalmol 1989; 73:502–511.

137. Baseler HA, Sutter EE. M and P components of the VEP and their visual field contribution. Vision Res 1997; 37:675–690.

138. Schimiti RB, Avelino RR, Kara-Jose N, et al. Full-threshold versus Swedish Interactive Threshold Algorithm (SITA) in normal individuals undergoing automated perimetry for the first time. Ophthalmology 2002; 109:2084–2092.

139. Holopigian K, Snow J, Seiple W, et al. Variability of the pattern electroretinogram. Doc Ophthalmol 1988; 70:103–115.

140. Birch DG, Anderson JL, Fish GE, et al. Pattern-reversal electroretinographic acuity in untreated eyes with subfoveal neovascular membranes. Invest Ophthalmol 1992; 33:2097–2104.

141. Trick GL. Retinal and cortical evoked potentials in diabetics with minimal retinopathy. Clin Vis Sci 1991; 6:209–218.

142. Goldberg I, Graham SL, Klistorner A. Multifocal objective perimetry in the detection of glaucomatous field loss. Am J Ophthalmol 2002; 133:29–39.

143. Graham SL, Klistorner A, Grigg JR, et al. Objective VEP perimetry in glaucoma – asymmetry analysis to identify early deficits. J Glaucoma 2000; 9:10–19.

144. Currie AD, Wen Y, Koeppens J, et al. Correlation between Humphrey visual field (HVF) multifocal electroretinogram, (mf VEP) multifocal visually evoked potentials (mf VEP) and Heidelberd retinal tomograph (HRT) optic disk topography in patient with glaucoma. Invest Ophthalmol Vis Sci 2003; 42.

145. Fortune B, Demirel S, Zhang X, et al. Comparing multifocal VEP and standard automated perimetry in high-risk ocular hypertension and early glaucoma. Invest Ophthalmol Vis Sci 2007; 48:1173–1180.

146. Klistorner A, Balachandran C, Graham SL, et al. Multifocal VEP latency in glaucoma. Invest Ophthalmol Vis Sci 2002; 43; ARVO abstract 2165.

147. Rodarte C, Hood DC, Yang EB, et al. The effects of glaucoma on the latency of the multifocal visual evoked potential. Br J Ophthalmol 2006; 90:1132–1136.

148. Hood DC, Zhang X, Greenstein VC, et al. An interocular comparison of the multifocal VEP: a possible technique for detecting local damage to the optic nerve. Invest Ophthalmol Vis Sci 2000; 41:1580–1587.

149. Hood DC, Odel JG, Zhang X. Tracking the recovery of local optic nerve function after optic neuritis: a multifocal VEP study. Invest Ophthalmol Vis Sci 2000; 41:4032–4038.

150. Fraser C, Klistorner A, Graham SL, et al. Multifocal visual evoked potential analysis of inflammatory or demyelinating optic neuritis. Ophthalmology 2006; 113:315–323.

151. Fraser C, Klistorner A, Graham SL, et al. Multifocal VEP latency analysis – predicting progression to multiple sclerosis. Arch Neurology 2006; 63:847–850.

152. Klistorner A, Graham SL, Grigg JR. Objective perimetry using mVEP in central visual pathway lesions. Br J Ophthalmol 2005; 89:739–744.

153. Betsuin Y, Mashima Y, Ohde H, et al. Clinical application of the multifocal VEPs. Curr Eye Res 2001; 22:54–63.

154. Miele DL, Odel JG, Behrens MM, et al. Functional bitemporal quadrantopia and the multifocal visual evoked potential. J Neuro-Ophthalmol 2000; 20:159–162.

155. Balachandran C, Klistorner A, Billson FA. Multifocal VEP perimetry in children: its maturation and clinical application. Br J Ophthalmol 2004; 88:226–232.

156. Martins A, Balachandran C, Klistorner A, et al. Effect of pupil size on multifocal pattern visual evoked potentials. Clin Exp Ophthalmol 2003; 31:354–356.

157. Whitehouse GM. The effect of cataract on AccuMap multifocal objective perimetry. Am J Ophthalmol 2003; 136:209–212.

158. Arvind H, Klistorner A, Graham SL, et al. Multifocal visual evoked responses to dichoptic stimuli using virtual reality goggles. Doc Ophthalmol 2006; 112(3):189–199.

159. Fortune B, Zhang X, Hood DC, et al. Normative ranges and specificity of the multifocal VEP. Doc Ophthalmol 2004; 109:87–100.

160. Martus P, Junemann A, Wisse M, et al. Multivariate approach for quantification of morphologic and functional damage in glaucoma. Invest Ophthalmol Vis Sci 2000; 41:1099–1110.

161. Hood DC, Thienprasiddhi P, Greenstein VC, et al. Detecting early to mild glaucomatous damage: a comparison of the multifocal VEP and automated perimetry. Invest Ophthalmol Vis Sci 2004; 45:492–498.

162. Thienprasiddhi P, Greenstein VC, Chu DH, et al. Detecting early functional damage in glaucoma suspect and ocular hypertensive patients with the multifocal VEP technique. J Glaucoma 2006; 15:321–327.

163. Balachandran C, Graham SL, Klistorner A, et al. Comparison of objective diagnostic tests in glaucoma: Heidelberg retinal tomography and multifocal visual evoked potentials. J Glaucoma 2006; 15:110–116.

164. Fortune B, Demirel S, Zhang X, et al. Repeatability of normal multifocal VEP: implications for detecting progression. J Glaucoma 2006; 15:131–141.

165. Bjerre A, Grigg JR, Parry NRA, et al. Test-retest variability of multifocal visual evoked potential and SITA standard perimetry in glaucoma. Invest Ophthalmol Vis Sci 2004; 45:4035–4040.

166. Klistorner A, Graham SL. Intertest variability of the mfVEP amplitude: reducing its effect on the interpretation of sequential tests. Doc Ophthalmol 2006; 111:159–167.

167. Martins A, Klistorner A, Graham SL, et al. Effect of fixation tasks on multifocal visual evoked potentials. Clin Exp Ophthalmol 2005; 33:499–504.

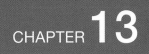

CHAPTER 13

Gonioscopy

John F Salmon

INTRODUCTION

Gonioscopy is the clinical technique that allows the structures in the anterior chamber angle to be visualized. The angle between the posterior corneal surface and the anterior surface of the iris constitutes the angle of the anterior chamber. Gonioscopy enables the glaucomas to be divided into two main groups: angle-closure glaucoma and open-angle glaucoma.[1] Because the therapy for each type of glaucoma must be specific to be effective, it is important to determine the mechanism responsible for the impedance of aqueous flow through the trabecular meshwork.

Gonioscopy is a demanding skill and an essential part of the examination of a glaucoma patient. If the correct diagnosis is to be made and successful management instituted, it is essential to be able to visualize the anterior chamber angle. A common cause of an incorrect diagnosis in a patient with glaucoma is the omission of gonioscopy by the clinician who concludes that the patient must have an open-angle mechanism because the slit lamp examination of the anterior chamber does not suggest a narrow angle, ocular inflammation, new vessel formation, or signs of previous trauma. Chronic angle-closure glaucoma and other forms of secondary glaucoma can be overlooked if gonioscopy is not undertaken. It is only by undertaking gonioscopy on every glaucoma patient that the clinician will become familiar with the variety of normal and abnormal findings that may be present.

HISTORICAL BACKGROUND OF GONIOSCOPY

The angle was first visualized in 1907 by Trantas, who was able to examine the angle of a patient with keratoglobus, by indenting the limbus. Salzmann[2] described the first gonioscopy lens in 1914, followed by Koeppe[3] with an improved design, 5 years later. Troncoso[4] contributed to gonioscopy by developing a gonioscope which allowed magnification and illumination of the angle. In 1968, Goldmann[5] introduced the gonioprism

which is used today. The modern gonioscopic classification was originally suggested by Barkan[1] in 1938 and elaborated by Sugar[6] in 1949.

OPTICAL PRINCIPLES

The angle of the anterior chamber cannot be visualized directly through the intact cornea because light emitted from angle structures undergoes total internal reflection at the anterior surface of the precorneal tear film (Fig. 13.1). A goniolens eliminates total internal reflection by replacing the tear film–air interface with a new tear film–goniolens interface. There are two basic forms of gonioscopy: direct gonioscopy, which provides a direct view of the angle; and indirect gonioscopy, which provides a mirror image of the opposite angle and is by far the most common technique in use.

GONIOLENSES

GOLDMANN

This is an indirect goniolens with a contact surface diameter of approximately 12 mm. The mirror is inclined at 62° for gonioscopy. Relatively easy to master, it affords an excellent view of the angle. It also stabilizes the globe and is therefore suitable for argon laser trabeculoplasty. Because the curvature of the contact surface of the lens is steeper than that of the cornea, a viscous coupling substance with the same refractive index as the cornea is required to bridge the gap between the cornea and the goniolens. Following the use of the coupling substance, the patient's vision is blurred and fundus examination impaired. Perimetry, ophthalmoscopy, or photography of the discs should therefore be performed before gonioscopy. The original Goldmann lens has three mirrors. Modifications with one mirror (Fig. 13.2) and two mirrors with an antireflective coating have been designed for laser trabeculoplasty, enabling simultaneous visualization of a wider circumference of the angle.

ZEISS

This, and the similar Posner and Sussman, are indirect four-mirror goniolenses mounted on a handle (Fig. 13.3). The contact surface of the lens has a diameter of 9 mm and a curvature flatter than that of the cornea, avoiding the need for a coupling substance. All four mirrors are inclined at 64°. Tears provide adequate contact material and lubrication for the lens. This permits quick and comfortable examination of the angle and, importantly, does not interfere with the subsequent examination of the fundus. The four mirrors enable the entire circumference of the angle to be visualized with minimal rotation. The lens is useful for indentation gonioscopy (see later) but, because it does not stabilize the globe, it cannot be used for laser trabeculoplasty.

KOEPPE

This is a dome-shaped direct diagnostic goniolens which comes in several sizes (Fig. 13.4). It is easy to use and provides a panoramic view of the angle. It is

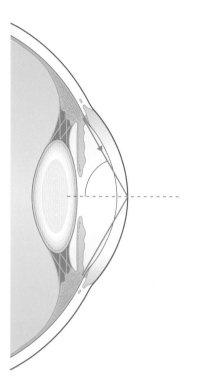

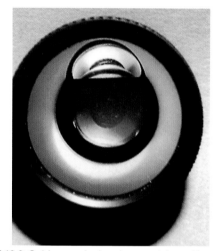

FIGURE 13.2 Goldmann single-mirror goniolens. (Reproduced from Salmon JF, Kanski JJ, eds. Glaucoma. A colour manual of diagnosis and treatment. 3rd edn. Edinburgh: Butterworth-Heinemann; 2004.)

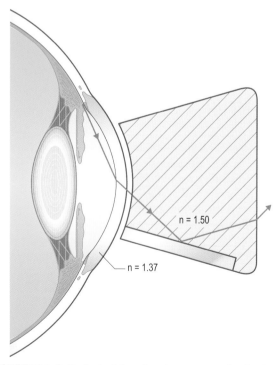

n = 1.50

n = 1.37

FIGURE 13.1 Optical principles of gonioscopy; n, refractive index; I, angle of incidence. (Reproduced from Salmon JF, Kanski JJ, eds. Glaucoma. A colour manual of diagnosis and treatment, 3rd edn. Edinburgh: Butterworth-Heinemann; 2004.)

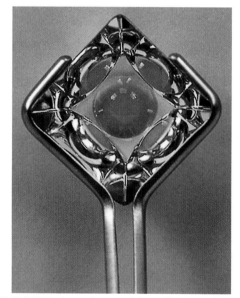

FIGURE 13.3 Zeiss four-mirror goniolens. (Reproduced from Salmon JF, Kanski JJ, eds. Glaucoma. A colour manual of diagnosis and treatment. 3rd edn. Edinburgh: Butterworth-Heinemann; 2004.)

therefore particularly useful for simultaneous comparison of one portion of the angle with another. Moreover, with the patient in a supine position the anterior chamber may deepen slightly and the angle may become easier to visualize. When used in conjunction with a hand-held microscope, it offers greater flexibility, allowing detailed inspection of the various subtleties of the angle structures by both direct and retroillumination. It cannot be used in conjunction with a slit lamp and therefore does not provide the same clarity, illumination, and variable powers as slit lamp goniolenses.

GONIOSCOPIC TECHNIQUES

GENERAL

Gonioscopy should be performed with minimal illumination in order to prevent artifactual opening of the drainage angle. Where possible, the room lights should be switched off and the slit lamp beam shortened to avoid light entering through the pupil. Unintended

corneal indentation may also artificially open the angle. The presence of corneal striation may alert the observer that he or she is indenting the cornea.

Goldmann gonioscopy The patient should be advised that the lens will touch the eye but not cause more than slight discomfort. The patient should also be requested to keep both eyes open at all times and not to move the head backwards when the lens has been inserted. Topical anesthetic is instilled into the lower fornix. A coupling fluid (e.g. a carbomer gel) is inserted into the cup of the lens. The patient is instructed to look up and the inferior rim of the lens is inserted into the lower fornix (Fig. 13.5) and then pressed quickly against the cornea so that the coupling substance does not escape (Fig. 13.6). The patient is then asked to gaze ahead with the other eye. The angle is visualized with a gonioscopic mirror. Initially, the mirror is placed at the 12 o'clock position to visualize the inferior angle and then rotated clockwise. The slit beam should be 2 mm wide, and when viewing different positions it is

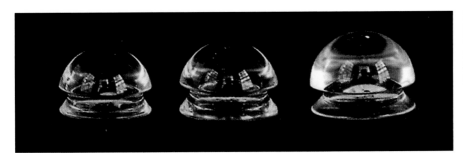

FIGURE 13.4 Koeppe goniolenses. (Reproduced from Salmon JF, Kanski JJ, eds. Glaucoma. A colour manual of diagnosis and treatment. 3rd edn. Edinburgh: Butterworth-Heinemann; 2004.)

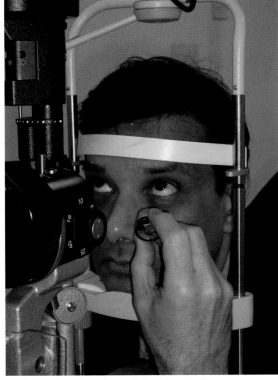

FIGURE 13.5 Insertion of a goniolens (see text).

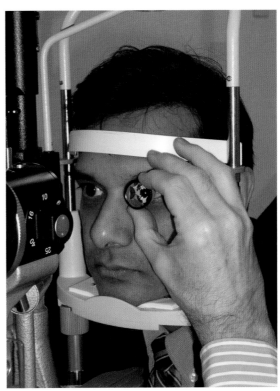

FIGURE 13.6 Insertion of a goniolens (see text).

usually best to rotate the beam so that its access is at right angles to the mirror. The mirror arrangement of this lens causes the observed image of the angle to be reversed, but not crossed. (The structures seen in the mirror are 180° away, but the detail is not altered with respect to the right and left). When the view of the angle is obscured by a convex iris, it is possible to 'see over the hill' by asking the patient to look in the direction of the mirror. When the plane of the iris is flat, the patient should be asked to look away from the mirror in order to obtain a view parallel to the iris with optimal image quality. This is particularly important when performing laser trabeculoplasty.

In individuals who cannot be examined at the slit lamp, the angle can be visualized with the gonioscope by using a direct ophthalmoscope.[7]

Zeiss gonioscopy The preliminary steps are the same as for Goldmann gonioscopy but a coupling fluid is not required. The patient looks straight ahead. Under slit lamp visualization the lens is placed directly on the center of the cornea. Only gentle contact with the cornea is needed because excessive pressure will inadvertently distort angle structures. Each quadrant of the angle is visualized with the opposite mirror (Fig. 13.7). The central fundus can be viewed through the center of the lens. Indentation gonioscopy may be performed by pressing posteriorly against the cornea (Fig. 13.8). This will force aqueous into the angle of the anterior chamber, forcing the peripheral iris posteriorly. If the angle is closed by mere apposition between iris and cornea, the angle will be forced open, allowing visualization of the angle recess (Fig. 13.9).[8] If the angle is completely closed by adhesions between the peripheral iris and cornea (synechial closure), it will remain closed. If synechial closure is partial, part of the angle will open and part will remain closed.

Koeppe gonioscopy The patient lies in a supine position, with the head turned towards the examiner and eyes looking at the examiner's nose. The examiner holds the lens between the right thumb and index finger for the right eye and between the left thumb and index finger for the left eye and inserts the lens between the lids. Saline or viscous 1% methylcellulose is used to bridge the gap between the Koeppe lens and the cornea. The angle is examined using a counterbalanced biomicroscope and Barkan illuminator.

STERILIZATION OF GONIOLENSES

Goniolenses are a potential source of infection and should be disinfected in the same way as tonometer heads. A container has been developed that allows the diagnostic lens to stay in contact with the disinfectant solution.[9]

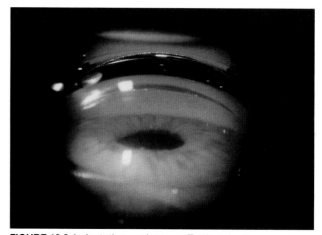

FIGURE 13.8 Indentation gonioscopy. Total angle closure prior to indentation. (Reproduced from Salmon JF, Kanski JJ, eds. Glaucoma. A colour manual of diagnosis and treatment. 3rd edn. Edinburgh: Butterworth-Heinemann; 2004.)

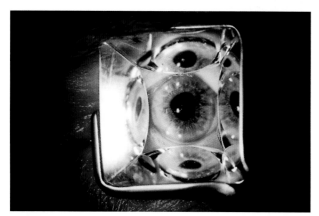

FIGURE 13.7 Zeiss four-mirror goniolens in place. (Reproduced from Salmon JF, Kanski JJ, eds. Glaucoma. A colour manual of diagnosis and treatment. 3rd edn. Edinburgh: Butterworth-Heinemann; 2004.)

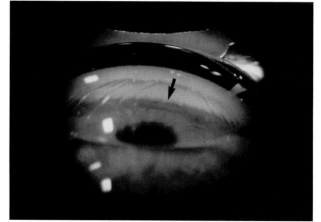

FIGURE 13.9 Indentation gonioscopy. Following indentation, the entire trabecular meshwork becomes visible (arrow): note the folds in the cornea. (Reproduced from Salmon JF, Kans ki JJ, eds. Glaucoma. A colour manual of diagnosis and treatment. 3rd edn. Edinburgh: Butterworth-Heinemann; 2004.)

IDENTIFICATION OF ANGLE STRUCTURES

It is important that the examiner is familiar with the normal anatomy of the angle. Each structure should be identified (Figs 13.10 and 13.11; see also Fig. 13.8).

CILIARY BODY BAND

The most posterior structure appears pink to dull-brown to slate-gray in color. Its width depends on the position of the iris insertion, tending to be narrower in hypermetropic eyes and wider in myopic eyes. The angle recess represents the dipping of the iris as it inserts into the ciliary body.

SCLERAL SPUR

This is the most anterior projection of the sclera and the site of attachment of the longitudinal muscle of the ciliary body. Gonioscopically, the scleral spur is situated just posterior to the trabecular meshwork and appears as a narrow dense, often shiny, whitish band. It is the most important landmark because it has a relatively consistent appearance in different eyes.

TRABECULAR MESHWORK

This extends from the scleral spur to Schwalbe's line. The posterior functional pigmented part lies adjacent to the scleral spur and has a grayish-blue translucent appearance. The anterior nonfunctional part lies adjacent to Schwalbe's line and has a whitish color. Trabecular pigmentation is rare prior to puberty. In aging eyes it involves the posterior trabecula to a variable extent, especially inferiorly. Trabecular pigmentation is more marked in brown eyes.

SCHWALBE'S LINE

This is the most anterior structure and appears as an opaque line. Anatomically, it represents the peripheral termination of Descemet's membrane and the anterior limit of the trabecula. In normal eyes it often can be seen in the limbal circumference as a hazy zone at the inner corneal surface. With an indirect contact lens the corneal parallelepiped of the slit lamp beam comes together at this point.

SCHLEMM'S CANAL

This may be identified in the nonpigmented angle as a slightly darker line deep to the posterior trabecular meshwork. Blood can sometimes be seen in this canal if the goniolens compresses the episcleral veins such that the episcleral venous pressure exceeds the intraocular pressure (IOP).

IRIS PROCESSES

These are small extensions of the anterior surface of the iris which insert at the level of the scleral spur and

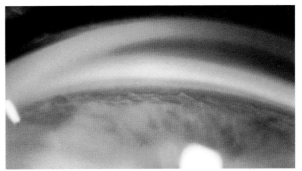

FIGURE 13.11 Normal wide-open angle. (Reproduced from Salmon JF, Kanski JJ, eds. Glaucoma. A colour manual of diagnosis and treatment, 3rd edn. Edinburgh: Butterworth-Heinemann; 2004.)

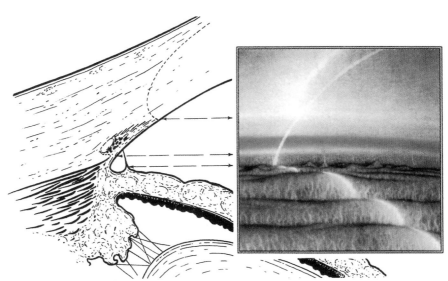

FIGURE 13.10 Normal angle structures. (Courtesy of Wallace LM Alward. From Color atlas of gonioscopy. San Francisco CA. AAO; 2001.)

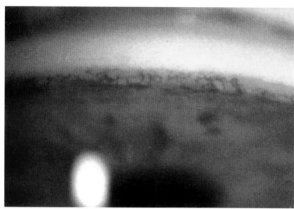

FIGURE 13.12 Iris processes are a normal variant.

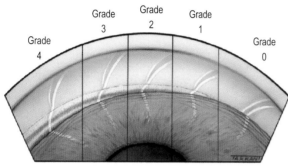

FIGURE 13.13 Shaffer grading system (see text). (Reproduced from Salmon JF, Kanski JJ, eds. Glaucoma. A colour manual of diagnosis and treatment. 3rd edn. Edinburgh: Butterworth-Heinemann; 2004.)

cover the ciliary body to a varying extent (Fig. 13.12). They are present in about one-third of normal eyes, and are most prominent during childhood and in brown eyes. With increasing age, they tend to wither and lose their continuity. Iris processes should not be confused with peripheral anterior synechiae, which are broader and represent adhesions between the iris and angle structures. However, fine stellate peripheral anterior synechiae introduced by inappropriate laser trabeculoplasty may easily be mistaken for iris processes.

BLOOD VESSELS

Blood vessels running in a radial pattern at the base of the angle recess are often seen in normal eyes. Angle vessels are gonioscopically visible in approximately two-thirds of individuals with blue eyes and in 10% with brown eyes. As a general principle, any blood vessel that crosses the scleral spur onto the trabecular meshwork is abnormal.

GRADING OF ANGLE WIDTH

The grading of angle width is an essential part of the ocular examination. The main aims are to evaluate the functional status of the angle, the degree of closure, and the risk of further closure. It is important to determine:

* the geometrical angle width in degrees
* the shape and contour of the peripheral iris
* the most posterior structure seen
* the presence of peripheral anterior synechiae
* the amount of trabecular pigmentation.

SHAFFER GRADING SYSTEM

The Shaffer system (Fig. 13.13) records the angle in degrees of arc subtended by two imaginary tangential lines drawn to the inner surface of the trabecula and the anterior surface of the iris about one-third of the distance from its periphery.[10] In practice, the angle is graded according to the visibility of various angle structures. The system assigns a numerical grade (4–0) to each angle with associated anatomical description, angle width in degrees, and implied clinical interpretation.

* Grade 4 (35–45°) is the widest angle characteristic of myopia and aphakia in which the ciliary body can be visualized with ease; it is incapable of closure.
* Grade 3 (25–35°) is an open angle in which at least the scleral spur can be identified; it is also incapable of closure.
* Grade 2 (20°) is a moderately narrow angle in which only the trabecula can be identified; angle closure is possible but unlikely.
* Grade 1 (10°) is a very narrow angle in which only Schwalbe's line, and perhaps also the top of the trabecula, can be identified; angle closure is not inevitable but the risk is high.
* Slit angle is one in which there is no obvious iridocorneal contact but no angle structures can be identified; this angle has the greatest danger of imminent closure.
* Grade 0 (0°) is a closed angle due to iridocorneal contact and is recognized by the inability to identify the apex of the corneal wedge. Indentation gonioscopy with a Zeiss goniolens is necessary to differentiate 'appositional' from 'synechial' angle closure.

SCHEIE GRADING SYSTEM

The Scheie grading system is based on the extent of visible angle structures and is not commonly used these days. The scale of I–IV is the reverse of the Shaffer grading system.[11]

* Grade I is the widest angle in which the ciliary body can be visualized with ease.
* Grade II is an open angle in which at least the scleral spur can be identified.
* Grade III is a moderately narrow angle in which only the anterior trabecular meshwork is visible.
* Grade IV angle is closed.

SPAETH SYSTEM

Although the Shaffer system is extremely useful, the configuration of the angle recess may be too complex

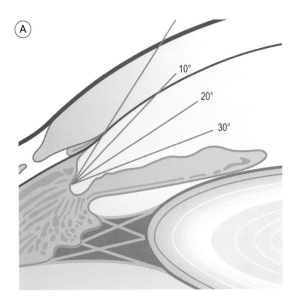

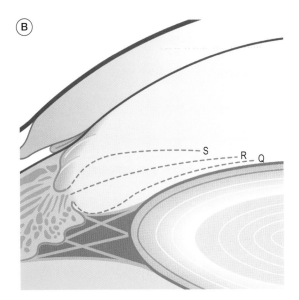

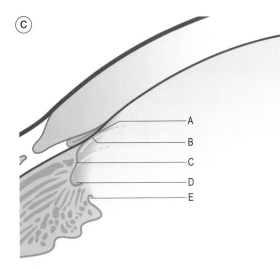

FIGURE 13.14 Spaeth grading system (see text). (Reproduced from Salmon JF, Kanski JJ, eds. Glaucoma. A colour manual of diagnosis and treatment. 3rd edn. Edinburgh: Butterworth-Heinemann; 2004.)

and varied to permit valid description by a single characteristic.[12] At least three different aspects of the configuration should be identified (Fig. 13.14):

* the angle approach
* the curvature of the peripheral iris
* the point of insertion of the iris.

Because these characteristics vary independently, each is described separately.

* *The angle* approach to the recess is a function of the depth of the anterior chamber. The point of reference is a line tangential to the inner surface of the trabecular meshwork. The angle width is then estimated by constructing a tangent to the anterior iris surface approximately one-third of the distance from the most peripheral portion of the iris. The angle width is then expressed in degrees.
* *The curvature of the peripheral iris* is graded as follows:
  - R = Regular, in which the iris courses regularly from its root without significant anterior or posterior bowing
  - S = Steep, in which the iris rises from its root with a sudden, steep, convex curve; eyes with marked anterior iris convexity are at increased risk of developing angle closure
  - Q = Queer, in which there is marked posterior concavity of the peripheral iris as may occur in aphakia, lens subluxation, high myopia, and pigment dispersion syndrome.
* *The iris insertion* may be in five different locations indicated by the letters A to E as follows:
  - A = Above Schwalbe's line, in which the angle is totally occluded by contact between the peripheral iris and cornea above Schwalbe's line
  - B = Behind Schwalbe's line, in which the peripheral iris is in contact with the trabecular meshwork behind Schwalbe's line
  - C = sCleral spur, in which the iris root is at the level of the scleral spur
  - D = Deep, which signifies a deep angle recess in which the anterior ciliary body is visible
  - E = Extremely deep, which allows an unusually large part of the ciliary body to be visualized.

Only, C, D, and E are normal while A and B are always pathological.

PATHOLOGICAL FINDINGS

It is important that gonioscopy is undertaken on all patients with glaucoma and glaucoma suspects. Abnormal gonioscopic findings and their causes are:

* peripheral anterior synechiae
* excessive pigmentation
* abnormal blood vessels
* angle recession.

PERIPHERAL ANTERIOR SYNECHIAE

Peripheral anterior synechiae (PAS) are adhesions of the iris root to the trabecular meshwork (Fig. 13.15).

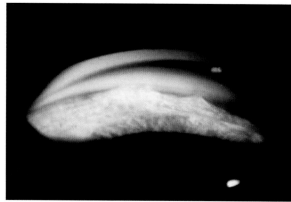

FIGURE 13.15 Peripheral anterior synechiae.

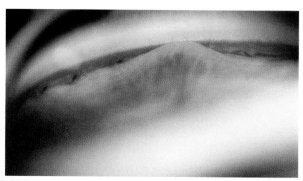

FIGURE 13.17 Inflammatory peripheral anterior synechiae formed preferentially in the inferior angle.

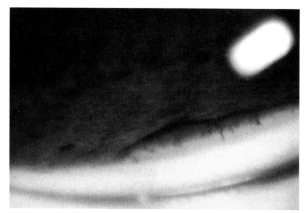

FIGURE 13.16 The angle appearance in chronic angle-closure glaucoma. The transition between open and closed angle is clearly visible.

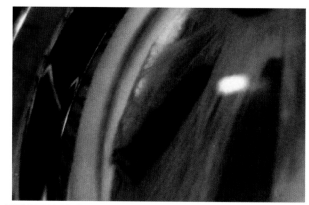

FIGURE 13.18 Peripheral anterior synechiae in ICE syndrome can advance anterior to Schwalbe's line.

It is important to distinguish between PAS, which are tented-up portions of the iris held by adhesions to the trabecular meshwork, and iris processes, which are a normal variant. PAS may be caused by appositional angle closure, creeping angle closure, inflammation, neovascular membranes, migrating corneal endothelial cells (ICE syndrome), and trauma.

Primary angle closure is an anatomical disorder of the anterior segment of the eye characterized by permanent closure of part of the filtration angle as a result of iris apposition to the trabecular meshwork (Fig. 13.16). The subsequent rise in intraocular pressure can cause optic nerve damage that is indistinguishable from that found in chronic open-angle glaucoma. This form of glaucoma is more prevalent than open-angle glaucoma in Sino-mongoloid populations and is the most important cause of preventable blindness in elderly East and Southeast Asians.[13] The treatment of chronic angle-closure glaucoma is significantly different from that of chronic open-angle glaucoma.

Inflammatory peripheral anterior synechiae tend to be broad-based and form preferentially in the inferior angle because of settling of white blood cells (Fig. 13.17). The peripheral anterior synechiae in ICE syndrome can advance anterior to Schwalbe's line, an unusual finding in other conditions (Fig. 13.18).

PIGMENT DISPERSION

Excessive pigment can be found in the trabecular meshwork in pigment dispersion syndrome, pigmentary glaucoma, pseudoexfoliation syndrome, uveitis and trauma, secondary to melanoma and pigment epithelial cysts, and may be a feature of pseudophakic pigment dispersion.

Pigment dispersion syndrome is usually a bilateral condition characterized by the liberation of pigment granules from the iris pigment epithelium and their deposition throughout the anterior segment including the zonules and ciliary body. Elevation of IOP is caused by pigmentary obstruction of the intertrabecular spaces and damage to the trabecular meshwork. Gonioscopy shows a wide-open angle, with a concavity of the peripheral iris near its insertion and trabecular hyperpigmentation (Fig. 13.19). The pigmentation is most marked over the posterior trabecula and forms a dense band involving the entire circumference of the meshwork uniformly. Schwalbe's line is heavily pigmented in most cases, with the pigment heaviest inferiorly, diminishing to no pigmentation superiorly. Occasionally, fine additional deposits of pigmentation can be seen anterior to Schwalbe's line in the inferior angle.[14]

In pseudoexfoliation syndrome, gonioscopy shows trabecular hyperpigmentation, which is usually most marked inferiorly (Fig. 13.20). The pigment lies on the

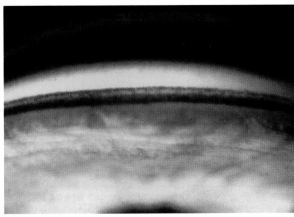

FIGURE 13.19 Trabecular hyperpigmentation in pigment dispersion syndrome.

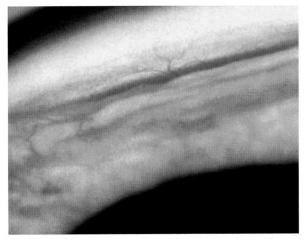

FIGURE 13.21 Fine vessels in the angle but not at the pupil margin.

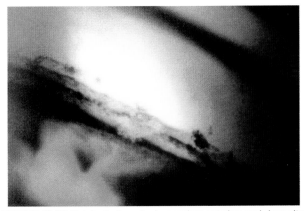

FIGURE 13.20 Patchy trabecular hyperpigmentation and deposits of pseudoexfoliation material. (Courtesy of E Michael Van Buskirk. From Clinical atlas of glaucoma, Philadelphia: WB Saunders; 1986.)

surface of the trabecula and has a patchy distribution. A scalloped band of pigment running onto or anterior to Schwalbe's line (Sampaolesi line) is also frequently seen. Pseudoexfoliation material may be seen within the trabecular meshwork and the angle may be narrow in some cases. As this form of glaucoma progresses more rapidly than primary open-angle glaucoma, gonioscopy may provide an early clue to the diagnosis because the signs of pigment dispersion may precede the detection of pseudoexfoliation material.[15]

NEW VESSEL FORMATION

Blood vessels may be seen normally in the filtration angle. However, as a general rule, any blood vessel that crosses the scleral spur onto the trabecular meshwork is usually abnormal. There is a significant risk of missing anterior segment neovascularization by omitting screening gonioscopy in patients with acute central retinal vein occlusion.[16] In patients with early new vessel formation, even light pressure on the lens is sufficient to collapse these neovascular tufts and render them clinically invisible. It is significantly less common

for angle new vessels to precede iris new vessels in diabetes. In Fuchs' heterochromic cyclitis, fine new vessels may be seen in the angle.[17] These vessels may cross the scleral spur onto the trabecular meshwork (Fig. 13.21).

Blood can sometimes be seen in the canal of Schlemm if the goniolens compresses the episcleral veins, such that the episcleral venous pressure exceeds the IOP. Pathological causes of blood in the canal include carotid-cavernous fistula and dural shunt, Sturge-Weber syndrome, and obstruction of the superior vena cava.

TRAUMA

Gonioscopy is particularly important in patients who have suffered previous blunt trauma. Angle recession, trabecular dialysis, and a cyclodialysis cleft can only be determined by using gonioscopy. In addition, the presence of a small foreign body in the angle may be seen by using this technique. These findings have significant medicolegal implications.

Angle recession is characterized by marked widening of the ciliary band. Bare sclera can be visualized and the scleral spur stands out as a glistening white line (Fig. 13.22). It is important to compare the abnormal areas with normal areas of angle within the same eye and to compare the abnormal eye with the opposite normal eye. Angle recession is the commonest sign of postcontusional eye injury and approximately 9% of patients will develop glaucoma as a late complication.[18] It is important to make the diagnosis of post-traumatic angle-recession glaucoma because argon laser trabeculoplasty is usually unsuccessful in controlling the intraocular pressure in these cases. In addition, angle-recession glaucoma is a significant risk factor for bleb failure after trabeculectomy and the presence of angle recession usually means that an antimetabolite should be used at the time of filtration surgery.[19]

In a patient with a post-traumatic cyclodialysis cleft, the anterior chamber is shallow and the intraocular

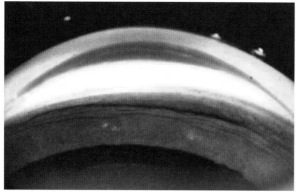

FIGURE 13.22 Angle recession showing irregular widening of the ciliary body band.

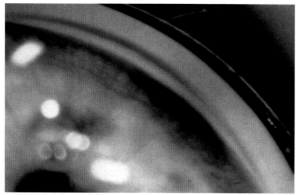

FIGURE 13.23 Post-traumatic cyclodialysis cleft.

<u>pressure is low</u> (Fig. 13.23). By using indentation gonioscopy the exact position of the cleft can be determined. All the methods currently employed to close a cyclodialysis cleft depend on a knowledge of the exact position of the cleft.

Summary

Gonioscopy is the clinical technique that allows the structures in the anterior chamber to be visualized. It is an essential part of the examination of a glaucoma patient. Primary angle closure and secondary causes of raised intraocular pressure can be overlooked if gonioscopy is not undertaken. Indirect

gonioscopy, which provides a mirror image of the opposite angle, is the most commonly used technique. Individual angle structures need to be identified, with the scleral spur being the most important landmark, as it has a constant appearance in different eyes. Grading of the angle width is an essential part of the examination. The Shaffer grading system is most commonly used. Indentation gonioscopy allows a distinction to be made between appositional closure of the angle and permanent peripheral anterior synechiae. Pathological findings, which may not be obvious on slit lamp examination of the anterior segment, include peripheral anterior synechiae, neovascularization, hyperpigmentation, and angle recession.

Key points

- Gonioscopy needs to be undertaken on all patients with glaucoma.
- Failure to examine the filtration angle is one of the most common causes of a missed diagnosis in patients with glaucoma or ocular hypertension.
- The examiner needs to be familiar with the normal angle anatomy.
- Individual angle structures need to be identified. The scleral spur is the most important landmark, as it has a constant appearance in different eyes.
- Indentation gonioscopy allows a distinction to be made between appositional closure of the angle and permanent peripheral anterior synechiae.
- Iris processes are normal and should not be confused with peripheral anterior synechiae.
- As a general principle, any blood vessel that crosses the scleral spur onto the trabecular meshwork is abnormal.
- The Shaffer system of grading the angle width assigns a numerical grade (4–0) to each angle with associated anatomical description, angle width in degrees, and implied clinical interpretation.
- The Spaeth system describes the angle approach, the curvature of the peripheral iris, and the point of insertion of the iris.
- Pathological findings, which may not be obvious on slit lamp examination of the anterior segment, include peripheral anterior synechiae, neovascularization, hyperpigmentation, and angle recession.

REFERENCES

1. Barkan O. Glaucoma: classification, causes and surgical control. Am J Ophthalmol 1938; 21:1099–1113.

2. Salzmann M. Die Oftalmoskopie der Kammerbucht. J Augenheilk 1914; 31:1–19.

3. Koeppe A. Das stereo-mikroskopische Bild des lebenden Kammerwinkels an der Nernstspaltlampe bein Glaukom. Klin Monatsbl Augenheilk 1920; 65:389–391.

4. Troncoso MU. Gonioscopy and its clinical applications. Am J Ophthalmol 1925; 8:433–449.

5. Goldmann H. Biomicroscopy of the eye. Am J Ophthalmol 1968; 66:789–804.

6. Sugar HS. Newer conceptions in the classification of the glaucomas. Am J Ophthalmol 1949; 32:425–433.

7. Shaw AD, Burnett CA, Eke T. A simple technique for indirect gonioscopy for patients who cannot be examined at the slit lamp. Br J Ophthalmol 2006; 90:1209.

8. Forbes M. Gonioscopy with corneal indentation: a method for distinguishing between appositional closure and synechial closure. Arch Ophthalmol 1966; 76:488–492.

9. Vijfvinkel G, de Jong PT. Disinfectant container for diagnostic lenses. Am J Ophthalmol 1985; 99:600–601.

10. Shaffer RN. Symposium: Primary glaucomas III. Gonioscopy, ophthalmoscopy and perimetry. Trans Am Acad Ophthalmol Otolaryngol, 1960; 64:112–127.

11. Scheie HG. Width and pigmentation of the angle of the anterior chamber; a system of grading by gonioscopy. Arch Ophthalmol 1957; 58:510–512.

12. Spaeth GL. The normal development of the human anterior chamber angle: a new system of descriptive grading. Trans Ophthalmol Soc UK 1971; 91:709–739.

13. Congdon N, Wang F, Tielsch JM. Major review. Issues in the epidemiology and population-based screening of primary angle-closure glaucoma. Surv Ophthalmol 1992; 36:411–423.

14. Lehto I, Vesti E. Diagnosis and management of pigmentary glaucoma. Curr Opin Ophthalmol 1998; 9(II):61–65.

15. Prince AM, Streeten BW, Ritch R, et al. Preclinical diagnosis of pseudoexfoliation syndrome. Arch Ophthalmol 1987; 105:1076–1082.

16. Browning DJ, Scott AQ, Peterson CB, et al. The risk of missing angle neovascularisation by omitting screening gonioscopy in acute central retinal vein occlusion. Ophthalmology 1998; 105:776–784.

17. Perry HD, Yanoff M, Scheie HG. Rubeosis in Fuchs' heterochromic irido-cyclitis. Arch Ophthalmol 1975; 93: 337–339.

18. Kaufman JH, Tolpin DW. Glaucoma after traumatic angle recession. A ten-year prospective study. Am J Ophthalmol 1974; 78:648–654.

19. Mermoud A, Salmon JF, Murray ADN. Post-traumatic angle recession glaucoma: a risk factor for bleb failure after trabeculectomy. Br J Ophthalmol 1993; 77:61–64.

Ultrasound Biomicroscopy

Giorgio Marchini, Robero Tosi, and Piero Ceruti

INSTRUMENTATION FOR ULTRASOUND BIOMICROSCOPY

Clinical echographic examinations usually require frequencies in the range of 1 to 10 MHz. The wavelengths produced by these lower frequencies are longer, allowing much deeper penetration of tissue to the detriment of a lower resolution. The current limitations of clinical imaging arise from the need to provide maximum resolution versus the need for ultrasound beams to penetrate the tissue. The critical parameter in clinical echography is the frequency of the ultrasound beam. As the frequency increases, the ultrasound is more strongly attenuated, reducing penetration but increasing resolution. The development of transducers for very-high-frequency (40–100 MHz) ultrasound imaging encouraged the origin of the technique called ultrasound biomicroscopy (UBM). The commercial instrument (Fig. 14.1) uses a 50 MHz transducer which provides a good compromise between resolution (axial resolution, 25 μm; lateral resolution, 50 μm) and penetration depth (5 mm). The probe (Fig. 14.2) is supported by an articulated arm which aids the operator in controlling the weight of the scanning head. Moreover, the probe is held close to the transducer end to improve fine control. The instrument is provided with: (1) an operating screen, which visualizes the image display section (5 × 5 mm image at a scan rate of 8 frames per second) and the preferred setting;[1] (2) the controlling devices, such as the hand controller, the light pen, the foot switch; and (3) an image storage option.

EXAMINATION TECHNIQUES

The technique of eye examination using UBM is similar to the conventional B-scan examination of the anterior segment with an immersion technique. The patient is usually examined in a supine position looking at the ceiling. The patient can be lying in a type of bed that allows the operator to sit near the head of the bed and approach the eye at a comfortable level. A series of eyecups are used to hold the eyelid open and allow more rapid patient preparation. Topical anesthesia is instilled, and the eyecup is placed under the eyelid and then is filled with the

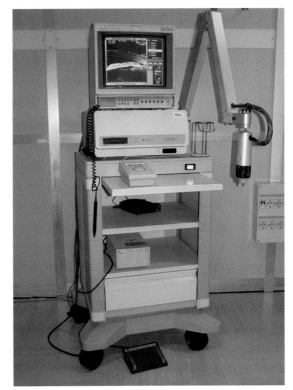

FIGURE 14.1 Ultrasound biomicroscope model 840 (Zeiss-Humphrey, San Leandro, CA).

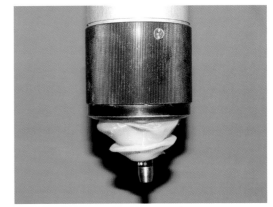

FIGURE 14.2 Detail of the tip of the transducer.

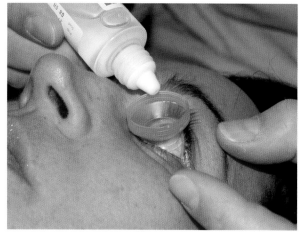

FIGURE 14.3 Methylcellulose is poured into the eyecup following instillation of topical anesthetic.

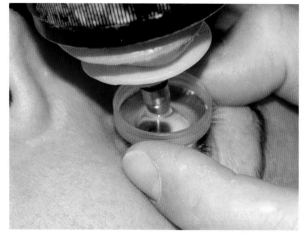

FIGURE 14.4 The transducer tip is placed in the fluid.

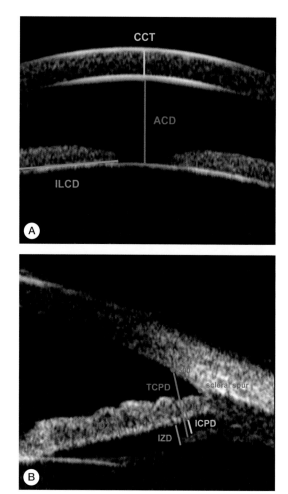

FIGURE 14.5 Main linear measurement parameters. **(A)** CCT, central corneal thickness; ACD, anterior chamber depth; ILCD, iris lens contact distance. **(B)** ID1, ID2, iris distance; IZD, iris zonule distance; ICPD, iris ciliary process distance; TCPD, trabecular ciliary process distance.

fluid coupling medium (1–2.5% methylcellulose) (Fig. 14.3). When the transducer is placed into the water bath the examination begins (Fig. 14.4). The examination of the eye is performed using both radial sections and transverse sections. The ultrasound operator is constantly making fine adjustments to aim the beam accurately and produce sections that show the best images that explain the pathological process clearly. It is important to note that the best images are obtained when the ultrasound beam strikes an interface in a perpendicular manner, so that the echo is reflected back toward the direction from which it originated. This orientation produced the greatest return of reflected sound to the transducer. A simple twist of the wrist can produce a very distorted appearance of an image and this is especially critical in the measurement of intraocular structures.

MEASUREMENT PARAMETERS

MEASUREMENT PARAMETERS IN GLAUCOMA RESEARCH AND CLINICAL PRACTICE

The high resolution of UBM images significantly contributes to the qualitative comprehension of the pathogenic mechanism involved in various ocular diseases.

Furthermore, ultrasound biomicroscopy provides an accurate measurement of ocular structures. This technique thus provides a good quantitative estimate, unlike the qualitative estimate of gonioscopy.

Measurement parameters[1] that can be obtained include:

- corneal thickness (CT), the distance between epithelium and endothelium (Fig. 14.5A)
- scleral distance (SD), the scleral thickness measured on the scleral spur (Fig. 14.6C)
- anterior chamber depth (ACD), measured from the corneal endothelial surface to the lens surface (Fig. 14.5A)
- angle opening distance (AOD 250 and AOD 500), the length of a perpendicular from the trabecular meshwork to the iris at points 250 or 500 μm from the scleral spur (Fig. 14.6A)
- trabecular ciliary process distance (TCPD), measured on a line extending from a point 500 μm from the scleral spur perpendicularly through the iris to the ciliary process (Fig. 14.5B)
- iris ciliary process distance (ICPD), representing the ciliary sulcus and measured from the posterior iris surface to the ciliary process, through the same line used for TCPD (Fig. 14.5B)

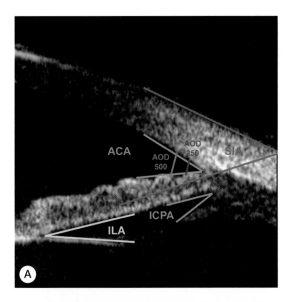

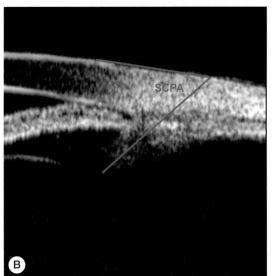

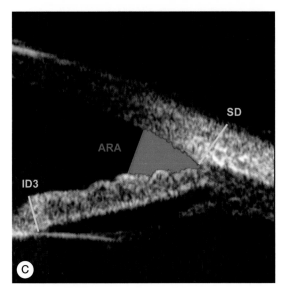

FIGURE 14.6 (A,B,C) Main angular measurement parameters.
(A) SIA, scleral-iris angle; AOD 250, AOD 500, angle opening distance; ACA, anterior chamber angle; ILA, iris–lens angle.
(B) SCPA, scleral ciliary process angle. **(C)** ID3, iris distance; ARA, angle recess area; SD, scleral distance.

TABLE 14.1 Coefficients of variation determined in two studies[3,4] for the 10 UBM parameters examined

	CV VALUES (%)	
UBM PARAMETER	TELLO et al.[3]	MARCHINI et al.[4]
ACD	0.3–0.5	1.4
ACA	4.5–11.1	12.4
TCPD	1.8–4.7	5.9
AOD 500	5.1–9.2	8.0
ID1	3.7–8.3	10.5
ICPD	3.7–6.7	15.6
IZD	2.6–7.1	6.6
ILCD	2.9–3.3	14.2
SCPA		8.6
SIA		7.5

CV, coefficients of variation; UMB, ultrasound biomicroscopy. A CV <10% is considered indicative of good reproducibility.

- iris distance (ID1, ID2, and ID3); ID1 is located on a line perpendicular to the iris connecting a point on the trabecular meshwork 500 μm from the scleral spur to the ciliary process (TCPD); ID2 is measured 2 mm from the scleral spur; ID3 is measured at the thickest point near the iris margin (Figs 14.5B and 14.6C)
- iris zonule distance (IZD), measured at a point just clearing the ciliary process (Fig. 14.5B)
- iris–lens contact distance (ILCD), the length of the iris–lens contact area (Fig. 14.5A)

Iridocorneal drainage angle measurement parameters[1] that can be obtained are:

- anterior chamber angle (ACA), measured with the apex of the iris sulcus and the arms passing through the point 500 μm from the scleral spur and the point perpendicularly opposite on the iris (Fig. 14.6A)
- iris–lens angle (ILA), the angle that the iris makes in relation to the lens (Fig. 14.6A)
- scleral–iris angle (SIA), the angle that the iris makes to a tangent to the scleral surface (Fig. 14.6A)
- scleral ciliary process angle (SCPA), the angle that the ciliary body makes to a tangent to the scleral surface (Fig. 14.6B)
- angle recess area (ARA),[2] the triangular area demarcated by the anterior iris surface, corneal endothelium, and a line perpendicular to the corneal endothelium drawn from a point 750 μm anterior to the scleral spur to the iris surface (Fig. 14.6C)

RELIABILITY OF THE MEASUREMENTS

The reliability of the UBM measurements has been analyzed by different authors who considered intraobserver and interobserver agreement for different measurement parameters. Considering existing literature, the reproducibility of the measurements increases when these are obtained by a single examiner (Table 14.1), but results show unacceptable variance when the same measurements are taken by different operators.

The choice of different anatomic landmarks between different examiners could explain the limited interobserver reliability of the measurements. Furthermore, the reproducibility of different measurements obtained by the same investigator on the same image is high, but it decreases when the same operator analyzes different images of the same ocular sector.[3,4]

ULTRASOUND BIOMICROSCOPY AND GLAUCOMA

PRIMARY OPEN-ANGLE GLAUCOMA

The main role of UBM in glaucoma is to provide a quantitative measurement of the anterior chamber angle width and to produce additional information to the qualitative estimate of gonioscopy (Fig. 14.7). The evaluation of the angle width is obtained using the ACA. Measurements of angle opening can vary with change in the state of iris dilation. Moreover, subtle and subjective variations in iris curvature around the periphery will induce small differences in measurements at various locations. Quantitative linear measurements of the angle (AOD 250 and 500) have been designed to control the variables such as iris dilation and to improve the reproducibility and the precision of a qualitative estimate of angle opening. Even using the quantitative approach, the evaluation of the angle is susceptible to low reliability when the UBM examination is performed using a small eyecup. The inadvertent corneal indentation due to the cups can cause artifactitious widening of the iridocorneal angle on UMB.[5]

PIGMENTARY DISPERSION SYNDROME AND PIGMENTARY GLAUCOMA

In pigmentary dispersion syndrome (PDS) and pigmentary glaucoma the high-resolution images obtained with the ultrasound biomicroscopy provide important data relating to the pathogenesis of this type of glaucoma. UBM provides a method of determining iris curvature, defining the relationship of the posterior surface of the iris to the zonule and lens, and documenting changes that take place after therapeutic intervention. Most patients with PDS show a posterior concavity of the peripheral iris, the ILCD measurement is usually large, the ciliary processes are located immediately behind the peripheral iris, and the zonule is likely to be in contact with the iris pigment epithelium (Fig. 14.8).[6] On the contrary, some patients with PDS present an absence of the concavity of the iris and small ILCD. It is possible that these examinations are taking place at a time when the forces that produce posterior iris bowing are not active. Recently, a new mechanism producing pigment loss has been proposed, which is the result of long anterior zonules that are inserted centrally on the lens capsule, without iris concavity. This particular anatomical variant would justify the presence of radial transillumination defects of the pupillary margin and central iris.[7] UBM confirmed the theory of the reverse pupillary block, which implies temporary reversal of the pressure differential in the anterior and posterior chambers, producing posterior bowing of the iris and leading to iris–zonule contact with mechanical pigment loss. The theory implies that peripheral iridotomy and miotic topical drugs could produce equalization of pressure in the two chambers. It has been observed clinically and by UBM that the iris concavity and iridolenticular contact decreases following laser peripheral iridotomy (Fig. 14.9).[8] Furthermore, UBM has shown that accommodation,[9] blinking,[10] and exercise[11] can produce posterior bowing of the iris and should be considered as possible mechanisms of PDS.

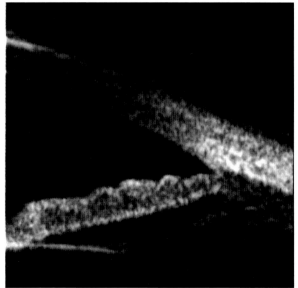

FIGURE 14.7 A typical UBM section through the angle in a patient with open-angle glaucoma.

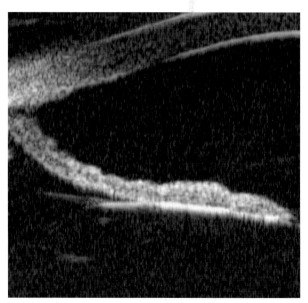

FIGURE 14.8 Posterior concavity of the peripheral iris and increased ILCD in a patient with PDS.

PSEUDOEXFOLIATION SYNDROME AND PSEUDOEXFOLIATIVE GLAUCOMA

Regarding glaucoma associated with pseudoexfoliation syndrome (PXF), the ultrasound biomicroscopy examination allows the observation of pseudoexfoliative material. It appears as small high reflective areas which are limited to the pupillary margin, on the anterior surface of the lens, in the anterior chamber angle, and under the corneal endothelium.[12] The pathogenesis of ocular hypertension associated with PXF is a consequence of the occlusion of the trabecular meshwork from the material and pigment. Considering the small percentage of PXF glaucoma which presents itself as an acute angle-closure form, UBM examination suggests a pupillary block due to the pseudoexfoliative material, with or without iridolenticular synechiae, or lens dislocation with zonule laxity.[13] Furthermore, UBM provides particularly useful information in the diagnosis of the rare capsular delamination (true exfoliation) of the crystalline lens.[14]

MECHANISMS UNDERLYING ANGLE-CLOSURE GLAUCOMA

Ultrasound biomicroscopy represents a helpful aid in the analysis of angle-closure glaucoma and the mechanisms that produce it. UBM contributed significantly to the comprehension of the pathogenesis of plateau iris syndrome and angle closure due to supraciliary uveal effusion. At the end of the 1960s, biometric studies showed the great differences between the anatomical characteristics of the anterior segment of healthy eyes compared to eyes with primary angle-closure glaucoma (PACG). Glaucomatous eyes present a smaller corneal diameter, smaller anterior corneal radius of curvature, smaller posterior corneal radius of curvature, shallower central and peripheral anterior chamber depth, greater lens thickness, smaller anterior lenticular radius of curvature, a more anterior lens position, shorter total axial length, and greater lens thickness:axial length ratio.[4] Only a small percentage of eyes with anatomically predisposing factors will develop a PACG during a lifetime. These biometric characteristics constitute the critical element in the absence of which the angle closure cannot take place. The importance of the biometric factors in glaucoma research has been further confirmed with ultrasound biomicroscopy, allowing precise measurements of the anterior chamber angle area to be obtained. The authors' studies with A-scan biometry and UBM in healthy eyes, patients with acute-intermittent PACG, and chronic PACG showed interesting results.[4] The measurement of the angle width in degrees pointed out a very narrow angle in the acute forms of the pathology (mean value of 11.7°) and this is concordant with the Shaffer classification, which identifies 10° as the dangerous edge for angle closure (Fig. 14.10). In the chronic forms, on the contrary, the angle is less tight, with a mean value of 19.8° compared to 31.2° of healthy eyes. Furthermore, the

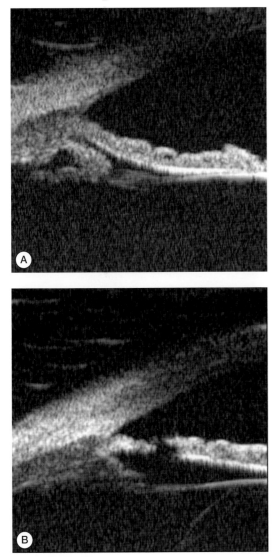

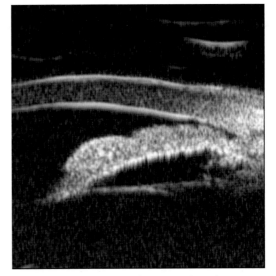

FIGURE 14.9 Iris concavity and iridolenticular contact **(A)** decrease following laser peripheral iridotomy **(B)** in a patient with PDS.

FIGURE 14.10 Ultrasound biomicroscopy view of a narrow angle in a patient with acute-intermittent PACG due to pupillary block.

189

considerations about the TCPD and SCPA are very interesting. The TCPD represents the width of the area which contains the iris and it is a characteristic parameter of each eye. The TCPD is directly influenced by the position of the ciliary processes, which can be obtained by measuring the SCPA. The SCPA has been found to be more acute in the eyes with PACG than in healthy subjects. That means that the ciliary processes of these patients are structurally rotated forward and the lens is placed in a more anterior position. Moreover, this anatomical condition influences the TCPD, the ICPD, the IZD, and the AOD 500, which are all particularly small in PACG eyes. The authors did not find any significant difference relating to the iris thickness between healthy and glaucomatous eyes; considering the study population, the iris thickness does not seem to reduce the angle width and increase the risk of angle closure. The analysis of the SIA demonstrates a progressive decrease of the value ranging from normal eyes, PACG eyes with chronic form, and those with acute-intermittent phenotype. This finding is in agreement with the pathogenesis of pupillary block, the probability of which is proportional to the degree of forward curvature of the iris plane. Consequently, patients with PACG present also a larger ILCD which is due to the great lens thickness, the more anterior lens position, and the forward rotation of the ciliary processes.[15] The anterior chamber angle closes when the iris root touches the trabecular meshwork. Three main mechanisms are responsible for the angle closure which is involved in the pathogenesis of the primary forms: PACG due to pupillary block, PACG due to direct crowding of the angle (plateau iris syndrome), and PACG due to ciliary block (posterior block glaucoma).

Pupillary block Ultrasound biomicroscopy allowed the confirmation of the hypothesis on the angle closure in two instances according to the theory of Mapstone (Fig. 14.11).[16] First, the shape of the iris root due to its anterior convexity profile would touch the peripheral cornea ahead of the trabecula (Fig. 14.12). Behind this contact area the angular recess would create an open tunnel, which is located between the iris and the trabecula (Fig. 14.13). Then, the contact would become more complete and the iris root would be pushed against the trabecular meshwork, determining the occlusion (Fig. 14.14).

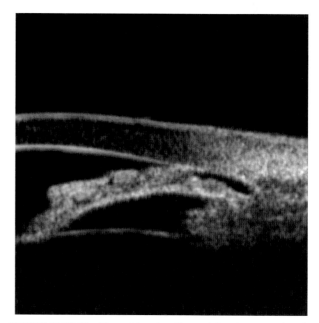

FIGURE 14.12 The iris root touches the peripheral cornea ahead of the trabecula.

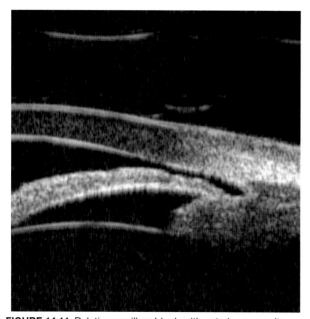

FIGURE 14.11 Relative pupillary block with anterior convexity profile of the iris.

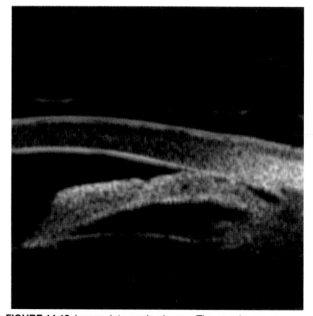

FIGURE 14.13 Incomplete angle closure. The angular recess creates an open tunnel, which is located between the iris and the trabecula.

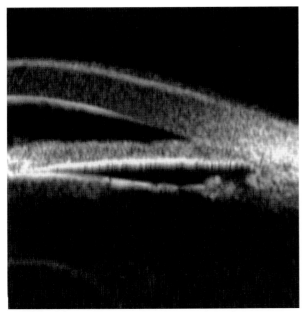

FIGURE 14.14 Complete occlusion of the trabecular meshwork.

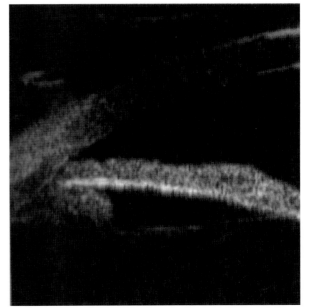

FIGURE 14.16 Plateau iris syndrome with a particularly narrow angular recess. The forward position and rotation of the ciliary processes, which are in contact with the peripheral portion of the iris, cause the closure of the ciliary sulcus and the creation of a support for the iris root, which therefore cannot detach itself from the trabecula even in the presence of an iridotomy.

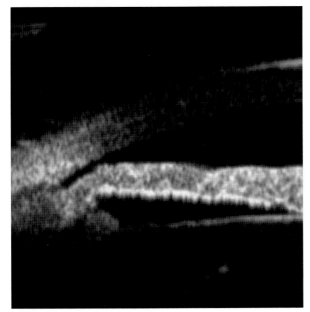

FIGURE 14.15 Plateau iris syndrome.

Plateau iris syndrome Ultrasound biomicroscopy has been used to elucidate the etiology of plateau iris syndrome. Considering the PACG due to direct crowding of the angle, this angle-closure mechanism occurs more rarely as a result of mydriasis in eyes that present the so-called 'iris plateau' (Fig. 14.15). In these eyes, the iris is characterized by a flat configuration, with a sharp bending back at the level of the trabecula which gives rise to the creation of a particularly narrow angular recess. When the pupil dilates, the volume of iris tissue builds up in the restricted angular space and closes the angle. Contrary to the angle closure due to pupillary block, the mechanism of the crowding of the angle produces directly a complete occlusion or it starts from the apex of the angular recess proceeding to the

trabecula. The most distinctive feature of eyes with a plateau iris is clearly demonstrated by UBM and consists in the forward position and rotation of the ciliary processes, which are in contact with the peripheral portion of the iris. This causes the closure of the ciliary sulcus and the creation of a support for the iris root, which therefore cannot detach itself from the trabecula even in the presence of an iridectomy (or YAG-laser iridotomy) (Fig. 14.16).[17] UBM also confirmed that the iridociliary apposition in plateau iris syndrome persists after cataract extraction.[18] In studies of plateau iris in the dark and after pilocarpine administration, it was demonstrated that the TCPD remained constant with iris thickness being the only variable contributing to angle narrowing. Finally, UBM contributed to reveal the pseudoplateau iris configuration due to the presence of multiple iris cysts that elevate the iris and produce varied angle narrowing (Fig. 14.17).[19]

Malignant glaucoma Malignant glaucoma is defined as a condition in which shallowing of the anterior chamber with elevated pressures occurs in spite of patent iridotomy. Ciliary block represents the main mechanism involved in the pathogenesis of malignant glaucoma. This condition rarely constitutes a primary event and frequently follows filtering surgery, especially in eyes with narrow angles. The pathogenetic mechanisms of the phakic and pseudophakic malignant glaucoma are based on a block to the outflow of aqueous humor in the area of lens equator, zonule, and ciliary processes, with misdirection of the flow towards the vitreous. The ciliary processes, which appear edematous and dislocated anteriorly, are of decisive importance in the genesis of ciliolenticular block. As a result of these phenomena, the lens or the intraocular lens (IOL) is pushed forward, the depth of the anterior chamber is reduced and ultimately abolished, and the angle closed.[20] For these reasons malignant glaucoma is also referred to as posterior block glaucoma. UBM allows the observation of the shallowing of the anterior chamber, the anterior rotation of the ciliary processes to a position just behind the iris, and the closure of the trabecula by either the lens margin (Fig. 14.18)[21] or ciliary processes (Fig. 14.19).[22]

Ciliochoroidal effusion and glaucoma Angle-closure glaucoma due to ciliochoroidal effusion represents a clinical condition that can be well detected by UBM. This complication occurs in a variety of conditions including inflammatory disease, retinal detachment surgery, central retinal vein occlusion, and glaucoma surgery. UBM allows the detection of the precise mechanism of the angle closure, which is caused by an anterior rotation of the ciliary processes and iris around the scleral spur (Fig. 14.20).[23,24] The high resolution of the

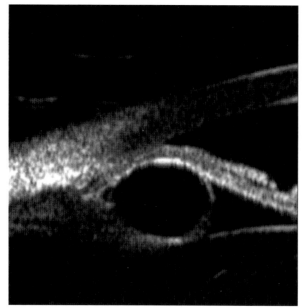

FIGURE 14.17 Iridociliary cystic angle closure with a pseudo-plateau iris configuration.

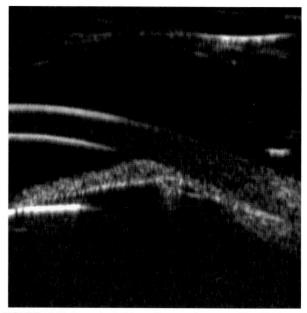

FIGURE 14.19 Pseudophakic malignant glaucoma. The IOL is located forward and pushes the peripheral iris against the cornea. The ciliary processes are dislocated anteriorly and the ciliary sulcus is abolished.

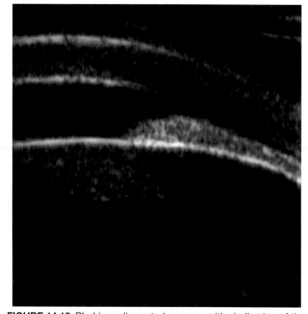

FIGURE 14.18 Phakic malignant glaucoma, with shallowing of the anterior chamber, anterior rotation of the ciliary processes, and closure of the trabecula by the lens margin.

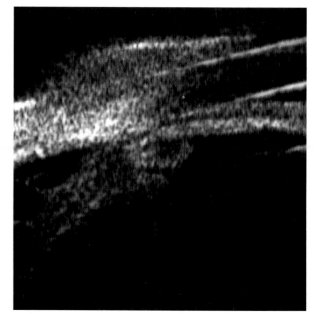

FIGURE 14.20 Angle-closure glaucoma due to ciliochoroidal effusion. The uveal effusion causes the detachment of the ciliary body, an anterior rotation of the ciliary processes and iris around the scleral spur.

images allows the identification of a very small effusion over the ciliary body without choroidal detachment. These conditions cannot usually be detected by conventional ultrasound or by clinical examination.

ULTRASOUND BIOMICROSCOPY USE IN GLAUCOMA RESEARCH

In spite of the well-known potentiality relating to the diagnosis of various diseases, UBM is a helpful aid in the management of parasurgical treatments. Many glaucomatous patients also undergo other forms of treatment such as laser iridotomy, peripheral iridoplasty, and cyclophotocoagulation. The efficacy of the above-mentioned techniques is frequently due to the precise localization of the anatomical structures that need to be treated.

IRIDOTOMY

Ultrasound biomicroscopy allows the accurate study of the internal relationship between the iris, the lens, and the ciliary processes. The knowledge of this data constitutes an important factor in the choice of the seat of the iridotomy. It should be performed more peripherally where the iridolenticular contact is larger, or centrally in the case of the ciliary processes are more resistant. UBM examination represents a useful tool in detecting the anatomical variations of the anterior segment, widening of the anterior chamber angle, lowering of the convexity of the iris profile, and increasing of the iridolenticular contact area (Fig. 14.21).[25] Furthermore, the high-resolution scans can differentiate the errors relating to the position or the efficacy of the procedures (Figs 14.22 and 14.23).[26]

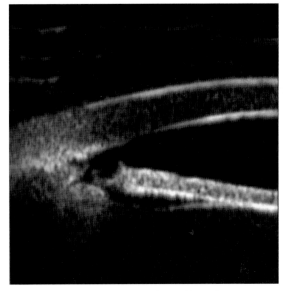

FIGURE 14.22 Patent iridotomy performed in an incorrect peripheral position.

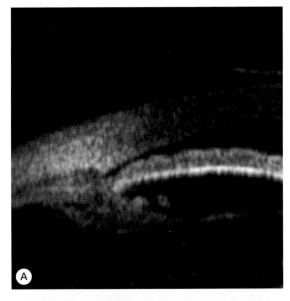

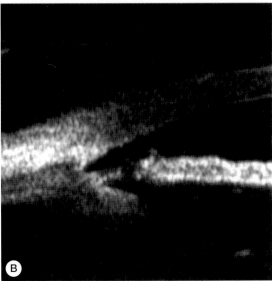

FIGURE 14.21 Ultrasound biomicroscopic assessment of the angle following laser iridotomy. **(A)** Narrow angle with relative pupillary block. **(B)** Widening of the anterior chamber angle and lowering of the convexity of the iris profile after laser iridotomy in the same eye.

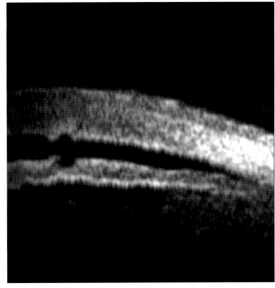

FIGURE 14.23 Incomplete iridotomy with endothelial damage due to inaccurate focusing of the laser beam.

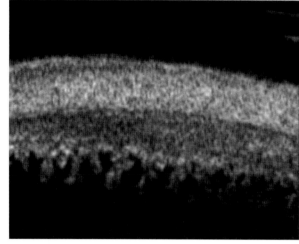

FIGURE 14.24 Transverse section through the ciliary processes.

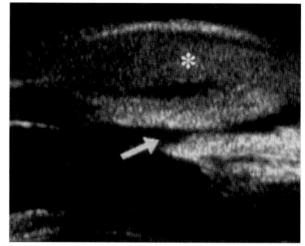

FIGURE 14.25 A functioning filtering surgery. UBM scan at the level of the peripheral iridectomy. The arrow indicates direct communication with the anterior chamber and the subconjunctival space in the area where the tissue containing the trabecula was removed. The filtering bleb (*asterisk*) is clearly visible.

IRIDOPLASTY

Regarding laser iridoplasty, which is used to produce flattening and thinning of the peripheral iris in conditions such as plateau iris, UBM has shown the effects of laser treatment on the structures forming the anterior segment. The high resolution of the ultrasound examination demonstrates the peripheral burns on the iris surface (high-reflective areas) and the partial opening of the angle.[1]

CYCLOPHOTOCOAGULATION

Ultrasound biomicroscopy constitutes a useful method in both ophthalmic research and clinical practice. The efficacy of the cyclophotocoagulation procedure is closely related to the positioning of the laser probe on the ciliary processes. However, this condition is not always so easy when the treatment is performed using the transscleral approach. UBM allows the detection of the correct position of the structures which must be treated (Fig. 14.24) and the avoidance of therapeutic failure due to an abnormal position of the ciliary processes.[27] Moreover, the method shows the morphological and structural modifications of the structures exposed to cyclophotocoagulation.[28]

ULTRASOUND BIOMICROSCOPY AND SURGICAL TREATMENT OF GLAUCOMA

FILTERING SURGERY

The high resolution of UBM makes it a useful tool for examination of filtering surgical techniques and causes of failure. Considering the trabeculectomy, UBM allows the detection of the precise scan of the new pathway of the aqueous humor: the internal ostium, the scleral dissection site, and the filtering bleb (Fig. 14.25).[29] Furthermore, UBM provides an important contribution in the analysis of the clinical results of filtering techniques. Considering the ultrabiomicroscopical internal reflectivity of the images obtained with UBM, a new classification system of the state of the filtering blebs has been proposed: type L (low-reflective), type H (high-reflective), type E (encapsulated) with a high reflective wall, and type F (flattened) with high conjunctival reflectivity.[30] This classification correlates well with the clinical functional result of the surgical procedure. The UBM analysis of the eyes which obtained a postoperative IOP value lower than 20 mmHg allowed the detection of common echographic elements: a low internal reflectivity of the subconjunctival bleb (type L) and the presence of an internal ostium which is continuous with a patent intrascleral pathway. The filtering blebs type H, E, and F have been observed especially in the eyes with moderate IOP-lowering effect (IOP = 20 mmHg with pharmacological antiglaucoma therapy) or poor (IOP > 20 mmHg in spite of pharmacological antiglaucoma therapy).[30,31] Furthermore, UBM can detect those complications of filtering surgery which are difficult to identify with the ophthalmoscopic approach: the closure of the internal ostium due to the apposition of iridociliary structures, the disappearance of the low-reflective space under the scleral split, and the presence of multiple cystic areas under the conjunctiva instead of spongy episcleral tissue.

NONPENETRATING SURGERY

The UBM analysis of eyes which have undergone deep sclerectomy, which represents the most common

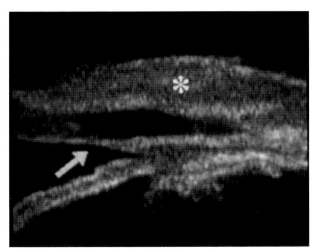

FIGURE 14.26 Nonpenetrating surgery. A UBM image of deep sclerectomy with hyaluronic acid implant. The trabeculo-Descemet's membrane (*arrow*) separates the anterior chamber from the decompression space, allowing the formation of a filtering bleb (*asterisk*).

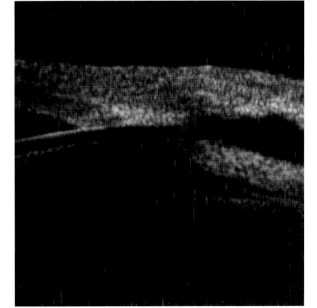

FIGURE 14.27 Baerveldt implant. UBM shows the drainage tube which creates a direct communication between the anterior chamber and the subconjunctival space.

nonpenetrating surgical treatment, allows the observation of the trabeculo-Descemet's membrane which separates the anterior chamber from the intrascleral decompression space (Fig. 14.26). Furthermore, the high resolution of UBM images significantly contributed to the comprehension of the mechanisms involved in aqueous drainage due to the nonpenetrating filtering technique. The echographic findings which have been detected with UBM are: the conjunctival bleb (subconjunctival filtering), the low reflectivity of the scleral tissue next to the space of decompression (intrascleral filtering), and the supraciliochoroidal hypoechoic area (uveal–scleral filtering pathways).[32]

GLAUCOMA DRAINAGE IMPLANT SURGERY

Glaucoma shunt implants are devices which achieve a self-controlled drainage, creating a direct pathway between the anterior chamber and the equatorial subconjunctival space. Glaucoma drainage implant surgery represents the therapeutic alternative to the conventional filtering surgical techniques and it is especially recommended in particular glaucoma forms or after surgical failure (wound healing) of the other filtering treatments. The high resolution of UBM makes it a useful tool for examination of the eyes which have undergone glaucoma drainage implant surgery. UBM allows the detection of the filtering subconjunctival bleb (Fig. 14.27), to check the close lodgement of the drainage tube into the anterior chamber, to verify the opening of the tube and its connection with the next anatomical structures (Fig. 14.28).[33] Furthermore, UBM provides an additional aid in the management of some rare complications due to the surgical placement of drainage shunts which would not be

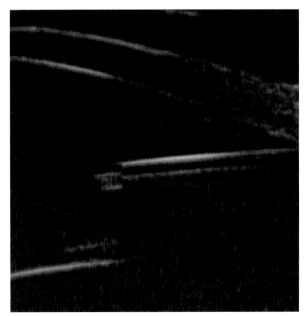

FIGURE 14.28 Baerveldt implant. UBM scan at the level of the drainage tube. UBM allows the detection of the close position of the tube into the anterior chamber and its connection with the next anatomical structures. The high resolution of the image shows the presence of an intraluminal suture. This technique is used to temporarily occlude the drainage tube and to prevent early postoperative hypotony.

detectable with the traditional echographic techniques, such as the postoperative hypotony due to peritubular filtering[34] or the late migration of an intraluminal ripcord suture.[35]

REFERENCES

1. Pavlin CJ, Foster FS. Ultrasound biomicroscopy of the eye. New York: Springer Verlag; 1995.

2. Radhakrishnan S, Goldsmith J, Huang D, et al. Comparison of optical coherence tomography and ultrasound biomicroscopy for detection of narrow anterior chamber angles. Arch Ophthalmol 2005; 123:1053–1059.

3. Tello C, Liebmann JM, Potash SD, et al. Measurement of ultrasound biomicroscopy images: intraobserver and interobserver reliability. Invest Ophthalmol Vis Sci 1994; 35:3549–3552.

4. Marchini G, Pagliarusco A, Toscano A, et al. Ultrasound biomicroscopic and conventional ultrasonographic study of ocular dimensions in primary angle-closure glaucoma. Ophthalmology 1998; 105:2091–2098.

5. Ishikawa H, Inazumi K, Liebmann JM, et al. Inadvertent corneal indentation can cause artifactitious widening of the iridocorneal angle on ultrasound biomicroscopy. Ophthalmic Surg Lasers 2000; 31:342–345.

6. Potash SD, Tello C, Liebmann J, et al. Ultrasound biomicroscopy in pigment dispersion syndrome. Ophthalmology 1994; 101:332–339.

7. Moroi SE, et al. Long anterior zonules and pigment dispersion. Am J Ophthalmol 2003; 136:1176–1178.

8. Breingan PJ, Esaki K, Ishikawa H, et al. Iridolenticular contact decreases following laser iridotomy for pigment dispersion syndrome. Arch Ophthalmol 1999; 117:325–328.

9. Balidis MO, Sandy CJ, Garway-Heath DF, et al. Iris configuration in accommodation in patients with pigment dispersion syndrome. Invest Ophthalmol Vis Sci 1998; 39:251.

10. Liebmann JM, Tello C, Chew SJ, et al. Prevention of blinking alters iris configuration in pigment dispersion syndrome and normal eyes. Ophthalmology 1995; 102:446–455.

11. Jensen PK, Nissen O, Kessing SV. Exercise and reversed pupillary block in pigmentary glaucoma. Am J Ophthalmol 1995; 120:110–112.

12. Bauzys RLM, Nishi M, Mello PAA, et al. Ultrasound biomicroscopy in pseudoexfoliation syndrome. Invest Ophthalmol Vis Sci 1995; 36:563.

13. Gohdo T, Takahashi H, Iijima H, et al. Ultrasound biomicroscopy of angle closure glaucoma with pseudoexfoliation syndrome. Br J Ophthalmol 1997; 81:706–707.

14. Hwang YS, Chang SH. Ultrasound biomicroscopy of capsular delamination (true exfoliation) of the crystalline lens. Chang Gung Med J 2003; 26:930–932.

15. Marchini G, Pagliarusco A, Tosi R, et al. In: Bonomi L, ed. I glaucomi da chiusura d'angolo. Relazione ufficiale LXXV Congresso S.O.I., Rome, December 7–10. Rome: I.N.C. Innovation-News-Comminication; 1995:29–62.

16. Mapstone R. The mechanism and clinical significance of angle closure. Glaucoma 1980; 2:249.

17. Pavlin CJ, Ritch R, Foster FS. Ultrasound biomicroscopy in plateau iris syndrome. Am J Ophthalmol 1992; 113:390–395.

18. Tran HV, Liebmann JM, Ritch R. Iridociliary apposition in plateau iris syndrome persists after cataract extraction. Am J Ophthalmol 2003; 135:40–43.

19. Inazumi K, Ishikawa H, Gurses-Odzen R, et al. 'Pseudo' plateau iris configuration caused by multiple iridociliary cysts. Invest Ophthalmol Vis Sci 1999; 40:835.

20. Trope GE, Pavlin CJ, Bau A, et al. Malignant glaucoma: clinical and ultrasound biomicroscopic features. Ophthalmology 1994; 101:1030–1035.

21. Marchini G, Tosi R, Ghilotti G, et al. Ultrasound biomicroscopy as decisive examination in resolving special glaucoma cases. Acta Ophthalmol Scand 1998; 76:30–31.

22. Tello C, Chi T, Shepps G, et al. Ultrasound biomicroscopy in pseudophakic malignant glaucoma. Ophthalmology 1993; 100:1330–1334.

23. Liebmann JM, Weinreb RN, Ritch R. Angle-closure glaucoma associated with occult annular ciliary body detachment. Arch Ophthalmol 1998; 116:731–735.

24. Postel EA, Assalian A, Epstein DL. Drug-induced transient myopia and angle-closure glaucoma associated with supraciliary choroidal effusion. Am J Ophthalmol 1996; 122:110–112.

25. Oh H, Hata N, Yamakawa R. Ultrasound biomicroscopic assessment of the angle following laser iridotomy. Invest Ophthalmol Vis Sci 1997; 38:165.

26. Marraffa M, et al. Ultrasound biomicroscopy and corneal endothelium in Nd:YAG laser iridotomy. Ophthalmic Surg Lasers 1995; 26:519–523.

27. Pavlin CJ, et al. Ultrasound biomicroscopic imaging of the effects of YAG laser cycloablation in post mortem eyes and living patients. Ophthalmology 1995; 102:334–341.

28. Carassa RG, Brancato R, Trabucchi G, et al. Ultrasound biomicroscopic and pathologic examination of eyes treated with contact transscleral cyclophotocoagulation. Invest Ophthalmol Vis Sci 1995; 36:564.

29. Chi T, Grayson DK, Potash S, et al. High resolution ultrasound biomicroscopy of filtration blebs. Invest Ophthalmol Vis Sci 1993; 34:733.

30. Yamamoto T, Sakuma T, Kitazawa Y. A new classification system for filtering blebs. Invest Ophthalmol Vis Sci 1995; 36:563.

31. Yamamoto T, Sakuma T, Kitazawa Y. An ultrasound biomicroscopic study of filtering blebs after mitomycin C trabeculectomy. Ophthalmology 1995; 102:1770–1776.

32. Marchini G, Marraffa M, Brunelli C, et al. Ultrasound biomicroscopy and intraocular-pressure-lowering mechanisms of deep sclerectomy with reticulated hyaluronic acid implant. J Cataract Refract Surg 2001; 27:507–517.

33. Crichton AC, McWhae JA, Reimer J. Ultrasound biomicroscopy for the assessment of Molteno valve tube position. Invest Ophthalmol Vis Sci 1993; 34:732.

34. Garcìa Feijòo J, Cuina Sardina R, Mèndez Fernàndez C, et al. Peritubular filtration as cause of severe hypotony after Ahmed valve implantation for glaucoma. Am J Ophthalmol 2001; 132:571–572.

35. Harasymowycz PJ, Katz LJ. Ultrasound biomicroscopy and management of late posterior migration of a ripcord suture after glaucoma drainage implant surgery. Ophthalmic Surg Lasers Imaging 2004; 30:826–831.

CHAPTER 15

Angle Imaging: Ultrasound Biomicroscopy and Anterior Segment Optical Coherence Tomography

Gus Gazzard and Winnie Nolan

INTRODUCTION

Imaging devices allow one to observe otherwise unseen structures in novel ways and to better quantify the already visible (Fig. 15.1). Anterior segment structures in the glaucoma patient may be obscured by blood or an opaque cornea and in these circumstances ultrasound biomicroscopy (UBM) or anterior segment optical coherence tomography (AS-OCT) may be helpful: for example, viewing obstructed drainage tubes through the edematous corneas of high-pressure eyes,[1] localization of hidden foreign bodies,[2] or the detection of ciliary body clefts in hypotony (Figs 15.2 and 15.3). Anterior segment imaging has also contributed to the assessment of trabeculectomy blebs[3] and glaucoma drainage device surgery (Fig. 15.4). Yet it is in angle-closure glaucoma that anterior segment imaging is having the greatest impact.

The diagnosis of angle closure depends entirely upon the reliable assessment of anterior chamber angle characteristics and the detection of iridotrabecular contact. Until recently, this has relied upon direct gonioscopic observation. Yet gonioscopy remains limited by an

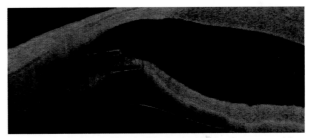

FIGURE 15.2 A Baerveldt tube blocked with iris after supramid removal seen by AS-OCT through a cloudy cornea. (Courtesy of Keith Barton, MD FRCP FRCOphth FRCS.)

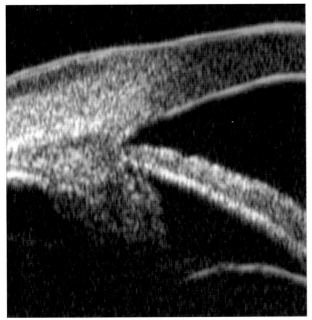

FIGURE 15.1 A normal UBM scan of an open angle.

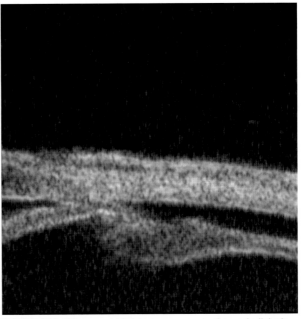

FIGURE 15.3 Ultrasound biomicroscopy scan of a cyclodialysis cleft that was obscured by PAS on gonioscopy.

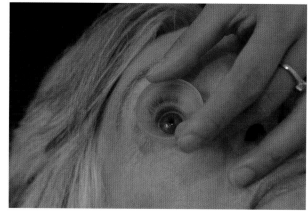

FIGURE 15.4 Water bath for supine UBM scanning.

inevitable subjectivity and poor interobserver reproducibility. A measure of the anterior chamber angle that is objective, quantifiable, and reproducible is the holy grail of angle-closure glaucoma. Numerous grading systems and techniques have been devised to derive numerical data from gonioscopy (such as eyepiece graticules) but all remain subject to poor reproducibility. Cross-sectional images obtained with both UBM and AS-OCT give novel views of angle structures. These allow objective image analysis and fuller descriptions of the complex angle morphology which subjective grading systems tend to simplify. These instruments ultimately *complement* rather than replace gonioscopy, which remains an essential tool in assessment of angle pigmentation, vessels, etc., and as a guide to interpretation of images.

ULTRASOUND BIOMICROSCOPY

MODE OF ACTION

All ultrasound (US) imaging relies upon the propagation of sound waves through tissues and their reflection from interfaces between tissues of different acoustic impedance. Sound pulse generation and detection of echoes are both performed by the transducer, the physical characteristics of which (diameter, focal length, etc.) partly determine the resolution available.[4,5]

Reflected sound waves obey the laws of geometric optics. Information about subsurface tissue interfaces is built up from the time taken for reflected and backscattered sound to be detected. The speed of sound is fairly constant in biological tissues (1540–1560 m/s) and so time can simply be converted into distance traveled. The resolution of the constructed image depends upon the frequency and pulse duration of the sound used: higher-frequency sound (hence shorter wavelength) allows more precise measurements. This leads to a fundamental trade-off between attainable resolution and depth of penetration. Higher-frequency sound is more attenuated by tissue absorption. A maximum penetration of 50 mm for a 10 MHz signal falls to 5 mm at 60 MHz but with an increase in *lateral* resolution from 600 μm to 60 μm. Axial resolution depends upon pulse duration, which is shorter with higher

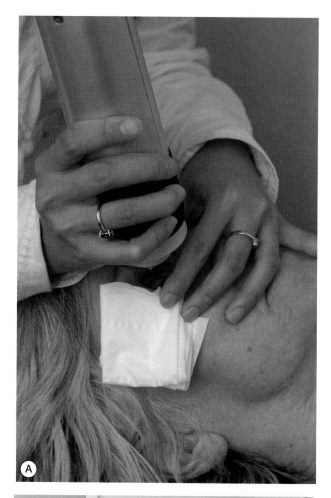

Ⓐ

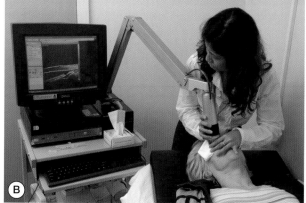

Ⓑ

FIGURE 15.5 Supine UBM scanning in progress.

wavelength machines (e.g. 190 μm at 10 MHz and 40 μm at 100 MHz). Signal attenuation also varies with tissue density, e.g. sclera attenuates more than iris, and intraocular lenses will cast acoustic shadows.[5]

The majority of medical US imaging uses wavelengths of between 3.5 and 5 MHz with conventional ophthalmic machines running at 10 MHz: in contrast, UBM uses 50–100 MHz. Practically, this means that detailed ciliary body and iris imaging is possible but that the posterior lens surface is not visible. Modern machines offer interchangeable probes with different wavelengths for imaging different structures, e.g. cornea at 100 MHz and angle at 50 MHz.

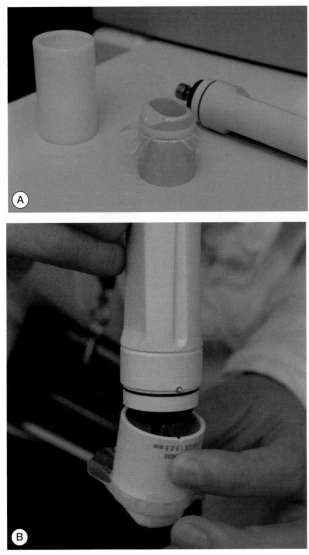

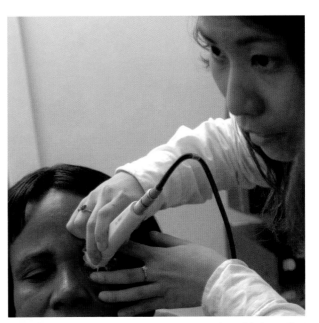

FIGURE 15.7 Ultrasound biomicroscopy scanning with the patient upright.

FIGURE 15.6 The new UBM probe from Paradigm for upright scanning.

The greatest signal intensity and hence best image quality is achieved when the probe is perpendicular to the tissue interface of interest. Different machines have used one of two approaches. 'Paradigm' and similar models originally used a supported mobile probe held in a water bath on a supine patient (Figs 15.4 and 15.5). More recent versions have incorporated a water bath around a smaller more mobile probe (Fig. 15.6). Using a viscous coupling gel between the eye and the taut rubber diaphragm of the probe, scanning in the upright position is now possible (Fig. 15.7), though it is still not truly noncontact.

An alternative, the 'Artemis,' places the patient facing downwards in a water bath with a probe that tracks the curve of the cornea for full limbus-to-limbus scans, but it is aimed more at the refractive market.

STRENGTHS AND LIMITATIONS

The greatest strengths of UBM are its high-resolution images, good tissue penetration (including the ciliary body), and a robust, established technology with automated image analysis software.[6] Scan acquisition time with UBM is short enough to give good real-time video that can be directly stored as digital video. Good ciliary body and iris penetration mean that deeper structures such as lens haptics or iridociliary cysts are clearly visible with UBM, although obscured on AS-OCT, and it can also be performed in near-darkness.

There are, however, limitations. A coupling medium is needed between the oscillating ultrasound transducer probe and the ocular surface, requiring topical anesthesia. Earlier machines relied upon a supine patient and a water bath retained by the eyelids, with the inherent risk of distorting the globe with the eyecup (see Fig. 15.4). It is not known how lens position and angle morphology change with lying supine.

Exact probe positioning is important for repeatable longitudinal comparisons. This can be tricky supine but even more difficult in the upright position, although it does avoid potential globe torsion on lying flat. There remains a significant dependence on user experience to obtain good-quality images with the UBM. Illumination is also an issue since angle opening may vary markedly with lighting (Fig. 15.8): scanning in the dark is difficult when direct observation of both subject and screen is required. In contrast, AS-OCT's greatest strength is the possibility of more physiological truly noncontact and even true in-the-dark scanning.

INTERPRETATION OF DATA, DATA STORAGE, AND INSTRUMENT PRINTOUTS

Image storage and archiving in early instruments was cumbersome, with software-specific data files. This is now much more convenient with the easy export of generic picture formats. Continuous improvements in

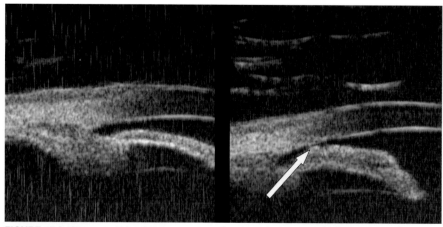

FIGURE 15.8 Ultrasound biomicroscopy scan of an open but narrow angle in bright light that closes in the dark.

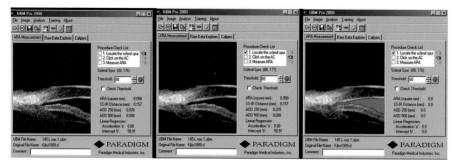

FIGURE 15.9 UBMPro 2000 image analysis software in use for angle assessment.

processing and storage have been accompanied by more flexible user interfaces.

Simple interpretation of the pictures generally requires no processing, but the real strengths of imaging lie in the possibility of deriving objective numerical measurements. On-screen calipers are straightforward but prone to observer error, particularly when attempting to measure angles between two curved surfaces. Various image analysis programs are available to automate the analysis of UBM angle images (e.g. UBMPro 2000[6]), some now incorporated into the instrument software (Fig. 15.9). These require the user to specify the scleral spur as a reliable landmark structure, so can be limited by poor image quality. Multiple measures of angle width have been derived, such as angle-recess area, angle opening distance, iris root to scleral spur distance, and iris–ciliary process distance,[6] although the importance and reliability of some of these is yet to be defined (e.g. iris–ciliary process distance).

Angle-recess area (ARA $x\mu m$) gives an overall measure of space between iris and trabecular meshwork (TM) out to a specified distance from the scleral spur, whereas the angle-opening distance (AOD $x\mu m$) is simply the distance between structures *at* a particular distance (usually defined as perpendicular to the TM/cornea). Similar ARAs may derive from quite different peripheral iris configurations. Ishikawa defined two measures of peripheral iris configuration by deriving the regression line on the AOD at successive distances from the scleral spur. These derived variables change differently in response to different stimuli, e.g. peripheral iridotomy versus pilocarpine.[6]

COMMON ARTIFACTS, HOW TO PREVENT THEM, AND TECHNICAL TIPS FOR USERS

Several common artifacts may degrade UBM images, the commonest being bubbles in the coupling medium. Larger bubbles cause significant reflections (Fig. 15.10)

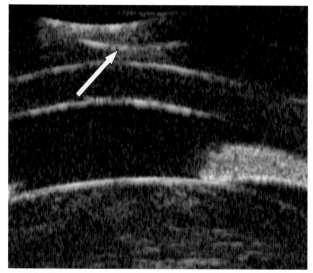

FIGURE 15.10 A large bubble causing an artifact in a UBM image of a phacomorphic lens.

and hence shadowing of distal structures due to signal attenuation, while with smaller bubbles there is an overall degradation of image quality. One particular cause of poor images is an air bubble trapped in the concave probe surface: this may be dislodged with a cotton bud. Intraocular lenses, tube drainage devices, and other echodense structures also lead to acoustic shadows, though this is rarely a problem in angle imaging.

The ultrasound transducer receives the strongest signal from tissue interfaces that are perpendicular to the probe. Oblique views give weaker signal and poorer definition. When several differently curved structures such as cornea and iris are of interest, areas at right angles will show clearly while off-axis parts will be blurred (Fig. 15.11). A series of images may be required to capture the full curves of the cornea or iris. To avoid this, the Artemis automatically tracks the probe across the arc of corneal surface, retaining a perpendicular scan position but sacrificing some user control.

Other potential sources of error arise from the scanning conditions. If an eyecup is used to retain coupling fluid, this may compress the globe and artifactually open a closed angle. This is reduced by use of a flexible silicon cup rather than one of rigid polypropylene. For small palpebral apertures as are often found in East Asian subjects it may be necessary to use 'pediatric' eyecups and occasionally it is not possible to image the superior angle at all. Illumination conditions can similarly affect the angle status; as with gonioscopy, a bright examination room will induce a pupillary miosis that can open a narrow angle. Miosis also occurs as part of the near triad with accommodation, so it would seem sensible to use a consistent distant fixation object where possible.

Full topical anesthesia is, of course, essential as any blepharospasm makes scanning without an eye-cup impossible; indeed, Bell's phenomenon may still prevent imaging of the superior angle. The most reliable technique for high-quality images still seems to be with a patient supine (and with the head supported and stable), an eyecup carefully placed to avoid globe compression, with a viscous tear substitute sealing the cup and saline as the prime coupling medium. It is usually easiest for the examiner to sit at the head of the couch, elbow supported, with a clear, direct view of the monitor.

ANTERIOR SEGMENT OPTICAL COHERENCE TOMOGRAPHY

MODE OF ACTION

Optical coherence tomography (OCT) technology employs low-coherence interferometry to obtain cross-sectional images of ocular tissues. Using light instead of sound (in contrast with UBM) a beam is shone on structures of the eye and reflections returning from the structures are analyzed to produce real-time images. Light of a wavelength of 830 nm is used to obtain images of posterior segment structures such as the macula, and anterior segment OCT (AS-OCT) imaging was at first done using this wavelength of light. Recently, this technology has been adapted for better visualization of the anterior segment by using a longer wavelength (1310 nm) light. At this wavelength increased penetration of nontransparent tissues such as sclera and high illumination power allow rapid, high-resolution imaging of the anterior segment with a capability similar to that of UBM. Images can be acquired at a rate of 8 frames per second (2000 A-scans per second) with lateral and axial resolutions of 15 μm and 8 μm, respectively.[7] Increased absorption of light by the water in ocular tissues at this wavelength protects the retina from light-induced damage of this high-power modality. In contrast with UBM, AS-OCT requires no contact with the eye. AS-OCT evolved primarily for use in refractive surgery and is used for the evaluation of the cornea and anterior segment dimensions prior to and following laser refractive procedures and phakic intraocular lens implantation.[8] However, its ability to obtain detailed cross-sectional images of the angle means it has great potential as a diagnostic tool in the detection and management of primary angle closure. Although anterior segment imaging cannot replace the direct visualization of angle structures possible with gonioscopy, it does provide a more comfortable and objective means of obtaining a qualitative and quantitative evaluation of the angle.

There are currently two commercially available AS-OCT machines, both of which have advantages and disadvantages: the Visante™ OCT (Carl Zeiss Meditec, Dublin CA) is a stand-alone AS-OCT machine (Fig. 15.12, right) and the slit lamp OCT (SL-OCT) (Heidelberg Engineering) is an AS-OCT attached to a

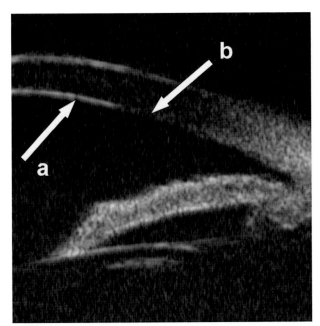

FIGURE 15.11 Structures give stronger signals when they are perpendicular to the probe (*arrow a*) than when they are not (*arrow b*).

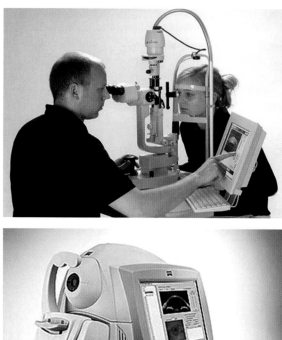

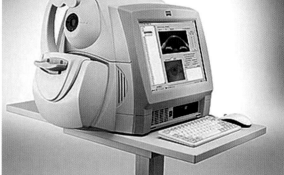

FIGURE 15.12 Heidelberg and Zeiss AS-OCT machines. Angles may be measured on-screen with both instruments.

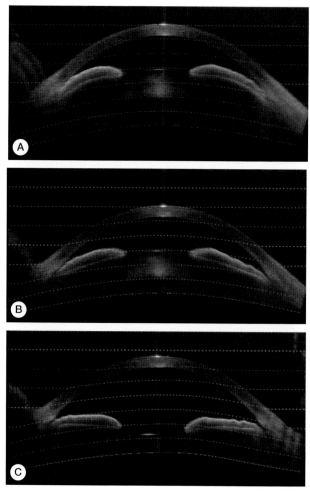

FIGURE 15.13 (A) Anterior segment ocular coherence tomography image showing appositional closure of nasal and temporal angle quadrants. (B) AS-OCT image of same eye as Fig. 15.13A following laser iridotomy. The nasal angle still looks narrow but wider than pre-iridotomy. (C) Image of same patient following phacoemulsification, showing further widening of the angle.

Haag-Streit slit lamp (Fig. 15.12, left). Both devices are capable of rapid noncontact imaging of the anterior segment with the patient sitting in the upright position.

STRENGTHS AND LIMITATIONS

The main advantages of AS-OCT are the fact that contact with the globe is not required, image acquisition time is rapid, and that the machines are easy to operate. It also provides a real-time cross-sectional view of the anterior chamber and angle structures, allowing clinicians to observe the dynamic relationships between the iris, lens, and angle wall. Quantitative and qualitative data can be collected and analyzed in an objective way that is much less observer dependent and more reproducible than gonioscopy. Because AS-OCT is a noncontact modality it is much more comfortable for the patient when compared with gonioscopy and ultrasound biomicroscopy. This means that frequent, repeat follow-up scans can be obtained at clinic visits without causing undue discomfort and distress to the patient.

There are two aspects of primary angle-closure management where AS-OCT technology will play an important role. The first is as a diagnostic tool; it can be used to diagnose or confirm appositional angle closure, and initial data show that it actually detects more cases of angle closure than gonioscopy (Fig. 15.13A).[8] Advantages of AS-OCT over gonioscopy are that no

visible light needs to be shone on the eye to obtain images and there is no pressure on the globe. Both these factors probably result in less distortion of resting angle anatomy. In populations where primary angle-closure glaucoma (PACG) prevalence is high, AS-OCT could potentially be used to screen for the disease within the hospital or community setting. The other application of AS-OCT is in evaluating the effect of laser iridotomy and other interventions on angle anatomy. A significant number of angle-closure patients demonstrate no widening of the angle following laser iridotomy[9] and may benefit from additional treatments such as iridoplasty or lens extraction. Although the ciliary body is not always visible (see below), changes in the anatomical relationships between the iris, trabecular meshwork, and lens under light and dark conditions are more easily seen in the cross-sectional images of the anterior chamber that are obtained with the AS-OCT. This helps clinicians plan further interventions if necessary (Figure 15.13A–C).

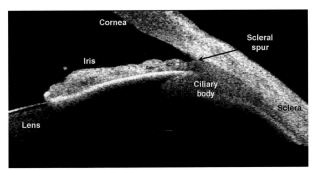

FIGURE 15.14 In this blue-eyed patient the ciliary body is partially visible.

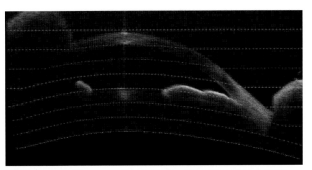

FIGURE 15.16 The upper lid often obscures the superior angle, especially in East Asian patients with small palpebral apertures.

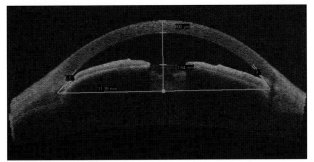

FIGURE 15.15 Quantitative analysis of anterior segment dimensions including corneal thickness, anterior chamber depth, angle-to-angle distance, and angle width in degrees (Visante™).

A significant limitation of AS-OCT is its poor ability to show details of the ciliary body and posterior surface of the iris (see Fig. 15.13). The posterior pigmented iris and ciliary epithelium block the passage of infrared light, so preventing a good view of these structures. In the diagnosis and management of angle closure (particularly postiridotomy residual angle closure) there is an advantage that UBM has over AS-OCT in determining nonpupil block mechanisms such as an anteriorly rotated ciliary body or iris/ciliary body cysts. Other pathology which may not be detectable using AS-OCT includes cyclodialysis clefts and ciliary body tumors. This limitation seems to be more of a problem in individuals with darkly pigmented brown eyes rather than blue eyes, where more of the light can be transmitted posteriorly (Fig. 15.14).

Other limitations include difficulty visualizing the superior angle quadrant due to the upper eyelid getting in the way and suboptimal quality of inferior quadrant images, possibly due to interference from the lower eyelid. With practice and experience, examiners can minimize interference from the lids. Landmarks such as scleral spur and Schwalbe's line are not always as clearly identifiable with AS-OCT as they are with UBM. This has important implications for obtaining quantitative measurements of angle width.

IMAGE ANALYSIS: STORAGE AND RETRIEVAL OF DATA

Both the Visante™ OCT and the SL-OCT are capable of capturing images of the entire anterior segment (so that opposing angle quadrants are visible simultaneously) in either the horizontal or vertical meridians, and also have a high-resolution corneal mode that can be used to give a more detailed single angle quadrant view (pictures of both). A number of images are captured and the operator can select the best-quality ones for further analysis. Selected scans are processed to adjust for image distortion arising from the effect of refraction at the air–cornea and cornea–aqueous interfaces. Scans can then be exported as JPEG or bitmap files to the desktop of the machine and undergo further analysis. Qualitative assessment of the anterior chamber and angle structures can be performed by viewing the cross-sectional and high-resolution scans. Quantitative analysis of anterior chamber measurement parameters is performed using in-built custom software present in both AS-OCT machines. Corneal thickness and anterior chamber depth measurements are provided by this software. Angle width can be measured in degrees using calipers, and the standard measures of angle width and volume devised for UBM are also provided by the AS-OCT software (angle-opening distance, angle-recess area, trabecular–iris surface area) (Fig. 15.15). Measurement of these parameters requires identification of scleral spur by the observer for the Visante™ machine, and is semiautomated, but can be adjusted for the SL-OCT machine.

COMMON ARTIFACTS AND TECHNICAL TIPS FOR USERS

Artifacts that cause most problem in AS-OCT angle imaging are interference from the eyelids and movement causing misalignment of the image (Fig. 15.16). The eyelids are more of a problem for imaging in the vertical meridian and particularly for the superior angle quadrant. However, with a cooperative patient and an assistant or the operator lifting the top eyelid out of the way, it is now possible to get good-quality cross-sectional images in the vertical meridian. Correct alignment of the patient's eye with the machine is essential for obtaining good-quality images. The Visante™ has an in-built fixation target which the patient is asked to focus on and the SL-OCT requires an external fixation point behind the operator. While the patient is fixing on these targets the operator can make fine adjustments to

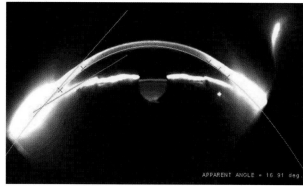

FIGURE 15.17 The traditional Scheimpflug images had obscured angles due to bright scleral reflections at the limbus.

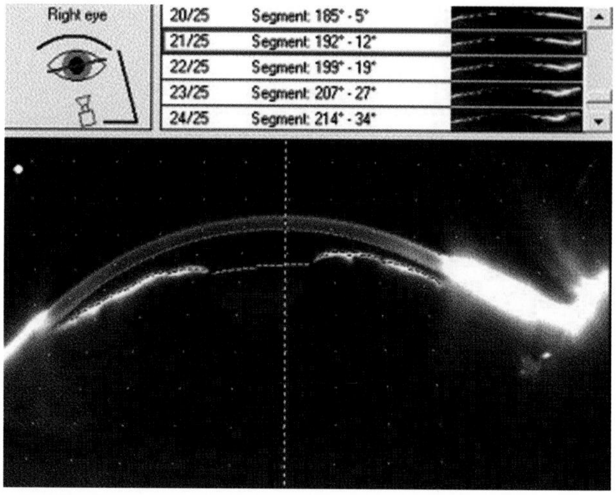

FIGURE 15.18 Preoperative Pentacam image of the right eye. (Reproduced from Sharan S, Grigg JR, Higgins RA. Nanophthalmos: ultrasound biomicroscopy and Pentacam assessment of angle structures before and after cataract surgery. J Cataract Refract Surg 2006; 32:1052–1055.)

align the eye until a bright axial beam is visible on the scan, confirming good alignment. The patient should then be asked to keep the eyes still and not blink while the scanning takes place.

UBM AND AS-OCT COMPARED

Both these angle-imaging technologies produce cross-sectional images of the anterior segment with different limitations. While UBM remains the only reliable noninvasive technology with which to determine ciliary body anatomy, the AS-OCT promises higher resolution of the iris and angle with greater ease of scanning in a more physiological setting. UBM is now a mature technology, whereas AS-OCT has great potential for further development. Being entirely noncontact, it is also likely that AS-OCT may prove to be more acceptable to patients. Nonetheless, with increasing emphasis on the importance of ciliary body angulation and insertion,[10] UBM retains a role.

OTHER TECHNOLOGIES

Several other techniques for anterior segment angle imaging exist but may have limitations compared to UBM or AS-OCT.

SCHEIMPFLUG AND PENTACAM

Scheimpflug photography gives an optical cross-sectional image of the anterior segment (Fig. 15.17) from which the iridocorneal angle can be inferred. Earlier machines such as the Nidek EAS-2000 took a single image at a variable angle about the visual axis. The newer 'Pentacam' uses five cameras rotating about the central axis to build up a composite three-dimensional map of corneal thickness and anterior chamber depth (Fig. 15.18).[11] Both devices are limited by the penetration of visible-wavelength light through limbal tissues, which obscures the true angle recess. Angle opening must be extrapolated from visible iris and cornea and this, along with the inherent variability of drawing an angle between the tangents to two curves, makes the Scheimpflug methods less useful.[12]

SCANNING PERIPHERAL ANTERIOR CHAMBER DEPTH ANALYZER

The new scanning peripheral anterior chamber (SPAC) depth analyzer machine automates the van Herick method of assessing anterior chamber depth with the aim of rapid noncontact screening of large populations for angle closure. It uses an oblique thin white illumination beam and has automatic image processing software that derives the iridocorneal distance. Concerns have been raised that the brightness of the visible-wavelength illuminating beam may cause pupil constriction and so artifactually open a closed or narrow angle. Validation studies and comparisons with AS-OCT are underway.

REFERENCES

1. Sarodia U, Sharkawi E, Hau S, et al. Visualization of aqueous shunt position and patency using anterior segment optical coherence tomography. Am J Ophthalmol. 2007; 143(6): 1054–1056.

2. Looi AL, Gazzard G, Tan DT. Surgical exploration minimised by ultrasound biomicroscopy localisation of intraocular foreign body. Eye 2001; 15:234–235.

3. Singh M, Chew PT, Friedman DS, et al. Imaging of trabeculectomy blebs using anterior segment optical coherence tomography. Ophthalmology 2007; 114:47–53.

4. Foster FS, Pavlin CJ, Harasiewicz KA, et al. Advances in ultrasound biomicroscopy. Ultrasound Med Biol 2000; 26:1–27.

5. Pavlin CJ, Foster FS. Ultrasound biomicroscopy of the eye. New York: Springer-Verlag; 1995; 13–14.

6. Ishikawa H, Ritch R, Liebmann J. Quantitative assessment of the anterior segment using ultrasound biomicroscopy. Curr Opin Ophthalmol 2000; 11:133–139.

7. Gazzard G, Friedman DS, Devereux JG, et al. A prospective ultrasound biomicroscopy evaluation of changes in anterior

segment morphology after laser iridotomy in Asian eyes. Ophthalmology 2003; 110:630–638.

8. Nolan WP, See JL, Chew PT, et al. Detection of primary angle closure using anterior segment optical coherence tomography in Asian eyes. Ophthalmology 2007; 114:33–39.

9. He M, Friedman DS, Ge J, et al. Laser peripheral iridotomy in primary angle-closure suspects, biometric and gonioscopic outcomes: the Liwan Eye Study. Ophthalmology 2007; 114: 494–500.

10. He M, Foster PJ, Johnson GJ, et al. Angle-closure glaucoma in East Asian and European people. Different diseases? Eye 2006; 20:3–12.

11. Sharan S, Grigg JR, Higgins RA. Nanophthalmos: ultrasound biomicroscopy and Pentacam assessment of angle structures before and after cataract surgery. J Cataract Refract Surg Eye 2006; 32:1052–1055.

12. Friedman DS, Gazzard G, Foster P, et al. Ultrasonographic biomicroscopy, Scheimpflug photography, and novel provocative tests in contralateral eyes of Chinese patients initially seen with acute angle closure. Arch Ophthalmol 2003; 121:633–642.

The Impact of Central Corneal Thickness and Corneal Biomechanics on Tonometry

James D Brandt, Cynthia Roberts, Mark B Sherwood, and Clinton W Sheets

INTRODUCTION

The measurement of intraocular pressure (IOP) has been a cornerstone of ophthalmology since the sixteenth century when Bannister first recognized that certain forms of blindness were associated with a firm eye. Numerous techniques for estimating IOP were developed through the nineteenth and twentieth centuries, culminating in the various electronic and mechanical devices in widespread use today. Introduced some 50 years ago, Goldmann applanation tonometry (GAT) was rapidly accepted by the ophthalmic community due to its perceived accuracy, reproducibility, ease of use at slit lamp examination, low cost, and easily understood physical principles. Because GAT is the technique most commonly used worldwide, this chapter will focus on GAT and aspects of the human cornea, such as central corneal thickness (CCT) and the material properties of the cornea, that impact GAT's estimation of IOP.

GAT arrives at an estimate of IOP based on the force needed to flatten the corneal apex to a given area. A flattened area with a diameter of 3.06 mm was chosen empirically to offset the surface tension of the tear film (which tends to draw the tonometer tip towards the eye) and both corneal and ocular rigidity (which resist applanation, independent of IOP). Goldmann and Schmidt acknowledged several limitations in their design.[1] They based their design on what they believed was a relatively constant CCT of 0.5 mm among normal individuals. Given the paucity of published data at the time and the limitations of optical pachymeters of the time, 500 μm seemed a reasonable assumption for the 'average' patient; nonetheless, they acknowledged that the accuracy of their device would be affected if CCT deviated from this value. We now know CCT varies greatly among the general population, to a degree that impacts the accuracy of most tonometry techniques in daily practice. Other sources of error include corneal material properties, Valsalva's maneuver, astigmatism, corneal curvature, inappropriate amount of fluorescein, eyelid squeezing, and indirect pressure on the globe.

It is beyond the scope of this chapter to review all tonometry techniques other than to state that many other widely used tonometers represent variants of applanation tonometry. The TonoPen (Reichert Instruments, DePew, NY, USA) and noncontact (air-puff) tonometry both applanate a defined area of central cornea to estimate IOP. The Maklakov tonometer, still used in parts of Eastern Europe, employs a series of fixed weights to applanate the cornea; using a nomogram the clinician determines IOP based on the diameter of the area applanated. Each of these techniques, along with GAT, has its advantages and disadvantages in terms of portability, positioning, patient acceptance, and varying accuracy under different conditions and extremes of IOP. All are affected, to some degree, by variations in CCT and the underlying material properties of the cornea.

THE IMPACT OF CENTRAL CORNEAL THICKNESS ON TONOMETRY

The theoretical effects of CCT on GAT were confirmed in 1975 when Ehlers cannulated otherwise normal eyes undergoing cataract surgery and correlated corneal thickness with errors in GAT.[2] He found that GAT most accurately reflected true intracameral IOP when the CCT was 520 μm. The table contained in his article has been widely interpreted to imply that with a ±100 μm deviation from this nominal value, IOP must be adjusted ±7 mmHg. It is not widely appreciated how limited Ehlers' data set was; it was based on only 29 eyes from a racially homogeneous population in Scandinavia with a limited range of CCTs.

Subsequent cannulation experiments performed with modern pressure transducers have confirmed Ehlers' basic findings.[3,4] Numerous investigators have since demonstrated that CCT varies far more among otherwise normal individuals than Goldmann and Schmidt ever dreamed; differences in CCT are seen among different racial and ethnic groups,[5–7] and may lead to misclassification of patients with normal-tension glaucoma and ocular hypertension.[8,9]

THE OCULAR HYPERTENSION TREATMENT STUDY

The importance of CCT in the management of glaucoma patients, particularly those with ocular hypertension, was brought to the forefront by findings from the Ocular Hypertension Treatment Study (OHTS)[10,11] Among the OHTS participants, African-American participants had thinner corneas than their Caucasian counterparts, and 25% of the overall OHTS cohort had CCT values above 600 μm.[7] If one uses Ehlers' correction of roughly 7 mmHg/100 μm deviation from the nominal value of 520 μm, then as many as 50% of OHTS subjects had 'corrected' IOP values upon entry equal to 21 mmHg! Most dramatically, a multivariate model of baseline characteristics found to be predictive of which OHTS subjects would develop glaucoma, CCT proved to be the most potent.[11] These findings have been confirmed independently in the European Glaucoma Prevention Study (EGPS),[12,13] and the merged OHTS/EGPS risk model features CCT as a major component of glaucoma risk.[14]

The OHTS and EGPS results suggest that many patients are being misclassified in terms of glaucoma risk on the basis of erroneous IOP estimates by GAT. Clearly, many individuals with elevated GAT measurements but no other findings suggestive of glaucoma probably have normal 'true' IOPs and do not need treatment or even increased glaucoma surveillance. CCT measurements in patients with diagnosed glaucoma also appear useful; following the OHTS publications, numerous investigators have explored the role of CCT in patients with existing glaucoma, and they have generally found CCT to have a significant impact in these patients as well.[15–22]

CENTRAL CORNEAL THICKNESS DIFFERENCES AMONG RACIAL GROUPS

In the OHTS' multivariate predictive model, racial differences in cup-to-disc ratios and CCT explained racial differences in disease risk, eliminating African-American race per se as a risk factor.[11] Several investigators provide further evidence that African-American subjects, as a group, tend to have thinner corneas than their Caucasian counterparts. Nemesure et al., following a CCT survey of participants in the Barbados Eye Survey, reported that black participants had thinner corneas (mean thickness 529.8 μm) than white participants (545 μm).[23] No relationship between IOP and CCT was found in this population-based survey. Shimmyo and colleagues performed a retrospective biometric review of patients at a large refractive surgery center, also finding that African-American patients had thinner corneas than Caucasian patients seeking refractive surgery; they found no difference in CCT among Caucasian, Asian, and Hispanic patients in their population.[24] This is in contrast to the findings of the population-based Los Angeles Latino Eye Study, which found CCTs among their Hispanic patients intermediate between values reported for African-American and Caucasian populations.[25]

CENTRAL CORNEAL THICKNESS – TONOMETRY ARTIFACT, OR SOMETHING MORE?

The results of the OHTS and other studies beg the question of whether CCT's influence on glaucoma risk is attributable solely to its known impact on tonometry, or to something else. Perhaps there is a biological link between aspects of the front of the eye that can be measured, such as the thickness or material properties of the cornea (e.g. corneal hysteresis), and the structure/deformability/physiology of the lamina cribrosa and peripapillary sclera.

The OHTS and other studies that demonstrate a link between CCT and either glaucoma risk or disease severity are unable to separate tonometry effect from underlying biological risk. In the OHTS, initial eligibility was based primarily on GAT; in the OHTS and in retrospective chart reviews of CCT and glaucoma it is also impossible to account for physician behavior in treatment decisions that are, to a large part, driven by GAT results.

In contrast to the OHTS, which studied patients initially enrolled *without* glaucoma damage, the Early Manifest Glaucoma Trial (EMGT) studied subjects *with* glaucomatous damage documented at enrollment.[26] Like the OHTS, the EMGT measured CCT in all participants shortly after enrollment was completed. Two fundamental differences between the OHTS and EMGT, at least from the standpoint of differentiating tonometry artifact from an underlying biological link related to CCT, are that the EMGT randomized patients without regard to entry IOP, and all subjects in the treatment arm received only laser trabeculoplasty and betaxolol. This design minimized the influence of tonometry artifact on physician behavior.

In a publication analyzing baseline risk factors for progression of glaucoma at 5 years among EMGT participants, Leske et al. reported that CCT was *not* a significant predictor of progression.[27] However, the EMGT was a relatively small sample (at least compared to the OHTS) and may not have the statistical power to find such a relationship. The EMGT investigators have published few details on the range and distribution of CCTs they measured in their racially homogeneous population; it is quite possible it was far narrower than what was found in the OHTS. If there is an effect of CCT on progression rates in established disease, the EMGT might be too small, the follow-up too short, and the range of IOPs and CCTs too narrow to detect an effect. In fact, in an analysis of longer-term EMGT data, Leske and colleagues more recently reported thinner CCT to be a significant risk factor for progression (HR = 1.42 [1.05, 1.92] per 40 μm lower) at higher baseline IOPs but not at lower baseline IOPs.[28,29] They report that the relationship between CCT and glaucoma progression may be stronger, or perhaps only found in patients with higher baseline IOP.

THE CORNEA IS NOT A PIECE OF PLASTIC – THE IMPACT OF MATERIAL PROPERTIES

The elasticity of the cornea, one measure of biomechanical properties, has been theoretically shown to have a greater effect on error in IOP measurement than either curvature or thickness.[30] The current scientific and clinical focus on corneal thickness is due to a large extent on the ability to readily measure central corneal thickness (CCT) in the clinic, compounded by the current lack of a commercial device with the ability to measure corneal elasticity in vivo. This can be considered analogous to Goldmann's focus in the 1950s on the potential error caused by variation in corneal curvature, since that could be measured in the clinic at the time he was developing his tonometer, whereas corneal thickness could not. CCT is likely positively correlated to corneal elasticity in normal populations, with a more complicated relationship in the case of pathology or after corneal surgery.

Young's modulus of elasticity is defined as the ratio of the stress (load per unit area) and the strain (displacement per unit length). Therefore, a material with low modulus will exhibit greater deformation for a given stress than a material with high modulus. The experimentally determined values of Young's modulus reported in the literature for the cornea vary widely, ranging from 0.01 to 10 MPa.[31–33] The variability in the reported experimental data is vast, most likely due to variation in experimental techniques. In addition, the majority of corneas available for experimental testing are postmortem corneas of advanced age, since pristine young corneas are generally used for transplantation rather than research. The distribution of elasticity in a normal population of wide age ranges has not been determined; however, it is known that in general, the cornea stiffens as it ages. Because glaucoma is a strongly age-related disease, it seems reasonable to assume that there is a strong relationship between age and IOP. IOP data from population-based studies are contradictory in this regard – the Baltimore Eye Survey did not find such a relationship,[34,35] whereas the Barbados Eye Study[36] and the Beaver Dam Eye Study did.[37] If 'true' IOP is generally stable across a population, perhaps increasing corneal stiffness is what drives the increased *measured* IOP observed in many studies, even in the absence of a change in CCT.

It is also important to distinguish elasticity from viscoelasticity. The elastic response of the cornea to an applied force has no time-dependent component. The response is a function only of the magnitude of the applied force. The viscoelastic response, on the other hand, has a time-dependent component, meaning that both the magnitude and the rate at which a force is applied will affect the corneal response. Although no commercial technology exists to measure corneal elasticity in vivo, there is technology available that reports to provide a measure of corneal viscoelasticity. The Ocular Response Analyzer outputs two parameters, corneal hysteresis (CH) and corneal resistance factor (CRF). Both of these parameters are viscoelastic in nature, and neither can be accurately interpreted as elasticity. However, CRF was empirically derived to correlate with central corneal thickness,[38] and is therefore 'weighted' by elasticity, even though it is still affected by the viscoelastic properties of the cornea. In addition, a material which exhibits low corneal hysteresis can have either high or low elastic modulus, depending on the associated viscosity. Therefore, it is not accurate to interpret low hysteresis as either low elasticity or low viscosity. Recently, Congdon and co-workers showed that corneal hysteresis as measured by the Ocular Response Analyzer was independently associated with glaucoma risk.[19]

THE CORNEA FOLLOWING REFRACTIVE SURGERY

The alteration in measured IOP after refractive surgery adds yet a further layer of complexity to tonometry and an understanding of the material properties of the cornea. Several studies have shown that the mean change in measured pressure after refractive surgery is negative, but that the range of measured change is extensive, from +10 mmHg to −10 mmHg, using multiple methodologies for measuring IOP.[39,40] Following myopic procedures, both curvature and thickness are reduced, and yet the measured pressure is often increased. Mathematically, this can only be explained using current models as an increase in elasticity, which is extremely unlikely and contradicts experimental evidence. Therefore, current models are inadequate to explain the case of refractive surgery. The specific assumption that is violated following refractive surgery is that of uniform thickness and homogeneous corneal properties in the measurement of IOP. Following refractive surgery, it is known that the thickness profile is dramatically altered and can no longer satisfy the mathematical assumptions used in existing models. In addition, the presence of a flap in a lamellar procedure divides the cornea into regions of varying properties. Chang and Stulting suggest that the lamellar corneal flap makes no contribution to the load-bearing characteristics of the post-LASIK cornea.[39] Combined with undoubted variability of wound healing among different patients, it seems clear that refractive surgery alters an already complicated biomechanical structure, and its effects will require much more study to understand.

IMPLICATIONS FOR CLINICAL PRACTICE

Confronted with the expanding evidence that CCT is an important ocular parameter that should be measured in clinical practice, most ophthalmologists acquire pachymetry measurements in their patients but then wonder what to do with the information. How to use CCT measurements in daily practice, is not straightforward – there is wide disagreement among investigators as to whether there is an adequately validated 'correction algorithm;' without a validated algorithm, the argument goes, clinicians cannot use the data. When the pachymetry protocol was added to the OHTS,[7] many believed that CCT's impact in the OHTS would be primarily through the effect of CCT as a confounder of GAT measurements. It is notable that attempts to model and adjust the OHTS IOP data using every published 'correction nomogram' for GAT and CCT have thus far failed to eliminate CCT as a predictive factor from the OHTS multivariate model.

As noted above, several engineering models of the cornea suggest that variations in the material properties of the cornea (both viscoelastic properties and/or Young's modulus) likely dwarf the effect of CCT on GAT measurements, as shown in Figures 16.1 and 16.2.[30,41] These models suggest that if the material properties of the cornea were constant, variations in CCT from the mid-400s to mid-600s with constant material properties might explain only some ±4 mmHg in variance from 'true' (directly measured) IOP, whereas variations in material properties of the cornea with constant CCT might explain ±10 mmHg in variance from 'true' IOP. For example, a 625 μm cornea that was born that way is likely to behave quite differently than one that was thickened by subclinical edema. In the latter case, a thicker, slightly edematous cornea may in fact cause an erroneously *lower* GAT estimate than true IOP. Since CCT and material properties vary together, the interdependence of these parameters on the measurement error of applanation tonometry generates variability in

any population study. For example, Figure 16.3 illustrates that IOP measurement in corneas with a lower elastic modulus is less affected by CCT than in corneas with a higher elastic modulus. This has implications for IOP measurement as a function of age, as well as with diseased or postsurgical corneas.

In the linear regression analyses generated by cannulation experiments, just as many data points lie above

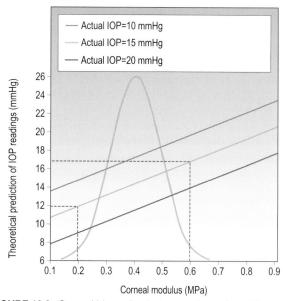

FIGURE 16.2 Corneal biomechanical properties – alone. The 'stiffer' the cornea, the greater the measured pressure. Potential error: huge ≥10 mm. (Liu J, Roberts CJ. Influence of corneal biomechanical properties on intraocular pressure measurement: quantitative analysis. J Cataract Refract Surg 2005; 31(1):146–155.)

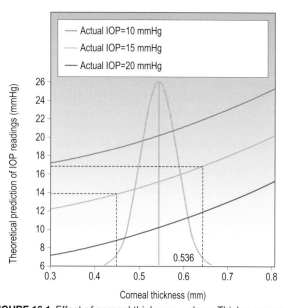

FIGURE 16.1 Effect of corneal thickness – alone. Thicker cornea equals higher measured pressure, whereas thinner cornea leads to lower measured pressure. Potential error: moderate. (Liu J, Roberts CJ. Influence of corneal biomechanical properties on intraocular pressure measurement: quantitative analysis. J Cataract Refract Surg 2005; 31(1):146–155.)

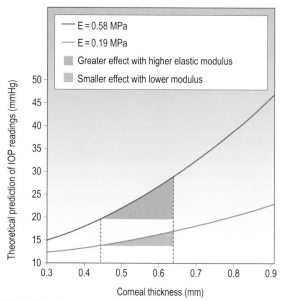

FIGURE 16.3 Corneal elasticity *and* corneal thickness. The effect of CCT depends on Young's modulus. (Liu J, Roberts CJ. Influence of corneal biomechanical properties on intraocular pressure measurement: quantitative analysis. J Cataract Refract Surg 2005; 31(1):146–155.)

the regression line as below; the data points above the line need to be 'corrected' downwards, those below 'corrected' upwards. In attempting to correct GAT measurements acquired in an individual patient by a fixed, linear correction nomogram, the ophthalmologist can be wrong both in the magnitude of the adjustment and also in its direction. A thick cornea gives rise to a greater probability of an IOP being overestimated (or in the case of a thin cornea, of IOP being underestimated) but the extent of measurement error in individual patients cannot be determined from CCT alone. No generalized 'correction nomogram' can ever adequately adjust IOP without knowing much more about the individual cornea being applanated.

Given our limited understanding of how CCT and corneal material properties affect both tonometry and glaucoma risk, how should the thoughtful clinician incorporate these measures into direct patient care? One practical recommendation is that one can take far better care of patients simply by categorizing corneas as 'thin,' 'average,' or 'thick,' just as it is important to recognize that optic discs come in 'small,'' medium,' and 'large,' allowing the clinician to interpret disc configurations accordingly. Measuring CCT leads to the discontinuation of therapy in many overtreated ocular hypertensives and escalation of therapy in patients with thin corneas in whom control is clearly inadequate. Ultimately, incorporating the measurement of CCT and corneal material properties (and recognizing the limitations of our present knowledge) into the glaucoma examination will allow the astute clinician to better target and titrate the treatment of glaucoma.

REFERENCES

1. Goldmann H, Schmidt T. Über applanationstonometrie. Ophthalmologica 1957; 134:221–242.

2. Ehlers N, Bramsen T, Sperling S. Applanation tonometry and central corneal thickness. Acta Ophthalmol (Copenh) 1975; 53(1):34–43.

3. Feltgen N, Leifert D, Funk J. Correlation between central corneal thickness, applanation tonometry, and direct intracameral IOP readings. Br J Ophthalmol 2001; 85(1):85–87.

4. Kohlhaas M, Boehm AG, Spoerl E, et al. Effect of central corneal thickness, corneal curvature, and axial length on applanation tonometry. Arch Ophthalmol 2006; 124(4):471–476.

5. La Rosa FA, Gross RL, Orengo-Nania S. Central corneal thickness of Caucasians and African Americans in glaucomatous and nonglaucomatous populations. Arch Ophthalmol 2001; 119(1):23–27.

6. Foster PJ, Baasanhu J, Alsbirkm PH, et al. Central corneal thickness and intraocular pressure in a Mongolian population. Ophthalmology 1998; 105(6):969–973.

7. Brandt JD, Beiser JA, Kass MA, et al. Central corneal thickness in the Ocular Hypertension Treatment Study (OHTS). Ophthalmology 2001; 108(10):1779–1788.

8. Ehlers N, Hansen FK. Central corneal thickness in low-tension glaucoma. Acta Ophthalmol (Copenh) 1974; 52(5):740–746.

9. Copt RP, Thomas R, Mermoud A. Corneal thickness in ocular hypertension, primary open-angle glaucoma, and normal tension glaucoma [see comments]. Arch Ophthalmol 1999; 117(1):14–16.

10. Kass MA, Heuer DK, Higginbotham EJ, et al. The Ocular Hypertension Treatment Study: a randomized trial determines that topical ocular hypotensive medication delays or prevents the onset of primary open-angle glaucoma. Arch Ophthalmol 2002; 120(6):701–713.

11. Gordon MO, Beiser JA, Brandt JD, et al. The Ocular Hypertension Treatment Study: baseline factors that predict the onset of primary open-angle glaucoma. Arch Ophthalmol 2002; 120(6):714–720.

12. Miglior S, Pfeiffer N, Torri V, et al. Predictive factors for open-angle glaucoma among patients with ocular hypertension in the European Glaucoma Prevention Study. Ophthalmology 2007; 114(1):3–9.

13. Pfeiffer N, Torri V, Miglior S, et al. Central corneal thickness in the European Glaucoma Prevention Study. Ophthalmology 2007; 114(3):454–459.

14. Gordon MO, Torri V, Miglior S, et al. Validated prediction model for the development of primary open-angle glaucoma in individuals with ocular hypertension. Ophthalmology 2007; 114(1):10–19.

15. Medeiros FA, Sample PA, Weinreb RN. Corneal thickness measurements and visual function abnormalities in ocular hypertensive patients. Am J Ophthalmol 2003; 135(2):131–137.

16. Medeiros FA, Sample PA, Weinreb RN. Corneal thickness measurements and frequency doubling technology perimetry abnormalities in ocular hypertensive eyes. Ophthalmology 2003; 110(10):1903–1908.

17. Herndon LW, Weizerm JS, Stinnett SS. Central corneal thickness as a risk factor for advanced glaucoma damage. Arch Ophthalmol 2004; 122(1):17–21.

18. Jonas JB, Stroux A, Velten I, et al. Central corneal thickness correlated with glaucoma damage and rate of progression. Invest Ophthalmol Vis Sci 2005; 46(4):1269–1274.

19. Congdon NG, Broman AT, Bandeen-Roche K, et al. Central corneal thickness and corneal hysteresis associated with glaucoma damage. Am J Ophthalmol 2006; 141(5):868–875.

20. Kniestedt C, Lin S, Choe J, et al. Correlation between intraocular pressure, central corneal thickness, stage of glaucoma, and demographic patient data: prospective analysis of biophysical parameters in tertiary glaucoma practice populations. J Glaucoma 2006; 15(2):91–97.

21. Hong S, Kim CY, Seong GJ, et al. Central corneal thickness and visual field progression in patients with chronic primary angle-closure glaucoma with low intraocular pressure. Am J Ophthalmol 2007; 143(2):362–363.

22. Rogers DL, Cantor RN, Catoira Y, et al. Central corneal thickness and visual field loss in fellow eyes of patients with open-angle glaucoma. Am J Ophthalmol 2007; 143(1):159–161.

23. Nemesure B, Wu SY, Hennis A, et al. Corneal thickness and intraocular pressure in the Barbados Eye Studies. Arch Ophthalmol 2003; 121(2):240–244.

24. Shimmyo M, Ross AJ, Moy A, et al. Intraocular pressure, Goldmann applanation tension, corneal thickness, and corneal curvature in Caucasians, Asians, Hispanics, and African Americans. Am J Ophthalmol 2003; 136(4):603–613.

25. Hahn S, Azen S, Ying-Lai M, et al. Central corneal thickness in Latinos. Invest Ophthalmol Vis Sci 2003; 44(4):1508–1512.

26. Leske MC, Heijl A, Hyman L, et al. Early Manifest Glaucoma Trial: design and baseline data. Ophthalmology 1999; 106(11):2144–2153.

27. Leske MC, Heijl A, Hussein M, et al. Factors for glaucoma progression and the effect of treatment: the Early Manifest Glaucoma Trial. Arch Ophthalmol 2003; 121(1):48–56.

28. Leske MC, Heijl A, Hyman L, et al. Predictors of long-term progression in the Early Manifest Glaucoma Trial. Ophthalmology 2007; 114(11):1965–1972.

29. Brandt JD. Central corneal thickness – tonometry artifact, or something more? Ophthalmology 2007; 114(11):1963–1964.

30. Liu J, Roberts CJ. Influence of corneal biomechanical properties on intraocular pressure measurement: quantitative analysis. J Cataract Refract Surg 2005; 31(1):146–155.

31. Jue B, Maurice DM. The mechanical properties of the rabbit and human cornea. J Biomech 1986; 19(10):847–853.

32. Hoeltzel DA, Altman P, Buzard K, et al. Strip extensiometry for comparison of the mechanical response of bovine, rabbit, and human corneas. J Biomech Eng 1992; 114(2):202–215.

33. Schwartz NJ, Mackay RS, Sackman JL. A theoretical and experimental study of the mechanical behavior of the cornea with application to the measurement of the intraocular pressure. Bull Math Biol 1966; 28:585–643.

34. Sommer A. Glaucoma risk factors observed in the Baltimore Eye Survey. Curr Opin Ophthalmol 1996; 7(2):93–98.

35. Sommer A, Tielsch JM, Katz J, et al. Relationship between intraocular pressure and primary open angle glaucoma among white and black Americans. The Baltimore Eye Survey. Arch Ophthalmol 1991; 109(8):1090–1095.

36. Leske MC, Connell AM, Wu SY, et al. Distribution of intraocular pressure. The Barbados Eye Study. Arch Ophthalmol 1997; 115(8):1051–1057.

37. Klein BE, Klein R, Linton KL. Intraocular pressure in an American community. The Beaver Dam Eye Study. Invest Ophthalmol Vis Sci 1992; 33(7):2224–2228.

38. Luce DA. Determining in vivo biomechanical properties of the cornea with an ocular response analyzer. J Cataract Refract Surg 2005; 31(1):156–162.

39. Chang DH, Stulting RD. Change in intraocular pressure measurements after LASIK: the effect of the refractive correction and the lamellar flap. Ophthalmology 2005; 112(6):1009–1016.

40. Pepose JS, Feigenbaum SK, Qazi MA, et al. Changes in corneal biomechanics and intraocular pressure following LASIK using static, dynamic, and noncontact tonometry. Am J Ophthalmol 2007; 143(1):39–47.

41. Orssengo GJ, Pye DC. Determination of the true intraocular pressure and modulus of elasticity of the human cornea in vivo. Bull Math Biol 1999; 61:551–572.

CHAPTER 17

Optic Disc Photography in the Diagnosis of Glaucoma

Jost B Jonas

INTRODUCTION

The photography of the optic disc consists of the clinical ophthalmoscopic examination of the optic nerve head, the peripapillary region, and the retinal nerve fiber layer under optimal examination conditions since the optic disc is not moving as in normal clinical situations and because the photographs can be examined for an unlimited amount of time. The photographic or clinical ophthalmoscopic examination of the optic nerve head includes the assessment of the classical morphologic signs of glaucomatous optic neuropathy. These characteristics can be evaluated using the optic nerve head variables: size and shape of the optic disc; size, shape, and pallor of the neuroretinal rim; size of the optic cup in relation to the area of the disc; configuration and depth of the optic cup; cup-to-disc diameter ratio and cup-to-disc area ratio; position of the exit of the central retinal vessel trunk on the lamina cribrosa surface; presence and location of splinter-shaped hemorrhages; occurrence, size, configuration, and location of peripapillary chorioretinal atrophy; diffuse and/or focal decrease of the diameter of the retinal arterioles; and visibility of the retinal nerve fiber layer.[1] The assessment of these variables is useful for the early detection of glaucomatous optic nerve damage, to follow up patients with glaucoma, to differentiate various types of the chronic open-angle glaucomas, and to get hints for the pathogenesis of glaucomatous optic nerve fiber loss.[2–27]

OPTIC DISC SIZE

The optic disc area is not constant among individuals but shows an interindividual variability of about 1:7 in a normal Caucasian population (Figs 17.1–17.3).[1,14,22] There are normal eyes with rather small optic discs, and there are normal eyes with very large optic discs. The optic disc area is mostly independent of age beyond an age of about 3 to 10 years, gender, and body length.[1] Within a range of −5 to +5 diopters of refractive error, optic disc size was statistically mostly independent of ametropia. Optic disc size is significantly larger in eyes with high myopia and it is significantly smaller in

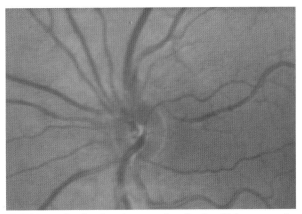

FIGURE 17.1 Small, otherwise normal, optic disc. Note: no cupping; due to the smallness of the optic disc physiologic unsharpness and slight prominence of the disc border; no parapapillary atrophy; unremarkable diameter of the retinal arterioles.

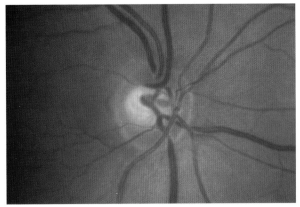

FIGURE 17.2 Medium-sized normal optic disc with circular steep cupping (also in the temporal disc region). Note: physiologic shape of the neuroretinal rim (ISNT rule); medium size of the optic cup in physiologic relation to the size of the optic disc; no parapapillary atrophy; unremarkable diameter of the retinal arterioles; good visibility of the retinal nerve fiber layer.

eyes with marked hyperopia (more than +5 D) than in eyes with a normal refractive error.[1] Size of the optic disc depends on race. Caucasians have relatively small optic discs, followed by Mexicans, Asians, and Afro-Americans.[1,22] One may infer that disc size increases

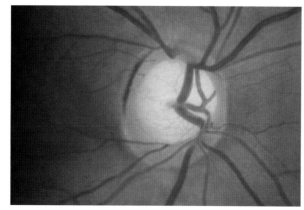

FIGURE 17.3 Large normal optic disc with circular steep cupping (also in the temporal disc region) ('primary macrodisc'). Note: physiologic shape of the neuroretinal rim (ISNT rule); large size of the optic cup in physiologic relation to the size of the optic disc; depth of the optic cup deep; no parapapillary atrophy; unremarkable diameter of the retinal arterioles; average visibility of the retinal nerve fiber layer.

with the ethnically determined pigmentation. A study on Caucasians did not find a relationship between disc size and iris color, suggesting that, within an ethnic group, disc size and pigmentation are not related with each other.[1]

Based on the Gaussian-like distribution curve of the optic disc area, very small discs or 'microdiscs' and very large discs or 'macrodiscs' can be defined morphometrically: a microdisc is smaller than the mean minus two standard deviations, and a macrodisc can be defined as being larger than the mean plus two standard deviations. Beyond each of these limits only 2.3% of a standard population are statistically expected. The macrodiscs can be divided into primary macrodiscs and secondary acquired macrodiscs. The size of primary macrodiscs is independent of age after the first years of life, and is independent or only slightly dependent on refractive error. The primary macrodiscs can be subclassified into 'asymptomatic primary macrodiscs' without any morphologic or functional defects, and 'symptomatic primary macrodiscs' with morphologic and functional defects such as pits of the optic disc and the 'morning glory syndrome.' Primary macrodiscs are marginally correlated with the size of the cornea: the larger the optic disc is, the larger is the cornea and the larger is the anterior corneal curvature radius. In contrast to the primary macrodiscs, the acquired or secondary macrodiscs increase in size after birth and occur in eyes with high myopia. They can further be subclassified into eyes with primary high myopia due to reasons yet unknown and eyes with secondary high myopia due to congenital glaucoma. In both subtypes of secondary macrodiscs, disc size is positively correlated with the myopic refractive error. Since the myopic refractive error can increase with age in highly myopic patients, the size of secondary macrodiscs in highly myopic eyes partially increases with age.[1]

The interindividual variability in optic disc size is morphogenetically and pathogenetically important. It is morphogenetically important because eyes with large optic discs as compared to eyes with small optic nerve heads have a larger neuroretinal rim area, more optic nerve fibers, less nerve fiber crowding per square millimeter of disc area, a higher count and a larger total area of lamina cribrosa pores, a higher ratio of interpore connective tissue area to total lamina cribrosa area, a higher count of cilioretinal arteries, and a higher count of retinal photoreceptors and retinal pigment epithelium cells in combination with a larger retinal surface area and longer horizontal and vertical diameters of the globe.[1,15] The optic disc size variability is pathogenetically important because some optic nerve anomalies and diseases are correlated with the optic disc size. Optic disc drusen, pseudopapilledema, and nonarteritic anterior ischemic optic neuropathy occur significantly more often in small optic discs. Pits of the optic disc and the morning glory syndrome are more common in large optic nerve heads. Eyes with arteritic anterior ischemic optic neuropathy and eyes with retinal vessel occlusions have optic discs with a statistically normal size.[1]

In glaucoma, the optic disc is normal in size in primary open-angle glaucoma, including the juvenile-onset type of primary open-angle glaucoma, the age-related atrophic type of primary open-angle glaucoma, and in secondary open-angle glaucoma due to primary melanin dispersion syndrome ('pigmentary glaucoma'). Two studies suggested that in secondary open-angle glaucoma due to pseudoexfoliation of the lens ('pseudoexfoliative glaucoma') the optic disc is slightly smaller than in primary open-angle glaucoma. This finding, however, can be due to a bias in the selection of the patients. In all glaucoma eyes with high myopia, including the highly myopic type of primary open-angle glaucoma, the optic disc is abnormally large. These secondary macrodiscs are considered to be acquired due to the myopic stretching of the posterior fundus pole.[1] In the diagnosis of glaucomatous optic neuropathy, assessment of the optic disc size is of utmost importance since the optic disc size is correlated with the size of the optic cup and neuroretinal rim. The larger the optic disc is, the larger are the optic cup and neuroretinal rim. A large cup in a large optic disc can, therefore, be normal, while a small optic cup in a very small optic disc suggests glaucomatous optic nerve damage.[1]

OPTIC DISC SHAPE

The optic disc has a slightly vertically oval form with the vertical diameter being about 7% to 10% larger than the horizontal one.[1] The maximal disc diameter is nearly identical with the vertical diameter and the horizontal diameter is almost equal to the minimal diameter. The ratio between minimal-to-maximal disc diameter ranged in previous investigations between 0.64 and 0.98, corresponding to an interindividual variability of 1:1.53. The ratio between the horizontal-to-vertical disc diameters varied between 0.70 and 1.37 (variability of 1:1.96). It shows that, just by numbers, the interindividual variability in optic disc shape measured by the ratio of horizontal-to-vertical disc diameter and the ratio of minimal-to-maximal disc diameter is less marked than the interindividual variability in area of the optic disc.

The disc form is not correlated with age, sex, and right and left eye, and body weight and height. An abnormal optic disc shape is significantly correlated with increased corneal astigmatism and amblyopia. In some studies, the amount of corneal astigmatism was significantly correlated ($p < 0.001$) with an increasingly elongated optic disc shape. Corneal astigmatism was significantly highest ($p < 0.01$) in eyes with tilted discs. It was significantly smallest ($p = 0.006$) in eyes with an almost circular disc shape. Amblyopia was significantly associated ($p < 0.05$) with an elongated optic disc shape and high corneal astigmatism. Especially in young children, if an optic disc with abnormal shape is found in routine ophthalmoscopy, keratometry or skiascopy should be performed to rule out corneal astigmatism and to prevent amblyopia. The orientation of the longest disc diameter can indicate the axis of corneal astigmatism. Furthermore, eyes with a tilted optic disc can exhibit visual field defects mimicking a temporal hemianopsia which may be due to, or may be associated with, a hypopigmentation of the fundus in the nasal inferior fundus region.[1]

In individuals with a myopic refractive error of less than -8 diopters, normal eyes and glaucoma eyes do not differ significantly in optic disc shape ($p > 0.20$).[1] Within the primary open-angle glaucoma group, optic disc shape is not correlated with neuroretinal rim area and mean perimetric defect, neither interindividually nor in an intraindividual bilateral comparison. It suggests that the glaucoma susceptibility is mostly independent of the shape of the optic disc. As a single variable, the optic disc shape is not markedly important for diagnosis and pathogenesis of glaucoma. This is valid for eyes with a myopic refractive error of less than -8 diopters. Considering the relationship between distance of the central retinal vessel trunk exit on the lamina cribrosa and location of glaucomatous neuroretinal rim loss, however, evaluation of the optic shape becomes important since the optic disc shape influences the distance between neuroretinal rim at the disc border and central retinal vessel trunk.[1]

In highly myopic eyes, the optic disc is significantly more oval and more elongated in configuration, and more obliquely oriented than in any other group (Fig. 17.4).[1] The abnormal shape of the optic disc is significantly more pronounced ($p < 0.05$) in eyes with a myopic refractive error of more than -12 diopters than in eyes with a refractive error ranging between -8 diopters and -12 diopters. It suggests that the myopic stretching leading to the secondary macrodisc in highly myopic eyes does not exert a similar traction on the optic disc in all directions but that the optic disc is drawn stronger in some meridians compared to others. One may speculate whether the marked and irregular stretching of the optic disc in highly myopic eyes is one of the factors why some of these eyes have a relatively high susceptibility for glaucomatous optic nerve fiber loss, as shown by glaucomatous optic nerve damage in the presence of normal intraocular pressure measurements.[1]

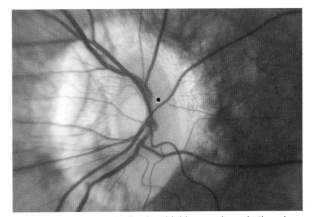

FIGURE 17.4 Large optic disc in a highly myopic and otherwise normal eye ('secondary macrodisc'). Note: abnormal disc shape; shallow disc cupping; physiologic shape of the neuroretinal rim (ISNT rule).

NEURORETINAL RIM SIZE

As the intrapapillary equivalent of the retinal nerve fibers and optic nerve fibers, the neuroretinal rim is one of the main targets in the ophthalmoscopic evaluation of the optic nerve.[1,3–6,12,22,25] The neuroretinal rim size is not interindividually constant but shows, similar to the optic disc and cup, a considerably high interindividual variability. It is correlated with the optic disc area: the larger the disc, the larger the rim. The increase of rim area with enlarging disc area is most marked for eyes with no disc cupping, medium pronounced for eyes with a temporal flat sloping of the optic cup, and it is least marked in eyes with a circular, steep disc cupping. The correlation between rim area and disc area corresponds with the positive correlation between optic disc size, optic nerve fiber count, and number and total area of the lamina cribrosa pores. It points towards a greater anatomic reserve capacity in eyes with large optic discs as compared to eyes with small optic discs.[1,15] Possible reasons for the interindividual size variability of the rim are a different nerve fiber count, a different relation between embryologically formed and regressed retinal ganglion cell axons, different density of nerve fibers within the optic disc, different lamina cribrosa architecture, different diameters of retinal ganglion cell axons, different proportion of glial cells on the whole intrapapillary tissue, and/or other factors. The nerve fibers within the neuroretinal rim are retinotopically arranged. Studies have shown that axons from ganglion cells close to the optic disc lie more centrally in the optic disc while axons from cells in the retinal periphery lie at the optic nerve head margins. It corresponds to the nerve fiber distribution in the retinal nerve fiber layer.

Due to its high interindividual variability of the rim area in the normal population, the overlap between normal subjects and patients with early glaucomatous optic nerve damage is high.[1,3–6,12,22,25] This is the disadvantage of many quantitative variables. To achieve a higher diagnostic power, the neuroretinal rim measured in the whole optic disc can be broken up into disc sectors, with the inferotemporal and superotemporal disc sectors having a higher predictive power than the neuroretinal rim as a whole. The reason is the preferential loss of neuroretinal rim in the inferior and superior disc regions in the early to medium-advanced stages of the disease.[1]

NEURORETINAL RIM SHAPE

In normal eyes, the neuroretinal rim shows a characteristic configuration (see Figs 17.1–17.3).[1] It is based on the vertically oval shape of the optic disc and the horizontally oval shape of the optic cup. The neuroretinal rim is usually broadest in the *Inferior* disc region, followed by the *Superior* disc region, the *Nasal* disc area, and finally the *Temporal* disc region (*ISNT* rule). The characteristic shape of the rim is of utmost importance in the diagnosis of early glaucomatous optic nerve damage in ocular hypertensive eyes prior to the development of visual field defects in white-on-white perimetry.[1] The physiologic shape of the neuroretinal rim is associated with the diameter of the retinal arterioles, which are significantly wider in the inferotemporal arcade than in the superotemporal arcade; the visibility of the retinal nerve fiber bundles that are significantly more often better detectable in the inferotemporal region than in the superotemporal region; the location of the foveola $0.53 \pm 0.34\,mm$ inferior to the optic disc center; the morphology of the lamina cribrosa with the largest pores and relatively the least amount of interpore connective tissue in the inferior and superior regions as compared to the temporal and nasal sectors; and the distribution of the thin and thick nerve fibers in the optic nerve just behind the globe with the thin fibers in the temporal part of the nerve. Although the neuroretinal rim is broadest in the inferior part of the optic disc, the neuroretinal rim area above a horizontal line drawn through the center of the foveola is larger than below this line. It is explainable by the location of the foveal center temporal inferior to the optic disc, and by the location of the blind spot temporal inferior to the fixation center in the visual field. It corresponds to the higher differential light sensitivity in perimetry in the inferior visual field than in the superior visual hemisphere.[1]

In glaucoma, neuroretinal rim is lost in all sectors of the optic disc with regional preferences depending on the stage of the disease (Fig. 17.5).[1,3–6,12,22,25] In eyes with modest glaucomatous damage, rim loss is found predominantly at the inferotemporal and superotemporal disc regions. In eyes with moderately advanced glaucomatous atrophy, the temporal horizontal disc region is the location with relatively the most marked rim loss. In very advanced glaucoma, the rim remnants are located mainly in the nasal disc sector, with a larger rim portion in the upper nasal region than in the lower nasal region. This sequence of disc sectors (inferotemporal – superotemporal – temporal horizontal – nasal

inferior – nasal superior) correlates with the progression of visual field defects with early perimetric changes in the nasal upper quadrant of the visual field and a last island of vision in the temporal inferior part of the visual field in eyes with almost absolute glaucoma. It indicates that for an early diagnosis of glaucoma, especially the temporal inferior and the temporal superior disc sectors should be checked for glaucomatous changes. It should be kept in mind, however, that the glaucomatous loss of neuroretinal rim is mostly diffuse, occurring in all sectors of the optic disc with some preferential locations for a slightly more pronounced damage depending on the stage of the disease.

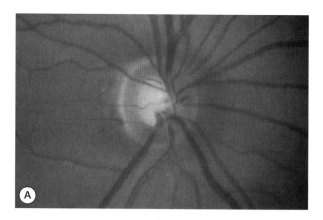

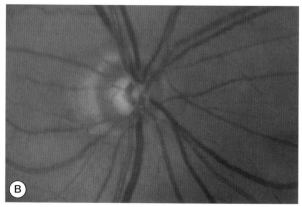

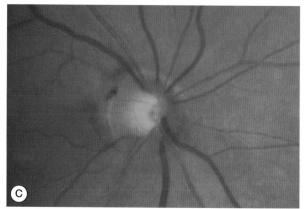

FIGURE 17.5 (A–C) Glaucomatous optic discs with abnormal shape of the neuroretinal rim: the rim width is more or less even in all disc sectors, which contradicts the ISNT rule. In **(C)**: additional localized retinal nerve fiber layer defect at 11 o'clock.

Previous studies have shown that factors which may be associated with the pattern of glaucomatous neuroretinal rim loss are:

- The physiologic configuration of the rim, being broader at the inferior and superior disc poles than at the nasal and temporal poles.
- The morphology of the inner surface of the lamina cribrosa with the larger pores and the higher ratio of pore to interpore connective tissue area in the inferior and superior regions as compared to the temporal and nasal regions; a high ratio of pore area to total area is considered to predispose to glaucomatous nerve fiber loss.
- The glaucomatous backward bowing of the lamina cribrosa to the outside mainly in the inferior and superior disc regions, as shown on scanning electron microscopic photographs of glaucomatous eyes.
- The anatomy of the lamina cribrosa, which is thicker in the disc periphery where the nerve fiber bundles have a slightly more bent course through the lamina cribrosa and where they are lost earlier than in the center of the optic disc.
- The regional distribution of thin and thick retinal nerve fibers with thin nerve fibers coming from the foveola, passing mainly through the temporal aspect of the optic disc and being less glaucoma susceptible than thick nerve fibers which originate predominantly in the fundus periphery, lead to the inferior, superior, and nasal disc regions and are more glaucoma sensitive. It may explain why glaucomatous rim loss occurs later in the temporal horizontal disc sector with predominantly thin nerve fibers than in the temporal inferior or temporal superior disc sectors containing thin and thick axons. It is a contradiction that in far advanced glaucoma, rim remnants are usually located in the nasal disc sector. There, preferentially thick retinal ganglion cell axons leave the eye.
- The distance from the central retinal vessel trunk exit on the lamina cribrosa is an additional parameter for the pattern of glaucomatous rim loss. The larger the distance to the central retinal vessel trunk exit on the lamina cribrosa, the more pronounced is the loss of neuroretinal rim and the perimetric defect in the corresponding visual field quadrant. Taking into account the slightly eccentric location of the retinal vessel trunk in the nasal upper quadrant of the vertically oval optic disc, one can infer that the progressive sequence of rim loss in glaucoma is partially dependent upon the distance of the region to the retinal vessel trunk; the further away the region from the retinal vessel trunk, the more likely it is to be affected by rim loss. As a corollary, glaucoma eyes with an atypical location of the retinal vessel trunk or an unusual optic disc form were found to exhibit an abnormal glaucomatous rim configuration.[1]

In contrast to glaucomatous optic neuropathy, nonglaucomatous optic nerve damage is not always associated with a loss of neuroretinal rim. Consequently, the shape of the neuroretinal rim is not markedly altered.[1]

NEURORETINAL RIM PALLOR

Increasing pallor of the optic disc, and especially of the neuroretinal rim, is a typical sign of optic nerve damage. The increase in pallor of the neuroretinal rim may be more marked in eyes with nonglaucomatous optic neuropathy than in eyes with glaucoma. In other words, if the neuroretinal rim looks rather pale, the probability for a nonglaucomatous optic neuropathy is higher than for glaucoma. Pallor of the neuroretinal rim is thus one among other variables to differentiate between glaucomatous versus nonglaucomatous optic neuropathy. In glaucoma, the overall pallor of the optic disc increases as the sum of optic cup and neuroretinal rim increases mainly due to the enlargement of the optic cup.

OPTIC CUP SIZE IN RELATION TO THE OPTIC DISC SIZE

Parallel to the optic disc and the neuroretinal rim, the optic cup also shows a high interindividual variability (Fig. 17.6; also see Figs 17.1–17.3).[1,3–6,12,22,25] In normal eyes, the areas of the optic disc and optic cup are correlated with each other: the larger the optic disc, the larger the optic cup. In the morphologic diagnosis of glaucoma, this feature has to be taken into account. Early or moderately advanced glaucomatous optic nerve damage may erroneously be overlooked in small optic discs with relatively low cup-to-disc ratios, if one does not take into account that small optic discs normally have no optic cup. The glaucomatous eyes with small optic discs and pseudonormal but glaucomatous minicups often show glaucomatous abnormalities in the peripapillary region such as a decreased visibility of the retinal nerve fiber layer, diffusely and/or focally diminished diameter of the retinal arterioles, and peripapillary chorioretinal atrophy. In contrast, a large optic cup in a large optic disc should not lead to the diagnosis of glaucoma, if the other intrapapillary variables are normal, the main configuration of the neuroretinal rim.

In contrast to glaucoma, the optic cup does not markedly enlarge in eyes with nonglaucomatous optic nerve

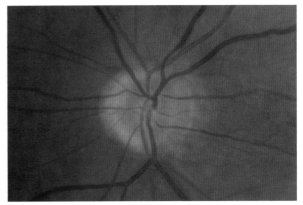

FIGURE 17.6 Small glaucomatous optic disc (left eye): pseudonormal but glaucomatous minicupping in minidisc. Note: small optic cup despite the smallness of the optic disc; abnormal shape of the neuroretinal rim (contradicting ISNT rule); decreased visibility of the retinal nerve fiber layer.

damage.[1] Correspondingly, the neuroretinal rim does not pronouncedly decrease in eyes with nonglaucomatous optic nerve damage. Besides peripapillary atrophy, disc pallor, and depth of the optic cup, the increase in cup area is thus an important marker to differentiate between glaucomatous and nonglaucomatous optic nerve damage.

CONFIGURATION AND DEPTH OF THE OPTIC CUP

In normal eyes, the shape of the optic cup is horizontally oval with the horizontal diameter being about 8% longer than the vertical diameter. Combining the horizontally oval shape of the optic cup and the vertically oval shape of the optic disc explains the configuration of the normal neuroretinal rim, which has its broadest parts in the inferior and superior disc regions and its smallest parts in the temporal and nasal region of the optic disc. Other than by its area, the optic cup is ophthalmoscopically described by its depth. In normal eyes, the optic cup depth depends on the cup area, and indirectly on the disc size. The larger the optic cup, the deeper it is. In glaucoma, the optic cup deepens dependent on the type of glaucoma and the level of intraocular pressure. Semiquantitative studies have shown that the deepest optic cups can be found in glaucoma eyes with high minimal values of intraocular pressure such as juvenile-onset primary open-angle glaucoma and secondary open-angle glaucoma due to traumatic recession of the anterior chamber angle. Considering all types of the open-angle glaucomas, the optic cup is most shallow in eyes with the highly myopic type of primary open-angle glaucoma and eyes with the age-related atrophic type of primary open-angle glaucoma. In glaucoma, the depth of the optic cup is slightly associated with the degree of peripapillary atrophy. The deeper the optic cup, the smaller is the peripapillary atrophy. This holds true especially for the juvenile-onset type of primary open-angle glaucoma with high minimal and maximal intraocular pressure measurements, and for the focal type of normal-pressure glaucoma. Both types of glaucoma can show relatively steep and deep disc cupping and an almost unremarkable peripapillary atrophy.

CUP-TO-DISC RATIOS

Due to the vertically oval optic disc and the horizontally oval optic cup, the cup-to-disc ratios in normal eyes are significantly larger horizontally than vertically (see Figs 17.1–17.3, 17.5).[1,3–6,12,22,25] In less than 7% of normal eyes the horizontal cup-to-disc ratio is smaller than the vertical one, i.e. the quotient of the horizontal-to-vertical cup-to-disc ratios is usually higher than 1.0. It is important for the diagnosis of glaucoma, in which, in the early to medium-advanced stages, the vertical cup-to-disc diameter ratio increases faster than the horizontal one, leading to an increase of the quotient of horizontal-to-vertical cup-to-disc ratios to values lower than 1.0.

As ratio of cup diameter to disc diameter, the cup-to-disc ratios depend on the size of the optic disc and cup. The high interindividual variability of the optic disc and cup diameters determines that the cup-to-disc ratios range in a normal population between 0.0 and almost 0.9. Due to the correlation between disc area and cup area, they are low in small optic nerve heads, and they are high in large optic discs. An unusually high cup-to-disc ratio, therefore, can be physiologic in eyes with large optic nerve heads, while an average cup-to-disk ratio is uncommon in normal eyes with small optic discs. In the diagnosis of glaucomatous optic nerve damage, this interindividual variability of cup-to-disc ratios and their dependence on the optic disc size has to be taken into account. Eyes with physiologically high cup-to-disc ratios in macrodiscs should not be overdiagnosed and should not be considered to be glaucomatous, and eyes with increased intraocular pressure, small optic nerve heads, and average or low cup-to-disc ratios should not be underdiagnosed and regarded to be only 'ocular hypertensive.' Using an optic disc grid may be helpful for the estimation of the cup-to-disc ratios.

As ratio of cup diameter to disc diameter, the cup-to-disc ratios are independent of the magnification by the optic media of the examined eye and of the fundus camera or other instrument. It indicates that methods to correct for the ocular and camera magnification do not have to be applied. The quotient of the horizontal-to-vertical cup-to-disc ratios is additionally independent of the size of the optic cup and disc.

POSITION OF THE EXIT OF THE CENTRAL RETINAL VESSEL TRUNK ON THE LAMINA CRIBROSA SURFACE

As already pointed out, the local susceptibility for glaucomatous neuroretinal rim loss partially depends on the distance to the exit of the central retinal vessel trunk on the lamina cribrosa surface.[1] The longer the distance to the central retinal vessel trunk exit, the more marked can be the glaucomatous loss of neuroretinal rim and the loss of visual field in the corresponding visual field quadrant (Fig. 17.7). The location of the central retinal

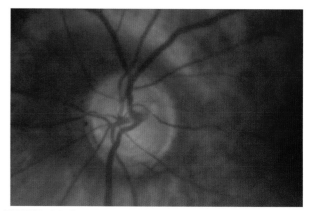

FIGURE 17.7 Glaucomatous optic disc (left eye) with abnormal shape of the neuroretinal rim (broadest part in the temporal superior disc region) and abnormal position of the central retinal vessel trunk exit in the temporal superior disc sector. Note: parapapillary atrophy is largest in the nasal region in spatial correlation to the most marked neuroretinal rim loss in the nasal disc sector.

vessel trunk exit can therefore be one of several factors influencing the local susceptibility for glaucomatous optic nerve fiber loss within the region of the optic disc. In a parallel manner, another investigation showed that open-angle glaucoma eyes with a temporal cilioretinal artery retained longer central visual field (and temporal neuroretinal rim) than open-angle glaucoma eyes without a temporal cilioretinal artery. The location of the central retinal vessel trunk exit on the lamina cribrosa and an abnormal shape of the optic disc should therefore be noted in glaucomatous eyes with an unusual configuration of the neuroretinal rim.[1]

The relationship between distance to the central retinal vessel trunk exit and location of glaucomatous damage may be valid also for peripapillary atrophy. A recent study found that the longer was the distance to the central retinal vessel trunk exit, the more enlarged was peripapillary atrophy in glaucomatous eyes compared with normal eyes. These findings agree with the spatial relationship between glaucomatous neuroretinal rim loss inside of the optic disc and enlargement of peripapillary atrophy outside of the optic disc border.[1]

OPTIC DISC HEMORRHAGES

Splinter-shaped or flame-shaped hemorrhages at the border of the optic disc are a hallmark of glaucomatous optic nerve atrophy.[1,12] Rarely or very rarely found in normal eyes, disc hemorrhages are detected in about 4–7% of eyes with glaucoma. Their frequency increases from an early stage of glaucoma to a medium-advanced stage and decreases again towards a far advanced stage. One study suggested that disc hemorrhages are not found in disc regions or eyes without detectable neuroretinal rim. In early glaucoma, they are usually located in the inferotemporal or superotemporal disc regions. They are associated with localized retinal nerve fiber layer defects, neuroretinal rim notches, and circumscribed perimetric loss.

In recent population-based studies, optic disc hemorrhages were detected in about 1.2% of subjects. The occurrence of disc hemorrhages was significantly associated with glaucomatous optic nerve damage ($p < 0.001$) and age ($p = 0.008$). About 19% of the disc hemorrhages were found in glaucomatous eyes, and about 9% of the glaucomatous eyes showed a disc hemorrhage. Hypertensive glaucoma eyes and normotensive glaucoma eyes did not vary significantly in frequency of disc hemorrhages ($p = 0.44$).[28]

Since frequency of optic disc hemorrhages differs between the various types of the open-angle glaucomas, assessment of disc bleedings can be helpful for classification of the glaucoma type. Disc hemorrhages were found most often in patients with focal normal-pressure glaucoma. Frequency of detected disc bleedings was lower in patients with juvenile-onset primary open-glaucoma, age-related atrophic primary open-angle glaucoma, and highly myopic primary open-angle glaucoma. Disc hemorrhages, however, can be found in all types of the chronic open-angle glaucomas, suggesting that the pathomechanism associated with disc hemorrhages may be present in all these glaucoma types.

PERIPAPILLARY CHORIORETINAL ATROPHY

Ophthalmoscopically, the peripapillary chorioretinal atrophy can be divided into a central beta zone and a peripheral alpha zone (Fig. 17.8).[1,10,21,25,27] The peripheral zone (alpha zone) is characterized by an irregular hypopigmentation and hyperpigmentation and intimated thinning of the chorioretinal tissue layer. On its outer side it is adjacent to the retina, and on its inner side it is in touch with a zone characterized by visible sclera and visible large choroidal vessels (beta zone), or with the peripapillary scleral ring, respectively. Features of the inner zone (beta zone) are marked atrophy of the retinal pigment epithelium and of the choriocapillaris,

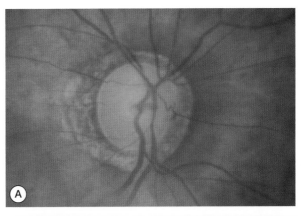

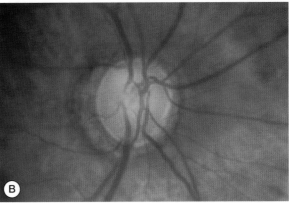

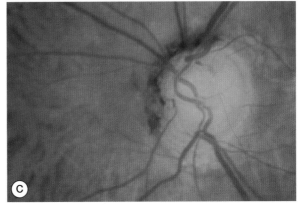

FIGURE 17.8 (A–C) Glaucomatous optic disc with parapapillary atrophy: alpha zone with irregular pigmentation (outer zone); beta zone with visible sclera and visible large choroidal vessels (adjacent to the peripapillary scleral ring).

good visibility of the large choroidal vessels and the sclera, thinning of the chorioretinal tissues, and round bounds to the adjacent alpha zone on its peripheral side and to the peripapillary scleral ring on its central side. If both zones are present, the beta zone is always closer to the optic disc than the alpha zone.

In indirect and direct clinical-histologic comparisons, the beta zone correlates with a complete loss of retinal pigment epithelium cells and a markedly diminished count of retinal photoreceptors.[1,13] The alpha zone is the equivalent of pigmentary irregularities in the retinal pigment epithelium. Correspondingly, the beta zone corresponds psychophysically to an absolute scotoma, and the alpha zone to a relative scotoma. It is unclear whether the observed thinning of the uvea in eyes with glaucoma suggesting a decreased uveal blood flow is pathogenetically connected with the development of peripapillary chorioretinal atrophy in glaucoma eyes. Indocyanine green angiography showed areas of hypofluorescence in the peripapillary region in late-phase angiograms in about two-third of eyes with glaucoma compared to 20% of control eyes. These hypofluorescent areas were theorized to be either the result of blockage of background fluorescence by pigment or caused by an absence of vascular tissue in the level of the choriocapillaris.

In normal eyes, both the alpha zone and the beta zone are largest and most frequently located in the temporal horizontal sector, followed by the inferior temporal area and the superior temporal region. They are smallest and most rarely found in the nasal peripapillary area. The alpha zone is present in almost all normal eyes and is thus more common than the beta zone (mean frequency in normal eyes: about 15–20%). The alpha zone and the beta zone have to be differentiated from the myopic scleral crescent in eyes with high myopia and from the inferior scleral crescent in eyes with 'tilted optic discs.' The myopic scleral crescent present in highly myopic eyes differs histologically from the glaucomatous beta zone in non-highly myopic eyes. In the region of the myopic crescent, only the inner limiting membrane and underlying retinal nerve fiber layer or its remnants cover the sclera while in the glaucomatous beta zone, Bruch's membrane and the choroid is interposed between the remnants of the retina and the sclera.[1]

Size, shape, and frequency of the alpha zone and the beta zone do not differ significantly between normal eyes and eyes with nonglaucomatous optic nerve atrophy. Both zones are significantly larger and the beta zone occurs more often in eyes with glaucomatous optic nerve atrophy than in normal eyes. Size of both zones and frequency of the beta zone are significantly correlated with variables indicating the severity of the glaucomatous optic nerve damage such as neuroretinal rim loss, decrease of retinal vessel diameter, reduced visibility of the retinal nerve fiber bundles, and perimetric defects. A large beta zone, also called 'halo glaucomatosus' when encircling the optic disc, is often associated with a marked degree of fundus tessellation, a shallow glaucomatous disc cupping, a relatively low frequency of disc hemorrhages and detectable localized defects of

the retinal nerve fiber layer, a mostly concentric loss of neuroretinal rim, and normal or almost normal intraocular pressure measurements. The location of peripapillary chorioretinal atrophy is spatially correlated with the neuroretinal rim loss in the intrapapillary region. It is larger in that sector, with the more marked loss of neuroretinal rim.

In clinical studies as well as in investigations on experimental high-pressure glaucoma in monkeys, side differences in peripapillary atrophy were significantly correlated with side differences in neuroretinal rim area and mean visual field defect.[1,10,21,25,27] In unilateral glaucoma, peripapillary atrophy was significantly larger and the beta zone was found significantly more often in the affected eyes than in the contralateral nonglaucomatous eyes. Eliminating the effect of systemic parameters such as age, arthrosclerosis, and arterial blood pressure in these intraindividual intereye comparisons, these correlations suggest an association between peripapillary chorioretinal atrophy and the degree of glaucomatous optic nerve atrophy. It agrees with significant correlations of increasing frequency and enlarging area of peripapillary atrophy with decreasing area of neuroretinal rim, diminishing visibility of retinal nerve fiber layer, increasing visual field defect, decreased temporal contrast sensitivity as determined by a full-field flicker test, and decreasing diameter of the retrobulbar part of the optic nerve as measured sonographically. In recent follow-up studies, progression of peripapillary atrophy, especially the beta zone, was described as an early glaucomatous finding in some patients with ocular hypertension. Accordingly, presence and size of peripapillary atrophy were related to the development of subsequent optic disc or visual field damage in ocular hypertensive patients. In a study on patients with normal-pressure glaucoma, disc hemorrhages were closely associated with the size of peripapillary atrophy, underlining the importance of peripapillary atrophy in the morphologic diagnosis of glaucomatous optic neuropathy.

In contrast to glaucomatous optic neuropathy, nonglaucomatous optic nerve damage does not lead to an enlargement of peripapillary atrophy. It indicates that peripapillary atrophy is one among other optic disc variables to differentiate between glaucomatous and nonglaucomatous optic nerve damage.

Parallel to the spatial association between position of the central retinal vessel trunk and the local loss of neuroretinal rim in the optic disc, a spatial correlation between the position of the central retinal vessel trunk exit in the lamina cribrosa and the location of peripapillary atrophy has been reported. The longer the distance to the central retinal vessel trunk, the larger is the beta zone. The pathogenetic explanation for this finding has remained unclear so far.

DIAMETER OF RETINAL ARTERIOLES

Diffuse narrowing of the retinal vessels has been described for glaucomatous and nonglaucomatous optic neuropathies.[1] In glaucoma, the vessel diameter reduces with decreasing area of the neuroretinal rim, diminishing visibility of the retinal nerve fiber layer, and increasing visual field defects. Since the reduction of the vessel caliber is also found in eyes with nonglaucomatous optic nerve damage such as descending optic nerve atrophy and nonarteritic anterior ischemic optic neuropathy, one inferred that a generalized reduction of the vessel diameter is typical for optic nerve damage but not characteristic for glaucoma. From a pathogenetic point of view, it suggests that vessel reduction is not causative for glaucomatous optic nerve fiber loss but is, at least partially, secondary to a reduced demand in the superficial layers of the retina.[1]

Besides diffuse narrowing, the retinal arterioles additionally show focal narrowing of their caliber in eyes with optic nerve damage such as nonarteritic anterior ischemic optic neuropathy and glaucoma. The degree of focal narrowing of the retinal arterioles increased significantly with age in normal eyes. It was significantly higher in eyes with an optic nerve atrophy than in normal eyes. Eyes with glaucoma and eyes with nonglaucomatous optic nerve damage did not vary significantly in the severity of focal narrowing. Focal arteriole narrowing was slightly more pronounced in eyes with normal-pressure glaucoma and eyes with nonarteritic anterior ischemic optic neuropathy than in other groups. These differences, however, were not marked. In the glaucoma group, the degree of focal narrowing of the retinal arterioles was significantly more pronounced if the optic nerve damage was more advanced. A recent study comparing fundus photographs and fluorescein angiograms with each other showed that focal narrowing of the retinal arterioles in the peripapillary region of eyes with optic neuropathies represented a real stenosis of the vessel lumen and was not due to an ophthalmoscopic artifact.[1]

EVALUATION OF THE RETINAL NERVE FIBER LAYER

In normal eyes, visibility of the retinal nerve fiber layer (RNFL) is regionally unevenly distributed.[1,2,5,9,11,12,16,17,26] Dividing the fundus into eight regions, the nerve fiber bundles are most visible in the temporal inferior sector, followed by the temporal superior area, the nasal superior region, and finally the nasal inferior sector. It is least visible in the superior, inferior, temporal horizontal, and nasal horizontal regions. Correspondingly, the diameters of the retinal arterioles are significantly widest at the temporal inferior disc border, followed by the temporal superior disc region, the nasal superior area, and finally the nasal inferior disc region. It is in agreement with the location of the foveola below a horizontal line drawn through the center of the optic disc, and with the configuration of the neuroretinal rim that is broadest at the temporal inferior disc border, followed by the temporal superior disc region. The sequence of the sectors concerning the best visibility of the RNFL correlates with the sectors' sequence in respect to rim configuration and retinal artery caliber. Physiologically,

it points towards an anatomical and nutritional relationship. Visibility of the RNFL decreases with age. This correlates with an age-related reduction of the optic nerve fiber count, with an annual loss of about 4000 to 5000 fibers per year out of an original population of approximately 1.4 million optic nerve fibers. These features of the normal RNFL are important for diagnosis of RNFL changes secondary to optic nerve damage in the diseased eye.

In 1973, Hoyt and co-workers were the first to report on the significance of localized RNFL defects in glaucomatous eyes.[2] Localized defects of the RNFL are defined as wedge-shaped and not spindle-like defects, running towards or touching the optic disc border. If they are pronounced, they can have a broad basis at the temporal raphe of the fundus. Typically occurring in about 20% or more of all glaucoma eyes, they can also be found in eyes with an atrophy of the optic nerve due to other reasons such as optic disc drusen, toxoplasmotic retinochoroidal scars, ischemic retinopathies with cotton-wool spots of the retina, after long-standing papilledema or optic neuritis due to multiple sclerosis, to mention some examples. Since the localized RNFL defects are not present in normal eyes, they almost always signify a pathological abnormality. This is important for subjects with ocular hypertension in which a localized RNFL defect points to an optic nerve damage even in the absence of perimetric abnormalities. One has to take into account, however, that localized RNFL defects are not pathognomonic for glaucoma since they occur also in other types of optic nerve atrophy. Due to their relatively low frequency in eyes with optic nerve damage, their sensitivity to indicate optic nerve atrophy is not very high.

In glaucomatous eyes, the frequency of localized RNFL defects increases significantly from an 'early' glaucoma stage, to a stage with medium-advanced glaucomatous damage, and decreases again to a stage with very marked glaucomatous changes. In eyes with very advanced optic nerve damage, they are usually no longer detectable due to the pronounced loss of nerve fibers in all fundus sectors. Localized RNFL defects are detected more often in eyes with the focal type of normal-pressure glaucoma than in eyes with the age-related atrophic type of open-angle glaucoma and the highly myopic type of open-angle glaucoma. In their vicinity at the optic disc border, one often finds notches of the neuroretinal rim, sometimes an optic disc hemorrhage, and a peripapillary chorioretinal atrophy which is relatively more marked in that sector than in other sectors. Localized RNFL defects are often found 6 to 8 weeks after an optic disc bleeding. They point towards a localized type of optic nerve damage.

With respect to different sectors of the fundus, localized RNFL defects are most often found in the temporal inferior sector followed by the temporal superior sector. In the nasal fundus region, localized RNFL defects are only rarely seen. This may be due to the fact that the RNFL in normal eyes is less detectable in the nasal fundus than in the temporal inferior and temporal superior fundus areas. In fundus areas, in which the RNFL physiologically is thin, localized defects are also harder to find than in areas with a thick RNFL. It is unclear whether the morphology of the lamina cribrosa, with larger pores in the inferior and superior sectors and smaller pores in the temporal and nasal regions, plays a role for the development of localized RNFL defects.

The importance of localized defects of the RNFL for the diagnosis of glaucoma has been shown in many studies. Airaksinen described clearly detectable wedge-shaped defects of the RNFL in eyes with increased intraocular pressure and normal visual field. Later, these eyes showed localized perimetric changes when the area of concern was especially examined.

Experimental studies have shown that localized RNFL defects can be detected ophthalmoscopically if more than 50% of the thickness of the retinal nerve fiber layer is lost. This can be explained by the 'sandwich' arrangement of the retinal nerve fiber bundles in the RNFL. The first glaucomatous defects concern mainly retinal ganglion cells close at the temporal raphe of the retina. Their axons are located in the deep and middle layer of the RNFL. If these axons are lost, the configuration of the surface of the RNFL is only slightly changed because the axons over the lost fibers still cover the defect under them. The localized RNFL defects have to be differentiated from slitlike or groovelike (pseudo-) defects that often do not extend to the optic disc border and that do not have a broad base close at the temporal raphe of the fundus. This includes a so-called cleavage of the RNFL that can mimic a true defect of the RNFL, especially in high myopia.

Besides localized RNFL defects, a diffuse loss of retinal nerve fibers occurs in eyes with damage to the optic nerve.[1,2] It leads to a decreased visibility of the RNFL. After sectioning of the optic nerve in the orbit of monkeys, Quigley et al. observed a disappearing of the visibility of the RNFL starting 1 month after the operation, and being complete 4 weeks later. Ophthalmoscopically, the diffuse RNFL loss is more difficult to detect than a localized defect. It is helpful to use the variable 'sequence of fundus sectors concerning the best RNFL visibility.' If one detects that in an eye without fundus irregularities the RNFL is markedly better detectable in the temporal superior fundus region than in the temporal inferior sector, it points towards a loss of RNFL mainly in the temporal inferior fundus region. This variable can be examined upon ophthalmoscopy without applying sophisticated techniques. It is also helpful to evaluate whether the retinal vessels are clearly and sharply detectable. The retinal vessels are normally embedded into the RNFL. In eyes with a diffuse RNFL loss, the retinal vessels are covered only by the inner limiting membrane, resulting in a better visibility and a sharper image of the large retinal vessels. This is an important variable in the diagnosis of optic nerve damage.

Considering its great importance in the assessment of anomalies and diseases of the optic nerve and taking into account the feasibility of its ophthalmoscopical evaluation, the retinal nerve fiber layer should be examined during every routine ophthalmoscopy.[1,2,5,9,11,12,16,17,26] This holds true particularly for patients with an early damage of the optic nerve. The importance to evaluate the RNFL is further exemplified in studies in which a glaucomatous damage of the optic nerve could be detected earlier by examination of the RNFL than by conventional computerized perimetry. It is of utmost importance for the detection of glaucoma in eyes with a pseudonormal but glaucomatous minicup in minidiscs, and it is useful to classify an eye with a pseudoglaucomatous but normal large cup in a large disc as normal. In eyes with advanced optic nerve atrophy, other examination techniques such as perimetry may be more helpful for the follow-up of the optic nerve damage.

REFERENCES

1. Jonas JB, Budde WM, Panda-Jonas S. Ophthalmoscopic evaluation of the optic nerve head. Surv Ophthalmol 1999; 43:293–320.

2. Hoyt WF, Frisén LL, Newman NM. Funduscopy of nerve fiber layer defects in glaucoma. Invest Ophthalmol 1973; 12:814–829.

3. Hitchings RA, Spaeth GL. The optic disc in glaucoma. I. Classification. Br J Ophthalmol 1976; 60:778–785.

4. Hitchings RA, Spaeth GL. The optic disc in glaucoma. II. Correlation of the appearance of the optic disc with the visual field. Br J Ophthalmol 1977; 61:107–113.

5. Sommer A, Pollack I, Maumenee AE. Optic disc parameters and onset of glaucomatous visual field loss. I. Methods and progressive changes in disc morphology. Arch Ophthalmol 1979; 97:1444–1448.

6. Airaksinen PJ, Mustonen E, Alanko HI. Optic disc haemorrhages – an analysis of stereophotographs and clinical data of 112 patients. Arch Ophthalmol 1981; 99:1795–1801.

7. Quigley HA, Addicks EM, Green WR, et al. Optic nerve damage in human glaucoma. II. The site of injury and susceptibility to damage. Arch Ophthalmol 1981; 99:635–649.

8. Quigley HA, Addicks EM, Green WR, et al. Optic nerve damage in human glaucoma. III. Quantitative correlation of nerve fiber loss and visual field defect in glaucoma, ischemic optic neuropathy, papilledema and toxic neuropathy. Arch Ophthalmol 1981; 100:135–146.

9. Quigley HA, Addicks EM. Quantitative studies of retinal nerve fiber layer defects. Arch Ophthalmol 1982; 100:807–814.

10. Anderson DR. Correlation of the peripapillary damage with the disc anatomy and field abnormalities in glaucoma. Doc Ophthalmol 1983; 35:1–10.

11. Airaksinen PJ, Drance SM, Douglas GR, et al. Diffuse and localised nerve fiber loss in glaucoma. Am J Ophthalmol 1984; 98:566–571.

12. Airaksinen PJ, Drance SM. Neuroretinal rim area and retinal nerve fiber layer in glaucoma. Arch Ophthalmol 1985; 103:203–204.

13. Fantes FE, Anderson DR. Clinical histologic correlation of human peripapillary anatomy. Ophthalmology 1989; 96:20–25.

14. Dandona L, Quigley HA, Brown AE, et al. Quantitative regional structure of the normal human lamina cribrosa. Arch Ophthalmol 1990; 108:393–398.

15. Quigley HA, Coleman AL, Dorman-Pease ME. Larger optic nerve heads have more nerve fibers in normal monkey eyes. Arch Ophthalmol 1991; 109:1441–1443.

16. Sommer A, Katz J, Quigely HA, et al. Clinically detectable nerve fiber atrophy precedes the onset of glaucomatous field loss. Arch Ophthalmol 1991; 109:77–83.

17. Tuulonen A, Airaksinen PJ. Initial glaucomatous optic disk and retinal nerve fiber layer abnormalities and the mode of their progression. Am J Ophthalmol 1991; 111:485–490.

18. Caprioli J. Discrimination between normal and glaucomatous eyes. Invest Ophthalmol Vis Sci 1992; 33:153–159.

19. Drance SM, King D. The neuroretinal rim in descending optic atrophy. Graefe's Arch Clin Exp Ophthalmol 1992; 230:154–157.

20. Liu D, Kahn M. Measurement and relationship of subarachnoidal pressure of the optic nerve to intracranial pressure in fresh cadavers. Am J Ophthalmol 1993; 116:548–556.

21. Derick RJ, Pasquale LR, Pease ME, et al. A clinical study of peripapillary crescents of the optic disc in chronic experimental glaucoma in monkey eyes. Arch Ophthalmol 1994; 12:846–850.

22. Varma R, Tielsch JM, Quigley HA, et al. Race-, age-, gender-, and refractive error-related differences in the normal optic disc. Arch Ophthalmol 1994; 112:1068–1076.

23. Spaeth GL. A new classification of glaucoma including focal glaucoma. Surv Ophthalmol 1994; 38:S9–S17.

24. Morgan WH, Dao-Yi Y, Cooper RL, et al. The influence of cerebrospinal fluid pressure on the lamina cribrosa tissue pressure gradient. Invest Ophthalmol Vis Sci 1995; 36:1163–1172.

25. Nicolela MT, Drance SM. Various glaucomatous optic nerve appearances: clinical correlations. Ophthalmology 1996; 103:640–649.

26. Weinreb RN, Shakiba S, Zangwill L. Scanning laser polarimetry to measure the nerve fiber layer of normal and glaucomatous eyes. Am J Ophthalmol 1995; 119:627–636.

27. Tezel G, Kass MA, Kolker AE, et al. Comparative optic disc analysis in normal pressure glaucoma, primary open-angle glaucoma, and ocular hypertension. Ophthalmology 1996; 103:2105–2113.

28. Wang Y, Xu L, Hu L, et al. Frequency of optic disc hemorrhages in adult Chinese in rural and urban China. The Beijing Eye Study. Am J Ophthalmol 2006; 142:241–246.

CHAPTER 18

Optic Disc Imaging

Linda M Zangwill, Christopher Bowd, and Felipe A Medeiros

INTRODUCTION

Glaucoma is a progressive optic neuropathy typified by characteristic optic disc and retinal nerve fiber layer (RNFL) change that often precedes characteristic visual field loss. Although assessment of the optic disc is the cornerstone of glaucoma management, clinical examination of the optic disc is subjective and can be imprecise. Moreover, there is evidence that many ophthalmologists do not routinely examine the optic disc or obtain optic disc photographs in clinical practice. Imaging instruments have evolved to provide objective and reproducible information that can be used to assist the clinician in diagnosing and monitoring glaucomatous structural changes. It is essential that clinicians understand the strengths and limitations of the techniques used. This chapter will update recent reviews[1,2] of optic disc topography imaging techniques using the Heidelberg Retina Tomograph (HRT; Heidelberg Engineering, Heidelberg Germany) and the Optical Coherence Tomograph (Stratus OCT, Zeiss Meditec Inc., Dublin, CA) with an emphasis on how to appropriately apply these techniques in clinical practice.

HEIDELBERG RETINA TOMOGRAPH

INTRODUCTION AND MODE OF ACTION

Confocal scanning laser technology has been available commercially for glaucoma detection since 1992. In brief, confocal optics (including a 670 nm diode laser) are used to obtain multiple measures of retinal height, each with a very shallow depth of field. Multiple confocal 'slices' (XY measurements in multiple Z planes), obtained at consecutive focal planes are combined to provide a three-dimensional reconstruction of retinal height extending from the lamina cribrosa to the anterior surface of the retina. For the current version of the Heidelberg Retina Tomograph (HRT II/HRT 3), the scan is centered on the optic disc and a variable number of slices are obtained at a rate of 16 per millimeter of scan depth. The depth of scanning ranges from 0.5 mm to 4 mm depending on the eye, and image field of view is 15°, yielding 384 × 384 picture elements. Three consecutive scans are obtained within approximately 2 seconds and automatically combined to improve reproducibility and to provide a measure of variability of retinal height at each examination.

REPRODUCIBILITY

Many studies have shown good reproducibility of the first-generation HRT instrument with coefficients of variability for stereometric parameters ranging from about 2% to 10%, with variability slightly higher in glaucomatous eyes than in healthy eyes.[1–3] Similar variation has been reported for HRT II.[4–6] With the recent addition of improved alignment techniques and informative image quality warnings, reproducibility using the current HRT 3 software should be as good or better, although this assumption has not yet been well tested. Recent studies have investigated advanced techniques for improving reproducibility including use of nonstandard references planes[7,8] and the use of image improvement techniques.[9] While effective, these techniques have not been incorporated into current HRT software.

AVAILABLE ANALYSES, PRINTOUTS, AND INTERPRETATION OF DATA

Comprehensive software is provided that facilitates image acquisition, storage, retrieval, and analysis. Stereometric parameters are provided to describe the retinal topography of each image. These stereometric parameters utilize information within the optic disc margin, which is defined manually by placing a contour line along the inner edge of the scleral ring at the baseline examination. The contour line is automatically transferred to all follow-up examinations. Many of the stereometric parameters are calculated based on a standard reference plane set 50 μm posterior to the average contour line height (i.e. retinal height) at a 5° sector along the temporal rim, an area thought to be least effected by glaucomatous progression and therefore

TABLE 18.1 Description of HRT stereometric parameters provided in printouts

PARAMETER	DESCRIPTION
Disc area (mm²)	Area of the optic disc (total area enclosed by contour line)
Cup area (mm²)	Area of optic disc cupping (area enclosed by the contour line and located beneath the reference plane)
Rim area (mm²)	Area of neuroretinal rim (area enclosed by the contour line and located above the reference plane)
Cup volume (mm³)	Volume of optic disc cupping (volume enclosed by the contour line and located beneath the reference plane)
Rim volume (mm³)	Volume of neuroretinal rim (volume enclosed by the contour line and located above the reference plane)
Cup-to-disc area ratio	Ratio between area of disc cupping and area of optic disc: (cup area) / (disc area)
Linear cup-to-disc ratio	Average cup-to-disc diameter ratio (square root of cup-to-disc area ratio)
Mean cup depth (mm)	Mean depth of optic disc cupping
Maximum cup depth (mm)	Maximum depth of optic disc cupping
Cup shape measure	Measure for the overall three-dimensional shape of optic disc cupping
Height variation contour (mm)	Height variation of the retinal surface along the contour line: height difference between the most elevated and most depressed point of the contour line
Mean RNFL thickness (mm)	Mean thickness of the RNFL along the contour line (measured relative to the reference plane)
RNFL cross-sectional area (mm²)	Total cross-sectional area of the RNFL along the contour line (measured relative to the reference plane)
Reference height (mm)	Location of the reference plane, relative to the mean height of the peripapillary retinal surface

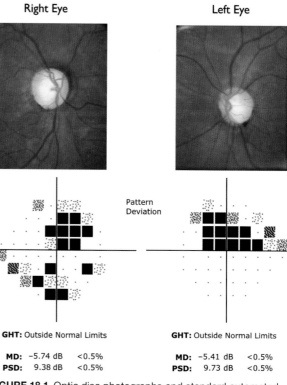

FIGURE 18.1 Optic disc photographs and standard automated perimetry pattern deviation probability plots from a 72-year-old female glaucoma patient (Glaucoma Patient 1). The right optic disc shows advanced rim thinning in the superior nasal and inferior temporal regions with an associated inferotemporal RNFL defect. The right visual field shows inferior arcuate and paracentral abnormalities. The left optic disc shows advanced inferotemporal rim thinning and the visual field shows a corresponding superior arcuate defect. HRT and OCT output from the same patient are shown in Figures 18.2–18.4, and 18.15.

thought to change minimally over time. Stereometric parameters include: disc area (area within contour), rim area (area within contour and above reference plane), cup area (area within contour and below reference plane), rim volume, cup volume, mean cup depth, mean height of contour, an indirect measure of retinal nerve fiber layer (RNFL) thickness, and cup shape (Table 18.1). Several of these parameters are reported and compared to a race-specific normative database. The examples that follow are from a female glaucoma patient, age 72 (Fig. 18.1). Figure 18.2 shows the standard 'OU Report' comparing stereometric measurements from both eyes of this patient.

In addition to descriptive stereometric measurements, the results from the Moorfields Regression Analysis (MRA) classification technique also are provided on the 'OU Report.' The MRA compares global and local rim area measurements (reference plane dependent) to a normative database taking into account disc area and age (Fig. 18.3).[10] The newer Glaucoma Probability Score (GPS) uses a geometric model to describe the shape of the optic disc/parapapillary retina (globally and locally) based on five parameters (cup size, cup depth, rim steepness, horizontal retinal nerve fiber layer curvature, and vertical retina nerve fiber layer curvature).[11] These parameters are then interpreted by a relevance vector machine classifier[12] and the resulting output describes the probability that the eye is glaucomatous (based on fit-to-training data from healthy and glaucoma eyes). This technique does not depend on an operator-drawn contour line or a reference plane and is

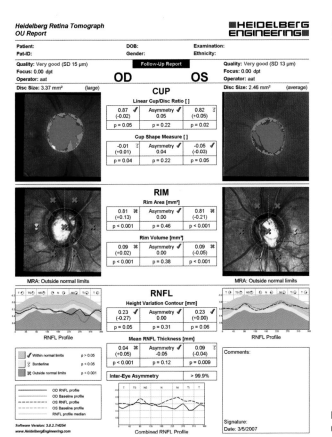

FIGURE 18.2 Glaucoma Patient 1. 'The OU report' provides examination information on both eyes in a concise and clear format. Measurements of three important features, the cup, neuroretinal rim, and RNFL, for documenting glaucomatous optic neuropathy are presented. The cup is represented by the linear cup-to-disc ratio and cup shape measure, the neuroretinal rim by rim area and rim volume, and the RNFL by height variation contour and mean RNFL thickness. For each of these parameters, classification as within normal limits (*green check*), borderline (*yellow exclamation point*), outside normal limits (*red check*) and the degree of asymmetry (difference between eyes) is provided. The black line on RNFL profile shows the individual's RNFL thickness along the contour line. The background on the profile shows the outside normal limits, borderline, and within normal limits values as well as the green line indicating the average values for the corresponding age, optic disc size, and ethnicity. In addition, regional MRA results are provided, with text describing the overall MRA result. For these eyes, rim area and volume are below normal limits, MRA results are outside of normal limits in most sectors and overall and, for the right eye, the RNFL profile shows an inferotemporal defect that corresponds with a defect visible in the stereophotograph (Fig 18.1).

therefore operator independent (Fig. 18.4). Results from both classification techniques are reported as 'within normal limits,' 'borderline,' or 'outside normal limits' globally, and for each of six disc sectors relative to the normative data.

Change over time can be measured in several ways using the commercially available HRT. First, a linear regression analysis can be obtained that describes the change in stereometric parameters from visit to visit. A variation on this technique normalizes all stereometric parameters to zero at baseline allowing observation of relative change in measurements over time

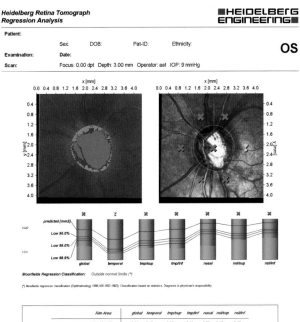

FIGURE 18.3 Glaucoma Patient 1. The HRT 'Regression Analysis' report shows the color-coded topography image, indicating optic disc and cup boundaries, the reflectance image with regional and global MRA assessment icons, and the rim area relative to the normative database (*bar graphs*). Regional and global rim area measurements also are presented as are various percentile cut-offs calculated from the normative database.

(Fig. 18.5, examples illustrating change are from a female glaucoma patient of African ancestry, age 42 at study enrollment, Glaucoma Patient 2). Second, the stereometric parameters from the baseline examination can be compared to a follow-up examination. With the 'Follow-up Report,' the Topographic Change Analysis (TCA) analysis, MRA analysis, and difference in stereometric parameters are displayed (Fig. 18.6). Third, a more sophisticated analysis based on local change in retinal height compared to baseline is available. The TCA compares the change in retinal height between baseline and follow-up images to the change in retinal height between the three images that compose the baseline image, using analysis of variance on a superpixel by superpixel basis (1 superpixel equals 4 pixels[2]) (Fig. 18.7).[13] With the HRT 3.0 software, three-dimensional alignment algorithms are used to align images to the baseline examination to facilitate this analysis. Superpixels that change significantly compared to baseline are flagged as red (decrease in retinal height) or green (increase in retinal height). Clusters of red contiguous pixels (either by raw count or by count as percentage of optic disc area) in areas most associated with glaucomatous change (e.g. superotemporal and inferotemporal neuroretinal rim) likely indicate glaucomatous progression. The volume and area of these clusters

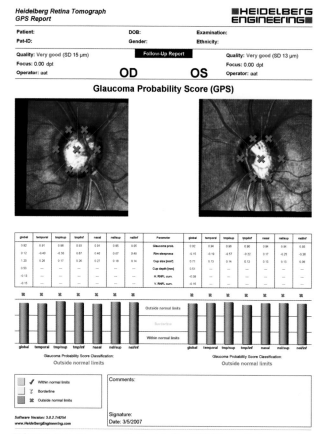

FIGURE 18.4 Glaucoma Patient 1. The 'GPS Report' documents the results of the Global GPS, and the GPS by region, as outside normal limits, borderline, or within normal limits, in a manner similar to the MRA report. In addition, the values for each of the five parameters that are used in the GPS model are provided globally and/or by each predefined segment, as appropriate. All GPS sectors and the GPS global result are outside normal limits for this eye.

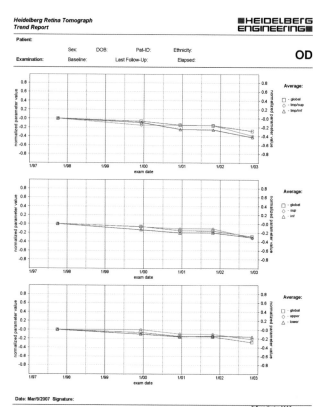

FIGURE 18.5 Glaucoma Patient 2. The 'Trend Report' presents the three graphs with time as the x-axis and the normalized 'average' parameter value as the y-axis. The average parameter is the mean value of all parameters. Each graph presents the global 'average' as a red box, and three different sector combinations. The top graph reports temporal superior (*green diamond*) and temporal inferior (*blue triangle*) sectors over time. The center graph reports superior (*green diamond*) and inferior (*blue triangle*) sectors while the bottom graph reports upper (*green diamond*) and lower (*blue triangle*) sectors over time. The baseline value for each graph is by definition zero with change consistent with glaucoma decreasing the parameter value below zero.

can be charted over time using the 'Cluster Change Analysis' printout (Fig. 18.8). The reason for the increase in retinal height shown as green superpixels is not always evident, and may represent a true increase in retinal height, a remodeling of the optic nerve head in response to glaucomatous change, an artifact, or a type 1 statistical error. An increase in retinal height has been shown to occur after surgery or administration of intraocular pressure (IOP)-lowering medication.[14,15]

Several alternate means of detecting change with HRT have been proposed over the past 5 years.[7,16-18] These techniques range from relatively simple comparisons of intra-image variability and inter-image variability of stereometric parameters[16] to simulation-based comparisons derived from techniques first developed for neuroimaging (statistical image mapping, SIM).[18] Because SIM analysis is contour line-independent, is based on measurements from the individual tested, and does not rely on population statistics that often show great variability, and because it exploits the whole image (and considers local spatial correlation), this technique currently appears the most promising. In one study, sensitivity and specificity of SIM analysis were compared to TCA analysis in simulated and real cases.[18] In simulated cases, specificity was approximately 95% for SIM and approximately 83% for TCA. Sensitivity ranged from 55% to 100% for SIM and from 28% to 95% for TCA, depending on the magnitude (change in retinal height) and type (gradual or sudden) of change simulated. In real cases, SIM identified change in more ocular hypertensive eyes that converted to glaucomatous visual fields and fewer healthy eyes than did TCA. At the time of writing, none of these newer techniques has been incorporated into commercially available HRT software.

DIAGNOSTIC ACCURACY

Numerous studies have estimated the diagnostic accuracy of the HRT I and HRT II for detecting early and moderate glaucoma.[1,2,19] In short, the area under the receiver operating characteristic curve (AUROC) for discriminating between eyes with and without visual field damage ranges from 0.86 to 0.96 depending on the HRT measurements evaluated, severity of glaucoma included, and other characteristics of the study. For example, AUROC may be considerably lower when trying to detect eyes with preperimetric glaucoma. Several recent studies have shown that the diagnostic accuracy

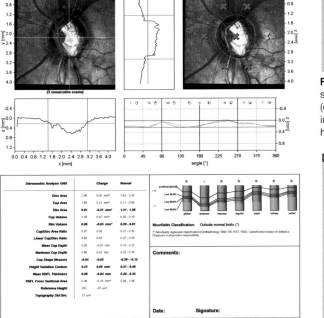

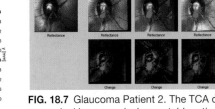

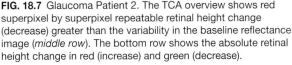

FIGURE 18.6 Glaucoma Patient 2. The Follow-up Report shows TCA significant change from baseline (*top left*), MRA results (*top right*), change over time of stereometric measurements, and compare the contour line height at follow-up to the baseline measurements. In addition, the normative values for the stereometric parameters are provided with the measurements of the current examination that are outside normal limits presented in bold.

FIG. 18.7 Glaucoma Patient 2. The TCA overview shows red superpixel by superpixel repeatable retinal height change (decrease) greater than the variability in the baseline reflectance image (*middle row*). The bottom row shows the absolute retinal height change in red (increase) and green (decrease).

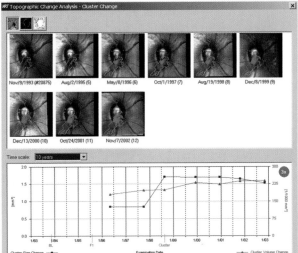

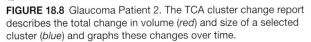

FIGURE 18.8 Glaucoma Patient 2. The TCA cluster change report describes the total change in volume (*red*) and size of a selected cluster (*blue*) and graphs these changes over time.

TABLE 18.2 Diagnostic accuracy of HRT Glaucoma Probability Score (GPS) and Moorfields Regression Analysis (MRA) for selected studies

STUDY	PARAMETER	SENSITIVITY (%)	SPECIFICITY (%)	ROC AREA	GL SAP MD (dB)
20	Global GPS	77.1	90.3	Not reported	−7.31
20	Worst MRA sector	71.1	91.8	Not reported	−7.31
21	Worst GPS sector	59.0	91.0	0.78	−3.60
21	Worst MRA sector	56.0	87.0	0.77	−3.60
24	Overall GPS	Not reported	Not reported	0.93	−6.03
24	Overall MRA	Not reported	Not reported	0.88	−6.03
22	Global GPS	71.7	82.3	0.70	−5.20
22	Global MRA	67.7	88.7	0.74	−5.20

of the GPS is similar to that of the MRA (Table 18.2). In one study, global MRA sensitivity and specificity were 71.1% and 91.8%, respectively, while global GPS sensitivity and specificity were 77.1% and 90.3%, respectively.[20] Sensitivity for detecting early glaucoma (standard automated perimetry mean deviation = −5.0 dB), was better for GPS (72.3%) than for MRA (59.6%).[20] In a similar study, MRA sensitivity and specificity were 56% and 87% when borderline results were

included in the within normal limits group (most specific criteria), and 78% and 66% when borderline results were included in the outside normal limits group (least specific criteria). Sensitivity and specificity for GPS were similar: 59% and 91% (specific criteria) and 78% and 63% (least-specific criteria).[21] Both studies reported that a significant percentage (2–5%) of eyes could not be analyzed using GPS (due to algorithm failure) and the latter study reported that both MRA and GPS were strongly affected by disc size, with both classifiers showing relatively poor sensitivity in eyes with small discs and relatively poor specificity in eyes with large discs (although this finding likely was partly attributable to sampling bias). The effect of disc size for both MRA and GPS was shown to be stronger regionally than globally in another study.[22] This study also described the effect of glaucoma severity on GPS and MRA. Predictably, sensitivity increased as a function of increases in disease severity (defined based on standard automated perimetry Advanced Glaucoma Intervention Study scores)[23] (see also reference 21). Finally, one study reported no effect of disc size on GPS or MRA sensitivity.[24] It is important to note that decreased diagnostic accuracy in eyes with smaller discs does not suggest decreased ability to detect change over time in these eyes.

Figure 18.9 highlights the clear detection of rim and RNFL changes with the TCA, while the MRA and GPS are consistently classified as borderline or within normal limits throughout the 10-year follow-up period of Glaucoma Patient 2. If one relied on the MRA or GPS analysis, clear glaucomatous changes would have been missed. The automated TCA analysis clearly identified repeatable glaucomatous changes, even when the MRA and GPS were not outside normal limits.

COMMON ARTIFACTS AND HOW TO PREVENT THEM

A good-quality HRT image has a well-centered optic disc, even illumination, minimal movement, and good focus. The HRT 3.0 software provides real-time information during image acquisition on the quality of the scan. The new image quality bar visible to the operator during the scanning session indicates potential problems if the bar is yellow or red; a green bar indicates a good-quality scan. The software automatically determines the scan depth, fine tunes the focus, and discards series that are problematic due to blinking or large eye movement. It continues to scan until three good-quality series are obtained. In addition, the 'Imaging Quality Score' is reported based on checks of the image series for accommodation, camera distance, blink and fixation loss, image brightness, eye movement, image illumination, and eye drift. Based on these checks, messages appear on the screen indicating whether the image quality is 'good,' 'acceptable,' or 'poor.' If flagged as 'poor,' suggestions are provided on how to improve image quality. Another calculation that is reported on the printout is the 'Image Quality Score' which classifies the scan according to the mean topographic standard deviation as 'excellent' ($<10\,\mu m$), 'very good' (between $11\,\mu m$ and $20\,\mu m$), 'good' (between $21\,\mu m$ and $30\,\mu m$), 'acceptable' (between $31\,\mu m$ and $40\,\mu m$), 'poor, try to improve' (between $41\,\mu m$ and $50\,\mu m$), and 'very poor – documentation only' (above $50\,\mu m$). 'Poor' and 'very poor' images should be retaken. It is recommended that images with a standard deviation above $30\,\mu m$ should also be retaken. If the quality of the image does not improve with repeat testing, then the optic disc measurements and analysis should be interpreted with caution. It is important to note that any automated image quality assessment is not foolproof and can miss poor-quality images. It is therefore essential that images are assessed subjectively for quality before they are utilized for clinical decision-making.

Figure 18.10 illustrates the effect of including a poor-quality scan in a TCA analysis. Because the poor-quality baseline scan results were inaccurate, the TCA identified 'significant repeatable change' from baseline. By excluding the poor-quality baseline scan, the change is no longer present.

Poor-quality scans with a high standard deviation will likely be identified by the automated image quality assessment, and messages to the operator will be provided to improve the scan However, the standard deviation can be $<40\,\mu m$ and the scan still be unuseable due to poor focus, uneven illumination, or doubling of vessels. Although the vast majority of eyes can be scanned without dilation, dilating the eyes and/or applying artificial tears can improve image quality. Figure 18.11 illustrates an example of a poor-quality scan with a high standard deviation (top) compared to a good-quality scan (bottom) of the same individual.

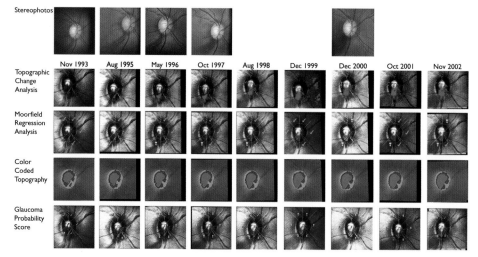

FIGURE 18.9 Glaucoma Patient 2. Stereophotographs show an increase in size of the inferotemporal RNFL defect that also is detected by TCA analysis. The color-coded topography suggests inferior rim thinning. MRA and GPS are primarily within normal and borderline limits throughout follow-up.

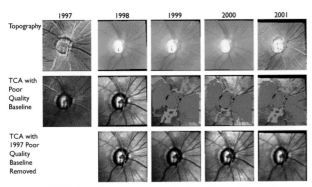

FIGURE 18.10 Including a poor-quality baseline in the TCA analysis resulted in the detection of spurious change. Removal of the poor-quality baseline decreases areas of significant change.

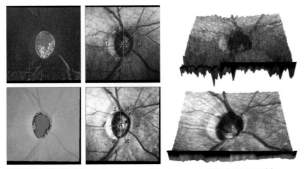

FIGURE 18.11 (Top) A poor-quality topographic image with a standard deviation >50 μm. Note grainy appearance of topography and reflectance images and irregular (noisy) retinal surface on 3-D plot. **(Bottom)** A good image from the same eye with standard deviation <20 μm.

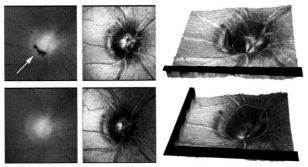

FIGURE 18.12 (Top) Topographic image with a dense floater over the contour line. Note spike in contour height on 3-D plot (*arrow*). **(Bottom)** Image from the same eye with floater displaced.

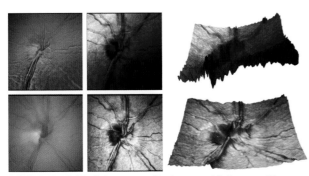

FIGURE 18.13 (Top) A poor-quality topographic image with uneven illumination, some framing in the lower right-hand corner, and a relatively high standard deviation of 40 μm. This standard deviation may be classified as 'acceptable' by the quality control but is clearly not useable for analysis. **(Bottom)** A good-quality image of the same eye, with a standard deviation of 12 μm.

Floaters appear as dark areas on the reflectance image and if located within the disc margin can cause errors in the calculation of the stereometric parameters. The automated image quality assessment will likely not identify floaters. Requesting the patient to blink several times and/or move his head to the left or right can often result in the floaters changing location or moving out of the HRT field of view (Fig. 18.12).

If a scan is very unevenly illuminated it should be retaken (Fig. 18.13). In some cases, framing occurs, with corners appearing darker due to too much distance between camera and eye. The automated image quality messages may be triggered, suggesting a way to improve the scan. In general, uneven illumination and framing can be eliminated by obtaining images with good focus at appropriate distances from the camera.

STRENGTHS AND LIMITATIONS

The primary limitation of HRT is that many measurements rely on a reference plane based on the placement of a user-defined contour line. This fact makes objective measurements subjective to some degree, because contour line placement can vary even among experienced users[25] (for conflicting results, see references 26 and 27). Introduction of the contour line- and reference plane-independent GPS classifier is a significant improvement because it allows user-independent analysis and tends to perform similarly to, or better than, the reference plane-dependent MRA.

An additional strength of the newest generation of HRT is the inclusion of a race-specific normative database. The previous MRA normative database was composed of 112 healthy eyes of European ancestry (EA), while the updated normative database is composed of 733 EA eyes, 215 eyes of African ancestry (AA), and 104 Indian eyes. The single study published to date[28] on race-specific normative databases indicates that use of the new normative data has improved HRT MRA sensitivity in EA eyes, likely because of the larger database and presumed corresponding decrease in variance. However, a decrease in sensitivity was observed for AA eyes using the new race-specific AA normative database. This finding was attributed to the homogeneity of AA eyes composing the new database and the presumed heterogeneity of AA eyes upon which it was tested. As explained, this discrepancy was due to evidence of regional variations in racial admixture.

Another possible limitation of HRT is that stereometric measurements can be influenced by moderate changes in IOP (e.g. reference 14). This finding suggests that IOP fluctuation be considered when assessing HRT images over time. However, a recent study of 23 subjects suggests that IOP fluctuation of 5 mmHg or 20% (on average) has no statistically significant effect on stereometric measurements and retinal height (assessed using TCA) compared to nonfluctuating control eyes.[29]

Strengths of the HRT include its real-time quality control during image acquisition, sophisticated analysis software for glaucoma detection and progression, and its large race-specific normative database.

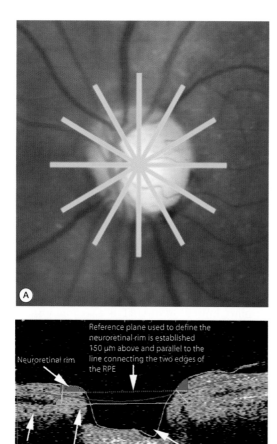

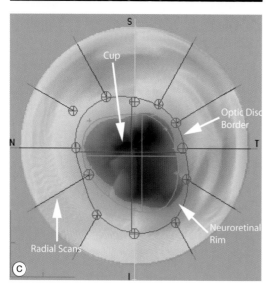

FIGURE 18.14 (A) The OCT optic nerve head scanning pattern of the video image. Six radial scans centered on the optic disc are acquired. **(B)** The retinal pigment epithelium (RPE) can be identified as the deep reflective red layer. A blue straight line connects the edges of the RPE. A reference plane is established, located 150 μm above and parallel to this line. The neuroretinal rim is identified as the red area located above the reference plane and the cup is the area located below this plane. **(C)** Two-dimensional representation of the optic disc topography. The optic disc margin is shown in red and the cup delimitation is shown in green.

OPTICAL COHERENCE TOMOGRAPHY

INTRODUCTION AND MODE OF ACTION

Optical coherence tomography (OCT) is an imaging technology able to provide cross-sectional images of ocular structures with high resolution both in vitro and in vivo.[30] The principle of OCT is analogous to that of ultrasonography, but uses light instead of sound to acquire high-resolution images of ocular structures. The distances and sizes of different tissue structures in the eye can be determined by measuring the time it takes for light to be reflected from the different structures.

The Optical Coherence Tomograph (Stratus OCT, Carl-Zeiss Meditec, Dublin, CA) now includes assessment of the optic nerve head (ONH) topography for glaucoma management. The ONH scan consists of six radial scans in a spokelike pattern centered on the ONH (Fig. 18.14A). To provide measurements throughout the ONH, the OCT interpolates between the scans with the disc margin automatically determined as the end of the retinal pigment epithelium (RPE)/choriocapillaris layer (Fig. 18.14B). A straight line connects the edges of the RPE and a parallel line, or reference plane, is constructed 150 μm (standard cup offset) anteriorly. The neuroretinal rim is identified as the area located above the reference plane, whereas the cup is the area located below this plane. A topographic image of the ONH (Fig. 18.14C) is constructed with the optic disc border, corresponding to the edges of the RPE, shown in red and the cup shown in green.

REPRODUCIBILITY

Few studies have evaluated the reproducibility of Stratus OCT ONH measurements. In one study, eight scan sessions were completed on glaucoma and normal eyes during two separate visits.[31] Reliability values, as measured by intraclass correlation coefficients (ICCs), were above 0.80 for most parameters with disc area tending to have lower ICC. In general, ICC values above 0.75 are considered to indicate good reproducibility. In another study of 10 normal subjects imaged six times per day on three different days, ICCs of undilated eyes ranged from 0.60 to 0.94, depending on the ONH parameter evaluated.[32] Cup-to-disc area ratio had the best ICCs (0.78 and 0.97, before and after dilation, respectively). Interestingly, this study reported higher reproducibility for the Fast Optic Disc Protocol than the high-density protocol, and no significant effect of dilation. This is probably explained by the shorter acquisition time and less influence of eye movements using the Fast Optic Disc Protocol, and that images are more easily acquired without dilation on healthy compared to glaucoma eyes.

AVAILABLE ANALYSES, PRINTOUTS, AND INTERPRETATION OF DATA

The OCT software facilitates image acquisition, storage, retrieval, and analysis. Several topographic optic disc parameters are automatically calculated and are

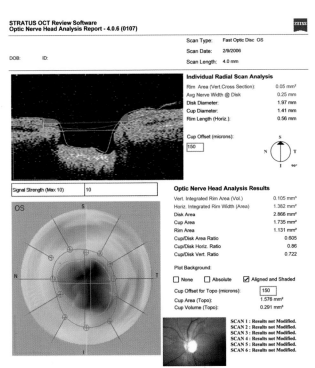

STRATUS OCT Review Software
Optic Nerve Head Analysis Report - 4.0.6 (0107)   ZEISS

DOB: ID:

Scan Type: Fast Optic Disc OS
Scan Date: 2/9/2006
Scan Length: 4.0 mm

Individual Radial Scan Analysis

Rim Area (Vert.Cross Section):	0.05 mm²
Avg Nerve Width @ Disk	0.25 mm
Disk Diameter:	1.97 mm
Cup Diameter:	1.41 mm
Rim Length (Horiz.):	0.56 mm

Cup Offset (microns): 150

Signal Strength (Max 10)   10

OS

Optic Nerve Head Analysis Results

Vert. Integrated Rim Area (Vol.)	0.105 mm³
Horiz. Integrated Rim Width (Area)	1.382 mm²
Disk Area	2.866 mm²
Cup Area	1.735 mm²
Rim Area	1.131 mm²
Cup/Disk Area Ratio	0.605
Cup/Disk Horiz. Ratio	0.86
Cup/Disk Vert. Ratio	0.722

Plot Background:

☐ None   ☐ Absolute   ☑ Aligned and Shaded

Cup Offset for Topo (microns):   150
Cup Area (Topo):   1.576 mm²
Cup Volume (Topo):   0.291 mm³

SCAN 1 : Results not Modified.
SCAN 2 : Results not Modified.
SCAN 3 : Results not Modified.
SCAN 4 : Results not Modified.
SCAN 5 : Results not Modified.
SCAN 6 : Results not Modified.

FIGURE 18.15 Glaucoma Patient 1. Optic Nerve Head Analysis Report showing the color-coded map (*above*), the topographic map (*below*), the Individual radial scan analysis (based on one individual scan analyzed on the printout shown as a yellow line on the topography map), and the Optic Nerve Head Analysis Results (based on all radial scans, and the interpolation between them represented by the topographic map). The five individual radial scan analysis parameters – rim area, average nerve width @ disk, disk diameter, cup diameter, and rim length (horizontal) – represent measurements along the radial scan chosen for analysis. The eight optic nerve head analysis results, described in Table 18.3, are generally more useful than those provided by the Individual Radial Scan Analysis.

reported along with a color-coded map and the ONH topographic map on the standard Optic Nerve Head Analysis Report (Fig. 18.15). Two sets of parameters are provided. One set of five parameters corresponds to the individual radial scan analysis and is calculated using one of the six cross-sectional radial scans chosen by the operator. The five parameters provided by the individual radial scan analysis are rim area (vertical cross-section), average nerve width @ disk, disk diameter, cup diameter, and rim length. The second set of eight parameters corresponds to the optic nerve head analysis results, which includes information from all the six radial scans as well as from the interpolation performed between them. Table 18.3 provides a description of the eight parameters from the optic nerve head analysis results – (vertical integrated rim area (VIRA), horizontal integrated rim area (HIRA), disk area, cup area, rim area, cup/disk area ratio – cup/disk horizontal ratio, and cup/disk vertical ratio) which are generally more useful for evaluation of the optic nerve head topography than those provided by the individual radial scan analysis.

OCT optic nerve head parameters are currently not compared to normative data and there is no automated method available for detecting progressive ONH changes with the Stratus OCT.

TABLE 18.3 Description of Stratus OCT optic nerve head parameters provided in the printout

PARAMETER	DESCRIPTION
Vertical integrated rim area (VIRA)	Estimate of the total volume of RNFL tissue in the rim calculated by multiplying the average of the individual rim areas times the circumference of the disc
Horizontal integrated rim area (HIRA)	Estimate of the total rim area calculated by multiplying the average of the individual nerve widths times the circumference of the disc
Disk area (mm²)	The area bounded by the red outline of the disc in the topographic map
Cup area (mm²)	The area bounded by the green outline of the cup in the topographic map
Rim area (mm²)	Disc area minus cup area
Cup-to-disk area ratio	Ratio of cup area to disc area
Cup-to-disk horizontal ratio	Ratio of the longest horizontal line across the cup to the longest horizontal line across the disc
Cup-to-disk vertical ratio	Ratio of the longest vertical line across the cup to the longest vertical line across the disc

DIAGNOSTIC ACCURACY

Several cross-sectional studies have evaluated the ability of Stratus OCT ONH parameters to detect glaucomatous damage.[33–38] These parameters have been shown to be significantly different between eyes with glaucomatous visual field loss and normal eyes. However, considerable overlap can be demonstrated in individual measurements from subjects in both groups. In one study, the analysis of AUROC curves revealed that all topographic parameters performed similarly (except for disc area), with areas ranging from 0.84 to 0.88. With 95% specificity, the parameter cup-to-disc area ratio had the highest sensitivity of 69%. For a moderate specificity, the sensitivity of this parameter was 80%. The cup-to-disc area ratio has also been demonstrated to have high reproducibility and, therefore, this parameter may be a useful one for diagnostic evaluation in glaucoma. It is expected that AUROC's sensitivities and specificities are affected by disease severity, as has been shown for OCT RNFL measurements.[39]

Comparisons among all Stratus OCT parameters have generally revealed that ONH parameters perform as well as RNFL thickness ones and better than macular thickness measures for detection of patients with glaucomatous visual field loss. More importantly, a few studies have suggested that a combination of selected ONH and RNFL thickness may improve detection of glaucoma with this instrument.[33–38]

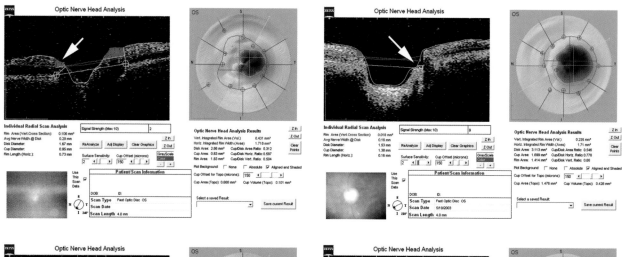

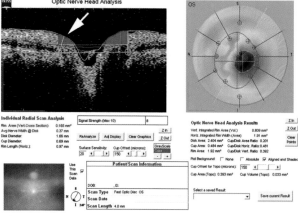

FIGURE 18.16 (Top) Poor-quality optic nerve head scan. Note the low signal strength value (2). The retinal layers, including the retinal pigment epithelium, are just barely visible and the optic disc margin is poorly defined. **(Bottom)** A subsequent scan with signal strength of 8. Note the larger rim area (*arrows*) with the good-quality scan.

FIGURE 18.17 (Top) The automatic algorithm incorrectly determined the optic disc margin. Because of a discontinuity in the RPE/choriocapillaris layer, the algorithm missed the true edge of the optic disc. Surface sensitivity is 2. **(Bottom)** Increasing the surface sensitivity to 20 resulted in a more appropriate automated delimitation of the optic disc margin/RPE.

COMMON ARTIFACTS AND HOW TO PREVENT THEM

A good-quality OCT scan should have adequate signal strength and be centered on the optic nerve head. Scans with signal strength of 7 are generally good, whereas scans with signal strength <5 are generally unacceptable (Fig. 18.16). For values in between, it is important to check the color-coded map for a clearly designated retinal pigment epithelial (RPE) layer which should appear red with some white speckles. To assess whether the scan is adequately centered on the optic nerve head, the examiner should look at the fundus image provided on the computer screen as well as on the printout. Off-center scans can result in incorrect measurements of the neuroretinal rim and cup dimensions.

In addition to assessing signal strength and centering, the operator should carefully search for failures in the algorithm that detects the retinal/ONH boundaries by reviewing each of the six color-coded maps (one for each radial scan). In general, a minimum of five out of the six maps should be acceptable after the necessary corrections have been performed for an ONH analysis to be useable. If an incorrect determination of the retinal/ONH boundaries is found on a particular map, the user can manually adjust the surface sensitivity. The surface sensitivity value (ranges from 0 to 20) determines the reflectivity threshold value considered to be the anterior surface. By increasing the surface sensitivity, potential artifacts and noise are better ignored when defining the surface (Figs 18.17 and 18.18). Alternatively, the location of the RPE edge can be modified by clicking and dragging the points on the computer screen. Review of the topographic map for unlikely optic nerve head shapes is also useful to determine whether the OCT algorithm correctly identified the optic disc margins.

One study comparing the automatic and manual methods of determining the optic disc margins has shown a good correlation between the two methods.[40] However, subsequent studies demonstrated that, although a good correlation could be demonstrated, their measurements did not agree in several cases. Specifically, one study reported that the automatic recognition software failed in 53% of 49 optic discs and misplaced margin points were more common in myopic eyes.[41] In another study, unsatisfactory automatic recognition of ONH edges was reported in 61.1% of the cases, indicating the importance of evaluating each ONH scan for appropriate placement of the optic disc margins.[42]

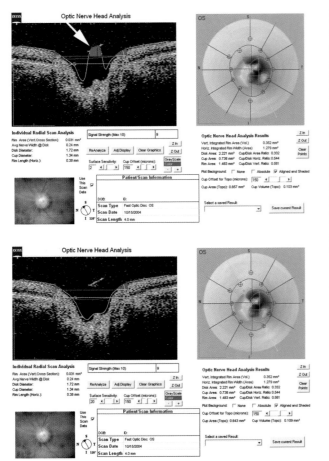

FIGURE 18.18 (Top) Incorrect determination of the surface of the optic nerve head due to the presence of an overlying vitreous opacity (*arrow*). **(Bottom)** Same scan after changing the sensitivity threshold.

Another source of error comes from the automatic delineation of the vitreoretinal/ONH surface shown as a blue line on the color-coded map of the OCT ONH scan. This boundary is associated with a sharp edge in each OCT scan because of the high contrast in optical reflectivity between the relatively nonreflective vitreous and the reflective neurosensory retina/ONH. Occasionally, the automatic OCT algorithm fails and incorrectly assigns an overlaying fibrous tissue or vitreous opacity as being the retinal or ONH surface (Fig. 18.18). Increasing the sensitivity threshold usually results in the algorithm ignoring the overlying tissue and correctly identifying the retinal/ONH surface. In some cases, adjustment of both the optic disc margins and the surface sensitivity are necessary to ensure correct evaluation of the optic disc topography.

STRENGTHS AND LIMITATIONS

Strengths of the Stratus OCT ONH analysis include the possibility of evaluation of optic nerve head topography and RNFL thickness analysis using a single instrument. As mentioned previously, a combination of parameters from these different scanning areas may result in improved ability to detect glaucomatous damage. The automatic demarcation of the optic nerve borders

is another potential advantage. However, the automatic algorithm frequently fails in correctly detecting the optic disc margins. Further, the automated demarcation of the optic disc margin can potentially be influenced by areas of parapapillary atrophy, which are often larger in glaucoma patients than normal subjects. These areas of parapapillary atrophy have been demonstrated to be associated with atrophy of the RPE and choriocapillaris. Therefore, as the RPE/choriocapillaris edges are used as landmarks for determination of the optic disc margins, progressive atrophy of this layer could potentially affect the demarcation of optic disc margins. Changes in the demarcation of the optic disc margin in the same patient would confound the interpretation of topographic optic disc measurements over time, potentially limiting the ability of this instrument to detect progressive glaucomatous optic disc damage.

It is also unclear how much effect the interpolation between the six radial scans has on the overall ONH analysis results. It is possible that localized neuroretinal rim or optic disc cup changes would be missed by the interpolation algorithm. In addition, in contrast to the Stratus OCT RNFL and macular analysis, the current Stratus OCT software does not include normative values for the ONH parameters so that it is difficult for the clinician to determine the probability of abnormality for a specific examination. Finally, the Stratus OCT does not provide automated analysis of change for any of its scan protocols, including the ONH scan.

COMPARISON OF HEIDELBERG RETINA TOMOGRAPH AND OPTICAL COHERENCE TOMOGRAPHY TO OTHER INSTRUMENTS

CORRELATION OF HEIDELBERG RETINA TOMOGRAPH AND OPTICAL COHERENCE TOMOGRAPHY MEASUREMENTS

In order to validate HRT and OCT optic nerve head measurements, several studies have compared them to each other and to other methods of ONH evaluation, such as stereophotography. A recent study comparing optic nerve head measurements obtained by HRT and OCT in glaucoma patients, glaucoma suspects, and normal individuals reported fair to moderate correlation for disc area, cup-to-disc area ratio, cup area, cup volume, and rim volume, with R^2 ranging from 12% to 72%.[40] It is important to emphasize that, although significant correlations were obtained, the absolute values for the optic nerve head parameters were generally different between the two instruments.

Statistically significant correlations between HRT and OCT measurements and stereophotograph assessment of vertical and horizontal cup-to-disc ratios and rim area have also been reported.[33,43,44] However, important disagreements were detected between automated imaging and qualitative stereophotographic methods. Specifically, for HRT, rim area measurements tended to be larger than those measured by planimetry of disc photographs. This is likely because the central vessel trunk of the optic nerve is measured as part of the rim because it lies within the contour line and above the reference plane. For OCT vertical cup-to-disc ratio assessment, discrepancies of up to 0.3 between the OCT and stereophotography were seen in some patients, although in the majority of cases the difference between the estimates from the two methods was within 0.2. The limited agreement with stereophotograph assessment does not preclude the use of optical imaging measurements for glaucoma diagnosis and follow-up as long as the same instrument is used consistently over time. Stereophotograph assessment of cup-to-disc ratio is a subjective measure and has a large interobserver variability.[45] In contrast, HRT and Stratus OCT ONH assessment provides objective measures of optic disc topography that have been shown to be reproducible. One should keep in mind, however, that topographic estimates from these techniques are not interchangeable.

COMPARISON OF DIAGNOSTIC ACCURACY

The overall diagnostic accuracy of HRT and OCT optic nerve head measurements is similar to that of RNFL measures obtained using scanning laser polarimetry (SLP) and Stratus OCT. In general, the best-performing parameters from each instrument yield similar sensitivities, specificities, and AUROC curves for discriminating between healthy and glaucoma eyes. For instance, one study showed that the AUROC for the best-performing parameters among instruments ranged from 0.86 to 0.92 (no significant differences) and sensitivities at specificities equal to 95% ranged from 59% to 64% (specificities ranged from 95% to 97%).[19] There are few studies directly comparing the diagnostic accuracy of the HRT and Stratus OCT optic nerve head parameters. In one recent study,[46] the AUROC of the best HRT II parameter, cup-to-disc ratio was similar to that of the best OCT parameter, vertical integrated rim area (0.86 and 0.85, respectively).

DETECTION OF PROGRESSION

No studies to date have compared the ability of HRT and other imaging techniques for detecting change over time. Studies investigating change over time with HRT TCA suggest that change is detectable in most eyes with known progression based on visual field testing or serial assessment of optic disc photographs. In addition, many eyes are identified as showing change with no accompanying evidence of change on other tests.[47] It is not clear if these observed changes are examples of false-positive change or if true change is detectable earlier using HRT compared to other techniques. It is likely that the answer is a combination of both because the HRT false-positive rate in healthy eyes tested over time is quite low.[13] More research is necessary in order to determine the best criteria for determining clinically

significant change in HRT images. This determination likely will be hampered somewhat by the current lack of a perfect reference standard for defining glaucomatous progression.

Several studies indicate that HRT measurements in glaucoma suspects (ocular hypertensives and/or eyes with suspicious-appearing optic discs) are predictive of the future development of repeatable glaucomatous visual field defects. In the Confocal Scanning Laser Ophthalmoscopy Ancillary Study to the Ocular Hypertensive Treatment Study (OHTS), baseline stereometric measurements were different in suspect eyes that later converted to visual field defects, and eyes with an MRA result outside of normal limits in any sector at baseline had a 2.4 times greater chance of converting from normal-appearing discs and normal visual field results to glaucomatous-appearing discs and/or repeatable abnormal visual field results compared to eyes with MRA within normal limits[48] (see also reference 49 and references 50 and 51 for similar results for RNFL measurements by scanning laser polarimetry and OCT1). However, not all subjects with baseline MRA outside of normal limits developed glaucoma during the follow-up period studied. Specifically, in the OHTS the positive predictive value (the probability of developing glaucoma during follow-up with a baseline MRA outside of normal limits) ranged from 14% to 40% depending on the MRA sector selected. The negative predictive value (probability of not developing glaucoma with a baseline MRA within normal limits or borderline), on the other hand, was as high as 93%. A very recent study suggests that in glaucoma suspect eyes, a baseline GPS outside of normal limits is as predictive of future repeatable visual field defects as a baseline suspect optic disc by stereophotograph assessment.[52] No studies are available evaluating the ability of Stratus OCT ONH measurements for predicting the development of glaucomatous changes.

Summary

Optic nerve imaging instruments provide reproducible, objective measurements of the optic nerve head that can assist the clinician in detecting glaucomatous damage and change. It is important that the clinician understands the specific strengths and weaknesses of each instrument so that the best-quality information will be used for glaucoma management decisions. Instruments that provide automated assessment of significant glaucomatous change are particularly useful. As illustrated in Figure 18.9, glaucomatous changes can be missed if one relies solely on whether an examination is outside normal limits. Because of the limited ability of any one test to detect glaucomatous damage and change, these techniques should be utilized in conjunction with careful clinical examination and visual function testing.

ACKNOWLEDGEMENTS

Supported in part by NIH grant EY11008 (LMZ).

Financial Disclosure: Dr Zangwill has received research support (equipment) from Heidelberg Engineering and Carl Zeiss Meditec Inc.

REFERENCES

1. Susanna R Jr., Medeiros FA. The optic nerve in glaucoma. Rio de Janeiro: Cultura Medica; 2006: 392.

2. Zangwill LM, Medeiros FA, Bowd C, et al. Optic nerve imaging devices: recent advances. In: Grehn F, Stampher R, eds. Essentials in ophthalmology: glaucoma. Heidelberg: Springer-Verlag; 2004.

3. Zangwill LM, Bowd C, Weinreb RN. Evaluating the optic disc and retinal nerve fiber layer in glaucoma II: optical image analysis. Semin Ophthalmol 2000; 15:206–220.

4. Arthur SN, Aldridge AJ, De Leon-Ortega J, et al. Agreement in assessing cup-to-disc ratio measurement among stereoscopic optic nerve head photographs, HRT II, and Stratus OCT. J Glaucoma 2006; 15(3):183–189.

5. Jampel HD, Vitale S, Ding Y, et al. Test-retest variability in structural and functional parameters of glaucoma damage in the glaucoma imaging longitudinal study. J Glaucoma 2006; 15(2):152–157.

6. Sihota R, Gulati V, Agarwal HC, et al. Variables affecting test-retest variability of Heidelberg Retina Tomograph II stereometric parameters. J Glaucoma 2002; 11(4):321–328.

7. Strouthidis NG, White ET, Owen VM, et al. Improving the repeatability of Heidelberg Retina Tomograph and Heidelberg Retina Tomograph II rim area measurements. Br J Ophthalmol 2005; 89(11):1433–1437.

8. Strouthidis NG, White ET, Owen VM, et al. Factors affecting the test-retest variability of Heidelberg Retina Tomograph and Heidelberg Retina Tomograph II measurements. Br J Ophthalmol 2005; 89(11):1427–1432.

9. Patterson AJ, Garway-Heath DF, Crabb DP. Improving the repeatability of topographic height measurements in confocal scanning laser imaging using maximum-likelihood deconvolution. Invest Ophthalmol Vis Sci 2006; 47(10):4415–4421.

10. Wollstein G, Garway-Heath DF, Hitchings RA. Identification of early glaucoma cases with the scanning laser ophthalmoscope. Ophthalmology 1998; 105(8):1557–1563.

11. Swindale NV, Stjepanovic G, Chin A, et al. Automated analysis of normal and glaucomatous optic nerve head topography images. Invest Ophthalmol Vis Sci 2000; 41(7):1730–1742.

12. Tipping ME. Sparse Bayesian learning and the relevance vector machine. J. Machine Learning Res 2001; 1:211–244.

13. Chauhan BC, Blanchard JW, Hamilton DC, et al. Technique for detecting serial topographic changes in the optic disc and peripapillary retina using scanning laser tomography. Invest Ophthalmol Vis Sci 2000; 41(3):775–782.

14. Bowd C, Weinreb RN, Lee B, et al. Optic disk topography after medical treatment to reduce intraocular pressure. Am J Ophthalmol 2000; 130(3):280–286.

15. Irak I, Zangwill L, Garden V, et al. Change in optic disk topography after trabeculectomy. Am J Ophthalmol 1996; 122(5):690–695.

16. Tan JC, Hitchings RA. Approach for identifying glaucomatous optic nerve progression by scanning laser tomography. Invest Ophthalmol Vis Sci 2003; 44(6):2621–2626.

17. Artes PH, Chauhan BC. Longitudinal changes in the visual field and optic disc in glaucoma. Prog Retin Eye Res 2005; 24(3):333–354.

18. Patterson AJ, Garway-Heath DF, Strouthidis NG, et al. A new statistical approach for quantifying change in series of retinal and optic nerve head topography images. Invest Ophthalmol Vis Sci 2005; 46(5):1659–1667.

19. Medeiros FA, Zangwill LM, Bowd C, et al. Comparison of the GDx VCC scanning laser polarimeter, HRT II confocal scanning laser ophthalmoscope, and Stratus OCT optical coherence tomograph for the detection of glaucoma. Arch Ophthalmol 2004; 122(6):827–837.

20. Harizman N, Zelefsky JR, Ilitchev E, et al. Detection of glaucoma using operator-dependent versus operator-independent classification in the Heidelberg Retinal Tomograph-III. Br J Ophthalmol 2006; 90(11):1390–1392.

21. Coops A, Henson DB, Kwartz AJ, et al. Automated analysis of Heidelberg Retina Tomograph optic disc images by glaucoma probability score. Invest Ophthalmol Vis Sci 2006; 47(12):5348–5355.

22. Zangwill LM, Jain S, Racette L, et al. The effect of disc size and severity of disease on the diagnostic accuracy of the Heidelberg Retina Tomograph (HRT) Glaucoma Probability Score and Moorfields Regression Analysis. Invest Ophthalmol Vis Sci 2007; 48(6):2653–2660.

23. Advanced Glaucoma Intervention Study:2. Visual field test scoring and reliability. Ophthalmology 1994; 101(8): 1445–1455.

24. Bergansky-Eliash Z, Wollstein G, Bilonick RA, et al. Glaucoma detection with the Heidelberg Retina Tomograph 3. Ophthalmology 2007; 114:466–471.

25. Garway-Heath DF, Poinoosawmy D, Wollstein G, et al. Inter- and intraobserver variation in the analysis of optic disc images: comparison of the Heidelberg Retina Tomograph and computer assisted planimetry. Br J Ophthalmol 1999; 83(6):664–669.

26. Hatch WV, Flanagan JG, Williams-Lyn DE, et al. Interobserver agreement of Heidelberg Retina Tomograph parameters. J Glaucoma 1999; 8(4):232–237.

27. Miglior S, Albe E, Guareschi M, et al. Intraobserver and interobserver reproducibility in the evaluation of optic disc stereometric parameters by Heidelberg Retina Tomograph. Ophthalmology 2002; 109(6):1072–1077.

28. Zelefsky JR, Harizman N, Mora R, et al. Assessment of a race-specific normative HRT-III database to differentiate glaucomatous from normal eyes. J Glaucoma 2006; 15(6): 548–551.

29. Nicolela MT, Soares AS, Carrillo MM, et al. Effect of moderate intraocular pressure changes on topographic measurements with confocal scanning laser tomography in patients with glaucoma. Arch Ophthalmol 2006; 124(5):633–640.

30. Huang D, Swanson EA, Lin CP, et al. Optical coherence tomography. Science 1991; 254(5035):1178–1181.

31. Olmedo M, Cadarso-Suarez C, Gomez-Ulla F, et al. Reproducibility of optic nerve head measurements obtained by optical coherence tomography. Eur J Ophthalmol 2005; 15(4):486–492.

32. Paunescu LA, Schuman JS, Price LL, et al. Reproducibility of nerve fiber thickness, macular thickness, and optic nerve head measurements using Stratus OCT. Invest Ophthalmol Vis Sci 2004; 45(6):1716–1724.

33. Medeiros FA, Zangwill LM, Bowd C, et al. Evaluation of retinal nerve fiber layer, optic nerve head, and macular thickness measurements for glaucoma detection using optical coherence tomography. Am J Ophthalmol 2005; 139(1):44–55.

34. Anton A, Moreno-Montanes J, Blazquez F, et al. Usefulness of optical coherence tomography parameters of the optic disc and the retinal nerve fiber layer to differentiate glaucomatous, ocular hypertensive, and normal eyes. J Glaucoma 2007; 16(1):1–8.

35. Huang ML, Chen HY. Development and comparison of automated classifiers for glaucoma diagnosis using Stratus optical coherence tomography. Invest Ophthalmol Vis Sci 2005; 46(11):4121–4129.

36. Burgansky-Eliash Z, Wollstein G, Chu T, et al. Optical coherence tomography machine learning classifiers for glaucoma detection, a preliminary study. Invest Ophthalmol Vis Sci 2005; 46(11):4147–4152.

37. Wollstein G, Ishikawa H, Wang J, et al. Comparison of three optical coherence tomography scanning areas for detection of glaucomatous damage. Am J Ophthalmol 2005; 139(1):39–43.

38. Chen HY, Huang ML. Discrimination between normal and glaucomatous eyes using Stratus optical coherence tomography

in Taiwan Chinese subjects. Graefe's Arch Clin Exp Ophthalmol 2005; 243(9):894–902.

39. Medeiros FA, Zangwill LM, Bowd C, et al. Influence of disease severity and optic disc size on the diagnostic performance of imaging instruments in glaucoma. Invest Ophthalmol Vis Sci 2006; 47(3):1008–1015.

40. Schuman JS, Wollstein G, Farra T, et al. Comparison of optic nerve head measurements obtained by optical coherence tomography and confocal scanning laser ophthalmoscopy. Am J Ophthalmol 2003; 135(4):504–512.

41. Iliev ME, Meyenberg A, Garweg JG. Morphometric assessment of normal, suspect and glaucomatous optic discs with Stratus OCT and HRT II. Eye 2006; 20(11):1288–1299.

42. Savini G, Zanini M, Carelli V, et al. Correlation between retinal nerve fibre layer thickness and optic nerve head size: an optical coherence tomography study. Br J Ophthalmol 2005; 89(4): 489–492.

43. Jonas JB, Mardin CY, Grundler A,E. Comparison of measurements of neuroretinal rim area between confocal laser scanning tomography and planimetry of photographs. Br J Ophthalmol 1998; 82(4):362–366.

44. Zangwill LM, Chang CF, Williams JM, et al. New technologies for diagnosing and monitoring glaucomatous optic neuropathy. Optom Vis Sci 1999; 76(8):526–536.

45. Tielsch JM, Katz J, Quigley HA, et al. Intraobserver and interobserver agreement in measurement of optic disc characteristics. Ophthalmology 1988; 95(3):350–356.

46. Deleon-Ortega JE, Arthur SN, McGwin G Jr, et al. Discrimination between glaucomatous and nonglaucomatous eyes using quantitative imaging devices and subjective optic nerve head assessment. Invest Ophthalmol Vis Sci 2006; 47(8):3374–3380.

47. Chauhan BC, McCormick TA, Nicolela MT, et al. Optic disc and visual field changes in a prospective longitudinal study of patients with glaucoma: comparison of scanning laser tomography with conventional perimetry and optic disc photography. Arch Ophthalmol 2001; 119(10):1492–1499.

48. Zangwill LM, Weinreb RN, Beiser JA, et al. Baseline topographic optic disc measurements are associated with the development of primary open-angle glaucoma, the Confocal Scanning Laser Ophthalmoscopy Ancillary Study to the Ocular Hypertension Treatment Study. Arch Ophthalmol 2005; 123(9):1188–1197.

49. Bowd C, Zangwill LM, Medeiros FA, et al. Confocal scanning laser ophthalmoscopy classifiers and stereophotograph evaluation for prediction of visual field abnormalities in glaucoma-suspect eyes. Invest Ophthalmol Vis Sci 2004; 45(7):2255–2262.

50. Mohammadi K, Bowd C, Weinreb RN, et al. Retinal nerve fiber layer thickness measurements with scanning laser polarimetry predict glaucomatous visual field loss. Am J Ophthalmol 2004; 138(4):592–601.

51. Lalezary M, Medeiros FA, Weinreb RN, et al. Baseline optical coherence tomography predicts the development of glaucomatous change in glaucoma suspects. Am J Ophthalmol 2006; 142(4):576–582.

52. Alencar LM, Medeiros FA, Bowd C, et al. HRT 3 glaucoma probability score results are predictive of development of glaucomatous visual field defects in glaucoma suspects. Invest Ophthalmol Vis Sci 2008; In Press.

CHAPTER 19

Retinal Nerve Fiber Layer Photography and Computer Analysis

Neil T Choplin, E Randy Craven, Toni T Meyers, Nic J Reus, and Hans G Lemij

INTRODUCTION

Primary open-angle glaucoma is a progressive, chronic optic neuropathy in which there is characteristic acquired atrophy of the optic nerve and loss of retinal ganglion cells and their axons.[1] Both initial evaluation and monitoring of patients with glaucoma or suspected of having glaucoma includes measurement of intraocular pressure, evaluation of the optic nerve head (structure), and performance of psychophysical tests such as automated perimetry (function). The axons of the optic nerve fibers are contained in the retinal nerve fiber layer (RNFL), and the process of glaucomatous optic neuropathy involves loss of these axons. Damage to the RNFL precedes observable changes in the optic nerve head ('cupping'), and significant RNFL loss can occur before reproducible functional loss can be demonstrated.[2,3] Thus, examination and documentation of the RNFL is an essential component of the glaucoma examination,

and is most important for the detection of structural damage before functional loss occurs, allowing appropriate therapeutic intervention.

A number of different methods are available to evaluate the RNFL, and will be discussed in this chapter. These techniques rely on the anatomy and physical properties of the RNFL to provide qualitative and/or quantitative information. Table 19.1 summarizes some of these methods for evaluating the RNFL.

RED-FREE OPHTHALMOSCOPY AND PHOTOGRAPHY

The RNFL can be examined clinically and glaucomatous defects identified.[4–6] The examination is facilitated by the use of red-free or green light, as the RNFL is invisible to red light but more easily visualized with shorter-wavelength light which does not penetrate the RNFL and is reflected by the superficial layers of

TABLE 19.1 Summary of RNFL analysis techniques				
TECHNIQUE	**EQUIPMENT**	**PRINCIPLE**	**ADVANTAGES**	**DISADVANTAGES**
Ophthalmoscopy	Direct ophthalmoscope or slit lamp with hand-held lens	Utilizes RNFL reflectivity; visibility is enhanced with red-free (green) light	Equipment readily available, defects may be visible in clear media and darker (high-contrast) fundi	Difficult to visualize RNFL through media opacities or lightly pigmented (low-contrast) fundi
Photography	Fundus camera with red-free filter, high-contrast film or digital capture	Same as ophthalmoscopy	Defects may be visible in clear media and darker (high-contrast) fundi	Requires skilled photographer, dilation, clear media, high contrast
Retinal contour analysis (topography)	Heidelberg Retinal Tomograph (HRT, Heidelberg Engineering)	Confocal scanning laser ophthalmoscopy, uses reflected light	Easy to perform, no dilation, does not require marking of disc edge, good specificity	Expensive equipment, poor sensitivity
Optical coherence tomography	Stratus OCT (Carl Zeiss Meditec)	Analysis of reflected and backscattered light by interferometry	Differentiates retinal layers, correlates with histology	Operator dependent, expensive equipment, difficult to reproduce
Scanning laser polarimetry	GDx VCC (Carl Zeiss Meditec)	Measures retardation of polarized laser light passing through naturally birefringent RNFL	Easy to operate, no dilation, large normative database, only technology specific for RNFL, high resolution and reproducibility	Expensive equipment, requires compensation for anterior segment birefringence, relative measure of RNFL

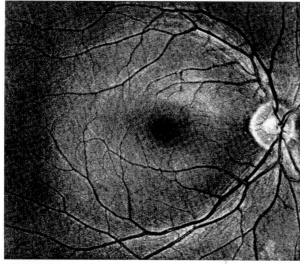

FIGURE 19.1 Red-free photograph of the normal retinal nerve fiber layer. Note the bright reflections from the arcuate bundles emanating from the optic disc. (From Airaksinen PJ, Nieminen H. Retinal nerve fiber layer photography in glaucoma. Ophthalmology 1985; 92:877–879.)

the retina.[7] Further, good visualization of the RNFL requires relatively clear media and high contrast, making examination difficult in patients with cataract and lightly pigmented fundi. Ophthalmoscopy can be performed through the dilated pupil with the red-free light of the direct ophthalmoscope or (preferably) with a hand-held lens at the slit lamp; the latter offers the advantage of stereo viewing and a slightly larger field of view, even with magnification.

The RNFL may be difficult to visualize on clinical examination, even with clear media and a dark fundus. Photography offers an opportunity to maximize the visualization of the RNFL and study it even for subtle defects. The technique of RNFL photography has been well described by Airaksinen and Nieminen.[8] Their technique utilized either a Canon CF-60Z wide-angle camera with a 60° picture angle and a built-in blue exciter filter or a Zeiss fundus camera with an Allen stereoseparator and 2.5× magnification with a Kodak Wratten no. 58 filter. Images were captured with high-resolution black-and-white Kodak Panatomic-X film, developed for high contrast, and printed with approximately 9× (print to negative) magnification. Similarly, with currently available camera backs, images may be captured digitally and enhanced with various available software packages to maximize contrast.

However the RNFL is visualized, its reflectivity relative to deeper structures as well as the orientation of the fibers gives the RNFL its characteristic appearance. A healthy RNFL will appear slightly opaque with visible, radially oriented striations emanating from the optic nerve head. As expected based upon the anatomy, the striations will appear arcuate in nature on the temporal side of the disc (Fig. 19.1). Glaucomatous defects will manifest in three different ways: slit, groove, or wedge-shaped defects (Fig. 19.2), or diffuse (generalized)

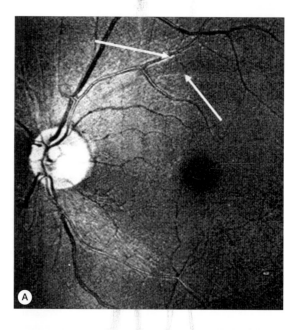

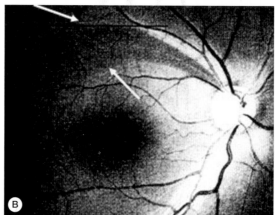

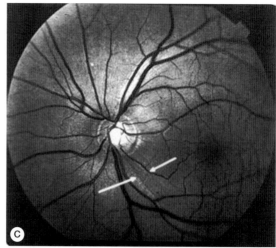

FIGURE 19.2 Examples of focal RNFL defects: **(A)** slitlike defect; **(B)** and **(C)** groove- or wedge-shaped defects. The middle example **(B)** is highly digitally enhanced to bring out the contrast. The example on the right **(C)** was captured with a digital color camera and converted to black and white. Defects in the RNFL appear dark (*between the white arrows*) in contrast to the more reflective normal nerve fibers. (**(A)** From Airaksinen PJ, Nieminen H. Retinal nerve fiber layer photography in glaucoma. Ophthalmology 1985; 92:877–879.)

loss (Fig. 19.3). The focal defects are easier to detect since they will appear 'dark' relative to the healthier, more reflective surrounding tissue.

A number of published studies have addressed the clinical utility of RNFL photography in the assessment of glaucoma damage. Quigley et al.[6] detected RNFL damage in 84% of eyes with visual field loss but only in 3% of normal eyes. They also demonstrated defects in 13% of glaucoma-suspect eyes (with no visual field loss), which tended to be more localized as opposed to more diffuse loss in eyes with visual field loss. In a similar study, Airaksinen and co-workers[9] demonstrated RNFL abnormalities in 48 of 51 patients with glaucoma (tending to be diffuse), 27 of 52 patients with ocular hypertension (tending to be more focal), and 5 of 29 normals. In an evaluation of RNFL assessment, Sommer et al.[10] demonstrated RNFL photography to have a sensitivity of about 80% with a specificity of 94%. These studies underscore the importance of RNFL assessment as an indicator for early (preperimetric) glaucomatous damage.

SCANNING LASER POLARIMETRY

Scanning laser polarimetry (SLP) is a technique designed to evaluate the RNFL based on the presumed form a birefringence of microtubules,[11] very small cylindrical structures that support the nerve fibers. The parallel arrangement of these microtubules in the RNFL produces a phase shift between orthogonal waves of polarized laser light passing through the structures; this is known as retardation. The greater the number of microtubules, the larger the amount of retardation measured by SLP, thus indicating the presence of more nerve fibers. Although retardation is measured in angular degrees (theta), for clinical purposes retardation is expressed in microns (μm) based upon a primate study that showed one degree of angular shift corresponds to approximately 7.4 μm of RNFL thickness.[12]

Two structures in the anterior segment, i.e. the cornea and, to a lesser extent, the lens, are also birefringent. The total retardation signal detected by scanning laser polarimetry thus consists of contributions from the anterior segment and the RNFL. In order to quantitate the RNFL, the anterior segment signal must be removed. The latest commercially available scanning laser polarimeter is the GDx VCC (Carl Zeiss Meditec, Inc., Dublin, California, USA). This instrument is equipped with a variable corneal compensation (VCC) that allows eye-specific compensation of the birefringent effects of the anterior segment. Equipped with VCC, RNFL measurements have been shown to match the appearance of the RNFL in red-free fundus photographs of glaucoma patients[13] and in stereoscopic optic disc photographs of monkey eyes with and without glaucoma.[14]

When taking a measurement with the GDx VCC, the imaged subject rests his head in a facemask and looks at an internal fixation light. Pupils are preferably not dilated and the room lights are left on. A near-infrared laser (wavelength, 785 nm) scans the fundus at a 40° × 20° scanning angle (horizontal × vertical). Two imaging trials per eye are run successively, the first to determine anterior segment birefringence, the second to image the retina with adjusted compensation. Anterior segment birefringence is assessed with the method described by Zhou and Weinreb.[15] In this method, the instrument's compensator is first set to zero retardance and the fundus is scanned. The interaction between the birefringence of the radially oriented axons of the photoreceptors that constitute Henle's fiber layer in the macula and the birefringence of the anterior segment results in a bow-tie shaped pattern in the retardation image (Fig. 19.4). A dedicated algorithm determines the anterior segment birefringence (described in terms of slow polarization axis and magnitude) from this profile. The software then automatically adjusts the anterior segment compensator.

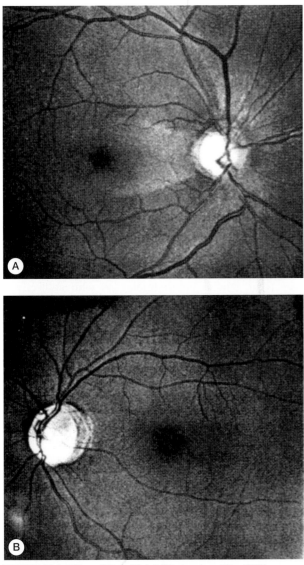

FIGURE 19.3 Diffuse **(A)** and total **(B)** atrophy of the RNFL. Note in **(A)** preservation of the papulomacular bundle. (From Airaksinen PJ, Nieminen H. Retinal nerve fiber layer photography in glaucoma. Ophthalmology 1985; 92:877–879.)

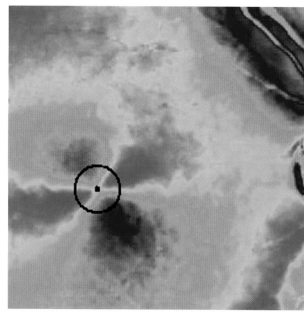

FIGURE 19.4 Determination of anterior segment birefringence. In the first phase of scanning laser polarimetry, the anterior segment compensator is set to zero retardance and the software analyzes the birefringence pattern of the macula. Warmer colors (red, orange, yellow) represent areas of higher retardation while cooler colors (blue, black) represent areas of lesser retardation. The Henle layer, consisting of extensions of photoreceptors around the fovea, is normally uniformly birefringent. In this macular retardation image, the 'bow-tie' appearance is due to uncompensated anterior segment birefringence. The software analyzes the pattern, determines the magnitude and orientation of the anterior segment birefringence, and automatically sets the compensator to remove that portion of the signal. Once the proper compensation is in place, the observed macular pattern would be uniformly blue. (Reproduced from Airaksinen PJ, Nieminen H. Retinal nerve fiber layer photography in glaucoma. Ophthalmology 1985; 92: 877–879.)

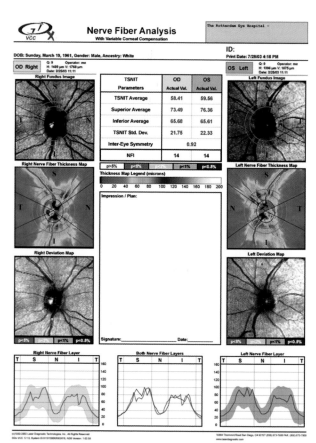

FIGURE 19.5 Printout from GDx VCC, both eyes normal. See text for full discussion.

A second scan is then obtained and the patient's RNFL thickness can then be estimated with eye-specific corneal compensation in a 20° × 20° field of view at a resolution of 128 pixels × 128 pixels. The margin of the optic disc is marked by the instrument's software with an ellipse that can be manually adjusted in a reflection image of the fundus. The software positions a measurement circle, 8 pixels wide (≈0.4 mm in an emmetropic eye) and with an inner diameter of 54 pixels (≈2.5 mm in an emmetropic eye), centered on this ellipse. Based on the retardation values beneath this band, the software calculates six parameters.

Of all GDx VCC parameters, the NFI (nerve fiber indicator) is the best one.[16] It has been trained specifically to discriminate between healthy and glaucomatous eyes with varying degrees of disease severity.[11] The NFI provides a single number (range, 1–100) representing the overall integrity of the RNFL. The score is the output of a machine learning classifier based on a linear support vector machine. The higher the score, the more likely the scan comes from a glaucomatous eye. The diagnostic accuracy of the GDx VCC's NFI parameter for glaucoma has been shown to be very good, with a sensitivity of 91.7%, a specificity of 95.0%,

and an overall accuracy of 93.2%.[17] The Heidelberg Retina Tomograph (HRT) and the Optical Coherence Tomograph (OCT) have been shown to provide similar accuracies for discriminating between healthy and glaucomatous eyes.[14,18,19] Interestingly, automated analysis of measurements with the GDx VCC and HRT may better discriminate between healthy and glaucomatous eyes than general ophthalmologists who subjectively grade the appearance of the optic nerve head in stereoscopic optic disc photographs.[20]

In daily practice, clinicians are not limited to evaluating GDx VCC data solely expressed as NFI. In contrast, the entire printout may be assessed subjectively, which presumably allows for an even better discrimination between healthy and glaucomatous eyes than the NFI by itself. Analysis of progressive glaucomatous loss is done subjectively by evaluating retardation maps in chronological order. There have been few publications to date describing the detection of progression of glaucoma with the GDx VCC. Work is being done to allow automated statistical analysis of changes in RNFL retardation over time with the GDx VCC.

With the GDx VCC, the RNFL information is provided to the user through an OU printout (Fig. 19.5). In the printout, data of the right eye are shown on the left, and data of the left eye on the right. The printout features a *reflectance image* of the fundus at the top that is used for orientation and assessment of image quality. Below that, the *retardation image* (named Nerve Fiber

Thickness Map) presents the measurements of retardation in a 20° × 20° field of view. Bright, warm colors represent thicker areas; dark, cool colors represent thinner areas. In healthy eyes, larger amounts of retardation (and thus brighter colors) are present adjacent to the thicker blood vessels superior and inferior to the optic disc. There is a large variability in the appearance of the RNFL in healthy eyes. In glaucomatous eyes, retardation is lost adjacent to the thicker blood vessels, especially superotemporal and inferotemporal to the optic disc. The *deviation map* shows the measurements compared to a normative database. Measurements that are below normal limits are flagged. This map is comparable to the Humphrey Field Analyzer's total deviation probability plot. The *TSNIT plot* (named Nerve Fiber Layer in the printout) at the bottom of the printout represents the amount of retardation around the optic disc (shown as a colored dark line). These data are taken from the measurement circle that had been centered on the optic disc, which is shown in both the reflection and retardation image. In the TSNIT plot, the normal 95% range is shown as a shaded area. The graph at the bottom in the middle named 'Both Nerve Fiber Layers' shows the TSNIT plots of both eyes superimposed, allowing an inter-eye comparison. The green and the purple graphs represent the right and left eye, respectively. The so-called *TSNIT parameters* are shown in the center at the top of the printout. Parameters that are within normal limits are presented in green print; those that are outside normal limits are shown in white print on a colored background. The TSNIT Average parameter represents the average retardation beneath the entire measurement circle. The Superior Average and Inferior Average parameters represent the average retardation beneath the measurement circle in the superior and inferior sectors, respectively. The parameter TSNIT Std. Dev. presents the standard deviation of the average of the retardation beneath the measurement circle. The Inter-Eye Symmetry parameter describes the amount of symmetry between the TSNIT plots of the right and the left eye. Finally, the NFI is presented at the bottom of this parameter table. This parameter is presented as a number between 1 and 100 and, unlike the other parameters, is not color-coded.

In the retardation images of healthy eyes, larger amounts of retardation are always present around the thicker blood vessels superior and inferior to the optic disc. This is illustrated in the printout of a healthy subject shown in Fig. 19.5. The deviation map is generally without areas of flagged pixels. Occasionally, some areas with false-positively flagged pixels may occur in the nasal half of the map in healthy subjects, and are usually not clinically significant. The TSNIT plot typically shows a double-hump pattern. Although the appearance of the TSNIT plot may vary considerably between subjects, the plot is usually within the normal range (indicated by the shaded band). The TSNIT plots of the two eyes are symmetrical, as can be observed in the 'Both Nerve Fiber Layers' graph. In healthy eyes, the NFI usually is below 35; in this case it is 14 in both eyes.

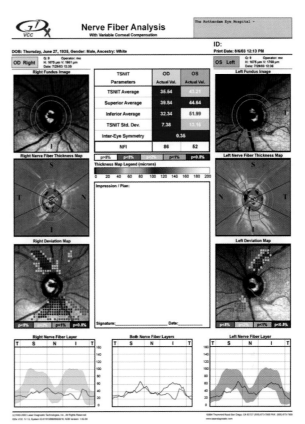

FIGURE 19.6 Printout from GDx VCC, showing extensive glaucoma damage in the right eye and moderate damage in the left.

In glaucoma patients, defects of the RNFL often develop superotemporal and inferotemporal to the optic disc. Loss may be localized, sometimes visible as a clear wedge-shaped defect, and diffuse. In the retardation maps of glaucomatous eyes, retardation is lost adjacent to the thicker blood vessels, especially superotemporal and inferotemporal to the optic disc. The deviation maps show areas of flagged pixels (with $p < 0.5\%$ and $p < 1\%$) superotemporal and inferotemporal to the optic disc. The TSNIT plots are often below the normal range in the temporal part of the superior and inferior bundles in mild to moderate glaucoma. In addition, TSNIT plots are often asymmetrical between eyes in the superotemporal and inferotemporal regions, as glaucoma is frequently more advanced in one eye compared to the fellow one. Asymmetries in the nasal sectors are less specific, as they occur in healthy subjects as well. In patients with severe glaucomatous damage, the TSNIT plot may be flat. In glaucoma patients, the NFI is usually 35 or higher. However, some localized defects may not be picked up by this parameter, as the NFI parameter was only trained to detect and characterize the pattern of global RNFL loss caused by glaucoma; such RNFL abnormalities may be easily detected in the raw RNFL measurements and often also in the deviation and TSNIT plots (especially when compared with the fellow eye).

Figures 19.6 and 19.7 show printouts from patients with glaucoma. The right eye of the patient in Figure 19.6

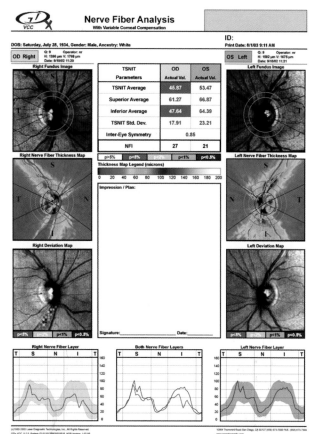

FIGURE 19.7 Printout from GDx VCC, showing a wedge-shaped inferior focal defect in the right eye. Note the retardation map and the deviation map.

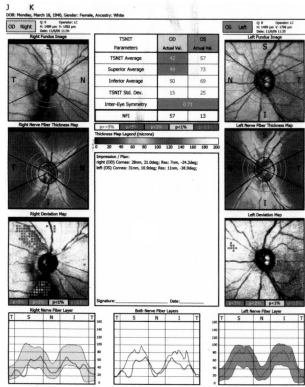

FIGURE 19.8 Printout from GDx VCC, showing moderate glaucomatous damage in the right eye. This is from the same patient as Figure 19.4, and corroborates the RNFL loss superiorly that is responsible for the inferior arcuate scotoma seen on the visual field examination. Interestingly, the GDx shows inferior loss as well, although the superior visual field shows no defect, supporting the concept that structural damage may be seen prior to functional loss in glaucoma.

shows a general loss of retardation: the bright colors have become attenuated. In addition, many pixels in the superior and inferior region have been flagged by the software. The TSNIT plot shows that the RNFL signal has decreased markedly both superiorly and inferiorly as it falls below the normative data. Parameters are all flagged in red. The NFI is 86, significantly higher than 35. The left eye shows a loss of retardation around the thicker blood vessels superotemporal to the optic disc. The same region is flagged in the deviation map. The TSNIT plot falls below the normative data in the superotemporal region. The plots of the right and left eye are asymmetrical. In addition, several parameters are flagged and the NFI is 52.

Figure 19.7 is from a patient who has a localized, wedge-shaped, defect of the RNFL inferotemporal to the optic disc in the right eye. Note the sharp edges of the defect in the retardation map. The loss of RNFL has been flagged in the deviation map. The TSNIT plot shows the localized loss of retardation as a sudden drop in retardation, thereby falling below the normal range. However, parameters are at most borderline ($p < 5\%$) and the NFI is only 27. The left eye does not show any sign of RNFL loss. In this eye, retardation is apparent adjacent to the thicker blood vessels superior and inferior to the optic disc, there are no flagged areas in the

deviation map, the TSNIT plot is within the normal range, and all parameters are within normal limits.

Figure 19.8 shows another example of a glaucomatous defect as shown by scanning laser polarimetry.

The normative data in the GDx VCC includes 540 healthy subjects and 271 glaucoma patients with varying degrees of disease severity.[21] Included subjects are of Asian, African-American, Caucasian, and Hispanic descent. Their age and refractive error ranged from 18 to 80 years old and from −8.4 to +5.5 diopters, respectively. These normal values are used to compare a patient's measurements to that of healthy and glaucoma patients, stratified by age. The result of this comparison is shown in the deviation plots and in the parameter section. In addition, the normative data, as well as data from glaucomatous eyes, have been used to train the NFI parameter.

As is true for all imaging techniques, images obtained with the GDx VCC should be of high quality, i.e. with a centered optic disc, well focused, even and just illuminated throughout the image, and without motion artifacts. The scan quality check that is performed automatically by the GDx VCC may assist one in assessing good image quality. Centration of the optic disc is necessary for optimal assessment of the peripapillary RNFL in the diagnosis of glaucoma and its follow-up.

In addition, the image should be well focused, as a defocused measurement may influence the amount of retardation that is measured by the GDx VCC. Suboptimal illumination may also negatively affect image quality and measurements in areas without good illumination may show more noise and sometimes no measurement of retardation at all. If images with even and just illumination cannot be obtained, one may check whether the upper eyelid is in front of the pupil or the patient's head is not properly positioned at the facemask. Although a measurement with the GDx VCC takes only 0.7 second to obtain, eye movements within a measurement do occur. In general, small eye movements have a negligible impact on the measurement. However, larger eye movements (resulting in black bars at the side of a picture due to registration of the misaligned images) do affect the measurement. Such images should be retaken.

Cataract may also affect image quality, especially posterior subcapsular cataract and dense nuclear cataract which may have an impact on the measurement. In some cases, reliable measurements cannot be obtained. When cataract surgery has been performed, one should always reassess anterior segment birefringence, as this may have changed. Eyes with a refractive error below -10 diopters or exceeding $+5$ diopters cannot be directly measured with the GDx VCC due to a mechanical limit. In such cases, a soft contact lens may be used to bring the eye into the measurement range of the instrument.

Large areas of peripapillary atrophy may preclude a correct assessment of the RNFL, as it generally leads to an apparent large amount of retardation due to reflectivity of the peripapillary crescent which is misread by the detector as birefringence signal. In most cases, the diameter of the measurement circle may be enlarged in the GDx VCC software beyond the area of parapapillary atrophy in order to allow calculation of the parameters and drawing of the TSNIT plot outside the area of atrophy. Normative data are automatically adjusted for a larger-diameter measurement circle.

Floaters in the vitreous may absorb the scanning laser light and therefore preclude a measurement of the RNFL posterior to the floater. In the retardation image, such an artifact may show as a dark area, which, of course, may be flagged in the deviation plot as being below normal limits.

In approximately 7% of cases, an atypical pattern of retardation may be observed in SLP-VCC images. The source of these patterns is unknown, although it appears to occur more frequently in eyes with lightly pigmented fundi, in myopes, and in eyes of elderly subjects. In these eyes, the signal-to-noise ratio of the SLP images is relatively poor. A new algorithm, called enhanced cornea compensation (ECC), has been shown to improve assessment of RNFL morphology in these eyes.[21] This algorithm is based on a preset measurement bias that is introduced in the measurement beam, thereby shifting the measurements into a more sensitive detection range of the instrument. Afterwards, this bias is mathematically removed from the measurements. In addition to a better assessment of the RNFL, the discrimination between healthy and glaucomatous eyes also appears to be better with ECC than with regular VCC.

CONFOCAL SCANNING LASER OPHTHALMOSCOPY: TOPOGRAPHIC ANALYSIS OF THE RETINAL NERVE FIBER LAYER

Confocal scanning laser ophthalmoscopy is a technique designed to evaluate the three-dimensional structure of the optic disc. The commercially available scanning laser ophthalmoscope is made by Heidelberg Engineering, and is called the Heidelberg Retinal Tomograph (HRT). The latest version, the HRT 3, is a confocal scanning laser ophthalmoscope that provides objective and quantifiable measurements of the optic disc cup, neuroretinal rim, and RNFL. The HRT 3 uses reflected light imaged on the optic nerve and peripapillary region at numerous depths in order to create a three-dimensional composite image over a $15° \times 15°$ degree field of view (approximately $4.1\,mm \times 4.1\,mm$ in an emmetropic eye). The HRT 3 captures the RNFL information by analyzing the height values that fall on the edge of the optic disc margin, which is marked by the user and is called the contour line. Once the contour line is drawn around the optic disc, the height values on the contour line are used to determine the RNFL integrity. Because the RNFL is thicker in the superior and inferior poles of the disc, the height values are correspondingly greater compared to the nasal and temporal sides of the optic disc. Moving around the optic nerve, starting temporally and progressing superiorly, nasally, inferiorly, and back temporally, a double-hump pattern of the RNFL is observed in a healthy eye. This double-hump pattern is caused by the path the axons take as they move toward the optic nerve. This double-hump pattern is captured by the height values of the HRT 3 in the contour line. In addition to providing the height values on the disc margin, the HRT 3 also provides RNFL thickness estimates by subtracting a reference plane from the height values. The reference plane is a plane that runs parallel to the surface of the image, and is located $50\,\mu m$ below the contour line height at the temporal side of the optic disc. Once the contour line is drawn, the reference plane is automatically determined and is used to calculate the various HRT 3 stereometric parameters, including the RNFL thickness values and the RNFL cross-sectional area values.

Yucel and colleagues[22] compared histologically measured RNFL density in 10 monkey eyes to values obtained with the HRT in the same eyes. They found that numerous HRT measures significantly correlated with the optic nerve fiber number counts. In particular, they showed that both RNFL thickness values and RNFL cross-sectional area correlated very strongly with the nerve fiber counts. A more recent study by Zangwill and colleagues[23] investigated the diagnostic accuracy of HRT RNFL measurements. They found that both the mean height values and the RNFL values were highly accurate at distinguishing normal controls from glaucoma patients.

The RFNL information is provided to the user through displays in the software as well as on the new OU printout available with the HRT 3. Figure 19.9 is an example of the printout from the HRT 3. The OU printout is divided into 3 main sections, with Cup analysis at the top, Rim analysis in the middle, and RNFL analysis at the bottom. The information from the right eyes is presented on the left of the printout, and the information from the left eye is on the right. In the middle of the printout is an Asymmetry analysis for all HRT measures, including the RNFL. In the RNFL section, there is a graph of the height values going around the optic nerve, beginning temporally, and moving around the disc superiorly, nasally, inferiorly, and back temporally (TSNIT plot). This graph is called the RNFL profile graph. In healthy eyes this typically has the double-hump appearance. In glaucoma, as ganglion cells and their axons are lost, the curve becomes flatter. To aid in the evaluation of the RNFL, the normal range of healthy eyes is superimposed over the graph. This is shown as a green-shaded area, and in healthy eyes the height values on the graph will fall within this region. This region shows the 95% normal range according to the normal database used for comparison. Values that fall outside the green area are likely to have RNFL loss.

In addition to the RNFL profile graph, two RNFL parameters are provided: the mean RNFL thickness parameter and the Height Variation parameter. The mean RNFL thickness is the average RNFL thickness from the graph, using the reference plane to calculate RNFL thickness values. The Height Variation is calculated by taking the difference between the maximum value from the graph and subtracting the minimum value. This height difference (max − min) is usually large in healthy eyes because of the double-hump pattern of the RNFL. In glaucoma as the RNFL pattern becomes flatter, the Height Variation is reduced. Along with the parameter value, the probability value (p value) of the comparison to the normative database is presented and a symbol is provided to flag the clinician as to whether or not the parameter is normal. If the parameter value falls within the 95% normal range, a green check is presented to signal the parameter value is within the normal range. If the p value is below 5%, then a yellow exclamation point is presented to signal a 'Borderline' result. If the p value is below the 0.1%, a red X is presented to signal that the value is outside normal limits. As with the RNFL profile graph, all comparisons to the normative database are adjusted for age, optic disc size, and use the appropriate ethnic database. There is also a graph in the middle of the printout showing both the RNFL profile graphs of the right eye and the left eye together. The amount of symmetry between eyes can be determined from this graph. Although glaucoma is a bilateral disease, one eye is often more advanced than the fellow eye and

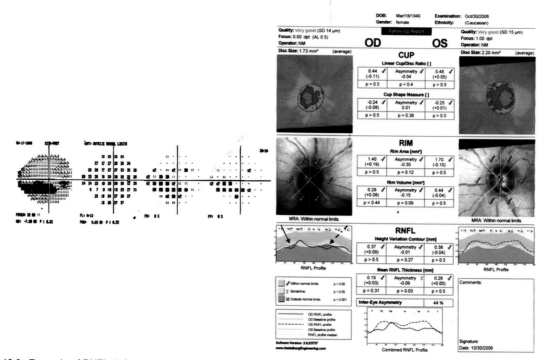

FIGURE 19.9 Example of RNFL defect visualized by scanning laser topography with the HRT 3. This patient with glaucoma has a well-established inferior arcuate scotoma (*left*). The optic nerve head analysis shows essentially normal parameters. The RNFL contour at the bottom of the printout shows that the superior RNFL values are outside of normal limits (*solid black arrow*), corresponding to the visual field defect. In addition, the inferior RNFL is also abnormal (*dotted arrow*), while the corresponding visual field area does not show a defect.

symmetry comparisons can be helpful in identifying early disease.

The HRT 3 allows the user to select an ethnic-specific normal database to use for comparison. By selecting the ethnicity of the patient, the comparison to the normal database will use individuals from the same ethnic group. This will likely improve diagnostic accuracy. In addition to using ethnic-specific databases, all HRT values are adjusted for other factors that affect the normal range such as age and optic disc size. By factoring in age, optic disc size, and ethnicity, the normal ranges of the HRT 3 databases are improved, which will likely increase sensitivity for detecting glaucoma. Currently, there are three databases available with the HRT 3, including over 700 healthy Caucasian eyes, an African-American database of over 200 healthy eyes, and an Asian Indian database consisting of over 100 healthy eyes. Ethnic-specific databases will be part of the software, if not already added by the time of this publication. The age range of the subjects in these databases is from 18 to 80 years old, and includes eyes with ±6 diopters of refractive error. The incorporation of age- and race-specific normative databases allows comparison of patient values to expected norms as a measure of probability of abnormality. The previous version of the HRT (HRT 2) utilized this concept in the Moorfield's Regression Analysis (MRA), in which the disc was divided into six sectors and thickness of the rim in each sector was compared to the database as an indirect measure of RNFL. This analysis is highly dependent upon where the operator places the contour line, which the software uses in determining where the disc edge lies. This analysis is still available on the HRT 3. New to the HRT 3 is the calculation of the Glaucoma Probability Score (GPS). This algorithm evaluates three measures of the optic nerve head shape (cup size, cup depth, and rim steepness) and two measures of parapapillary RNFL shape (horizontal and vertical RNFL curvature) and estimates the probability of the measured eye having glaucoma. The GPS calculation is independent of any operator-placed contour line or reference plane. In a study comparing the MRA to the GPS in eyes with glaucoma with visual field defects,[24] values were similar: sensitivity was 77% for the GPS and 71% for the MRA; specificity was 90% for GPS and 92% for MRA.

Work has been done on progression of cupping, as determined by contour analysis on the HRT 2, and is discussed elsewhere in this text. To date, there has been no information on follow-up of RNFL contour with the HRT 3.

OPTICAL COHERENCE TOMOGRAPHY

Optical coherence tomography (OCT) is based upon the principle of low-coherence interferometry, which allows a direct cross-sectional image analogous to an ultrasound. OCT uses a Michelson Interferometer, a superluminescent diode creates light that is split, reflects off the retina, and is compared to its unaltered form. The light is captured by a photodetector, which converts the signal into an A-scan or OCT image. This enables a cross-section of the tissue, in this case the retina and retinal nerve fiber layer, to a very precise scale. The time-of-flight delay information is then used to determine the actual thickness of the nerve fiber layer, based upon reflectivity of the individual retinal layers. OC differs from the confocal scanning laser tomography in that it provides histological representation of the tissue and is also not as subject to anterior segment polarization issues as seen with scanning laser polarimetry.

The OCT III imaging system (Stratus OCT, Carl Zeiss Meditec, Dublin, California, USA) uses a low-coherence light to penetrate the tissue and a camera analyzes the reflected image. This 40-nm broadband light differs from highly coherent light used in other imaging devices. The image acquired represents some 500 points of information from the depth at a single point. One hundred scans are put together to create a linear cross-section of the tissue. The cross-sectional image is color-coded, corresponding to the strength of the reflected signal. 'Hot' colors such as red and white correspond to highly reflective areas such as the retinal pigment epithelium (RPE) and retinal nerve fiber layer (RNFL). 'Cool' colors such as blue and black are less reflective, indicating ganglion cells, photoreceptors, and choroid. Reproducibility is on the order of $10\,\mu m$. Dilation is not always required for a good image. Image quality is affected by operator technique, corneal dryness, lens surface, and media opacities.

Retinal applications of OCT usually involve linear scans across the area of interest, such as the macula. For glaucoma, the peripapillary RNFL can be imaged. The OCT III takes three (or more) circular scans centered on the optic nerve head to produce a cylinder of information, which is 'straightened' and viewed in cross-section. This 360° circumpapillary scan evaluates nerve fibers from the entire retina entering the ONH. The printout depicts the thickness of the patient's RNFL in a cross-sectional pattern plotted along the temporal, superior, nasal, inferior, and again temporal regions, which is called the TSNIT graph. The graph also displays the RNFL normative database information as bands of red, yellow, green, and white, corresponding to the normal distribution percentiles. This allows for an easy assessment of the RNFL. Both eyes are also compared in the RNFL overlay, which allows for cross-comparison of bilateral RNFL heights in the same graph. Also included are sector averages and quadrant averages with the normative data color scheme. Statistical values are displayed in a table comparing the two eyes with a red and green color scheme indicating deviation from the normative database.

Figure 19.10 is an example of a normal RNFL as imaged by OCT. Patients with a normal RNFL distribution demonstrate a double-hump pattern with the peaks of the humps at the superior and inferior poles. There is often variance from this double-hump pattern within the normal population. For example, normal patients can exhibit 'split' nerve fiber bundles, which show up as a three- or four-hump pattern. Most papers show the average RNFL height is in the $100–120\,\mu m$ range. By the time a patient develops early glaucoma, the RNFL thickness usually falls below $80\,\mu m$. Patients with end-stage or

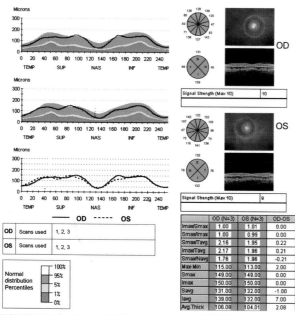

FIGURE 19.10 Normal RNFL as imaged by OCT. Both eyes from this patient demonstrate peripapillary RNFL values well within the green 'normal' range. All of the quadrant, clock hour segments, and parameter values for both eyes are likewise color-coded green, indicating that their values are above the fifth percentile. There is also a high degree of symmetry between the values from both eyes seen in the overlay of the TSNIT plots of the two eyes and the differences between parameter values.

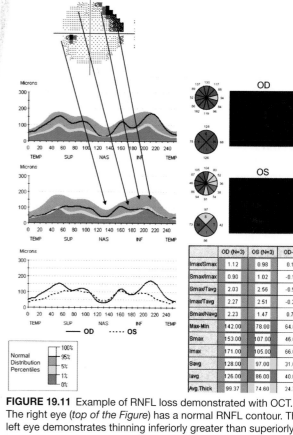

FIGURE 19.11 Example of RNFL loss demonstrated with OCT. The right eye (*top of the Figure*) has a normal RNFL contour. The left eye demonstrates thinning inferiorly greater than superiorly. Note the correlation between the inferior RNFL loss and the superior visual field defect; the arrows show the corresponding RNFL and visual field areas.

absolute glaucoma demonstrate RNFL thicknesses in the forties. Several papers have evaluated the maximum superior RNFL thickness (Smax) and the maximum inferior RNFL thickness (Imax). Normal Smax and Imax values are usually greater than 125μm. As the RNFL changes, abnormalities are observed in the TSNIT plots in glaucoma patients and include: a loss of a portion of a peak (e.g. an inferotemporal depression indicating a superonasal step on VF analysis), loss of the top of the superior or inferior peaks indicating a loss of the superior or inferior RNFL (look for arcuate defects on VF analysis), or generalized thinning or diffuse loss of the RNFL, which may appear as a lower height of the peaks or an overall straighter line (correlates as significant generalized depression or superior and inferior arcuate defects on VF analysis). Superior thinning correlates with inferior visual field defects, and vice versa. Normal eyes usually display RNFL symmetry, whereas pathologic eyes display asymmetry; thus, it is very important to look at the RNFL overlay to make a bilateral comparison. Loss of the inferior RNFL has been found more sensitive for detecting glaucoma.[16,25,26] Figure 19.11 is an example of RNFL loss as shown with OCT, correlating nicely with the visual field.

There is a suggestion that, between individuals, there is a difference in the thickness of the RNFL as measured by the OCT. A study comparing monozygotic to dizygotic twins found that the monozygotic twins had a closer RNFL overall thickness than the dizygotic twins.[20] Furthermore, there is evidence that when the disk is larger, the ability to detect RNFL loss is reduced.[27] The biggest change in the RNFL thickness occurs between the normal and early glaucoma patients. The rate of loss of the overall RNFL thickness decreases as the glaucoma advances on visual fields.[28]

In addition to RNFL analysis, OCT has also been used to evaluate the optic nerve head and macular thickness, the latter being an indirect evaluation of glaucoma damage based upon the fact that more than 50% of the RNFL comes from the macula. These analyses are not the subject of this chapter. However, in a study done to review the best method for detecting glaucoma,[29] Manassakorn and co-workers found that if inferior quadrant RNFL thinning was below 92.5μm, there was a high correlation with glaucoma. If the RNFL was between 92.5 and 119.1μm, obtaining an optic nerve head analysis helped to determine if glaucoma was present. In these patients, if the vertical cup-to-disc ratio was over 0.59, the likelihood of glaucoma was 89% and if the cup was smaller, there was a 92% likelihood of being normal. If the RNFL thickness in the inferior quadrant was greater than 119.1μm, there was an 88% likelihood of being normal. Wollstein and Schuman[26] evaluated the RNFL, optic nerve head, and the macula in 37 patients with and 37 patients without glaucoma. They found the area under the receiver operator characteristic curve for the macula was 0.08, for the RNFL (mean and inferior) 0.93, for the cup rim area 0.97, for the horizontal integrated rim width 0.96, and for the vertical integrated rim width

0.95. So, for this population, the horizontal and vertical rim width were very sensitive for detecting glaucoma and the RNFL was close. The final selection of testing method varies based on the study; many practitioners perform both the optic nerve analysis and the RNFL.

OCT has been shown to have a high level of reproducibility in determining RNFL thickness. However, the value of OCT in detecting change over time is yet to be determined.

Summary

Retinal nerve fiber layer analysis is an essential part of the glaucoma evaluation, since, in reality, the RNFL is the tissue damaged by glaucoma. Structural damage almost always precedes functional damage, and the techniques described in this chapter can often detect the earliest damage. The early detection and treatment of glaucoma is becoming more and more important as the population ages and life expectancy increases.

Over the next 5–10 years computerized scanning laser imaging devices will be updated and improved, resulting in faster, more reliable, and more accurate assessments of the RNFL. New software enhancements are ready for release for scanning laser polarimetry, and include enhanced corneal compensation (ECC), a method for reducing the 'noise' present in areas of low signal or high reflectivity. Change analysis software based upon individualized repeatability of measurements is also due for release soon, as well as new normative databases, particularly for ECC. For optical coherence tomography, the current methodology is called 'time domain,' and is relatively slow and of low resolution. High-resolution OCT has been developed, but the laser used in the device is prohibitively expensive for commercial application. A new scanning method called Fourier domain OCT is on the horizon, with commercial instruments soon to be available. Fourier domain OCT uses a broad spectrum of light with the spectral domain to capture a high-speed image with the photodetector. Another Fourier domain OCT uses a narrow band of light with a continuous-wave light source to provide a sample of the optical frequency domain of the image. The standard time domain, on the other hand, uses light waves 40 nm wide. Fourier (or 'spectral') domain OCT allows much more rapid and higher-resolution imaging.

ACKNOWLEDGEMENTS

The authors gratefully acknowledge the assistance of Michael Sinai, PhD, Heidelberg Engineering, Inc., Carlsbad, California, USA, in the preparation of some of the material in this chapter.

REFERENCES

1. American Academy of Ophthalmology. Preferred practice patterns: primary open angle glaucoma. San Francisco: California; 2005:5.

2. Quigley HA, Addicks EM, Green WR. Optic nerve damage in human glaucoma III. Quantitative correlation of nerve fiber loss and visual field defect in glaucoma, ischemic neuropathy, papilledema, and toxic neuropathy. Arch Ophthalmol 1982; 100:135–146.

3. Sommer A, Katz J, Quigley HA, et al. Clinically detectable nerve fiber atrophy precedes the onset of glaucomatous field loss. Arch Ophthalmol 1991; 109:77–83.

4. Hoyt WF, Frisén L, Newman NM. Fundoscopy of nerve fiber layer defects in glaucoma. Invest Ophthalmol 1973; 12: 814–829.

5. Sommer A, Miller NR, Pollack I, et al. The nerve fiber layer in the diagnosis of glaucoma. Arch Ophthalmol 1977; 95: 2149–2156.

6. Quigley HA, Miller NR, George T. Clinical evaluation of nerve fiber layer atrophy as an indicator of glaucomatous optic nerve damage. Arch Ophthalmol 1980; 98:1564–1571.

7. Behrendt T, Wilson LA. Spectral reflectance photography of the retina. Am J Ophthalmol 1965; 59:1079–1088.

8. Airaksinen PJ, Nieminen H. Retinal nerve fiber layer photography in glaucoma. Ophthalmology 1985; 92:877–879.

9. Airaksinen PJ, Drance SM, Douglas GR, et al. Diffuse and localized nerve fiber loss in glaucoma. Am J Ophthalmol 1984; 98:566–571.

10. Sommer A, Quigley HA, Robin AL, et al. Evaluation of nerve fiber layer assessment. Arch Ophthalmol 1984; 102:1766–1771.

11. Laser Diagnostic Technologies I. RNFL analysis with GDx VCC: a primer and clinical guide. 251-0083B ed. San Diego, CA: Laser Diagnostic Technologies, Inc.; 2004.

12. Weinreb RN, Dreher AW, Coleman A, et al. Histopathologic validation of Fourier-ellipsometry measurements of retinal nerve fiber layer thickness. Arch Ophthalmol 1990; 108(4):557–560.

13. Reus NJ, Colen TP, Lemij HG. Visualization of localized retinal nerve fiber layer defects with the GDx with individualized and fixed compensation for anterior segment birefringence. Ophthalmology 2003; 110:1512–1516.

14. Medeiros FA, Zangwill LM, Bowd C, et al. Comparison of the GDx VCC scanning laser polarimeter, HRT II confocal scanning laser ophthalmoscope, and Stratus OCT optical coherence tomograph for the detection of glaucoma. Arch Ophthalmol 2004; 122(6):827–837.

15. Zhou Q, Weinreb RN. Individualized compensation of anterior segment birefringence during scanning laser polarimetry. Invest Ophthalmol Vis Sci 2002; 43(7):2221–2228.

16. Reus NJ, Lemij HG. Diagnostic accuracy of the GDx VCC for glaucoma. Ophthalmology 2004; 111(10):1860–1865.

17. Lalezary M, Zangwill LM. Baseline optical coherence tomography predicts the development of glaucomatous change in glaucoma suspects. Am J Ophthalmol 2006; 142(4):576e1–576e8.

18. Reus NJ, de Graaf M, Lemij HG. Accuracy of GDx VCC, HRT I, and clinical assessment of stereoscopic optic nerve head photographs for diagnosing glaucoma. Br J Ophthalmol 2007; 91(3):273–274.

19. Deleon-Ortega JE, Arthur SN, McGwin G, et al. Discrimination between glaucomatous and nonglaucomatous eyes using quantitative imaging devices and subjective optic nerve head assessment. Invest Ophthalmol Vis Sci 2006; 47(8):3374–3380.

20. Hougaard JL, Kessel L, Sander B, et al. Evaluation of heredity as a determinant of retinal nerve fiber layer thickness as measured by optical coherence tomography. Invest Ophthalmol Vis Sci 2003; 44(7):3011–3016.

21. Reus NJ, Zhou Q, Lemij HG. Enhanced imaging algorithm for scanning laser polarimetry with variable corneal compensation. Invest Ophthalmol Vis Sci 2006; 47(9):3870–3877.

22. Yucel YH, Gupta N, Kalichman MW, et al. Relationship of optic disc topography to optic nerve fiber number in glaucoma. Arch Ophthalmol 1998; 116(4):493–497.

23. Zangwill LM, Chan K, Bowd C, et al. Heidelberg retina tomograph measurements of the optic disc and parapapillary retina for detecting glaucoma analyzed by machine learning classifiers. Invest Ophthalmol Vis Sci 2004; 45(9):3144–3151.

24. Harizman N, Zelefsky JR, Ilitchev E, et al. Detection of glaucoma using operator-dependent versus operator-independent classification in the Heidelberg retinal tomography-III. Br J Ophthalmol 2006; 90:1390–1392.

25. Nouri-Mahdavi K, Caprioli J. Identifying early glaucoma with optical coherence tomography. Am J Ophthalmol 2004; 137(2):228–235.

26. Wollstein G, Schuman JS. Comparison of three optical coherence tomography scanning areas for detection of glaucomatous damage. Am J Ophthalmol 2005; 139(1):39–43.

27. Medeiros FA, Weinreb RN. Influence of disease severity and optic disc size on the diagnostic performance of imaging instruments in glaucoma. Invest Ophthalmol Vis Sci 2006; 47(3):1008–1015.

28. Sihota R, Singh R. Diagnostic capability of optical coherence tomography in evaluating the degree of glaucomatous retinal nerve fiber damage. Invest Ophthalmol Vis Sci 2006; 47: 2006–2010.

29. Manassakorn A, Nouri-Mahdavi K, Caprioli J. Comparison of retinal nerve fiber layer thickness and optic disk algorithms with optical coherence tomography to detect glaucoma. Am J Ophthalmol 2006; 141(1):105–115.

Structure and Function Relationships in Glaucoma

Marcelo T Nicolela, Lesya M Shuba, and Bettina K Windisch

INTRODUCTION

Functional loss in glaucoma is usually insidious and starts peripherally, leaving patients asymptomatic in the early stages of the disease. Currently, we do not have any clinically applicable direct way to measure neuronal loss in glaucoma and we use, instead, different surrogate measures to estimate the functional and structural loss in this disease. It is of paramount importance to have sensitive and specific tests to detect subtle optic nerve and/or visual field changes both for early diagnosis of the disease and for monitoring it. Optic disc and visual field assessments are complex tasks that have become an integral part of glaucoma management. Until recently, most studies have relied on subjective and nonquantitative ways to assess structural damage. With the advent of automated imaging techniques, we have, for the first time, the capability to reliably quantify structural loss in glaucoma. In addition, newer functional tests, such as short-wavelength automated perimetry (SWAP) and frequency double perimetry (FDT), are designed to measure function of specific subpopulations of retinal ganglion cells (RGCs). These tests often can detect early visual field loss even when function is normal on standard automated perimetry (SAP). It is fair to say that these new structural and functional tests are allowing us to reexamine the nature and the strength of structure–function correlation in glaucoma.

This chapter will concentrate on the structure and function correlation in glaucoma as determined with these new test modalities and will provide a critical appraisal of the published cross-sectional and longitudinal studies on this topic, from primate models to human studies.

STRUCTURE AND FUNCTION CORRELATION IN GLAUCOMA EVALUATED WITH CONVENTIONAL TESTING

The topographic relationship between arcuate scotoma and retinal nerve fiber layer (RNFL) anatomy was first studied by Bjerrum in 1889. With the advent of more sophisticated manual and automated perimetry, as well as photographic methods to document the status of the optic nerve and RNFL, several cross-sectional studies have better evaluated the correlation between structural and functional changes in glaucoma.[1,2] Drance and colleagues[3] were able to predict the presence of visual field defects by examining the optic disc with 85% specificity and 80% sensitivity, which was repeated by other authors.[4] These cross-sectional studies also suggested that structural changes at the optic nerve head (ONH) and/or RNFL tend to precede visual field changes early in the disease.

Over the years, some large longitudinal studies have better evaluated the temporal relationship between structural and functional changes utilizing conventional techniques. Sommer et al.[5] reported on a large cohort of ocular hypertensive patients ($n = 1344$) followed for an average of 6 years and showed that 50–85% of patients who developed visual field defects had RNFL defects prior to visual field loss, in some cases by as much as 6 years. The Ocular Hypertension Treatment Study (OHTS) showed that approximately half of patients converted to glaucoma on the basis of visual field changes and half on the basis of optic disc changes.[6] It should be noted that RNFL was not evaluated in the OHTS and that patients who converted to glaucoma had a larger baseline cup-to-disc ratio than those who did not convert, raising the possibility that perhaps some of converters already had some subtle structural damage at the onset of the study. Similar results were observed in the European Glaucoma Prevention Study, except that a slightly higher percentage of patients converted on the basis of visual field changes, but again these subjects had larger cup-to-disc ratios than non-converters.[7] Johnson et al.[8] followed 259 subjects (479 eyes) with elevated intraocular pressure (IOP) and normal SAP at baseline and showed that 75–80% of patients who developed abnormalities on SAP had optic discs that were judged glaucomatous at baseline.

These clinical observations, suggesting that structural changes often precede visual field changes, are confirmed by studies of Quigley and colleagues who first showed in human eyes from autopsy cases that a significant number of RGCs could be lost before a detectable visual field abnormality was present, on either Goldmann perimetry or on SAP.[9,10]

STRUCTURE AND FUNCTION CORRELATION IN GLAUCOMA EVALUATED WITH AUTOMATED IMAGING TECHNIQUES

The relation between structure and function is intimately linked to methods used to measure these parameters. The advent of automated imaging techniques allowed practitioners for the first time to objectively and reproducibly quantify glaucomatous structural losses in the ONH and RNFL. Some of the new imaging devices have been extensively studied and successfully incorporated in clinical practice: confocal scanning laser ophthalmoscopy (CSLO), ocular coherence tomography (OCT), and scanning laser polarimetry (SLP). CSLO (clinical device: Heidelberg Retina Tomograph) generates a topographic height map of the optic nerve and surrounding retina by analyzing the light peak reflectance off the retinal surface captured with a confocal photodetector. OCT (clinical device: Stratus OCT) uses interferometry of backscattered light to determine thickness of different structures in the retina and ONH. The basis of this device is similar to B-scan ultrasonography, but with much higher image resolution. This technique is used in glaucoma for either measurement of the RNFL thickness with circular scans, or measurement of the ONH topography with radial scans. Measurements of the RNFL thickness appear to be more promising and have been more extensively studied. SLP (clinical device: GDx VCC) also estimates RNFL thickness by measuring retardation of polarized light reflected back from the eye, which is correlated to the thickness of the RNFL due to its microtubular anatomy.

A number of studies evaluated the structure–function relationship using one or more of these automated devices with, sometimes, conflicting results. Most studies showed a significant but relatively poor correlation between optic disc stereometric parameters measured with CSLO and visual field indices measured with SAP.[11-15] The results from these studies suggest that, as expected, (1) the correlation is stronger if a wide range of individuals is included (from normal subjects to those with advanced disease), and (2) regional correlations are usually stronger than global ones. Studies performed with OCT and SLP correlating RNFL and visual field parameters showed similar pattern of results as the ones performed with CSLO.[13,14,16] Bowd et al.[13] correlated measures of all three automated imaging devices (CSLO, OCT, and SLP) with visual function (SAP) in normal subjects, glaucoma suspects, and individuals with glaucoma. The authors showed a significant but weak correlation (maximal R^2 with each device was 0.26, 0.38, and 0.21, respectively) between structural and functional parameters, with little difference between linear and logarithmic associations.

One problem introduced by the new automated imaging devices in understanding the structure and function correlation in glaucoma is that they all measure different structures in the eye using different techniques, and even the correlation between structural measures obtained by these devices is less than ideal.

STRUCTURAL CORRELATION WITH SELECTIVE FUNCTIONAL TESTS

The vast majority of studies evaluated structural correlation with visual function measured with SAP. SAP uses a differential contrast stimulus that consists of a small spot of white light briefly presented on a white background. Most RGC types can respond to this stimulus. Owing to the redundancy within the visual system, a considerable amount of RGC loss can occur in some cases before SAP is able to detect functional damage. Newer perimetric techniques such as SWAP and FDT have been designed to measure specific subpopulations of RGCs. There are two hypotheses explaining why these tests are believed to be more sensitive than SAP in detecting early functional losses: (1) they measure ganglion cells that are preferentially damaged in early glaucoma, and/or (2) by stimulating selective RGC subpopulations the redundancy of the visual system is reduced.[17]

SWAP isolates the short-wavelength-sensitive pathway throughout the retino-geniculo-cortical route which originates at the receptor level in the retina, with the short-wavelength (blue) cones. These cones send projections to the blue-cone bipolar cells, which in turn project to the small bistratified RGCs. Recent evidence suggests that the small bistratified RGCs are distinct from the parvocellular cells because their axons project to the intralaminar-koniocellular layers of the lateral geniculate nucleus (LGN).[18,19]

A number of studies have demonstrated that SWAP is able to detect glaucomatous damage earlier than SAP, in some cases even 3–5 years earlier.[20] SWAP field defects may correspond more closely to structural changes of the ONH than white-on-white field defects.[8] SWAP deficits have been found to correlate well with optic disc and RNFL damage.[21,22]

Frequency doubling technology (FDT) perimetry was introduced in 1997.[23] The frequency doubling effect is created by a low spatial frequency sinusoidal grating (<1 cycle/degree) undergoing high temporal frequency counterphase flicker (>15 Hz), thereby producing the appearance of twice as many light and dark bars than are physically present (i.e. the spatial frequency of the bars appears to be doubled). This phenomenon is believed to isolate a subset of M ganglion cells, the M_y cells.[24]

Several studies showed that FDT is able to detect glaucomatous damage before the SAP,[25,26] while others suggest that FDT and SAP detect different visual field defects.[27,28] Overall, FDT may be a good adjunct for diagnosis and follow-up of patients with glaucoma.[29,30] Few studies reported on correlation of FDT abnormalities to structural changes. In one study, rim area (measured with CSLO) was the stereometric parameter that best correlated to FDT indices.[31]

STRENGTH OF STRUCTURE–FUNCTION CORRELATION

Studies that examined in greater details the structure–function relationship in glaucoma have produced variable results.[32–35] The strength of the relationship seems to depend strongly on the stage of the disease, as well as on the techniques used to measure structure and function.[36] It is frequently believed that optic disc changes and, particularly, RNFL changes often occur before detectable visual field loss. Optic disc examination is more useful at earlier stages in glaucoma. As the disease progresses, and in end-stage glaucoma, visual field examinations become of greater value.[37]

Despite the clear statistical correlation between structure and function in cross-sectional studies, there is a significant spread of the results and some controversy regarding what type of mathematical function best explains this correlation (linear, logarithmic, or other mathematical functions). In a recent review article, Anderson outlined a number of limitations in the assessment of the relationship between structure and function in glaucoma: (1) problems related to variability of functional and structural measures; (2) the fact that stimulus size in automated perimetry is typically uniform across the visual field, leading to a mismatch between stimulus size and the receptive field size which increases with eccentricity; (3) the debate as to whether there is a selective loss of certain subpopulations of RGCs in glaucoma; (4) problems with background luminance in automated perimetry; and (5) peripheral optical defocus due to peripheral refractive errors.[38]

TOPOGRAPHIC STRUCTURE–FUNCTION CORRELATION

In order to topographically correlate structure and function in glaucoma, it is necessary to develop adequate functional maps that relate visual field test points to areas on the optic disc and/or RNFL. Weber and Ulrich produced a functional map with 21 retinal nerve fiber areas.[39] Garway-Heath and colleagues used RNFL images from glaucoma and glaucoma suspect patients to derive a map relating visual field test points in the Humphrey 24–2 to regions on the optic disc (Fig. 20.1).[40] Gardiner et al. found in their group of 166 subjects with early glaucoma or glaucoma suspects that the overall optic disc sectors often correlated with the visual field sensitivity in a way predicted by the map of Garway-Heath and colleagues.[15] It is clear that these functional maps work for most but not all individuals. Patients with tilted optic discs or severe myopia, for instance, might have altered or abnormal functional maps.

THE ISSUE OF SCALING OF FUNCTIONAL AND STRUCTURAL MEASURES

Studies by Garway-Heath and colleagues,[33,41] as well as other authors, suggested that there is an issue of scaling when correlating visual field sensitivity measured on a

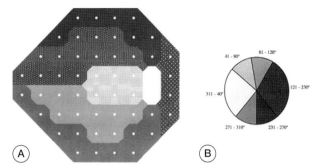

FIGURE 20.1 Example of topographic map correlating areas of the visual field **(A)** with areas of the optic disc **(B)**. (From Garway-Heath DF, et al. Mapping the visual field to the optic disc in normal tension glaucoma eyes. Ophthalmology 2000; 107:1809–1815.)

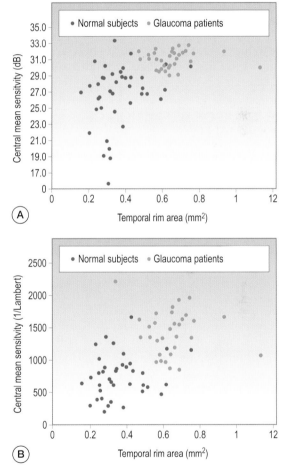

FIGURE 20.2 Correlation between mean sensitivity measured with SAP displayed on a logarithmic scale (dB in **(A)**); and on a linear scale (1/Lambert in **(B)**) and temporal rim area measured with CSLO. (Adapted from Garway-Heath DF, et al. Scaling the hill of vision: the physiological relationship between light sensitivity and ganglion cell numbers. Invest Ophthalmol Vis Sci 2000; 41:1774–1782.)

logarithmic scale (dB) with structural parameters measured on a linear scale, such as rim area, for example.[34] The logarithmic scale of visual function tests accentuates changes at low decibel levels while minimizing changes at high decibel levels, which could partly explain the typical curvilinear relationship between visual function and structural losses (Fig. 20.2A). When a linear scale is used for differential light sensitivity (such as 1/Lambert), the original curvilinear relationship becomes linear (Fig. 20.2B). Despite this scaling issue, it should be noted that a considerable scatter still remains when comparing two linear variables, even in the normal end of the curve, and the structure–function relationship is significant only because individuals with a wide range of losses are included, from normal to end-stage glaucoma (see Fig. 20.2A). Such large scatter was also observed in the experimental studies in monkeys performed by Harwerth and colleagues.[34,42] It underlies the fundamental fact that the strength of the correlation between structure and function in glaucoma is relatively weak.

Apart from the scaling issue, other important factors can weaken the structure–function correlation in glaucoma: variability in structural and functional measures, study design, definitions of abnormality, and even possible influence of non-RGC changes in structural measurements (for instance, changes in other cells, such as glial cells).

THE ISSUE OF DEFINITION OF ABNORMALITY

In cross-sectional studies abnormality is defined as a departure from normal levels. Normal limits, however, are usually fairly large, both for functional and particularly for structural measures.[43] For instance, individuals with large optic discs are known to have larger cups as well as larger neuroretinal rim area and can be easily misclassified as having structural damage if the size of the optic disc size is not taken into consideration during measurements. The opposite situation can occur in individuals with small optic discs. On the other hand, some individuals might be considered supernormals in terms of visual function and, in these cases, even a large amount of visual field loss can still fall within normal limits of cross-sectional data. This large interindividual variability complicates the identification of the precise nature of the structure–function correlation in glaucoma. This is particularly relevant when analyzing earlier changes, since the differentiation between true early losses and just a normal variant can be problematic. In such situations, longitudinal data are more helpful, since damage is defined as a change from baseline for a particular individual, and is, therefore, independent of interindividual variability.

THE ISSUE OF DETERMINING CHANGE (OR PROGRESSION) IN LONGITUDINAL STUDIES

Few longitudinal studies have evaluated the nature of the structure–function relationship in progressive glaucoma.

Most of the published studies have employed CSLO and SAP. One of the significant issues to be considered is lack of a universally accepted method for determining progression with CSLO (or any other imaging technique) or even with SAP. Several recent studies evaluated the ability of SAP to reliably determine progression using trend, event, or stratification type of analysis, concluding that each method has advantages and disadvantages and at any given time different subjects are identified as progressing with each analysis.[44,45] The same lack of accepted criteria occurs for structural progression.[30] One approach is to utilize empirical criteria for progression derived from long-term variability data obtained from normal controls.[46,47] One problem with this type of method is that the variability characteristics of normal and glaucomatous optic discs are intrinsically different.

An additional factor that might complicate longitudinal comparisons of structure and function is that the relative change that is detectable with each technique might vary. In a recent study, Artes and Chauhan proposed an analysis termed 'evidence of change' (EOC) which was developed to enable a fair comparison of the utility of functional and structural tests in detecting progression.[35] This analysis compares the strength of the statistical evidence that the measurements have changed over time, as opposed to comparing absolute changes. In their article, the authors conclude that in their population of early to moderate glaucoma individuals, indicators of visual function (measured with SAP) and of optic disc structure (measured with CSLO) provided largely independent measures of progression.

Summary

There is no question that structure and function are correlated in glaucoma and both are important for making the diagnosis of the disease and/or for monitoring it. Having said that, several studies have demonstrated that there is a large scatter in this correlation, representing the large interindividual variability that exists for both structural and functional measures. With the advent of automated imaging devices and new functional techniques, the nature of the structural–functional relationship in glaucoma is being reassessed. In practical terms, however, it remains true in the majority of cases that structural deficits of the optic disc and/or RNFL tend to precede detectable visual field changes. However, this is not necessarily always true, particularly in cases with small optic discs. In individuals with well-established glaucoma, both structural and functional tests are important for monitoring the disease, but there is often a disconnection between structural and functional progression, due in part to limitations in our ability to determine progression with current clinical measures. As the disease progresses, visual function tests become increasingly important in monitoring glaucoma, since often in advanced glaucoma the tests measuring structure do not have any dynamic range left to allow for meaningful clinical decisions.

REFERENCES

1. Caprioli J, Miller JM. Correlation of structure and function in glaucoma. Quantitative measurements of disc and field. Ophthalmology 1988; 95(6):723–727.

2. Drance SM, et al. The correlation of functional and structural measurements in glaucoma patients and normal subjects. Am J Ophthalmol 1986; 102(5):612–616.

3. Drance SM. The disc and the field in glaucoma. Ophthalmology 1978; 85(3):209–214.

4. Hitchings RA, Spaeth GL. The optic disc in glaucoma II: correlation of the appearance of the optic disc with the visual field. Br J Ophthalmol 1977; 61(2):107–113.

5. Sommer A, et al. Clinically detectable nerve fiber atrophy precedes the onset of glaucomatous field loss. Arch Ophthalmol 1991; 109(1):77–83.

6. Gordon MO, et al. The Ocular Hypertension Treatment Study: baseline factors that predict the onset of primary open-angle glaucoma. Arch Ophthalmol 2002; 120(6):714–720; discussion 829–830.

7. Miglior S, et al. Predictive factors for open-angle glaucoma among patients with ocular hypertension in the European Glaucoma Prevention Study. Ophthalmology 2007; 114(1):3–9.

8. Johnson CA, et al. Structure and function evaluation (SAFE): II. Comparison of optic disk and visual field characteristics. Am J Ophthalmol 2003; 135(2):148–154.

9. Quigley HA, et al. Optic nerve damage in human glaucoma. II. The site of injury and susceptibility to damage. Arch Ophthalmol 1981; 99(4):635–649.

10. Quigley HA, Dunkelberger GR, Green WR. Retinal ganglion cell atrophy correlated with automated perimetry in human eyes with glaucoma. Am J Ophthalmol 1989; 107(5):453–464.

11. Danesh-Meyer HV, et al. Regional correlation of structure and function in glaucoma, using the Disc Damage Likelihood Scale, Heidelberg Retina Tomograph, and visual fields. Ophthalmology 2006; 113(4):603–611.

12. Lan YW, Henson DB, Kwartz AJ. The correlation between optic nerve head topographic measurements, peripapillary nerve fibre layer thickness, and visual field indices in glaucoma. Br J Ophthalmol 2003; 87(9):1135–1141.

13. Bowd C, et al. Structure–function relationships using confocal scanning laser ophthalmoscopy, optical coherence tomography, and scanning laser polarimetry. Invest Ophthalmol Vis Sci 2006; 47(7):2889–2895.

14. Reus NJ, Lemij HG. Relationships between standard automated perimetry, HRT confocal scanning laser ophthalmoscopy, and GDx VCC scanning laser polarimetry. Invest Ophthalmol Vis Sci 2005; 46(11):4182–4188.

15. Gardiner SK, Johnson CA, Cioffi GA. Evaluation of the structure–function relationship in glaucoma. Invest Ophthalmol Vis Sci 2005; 46(10):3712–3717.

16. Ajtony C, et al. Relationship between visual field sensitivity and retinal nerve fiber layer thickness as measured by optical coherence tomography. Invest Ophthalmol Vis Sci 2007; 48(1):258–263.

17. Johnson CA, The Glenn A. Fry Award Lecture. Early losses of visual function in glaucoma. Optom Vis Sci 1995; 72(6):359–370.

18. Dacey DM, Lee BB. The 'blue-on' opponent pathway in primate retina originates from a distinct bistratified ganglion cell type. Nature 1994; 367(6465):731–735.

19. Martin PR, et al. Evidence that blue-on cells are part of the third geniculocortical pathway in primates. Eur J Neurosci 1997; 9(7):1536–1541.

20. Johnson CA, et al. Blue-on-yellow perimetry can predict the development of glaucomatous visual field loss. Arch Ophthalmol 1993; 111(5):645–650.

21. Mok KH, Lee VW. Nerve fiber analyzer and short-wavelength automated perimetry in glaucoma suspects: a pilot study. Ophthalmology 2000; 107(11):2101–2104.

22. Ugurlu S, et al. Relationship between structural abnormalities and short-wavelength perimetric defects in eyes at risk of glaucoma. Am J Ophthalmol 2000; 129(5):592–598.

23. Johnson CA, Samuels SJ. Screening for glaucomatous visual field loss with frequency-doubling perimetry. Invest Ophthalmol Vis Sci 1997; 38(2):413–425.

24. Shabana N, et al. Motion perception in glaucoma patients: a review. Surv Ophthalmol 2003; 48(1):92–106.

25. Sample PA, et al. Visual function-specific perimetry for indirect comparison of different ganglion cell populations in glaucoma. Invest Ophthalmol Vis Sci 2000; 41(7):1783–1790.

26. Medeiros FA, Sample PA, Weinreb RN. Frequency doubling technology perimetry abnormalities as predictors of glaucomatous visual field loss. Am J Ophthalmol 2004; 137(5):863–871.

27. Haymes SA, et al. Glaucomatous visual field progression with frequency-doubling technology and standard automated perimetry in a longitudinal prospective study. Invest Ophthalmol Vis Sci 2005; 46(2):547–554.

28. Leeprechanon N, et al. Frequency doubling perimetry and short-wavelength automated perimetry to detect early glaucoma. Ophthalmology 2007; 114(5):931–937.

29. Alward WL. Frequency doubling technology perimetry for the detection of glaucomatous visual field loss. Am J Ophthalmol 2000; 129(3):376–378.

30. Artes PH, et al. Threshold and variability properties of matrix frequency-doubling technology and standard automated perimetry in glaucoma. Invest Ophthalmol Vis Sci 2005; 46(7):2451–2457.

31. Iester M, et al. Sector-based analysis of frequency doubling technology sensitivity and optic nerve head shape parameters. Eur J Ophthalmol 2007; 17(2):223–229.

32. Strouthidis NG, et al. Structure and function in glaucoma: the relationship between a functional visual field map and an anatomic retinal map. Invest Ophthalmol Vis Sci 2006; 47(12):5356–5362.

33. Garway-Heath DF, et al. Relationship between electrophysiological, psychophysical, and anatomical measurements in glaucoma. Invest Ophthalmol Vis Sci 2002; 43(7):2213–2220.

34. Harwerth RS, et al. Neural losses correlated with visual losses in clinical perimetry. Invest Ophthalmol Vis Sci 2004; 45(9):3152–3160.

35. Artes PH, Chauhan BC. Longitudinal changes in the visual field and optic disc in glaucoma. Prog Retin Eye Res 2005; 24(3):333–354.

36. Girkin CA. Relationship between structure of optic nerve/nerve fiber layer and functional measurements in glaucoma. Curr Opin Ophthalmol 2004; 15(2):96–101.

37. Blumenthal EZ, et al. Correlating structure with function in end-stage glaucoma. Ophthalmic Surg Lasers Imaging 2006; 37(3):218–223.

38. Anderson RS. The psychophysics of glaucoma: improving the structure/function relationship. Prog Retin Eye Res 2006; 25(1):79–97.

39. Weber J, Ulrich H. A perimetric nerve fiber bundle map. Int Ophthalmol 1991; 15(3):193–200.

40. Garway-Heath DF, et al. Mapping the visual field to the optic disc in normal tension glaucoma eyes. Ophthalmology 2000; 107(10):1809–1815.

41. Garway-Heath DF, et al. Scaling the hill of vision: the physiological relationship between light sensitivity and ganglion cell numbers. Invest Ophthalmol Vis Sci 2000; 41(7):1774–1782.

42. Harwerth RS, et al. Visual field defects and neural losses from experimental glaucoma. Prog Retin Eye Res 2002; 21(1):91–125.

43. Jonas JB, Gusek GC, Naumann GO. Optic disc, cup and neuroretinal rim size, configuration and correlations in normal eyes. Invest Ophthalmol Vis Sci 1988; 29(7):1151–1158.

44. Spry PG, Johnson CA. Identification of progressive glaucomatous visual field loss. Surv Ophthalmol 2002; 47(2):158–173.

45. Vesti E, Johnson CA, Chauhan BC. Comparison of different methods for detecting glaucomatous visual field progression. Invest Ophthalmol Vis Sci 2003; 44(9):3873–3879.

46. Chauhan BC, et al. Optic disc and visual field changes in a prospective longitudinal study of patients with glaucoma: comparison of scanning laser tomography with conventional perimetry and optic disc photography. Arch Ophthalmol 2001; 119(10):1492–1499.

47. Tan JC, Hitchings RA. Optimizing and validating an approach for identifying glaucomatous change in optic nerve topography. Invest Ophthalmol Vis Sci 2004; 45(5):1396–1403.

Techniques Used for Evaluation of Ocular Blood Flow

Ali S Hafez and Mark R Lesk

INTRODUCTION

Vascular disorders in the eye may have an important role in the pathogenesis of glaucomatous optic neuropathy. A primary requirement for understanding such vascular disorders is the ability to precisely and reliably evaluate the state of ocular perfusion in health and disease. This has led to the exploration of many innovative and diverse techniques. The fact that the different methods available measure different aspects of ocular circulation and at different locations in the eye complicates direct comparisons between techniques. In this chapter, the authors review the principle, validity, advantages, and limitations of the various methods used to measure ocular blood flow.

COLOR DOPPLER IMAGING

Color Doppler imaging (CDI) combines ultrasound imaging with Doppler shift analysis to measure blood flow in the retrobulbar vasculature. The technique evaluates blood flow velocity by detecting shifts in the frequency of sound reflected from the flowing blood.

CDI focuses primarily on velocities in the ophthalmic artery (OA), central retinal artery (CRA), and short posterior ciliary arteries (SPCAs), specifically those feeding the nasal and temporal sides of the optic nerve head (ONH). From knowledge of retrobulbar vascular landmarks as well as an understanding of the characteristic waveform and sound of velocities, specific retrobulbar vessels can be located. From the Doppler spectrum of these vessels the direction of blood flow is identified;[1] blood flowing away from the center of the body towards the CDI probe is generally arterial and is displayed in red, whereas blood flowing towards the center of the body and away from the probe is venous and is displayed in blue. Flow velocities data are plotted against time. The peak and trough of the waves are then identified by the operator. From these points, peak systolic velocity (PSV) and end diastolic velocity (EDV) are measured. These parameters can be used to calculate the resistivity index (RI) (Fig. 21.1). RI is the most reproducible parameter of the CDI and is calculated as RI = (PSV − EDV)/PSV.

CDI studies have found reduced peak systolic velocity and end diastolic velocity and an increased resistivity index in the retrobulbar vessels of open-angle glaucoma (OAG) patients[2] and normal-tension glaucoma (NTG) patients[3] when compared with normal controls. Lower baseline retrobulbar blood flow velocities were found in eyes with progressive visual field damage and uncontrolled intraocular pressure (IOP).[4] Conversely, reduction of IOP after trabeculectomy was shown to result in a significant improvement in retrobulbar blood flow parameters.[5]

ADVANTAGES

The technique is attractive and relatively easy to understand. Results can be obtained reliably from the larger vessels such as the ophthalmic or central retinal arteries. The widespread presence of color Doppler machines further encourages pursuing it as a useful investigative tool for the retrobulbar vasculature.

LIMITATIONS

1. CDI allows measurement of velocity rather than blood flow. With no information about vessel diameter, it is not possible to determine the blood flow

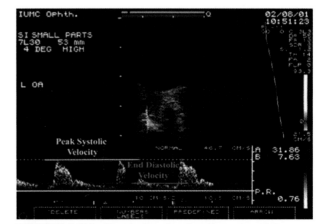

FIGURE 21.1 Color Doppler imaging showing peak systolic (*yellow arrow*) and end diastolic velocities (*red arrow*) in the ophthalmic artery. (Courtesy Dr Alon Harris.)

in a particular vessel. Localized narrowing of vessels was also reported to produce an increase in velocity despite a decrease in blood flow.[6]

2. The reliability of CDI results depends on the caliber of the vessel imaged and the angulation of the Doppler probe relative to it. A high level of location-dependent variability has been reported for measurements from the CRA.[7] Reproducible probe positioning is subject to the skill and experience of the user and comes after a relatively long learning curve.

3. It is not clear whether the calculated resistivity index (RI) correlates with true vascular resistance in vivo.

4. The resolution of CDI might not allow precise measurement of the blood velocity within the small vessels supplying the ONH (e.g. short posterior ciliary arteries).[8] The variability of measurements in these arteries was reported to be higher compared to the OA or the CRA.

5. In the retrobulbar region, short posterior ciliary arteries are varied in their number, size, and position from eye to eye[9] and lie intertwined with one another, which makes it difficult to detect by CDI which of those short posterior ciliary arteries is being measured and which actually supplies the ONH.

6. Abnormal velocities and resistivity in the ophthalmic artery do not mean reduced blood flow in the ONH, because blood flow in the ophthalmic artery does not necessarily correlate with that in the short posterior ciliary arteries.[6]

PULSATILE OCULAR BLOOD FLOW AND FUNDUS PULSATION AMPLITUDE

Arterial blood flow to the eye varies with the heart cycle. Blood flow with each pulse causes a change in intraocular volume, primarily via filling of the choroid and, in turn, results in modulation of IOP. Correspondingly, the intraocular volume and the pressure are highest during systole and lowest during diastole.

Pulsatile ocular blood flow (POBF) quantifies the pulsatile component of the ocular blood measured during systole, which was reported to account for as much as 75–85% of the total blood flow.[10] Pulsatile blood flow mainly reflects the choroidal circulation, with some contribution from retrobulbar pulsations, while the role of the retinal circulation is minimal.

The Langham POBF technique[11,12] is based on continuous IOP recording, which allows measurement of the pulsatile change in IOP during the cardiac cycle. The instrument consists of an applanation pneumotonometer interfaced with a microcomputer that records the ocular pulse. The amplitude of the IOP pulse wave is used to calculate the change in ocular volume and thereby to calculate the pulsatile component of ocular blood flow. Another method for quantification of choroidal pulsation is by means of interferometry.[13,14] A beam of a diode laser (783 nm) is reflected at both the front surface of the cornea and the fundus. The two re-emitted waves produce interference fringes from which the changes in distance between cornea and retina during the cardiac cycle

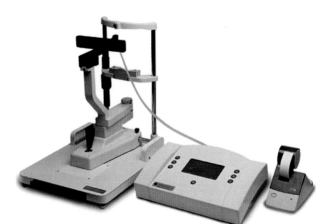

FIGURE 21.2 Pulsatile ocular blood flowmeter. (Courtesy Dr Alon Harris.)

can be calculated. The maximum change in distance is called fundus pulsation amplitude (FPA) and corresponds to the pulsatile displacement of the retinal surface caused primarily by the filling of the underlying choroid during systole.

POBF studies reported a significantly reduced POBF in OAG patients compared to normal subjects and ocular hypertensives.[15,16] Lower POBF was also shown in high-risk versus low-risk ocular hypertensives.[17]

ADVANTAGE

Pulsatile ocular blood flow is relatively inexpensive and noninvasive, and is simple to perform. Neither clear media nor good fixation is required for accurate measurements. The latest POBF machine (Fig. 21.2) is compact, portable, and more reliable than its predecessors. FPA gives an estimation of the choroidal pulsations and has good reproducibility.

LIMITATIONS

1. Interpretation of the results derived by POBF is based on a number of assumptions:[18] first, the change of IOP is solely caused by volume change due to the blood bolus entering the eye with each pulse; second, retrograde blood flow does not occur; third, the pressure–volume relationship (ocular rigidity) is standard for all persons; and fourth, the outflow to the venous system is constant and not pulsatile.

2. POBF can only detect the pulsatile component of ocular blood flow and cannot estimate the nonpulsatile component. It is not precisely known what proportions of the total ocular blood flow are pulsatile and nonpulsatile and whether this proportion might vary from eye to eye.

3. The ratio of pulsatile to nonpulsatile blood flow is unlikely to be constant, especially with changes of systemic blood pressure or IOP. Changes in pulsatile blood flow are therefore not necessarily representative of changes in total blood flow.

4. POBF measurements were shown to be significantly influenced by factors such as posture,[15,16] axial

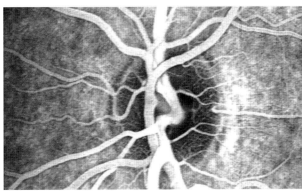

FIGURE 21.3 Fluorescein fundus angiogram of the optic nerve head and peripapillary retina.

length of the eye,[19] and heart rate.[20] This might have an impact on comparisons between different groups.

5. Measurements of FPA include the displacement of the cornea, thought to contribute as much as 20% of the signal. Like POBF, FPA measures only the pulsatile component of ocular blood flow.

FLUORESCEIN AND INDOCYANINE GREEN ANGIOGRAPHY

In fluorescein fundus angiography, fluorescein is injected into the cubital vein and the passage of the dye is visualized through the ocular vessels (Fig. 21.3). Under normal conditions the blood–retinal barrier prevents free passage of fluorescein into the tissues. Tight junctions are present both at the endothelial level of the retinal vessels and between the cells of the retinal pigment epithelium.

Fluorescein makes it possible to study the retinal circulation in great detail and the ONH circulation to some extent, while analysis of the choroidal circulation remains more difficult as the endothelium of the choriocapillaris has fenestrations through which fluorescein molecules can pass.[21] Indocyanine green (ICG) is thus used for better visualization of the choroidal circulation. ICG is a dye that binds rapidly and completely to certain plasma proteins, preventing the dye from leaving the fenestrated endothelium of the choriocapillaris.

Some of the main evidence implicating blood flow deficits in glaucoma is derived from fluorescein and ICG angiography.[22–27] In the ONH, filling defects seen on angiography were found to represent areas of ischemia.[23,24] Such filling defects were more marked in glaucomatous discs than in ocular hypertensives and were least marked in normal discs.[25] Delayed filling and prolonged arteriovenous passage time have also been described in both the retina and the choroid of glaucoma patients. The reduction in retinal circulation was reported primarily in OAG patients, whereas choroidal blood flow was primarily reduced in NTG patients.[27]

ADVANTAGE

Through computerized frame-by-frame analysis of fluorescein or ICG angiograms, quantification of ONH, peripapillary retinal, and choroidal hemodynamics is possible. Confocal imaging techniques help measure filling rates and areas of fluorescein filling defects.[28]

LIMITATIONS

1. Inadequate quality of fluorescein or ICG angiograms to outline circulation in the ONH and choroid as well as inadequate resolution to visualize disc vessels arranged in multiple superimposed layers.
2. Reliability of a single angiographic examination in providing information about the ocular circulation.
3. Difficulty in outlining the deeper ONH capillaries. Capillaries of posterior ciliary arteries (PCAs) origin are completely masked by capillaries of retinal origin in the surface nerve fiber layer of the disc.
4. Variation in the sources of optic disc fluorescence. Fluorescence of the disc is essentially caused by retinal vessels with little contribution from the deeper ciliary vessels as well as staining from the adjacent peripapillary choroid.[29]
5. Significance of the presence or absence of filling defects. Angiography may fail to demonstrate filling defects in cases of transient ischemia caused by temporary fall in ocular perfusion pressure.[30]
6. Transient systemic hypotensive changes demonstrated by some patients following the injection of dye might affect the arteriovenous passage time measurements. These measurements may thus not reflect the subject's true ocular hemodynamics.

LASER DOPPLER VELOCIMETRY

The Doppler effect was first described by the Austrian physicist Christian Doppler in 1842. It describes the frequency shift that a sound or light wave undergoes when emitted from an object, which is moving away from or towards an observer. Measurement of red blood cell velocity using this technique was first described in 1972 by Riva and co-workers.[31]

In laser Doppler velocimetry (LDV), the laser beam is directed at a specific vessel. The backscattered light contains two components: light scattered by stationary structures such as the vessel wall, and light scattered by red blood cells flowing through this vessel. The interference of these two components leads to an alternating signal at the photodetector. This signal is then subjected to a fast Fourier transform algorithm to obtain a Doppler shift frequency spectrum (DSFS) which is found to be proportional to blood velocities within the vessel measured.[32]

Laser Doppler velocimetry was found to vary with variations of IOP. The return of the red blood cell velocity towards normal after an IOP increase above normal or an IOP decrease below normal was reported and attributed to autoregulatory mechanisms.[33]

ADVANTAGE

This method provides noninvasive, fast, and quantitative measurement of red blood cell velocity at the center of a single major vessel of the optic nerve head and retina.

With bidirectional LDV, red, blood cell velocity is calibrated in absolute values whereas with unidirectional LDV only relative measurements of velocity are possible.

LIMITATIONS

1. Laser Doppler velocimetry provides data on velocity, whereas assessment of blood flow requires taking into account the diameter of the measured vessel.
2. LDV measurements can also be affected by a change in the aggregability of the red blood cells within the vessel.

LASER DOPPLER FLOWMETRY

In 1992, Riva et al.[34] described single-point laser Doppler flowmetry (LDF). Unlike velocimetry, the LDF measures blood flow in capillary beds with the laser directed at areas between larger vessels.

The technique is similarly based on the Doppler effect with a laser beam of 160 μm focused on a selected location of the ONH or choroid. The LDF allows continuous measurement over several minutes and the Doppler shift frequency spectrum is then identified by a photodetector. The analysis yields information about relative velocity of the red blood cells and relative volume of moving red blood cells, and from these parameters blood flow through the tissue is calculated (Fig. 21.4).

The technique is used to measure microcirculation in the neuroretinal rim or lamina cribrosa. By directing the beam into the fovea (which is not perfused by the inner retinal circulation) subfoveolar choroidal blood flow can be measured. Using a different laser wavelength, measurements can be also performed on the retina, between large retinal vessels.

Several physiological studies have been undertaken using LDF in the ONH,[35,36] retina,[37] and choroid.[38,39] These studies showed that the technique was able to detect a change in blood flow induced by breathing of various gases, neuronal stimulation, and pharmacologic agents. LDF also reported reduced ONH blood flow in glaucoma patients[40] and glaucoma suspects with no manifest visual field defects[41] compared to control subjects. Lower optic nerve LDF measurements were also reported to correlate well with glaucomatous visual field progression.[42]

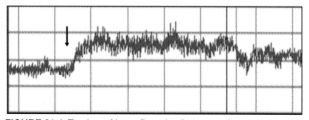

FIGURE 21.4 Tracing of laser Doppler flowmetry for neuroretinal rim blood flow in a normal subject. The arrow marks the onset of a flickering light and the purple line marks the end of the flicker. The recording duration was 80 seconds and flow is in arbitrary units. (Courtesy of Drs Wajszilber, Hafez, and Lesk.)

ADVANTAGE

Laser Doppler flowmetry is a powerful technique to investigate intraindividual changes of blood flow at a selected location over a fixed period of time. The technique is highly sensitive, reproducible, and has a fast response time. The device is well suited to look at perfusion changes during one imaging session, i.e. changes provoked by flickering light or inhaled gases, acute pressure changes, and acute drug treatments.

LIMITATIONS

1. It is not possible to calibrate the device, and the measurements are made in relative units.
2. Although the reported theoretical depth of penetration of the LDF is 1000 μm, the device may have a true penetration depth of approximately 400 μm. Therefore, in normal optic discs it may measure predominantly the retinal circulation in the surface nerve fiber layer of the disc.[6] However, in glaucomatous optic discs, since the neuroretinal rim is much thinner, it is more likely to detect a greater proportion of flow values from the deeper SPCA circulation.
3. Measurements are limited to a small selected area and the exact volume of tissue being measured is unknown. Therefore, the technique does not allow easy comparison between individuals and is best suited for looking at changes from one time-point to another or at vascular response to a stimulus within the same individual.

SCANNING LASER DOPPLER FLOWMETRY

The scanning laser Doppler flowmetry (SLDF) (Heidelberg retinal flowmeter, HRF, Heidelberg Engineering GmbH, Heidelberg, Germany) is a noninvasive instrument combining both a laser Doppler flowmeter with a scanning laser technique (Fig. 21.5).

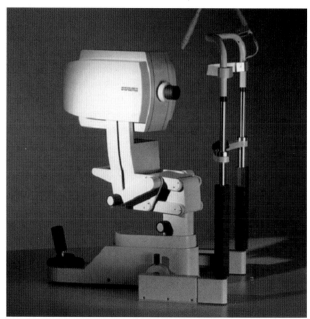

FIGURE 21.5 Heidelberg retinal flowmeter (HRF).

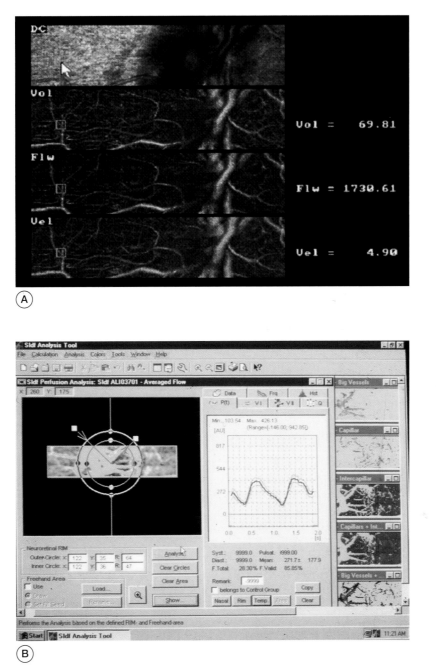

FIGURE 21.6 Heidelberg retinal flowmeter perfusion map showing the standard 10 × 10 pixel measurement box and the relative values for volume, flow, and velocity **(A)**, and SLDF full-field perfusion image analysis of the neuroretinal rim area after exclusion of vessels with a diameter of >30 μm and outlining of the ONH and the neuroretinal rim **(B)**.

SLDF measures the amount of backscattered light at different locations in the tissue of interest in a short period of time. The imaging system contains a scanning beam and so hemodynamic parameters at multiple discrete locations can be obtained. The imaging system is also confocal and thus signals from axial planes other than the focal plane of the laser are suppressed.[43,44]

The SLDF utilizes an infrared diode laser with wavelength of 780 nm and a power of 200 mW focused at the retina. The laser scans an area of 2.7 mm × 0.7 mm composed of 64 horizontal lines, each with 256 points and an approximate spatial resolution of 10 μm. Each line is scanned sequentially a total of 128 times with a total acquisition time of 2.05 seconds.

Each of the points (pixels) is then subjected to a fast Fourier transform to convert the 128 intensity values (as a function of time) to a power spectrum (as a function of frequency).[43,44] The result is a two-dimensional map of microvascular perfusion from which the parameters velocity, volume, and flow are calculated in arbitrary units (Fig. 21.6).

SLDF automatic full-field perfusion image analysis (AFFPIA) is an analysis technique designed to reduce the influence of heterogeneity in the perfusion map, correct for heartbeat-associated pulsations, as well as enhance the computations generated by the HRF.[45] The technique eliminates pixels with incorrect brightness as well as marks saccades that lead to erroneous perfusion data. It also excludes pixels of retinal vessels with a diameter greater than 30 μm, whose flow velocities are too high for the sampling frequency afforded by this technique (4000 Hz). The analysis is based on the average of all valid pixels in the entire scan area rather than from a discrete target square (see Fig. 21.6).

The potential effective measuring depth into a tissue using the SLDF has been estimated at between 300 and 400 μm when the laser is focused on the tissue surface. Wang et al.[46] estimated using microspheres the depth of penetration of scanning laser Doppler flowmetry in the anterior optic nerve of monkeys. They concluded that the when focused on the surface of the neuroretinal rim of the ONH, SLDF measures perfusion mainly from the superficial region of the ONH where the vascular supply is primarily from the CRA. However, in glaucomatous optic discs, since the rim layers are much thinner, it is likely to detect a greater proportion of flow values from the PCA circulation.

VALIDITY AND REPRODUCIBILITY

Several authors have investigated the validity of the HRF for quantitative evaluation of retinal and ONH perfusion.

Michelson and Schmauss[43] reported a significant linear relationship between SLDF flow and ocular perfusion pressure while varying the IOP by a suction cup in normal volunteers. Furthermore, the authors compared measurements of corresponding retinal points by SLDF and single-point laser Doppler flowmeter and reported a significant linear relationship in normal and glaucomatous eyes.[44] Using a model flow system of glass capillaries perfused with skimmed milk over a range of pump flow rates, Chauhan and Smith[47] and Tsang and colleagues[48] reported a high significant linear correlation between the HRF-measured flow and actual flow within a given operating range. Other investigators[49,50] have also shown that the SLDF is appropriate for description of the effect of graded changes in blood gases on retinal hemodynamics. They noted that changes in measured blood flow at the ONH occurred in the expected direction in response to blood gas perturbations.

The reproducibility of HRF measurements has also been shown within certain limits. The technical design and anatomy of ocular blood flow has imposed some limitations on the technology.

Using the 10×10 pixel measurement box, reported intrasession reliability for flow in a retinal location of normal subjects was 0.84[41] while intersession reliability ranged between 0.62 and 0.82.[42] However, in a rim location, the reported intersession reliability was 0.47 in normal subjects and 0.36 in glaucoma patients.[51]

In one study, using flow histograms and pixel-by-pixel analysis of the entire perfusion image, the intersession coefficient of variation for retinal flow decreased from 30.1% to 16.3%.[52] Using AFFPIA, Michelson and associates reported intersession reliability of 0.74 for flow in the retina of normal subjects.[45] Iester et al.[53] used this technique to analyze superior and inferior sectors of the ONH and peripapillary retina and reported a significantly better reproducibility in the retina compared to the rim, whereas Hafez et al.,[54] using mean data from the analysis of five perfusion images acquired sequentially, reported mean intersession coefficient of variation of 9.7% in the neuroretinal rim of glaucoma patients.

Studies using SLDF have reported reduced ONH and peripapillary retinal perfusion in OAG patients compared to normal subjects[55–57] and ocular hypertensives.[58,59] Sustained therapeutic reduction of IOP was also shown to result in significant improvement in neuroretinal rim blood flow in glaucoma patients.[60]

ADVANTAGE

Scanning laser Doppler flowmetry is a noninvasive and fast technique. It provides microvascular mapping of the retinal and ONH perfusion for the selected location of interest. AFFPIA facilitates analysis of blood flow in relatively large areas of the neuroretinal rim and the peripapillary retina.

LIMITATIONS

1. Total time of image acquisition is 2 seconds and microsaccades during measurement create artifacts by disturbing the Doppler shift signal. Microsaccades can be removed using the AFFPIA software.
2. Clinically insignificant media opacities, particularly posterior nuclear cataracts, degrade the image quality.
3. Uniocular patients cannot be tested because fixation with the fellow eye is essential for the 2–second duration of the test.
4. The subjective choice of the area to be measured can be an important source of variation. The slightest difference in the location of the measurement box in relation to retinal or ONH vessels may lead to considerable variation of perfusion values between images. This problem is considerably overcome with the AFFPIA software.
5. The technique is sensitive to illumination differences of the ocular tissue during image acquisition as well as to the low reflectivity of the ONH compared to the peripapillary retina.
6. Since there are differences in focusing between the neuroretinal rim and peripapillary retina versus the lamina cribrosa, different focal planes should be used for evaluation of cup and rim perfusion.
7. Accurate image analysis is time consuming and requires considerable experience.

LASER SPECKLE TECHNIQUE

The technique is based on the principle that a random speckle pattern is created when laser light is focused on a matte surface such as the fundus. The effect is caused by light interference[61] and the image speckle is detected by a sensor. The variation between successive scans of the image speckles is calculated and integrated for each pixel to obtain the normalized blur, a quantitative index of blood velocity.

Laser speckle flowgraphy demonstrated little change in the superficial ONH circulation following trabeculectomy in a Japanese population of glaucoma patients.[62] The technique showed a significant correlation between changes in ONH circulation and visual field damage in NTG but not in OAG.[63]

ADVANTAGE

The technique provides noncontact, two-dimensional, and valid measurements for retinal and superficial ONH blood velocities, which can then be used for the quantification of flow.

LIMITATIONS

1. The technique measures the superficial blood velocity of the ONH. Such measurements reflect the CRA circulation with no contribution from the SPCAs.
2. To date, most studies have mainly focused on the validation of the technique and the study of treatment effects.

RETINAL VESSEL ANALYZER

The Retinal Vessel Analyzer (RVA; Imedos, Jena, Germany) comprises a fundus camera (FF 450; Carl Zeiss Meditec), a video camera, a real-time monitor, and a computer with vessel diameter analysis software. It allows continuous and on-line measurement of the diameter of a segment of a retinal blood vessel with a temporal resolution of 25 readings/second.[64]

The subject's fixation is adjusted to position the ONH in the center of the monitor. A square box is then placed by the examiner over the retinal region of interest (ROI) containing the vessel to be analyzed. A rectangular cursor is then placed over the vessel of interest to identify the vessel length (approximately 0.5 mm) to be analyzed for changes in caliber throughout experimentation. The RVA program then initiates analysis of vessel diameter over the length of the vessel within the rectangular cursor (Fig. 21.7).

The RVA has been shown to have high short-term as well as day-to-day reproducibility with coefficients of variation between 1.3–2.6% and 4.4–5.2%, respectively.[64]

The technique demonstrates sensitivity to pharmacologic interventions[65] and reflects changes in vessel caliber consistent with physiological provocation after breathing 100% oxygen.[65,66]

ADVANTAGES

1. The technique enables continuous monitoring of the vessel diameter, both as a function of location and time.

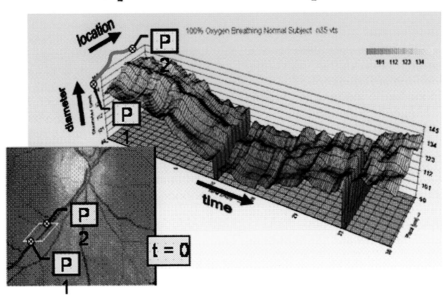

FIGURE 21.7 Retinal Vessel Analyzer. Fundus image as seen on the device's monitor showing the cursor aligned over the vessel of interest (P1 and P2) (*bottom left*) and retinal vessel diameter data collected over 38 seconds (t). (Courtesy of Dr Ines Lanzl, Munich, Germany.)

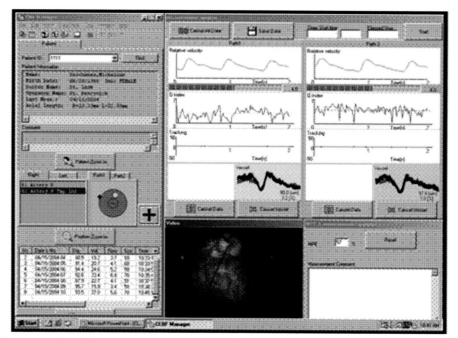

FIGURE 21.8 The Canon laser blood flowmeter measurement of the inferior temporal retinal artery showing the tracking stripe (*fundus image, bottom center*). The display shows a plot of the velocity variation during the cardiac cycle (*green line, top center and top right*; plot is over 2 seconds) and the vessel diameter (*V-shaped plots, center and right*) as well as a tabulation of the data analysis with values for blood column diameter, centerline blood velocity, and blood flow from successive measurements (*table, bottom left*). (Courtesy of Drs D Descovich, A Hafez, and M Lesk.)

2. Using this technique, different vessel segments as well as different retinal vessels can be investigated simultaneously.
3. The system is largely independent of alterations in luminance induced by slight eye movements. Sections of recordings contaminated by eye movements or blinks are automatically eliminated from the analysis.
4. Fundus images are stored on a videotape recorder for off-line measurement of other vessels within the captured field of view.

LIMITATIONS

1. The retinal vessel analyzer does not allow absolute retinal vessel diameter measurements, which may limit its use in cross-sectional studies.
2. While giving a reproducible assessment of vessel diameter, the technique does not evaluate blood velocity.

CANON LASER BLOOD FLOWMETER

The Canon laser blood flowmeter (CLBF 100, Canon, Tokyo, Japan) measures the blood column diameter, blood velocity, and blood flow in major retinal vessels.

The technique is based on the principle of bidirectional laser Doppler velocimetry.[67] It utilizes a fundus camera and two low-intensity lasers, one for measuring retinal artery blood velocity and the other for measuring vessel diameter. A beam from a red 675 nm diode laser is used for velocity measurement and is emitted from a fundus camera measuring head. The Doppler-shifted light scattered from the flowing blood cells in the target vessel is detected simultaneously in two directions separated by a fixed angle. The signals from the two tube detectors undergo computer-controlled spectrum analysis and sequential measurements of velocity are performed automatically. Results are acquired at 50 measurements per second for 2 seconds. A stripe provided by a green 543 nm HeNe laser oriented perpendicular to the target vessel is used to measure the diameter of the retinal vessel. The diameter is determined by computer analysis of the captured image of the vessel. From these two measurements, flow is accurately calculated by the instrument's software in actual units of microliters per minute (Fig. 21.8).[67] The CLBF is equipped with an internal fixation target, a vessel tracking system, and a pupil centration device. These elements help to monitor the target vessel and maintain centration of the laser beam at all times during measurement and thus improve the accuracy of the technique.

CLBF measurements have been shown to be valid as well as reproducible.[68,69] Mean intersession coefficients of variability for the technique have been reported to range between 16.4%[70] and 19.3%[71] for flow in vessels of normal subjects. The technique is well suited for evaluating changes in retinal blood flow during or between sessions. However, comparisons between retinal vessels in OAG patients and OHT patients or normal subjects have not been reported to date.

ADVANTAGES

1. Vessel diameter measurements are corrected for the axial length of the eye (operator input) and refractive error of the eye (measured by the CLBF).
2. The position of the measurement is recorded on the captured fundus image for subsequent comparisons.

3. Only Doppler curves with a high-quality 'Q-index,' as determined by the instrument's software, are accepted.

4. Because it measures both vessel diameter and blood velocity, the CLBF is the only existing technique that gives quantitative measurements of retinal blood flow in absolute units.

LIMITATIONS

1. Comparisons between populations may be difficult to make because of the intersubject variation in the location of measurement in relation to the vascular tree.

2. When the targeted vessel segment is very close to another vessel, the tracking device sometimes skips to the other vessel.

BLUE FIELD ENTOPTICS

The technique is based on the flow of white blood cells to assess retinal blood flow. Subjects can perceive the presence of leukocytes in the capillaries around the macula when looking at diffuse blue light of 430 nm. Similar patterns are created by computer simulation and subjects are then asked to match the speed of the computer-generated particles with those that they see in the blue field. The pattern match can then be used to draw conclusions about perifoveal perfusion. The method was developed by Riva and Petrig[72] for subjective evaluation of perimacular leukocyte velocity and density.

Using blue field entoptics, studies reported abnormal autoregulation of macular blood flow in OAG[73] as well as a significant positive correlation between loss of visual function and reduced leukocyte velocity.[74]

LIMITATIONS

1. The technique is based on the assumption that macular capillaries have a fixed diameter.

2. The patient must estimate the number of moving white blood cells. However, the accuracy of such estimations may be affected by the physiologic and pathophysiologic state of the retina.

3. The conclusions that can be drawn from the technique are limited, as the quality of the data depends on the patient's cooperation and perception.

4. Large variations between patients exist and only data from perifoveal capillaries are provided.

PERIPHERAL BLOOD FLOW

Blood flow disturbances in glaucoma patients point to some correlation between ocular blood flow and peripheral blood flow. Since vasospasticity and vascular dysregulation have been linked to glaucoma, the authors will briefly review the methods of assessment of peripheral blood flow.

Evaluation of peripheral blood flow has been performed using two methods: microscopy of the nail-fold capillaries of the fingers,[75] and LDF measurement of bulk blood flow at selected locations of the fingers.[76]

Using microscopic examination of the cellular elements in the nail-fold capillaries, blood flow velocity can be monitored and videotaped for analysis. A provocation test with local cold exposure of the nail-fold area to cold air ($-15°C$ for 60 seconds) results in a significant reduction of the velocity of erythrocytes in patients with vasospasm. The reduction can be so marked that a cessation of blood flow in the nail-fold capillaries can be observed. Digital vasospasm is defined as a closing of one or more visible capillaries, with a mean stoppage time of longer than 12 seconds.

Laser Doppler flowmetery (LDF, Transonic Systems Inc., Ithaca, NY) is another technique that uses a low-intensity laser beam to illuminate the nail-fold capillaries of the finger. A receiver detects light reflected by both stationary structures and moving particles (mainly red blood cells). The latter portion of reflected light undergoes a Doppler frequency shift, allowing the computation of blood flow. The methodology used for LDF finger blood flow measurements as well as the definition of a positive vasospastic response were both based on a leading study by Drance et al.[77] Baseline flow was measured on the underside of the end of the middle finger of a randomly selected hand. After a stable flow reading was obtained, the hand was immersed in warm water (40°C) for 2 minutes. The hand was then immersed in ice-cold water (4°C) for 10 seconds and then finally placed at room temperature for 10 minutes (recovery period). Finger flow measurements were made continuously by the laser Doppler flowmeter and transmitted in real-time to a computer via an interface. Drance et al.[77] defined a ratio of maximum to minimum flow of more than 7 as vasospastic, but low baseline flow and low flow upon cold exposure may also be signs of vasospasticity.

Studies of peripheral blood flow have suggested the possible role of vasospastic phenomena in the development and progression of glaucomatous optic neuropathy. Blood flow in both the nail-fold capillaries of the fingers[78] and the microcirculation of the skin[79] was reported to be reduced in glaucoma patients (Fig. 21.9).

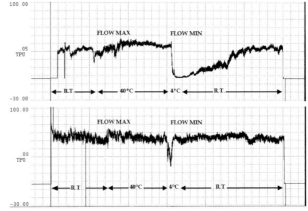

FIGURE 21.9 Tracings of laser Doppler flowmetry (LDF) showing response to cold water immersion in vasospasm (*above*) versus normal (*below*). (Courtesy of Drs R Bizzarro, A Hafez, and M Lesk.)

ADVANTAGE

Patients do not need to fixate or have clear media.

LIMITATIONS

Finger LDF measurements are sensitive to movement by the patient and distractions such as talking, so measurements have to be performed under controlled conditions.

ANIMAL EXPERIMENTAL METHODS

Most of these methods are invasive and are briefly mentioned to give the reader a full picture of the field of measurement of ocular blood flow.

1. *Oxygen tension method*: based on measurement of intravascular PO_2 using a phosphorescence imaging technique as well as measurement of extravascular PO_2 using microelectrodes placed in front of or within the ONH.[80]
2. *Microspheres method*: unlabeled or radioactive labeled or nonradioactive colored microspheres have been used to study ocular and ONH blood flow in animals.[67]
3. *Autoradiographic methods using iodoantipyrine*: the method has been used in animals to evaluate blood flow in the retina, choroid, and ONH[68,81] as well as to demonstrate autoregulation in the ONH and lamina cribrosa.
4. *Labile liposomes method*: encapsulated heat-sensitive liposomes containing fluorescent dye have been injected intravenously and lysed by a heat pulse delivered by laser.[82]
5. *Hydrogen clearance method*: optic disc blood flow has been measured in rhesus monkeys by inserting a microelectrode in the lamina cribrosa and determining the half-time for clearance of hydrogen gas from the saturated tissue.[83]
6. *Krypton washout method*: used to measure blood flow in the retinal vessels and in the choriocapillaris but not in the ONH.[84]
7. *An innovative 40 MHz ultrasound biomicroscope pulsed Doppler probe*: can measure blood flow in various ocular tissues but has a depth of penetration that is suitable for rodent but not human eyes.[85]

LIMITATIONS OF OCULAR BLOOD FLOW ASSESSMENT TECHNIQUES AND THEIR INTERPRETATIONS

The difficulties involved in the assessment of ocular blood flow have led to a variety of innovative techniques. These techniques have been used in both experimental animal models and human clinical investigations. While each technique may provide valuable information about the status of a particular vascular bed within the eye, each also has its limitations and restrictions that must be taken into account when interpreting their measurements.

Many of the techniques available measure either velocity of blood cells or transit times for fluorescein in the vascular bed. These measurements cannot be translated directly into flow measurements, unless the precise diameters of the blood vessels measured or information about the total volume of the vascular bed is known. Other techniques examine physiological parameters such as the oxygen profile in the retina. These are not direct measurements of blood flow but rather estimates of alterations in oxygen delivery and metabolic demands and have proven useful for studying the effects of increased IOP on the retina and ONH.

Fluorescein angiography (FA) remains the basic technique for studies of retinal blood flow in clinical practice. In its basic form FA provides qualitative information, though recent attempts have been made to obtain quantitative information as well. Major limitations still exist in quantitative interpretation. Both *color Doppler imaging* and *ocular pulse amplitude* provide useful information. However, it is important to understand what aspect of ocular hemodynamics each method measures so that their relevance in glaucoma is understood. CDI provides its most reproducible measurements for the ophthalmic artery and CRA and the resistivity index is calculated from the velocities measured. Information provided from the SPCAs, the most important source for ONH perfusion, is significantly less reproducible. Ocular pulse amplitude is a measure of the pulsatile component of choroidal blood flow, which does not correlate necessarily with total blood flow and which is a poor estimate of blood flow in other ocular tissues.

The principle of frequency shift induced by moving objects (Doppler shift) has been widely used in the estimation of ocular blood flow in the ONH, retina, and choroid. These techniques have been arguably most successful when applied to the retinal arteries where both velocity and diameter can be measured with reasonable accuracy. When applied to the ONH, the techniques of *laser Doppler flowmetry* and *SLDF* remain sensitive to blood flow changes in the superficial layers of the ONH with an estimated depth of penetration of 400 μm according to some authors. A highly accurate and reproducible technique for the measurement of blood flow in the prelaminar and laminar ONH remains elusive.

Ocular blood flow techniques will continue to evolve. There are recent and promising advances in Doppler ultrasound and spectral domain OCT coupled with Doppler technology. Several research groups are making advances in fundus spectroscopy. Detection of metabolic by-products, the consequences of relative ischemia, may soon be realizable. Most of these advances are currently research tools with too little known to assess which ones will find a practical clinical application. The prospects for the continued evolution of such technologies and for the knowledge obtained from their application is promising, although successful use will always depend on a thorough understanding of the limitations of the data obtained.

REFERENCES

1. Williamson T, Baxter GM, Datton GN. Color Doppler velocimetry of the retinal vasculature of the optic nerve head and orbit. Eye 1993; 7:74–79.

2. Galassi F, Nuzzaci G, Sodi A, et al. Color Doppler imaging in evaluation of optic nerve blood supply in normal and glaucomatous subjects. Int Ophthalmol 1992; 16:273–276.

3. Harris A, Sergott RC, Spaeth GL, et al. Color Doppler analysis of ocular vessel blood velocity in normal-tension glaucoma. Am J Ophthalmol 1994; 118:642–649.

4. Galassi F, Nuzzaci G, Sodi A, et al. Possible correlation of ocular blood flow parameters with intraocular pressure and visual field alterations in glaucoma: a study by means of color Doppler imaging. Ophthalmologica 1994; 208: 304–308.

5. Trible JR, Sergott RC, Spaeth GL, et al. Trabeculectomy is associated with retrobulbar hemodynamic change: a color Doppler analysis. Ophthalmology 1994; 101:340–351.

6. Hayreh SS. Evaluation of optic nerve head circulation: review of the methods used. J Glaucoma 1997; 6:319–330.

7. Dennis KJ, Dixon RD, Winsberg F, et al. Variability in measurement of central retinal artery velocity using color Doppler imaging. J Ultrasound Med 1995; 14:463–466.

8. Hayreh SS, Beach KW. Optic nerve sheath decompression: discussion. Ophthalmology 1993; 100:303–305.

9. Hayreh SS. The ophthalmic artery. III. Branches. Br J Ophthalmol 1962; 46:212–247.

10. Langham ME, Farell MA, O'Brien V, et al. Non-invasive measurement of pulsatile blood flow in the human eye. In: Lambrou GN, Greve EL, eds. Ocular blood flow in glaucoma. Amsterdam: Kugler and Ghedini; 1989:93–99.

11. Langham ME, To'mey K. A clinical procedure for measuring the ocular pulse–pressure relationship and the ophthalmic arterial pressure. Exp Eye Res 1987; 27:17–25.

12. Langham ME, Farrell RA, O'Brien V, et al. Blood flow in the human eye. Acta Ophthalmol 1989; 67:9–12.

13. Schmetterer L, Dallinger S, Findl O, et al. A comparison between laser interferometric measurement of fundus pulsation and pneumotonometric measurement of pulsatile ocular blood flow. 1. Baseline considerations. Eye 2000; 14:39–45.

14. Schmetterer L, Dallinger S, Findl O, et al. A comparison between laser interferometric measurement of fundus pulsation and pneumotonometric measurement of pulsatile ocular blood flow. 2. Effects of changes in pCO_2 and pO_2 and of isoproterenol. Eye 2000; 14:46–52.

15. Trew DR, Smith SE. Postural studies in pulsatile ocular blood flow: I: ocular hypertension and normotension. Br J Ophthalmol 1991; 75:66–70.

16. Trew DR, Smith SE. Postural studies in pulsatile ocular blood flow: II: chronic open-angle glaucoma. Br J Ophthalmol 1991; 75:71–75.

17. Kerr J, Nelson P, O'Brian C. Pulsatile ocular blood flow in primary open angle glaucoma and ocular hypertension. Am J Ophthalmol 2003; 136:1106–1113.

18. Williamson TH, Harris A. Ocular blood flow measurements. Br J Ophthalmol 1994; 78:939–945.

19. James CB, Trew DR, Clark K, et al. Factors influencing the ocular pulse – axial length. Graefe's Arch Clin Exp Ophthalmol 1991; 229:341–344.

20. Trew DR, James CB, Thomas SH, et al. Factors influencing the ocular pulse – the heart rate. Graefe's Arch Clin Exp Ophthalmol 1991; 229:553–556.

21. Hayreh SS, Walker WM. Fluorescent fundus photography in glaucoma. Am J Ophthalmol 1967; 63:982–989.

22. Schwartz B. Circulatory defects of the optic disc and retina in ocular hypertension and high pressure open-angle glaucoma. Surv Ophthalmol 1994; 38:23–24.

23. Spaeth GL. Fluorescein angiography: its contributions towards understanding the mechanisms of visual loss in glaucoma. Trans Am Ophthalmol Soc 1975; 73:491–553.

24. Talusan E, Schwartz B. Specificity of fluorescein angiographic defects of the optic disc in glaucoma. Arch Ophthalmol 1977; 95:2166–2175.

25. Nanba K, Schwartz B. Nerve fiber layer and optic disc fluorescein defects in glaucoma and ocular hypertension. Ophthalmology 1988; 95:1227–1233.

26. Plange N, Kaup M, Huber K, et al. Fluorescein filling defects of the optic nerve head in normal tension glaucoma, primary open angle glaucoma, ocular hypertension and healthy controls. Ophthalmic Physiol Opt 2006; 26:26–32.

27. Duijm HF, van den Berg, Greve EL. A comparison of retinal and choroidal hemodynamics in patients with primary open angle glaucoma and normal pressure glaucoma. Am J Ophthalmol 1997; 123:644–656.

28. Nagin P, Schwartz B, Reynolds G. Measurement of fluorescein angiograms of the optic disc and retina using computerized image analysis. Ophthalmology 1985; 92:547–552.

29. Greve EL, Duijm FA, Geijssen HC. Simultaneous retinal and choroidal angiography and its relationship to other measurements. In: Pillunat LE, Harris A, Anderson DR, et al, eds. Current concepts on ocular blood flow in glaucoma. The Hague: Kugler; 1999:153–158.

30. Hayreh SS. Pathogenesis of optic nerve damage and visual field defects. In: Heilmann K, Richardson KT, eds. Glaucoma. Conceptions of a disease. Stuttgart: Georg Thieme; 1978: 103–138.

31. Riva CE, Ross B, Benedek GB. Laser Doppler measurements of blood flow in capillary tubes and retinal arteries. Invest Ophthalmol 1972; 11:936–944.

32. Logean E, Geiser MH, Petrig BL, et al. Portable ocular laser Doppler red blood cell velocimeter. Rev Sci Instrum 1997; 68:2878.

33. Riva CE, Grunwald JE, Sinclair SH. Laser Doppler measurement of relative blood velocity in the human optic nerve head. Invest Ophthalmol Vis Sci 1982; 22:241–248.

34. Riva CE, Harino S, Petrig BL, et al. Laser Doppler flowmetry in the optic nerve. Exp Eye Res 1992; 55:936–944.

35. Harino S, Riva CE, Petrig BL. Intravenous nicardipine in cats increases optic nerve head but not retinal blood flow. Invest Ophthalmol Vis Sci 1992; 33:2885–2890.

36. Harris A, Anderson DR, Pillunet L, et al. Laser Doppler flowmetry measurement of changes in human optic nerve head blood flow in response to blood gas perturbations. J Glaucoma 1996; 5:258–265.

37. Riva CE, Cranstoun SD, Grunwald JE, et al. Choroidal blood flow in the foveal region of the human ocular fundus. Invest Ophthalmol Vis Sci 1994; 35:4273–4281.

38. Riva CE, Cranstoun SD, Mann RN, et al. Local choroidal blood flow in the cat by laser Doppler flowmetry. Invest Ophthalmol Vis Sci 1994; 35:608–618.

39. Mann RM, Riva CE, Stone RA, et al. Nitric oxide and choroidal blood flow regulation Invest Ophthalmol Vis Sci 1995; 36: 925–930.

40. Grunwald JE, Piltz J, Hariprasad SM, et al. Optic nerve and choroidal circulation in glaucoma. Invest Ophthalmol Vis Sci 1998; 39:2329–2336.

41. Piltz-Seymour JR, Grunwald JE, Hariprasad SM, et al. Optic nerve blood flow is diminished in eyes of primary open-angle glaucoma suspects. Am J Ophthalmol 2001; 132:63–69.

42. Zink JM, Grunwald JE, Piltz-Seymour J, et al. Association between lower optic nerve laser Doppler blood volume measurements and glaucomatous visual field progression. Br J Ophthalmol 2003; 87:1487–1491.

43. Michelson G, Schmauss B. Two-dimensional mapping of the perfusion of the retina and optic nerve head. Br J Ophthalmol 1995; 79:1126–1132.

44. Michelson G, Schmauss B, Langhans MJ, et al. Principle, validity, and reliability of scanning laser Doppler flowmetry. J Glaucoma 1996; 5:99–105.

45. Michelson G, Welzenbach J, Pal I, et al. Automatic full field analysis of perfusion images gained by scanning laser Doppler flowmetry. Br J Ophthalmol 1998; 82:1294–1300.

46. Wang L, Cull G, Cioffi GA. Depth of penetration of scanning laser Doppler flowmetry in the primate optic nerve. Arch Ophthalmol 2001; 119:1810–1814.

47. Chauhan BC, Smith FM. Confocal scanning laser Doppler flowmetry: experiments in a model flow system. J Glaucoma 1997; 6:237–245.

48. Tsang AC, Harris A, Kagemann L, et al. Brightness alters Heidelberg retinal flowmeter measurements in an in vitro model. Invest Ophthalmol Vis Sci 1999; 40:795–799.

49. Strenn K, Menapace R, Rainer G, et al. Reproducibility and sensitivity of scanning laser Doppler flowmetry during graded changes in PO_2. Br J Ophthalmol 1997; 81:360–364.

50. Lietz A, Hendrickson P, Flammer J, et al. Effect of carbogen, oxygen and intraocular pressure on Heidelberg retinal flowmeter parameter flow measured at the papilla. Ophthalmologica 1998; 212(3):149–152.

51. Nicolela MT, Hnik P, Schulzer M, et al. Reproducibility of retinal and optic nerve head blood flow measurements with scanning laser Doppler flowmetry. J Glaucoma 1997; 6:157–164.

52. Kagemann L, Harris A, Chung HS, et al. Heidelberg retinal flowmetry: factors affecting blood flow measurement. Br J Ophthalmol 1998; 82:131–136.

53. Iester M, Altieri M, Michelson G, et al. Intraobserver reproducibility of a two-dimensional mapping of the optic nerve head perfusion. J Glaucoma 2002; 11:488–492.

54. Hafez AS, Bizzarro RLG, Rivard M, et al. Reproducibility of retinal and optic nerve head perfusion measurements using scanning laser Doppler flowmetry. Ophthalmic Surg Lasers Imaging 2003; 34(5):422–432.

55. Michelson G, Langhans MJ, Groh MJM. Perfusion of the juxtapapillary retina and the neuroretinal rim area in primary open angle glaucoma. J Glaucoma 1996; 5:91–98.

56. Nicolela MT, Hnik P, Drance SM. Scanning laser Doppler flowmeter study of retinal and optic disk blood flow in glaucomatous patients. Am J Ophthalmol 1996; 122:775–783.

57. Findl O, Rainer G, Dallinger S, et al. Assessment of optic disk blood flow in patients with open-angle glaucoma. Am J Ophthalmol 2000; 130:589–596.

58. Kerr J, Nelson P, O'Brian C. A comparison of ocular blood flow in untreated primary open-angle glaucoma and ocular hypertension. Am J Ophthalmol 1998; 126:42–51.

59. Hafez AS, Bizzarro RLG, Lesk MR. Optic nerve head blood flow in glaucoma patients, ocular hypertensives and normal subjects measured by scanning laser Doppler flowmetry. Am J Ophthalmol 2003; 136(6):1022–1031.

60. Hafez AS, Bizzarro RLG, Rivard M, et al. Changes in optic nerve head blood flow after therapeutic intraocular pressure reduction in glaucoma patients and ocular hypertensives. Ophthalmology 2003; 110(1):201–210.

61. Tamaki Y, Araie M, Kawamoto E, et al. Noncontact, two-dimensional measurement of retinal microvasculature using laser speckle phenomenon. Invest Ophthalmol Vis Sci 1994; 35:3825–3834.

62. Tamaki Y, Araie M, Hasegawa T, et al. Optic nerve head circulation after intraocular pressure reduction achieved by trabeculectomy. Ophthalmology 2001; 108:627–632.

63. Yaoeda K, Shirakashi M, Fukushima A, et al. Relationship between optic nerve head microcirculation and visual field loss in glaucoma. Acta Ophthalmol Scand 2003; 81:253–259.

64. Polak K, Dorner G, Kiss B, et al. Evaluation of the Zeiss retinal vessel analyzer. Br J Ophthalmol 2000; 84:1285–1290.

65. Jean-Louis S, Lovasik JV, Kergoat H. Systemic hyperoxia and retinal vasomotor responses. Invest Ophthalmol Vis Sci 2005; 46:1714–1720.

66. Lanzl IM, Witta B, Kotliar K, et al. Retinal vessel reaction to 100% O_2-breathing: functional imaging using the retinal vessel analyzer with 10 volunteers. Klin Monatsbl Augenheilkd 2000; 217:231–235.

67. Garcia JPS, Garcia PT, Rosen RB. Retinal blood flow in the human eye using the Canon laser blood flowmeter. Ophthalmic Res 2002; 34:295–299.

68. Alm A, Lambrou GN, Mäepea O, et al. Ocular blood flow in experimental glaucoma: a study in cynomolgus monkeys. Ophthalmologica 1997; 211:178–182.

69. Sossi N, Anderson DR. Effect of elevated intraocular pressure on blood flow: occurrence in cat optic nerve head studied with iodoantipyrine I125. Arch Ophthalmol 1983; 101:98–101.

70. Yoshida A, Feke GT, Mori F, et al. Reproducibility and clinical application of a newly developed stabilized retinal laser Doppler instrument. Am J Ophthalmol 2003; 135:356–361.

71. Guan K, Hudson C, Flanagan JG. Variability and repeatability of retinal blood flow measurements using the Canon laser blood flowmeter. Microvasc Res 2003; 65:145–151.

72. Riva CE, Petrig B. Blue field entoptic phenomenon and blood velocity in the retinal capillaries. J Opt Soc Am 1980; 70:1234–1238.

73. Grunwald JE, Riva CE, Stone RA, et al. Retinal autoregulation in open angle glaucoma. Ophthalmology 1984; 91:1690–1694.

74. Sponsel WE, DePaul KL, Kaufman PL. Correlation of visual function and retinal leukocyte velocity in glaucoma. Am J Ophthalmol 1990; 90:49–54.

75. Mahler F, Saner H, Wurbel H, et al. Local cooling test for clinical capillaroscopy in Raynaud's phenomenon, unstable angina, and vasospastic visual disorders. Vasa 1989; 18:201–204.

76. Gasser P, Muller P, Mauli D, et al. Evaluation of reflex cold provocation by laser Doppler flowmetry in clinically healthy subjects with a history of cold hands. Angiology 1992; 43:389–394.

77. Drance SM, Douglas GD, Wijsman K, et al. Response of blood flow to warm and cold in normal and low-tension glaucoma patients. Am J Ophthalmol 1988; 105:35–39.

78. Flammer J. To what extent are vascular factors involved in the pathogenesis of glaucoma? In: Kaiser HJ, Flammer J, Hendrickson P, eds. Ocular blood flow: new insights into the pathogenesis of ocular diseases. Basel: Karger; 1995:13–39.

79. O'Brian C, Butt Z. Blood flow velocity in the peripheral circulation of glaucoma patients. Ophthalmologica 1999; 213:150–153.

80. Riva CE. Noninvasive measurement of oxygen tension in the optic nerve head. Curr Opin Ophthalmol 1998; 9:56–60.

81. Weinstein JM, Duckrow B, Beard D, et al. Regional optic nerve blood flow and its autoregulation. Invest Ophthalmol Vis Sci 1983; 24:1559–1565.

82. Khoobehi B, Schuele KM, Ali OM, et al. Measurement of circulation time in the retinal vasculature using selective angiography. Ophthalmology 1990; 97:1061–1070.

83. Ernest JT. Optic disc blood flow. Trans Ophthalmol Soc UK 1976; 96:348–351.

84. Friedman E, Kopald HH, Smith TR. Retinal and choroidal blood flow determined with krypton-85 anesthetized animals. Invest Ophthalmol 1964; 3:539–547.

85. Brown AS, Leamen L, Cucevic V, et al. Quantitation of hemodynamic function during developmental vascular regression in the mouse eye. Invest Ophthalmol Vis Sci 2005; 46:2231–2237.

CHAPTER 22

Genetics of Glaucoma

Mohammed K ElMallah and R Rand Allingham

INTRODUCTION

A genetic predisposition for glaucoma has long been observed in certain families. This has led to the search for specific genes for glaucoma. Over the last two decades, some of these genes have been identified and each new discovery has brought with it more questions. It is now clear that the glaucomas have wide genetic heterogeneity with no single gene accounting for all cases of any single glaucoma phenotype. In other words, alterations in different genes can lead to the same phenotype while in other cases variants in the same gene may lead to different phenotypes.

Despite these hurdles, significant advances have been made in understanding the genetic basis of glaucoma. What follows is a description of the genes discovered thus far that are associated with glaucoma as well as a discussion of some glaucoma subtypes that may be genetically inherited but for which no specific gene has yet been found.

PRIMARY OPEN-ANGLE GLAUCOMA

Primary open-angle glaucoma (POAG) is the prevalent form of glaucoma in most populations studied. Over 20 chromosomal loci have been associated with POAG (Table 22.1). Mutations in three disease-associated genes have been identified among these loci: they are myocilin (MYOC), optineurin (OPTN), and WD repeat domain 36 (WDR36).[1]

Primary open-angle glaucoma does not display simple mendelian inheritance; rather, it is inherited as a complex trait. Environmental as well as genetic factors have been associated with the development of glaucoma. The genetic factors that contribute to the phenotype in most cases are the result of interactions between several different genes. In fact, of the three genes identified, only myocilin is established as a directly causative glaucoma gene.

The three genes discovered thus far only contribute to approximately 5–6% of all POAG cases. The genetic source of the vast majority of POAG cases remains to be discovered.

TABLE 22.1 Reported genetic loci for primary open-angle glaucoma

CHROMOSOMAL LOCATION	LOCUS NAME	GENE IDENTIFIED
1q21-q31	GLC1A	MYOC
2p14		
2p16.3-p15	GLC1H	
2cen-q13	GLC1B	
2q33-q34		
3p21-p22		
3q21-q24	GLC1C	
5q22.1	GLC1G	WDR36
7q35-q36	GLC1F	
8q23	GLC1D	
9q22	GLC1J	
10p12-p13		
10p15-p14	GLC1E	OPTN
14q11		
14q21-q22		
15q11-q13	GLC1I	
17p13		
17q25		
19q12-q14		
20p12	GLC1K	
3p22-p21	GLC1L	
5q22.1-q32	GLC1M	
15q22-q24	GLC1N	

Adapted from Fan BJ, Wang DY, Lam DS, Pang CP. Gene mapping for primary open-angle glaucoma. Clin Biochem 2006; 39(3):249–258.

MYOCILIN

Myocilin (MYOC) was the first gene identified for POAG. Mutations in MYOC cause an autosomal dominant form of the disease. Disease-associated mutations in MYOC cause a juvenile or early-adult form of POAG that is associated with high intraocular pressures and a clinically severe form of POAG. The MYOC gene is located at chromosome 1q25, corresponding to the GLC1A locus. Its protein product, myocilin, was previously also known as the trabecular meshwork inducible-glucocorticoid response protein (TIGR). The MYOC gene consists of three exons. Myocilin, the encoded protein, has sequence similarity to the muscle protein myosin at the N-terminus, while at the C-terminus it has a conserved olfactomedin-like domain. Most glaucoma-associated mutations in the MYOC gene are in the third exon, which contains the olfactomedin-like domain. Myocilin is found not only in most tissues of the eye but also in most tissues of the body.[2]

To date, there have been over 70 disease-associated mutations identified in MYOC. Taken together these mutations account for approximately 3–5% of POAG cases worldwide. The mechanism by which these mutations cause POAG is an area of intense study and several different hypotheses exist.

Fundamentally, the function of myocilin in normal physiology is not understood. In trabecular meshwork cell cultures, myocilin expression increases dramatically in response to steroid exposure.[3] Steroid administration also increases intraocular pressure. Therefore, one theory is that increased wild-type myocilin expression may be responsible for the increased intraocular pressure seen in steroid-induced ocular hypertension. However, a mouse model where myocilin expression was increased 15-fold failed to develop glaucoma.[4] Therefore, increased myocilin does not appear to cause elevated pressure.

Another theory for the function of myocilin is that wild-type myocilin protects against increased intraocular pressure. However, null mice that lack myocilin protein do not develop increased intraocular pressure (IOP) or glaucoma.[4]

Since neither the overexpression of myocilin nor the total lack of myocilin causes glaucoma, mutations in MYOC likely lead to increased IOP and glaucoma through a gain-of-function mechanism. One such hypothesis is that mutated myocilin is misfolded, accumulates in trabecular meshwork cells, is not secreted, and also impedes the secretion of normal myocilin. These accumulated misfolded proteins can cause dysfunction of cellular organelles responsible for removal of unneeded protein products, resulting in further accumulation of proteins and, ultimately, cell apoptosis. In vitro, this has occurred through overactivation of a normally cell-protective mechanism called the unfolded protein response (UPR). In a transgenic animal model with a glaucoma-associated mutation in myocilin, mutant myocilin accumulated in the anterior chamber angle, inhibited normal myocilin secretion, but ultimately did not affect IOP when compared to controls without mutations.[4] However, other investigators examining the same mutation in the mouse model found a modest IOP elevation (approximately 2 mmHg) associated with retinal ganglion cell loss and axonal degeneration in the optic nerve which was felt to be consistent with glaucoma.[5]

More recently, myocilin has been shown to associate with the shedding of small vesicles called exosomes. In other tissues exosomes contain ligands that participate in autocrine/paracrine signaling, and thus serve as vehicles that may potentially play a role in trabecular meshwork homeostasis.[6,7] It is known that disease-associated mutations in myocilin prevent the release of myocilin from cells as well as decrease myocilin's presence in the aqueous humor where it is normally found.[8] It remains to be determined whether myocilin mutations cause trabecular meshwork dysfunction by interfering with myocilin-associated exosome release and associated paracrine signaling in the conventional outflow pathway. However, regardless of its mechanism, it is clear that elucidating the role of myocilin in the pathogenesis of POAG will be critical to our understanding of the pathophysiology of this disorder.

OPTINEURIN

Optineurin (OPTN) is the second gene discovered in which variations are associated with an autosomal dominant form of primary open-angle glaucoma. This form of glaucoma occurs in mid-life and is often associated with a normal-tension form of POAG. Located on chromosome 10p14, it corresponds to the GLC1E locus. The gene consists of 3 noncoding exons and 13 coding exons which produces a 577-amino acid protein product. Optineurin has been found in the trabecular meshwork, nonpigmented ciliary epithelium, retina, and numerous nonocular tissues.[9]

Many studies have examined the prevalence of optineurin mutations in glaucoma populations. The original paper which described optineurin reported that 16.7% of 54 families with hereditary POAG had sequence alterations in OPTN.[9] In a subsequent study looking at 1048 patients, one sequence variation, E50K, was found in a patient with familial normal-tension glaucoma. However, given the rarity of familial normal-tension glaucoma, it was estimated that this variant would account for less than 0.1% of all primary open-angle glaucoma cases. There was also an association found between another variant, M98K, and 20% of Japanese normal-tension glaucoma patients. Although this variant was also found in 9% of Japanese controls, this difference was statistically significant.[10] Most other studies have not found a significant association between OPTN mutations and POAG. At most, mutations in this gene account for 1% of POAG patients.

Mutations in the OPTN gene are associated with familial normal-tension glaucoma. The first mutation reported, E50K, remains the most consistently found in association studies. At the time of glaucoma diagnosis, normal-tension glaucoma patients who possess this mutation are younger, have a larger cup-to-disc ratio, and have less neuroretinal rim than normal-tension glaucoma patients without this mutation. They also have a higher rate of filtration surgery and are more likely to have progression on visual field testing.[11]

Current evidence as to the function of optineurin in glaucoma points to a neuroprotective role. It has been found to protect cells from tumor necrosis factor (TNF)-α-mediated apoptosis in vitro. However, in vivo, in a transgenic mouse model, optineurin failed to protect against transforming growth factor (TGF)-β_1-induced apoptosis. It was also found to be a cytoplasmic rather than a secretory protein and was located in greatest amount in retinal ganglion cells.[12]

Recently, optineurin has been shown to play a central role in maintaining Golgi body morphology as well as in the cell's ability to perform exocytosis.[13] It has not been defined what role, if any, this would play in the pathophysiology of glaucoma.

Other investigators have found evidence of a role in apoptosis prevention. Overexpression of optineurin protected cells from hydrogen peroxide-induced cell death whereas overexpression of protein with the E50K mutation resulted in cells that were less likely to survive stress conditions.[14]

While the function of optineurin is still under investigation, it appears to play a neuroprotective role.

WDR36

The most recently discovered gene associated with primary open-angle glaucoma is WDR36, a 23-exon gene which encodes for a 951-amino acid protein product.[15] It is located at chromosome 5q22.1 in the GLC1G locus. The mRNA transcripts of this gene have been found in various tissues of the body including the heart, placenta, liver, and kidney, as well as throughout the structures of the eye.

It is not clear whether variants of WDR36 are causative for POAG or whether they may be better described as modifiers for glaucoma. The mutation found in the original family studied (D658G) was not associated with glaucoma in an Australian population where it was found at equal levels in POAG patients as well as controls.[16] In a separate study, 32 WDR36 sequence variants were found, but these variants did not segregate consistently between patients and controls. However, variants in WDR36 were associated with greater clinical severity, suggesting that WDR36 may play a role as a modifier gene.[17]

In addition, there is evidence to suggest that the WDR36 gene may not be the only glaucoma-associated gene within the GLC1G locus. The original POAG family used to establish linkage of the GLC1G locus to chromosome 5q did not have any of the subsequently discovered WDR36 disease-causing mutations. This raises the possibility that there may be two genes associated with POAG within this locus.[18]

PIGMENT DISPERSION SYNDROME AND GLAUCOMA

First described in 1949 by Sugar and Barbour,[19] pigment dispersion syndrome is characterized by deposition of pigment throughout the anterior segment, including the cornea, iris, trabecular meshwork, and lens, with associated mid-peripheral iris transillumination defects

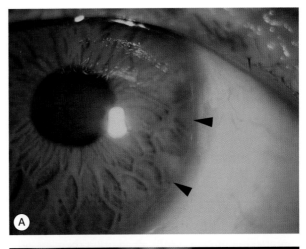

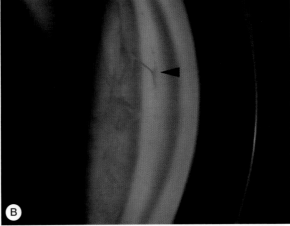

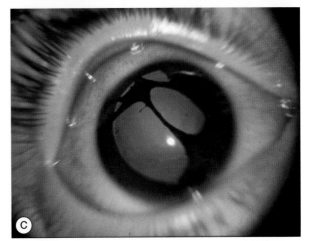

FIGURE 22.1 Axenfeld-Reiger syndrome. Spectrum of disease. **(A)** Posterior embryotoxin (*arrowheads*). **(B)** Iris–cornea adhesion with iris strand to posterior embryotoxin on gonio photo (*arrowhead*). **(C)** A more advanced case with iris hypoplasia and corectopia. (**(A)** and **(B)** Courtesy of Joseph Halabis, OD.)

(Fig. 22.1). Onset is typically in early- to mid-adult life with males more often affected than females. It is usually associated with myopia and, when it occurs, is most often bilateral.[20]

Pigment dispersion syndrome in humans may be sporadic or inherited as an autosomal dominant trait.[21] In four families with an autosomal dominant form of disease, genetic linkage analysis demonstrated linkage with a marker at chromosome 7q35-q36.[22] The gene for pigment dispersion syndrome has not been identified.

It has an incomplete autosomal dominant pattern of inheritance. It has been suggested that up to 50% of patients with pigmentary dispersion may go on to develop associated glaucoma. However, this may an overestimation given that the prevalence of pigment dispersion syndrome is likely underestimated.[23] It is likely that the mechanism of glaucoma is through pigment release into the aqueous humor that causes damage to the trabecular meshwork and resultant elevated IOP.

An animal model of pigmentary glaucoma has been identified, the DBA/2J mouse. In this model of pigment dispersion at least two genes interact to cause glaucoma, TYRP1 (tyrosinase-related protein 1) and Gpnmb (glycoprotein NMB); in addition there are other genes, as yet undefined, that modify the severity of the glaucoma in these mice.[24] The protein products of the two identified genes, TYRP1 and Gpnmb, are involved in melanosome stabilization. Interestingly, neither of these genes appears to play a role in the human form of this pigmentary glaucoma.[25]

PSEUDOEXFOLIATION SYNDROME

Pseudoexfoliation syndrome is characterized by the deposition of fibrillar material throughout the anterior segment, particularly on the lens, iris, trabecular meshwork, and ciliary body (Fig. 22.2). The incidence of pseudoexfoliation varies, based on the population studied. In one population studied in Minnesota, the incidence of the pseudoexfoliation syndrome was approximately 26 per 100 000 whereas the incidence of pseudoexfoliation glaucoma was approximately 10 per 100 000. Based on these data, 40% of patients with pseudoexfoliation syndrome have pseudoexfoliation glaucoma. The incidence of pseudoexfoliation was higher in females (76% of those diagnosed with pseudoexfoliation were female) and the disease showed increasing incidence with advancing age.[26]

Although the mechanism by which pseudoexfoliation syndrome results in pseudoexfoliation glaucoma is not clear, there is a correlation between the severity of the glaucoma and the amount of pseudoexfoliation material found in the trabecular meshwork and the inner wall of Schlemm's canal.[27]

In a groundbreaking study, the genetic etiology of pseudoexfoliative syndrome and glaucoma was identified.[28] Two polymorphisms in the coding region of the gene lysil oxidase-like 1 gene (LOXL1) are associated with pseudoexfoliative syndrome and glaucoma in the Icelandic and Swedish populations. LOXL1, located on chromosome region 15q24, is one of many enzymes that are essential for the formation of elastin fibers; they modify tropoelastin, the basic building block of elastin and catalyze the process for monomers to cross-link and form elastin. Interestingly, many components of the fibrillar material found in pseudoexfoliation are from the elastic fiber system and include elastin and tropoelastin.[29]

The disease-associated polymorphisms appear to account for all pseudoexfoliation within the studied populations. Those individuals carrying both copies of the high-risk haplotype were estimated to have a 700-fold increased risk of developing pseudoexfoliation glaucoma compared to those with the lower-risk haplotype.[28] These LOXL1 variants do not appear to confer genetic risk for primary open-angle glaucoma in the studied populations. Whether other risk-associated polymorphisms account for pseudoexfoliation syndrome in non-Scandinavian populations remains to be determined. Furthermore, it is not known if other genes may increase susceptibility for conversion from pseudoexfoliation syndrome to glaucoma.

Identification of the genetic component of pseudoexfoliation syndrome is a major achievement and will be instrumental in improving our understanding of pseudoexfoliation syndrome as well as in providing critical insights into its pathophysiology, thus permitting the development of novel treatment approaches for this common form of secondary glaucoma.

CONGENITAL GLAUCOMA

Glaucoma present at birth is termed congenital glaucoma. Typically, infants or young children present with an enlarged eye (buphthalmos), cloudy corneas, photophobia and epiphora (Fig. 22.3). Physical examination may also reveal the presence of breaks in Descemet's membrane termed Haab's striae. Classically, boys are affected twice as often as girls and the majority of cases have bilateral involvement. The inheritance pattern in most pedigrees is

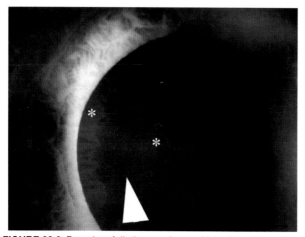

FIGURE 22.2 Pseudoexfoliation syndrome. Note deposition of pseudoexfoliation material on anterior lens surface (*asterisks*). Clear zone caused by iris movement (*arrowhead*).

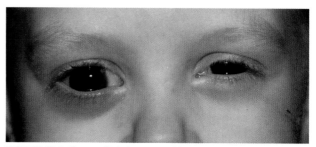

FIGURE 22.3 Congenital glaucoma. Note asymmetric buphthalmos. (Courtesy of Sharon Freedman, MD.)

autosomal recessive and thus there is increased incidence in populations with consanguineous marriages. The average incidence in Europe is 1:10 000; the highest reported incidence, 1:1250, is in an Eastern European ethnic group, the Roms, found predominantly in Slovakia.[30]

Two genetic loci have been associated with primary congenital glaucoma in published reports, GLC3A and GLC3B. A third locus, GLC3C, was presented in 2002 but has yet to be published at the time of this printing. CYP1B1, located in the GLC3A locus on chromosome 2p21, codes for the cytochrome P450 protein, cytochrome P4501B1. The nomenclature of the protein cytochrome P4501B1 refers to family 1, subfamily B, polypeptide 1 of the P450 superfamily. The cytochrome P450 proteins make up a superfamily of proteins that are involved in the metabolism of a wide range of endogenous and exogenous compounds.

The incidence of CYP1B1 mutations in populations with primary congenital glaucoma varies based on the population being studied. In Saudi Arabian and Slovakian Rom families, CYP1B1 mutations were found in almost 100% of primary congenital glaucoma patients. The prevalence of mutations in Brazil is 50%, in Indonesia 30%, and in Japan 20%.[30] This clearly indicates that other major genetic factors for congenital glaucoma remain to be identified.

CYP1B1 is involved in estrogen metabolism, namely in the metabolism of 17β-estradiol. Therefore, it acts to decrease estrogenic activity. In the body, it is mainly expressed in endocrine-regulated tissues such as in mammary tissue, the uterus, and the ovary.[31] In the eye, it is expressed in inner ciliary epithelium, lens epithelium, retinal ganglion, and inner nuclear layers, as well as the corneal epithelium.

The variety of mutations in CYP1B1 as well as a knockout mouse model point to a loss-of-function mechanism. That is, lack of the normal CYP1B1 gene results in the phenotype of primary congenital glaucoma. Since this protein is involved in estrogen metabolism, it is possible that increased estrogenic activity resulting from these mutations may cause failure of the anterior chamber angle to develop normally.[21]

Interestingly, CYP1B1 mutations have also been found in patients with juvenile open-angle glaucoma; in one study, the incidence was 5%. This suggests that primary congenital glaucoma and juvenile open-angle glaucoma are both within the phenotypic spectrum of CYP1B1 mutations.[32]

Further pointing to the heterogeneity of the glaucomas, CYP1B1 has also been described as a modifier gene for myocilin-associated glaucoma. In one autosomal dominant family with myocilin glaucoma, the presence of CYP1B1 correlated with an earlier onset of disease. Patients with only the MYOC mutation had an average age of onset of 51 years whereas patients in this same family with both MYOC and CYP1B1 mutations had an age of onset of 27 years.[32]

Incomplete penetrance has also been described for CYP1B1 mutations. In a minority of Saudi families studied, half of patients carrying CYP1B1 mutations did not have the primary congenital glaucoma phenotype whereas the other half that carried the same CYP1B1 mutations did have primary congenital glaucoma. This suggests the presence of a modifier locus. Since half of the patients with the 'affected' genotype manifested the disease phenotype, this would suggest that this modifier locus behaves in an autosomal dominant fashion.[33]

A CYP1B1 knockout mouse model did confirm the presence of a modifier locus. CYP1B1 knockout mice in which the tyrosinase gene was also defective had severe dysgenesis of ocular drainage structures compared to CYP1B1 knockout mice with normal tyrosinase. Administration of the tyrosinase product, L-dopa, resulted in less severe dysgenesis in tyrosinase defective mice. This would suggest that the tyrosinase gene is a modifier for the CYP1B1 gene in mice.[34] However, tyrosinase was not found to be a modifier for the CYP1B1 gene in humans.[35]

DEVELOPMENTAL GLAUCOMAS

Glaucoma can be associated with developmental defects of the eye. Anterior segment dysgenesis (ASD) is a broad term encompassing many developmental defects of the eye. There are three main categories within anterior segment dysgenesis – Axenfeld-Reiger syndrome, aniridia, and Peters anomaly. From a glaucoma standpoint, these disorders can be grouped together as they all result in glaucoma secondary to developmental defects in the drainage structures of the eye: the trabecular meshwork and Schlemm's canal. Generally, these disorders have autosomal dominant inheritance.

Axenfeld-Reiger syndrome itself refers to a spectrum of disorders with ocular findings of anteriorly displaced Schwalbe's line (posterior embryotoxon), peripheral iris–cornea adhesions, iris stromal hypoplasia, and corectopia (Fig. 22.4). Systemic findings include dental and skeletal anomalies.

Aniridia refers to bilateral partial or complete absence of the iris (Fig. 22.5). In addition, patients may have corneal and lenticular anomalies as well as foveal hypoplasia. Peters anomaly patients have a central corneal opacity which is associated with iridocorneal or lenticulocorneal adhesions, and absence of Descemet's membrane (Fig. 22.6).

In addition to these anterior segment dysgenesis syndromes, a systemic developmental disease, nail-patella syndrome (NPS) is also associated with primary open-angle glaucoma. Systemic manifestations include nail dysplasia, hypoplastic or absent patellae, and renal disease. Although glaucoma is associated with this condition, there are no pathognomonic ocular findings. The phenotype can include multiple iris processes, increased corneal thickness, and/or increased retinal nerve fiber layer thickness.[36]

These rare forms of glaucoma are more amenable to traditional forms of genetic analysis than POAG due to an earlier age of onset and clearly identifiable ocular and nonocular phenotypes. Thus, several genes have been identified that cause developmental glaucomas in humans. These include PITX2, FOXC1, PAX6, LMX1B,

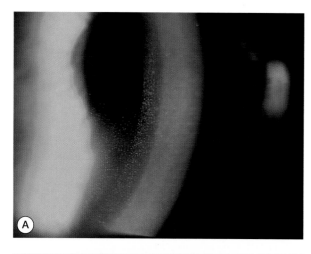

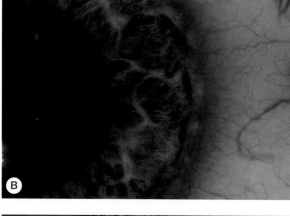

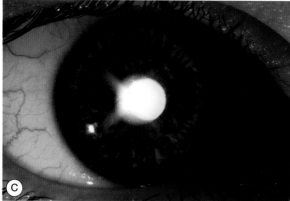

FIGURE 22.4 Pigment dispersion syndrome. **(A)** Krukenberg spindle – pigment deposition on corneal endothelial surface. **(B)** Pigment deposition on anterior iris. **(C)** Iris mid-peripheral transillumination defects. **(A)** Courtesy of Joseph Halabis, OD.)

PITX3, and FOXE3. Many of these genes are transcription factors. Mutations in these genes interfere with the cell signaling as well as the extracellular matrix signaling that is necessary for the normal development of the eye.[37]

ANGLE-CLOSURE GLAUCOMA

No gene has been identified for primary angle-closure glaucoma. However, a locus has been mapped for autosomal dominant nanophthalmos, a condition which predisposes to a frequently severe, early-onset form of

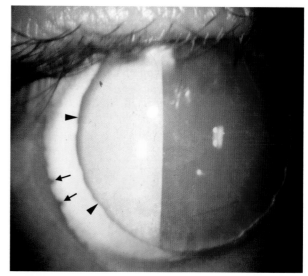

FIGURE 22.5 Aniridia. Absence of iris with visible ciliary processes (*arrows*). Note edge of lens (*arrowheads*).

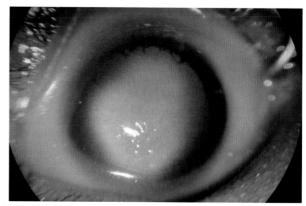

FIGURE 22.6 Peters anomaly. Central corneal opacity. Note iridocorneal adhesions superiorly.

angle closure. This locus, NNO1, is located on chromosome 11. Nanophthalmos has also been associated with the gene VMD2 in autosomal dominant vitreo-retinochoroidopathy.[21] More recently, acute primary angle-closure glaucoma has been associated with a single nucleotide polymorphism in the MMP-9 gene.[38]

Thus, one locus, NNO1, and one gene, VMD2, have been associated with nanophthalmos. For angle-closure glaucoma specifically, an association has been made with a single nucleotide polymorphism in the MMP-9 gene. The mechanism by which this would cause angle closure has not been elucidated.

Summary

Significant inroads have been made in gene discovery for glaucoma. Also, a molecular understanding for how some of these defects result in glaucoma is beginning to unfold. Genetic studies of the glaucomas will ultimately change glaucoma classification systems as patients are grouped together based on gene variations rather than clinical descriptions. Genetic and molecular studies will continue to enhance our understanding of the pathophysiology of glaucoma, ultimately resulting in earlier diagnosis as well as new treatments.

REFERENCES

1. Fan BJ, Wang DY, Lam DS, et al. Gene mapping for primary open angle glaucoma. Clin Biochem 2006; 39(3):249–258.

2. Fingert JH, Stone EM, Sheffield VC, et al. Myocilin glaucoma. Surv Ophthalmol 2002; 47(6):547–561.

3. Polansky JR, Fauss DJ, Chen P, et al. Cellular pharmacology and molecular biology of the trabecular meshwork inducible glucocorticoid response gene product. Ophthalmologica 1997; 211(3):126–139.

4. Gould DB, Reedy M, Wilson LA, et al. Mutant myocilin nonsecretion in vivo is not sufficient to cause glaucoma. Mol Cell Biol 2006; 26(22):8427–8436.

5. Senatorov V, Malyukova I, Fariss R, et al. Expression of mutated mouse myocilin induces open-angle glaucoma in transgenic mice. J Neurosci 2006; 26(46):11903–11914.

6. Hardy KM, Hoffman EA, Gonzalez P, et al. Extracellular trafficking of myocilin in human trabecular meshwork cells. J Biol Chem 2005; 280(32):28917–28926.

7. Fevrier B, Raposo G. Exosomes: endosomal-derived vesicles shipping extracellular messages. Curr Opin Cell Biol 2004; 16(4):415–421.

8. Jacobson N, Andrews M, Shepard AR, et al. Non-secretion of mutant proteins of the glaucoma gene myocilin in cultured trabecular meshwork cells and in aqueous humor. Hum Mol Genet 2001; 10(2):117–125.

9. Rezaie T, Child A, Hitchings R, et al. Adult-onset primary open-angle glaucoma caused by mutations in optineurin. Science 2002; 295(5557):1077–1079.

10. Alward WL, Kwon YH, Kawase K, et al. Evaluation of optineurin sequence variations in 1,048 patients with open-angle glaucoma. Am J Ophthalmol 2003; 136(5):904–910.

11. Aung T, Rezaie T, Okada K, et al. Clinical features and course of patients with glaucoma with the E50K mutation in the optineurin gene. Invest Ophthalmol Vis Sci 2005; 46(8):2816–2822.

12. Kroeber M, Ohlmann A, Russell P, et al. Transgenic studies on the role of optineurin in the mouse eye. Exp Eye Res 2006; 82(6):1075–1085.

13. Sahlender DA, Roberts RC, Arden SD, et al. Optineurin links myosin VI to the Golgi complex and is involved in Golgi organization and exocytosis. J Cell Biol 2005; 169(2):285–295.

14. De Marco N, Buono M, Troise F, et al. Optineurin increases cell survival and translocates to the nucleus in a Rab8-dependent manner upon an apoptotic stimulus. J Biol Chem 2006; 281(23):16147–16156.

15. Monemi S, Spaeth G, DaSilva A, et al. Identification of a novel adult-onset primary open-angle glaucoma (POAG) gene on 5q22.1. Hum Mol Genet 2005; 14(6):725–733.

16. Hewitt AW, Dimasi DP, Mackey DA, et al. A glaucoma case-control study of the WDR36 gene D658G sequence variant. Am J Ophthalmol 2006; 142(2):324–325.

17. Hauser MA, Allingham RR, Linkroum K, et al. Distribution of WDR36 DNA sequence variants in patients with primary open-angle glaucoma. Invest Ophthalmol Vis Sci 2006; 47(6):2542–2546.

18. Kramer PL, Samples JR, Monemi S, et al. The role of the WDR36 gene on chromosome 5q22.1 in a large family with primary open-angle glaucoma mapped to this region. Arch Ophthalmol 2006; 124(9):1328–1331.

19. Sugar H, Barbour F. Pigmentary glaucoma: a rare clinical entity. Am J Ophthalmol 1949; 32:90–92.

20. Ritch R. Pigment dispersion syndrome. Am J Ophthalmol 1998; 126(3):442–445.

21. Wiggs JL. Genes associated with human glaucoma. Ophthalmol Clin North Am 2005; 18(3):335–343.

22. Andersen JS, Pralea AM, DelBono EA, et al. A gene responsible for the pigment dispersion syndrome maps to chromosome 7q35-q36. Arch Ophthalmol 1997; 115(3):384–388.

23. Ritch R, Steinberger D, Liebmann JM. Prevalence of pigment dispersion syndrome in a population undergoing glaucoma screening. Am J Ophthalmol 1993; 115(6):707–710.

24. Anderson MG, Libby RT, Mao M, et al. Genetic context determines susceptibility to intraocular pressure elevation in a mouse pigmentary glaucoma. BMC Biol 2006; 4:20.

25. Anderson MG, Smith RS, Hawes NL, et al. Mutations in genes encoding melanosomal proteins cause pigmentary glaucoma in DBA/2J mice. Nat Genet 2002; 30(1):81–85.

26. Karger RA, Jeng SM, Johnson DH, et al. Estimated incidence of pseudoexfoliation syndrome and pseudoexfoliation glaucoma in Olmsted County, Minnesota. J Glaucoma 2003; 12(3):193–197.

27. Gottanka J, Flugel-Koch C, Martus P, et al. Correlation of pseudoexfoliative material and optic nerve damage in pseudoexfoliation syndrome. Invest Ophthalmol Vis Sci 1997; 38(12):2435–2446.

28. Thorleifsson G, Magnusson KP, Sulem P, et al. Common sequence variants in the LOXL1 gene confer susceptibility to exfoliation glaucoma. Science 2007; 317(5843):1397–1400.

29. Ritch R, Schlotzer-Schrehardt U, Konstas AG. Why is glaucoma associated with exfoliation syndrome? Prog Retin Eye Res 2003; 22(3):253–275.

30. Chakrabarti S, Kaur K, Kaur I, et al. Globally, CYP1B1 mutations in primary congenital glaucoma are strongly structured by geographic and haplotype backgrounds. Invest Ophthalmol Vis Sci 2006; 47(1):43–47.

31. Tsuchiya Y, Nakajima M, Kyo S, et al. Human CYP1B1 is regulated by estradiol via estrogen receptor. Cancer Res 2004; 64(9):3119–3125.

32. Vincent AL, Billingsley G, Buys Y, et al. Digenic inheritance of early-onset glaucoma: CYP1B1, a potential modifier gene. Am J Hum Genet 2002; 70(2):448–460.

33. Bejjani BA, Stockton DW, Lewis RA, et al. Multiple CYP1B1 mutations and incomplete penetrance in an inbred population segregating primary congenital glaucoma suggest frequent de novo events and a dominant modifier locus. Hum Mol Genet 2000; 9(3):367–374.

34. Libby RT, Smith RS, Savinova OV, et al. Modification of ocular defects in mouse developmental glaucoma models by tyrosinase. Science 2003; 299(5612):1578–1581.

35. Bidinost C, Hernandez N, Edward DP, et al. Of mice and men: tyrosinase modification of congenital glaucoma in mice but not in humans. Invest Ophthalmol Vis Sci 2006; 47(4):1486–1490.

36. Milla E, Hernan I, Gamundi MJ, et al. Novel LMX1B mutation in familial nail-patella syndrome with variable expression of open angle glaucoma. Mol Vis 2007; 13:639–648.

37. Gould DB, Smith RS, John SW. Anterior segment development relevant to glaucoma. Int J Dev Biol 2004; 48(8–9):1015–1029.

38. Wang IJ, Chiang TH, Shih YF, et al. The association of single nucleotide polymorphisms in the MMP-9 genes with susceptibility to acute primary angle closure glaucoma in Taiwanese patients. Mol Vis 2006; 12:1223–1232.

Genetic Epidemiology

Leonieke ME van Koolwijk, Catey Bunce, and Ananth C Viswanathan

INTRODUCTION

In 1869, Von Graefe described a heritable form of glaucoma and noted that the accurate etiology of this disease remained to be investigated.[1] In 2007, investigation is still ongoing. Although the presence of a genetic component has since been confirmed, unraveling this genetic component has proven difficult. Therefore, human geneticists, laboratory scientists, epidemiologists, and clinicians have currently integrated their expertise in a branch of science called genetic epidemiology.

Genetic epidemiology investigates how genes produce disease in human populations. It is distinct from two closely allied fields of study: it differs from classic epidemiology by its explicit consideration of genetic factors and it differs from medical genetics by its emphasis on population-based studies. Genetic epidemiology also studies the joint effects of genes and the environment and includes an incorporation of the underlying biology of the disease into its conceptual models. Genetic epidemiology is increasingly focusing on common diseases. Examples of common diseases in ophthalmology include age-related macular degeneration, myopia, and primary open-angle glaucoma (POAG).

Here we consider the methodologies used in genetic epidemiology, and discuss current and future perspectives on POAG genetics.

Genetic studies of POAG are important for two reasons. First, the identification of genes and of their biological pathways may elucidate the pathophysiological mechanisms that are presently little understood. This may then provide new directions for the development of glaucoma therapy. Second, by knowing the genes and how they predict the onset or progression of POAG, we may be able to create diagnostic and prognostic DNA tests. This may be especially valuable for POAG, as many patients are diagnosed only after significant and irreversible visual field damage has occurred. Early treatment may prevent or delay this damage. In addition, many 'suspects' who repeatedly attend the glaucoma clinic unnecessarily might be dismissed from regular surveillance based on their DNA test.

The route to a better understanding of POAG etiology starts by investigating whether susceptibility has a genetic basis and assessing the magnitude and type of this genetic susceptibility. These issues will be discussed in the first section of this chapter. When a genetic component has been established, the next step is searching for the genes that cause or contribute to POAG. The two approaches for this are *linkage* and *association*. Gene-finding has been the chief purpose of genetic epidemiology studies up to now. Linkage and association studies therefore take the lion's share of this chapter. In the second and third sections the authors address the basic principles of these approaches and evaluate how they have contributed to our current knowledge of POAG genetics. Before any results of these gene-finding studies can be usefully translated into ophthalmic practice the significance of the identified genes in the population and in the etiology of POAG need to be determined. Studies addressing these issues are still in their infancy and will be briefly discussed in the last section.

GENETIC SUSCEPTIBILITY TO PRIMARY OPEN-ANGLE GLAUCOMA

IS PRIMARY OPEN-ANGLE GLAUCOMA A GENETIC DISEASE?

Support for a genetic basis of POAG comes from numerous familial cases, epidemiological studies, and twin analyses. Family history has been reported to be an important risk factor for the development of POAG. First-degree family members of POAG patients are estimated to have as much as a tenfold increased risk of the disease compared to the general population.[2] Prevalence studies of POAG have shown significant racial variation.[3–7] Although environmental factors may partly account for this variation, genetic factors are likely to play an important role. This is substantiated by a recent meta-analysis demonstrating no significant differences in POAG prevalence among black populations from America, Europe, West Indies, or Africa.[8]

A high concordance of POAG in monozygotic twin pairs further supports a genetic predisposition for POAG.[9]

Except for the rare familial cases with clear mendelian patterns of inheritance, POAG is generally considered a complex disease: it most likely results from multiple genetic and environmental factors, and from interactions between them. No single factor is necessary or sufficient to cause the disease. A clue to understanding the etiology of complex diseases is provided by the liability threshold theory. Figure 23.1 shows the distribution of a theoretical variable that represents the liability to get the disease. Genetic and environmental factors determine someone's position on this liability distribution. A person with a favorable combination of protective factors in the absence of many risk factors will be at the left side of the distribution. A person with an unfavorable combination of genetic and environmental risk factors will be at the right side. A person whose liability variable exceeds a critical threshold will develop the disease.

GENETIC CONTRIBUTION TO QUANTITATIVE PRIMARY OPEN-ANGLE GLAUCOMA TRAITS

The etiological complexity of POAG may be reduced by discretely studying quantitative features of the phenotype: cup-to-disc ratio, rim area, retinal nerve fiber layer (RNFL) thickness, or risk factors such as intraocular pressure (IOP) and central corneal thickness (CCT). These quantitative traits may have simpler genetic origins and may therefore be easier to unravel. Moreover, they do not require an individual to be arbitrarily categorized as 'affected' or 'nonaffected' and are therefore not susceptible to misclassification, which has been a major problem in POAG studies. Another advantage is

that quantitative traits can also be studied in individuals without glaucoma, which means that this approach greatly increases the number of individuals available for genetic studies.

The genetic contribution to quantitative traits can be estimated by means of variance component analyses. These analyses separate the total variance of a trait into components attributable to different causes (Fig. 23.2). The first theoretical division entails a component explained by the effects of genotype and a component explained by the effects of environment. The genotype component represents everything that relates to the particular composition of genes possessed by the individual. The environment refers to all the nongenetic conditions that influence the phenotype. The genotype component can be subdivided into a segment that includes the cumulative effects of the individual alleles (*additive genetic variance*) and a segment that represents the effects of interactions. The latter may include interactions between the two alleles of one gene (*dominance*), interactions between the alleles of different genes (*epistasis*), and interactions between genes and environmental factors.

Separating the total variance into its components allows us to estimate the relative contribution of the different determinants to the phenotype. The relative contribution of heredity to the phenotype is called *heritability*: it is the proportion of the total variance that is explained by additive genetic effects. The heritability ranges from 0, indicating that additive genetic effects do not contribute to the phenotype, to 1, indicating that the phenotype is completely explained by additive effects of genes. Heritability can be estimated from the resemblance between family members.

Additive genetic effects have been reported to contribute significantly to the variances of quantitative POAG traits. Heritability estimates range from 0.29 to 0.50 for IOP, from 0.48 to 0.80 for cup-to-disc ratio, and from 0.48 to 0.82 for RNFL thickness.[10–15] CCT showed a heritability estimate of 0.95, which suggests that 95% of its variance is explained by the effects of genes.[16] These high heritability estimates support quantitative trait strategies to discover new genes for POAG.

However, the analyses described above only provide information on the combined additive effects of all genes. If there is a very large number of contributing genes, each with a very small effect on the phenotype, gene-finding studies would have very little chance of success. To assess gene-finding feasibility, a quantitative trait can be investigated for the presence

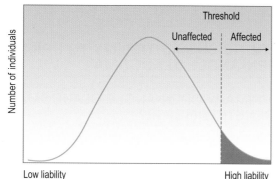

FIGURE 23.1 Liability threshold model for complex diseases.

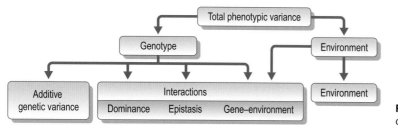

FIGURE 23.2 Partitioning of variance in a variance components analysis.

of a major gene accounting for its variance. A suitable method for this is by the use of commingling analysis. This analysis applies a maximum likelihood method to assess the strength of evidence for the effect of a major gene compared with the null model of no major gene. Furthermore, it estimates the contribution of the major gene to the total variance of the phenotype.

Commingling analysis was performed on IOP data of 3654 persons attending the Blue Mountains Eye Study.[17] The best fitting model for the dataset consisted of a mixture of three distributions (Fig. 23.3), which would be consistent with the presence of a major gene in the determination of IOP. This major gene was estimated to account for 18% of the total variance in IOP. The parameters of the best fitting distribution provide some guidance for the planning of future genetic studies. The middle distribution in Fig. 23.3 contains the heterozygotes, i.e. the individuals that carry one copy of the wild-type ('normal') allele and one copy of the rare ('IOP-increasing') allele. It is likely that values of IOP more extreme than three residual standard deviations (blue lines in Fig. 23.3) from the mean of this distribution will be from homozygotes: IOP values less than 18 mmHg will be from persons with two copies of the wild-type allele, and IOP values greater than 33 mmHg will be from persons with two copies of the rare allele. For the purposes of association studies, it would be desirable to compare individuals having at least one copy of the rare allele with individuals having no copies. The former group would be those with IOPs higher than three residual standard deviations (green line) from the mean of the leftmost distribution in Figure 23.3, which corresponds to IOP values greater than 23.5 mmHg. The latter group would be those with IOPs of less than 18 mmHg, for reasons already discussed.

LINKAGE STUDIES

Having established a likely genetic component in the etiology of a complex disease, the next step is to localize any disease genes. Linkage analysis provides a means to identify the chromosomal location (*locus*) of a disease gene without any prior knowledge about possible biological mechanisms. Linkage analysis has traditionally been performed to study monogenic diseases in large families with multiple affected members. This approach is called parametric or model-based linkage analysis. It requires an assumption of the genetic model, in which the mode of inheritance, the disease and marker allele numbers and frequencies, and the penetrance of the disease genotype need to be specified. As long as an adequate model can be assumed, parametric linkage provides a powerful method to locate a disease gene. However, it has failed to find the more common genes underlying complex diseases, for which a valid gene model cannot be specified. The shift towards the genetics of complex diseases has therefore led to the development of new methods of linkage analysis that are nonparametric, or model-free.

Both parametric and nonparametric linkage approaches have been used to identify the chromosomal locations of POAG susceptibility genes. The authors explain the principles of these methods and consider their roles in POAG genetics.

LINKAGE ANALYSIS OF MONOGENIC FORMS OF GLAUCOMA

Parametric linkage analyses investigate the co-segregation of genetic loci in pedigrees. The rationale is that two loci that lie very close together on a chromosome have a high

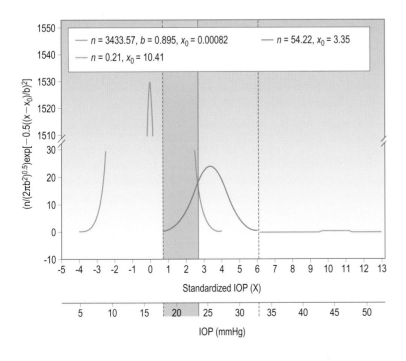

FIGURE 23.3 Commingling analysis of IOP in the Blue Mountains Eye Study.[17] This figure shows the model which, after commingling analysis, fitted the population IOP data best. It consists of three normal distributions, each containing n individuals, with mean x_0, and with common standard deviation b. The blue lines are placed at three standard deviations from the mean of the middle distribution, which contains the heterozygotes. More extreme IOP values (IOP < 18 mmHg or IOP > 33 mmHg) are likely to be from homozygotes. The green line is placed at three standard deviations from the mean of the leftmost distribution (IOP = 23.5 mmHg). For the purposes of association studies, it would be desirable to compare individuals having at least one copy of the risk allele (right from the green line, i.e. IOP > 23.5 mmHg) with individuals having no copies (left from the leftmost blue line, i.e. IOP < 18 mmHg).

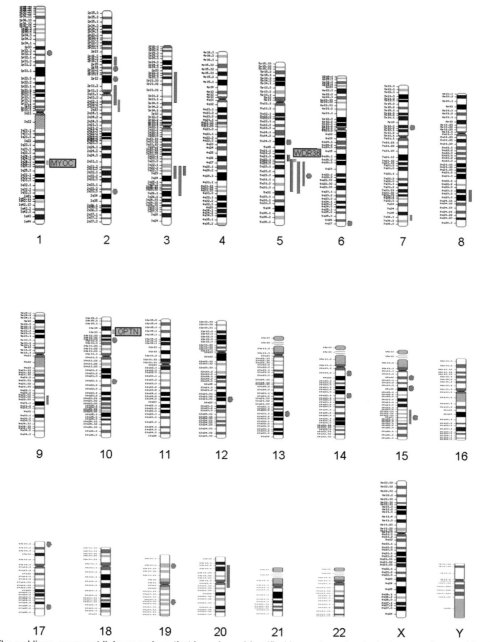

FIGURE 23.4 The red lines represent linkage regions that have been identified by analyses in single, large pedigrees. Line boundaries have been determined by haplotype analyses. Purple lines correspond to replicated or refined loci in the same population. Red dots represent maximum LOD scores from population-based (family) studies. The three identified genes are shown in blue. References are listed per chromosome in top-down order, and for chromosomes 3, 5, and 15 also in left-to-right order. See Table 23.1.

probability of being inherited together. The further apart two loci are on a chromosome, the higher the chance of a recombination event occurring between them during meiosis. This will put an end to their co-segregation. Loci on different chromosomes segregate independently. Thus, the probability of two loci segregating together is a measure of the genetic distance between them. Similarly, the probability of a genetic marker and the disease segregating together is a measure of the genetic distance between that marker and the disease gene. Designating the whole genome with genetic markers and observing their co-segregation with the disease in a pedigree can subsequently lead to localization of the disease gene.

The likelihood of genetic linkage (compared with the null-hypothesis of no linkage) between a genetic marker and the disease is usually expressed as an LOD (logarithm of the odds) score. High, positive LOD scores (traditionally >3) are evidence for linkage, and low, negative scores (<-2) are evidence against.

Why should we study monogenic forms of POAG while the large majority of POAG cases are considered of complex etiology? The loci and the genes that have been identified in these monogenic forms may also determine susceptibility for the more common forms of POAG. Moreover, they may provide a clue to the pathology, disease mechanisms, and signaling pathways in

TABLE 23.1 Primary open-angle glaucoma loci references belonging to Figure 23.4

CHROMOSOME	GENE/LOCUS NAMES AND REFERENCES
1	27, MYOC[89,90]
2	GLC1H[91, 19, 24], GLC1B[92,93, 20]
3	GLC1L[21], GLC1C[94–96]
5	24, GLC1G[97,98], WDR36[98], GLC1M[88,99,100]
6	23,24
7	24,GLC1F[101]
8	GLC1D[102]
9	GLC1J[103]
10	OPTN[104,105, 20, 27]
12	24
13	23
14	19, 100
15	GLC1I[106,107], GLC1N[24,108]
17	19, 19
19	24, 19
20	GLC1K[103]

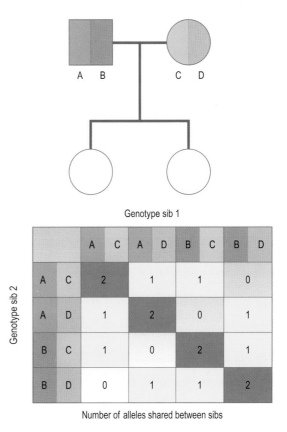

Genotype sib 1

		A C	A D	B C	B D
A	C	2	1	1	0
A	D	1	2	0	1
B	C	1	0	2	1
B	D	0	1	1	2

Number of alleles shared between sibs

P (sharing 0 alleles) = 4/16 = ¼
P (sharing 1 allele) = 8/16 = ½
P (sharing 2 alleles) = 4/16 = ¼

FIGURE 23.5 Allele sharing in sib pairs.

POAG. The advantage of dealing with monogenic forms of POAG is that methods of parametric linkage are more straightforward and well established than the methods used for complex diseases. However, parametric linkage analysis in pedigrees can be complicated by the late onset of POAG: the patients' parents are often deceased, while their children are too young to manifest the disease.

Fourteen POAG loci have been assigned a GLC1 symbol (GLC1A to GLC1N) by the HUGO Genome Nomenclature Committee (Fig. 23.4, Table 23.1). Most studies involved small numbers of large families in which the disease segregated as an autosomal dominant trait. GLC1A, GLC1J, GLC1K, GLC1M, and GLC1N were identified in families with the rare, juvenile onset form of POAG (JOAG). JOAG typically manifests before the age of 35 years and exhibits high IOP that often requires surgical therapy. It usually shows autosomal dominant rather than complex inheritance. The JOAG loci may contribute to susceptibility to the common, adult-onset form of POAG. This has already been established for the MYOC gene at the GLC1A locus. The role of the other JOAG loci has yet to be fully assessed in adult cases.

LINKAGE ANALYSIS OF COMPLEX FORMS OF GLAUCOMA

Nonparametric linkage methods investigate the degree of allele sharing by affected family members without assuming a particular mode of inheritance. The idea is that, in the region of the disease gene, affected relative pairs share copies of the same ancestral alleles more frequently than would be expected based on the degree of their relationship.

The most commonly used method of nonparametric linkage is the *sib pair analysis*, in which pairs of affected siblings from a large number of families are genotyped for markers along the whole genome. If a marker is not linked to the disease, each pair of siblings has a probability of 1/4 of sharing no parental alleles, 1/2 of sharing 1 parental allele, and 1/4 of sharing 2 parental alleles (Fig. 23.5). According to the null hypothesis of no linkage, therefore, a 1:2:1 ratio of sib pairs sharing 0, 1, or 2 marker alleles would be expected. For each marker, the observed number of pairs sharing 0, 1, or 2 alleles can be compared with this 1:2:1 ratio. Linkage would be suggested if this ratio is significantly shifted towards a higher extent of allele sharing.

A disadvantage of sib pair analysis is that it does not include other affected family members. Potentially important information from, for example, affected aunts, cousins, or grandparents could therefore be lost. To take greater advantage of extended pedigrees, several methods have been developed that do include this additional information. These *affected relative pair analyses* calculate the extent to which affected relatives share copies of the same ancestral marker alleles and compare this with the null hypothesis of random segregation of the marker. Some programs analyze each possible pair of affected individuals; others consider the total group of relatives.

Affected sib pair and relative pair analyses usually produce nonparametric LOD (NPL) scores. Interpreting these scores has been challenged by the question of where to put the threshold of statistical significance.

In 1995, Lander and Kruglyak in their guidelines for reporting linkage results proposed LOD score thresholds of 2.2 for suggestive linkage and 3.6 for significant linkage in affected sib pair analyses.[18] Their significance criteria have been commonly applied. Alternatively, linkage studies perform computer simulations to estimate significance thresholds that are specific for the particular population and circumstances (allele frequencies, missing data, etc.) under study.

In 2000, Wiggs et al. published the first genome screen of sib pairs with adult-onset POAG.[19] They initially studied 113 affected sib pairs originating from 41 mainly Caucasian families. Family sizes ranged from a single affected sib pair to nine affected individuals. Because of this variety in pedigree structures, they used three different analytical methods to assess linkage: a parametric LOD score analysis, a nonparametric affected relative pair method, and a nonparametric sib pair analysis. They revealed 25 chromosomal regions with positive results for at least one analysis. These regions were followed up with extra markers and 69 additional sib pairs. Sib pair analysis using the combined pedigree set of 182 affected sib pairs identified suggestive linkage at chromosomes 2, 14, 17, and 19 (see Fig. 23.4).

A genome-wide scan as part of the Barbados Family Study of Open-Angle Glaucoma (BFSG) was performed in 146 families of African descent.[20] As in Wiggs' study, a multianalytical approach was chosen to evaluate the results. Significance levels were estimated by simulation studies. Parametric linkage analysis indicated possible POAG gene regions on chromosomes 2 and 10, with LOD scores >3.0. Nonparametric affected relative pair analysis supported linkage on chromosome 2, but did not show any evidence for linkage on chromosome 10. The chromosome 2 locus had not previously been associated with POAG. The locus on chromosome 10 was close to the OPTN gene. Sequencing of this gene, however, did not reveal any pathogenic alterations, suggesting that another gene in this region had caused the linkage result.

One POAG locus (GLC1L) has been identified by means of nonparametric linkage analysis in a single, large pedigree.[21] Previous studies of this six-generation Tasmanian family had detected a mutation in the MYOC gene. However, only nine of the 24 affected family members presented with this mutation. This suggested genetic heterogeneity, indicating that at least one other gene would be expected to determine POAG susceptibility in this family. Parametric linkage methods failed to localize chromosomal POAG regions, probably due to the genetic heterogeneity and incomplete family information. Nonparametric strategies were subsequently employed. These identified a disease locus on the short arm of chromosome 3, where 11 affected family members shared the same ancestral allele. Interestingly, seven of them also carried the MYOC mutation. The results of this study suggested possible interaction between the MYOC gene and the chromosome 3 locus, although the numbers were too small to substantiate this with significant evidence.

LINKAGE ANALYSIS OF QUANTITATIVE TRAITS

Nonparametric linkage analyses can also be used to study the genetic mechanisms underlying quantitative traits. The most commonly employed methods are based on a strategy developed by Haseman and Elston in 1972.[22] They compared the resemblance of sib pairs for a particular trait with the amount of allele sharing. If a marker is linked to a gene that determines the quantitative trait (usually called a quantitative trait locus, or QTL), sib pairs who carry the same ancestral marker alleles would be expected to be more similar for that trait. Haseman and Elston regressed the squared sib pair difference for the trait on their extent of allele sharing at the marker locus. A significantly negative slope of the regression line would indicate significant linkage. This method has since been modified to increase power, but the basic concept has not changed.

Other methods for analyzing QTLs are based on variance components partitioning. The total phenotypic variance is separated into components attributable to the effects of a specific chromosomal region (the QTL), residual additive genetic effects, covariate effects, and remaining (environmental, interaction) effects. The parameter of interest is the proportion of the total variance that is explained by a QTL in the region spanned by the tested markers. A maximum likelihood approach can be used to estimate which value of this parameter fits the data best. The likelihood of this model is then compared with the likelihood of a null model, where the effect of the QTL is fixed at 0, and an LOD score is produced by the logarithm of the ratio of these likelihoods.

The authors have shown above that quantitative POAG traits are highly heritable. This suggests that a quantitative trait linkage analysis may be a powerful strategy for identifying new POAG genes. In 2005, Duggal et al. performed a genome-wide linkage analysis for IOP in a subpopulation of the Beaver Dam Eye study.[23] With a modified Haseman-Elston regression method in 218 sibling pairs, they revealed two loci as potential (although not statistically significant) linkage regions for IOP on chromosomes 6 and 13. Neither locus had previously been identified in a genome-wide scan for POAG. When they repeated the genome-wide IOP analysis in a larger sample ($n = 1979$) of the same population, the linkage result on chromosome 13 could not be replicated.[24] The genome-wide linkage analysis in the expanded cohort of the Beaver Dam Eye Study identified seven regions of interest on chromosomes 2, 5, 6, 7, 12, 15, and 19. The region with the strongest evidence for linkage, on the short arm of chromosome 19, had previously been identified in four genome-wide studies on blood pressure. This may suggest a common gene regulating both IOP and blood pressure, two quantitative traits that have already been shown to correlate. Alternatively, this region on chromosome 19 may contain two nearby genes that control IOP and blood pressure independently. The linkage peak on chromosome 2 was very close to the glaucoma locus GLC1B.

This locus had been identified in 1996 through classic linkage in six glaucoma families.[25] A recent study confirmed the locus in an extended pedigree from the Glaucoma Inheritance Study in Tasmania.[26] Paradoxically, the glaucoma patients in both studies had normal to slightly elevated IOPs.

Quantitative traits have also been analyzed in the extended Tasmanian POAG pedigree that had previously revealed a mutation in the MYOC gene and linkage to the 3p21-22 (GLC1L) region in some, but not all, affected family members.[21] Variance components linkage analyses identified a new locus for IOP on chromosome 10, with a significant LOD score of 3.3.[27] This study was the first to report a locus for cup-to-disc ratio. Suggestive linkage for this trait was found on chromosome 1, with a maximum LOD score of 2.3. The linkage peaks for both IOP and cup-to-disc ratio were substantially reduced after including the MYOC mutation status as a covariate in the variance components analysis. This may indicate that the MYOC gene interacts with the quantitative trait loci. The different studies in this single family nicely outline the complexity of gene-finding in POAG: they clearly show the heterogeneity, they illustrate that genes that contribute to the phenotype in a different way are likely to be identified by different gene-finding strategies, and they touch upon gene interactions, which may have an important role in the etiology of POAG.

The authors have already considered that quantitative traits may be beneficial in gene-finding studies of POAG for the reason that they may have simpler genetic backgrounds, are not prone to misclassification, and can be studied population-wide. A potential drawback, however, may concern their clinical relevance. Does a gene that has been found to mediate IOP in the general population really contribute to the development of POAG? Evidently, after a QTL has been identified, its role in disease pathogenesis needs to be thoroughly assessed. A weakness of the currently published quantitative trait linkage studies of IOP is that none has been able to adjust for central corneal thickness (CCT). CCT is a potential confounder of IOP measurements[28] as well as a potential risk factor for POAG[29] and has been shown to be highly heritable.[16] The identified loci may therefore, at least to some extent, control CCT rather than IOP.

Linkage studies have so far revealed more than 25 genetic loci for POAG, thereby clearly supporting its complex nature (see Fig. 23.4). For the vast majority of these loci, however, a gene has not yet been identified. How should we interpret these linkage results? And, how could they guide future gene-finding research? In this respect we can learn from other complex diseases, for which it has turned out successful to concentrate on gene-finding within loci that had been replicated. The CFH gene and the LOC387715 gene for age-related macular degeneration have thus been identified in two repeatedly detected loci on chromosomes 1 and 10, respectively.[30–33]

Many linkage regions for POAG have not been replicated. This may be due to the multiple genes that are involved in the pathogenesis of POAG. It may also be explained by the different study designs: mendelian linkage approaches are likely to identify loci with rare, highly penetrant mutations whereas nonparametric methods aim for loci with common, low penetrant variants. These loci may or may not be the same. Furthermore, the studies have been performed in different populations, in which different genes may account for POAG. Finally, some loci may have been false-positive findings, and other nonconfirmatory studies may have been false negatives.

GENETIC ASSOCIATION STUDIES

In contrast to the typically genetic concept of linkage, association is an established approach in traditional epidemiology. An association study assesses whether a disease is significantly related to a potential risk factor in a population. A *genetic* association study assesses whether a disease is significantly related to a *genetic variant* in a population. This association exists when individuals with the disease have a significantly higher frequency of a particular risk allele than would be expected from the disease and allele frequencies in the population.

Association between a disease and a genetic variant may occur for two reasons: (1) direct biological action of the genetic variant causes the association; and (2) the genetic variant does not have a direct role, but is associated with a causal variant in close proximity due to linkage disequilibrium. Linkage disequilibrium occurs when two loci are so close that the same alleles will be inherited together over many generations, thereby leading to an association at the population level. This is different from linkage, where the alleles are further apart and − although segregating together within one family − show a variety of combinations across different families.

CANDIDATE GENE ANALYSES

Many genetic association studies for POAG have been performed. They have either investigated associations with genetic variants in the known, causative genes (as has been discussed in Ch. 22, Genetics of Glaucoma), or have searched for risk alleles in potentially predisposing candidate genes. These candidate genes have been selected through different strategies. Most commonly, the selection is made through reasoning backwards from the mechanisms that are (assumed to be) involved in the pathogenesis of POAG. This has led to association studies of genes regulating ocular blood flow (nitric oxide synthase and endothelin-1-related genes),[34–36] aqueous humor outflow (renin–angiotensin system genes),[37,38] apoptosis (tumor-protein p53 gene),[39,40] immune system (interleukin-1β and tumor necrosis factor-α genes),[41,42] and neurodegeneration (apolipoprotein E gene).[43–46] Many of these studies have had inconsistent results and the role of these genes in the etiology of POAG is still controversial. A potential disadvantage of this approach is that each (patho)physiological mechanism probably results from many genes, the effects of which may be influenced by the environment, other genes, or complex gene networks. Working backwards from such a mechanism to one or a set of potential genes may therefore be based on too simplistic a model.

Alternatively, a candidate gene may be selected because of its homology with other disease-causing genes. More than 90% of the mutations in the MYOC gene are located in the so-called olfactomedin domain in the third exon. Mukhopadhyay et al. used a bioinformatics approach to search for myocilin-related proteins that had a conserved olfactomedin domain and were expressed in the eye.[47] They thus identified the Noelin 1 and 2 genes as potential candidates for POAG. One association study has since been performed for the Noelin 2 gene (OLFM2) in Japanese subjects.[48] A possible disease-causing mutation was identified and common genetic variants were suggested to contribute to the glaucoma phenotype by interacting with the optineurin gene. These results still need to be replicated, both in the Japanese and in other populations.

A third group of potential candidates are genes involved in the pathogenesis of related diseases. These diseases could either be complex syndromes of which glaucoma is one of the features, or diseases which show phenotypic similarities to glaucoma. An example is OPA1, the gene responsible for autosomal dominant optic atrophy.[49,50] Like glaucoma, optic atrophy is a progressive optic neuropathy caused by degeneration of retinal ganglion cells. The clinical similarities, together with the finding that OPA1 is expressed in retinal ganglion cells and in the optic nerve, made OPA1 a promising candidate gene.[51] Due to the absence of raised IOP, OPA1 was hypothesized to be most likely associated with normal-tension glaucoma. Genetic variants in the OPA1 gene have indeed been associated with normal-tension glaucoma, but not with high-tension glaucoma in Caucasian patients.[52,53] A study in Japanese subjects confirmed this, but showed that within the group of high-tension glaucoma patients an OPA1 variant was significantly related to the age at the time of diagnosis.[54] The association between OPA1 variants and normal-tension glaucoma could not be replicated in Korean and African-American subjects.[55,56] A second example in this category is CYP1B1. Genetic association studies have shown that this gene is not only involved in congenital glaucoma but also in high-tension POAG with juvenile or adult onset.[57,58]

ASSOCIATION ANALYSES FOLLOWING LINKAGE

Association analyses can be used to further investigate previously identified linkage regions. Candidate genes within a linkage region can be selected by means of the methods described above. Association studies for the ACE gene[37] (located in a region identified by a genome-wide sib pair analysis)[19] and the NOS3 gene[35] (located nearby the GLC1F locus)[59] have thus been performed. Alternatively, a dense marker set along the total linkage region can be analyzed for association. This method

has successfully identified variants in the complement factor H and LOC387715 genes as risk factors for age-related macular degeneration.[30–33]

GENOME-WIDE ASSOCIATION ANALYSES

To date, association studies of POAG have focused on candidate genes. With the identification of highly dense and easily genotyped markers called single nucleotide polymorphisms (SNPs), the increasing knowledge of the distribution of linkage disequilibrium throughout the genome, and reducing genotyping costs, a shift is rapidly being made towards genome-wide association studies. Although this approach still has its limitations (as discussed below), successes from other complex diseases support the application of genome-wide association studies to gene-finding in glaucoma.[60]

CONFOUNDING IN GENETIC ASSOCIATION STUDIES

As in traditional epidemiology, confounding factors lie in wait to either generate false positives or hide true results. One possible source of confounding in genetic association studies is population stratification. Due to increased migration and integration, each apparently homogeneous population may consist of multiple genetically distinct subpopulations. Different disease and allele frequencies between the subpopulations can lead to spurious association because cases and controls may not be properly matched (i.e. may derive from different subpopulations). To get round this problem, family-based association methods have been developed. The most widely used is the transmission disequilibrium test (TDT),[61] in which the frequencies of alleles that are transmitted from a parent to an affected child are compared to the frequencies of alleles that are not transmitted. This 'internal control' approach is independent of population stratification. Another option is to test the data for possible stratification effects by comparing allele frequencies of several unlinked loci in cases and controls.[62]

A second issue in genetic association studies is that of multiple comparisons. Typically, a large number of genetic markers are tested, each with a small a priori probability of association. Even without any true effect, 5% of the markers will show significant association if the usual p-value of 0.05 is respected. The significance level should thus be adjusted but there is no clear consensus about exactly how. The common post hoc corrections, such as the Bonferroni approach, seem to be too conservative: they assume independence of each test while many markers will actually be correlated owing to linkage disequilibrium. Although new methods to deal with possibly false-positive results come into view, the best approach still is to replicate the findings in a second, independent sample.

CHAPTER 23

ASSOCIATION AND LINKAGE

Association and linkage are complementary approaches. The choice to use one or the other depends on the availability of study subjects, expected genetic effects and allele frequencies, technical capacities, and funding. Association is assumed to be more powerful than linkage for identifying susceptibility alleles with a small effect, as is often the case in complex diseases. In addition, association studies do not require the recruitment of families with multiple affected cases or special family structures and are therefore easier to conduct. The technical demands and the costs for a genome-wide association study are, on the other hand, much higher than for a genome-wide linkage study, as more markers need to be genotyped. Furthermore, linkage studies probably have more power to detect susceptibility alleles with low frequencies.

FUTURE PERSPECTIVES

The unambiguous conclusion of the above-discussed gene-finding studies is that POAG is a complex disease. Many loci have been identified. The process of identifying genes related to these loci, however, is lagging. Moreover, the currently known genes (MYOC,[63] OPTN,[64] WDR36[65]) probably contribute to the pathogenesis of POAG in less than 5% of cases in the general population.[66–69] Genes accounting for a more significant proportion of the known heritable component of POAG remain to be identified.

How can we improve and accelerate the gene-finding process of POAG? Can we copy the art from other complex diseases? Recent successes have emphasized the potential value of association studies.[60] This seems a reasonable approach for POAG, as the effect sizes of the susceptibility alleles are expected to be small. In addition, this method has recently become more feasible as a result of emerging high-throughput and affordable genotyping technologies and increasing knowledge of the genome. Association studies may benefit from previous linkage analyses; loci that have repeatedly identified by linkage may be promising association targets.[30–33]

One of the keys to future success in gene-finding is collaboration. Insufficient power has been a common limitation of genetic association studies. Very large cohorts are needed to identify weak susceptibility genes and second cohorts to replicate any findings. Collaboration between research groups is therefore necessary to make progress, as has been realized by the currently increasing numbers of joint initiatives. Inaccurate or incomplete phenotyping has been a second limitation of genetic studies. The complex diagnosis and the insidious onset of POAG have often led to misclassification. Currently improving diagnostic techniques and the opportunity to study quantitative traits may partly solve this problem. A thorough understanding of the phenotype is a prerequisite for a fruitful study design. It is essential to know what clinical features are important

and how these can be accurately, efficiently, and reliably assessed. Therefore, close collaboration between scientists and clinicians is necessary.

Future studies will not only be directed at finding new genes but also at elucidating the role of already identified genes. Which gene variants cause disease? How does the gene interact with other genes and with environmental factors? How does the genotype predict the clinical course? And how can we use this information in effectively managing and treating POAG in a particular patient? Before any successful application to clinical practice can be made, these issues need to be resolved.

There is growing support for the role of gene–gene interactions in the pathogenesis of POAG. In a Japanese study of 194 patients with POAG, 217 patients with NTG, and 218 control subjects, Funayama and colleagues showed a possible interaction between the OPTN and TNF-α genes: genetic variants in OPTN were significantly associated with POAG or NTG in individuals carrying particular risk variants in the TNF-α gene, but not in individuals without these TNF-α risk variants.[70] Other genes that have been suggested to interact with OPTN include OLFM2, APOE, and MYOC.[48,71] For MYOC, genetic interactions with APOE and CYP1B1 have been described.[43,58,71] Knowledge of genetic interactions may give insight into the complex pathophysiological mechanisms and into potential targets for glaucoma therapy.

Interactions between genes and environmental factors are also assumed to contribute to the onset and progression of POAG. These interactions have already been demonstrated in other late-onset, complex diseases. In age-related macular degeneration, for example, risk alleles of the CFH and LOC387715 genes have been shown to significantly interact with cigarette smoking.[72,73] For POAG, in which still little is known about environmental risk factors, such interactions have not yet been revealed. Elucidating these may be of significant importance from a public health perspective for developing blindness-prevention programs.

After a gene has been identified, its role in the etiology of POAG in the population needs to be established. Genetic epidemiology studies have shown mutations in the MYOC gene in 3–4% of sporadic POAG patients.[67,74] More than 50 MYOC mutations have been identified in different ethnic groups worldwide. Some (e.g. the Pro370Leu, Tyr437His, and Ile477Asn mutations) are particularly associated with severe, early-onset forms of POAG.[75,76] Others are likely to predict a milder clinical course with a later onset. An example is Gln368stop, which is the most common glaucoma-causing MYOC mutation across populations.[67,74,77] For many mutations, the correlating phenotype still needs to be fully assessed.

OPTN mutations were initially identified in 16.7% of families with predominantly low-tension glaucoma.[78] Subsequent studies in nonfamilial cases, however, have reported much lower rates, and OPTN mutations are now assumed to be rare causes of low-tension glaucoma.[66,79,80] Associations with high-tension glaucoma have also been suggested, although several studies have not supported this.[66,70,80–82] The prevalence and pathogenicity of genetic variants differ substantially between populations of different ethnicity.[66,70,81,83] Genotype–phenotype correlations for OPTN have not been widely studied yet, except for the Glu50Lys mutation, which has been associated with an earlier onset and a more progressive disease course.[79,84] Information on mutation prevalences and genotype–phenotype correlations of all POAG-related genes will be very valuable to create prognostic and diagnostic DNA tests which may assist clinicians in disease management.

WDR36 has been reported to be the third POAG gene, but convincing evidence for its causative role has not yet been produced by population-based studies. The four mutations that had initially been reported by Monemi and colleagues were not found to cause POAG in four independent cohorts.[68,69,85,86] One study of POAG families rather revealed WDR36 to act as a modifier gene, with gene variants contributing to disease severity.[68] Interestingly, several POAG families have been reported that are linked to this region but do not show any WDR36 alterations.[86–88] POAG in these families may be caused by WDR36 variants outside the exons (within the promoter or introns) or by another gene within this region.

CONCLUSION

The complex genetic etiology of POAG is a hard nut for genetic epidemiologists to crack. Although more than 25 chromosomal regions have been linked to the disease, only three genes have currently been identified. These genes contribute to POAG in <5% of the cases in the general population. Hence, genes that explain a more significant fraction remain to be identified.

Genetic linkage and association analyses are the two main methods to search for new genes. These methods may yield more success in the near future due to more accurate and standardized phenotyping together with more sophisticated and cheaper genotyping. Molecular and biological studies will subsequently be needed to resolve the pathophysiological mechanisms, and gene prevalence, and genotype–phenotype correlation studies to sensibly translate these findings into ophthalmic practice.

Summary

- It is clear that there is a genetic component to development of POAG.
- There is consensus that the majority of POAG is inherited as a complex disorder.
- Linkage and association studies have helped identify loci involved but there is inconsistency between study results and much remains to be elucidated.
- Further work requires large-scale collaborative work involving numerous scientific disciplines and may focus on quantitative traits.
- Unraveling the genetic component of POAG might clarify the pathophysiology of the disease and greatly assist in treatment and prevention of visual loss of many thousands of individuals.

ELECTRONIC DATABASE INFORMATION

Online Mendelian Inheritance in Man (OMIM). Available: http://www.ncbi.nlm.nih.gov/sites/entrez?db=omim, for MYOC [MIM 601652], OPTN [MIM 602432], WDR36 [MIM 609669], OPA1 [MIM 605290], CYP1B1 [MIM 601771], ACE [MIM 106180], NOS3 [MIM 163729], APOE [MIM 107741], CFH [MIM 134370], and LOC387715 [MIM 611313].

REFERENCES

1. von Graefe A. Beitrage zur Pathologie, und Therapie des Glaukoms. Arch Ophthalmologie 1869; 15:108–252.

2. Wolfs RC, Klaver CC, Ramrattan RS, et al. Genetic risk of primary open-angle glaucoma. Population-based familial aggregation study. Arch Ophthalmol 1998; 116:1640–1645.

3. Tielsch JM, Sommer A, Katz J, et al. Racial variations in the prevalence of primary open-angle glaucoma. The Baltimore Eye Survey. JAMA 1991; 266:369–374.

4. Mitchell P, Smith W, Attebo K, et al. Prevalence of open-angle glaucoma in Australia. The Blue Mountains Eye Study. Ophthalmology 1996; 103:1661–1669.

5. Leske MC, Connell AM, Schachat AP, et al. The Barbados Eye Study. Prevalence of open angle glaucoma. Arch Ophthalmol 1994; 112:821–829.

6. Foster PJ, Oen FT, Machin D, et al. The prevalence of glaucoma in Chinese residents of Singapore: a cross-sectional population survey of the Tanjong Pagar district. Arch Ophthalmol 2000; 118:1105–1111.

7. Foster PJ, Baasanhu J, Alsbirk PH, et al. Glaucoma in Mongolia. A population-based survey in Hövsgöl province, northern Mongolia. Arch Ophthalmol 1996; 114:1235–1241.

8. Rudnicka AR, Mt-Isa S, Owen CG, et al. Variations in primary open-angle glaucoma prevalence by age, gender, and race: a Bayesian meta-analysis. Invest Ophthalmol Vis Sci 2006; 47:4254–4261.

9. Gottfredsdottir MS, Sverrisson T, Musch DC, et al. Chronic open-angle glaucoma, and associated ophthalmic findings in monozygotic twins, and their spouses in Iceland. J Glaucoma 1998; 8:134–139.

10. Hougaard JL, Kessel L, Sander B, et al. Evaluation of heredity as a determinant of retinal nerve fiber layer thickness as measured by optical coherence tomography. Invest Ophthalmol Vis Sci 2003; 44:3011–3016.

11. van Koolwijk LM, Despriet DD, van Duijn , et al. Genetic contributions to glaucoma, heritability of intraocular pressure, retinal nerve fiber layer thickness, and optic disc morphology. Invest Ophthalmol Vis Sci 2007; 48: 3669–3676.

12. Chang TC, Congdon NG, Wojciechowski R, et al. Determinants and heritability of intraocular pressure and cup-to-disc ratio in a defined older population. Ophthalmology 2005; 112:1186–1191.

13. Klein BE, Klein R, Lee KE. Heritability of risk factors for primary open-angle glaucoma: the Beaver Dam Eye Study. Invest Ophthalmol Vis Sci 2004; 45:59–62.

14. Levene RZ, Workman PL, Broder SW, et al. Heritability of ocular pressure in normal and suspect ranges. Arch Ophthalmol 1970; 84:730–734.

15. Schwartz JT, Reuling FH, Feinleib M. Size of the physiologic cup of the optic nerve head: Hereditary and environmental factors. Arch Ophthalmol 1975; 93:776–778.

16. Toh T, Liew SH, MacKinnon JR, et al. Central corneal thickness is highly heritable, the twin eye studies. Invest Ophthalmol Vis Sci 2005; 46:3718–3722.

17. Viswanathan AC, Hitchings RA, Indar A, et al. Commingling analysis of intraocular pressure and glaucoma in an older Australian population. Ann Hum Genet 2004; 68:489–497.

18. Lander E, Kruglyak L. Genetic dissection of complex traits: guidelines for interpreting and reporting linkage results. Nat Genet 1995; 11:241–247.

19. Wiggs JL, Allingham RR, Hossain A, et al. Genome-wide scan for adult onset primary open angle glaucoma. Hum Mol Genet 2000; 9:1109–1117.

20. Nemesure B, Jiao X, He Q, et al. A genome-wide scan for primary open-angle glaucoma (POAG): the Barbados Family Study of Open-Angle Glaucoma. Hum Genet 2003; 112:600–609.

21. Baird PN, Foote SJ, Mackey DA, et al. Evidence for a novel glaucoma locus at chromosome 3p21-22. Hum Genet 2005; 117:249–257.

22. Haseman JK, Elston RC. The investigation of linkage between a quantitative trait and a marker locus. Behav Genet 1972; 2:3–19.

23. Duggal P, Klein AP, Lee KE, et al. A genetic contribution to intraocular pressure: the Beaver Dam Eye Study. Invest Ophthalmol Vis Sci 2005; 46:555–560.

24. Duggal P, Klein AP, Lee KE, et al. Identification of novel genetic loci for intraocular pressure: a genomewide scan of the Beaver Dam Eye Study. Arch Ophthalmol 2007; 125:74–79.

25. Stoilova D, Child A, Trifan OC, et al. Localization of a locus (GLC1B) for adult-onset primary open angle glaucoma to the 2cen-q13 region. Genomics 1996; 36:142–150.

26. Charlesworth JC, Stankovich JM, Mackey DA, et al. Confirmation of the adult-onset primary open angle glaucoma locus GLC1B at 2cen-q13 in an Australian family. Ophthalmologica 2006; 220:23–30.

27. Charlesworth JC, Dyer TD, Stankovich JM, et al. Linkage to 10q22 for maximum intraocular pressure and 1p32 for maximum cup-to-disc ratio in an extended primary open-angle glaucoma pedigree. Invest Ophthalmol Vis Sci 2005; 46:3723–3729.

28. Kohlhaas M, Boehm AG, Spoerl E, et al. Effect of central corneal thickness, corneal curvature, and axial length on applanation tonometry. Arch Ophthalmol 2006; 124:471–476.

29. Gordon MO, Beiser JA, Brandt JD, et al. The Ocular Hypertension Treatment Study: baseline factors that predict the onset of primary open-angle glaucoma. Arch Ophthalmol 2002; 120:714–720; discussion 829–830,.

30. Edwards AO, Ritter R III, Abel KJ, et al. Complement factor H polymorphism and age-related macular degeneration. Science 2005; 308:421–424.

31. Haines JL, Hauser MA, Schmidt S, et al. Complement factor H variant increases the risk of age-related macular degeneration. Science 2005; 308:419–421.

32. Jakobsdottir J, Conley YP, Weeks DE, et al. Susceptibility genes for age-related maculopathy on chromosome 10q26. Am J Hum Genet 2005; 77:389–407.

33. Rivera A, Fisher SA, Fritsche LG, et al. Hypothetical LOC387715 is a second major susceptibility gene for age-related macular degeneration, contributing independently of complement factor H to disease risk. Hum Mol Genet 2005; 14:3227–3236.

34. Ishikawa K, Funayama T, Ohtake Y, et al. Association between glaucoma and gene polymorphism of endothelin type A receptor. Mol Vis 2005; 11:431–437.

35. Logan JF, Chakravarthy U, Hughes AE, et al. Evidence for association of endothelial nitric oxide synthase gene in subjects with glaucoma and a history of migraine. Invest Ophthalmol Vis Sci 2005; 46:3221–3226.

36. Motallebipour M, Rada-Iglesias A, Jansson M, et al. The promoter of inducible nitric oxide synthase implicated in glaucoma based on genetic analysis and nuclear factor binding. Mol Vis 2005; 11:950–957.

37. Bunce C, Hitchings RA, van Duijn CM, et al. Associations between the deletion polymorphism of the angiotensin 1-converting enzyme gene and ocular signs of primary open-angle glaucoma. Graefe's Arch Clin Exp Ophthalmol 2005; 243:294–299.

38. Hashizume K, Mashima Y, Fumayama T, et al. Genetic polymorphisms in the angiotensin II receptor gene and their association with open-angle glaucoma in a Japanese population. Invest Ophthalmol Vis Sci 2005; 46:1993–2001.

39. Dimasi DP, Hewitt AW, Green CM, et al. Lack of association of p53 polymorphisms and haplotypes in high and normal tension open angle glaucoma. J Med Genet 2005; 42:e55.

40. Lin HJ, Chen WC, Tsai FJ, et al. Distributions of p53 codon 72 polymorphism in primary open angle glaucoma. Br J Ophthalmol 2002; 86:767–770.

41. Lin HJ, Tsai SC, Tsai FJ, et al. Association of interleukin 1 beta and receptor antagonist gene polymorphisms with primary open-angle glaucoma. Ophthalmologica 2003; 217:358–364.

42. Lin HJ, Tsai FJ, Chen WC, et al. Association of tumour necrosis factor alpha-308 gene polymorphism with primary open-angle glaucoma in Chinese. Eye 2003; 17:31–34.

43. Copin B, Brezin AP, Valtot F, et al. Apolipoprotein E-promoter single-nucleotide polymorphisms affect the phenotype of primary open-angle glaucoma and demonstrate interaction with the myocilin gene. Am J Hum Genet 2002; 70:1575–1581.

44. Lam CY, Fan BJ, Wang DY, et al. Association of apolipoprotein E polymorphisms with normal tension glaucoma in a Chinese population. J Glaucoma 2006; 15:218–222.

45. Mabuchi F, Tang S, Ando D, et al. The apolipoprotein E gene polymorphism is associated with open angle glaucoma in the Japanese population. Mol Vis 2005; 11:609–612.

46. Vickers JC, Craig JE, Stankovich J, et al. The apolipoprotein epsilon4 gene is associated with elevated risk of normal tension glaucoma. Mol Vis 2002; 8:389–393.

47. Mukhopadhyay A, Talukdar S, Bhattacharjee A, et al. Bioinformatic approaches for identification and characterization of olfactomedin related genes with a potential role in pathogenesis of ocular disorders. Mol Vis 2004; 10:304–314.

48. Funayama T, Mashima Y, Ohtake Y, et al. SNPs and interaction analyses of noelin 2, myocilin, and optineurin genes in Japanese patients with open-angle glaucoma. Invest Ophthalmol Vis Sci 2006; 47:5368–5375.

49. Delettre C, Lenaers G, Griffoin JM, et al. Nuclear gene OPA1, encoding a mitochondrial dynamin-related protein, is mutated in dominant optic atrophy. Nat Genet 2000; 26:207–210.

50. Alexander C, Votruba M, Pesch UE, et al. OPA1, encoding a dynamin-related GTPase, is mutated in autosomal dominant optic atrophy linked to chromosome 3q28. Nat Genet 2000; 26:211–215.

51. Aung T, Ocaka L, Ebenezer ND, et al. A major marker for normal tension glaucoma: association with polymorphisms in the OPA1 gene. Hum Genet 2002; 110:52–56.

52. Aung T, Ocaka L, Ebenezer ND, et al. Investigating the association between OPA1 polymorphisms and glaucoma: comparison between normal tension and high tension primary open angle glaucoma. Hum Genet 2002; 110:513–514.

53. Powell BL, Toomes C, Scott S, et al. Polymorphisms in OPA1 are associated with normal tension glaucoma. Mol Vis 2003; 9:460–464.

54. Mabuchi F, Tang S, Kashiwagi K, et al. The OPA1 gene polymorphism is associated with normal tension and high tension glaucoma. Am J Ophthalmol 2007; 143:125–130.

55. Woo SJ, Kim DM, Kim JY, et al. Investigation of the association between OPA1 polymorphisms and normal-tension glaucoma in Korea. J Glaucoma 2004; 13:492–495.

56. Yao W, Jiao X, Hejtmancik JF, et al. Evaluation of the association between OPA1 polymorphisms and primary open-angle glaucoma in Barbados families. Mol Vis 2006; 12:649–654.

57. Melki R, Colomb E, Lefort N, et al. CYP1B1 mutations in French patients with early-onset primary open-angle glaucoma. J Med Genet 2004; 41:651–674.

58. Vincent AL, Billingsley G, Buys Y, et al. Digenic inheritance of early-onset glaucoma: CYP1B1, a potential modifier gene. Am J Hum Genet 2002; 70:448–460.

59. Wirtz MK, Samples JR, Rust K, et al. GLC1F, a new primary open-angle glaucoma locus, maps to 7q35-q36. Arch Ophthalmol 1999; 117:237–241.

60. Klein RJ, Zeiss C, Chew EY, et al. Complement factor H polymorphism in age-related macular degeneration. Science 2005; 308:385–389.

61. Spielman RS, McGinnis RE, Ewens WJ. Transmission test for linkage disequilibrium: the insulin gene region and insulin-dependent diabetes mellitus (IDDM). Am J Hum Genet 1993; 52:506–516.

62. Pritchard JK, Rosenberg NA. Use of unlinked genetic markers to detect population stratification in association studies. Am J Hum Genet 1993; 65:220–228.

63. Stone EM, Fingert JH, Alward WL, et al. Identification of a gene that causes primary open angle glaucoma. Science 1997; 275:668–670.

64. Rezaie T, Child A, Hitchings R, et al. Adult-onset primary open-angle glaucoma caused by mutations in optineurin. Science 2007; 295:1077–1079.

65. Monemi S, Spaeth G, DaSilva A, et al. Identification of a novel adult-onset primary open-angle glaucoma (POAG) gene on 5q22. 1. Hum Mol Genet 2005; 14:725–733.

66. Alward WL, Kwon YH, Kawase K, et al. Evaluation of optineurin sequence variations in 1,048 patients with open-angle glaucoma. Am J Ophthalmol 2003; 136:904–910.

67. Fingert JH, Heon E, Liebmann JM, et al. Analysis of myocilin mutations in 1703 glaucoma patients from five different populations. Hum Mol Genet 1999; 8:899–905.

68. Hauser MA, Allingham RR, Linkroum K, et al. Distribution of WDR36 DNA sequence variants in patients with primary open-angle glaucoma. Invest Ophthalmol Vis Sci 2006; 47:2542–2546.

69. Hewitt AW, Dimasi DP, Mackey DA, et al. A glaucoma case-control study of the WDR36 gene D658G sequence variant. Am J Ophthalmol 2006; 142:324–3245.

70. Funayama T, Ishikawa K, Ohtake Y, et al. Variants in optineurin gene and their association with tumor necrosis factor-alpha polymorphisms in Japanese patients with glaucoma. Invest Ophthalmol Vis Sci 2004; 45:4359–4367.

71. Fan BJ, Wang DY, Fan DS, et al. SNPs and interaction analyses of myocilin, optineurin, and apolipoprotein E in primary open angle glaucoma patients. Mol Vis 2005; 11:625–631.

72. Despriet DD, Klaver CC, Witteman JC, et al. Complement factor H polymorphism, complement activators, and risk of age-related macular degeneration. JAMA 2006; 296:301–309.

73. Schmidt S, Hauser MA, Scott WK, et al. Cigarette smoking strongly modifies the association of LOC387715 and age-related macular degeneration. Am J Hum Genet 2006; 78:852–864.

74. Alward WL, Kwon YH, Khanna CL, et al. Variations in the myocilin gene in patients with open-angle glaucoma. Arch Ophthalmol 2002; 120:1189–1197.

75. Alward L, Fingert JH, Coote MA, et al. Clinical features associated with mutations in the chromosome 1 open-angle glaucoma gene (GLC1A). N Engl J Med 1998; 338:1022–1027.

76. Shimizu S, Lichter PR, Johnson AT, et al. Age-dependent prevalence of mutations at the GLC1A locus in primary open-angle glaucoma. Am J Ophthalmol 2000; 130:165–177.

77. Angius A, Spinelli P, Ghilotti G, et al. Myocilin Gln368stop mutation and advanced age as risk factors for late-onset primary open-angle glaucoma. Arch Ophthalmol 2000; 118:674–679.

78. Rezaie T, Child A, Hitchings R, et al. Adult-onset primary open-angle glaucoma caused by mutations in optineurin. Science 2000; 295:1077–1079.

79. Hauser MA, Sena DF, Flor J, et al. Distribution of optineurin sequence variations in an ethnically diverse population of low-tension glaucoma patients from the United States. J Glaucoma 2006; 15:358–363.

80. Aung T, Ebenezer ND, Brice G, et al. Prevalence of optineurin sequence variants in adult primary open angle glaucoma: implications for diagnostic testing. J Med Genet 2003; 40:e101.

81. Leung YF, Fan BJ, Lam DS, et al. Different optineurin mutation pattern in primary open-angle glaucoma. Invest Ophthalmol Vis Sci 2003; 44:3880–3884.

82. Wiggs JL, Auguste J, Allingham RR, et al. Lack of association of mutations in optineurin with disease in patients with adult-onset primary open-angle glaucoma. Arch Ophthalmol 2007; 121:1181–1183.

83. Ayala-Lugo RM, Pawar H, Reed DM, et al. Variation in optineurin (OPTN) allele frequencies between and within populations. Mol Vis 2007; 13:151–163.

84. Aung T, Rezaie T, Okada K, et al. Clinical features and course of patients with glaucoma with the E50K mutation in the optineurin gene. Invest Ophthalmol Vis Sci 2005; 46:2816–2822.

85. Fingert JH, Alward WL, Kwon YH, et al. No association between variations in the WDR36 gene and primary open-angle glaucoma. Arch Ophthalmol 2007; 125:434–436.

86. Monemi S, Spaeth G, DaSilva A, et al. Identification of a novel adult-onset primary open-angle glaucoma (POAG) gene on 5q22.1. Hum Mol Genet 2005; 14:725–733.

87. Kramer PL, Samples JR, Monemi S, et al. The role of the WDR36 gene on chromosome 5q22.1 in a large family with primary open-angle glaucoma mapped to this region. Arch Ophthalmol 2006; 124:1328–1331.

88. Pang CP, Fan BJ, Canlas O, et al. A genome-wide scan maps a novel juvenile-onset primary open angle glaucoma locus to chromosome 5q. Mol Vis 2006; 12:85–92.

89. Sheffield VC, Stone EM, Alward WL, et al. Genetic linkage of familial open angle glaucoma to chromosome 1q21-q31. Nat Genet 1993; 4:47–50.

90. Stone EM, Fingert JH, Alward WL, et al. Identification of a gene that causes primary open angle glaucoma. Science 1997; 275:670–699.

91. Suriyapperuma SP, Child A, Desai T, et al. A new locus (GLC1H) for adult-onset primary open-angle glaucoma maps to the 2p15-p16 region. Arch Ophthalmol 2007; 125:86–92.

92. Stoilova D, Child A, Trifan OC, et al. Localization of a locus (GLC1B) for adult-onset primary open angle glaucoma to the 2cen-q13 region. Genomics 1996; 36:142–150.

93. Charlesworth JC, Stankovich JM, Mackey DA, et al. Confirmation of the adult-onset primary open angle glaucoma locus GLC1B at 2cen-q13 in an Australian family. Ophthalmologica 2006; 220:23–30.

94. Wirtz MK, Samples JR, Kramer PL, et al. Mapping a gene for adult-onset primary open-angle glaucoma to chromosome 3q. Am J Hum Genet 1997; 60:296–304.

95. Kitsos G, Eiberg H, Economou-Petersen E, et al. Genetic linkage of autosomal dominant primary open angle glaucoma to chromosome 3q in a Greek pedigree. Eur J Hum Genet 2001; 9:452–457.

96. Samples JR, Kitsos G, Economou-Petersen E, et al. Refining the primary open-angle glaucoma GLC1C region on chromosome 3 by haplotype analysis. Clin Genet 2004; 65:40–44.

97. Samples JR, Sykes R, Man J, et al. GLC1G: mapping a new POAG locus on chromosome 5. ARVO Annual Meeting 2004.

98. Monemi S, Spaeth G, DaSilva A, et al. Identification of a novel adult-onset primary open-angle glaucoma (POAG) gene on 5q22.1. Hum Mol Genet 2005; 14:725–733.

99. Fan BJ, Ko WC, Wang DY, et al. Fine mapping of new glaucoma locus GLC1M and exclusion of neuregulin 2 as the causative gene. Mol Vis 2007; 13:779–784.

100. Rotimi CN, Chen G, Adeyemo AA, et al. Genomewide scan and fine mapping of quantitative trait loci for intraocular pressure on 5q and 14q in West Africans. Invest Ophthalmol Vis Sci 2006; 47:3262–3267.

101. Wirtz MK, Samples JR, Rust K, et al. GLC1F, a new primary open-angle glaucoma locus, maps to 7q35-q36. Arch Ophthalmol 1999; 117:237–241.

102. Trifan OC, Traboulsi EI, Stoilova D, et al. A third locus (GLC1D) for adult-onset primary open-angle glaucoma maps to the 8q23 region. Am J Ophthalmol 1998; 126:17–28.

103. Wiggs JL, Lynch S, Ynagi G, et al. A genomewide scan identifies novel early-onset primary open-angle glaucoma loci on 9q22 and 20p12. Am J Hum Genet 2004; 74:1314–1320.

104. Sarfarazi M, Child A, Stoilova D, et al. Localization of the fourth locus (GLC1E) for adult-onset primary open-angle glaucoma to the 10p15-p14 region. Am J Hum Genet 1998; 62:641–652.

105. Rezaie T, Child A, Hitchings R, et al. Adult-onset primary open-angle glaucoma caused by mutations in optineurin. Science 2002; 295:1077–1079.

106. Allingham RR, Wiggs JL, Hauser ER, et al. Early adult-onset POAG linked to 15q11-13 using ordered subset analysis. Invest Ophthalmol Vis Sci 2005; 46:2002–2005.

107. Woodroffe A, Krafchak CM, Fuse N, et al. Ordered subset analysis supports a glaucoma locus at GLC1I on chromosome 15 in families with earlier adult age at diagnosis. Exp Eye Res 2006; 82:1068–1074.

108. Wang DY, Fan BJ, Chua JK, et al. A genome-wide scan maps a novel juvenile-onset primary open-angle glaucoma locus to 15q. Invest Ophthalmol Vis Sci 2006; 47:5315–5321.

TYPES OF GLAUCOMA

CHAPTER 24

Definitions: What is Glaucoma Worldwide?

George L Spaeth

INTRODUCTION

To discuss the impact of glaucoma worldwide, it is first necessary to understand what is meant by glaucoma. Unfortunately, there is little agreement in this regard.[1–18] This chapter will suggest commonalties intended to improve the situation. At the heart of the matter is the desired outcome. Surely, elimination of unnecessary misery must be at the top of almost any list of desired outcomes. As long as definitions of 'glaucoma,' including definitions of the desired outcomes are muddled or, worse, conflicting, it is not likely that progress will be made towards desired goals as rapidly as possible.

Considerations of the worldwide impact of glaucoma, to be meaningful, must include the debilitating aspects of the disease on individuals and communities. For the individual, the loss of sight can be devastating, causing loss of independence, isolation, loss of ability to be self-supportive, decreased income, lack of respect, loss or at least realignment of friends and support, and in varying ways disability and diminished quality of life. Some individuals such as the Argentinean author, Burgos, and others as well, have commented that a decrease in visual function helped them to be better artists or better people. It has been argued that Beethoven's loss of hearing was instrumental in his artistic growth, and loss of hearing can be likened to loss of sight. However, in their own words, these and others have made it clear they would not have chosen to have lost those sensory abilities. Many surveys have found that loss of vision is among mankind's most feared misfortunes. Having said that, however, it is also important to recall that the fear of misfortune may be seriously debilitating in itself. This fear and the associated decrease in quality of life associated with it need to be included in considerations of the impact of disease such as glaucoma. Additionally, and rarely considered, are the actions initiated by that fear, both by patients and those who are interested in preventing blindness or stand to benefit from its existence. When one considers, for example, why there is so much enthusiasm for treating individuals who have neither manifestations of disability nor certainty of developing disability, it is essential to recall that many millions of dollars will flow to those selling and providing treatments. The impact of 'glaucoma,' then, on individuals is complex and far more broadly reaching than usually considered.

From a societal point of view, the effects of glaucoma relate, of course, to the obvious socioeconomic considerations. These are difficult to calculate, because it is not just the direct costs, but the indirect costs such as the impact on the family and all those other aspects mentioned earlier, including loss of independence. Additionally, and also important, however, is the entire issue of society's priorities. Is health at the top or at the bottom? Is it important for society to care for its disabled?

This discussion of 'definitions' is intended to be considered in the broadest context. Specifically, what does glaucoma really mean for individuals and communities in the most specific, as well as the broadest, sense?

Any consideration of the definition of glaucoma must consider two different aspects: first, terminology related to the entity; and second, significance of the entity.

TERMINOLOGY

One reason why 'glaucoma' remains such a serious problem for mankind is the ambiguity of the word 'glaucoma' itself. Meanings change slowly over time. Old meanings tend to hang on for many generations. It is not possible to mandate a change in thinking even in a single individual, much less a population. For most current physicians, then, glaucoma continues to be thought of as it has been for over 100 years, specifically as a 'disease of elevated pressure.' Diagnosis is still made on the basis of the level of intraocular pressure (IOP), and treatments are still changed on the basis of the level of IOP. This is true worldwide. The worldwide definition of glaucoma was very clearly understood to be a condition in which the IOP is greater than a certain level of IOP, often 21 mmHg or 24 mmHg (as 21 mmHg is the upper limit of two standard deviations of IOP above the mean, and 24 mmHg the standard deviation of what is often considered the mean IOP in normals. This value, however, itself varies depending upon populations and measurement methods).

In the nineteenth century, disease came to be defined in terms of deviation from a mean value, such as blood sugar, blood pressure, body temperature, or IOP. This method of defining disease was clearly reflected in the words used by physicians and patients alike. 'Normal' was equated with average and 'abnormal' equated with deviation from average, usually a deviation of greater than two standard deviations. This method of defining disease allowed for statistical and quantitative analysis and was a step ahead from previous thinking of health and disease, in which illness was considered present when the person was unable to function properly, or felt sick. Disease, prior to the nineteenth century, was based on individual characteristics, such as fatigue, pain, or other symptoms, or signs which were characteristic of a particular entity, such as yellowing of the skin or conjunctiva. The new way of considering health and disease led to population surveys in Europe and America of many biological markers. Specifically, mean intraocular pressure was considered to be around 15 mmHg; consequently, this level was considered 'normal.' Because of the clear correlation between increasing level of IOP and increasing likelihood of the presence of a visual field loss that was characteristic of 'glaucoma,' it was concluded that glaucoma was caused solely by elevated IOP.[2,3,6] Massive surveys of around 10 000 or more persons were performed by Brau and Kirber[19] in the United States and Leydhecker et al.[6] in Germany, and concluding that an IOP of 28 mmHg was abnormal. Unfortunately, ophthalmologists, like everybody else, wanted a single figure they could call 'normal' and a cutoff point above which they were sure they were dealing with something that was abnormal. For a variety of reasons, these figures became 15 mmHg for normal and above 21 mmHg for abnormal. Definitions in a variety of sources such as medical texts and dictionaries all refer to glaucoma as a disease of elevated pressure, the manifestations of which were solely a consequence of the elevated pressure. The definition of glaucoma, as a result, was clear. Glaucoma was a condition in which the intraocular pressure was above 21 mmHg. The manifestations of this elevated pressure included varying levels of pain, varying amounts of inflammation of the eye, including corneal edema, dilation of the pupil in some individuals, or pacifications on the anterior surface of the lens in some individuals, 'cupping' of the optic nerve in most people, and visual loss in a variety of forms, related to the corneal edema or the loss of nerve fibers associated with cupping of the optic nerve.

As early as the early twentieth century, some questioned the closeness of the association between IOP and glaucoma, noting that in some individuals glaucomatous-like changes, especially in the optic nerve and visual fields, occurred in the absence of elevated pressure, whereas in others intraocular pressure was significantly and persistently elevated without causing optic nerve changes or visual field loss.[20] Around the turn of the twentieth century, studies done in a variety of centers should have definitively and permanently made ophthalmologists question the simple relationship that was believed to exist between the level of pressure and the development of the manifestations of glaucoma. The study led by Armaly at the University of Iowa, with the collaboration of the centers in St. Louis, Boston, and San Francisco, established the fact that individuals with elevated intraocular pressure, without apparent damage to the optic nerve or visual field, were not all likely to develop such manifestations of glaucoma within the 5 years that they were followed without treatment.[21] Indeed only about 5% of the subjects 'converted' from 'ocular hypertension' to 'glaucoma.' Other studies in Britain, Japan, and Scandinavia came up with similar findings,[22–24] and more recently so the United States.[25] In the study by Hollows and Graham of those over the age of 40 in Ferndale, Wales, individuals had their optic nerves and visual fields examined, as well as their intraocular pressures determined.[26] It was noted that around one-third of those who had the manifestations considered typical of glaucoma had intraocular pressures within the so-called 'normal range.' These studies demonstrated conclusively that it was not possible to use intraocular pressure to rule *out* glaucoma, regardless of the level of pressure, and that it was also not possible to use IOP to rule *in* glaucoma unless it was at a level far greater than previously considered to be required for the definition to be applied. The exact level required has still not been established, but certainly was not 21 mmHg. Perhaps it was 30, or perhaps 40, or perhaps even 50 mmHg.

When it became apparent that IOP was no longer the sole characteristic to be used to define the presence or absence of glaucoma, other definitive attributes were sought. These included a variety of provocative tests (water drinking, cycloplegia, fluorescein angiography, and response to various medications including corticosteroids[27–32]), the ease of outflow of aqueous humor (the so-called coefficient of aqueous outflow), the presence of a typical visual field defect,[33] or the observation of characteristic changes in the optic nerve and retina.[20,35–51] The winner was often the presence of a typical visual field defect. Indeed, many continue to believe that one cannot state that glaucoma is definitely present without the demonstration of a definitive visual field defect. Others challenge this, pointing out that most individuals' changes in the optic nerve precede changes in the visual field.[36,38] Were it not proper to say that a person had heart disease if it could be demonstrated that the electrocardiogram was unquestionably abnormal and the coronary arteries largely occluded, even if the person had no symptoms of pain or shortness of breath? Or should such a person be said to have heart disease? After all, disease takes its meaning from the prefix 'dis-' meaning wrong or away from; and the root '-ease' whose meaning is known to all. Thus, a disease is a condition in which a person does not feel well. Can one actually have a disease without having some kind of symptoms? The answer to that would clearly appear to be 'yes.' That is, the predecessors of the symptoms of an illness may be present without the symptoms manifesting themselves, and in those situations it makes sense to consider the person sick or, as the word has come to be used, diseased.

What changes in the optic nerve or retina are sufficiently characteristic that the person can be said to have glaucoma? This question can be answered relatively easily in the advanced stages of the disease. However, in the early phases, it is usually impossible to distinguish between the healthy and the minimally damaged nerve. How then can one meaningfully be sure that glaucoma is present when the findings in glaucoma can also be seen in those without glaucoma, and vice versa? Nevertheless, one of the definitions most frequently used in current textbooks is that glaucoma is an optic neuropathy.[11] Some authors require the addition of the phrase 'at least partially related to IOP,' and some do not add that qualifying comment. This distinction has probably been helpful in considering a condition such as the glaucoma associated with closure of the anterior chamber angle. Here, a distinction has come to be made between the narrow anterior chamber angle (that is, the angle which is narrower than average), the closed or partially closed anterior chamber angle, in which there is an adhesion of the iris to the inner wall of the eye, a so-called peripheral anterior synechiae, and angle-closure glaucoma, in which there is damage to the optic nerve in association with a peripheral anterior synechiae. Is there a name for a person who develops closure of the anterior chamber acutely whose intraocular pressure rapidly rises to 80 mmHg? Such a person would seem to have some type of illness, as manifested by severe pain, sudden loss of vision and, frequently, nausea and vomiting. But such a person does not have an optic neuropathy, and therefore current usage would suggest that the person should not be said to have angle-closure glaucoma. Merely saying that such a person has 'angle closure,' however, does not seem to describe adequately the situation.

The solution to the problem of how to define glaucoma may lie in considering glaucoma as a process in which ocular tissues become damaged in characteristic ways. The damage tends to be progressive and is always at least partially related to intraocular pressure. This definition would indicate that it is not the presence of any particular single finding, such as an IOP of 25 or even 30 mmHg, which allows attribution of the word 'glaucoma,' unless in the range where IOP is always abnormal. Furthermore, it would stress the progressive, evolutionary nature of the condition, indicating that nobody started with the manifestations of glaucoma and that they develop gradually or rapidly depending upon the particular individual. The author also suggests that it is not merely damage to the tissues which allows the diagnosis of glaucoma, but characteristic damage, such as a notch of the optic nerve head.

This subject deals with the definition of glaucoma worldwide. What is clear today is that there is no consensus in this regard. Within one city, different ophthalmologists will define glaucoma differently. The consequence of this is a confusion of epidemiological data, confusion regarding indications for treatment, confusion regarding desired outcomes, and confusion regarding the success or failure of various treatments. As the understanding of the glaucomatous process has increased over the years, new findings have been described. Those findings, such as IOP over 21 mmHg, were traditionally used as the new definition. As long as that method of defining glaucoma continues to be used, the definition of glaucoma will continue to change, and confusions regarding glaucoma, what it is and what it signifies, will continue to exist. In contrast, were it possible to accept the definition of glaucoma as a process in which characteristic findings are seen, then as the new findings are described, they can help refine the definition, but will not change its fundamental nature.

In summary, glaucoma is a process in which ocular tissues become damaged in characteristic ways; the damage is progressive at variable rates, and is always at least partially related to intraocular pressure; appropriate treatments are often effective. It is recognized that there is no consensus regarding the definition just given, and, more disturbingly, there is no consensus regarding any definition. For many, probably most, ophthalmologists in the world today, glaucoma means 'elevated intraocular pressure.' It is unlikely that this unfortunate situation will change until it is recognized that any particular attribute of glaucoma, such as pressure, coefficient of aqueous outflow, or damage to the optic nerve, is inadequate and will not be inclusive. Until we move away from defining glaucoma in terms of a single finding, it is unlikely that there will ever be a consensus.

A much more important consideration of the definition of glaucoma, however, relates to the significance of the entity. Physicians define glaucoma from the physicians' point of view. More pertinently, however, glaucoma needs to be defined from the patients' point of view – that is, from those who are afflicted by the condition – because the significance of glaucoma is that it can cause affliction and disability.[52,53] Figure 24.1 is a graphic depiction of this situation. What this graph demonstrates is that glaucoma is a condition which

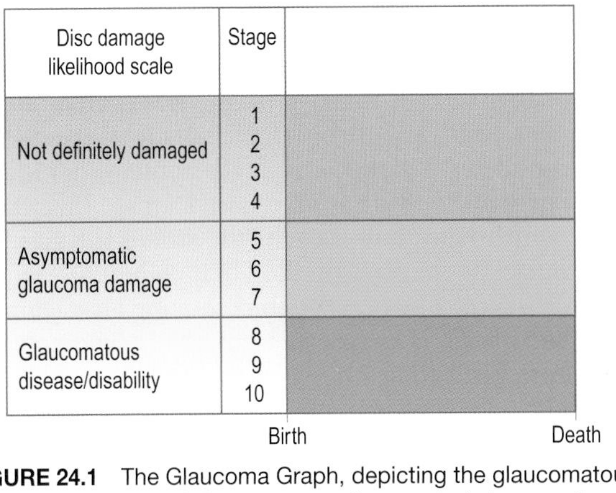

Disc damage likelihood scale	Stage	
Not definitely damaged	1 2 3 4	
Asymptomatic glaucoma damage	5 6 7	
Glaucomatous disease/disability	8 9 10	

Birth   Death

FIGURE 24.1 The Glaucoma Graph, depicting the glaucomatous process. On the y-axis is a measure of amount of glaucomatous damage from no damage to end stage. On the x-axis is the duration that the glaucomatous process will continue. In most cases, though not all, this is more simply thought of as life expectancy.

| DDLS stage | Narrowest width of rim (rim/disc ratio) | | | DDLS stage | Examples | | |
	For small disc <1.50 mm	For average size disc 1.50–2.00 mm	For large disc >2.00 mm		1.25 mm optic nerve	1.75 mm optic nerve	2.25 mm optic nerve
1	0.5 or more	0.4 or more	0.3 or more	0a			
2	0.4 to 0.49	0.3 to 0.39	0.2 to 0.29	0b			
3	0.3 to 0.39	0.2 to 0.29	0.1 to 0.19	1			
4	0.2 to 0.29	0.1 to 0.19	less than 0.1	2			
5	0.1 to 0.19	less than 0.1	0 for less than 45°	3			
6	less than 0.1	0 for less than 45°	0 for 46° to 90°	4			
7	0 for less than 45°	0 for 46° to 90°	0 for 91° to 180°	5			
8	0 for 46° to 90°	0 for 91° to 180°	0 for 181° to 270°	6			
9	0 for 91° to 180°	0 for 181° to 270°	0 for more than 270°	7a			
10	0 for more than 180°	0 for more than 270°		7b			

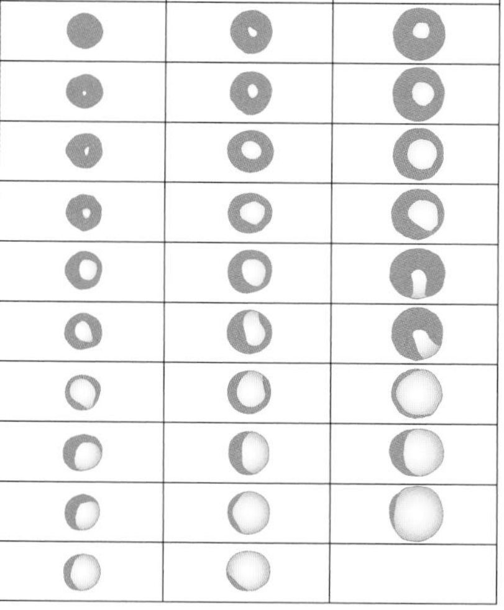

FIGURE 24.2 The Disc Damage Likelihood Scale (DDLS) can serve as the measure of glaucomatous nerve damage in the Glaucoma Graph (Fig. 24.1). The amount of nerve damage is based on the width of the optic disc at its narrowest point, or the circumferential extent of rim absence, corrected for the size of the optic disc. This is shown in this figure in terms of actual measurements in the columns for a small disc, an average-sized disc, and a large disc. The first column represents the stage of the DDLS, and the fifth column is the indication of the initial nomenclature in this regard. This is no longer appropriate, being replaced by the scale given in column one. The final three columns are graphic examples of the various 10 stages, indicating how the size of the disc affects the staging. For example, a cup:disc ratio of 0.6 in an average-sized disc depicted here with a cup that is slightly eccentric, so that the rim width is approximately 1.5 rim:disc ratios, would be graded a stage 4. A large disc with a similar appearance, that is a cup:disc ratio of around 0.6 in a slightly eccentric position, would be graded as a stage 3, whereas a similar appearance in a small disc would be graded as a stage 5. It is only necessary to know the characteristics of the 10 stages for an average-sized disc. For a disc which is larger than average, one subtracts one scale unit, and for a disc which is smaller than average, one adds one stage.

progresses, which progresses differently in different individuals, and which can, in some individuals, lead to disability. On the y-axis is an estimate of the amount of optic nerve damage. Ideally this would be in terms of number of retinal ganglion cells. Establishing this is not yet possible. The cup:disc ratio is not a suitable measure for the y-axis, because cup:disc ratio does not take into account disc size. A cup:disc ratio of 0.3 can be highly pathologic, and a cup:disc ratio of 0.8 can be entirely normal. Furthermore, cup:disc ratios do not take into account the position of the cup on the nerve. A concentric cup:disc ratio of 0.6 is more likely to be normal than abnormal, whereas an eccentric cup:disc ratio of 0.6, so that there is no rim remaining, is certainly abnormal, and highly characteristic of the change in the optic nerve that occurs in glaucoma. What is suggested here for the y-axis is the Disc Damage Likelihood Scale, which takes into account the size of the disc, the narrowness of the rim, or the circumferential amount of rim absence. The nomogram describing Disc Damage Likelihood Scale is shown in Figure 24.2. The x-axis is time from birth to death, which needs to be considered for each individual patient. Life expectancy is not the same for all and varies hugely from person to person, and markedly from region to region. An accurate way of estimating this easily has been shown by Lee et al.[54] The graph of the glaucoma process, then, allows visualizing and conceptualizing the fact that when a person has minimal disc damage, a Disc Damage Likelihood

Scale of 1 to 4, it is not possible to say whether or not the process is actually present, unless the disc has been previously examined and a change has been noted.[55,56]

In the yellow zone, however, there is no question that the glaucomatous process is present. Here, the person has unquestionable manifestations of glaucoma. Nevertheless, such a person is still unaware of the presence of the glaucomatous process, because the damage is not sufficiently marked that it causes recognizable symptoms. Finally, when a person gets into the red zone, the symptomatic manifestations of glaucoma are apparent to the patient. At this point, the patient notices some type of disability. The challenge is to prevent patients from progressing into the red zone before they die or, if already in the red zone, to prevent them from becoming any worse. Ideally the goals are: (1) to prevent symptomatic damage only, avoiding any treatment that is unnecessary to prevent the development of such symptoms; and (2) to restore any damage already present.

Figure 24.1 stresses the significance of the definition of glaucoma by emphasizing that the real concern with glaucoma is the disability that it can produce, in some individuals.

The next section of this chapter will deal with this particular aspect of the definition of glaucoma: specifically, its significance for the individuals and the cultures in which it causes deterioration in the quality of life of those individuals and of those cultures.

THE SIGNIFICANCE OF GLAUCOMA WORLDWIDE

The current situation regarding the impact of glaucoma on planet earth's people can largely be told in two sentences. Two additional sentences make that impact more poignant, yet suggest solutions.

1. Many people fear blindness more than death.
2. Glaucoma is the single largest cause of irreversible blindness in the world.
3. Most blindness caused by glaucoma could be prevented using diagnostic tests and treatments currently available.
4. Preventing blindness from glaucoma would improve socioeconomic conditions in the world.

BLINDNESS CAUSED BY GLAUCOMA

One of the fundamental problems with both the diagnosis of glaucoma and establishing an effective treatment for patients with glaucoma most likely to preserve their vision lies in the diversity of ways the condition manifests itself and is considered. Acute primary open-angle glaucoma can cause excruciating symptoms and blindness within hours and demands an approach to treatment totally different from that appropriate for the chronic open-angle glaucomas, where the time required to progress from the earliest stages of the condition is always years, and frequently many, many years. Finally, a finding which is frequently a precursor to the damage associated with glaucoma, specifically intraocular pressure (IOP) higher than the 'normal range,' is relatively common but does not commonly lead to blindness. Strategies of detection and treatment for one type of glaucoma, then, are not appropriate for other types, yet the singularity of the word betrays the fact that a multipronged approach to the condition is essential.

A similar difficulty relates to the biological differences in people both in macro and micro terms. For example, in Hispanics, IOP tends to increase with age, as does the incidence of glaucoma (from around 1% in those 40 years of age to 24% in octogenarians); in contrast, in Japanese, IOP tends to fall with increasing age. West Indians of African extraction appear to have an open-angle type of glaucoma in which control of intraocular pressure is extraordinarily difficult and progression to blindness usual, whereas such a situation does not appear to be typical of Scandinavians developing open-angle glaucoma. Primary angle-closure glaucoma in those of European extraction appears to have a different basic mechanism and to respond differently to peripheral iridotomy than the condition with the same name that occurs in the Chinese. It is essential to recognize these basic biological differences before generalizing conclusions regarding diagnosis, management, or public health strategies. The solution to the problem, however, is not to conclude that appropriate diagnosis and management are impossible, but rather to recognize that diversity of biology demands a diversity of biologically appropriate approaches to both diagnosis and management.

Cultural differences, superimposed on biological diversity, make the understanding of the significance of glaucoma even more complex. Where good self-care is the norm, and excellent facilities available, few go blind from glaucoma, whereas when self-care is not developed and facilities unavailable, blindness in glaucoma is common.

UNNECESSARY VISUAL LOSS

One hundred years ago, an individual who developed tuberculosis was destined to have a difficult time, with a likelihood of dying from the disease. Tuberculosis had different levels of severity, and those affected had different levels of resistance. Some succumbed. Some recovered relatively rapidly. But for all the condition was serious. Today, tuberculosis is also a serious disease, but the availability of drugs which are usually effective in killing the organism responsible for tuberculosis means that the overwhelming majority of those with tuberculosis will not succumb to that disease. This example is given because the situation is very similar when one considers glaucoma. Glaucoma comes in even more forms than tuberculosis; 100 years ago some of those with glaucoma went blind rapidly, whereas others never developed a significant visual loss despite the absence of effective treatments. There are still some types of glaucoma which rapidly lead to blindness, and there are many in whom glaucoma is mild or treatment effective.

Unfortunately, the fact that in the past glaucoma often led to blindness is still used today to excuse the fact that glaucoma is the leading cause of irreversible blindness in the world. The adverbial phrase 'unfortunate' is used because it is also a fact that appropriate use of currently available knowledge and facilities would prevent visual loss from glaucoma in most people. Specifically, no one of European extraction need lose vision from primary angle-closure glaucoma; all that is necessary is to diagnose the patient as having a narrow angle with a readily available and safe test, gonioscopy, and then properly perform an Nd:YAG laser iridotomy. That comment is probably also true for those of African extraction or Middle Eastern extraction though iridotomy is not as easily accomplished and the post-laser care has to be more careful. For those of Asian extraction, prevention of angle-closure appears to be more difficult, and may require lens extraction. The lens extraction is remarkably safe but is not without occasional complications. Given what we know and what we can do today, the percentage of Europeans that lose vision from angle-closure glaucoma should be less than 0.1%, whereas in Asians it may be as high as 5%. With regard to the commonest type of glaucoma, primary open-angle glaucoma, two recent randomized, controlled clinical trials have shown that, with proper care, almost all with early or moderate glaucoma can be prevented from getting worse.[54,57] Patients with far-advanced glaucoma were not included in either of those studies, and prevention of continuing deterioration in such cases is difficult and sometimes impossible. A third randomized, controlled trial provides strong support for the idea that the type of treatment matters. Specifically, the Early Manifest of a Glaucoma Treatment Study used a treatment program that was beneficial for only about half of those in the study.[58]

The juxtaposition of previously mentioned points number 1 and 2 with point number 3 is a disturbing commentary on how individuals, the medical profession, health departments, governments, and society in general approach the entire issue of health and disease, specifically glaucoma. Points number 1 and 2 note that a particular condition, in this instance glaucoma, causes huge amounts of personal, family, national, and societal misery; and point number 3 indicates that such misery is almost totally preventable. How can it be that a condition which is almost totally preventable continues to wreak such havoc in the world?

WHO BENEFITS FROM REDUCING BLINDNESS FROM GLAUCOMA?

Let us consider who benefits from reducing blindness from glaucoma. Let us consider the major players: the medical profession, the pharmaceutical industry, third-party payers, local and state governments, agencies for the blind, universities, teaching hospitals, research groups, and, finally, individual patients. The primary goal of most physicians, singly and corporately, is to care for those who are sick. Thus, a physician may say to Mr X, 'You are seriously overweight and you must lose weight or else your blood pressure is going to continue to be too high and your diabetes poorly controlled.' Few physicians, however, consider themselves responsible for eliminating the causes of sickness, except as they affect individual patients under their care. The physician is not likely to say, 'We have a population of individuals who are overweight, and how do we as a profession solve that problem?' Indeed, additionally, there is a fundamental conflict of interest with regards to physicians and illness, for if no people were sick, there would be no need for physicians. It is not surprising, then, that the medical profession concentrates its effort on caring for individual patients, rather than considering that it has the responsibility to eliminate illnesses. If that were to happen, the medical profession would be out of work.

The pharmaceutical industry makes products that truly benefit people. Certain companies have for many years made it clear that their reason for existence is to improve the health of those of who are ill. There is no reason to doubt the sincerity of those companies that make products that dramatically improve the quality of life of millions of people in every country in the world. However, the primary interest of the pharmaceutical company is not to eliminate the causes of illness. Indeed, were there no illnesses, there would be no need for pharmaceutical companies. Of course, the pharmaceutical industry does not purposely make people ill, but why would it want to eliminate disease? Why would it want to find a cure for glaucoma, specifically? Treatments, yes, but a cure – why?

In many parts of the world healthcare has evolved in a way that individuals are no longer responsible for paying for the costs of their care. So-called 'third-party payers' have developed in order to try to smooth the huge peaks and valleys related to the costs of healthcare. Because, by and large, people are healthy, healthcare costs for most are relatively small. But a serious illness may result in hundreds of thousands of dollars of expense that few can afford. One of the major justifications for healthcare 'insurance' is the possibility of damping those enormous costs for a few people by spreading them across many people. There are other reasons as well. Specifically, many individuals do not 'save money for a rainy day.' There are large cultural differences in this regard, and the issue is not solely one of amount of income. For example, in the United States the average income is much higher than in the Eastern European countries, yet the percentage of money saved by individuals living in Eastern European countries is greatly higher than that of those living in the United States. But worldwide, there is a tendency for healthy people to believe they will continue to be healthy and therefore not to consider that saving for a time when they might be ill is prudent. Furthermore, why should one save for a possible illness when, should one become ill, the state will pay for it? For many, however, incomes are so low that there is simply no possibility to put money aside for a possible illness in the future, or to afford the costs attendant by such an illness should it occur.

Any 'fee for service' system is flawed because of the self-interest of the person who will receive the fee. Consequently, the idea of a neutral group to protect patients by spreading costs, and advocating for the patients to assure that they do not get overcharged or exploited made and still makes very good sense. However, what was forgotten was that those running the allegedly neutral groups also had self-interest. This has become painfully apparent with regards to current insurance companies, where the profit for the shareholders takes precedence over the care provided to the policy holders, social service agencies, research groups, teaching hospitals, etc. These comments regarding insurance companies apply equally to all other groups in which the existence of the group comes to take precedence over the reason why the group was established. Patients might benefit by the spin-off that occurs from research, or teaching, but no institution will willingly bankrupt itself in pursuit of assuring that patients are put first.

Fundamental to the idea of every type of 'patient care' is that the person being consulted will act in the best interests of the 'patient.' This applies to the witch doctor, the shaman, the iatromant, the chiropractor, the midwife, and to the physician. But the guilds that developed around all of those who have been consulted for the purpose of helping others be healthy had as their primary goal the protection of the healer, not the well-being of the patient. Codes of behavior in formal or informal form were developed to assure 'patients' that they would be treated in a way that protected their best interests. But shamans also protected shamans, and physicians protected physicians.

Nevertheless, all of these groups flourish because of the existence of disease. None of these groups sees as its primary focus the elimination of disease, because to do so would be to work towards putting itself out of existence.

The impact of glaucoma, then, needs to be considered in two totally different ways: first, the effect on the individual who has developed an illness which may cause loss of sight; and second, the many groups who benefit from the existence of the disease, glaucoma. Until this complex duality is appreciated and evaluated realistically, the likelihood of the misery caused by glaucoma decreasing or disappearing is small, because patients as individuals are powerless compared to the groups whose well-being depends on the existence of the disease affecting the patients.

THE EFFECTS OF VISUAL LOSS DUE TO GLAUCOMA

The impact of visual loss caused by glaucoma on an individual depends upon the severity of visual damage, the type of visual loss, the various support systems that are available to that person, both internal and external, and the cultures in which that person lives. The interplay of these various factors is complex. What follows are discussions regarding the significance of glaucoma in several different parts of the world.

THE SIGNIFICANCE OF GLAUCOMA BY GEOGRAPHIC AREA

BRAZIL

Brazil is a country of contrasts. Among the 180 million Brazilians, only 20% have access to insurance paid/private healthcare. The remaining 80% depend on the public health system for assistance. Unfortunately, early detection of glaucoma is not being accomplished by the public health system. In a study performed at the University of Campinas, 52% of the patients first examined at the Glaucoma Service were unilaterally blind and 33% bilaterally blind from glaucoma.[59] This situation is a consequence of several factors:

1. Access to the public hospital is difficult. The mean distance between the University of Campinas and the patients' homes is 122 km, and they constantly rely on ambulances and buses that come once a week to Campinas. That explains why 68% of patients do not return for follow-up after being diagnosed with glaucoma.[59]
2. The population is not well educated about glaucoma. In 1996, the author interviewed 100 patients followed at the Glaucoma Service of the University of Campinas; 30% did not know they had glaucoma, 53% did not know what glaucoma was, 35% did not

know that glaucoma may cause blindness, and 94% did not know why visual field examinations were performed. Interestingly, the same interview was done with 183 patients followed at the Glaucoma Service of the Wills Eye Hospital. The results were also disappointing: 44% did not have an acceptable idea about what glaucoma is, 30% did not know the purpose of the medications they were taking, and 45% did not understand why visual fields were examined.[60]
3. Patients cannot afford the cost of treatment. Twenty-one percent of patients followed at the Glaucoma Service of the University of Campinas do not follow the prescribed treatment, the main reason being the lack of money.[59] In fact, the mean cost of treatment of glaucoma patients is equivalent to 16% of their family income.[61] Even with the arrival of new antiglaucoma medications, the number of glaucoma surgeries is still high in public hospitals, due to economic reasons.

Despite these difficulties, patients followed in a public hospital are gentle, humble, and rarely complain, even if they have to wait for 2–3 hours to be seen by a resident. A wide variety of gifts are frequently given to doctors as a proof of appreciation for their care. Communication is difficult, and patients have trouble understanding the instructions given by doctors. Efforts are directed towards the improvement in patient education,[62] simultaneously encouraging them to care for themselves properly.

Private patients represent a totally different group, extremely educated about the disease, using the Internet to gain information about the latest advances in glaucoma treatment. In this group, the number of antiglaucoma surgeries has significantly decreased due to the new, more efficacious medications. Cost of treatment for them does not represent a limiting factor. On the other hand, private patients in Brazil are demanding. They demand attention and time from their doctors, not only to discuss their disease but also to talk about their lives, families, and careers. In Brazil, private patients expect at least 20–30 minutes with their ophthalmologists, and do not appreciate it if they are seen by assistants or fellows.

THE INDIAN SUBCONTINENT

The author has made the assumption that data from India are likely to be applicable to the entire region. The Indian subcontinent comprises seven countries and, as home to about 1.5 billion people, is the most populous region in the world. An increase in the population, especially those aged over 60 years (12.3% of India's population in 1991), has resulted in an increase in the number of potentially blinding conditions. Projection of the Andhra Pradesh Eye Disease Study (APEDS) data estimated the number of blind people in India in 2000 to be 18.7 million (95% CI, 15.2–22.3); this number was expected to increase to 31.6 million (95% CI, 26.4–36.9) by 2020. Glaucoma is estimated to affect over 12 million Indians and is responsible for an estimated 8–13% of the 1.8% prevalence of blindness. It is also important to note that in India, at least, the prevalence of primary angle-closure disease is almost as common as primary open-angle glaucoma. Angle-closure disease certainly causes more blindness than open-angle glaucoma.

Economic burden of blindness In 2000, India had a gross domestic product (GDP) per capita of US$457. About 260 million (34.7%) of the Indian population fell below the international poverty level (defined as lower than the US$1 per day). The total expenditure on health is 5% of the GDP; 13% of this comes from the public sector and 87% from the private sector. The economic burden of blindness in India for the year 1997 (cost-of-illness methodology) was calculated to be US$4.4 billion; the cumulative loss over the lifetime of the blind was estimated at US$77.4 billion. Glaucoma accounts for 8–13% of the blindness (8–13% of US$77 billion is about US$10 billion). The direct loss of gross national product due to blindness in India (1997) was US$4.0 billion. The indirect loss for both adults and children was calculated to be US$0.70 billion. The cumulative loss due to preventable or curable blindness, for the lifespan of the blind, was estimated at US$52.5 billion; that is 67.8% of the total cumulative loss due to blindness. The government of India (GOI) is committed to the prevention of blindness: in 1976, India became the first country in the world to start a national program for control of blindness (NPCB). However, it is only very recently that diseases other than cataract have been included in the project. In theory, the government is committed to providing free healthcare to all its citizens. In practice, however, resources are not sufficient. A minority of the population can afford any expenditure for their healthcare. The private sector is readily available to the rich and perhaps to a small extent to the urban poor; but more than three-fourths of those below the poverty line reside in the rural areas. Any meaningful intervention (both ophthalmic and otherwise) has to target the rural poor. Under the circumstances, it is obvious that a chronic and potentially blinding condition such as glaucoma can be devastating.

Culture of ophthalmologists India's diversity and contradictions prompted the late Pope John Paul's statement that: 'Anything you say about India can be absolutely right and absolutely wrong at the same time.' The statement is probably true of Indian ophthalmology as well. Having said that, the author will hazard an opinion on the culture of ophthalmologists and their patients.

There are an estimated 12 000 ophthalmologists, including about 25 glaucoma specialists, in the country, located mainly in the cities. They work in their own clinics, privately owned hospitals, or medical schools (private or government). The patient can present initially at any of these settings. Several government and private hospitals provide state-of-the-art ophthalmic care; they, too, are mainly located in the large cities. There is also a regional variation in the quality of care from state to state.

The majority of Indian ophthalmologists do not perform the comprehensive eye examination suggested by the American Academy of Ophthalmology. As IOP, disc examination, and gonioscopy are not routine, even established glaucoma is inadvertently missed. There are about 140 medical schools in the country, the majority of which train residents in ophthalmology. The quality of the programs varies tremendously. While there are some residency training programs of excellent quality, these are few and far between. A survey of all the residency programs in one representative state performed 6 years ago revealed that none performed or taught a comprehensive ophthalmic examination. Despite two subsequent initiatives that followed the survey and provided modern equipment (and training), a repeat survey conducted last year showed hardly any change in teaching or practice. Specifically, an IOP (even Schiotz) was not routine but obtained only when glaucoma was suspected. The basis for that 'suspicion' was unclear. The disc was not examined routinely but only if glaucoma was 'suspected' and/or Schiotz tension was high. Most programs did not have a gonioscope; if they did, they did not perform routine gonioscopy. Perimetry of any type was rare: Humphrey perimeters that were being provided as part of the initiatives referred to earlier were either sparsely used (a total of six fields performed in the last year) or not used at all. Surgical training in glaucoma was nonexistent. The practice in the average clinic reflects this training and it is no wonder then that glaucoma, if detected, is generally far advanced.

Most training programs neither teach nor practice a discussion of the disease and management plan with the patient. A fully informed consent for procedures is rare. It follows then that most Indian ophthalmologists have not been exposed to, and hence do not discuss, management options or risks and benefits in detail with the patient. Informed consent, if obtained, is usually just a signature on the dotted line for legal purposes. In both the major academic departments the author headed, he faced an uphill task of implementing a policy of full discussion of benefits and risks with the patients. Informal discussions with other colleagues confirm this admittedly biased impression based on the author's own training and practices in the institutes that he has worked in. The increased activity of consumer courts in the country is forcing the ophthalmic community towards at least a signature on informed consent forms. Discussion of the disease and management is, however, rare. Government hospital departments, including most training programs (whose standards do not necessarily equal private clinics), do not come under the purview of such courts.

Patient culture Most patients in India consider physicians to be (next to) God and will usually blindly follow the treatment given to them. This applies to surgery, too. A minority of educated patients might seek information from other sources or further information from caregivers about the disease or management decisions. It is the author's impression that, for whatever reason, most Indian patients do not want to be part of the decision-making process. They certainly do not seem to want to know anything about possible risks. They would rather leave it to the doctor to make a decision; but in India, too, cognitive dissonance is real enough to be a potential problem later. All in all, the patients are very accepting and attribute poor outcomes to fate.

The areas for improvement are obvious.

NORTH AFRICA AND SAUDI ARABIA

The impact of a personal culture and the community's culture on how glaucoma manifests itself in North Africa is huge. These cultures affect detection, management, and how the disease progresses. Lack of proper health education, inappropriate and deficient health insurance systems, absent screening programs, and poorly trained and nonspecialized physicians hinder detection and treatment. Glaucoma is the third leading cause of blindness (5.7%) in the developing world after cataract (45.2%) and trachoma (25.7%).[67–70] That percentage increases with increasing age group. Epidemiological studies about glaucoma prevalence and incidence are lacking. For reasons that are not fully understood, congenital glaucoma is an especially great problem in the Middle East.[71,72] Glaucoma is a relatively common disease in this area, and in those above 60 years old there is a prevalence of around 15% and it is responsible for the blindness in almost one out of four individuals! The large number of patients presenting for the first time with visual loss or disability due to absolute or end-stage glaucoma is a reflection of the effect of socioeconomic factors and the absence of health programs to combat such a disease. In one private practice, over 40% of patients with glaucoma who are seeking medical advice for the first time have end-stage to absolute glaucoma in one or both eyes. The significance of this visual loss on lifestyle, life expectancy, and economic productivity of those affected is great. Many patients with glaucoma are no longer able to drive or work after their fifth decade.

Regarding diagnosis and management of glaucoma in the public and private hospitals, and the public and private clinics, there is a scarcity of the medical equipment and supplies needed to facilitate diagnosis and follow-up. Investment in a glaucoma clinic is much less attractive compared to a cataract or refractive surgery clinic. Glaucoma is a disease of bad reputation to patients (the terror of blindness) and to physicians (no visual gain and a lot of surgical complications). Many general ophthalmologists avoid treating glaucoma patients in their private clinics. Because of the absence of a referral strategy, many patients remain on eye medications regardless of being controlled or not. Oversimplification is the rule for many ophthalmologists: if the pressure is high, give drops; if the IOP does not respond, do a trabeculectomy. Remember to close the scleral and conjunctival flaps tightly to avoid hypotony and anterior chamber complications. If the IOP rises postoperatively, put the patient back on drops. In this way, the ophthalmologist is less likely to have to deal with horrible vision-threatening complications, and the patient apparently does not lose much.

The culture in which the patients and the doctors live has a major impact on how glaucoma is diagnosed and treated and on the outcomes of the treatment. Patients have many false beliefs, are influenced by rumors, and use nonscientific means for diagnosis and treatment. People get their information from where they can, and much of it is wrong. Patients ask relatives, friends, and paramedical personnel and one hears from patients many false ideas about glaucoma, its course, its causes, and its management.

In Egypt, many doctors and patients are reluctant to say, 'I do not know.' Egyptian patients do not want to hear the doctor say, 'I do not know, but I will find out.' Doctors are expected to know, and admitting lack of knowledge is a sign the doctor is incompetent. But it is essential for doctors and patients to learn when to say, 'I do not know.' When one is aware of one's limitations, one is less likely to make mistakes, and admitting those limitations, both to oneself and to others, is important. When aware of one's lack of knowledge, one is stimulated to ask and to search, and this applies to matters of health and vision as well.

What is to be done to improve the situation? Shall we focus our goal on treatment of glaucoma with drops, lasers, and surgery? Or shall we direct our main efforts towards education of individuals and communities about the problem of glaucoma and its disability effects, or improve awareness and diagnostic capabilities of general practitioners, optometrists, and ophthalmologists? In fact, the three routes all need to be pursued simultaneously in order to guarantee the most successful outcome.

The Egyptian Ministry of Health, as well as ophthalmic and glaucoma societies, need to feel responsible for improving awareness of communities about glaucoma. Glaucoma needs to be included in the programs for health education about diseases such as diabetes, hypertension, atherosclerosis, and rheumatoid arthritis. Educating individuals about health, what programs are available, changing false beliefs about glaucoma, and increasing the knowledge of physicians is essential. Screening programs and charity campaigns are helpful in detecting disease in its early stages before visual disability has occurred. Measurements of intraocular pressure and appropriate fundus examination should be a part of the routine physical examination for both ophthalmologists and optometrists. Patients who are at greater risk should be referred to more specialized centers for full glaucoma investigation and periodic follow-up. However, it is essential to be able to care for those who are detected, and that is not the case at the present time. Educating and then developing methods to assure periodic checkups and compliance with treatment recommendations and follow-up plans is an essential step to combat the devastating effects of glaucoma on both the individual and the community.

In Saudi Arabia, ophthalmic care is largely centered around major medical institutions such as the King Khaled Eye Specialist Hospital in Riyadh and the huge number of private hospitals and institutions such as Magrabi Eye Group (about 10 eye centers providing primary eye care and referral practice in the Kingdom). In these centers, ophthalmic care is of high quality. The impact of glaucoma on the population, however, is still massive, as not everybody can obtain care, and follow-up continues to be difficult.

In Saudi Arabia, glaucoma was responsible for blindness among 3% of the population above the age of 40 years.[67] In a clinic-based study, the author reviewed the medical records of newly diagnosed glaucoma patients from January till December 2006 in the Glaucoma and Cataract Unit at Magrabi Eye Center in Jeddah. Five hundred and fifty-three patients were identified. No light perception was noticed in 46 (8.2%) right and 46 left eyes, whereas unilateral legal blindness was seen in 35.5% of cases and bilateral legal blindness in 9.6%. Approximately one-third of patients (35.5%) did not show up after first examination compared to 33.5% with regular visits and 30.7% with inconsistent follow-up.[73]

The better economic status of the society and individuals and widespread private insurance systems ensure better healthcare in the Kingdom, with higher investment in the medical field from both the government and private organizations. However, the person and community culture largely affects healthcare programs and keep patients in the urban areas away from proper health service. A large part of the population in these areas is not insured and is usually directed to public hospitals with the same problems related to physicians, patients, administrations, and facilities as in Egypt and other countries in the Middle East.

SUB-SAHARAN AFRICA

Glaucoma remains a devastating and often neglected problem in sub-Saharan Africa. Epidemiologic data is inadequate, but we assume that findings are close to that found in the Caribbean.[74,75] Many patients walk into an eye clinic and are blind from glaucoma in at least one eye at time of diagnosis. There are regional variations in the type of glaucoma, but most patients have open-angle glaucoma.[75,76] In this population, glaucoma has been seen to occur at an earlier age and typically advances more rapidly with advanced glaucomatous vision loss compared with people of the same age elsewhere.[76,77] The diagnosis is made in people in their early 30s to 40s, which make up the main workforce in these communities.

The cost of blindness is borne specifically by the family unit as a loss of income and by the community as a loss of manpower. This just adds to the vicious circle of poverty that already exists.

Loss of vision remains a social stigma. There is inadequate social and rehabilitative support for people that are visually impaired. The management of glaucoma in this region is difficult.[78] Treatment is largely by surgery and medication, but long-term medication use is not advocated due to limited availability of medicines and its cost. Ophthalmologists are few, about 1 per 1 million of the population, and patients have to contend with cost and distance of traveling for eye care.

Trabeculectomy is effective with antimetabolite use but has shortcomings. Patient acceptance of surgery is poor even when it is free as a result of cultural and social barriers.[78] The other issues that have posed a problem include inadequate knowledge of available services and trust in outcome of surgery since this not quantifiable using vision as is the case with cataract surgery.[79,80]

In spite of the high incidence and prevalence of glaucoma in this population, only a limited amount of glaucoma management takes place in Africa. Glaucoma screening programs are not adequate and currently no local or international programs have allocated large resources to management and publicity of glaucoma. The WHO, in its *Vision 2020: The Right to Sight* program, does not mention glaucoma as one of its priorities at this time.[81] The human tragedy of the situation remains a large concern to ophthalmologists who have to deal with this problem every day.

EUROPE

There are 51 countries and more than 800 million people in Europe, covering an area from Greenland to the Pacific coast of the Russian Federation. Substantial political, socioeconomic, and cultural differences are observed. Regarding healthcare, the Western countries have high standards but still have pockets of underprivileged populations. The fall of socialist regimes in central and Eastern Europe has greatly influenced healthcare provision and, overall, the quality of care among these countries is variable. The central European region is showing a more successful economic transition.

There is a large number of ophthalmologists per population, although not evenly distributed. In many countries physicians employed by state healthcare institutions are underpaid, which may decrease their motivation. Both state and private healthcare services are available, and patients commonly pay a certain percentage of the cost of glaucoma treatment.[82]

Glaucoma is an important health problem in Europe, affecting approximately 1–2% of the adult population. With an aging population, the number of people with glaucoma will rise.[83] In 2010 more than 12 million people will have glaucoma,[84] and 1 person in 10 will eventually develop glaucoma.[85] In Western countries glaucoma is the second leading cause of blindness, after age-related macular degeneration. In Eastern Europe cataract is the most common cause of visual impairment.[82] The cost of direct medical care depends on the severity of glaucoma and, in developed countries, the average annual cost of patients with severe disease was found to be between 712 and 1065 Euros.[86] In the UK alone (with a population of approximately 60 million people), direct cost of glaucoma medical care is more than £150 million per year, and it is rising due to the use of new antiglaucoma medications.[87] However, the number of glaucoma surgeries is decreasing.[88] Indirect costs of glaucoma (e.g. residential care, social support, rehabilitation, disability benefits, provision of transport, loss of productivity, premature death) are even higher.[89,90]

The impact of glaucoma on quality of life is correlated with the severity of the disease. For example, impaired outdoor mobility and losing a driving license are common concerns in patients with early glaucoma. In patients with severe disease, the most concerning aspect is the possibility of losing central vision and the ability to read.[91] The level of social, economic, and family support greatly varies among European countries.

Healthcare systems and patients' characteristics (such as gender, age, educational level) influence doctor–patient communication.[92] In Eastern and Southern Europe a paternalistic type of medicine is still practiced, less information is given to patients, and written consent is not required (i.e. oral consent is accepted). Litigation is not a big problem in most countries.[93]

Late presentation[94] and poor socioeconomic background[95] are major risk factors for glaucoma blindness. More than half of the people with glaucoma are unaware of their condition. Thus, the feasibility and cost-effectiveness of screening for glaucoma is debated regularly in Western countries, though, at the moment, there are no screening programs in Europe.

In spite of the large regional variations in Europe, there is a political climate that facilitates cooperation among professionals. The European Glaucoma Society (www.eugs.org) is a good example of such collaboration.

JAPAN AND KOREA

Disability caused by blindness in Japan is a very major issue. One of the main reasons for this is that only 20% of those with glaucoma in Japan are diagnosed. Additionally, the prevalence of glaucoma associated with average pressure in Japan is much higher than in other regions where this has been studied. The prevalence in the Tajimi study was almost 4%. Also, the intraocular pressure in the Japanese tends to be lower, between 13 and 14 mmHg, and the rise of intraocular pressure with age is much less marked in the Japanese. These important differences need to be understood.[96–98]

The economic cost of glaucoma in Japan is estimated around US$920 million.[99]

In Korea, the care of patients with glaucoma is complicated by a medical system which makes spending time with patients difficult. Continuing follow-up with the same ophthalmologist is a challenge. The ability of the physician to help patients learn how to care for themselves is limited by time, money, and a culture in which patients tend to follow doctors' advice with little understanding. Physicians look for simple, quick methods of diagnosis.

Improvement in patient care would be enhanced by a medical care system that provided physicians more time with each patient and a culture that encouraged self-care.

Summary

This chapter has focused on two different issues related to the definition of glaucoma: first, definition in the classical sense; and second, definition in terms of the significance of glaucoma for the world's population. It makes no sense to define glaucoma in terms of the biological characteristics usually considered by physicians, such as intraocular pressure or the appearance of the optic nerve, without also considering the biological definition of glaucoma in terms of what glaucoma does.

Glaucoma is a process. It is not a finding such as a notched optic nerve or a nasal slip in the visual field. The process is progressive, though at variable rates. The causes for the onset of the process are multiple, from genetic defects[100,101] to small eyes, to topical corticosteroids, to trauma, to diabetes, to inherited syndrome, and various ocular diseases. The presence of the process is established by the presence of a finding which is never present except in a person with glaucoma, such as an acquired pit of the optic nerve, or a finding which is always a precursor of glaucoma, such as a specific gene defect, an intraocular pressure of 40 mmHg, or closure of the anterior chamber angle.

- Where a definitive finding is present the process is present and the patient is said to have *glaucoma*.
- When a definitive precursor is present, the patient is said to have pre-glaucoma.
- When findings are suggestive or the presence of the process definitive, the patient is called a glaucoma suspect.
- This terminology is an amalgam of current usage and new consensus meetings.[102]

There is a dramatic difference in the significance of glaucoma for different people, and this, too, varies from region to region, from time to time, and from individual to individual even in the same place. By and large, wealthy, educated individuals who know how to care for themselves find that glaucoma is a nuisance, but it is not likely to rob them of their sight. In contrast, those who are less educated and poor have a great likelihood of becoming bilaterally blind from glaucoma should the affliction strike them.

It is deeply disturbing that (1) over 50% of those with glaucoma are never even diagnosed, and (2) that many of those diagnosed lose sight because they live in cultures in all countries which do not place a high priority on health, even preservation of vision, which is of great personal and societal importance, or because they live in cultures or subcultures in which there are simply not enough resources to allow proper care to be provided. Until there is a change in the way the world's people allocate resources, the situation is not likely to improve significantly.

Additionally, and importantly, the only significance of the glaucomatous process is that it can – in some individuals – cause disability. Unfortunately, it still does this frequently in every country in the world. It is that disability which must be kept in mind when deciding how to allocate resources for research, training, and patient care. It is that disability which must be kept in mind when deciding on the risks and benefits of treatments.

ACKNOWLEDGEMENTS

The following individuals helped prepare this chapter: Myunk Douk Ahn, Professor of Ophthalmology, Catholic University, Seoul, Korea; Augusto Azuara-Blanco, MD, Queens Medical Centre University Hospital, Department of Ophthalmology, Nottingham, England; Thomas M Bosley, MD, Head of the Division of Neurology, Cooper University Hospital, New Jersey; Vital P Costa, MD, Director, Glaucoma Service, University of Campinas, Brazil; Associate Professor of Ophthalmology, University of Campinas and University of São Paulo, Brazil; Tarek Eid, MD, Associate Professor of Ophthalmology, Magrabi Eye & Ear Center, Jeddah, Saudi Arabia; Oluwatosin Smith, MD, Assistant Professor, University Medical Center, Department of Ophthalmology, Jackson, Mississippi; Professor Ravi Thomas, MD, Director, L V Prasad Eye Institute, L V Prasad Marg, Banjara Hills, Hyderabad, India; Shigeo Tsukahara, MD, Chairman Emeritus, Department of Ophthalmology, Yamanashi Medical University, Tamaho, Yamanashi, Japan.

REFERENCES

1. MacKenzie W. Practical diseases of the eye. Philadelphia: Lee & Blanchard; 1855.

2. Elliot RH. A treatise on glaucoma. London: Frowde and Hodden & Stoughton; 1918.

3. DeSchweinitz GE. Diseases of the eye. Philadelphia: Saunders; 1893.

4. The American College Dictionary. New York: Random House; 1956: 513.

5. Duke-Elder S, Jay B. Glaucoma and hypotony. In: Duke-Elder S, ed. System of ophthalmology. Mosby: St. Louis; 1969: 388.

6. Leydhecker W, Aikiyama K, Neumann HG. De intraokulare Druck gesunder menschlicher Augen. Klin Monatsbl Augenheilkd 1958: 133:662.

7. Chandler P, Grant M. Ocular hypertension or early glaucoma? Arch Ophthal 1977; 95:1083–1084.

8. Van Buskirk EM, Cioffi GA. Glaucomatous optic neuropathy. Am J Ophthalmol 1992; 113(4):447–452.

9. Spaeth GL. A new classification of glaucoma including focal glaucoma. Surv Ophthalmol 1994; 38(1):S9–SS17.

10. Bathija R, Gupta N, Zangwill L, et al. Changing definition of glaucoma. J Glaucoma 1998; 7(3):165–169.

11. Shields MB, Ritch R, Krupin T. Classification of the glaucomas. In: Ritch R, Shields MB, Krupin T, eds. The glaucomas: clinical science. 2nd edn. St. Louis: Mosby Yearbook; 1996: 717–725.

12. Shields MB. Textbook of glaucoma. 4th edn. Williams & Wilkins: Baltimore; 1998: 1–2.

13. Lee BL, Bathija R, Weinreb RN. The definition of normal-tension glaucoma. J Glaucoma 1998; 7(6):366–371.

14. Spaeth GL. Defining glaucoma, defining disease: the 1998 Dohlman Lecture. Int Ophthalmol Clin 1999; 39(1):1–14.

15. Wolfs RCW, Borger PH, Ramrattan RS, et al. Changing views on open-angle glaucoma: definitions and prevalances – The Rotterdam Study. Invest Ophthalmol Vis Sci 2000; 41(11):3309–3321.

16. Hitchings RS. Chronic glaucoma: definition of the phenotype. Eye 2000; 14(3):419–421.

17. Minckler D. Evidence-based ophthalmology series and content-based continuing medical education for the journal (editorial). Ophthalmology 2000; 107(1):9–11.

18. Tavares IM, Medeiros FA, Weinreb RM. Inconsistency of published definitions of ocular hypertension. J Glaucoma 2006:1529–1533.

19. Brau SS, Kirber HP. Mass screening for glaucoma. JAMA 1951; 147:1127–1134.

20. Elschnig A. Ueber physiologische, atrophische und glaucoma tose Excavation. Ber Dtsche Ophthalmol Ges 1907; 34:2–12.

21. Armaly MF. On the distribution of applanation pressure. 1. Statistical features and the effect of age, sex and family history of glaucoma. Arch Ophthalmol 1965; 73:11.

22. Bankes JLK, Perkins ES, Tsolokis S, et al. Bedford glaucoma survey. Br Med J 1968; 1:791–796.

23. E. Linnén, U. Strömberg. Ocular hypertension: a five-year study of the total population of a Swedish town. In: Leydhecker W, ed. Glaucoma: Tutzing Symposium. Basel: Karger. 187–193.

24. Kitazawa Y, Horie T, Aoki S, et al. Untreated ocular hypertension. Arch Ophthalmol 1977; 95:1180–1185.

25. Kass MA, Heuer DK, Higginbotham EJ, et al. The Ocular Hypertension Treatment Study, a randomized trial determines that topical ocular hypotensive medication delays or prevents the onset of primary open-angle glaucoma. Arch Ophthalmol 2002; 120:701–713.

26. Hollows FC, Graham PA. Intraocular pressure, glaucoma and glaucoma suspects in a defined population. Br J Ophthalmol 1966; 50:570–580.

27. Barany EH. A mathematical formulation of intraocular pressure as dependent on secretion, ultrafiltration, bulk outflow, and osmotic reabsorption of fluid. Invest Ophthalmol 1963; 2:584–590.

28. Fisher RF. Value of tonometry and tonography in the diagnosis of glaucoma. Br J Ophthalmol 1970; 9:42–46.

29. Becker B, Le Blanc RP. The glucose tolerance test and the response of intraocular pressure to topical corticosteroids. Diabetes 1970; 19:715–720.

30. Harris LS. Cycloplegic induced intraocular pressure elevation: a study of normal and open angle glaucomatous eyes. Arch Ophthalmol 1969; 68:973–980.

31. Philips BI, Leighton DA. Provocative test combining water drinking and homatropine eye drops: applanation versus tonography. Br J Ophthalmol 1971; 55:619–626.

32. Spaeth GL. The water drinking test. Arch Ophthalmol 1967; 76:77–85.

33. Spaeth GL, Vacharat N. Provocative tests and chronic simple glaucoma. I. Effect of atropine on the water drinking test: intimations of central regulatory control. II. Fluorescein angiography provocative test: a new approach to separation of the normal from the pathological. Br J Ophthalmol 1972; 56:205–216.

34. Reed H, Drance SM. The essentials of perimetry. 2nd edn. London: Oxford University Press; 1972.

35. Fuchs E. Textbook of ophthalmology. New York: D. Appleton; 1982: 334.

36. Kirsch RE, Anderson DR. Identification of the glaucomatous disc. Trans Am Acad Ophthalmol Otolaryngol 1973; 77:143–150.

37. Read R, Spaeth GL. The practical clinical appraisal of the optic disc in glaucoma: the natural history of cup progression and some specific disc-field correlations. Trans Am Acad Opthalmol Otolaryngol 1974; 78:255–265.

38. Schwartz B. The optic disc in glaucoma. Trans Am Acad Ophthamol Otolaryngol 1976; 81:227–237.

39. Quigley HA, Dunkelberger GR, Green WR. Retinal ganglion cell atrophy correlated with automated perimetry in human eyes with glaucoma. Am J Ophthalmol 1989; 107:453–464.

40. Spaeth GL. Clinical assessment of the optic nerve head. In: Van Buskirk EM, Shields MB, eds. 100 years of glaucoma. Philadelphia: Lippincott-Raven; 1997.

41. Cher I, Robinson LP. 'Thinning' of the neural rim of the optic nerve head. An altered state, providing a new ophthalmoscopic sign associated with characteristics of glaucoma. Trans Ophthalmol Soc UK 1973; 93:213.

42. Drance SM, Begg IS. Sector hemorrhage – a probable acute ischaemic disc change in chronic simple glaucoma. Can J Ophthalmol 1970; 5:137–141.

43. Jonas JB, Naumann GO. [Parapapillary region in normal and glaucoma eyes. II. Correlation of planimetric findings to intrapapillary, perimetry and general data]. Klin Monatsbl Augenheilkd 1988; 193:182–188.

44. Jonas JB. Clinical implications of peripapillary atrophy in glaucoma. Curr Opin Ophthalmol 2005; 15(2):84–88.

45. Airaksinen PF, Tuulonen A, Alanko HI. Rate and pattern of neuroretinal rim area decrease in ocular hypertension and glaucoma. Arch Ophthalmol 1992; 110(2):206–210.

46. Garway Heath DF, Wollstein G, Hitchings RA. Aging changes of the optic nerve head in relation to open angle glaucoma. Br J Ophthamol 1997; 81(10):840–845.

47. Radius RL, Maumenee AE, Green WR. Pit-like changes of the optic nerve head in open-angle glaucoma,. Br J Ophthalmol 1978; 62:389–393.

48. Javitt JC, Spaeth GL, Katz LJ, et al. Acquired pits of the optic nerve. Increased prevalence in patients with low-tension glaucoma. Ophthalmology 1990; 97(8):1038–1043.

49. Hoyt WF, Frisen L, Newman NM. Fundoscopy of nerve fiber layer defects in glaucoma. Invest Ophthalmol 1973; 12:814–829.

50. Quigley HA, Sommer A. How to use nerve fiber layer examination in the management of glaucoma. Trans Am Ophthalmol Soc 1987; 85:254–272.

51. Greenfield DS, Knighton RW, Feuer WF, et al. Correction for corneal polarization axis improves the discriminating power of scanning laser polarimetry. Am J Ophthalmol 2002; 134:27–33.

52. Choplin NT, Lundy DC, Dreher AW. Differentiating patients with glaucoma from glaucoma suspects and normal subjects by nerve fiber layer assessment with scanning laser polarimetry. Ophthalmology 1998; 105:2068–2076.

53. Spaeth GL. Glaucoma. In: Tasman W, Jaeger EE, eds. Wills Eye Hospital atlas of clinical ophthalmology. 2nd edn. Philadelphia. Lippincott, Williams and Wilkins; 2001: 91–167.

54. Lee SJ, et al. Development and validation of a prognostic index for 4-year mortality in older adults. JAMA 2006; 295:801–808.

55. Bayer A, Harasymowycz P, Henderer JD, et al. Validity of a new disk grading scale for estimating glaucomatous damage: correlation with visual field damage. Am J Ophthalmol 2002; 133:758–763.

56. Henderer JD, Liu C, Kesen M, et al. Reliability of the disk damage likelihood scale. Am J Ophthalmol 2003; 135:44–48.

57. The Advanced Glaucoma Intervention Study (AGIS). 1. Study design and methods and baseline characteristics of study patients. Controlled Clin Trials 1994; 15(4):299.

58. The Collaborative Initial Glaucoma Treatment Study. Study design, methods and baseline characteristics of enrolled patients. Ophthalmology 1999; 106(4):653–662.

59. Gullo RM, Costa VP, Bernardi L, et al. Condições visuais de pacientes glaucomatosos em um Hospital Universitário. Arq Bras Oftalmol 1996; 59:147–150.

60. Costa VP, Spaeth GL, Smith M, et al. What do patients know about glaucoma? Arq Bras Oftalmol, in press.

61. Magacho L, Vasconcelos JP, Temporini ER, et al. Tratamento clínico do glaucoma em um hospital universitário: custo mensal e impacto na renda familiar. Arq Bras Oftalmol 2002; 65:127–134.

62. Cintra FA, Costa VP, Tonussi JAG, et al. Avaliação de programa educativo para portadores de glaucoma. Rev Saúde Pública 1998; 32:172.

63. Dandona L, Dandona R, Srinivas M, et al. Blindness in the Indian state of Andhra Pradesh. Invest Ophthalmol Vis Sci 2001; 42:908–916.

64. Thomas R, Padma P, Rao GN, et al. Present status of eye care in India. Surv Ophthalmol 2005; 50(1):85–101.

65. Thomas R, Muliyil J, Paul P. Glaucoma in India. J Glaucoma 2003; 12:81–87.

66. Thomas R, Dogra M. An evaluation of medical college departments of ophthalmology in India and change following provision of modern instrumentation and training. IJO. In press.

67. Tabbara KF. Blindness in the eastern Mediterranean countries. Br J Ophthalmol 2001; 85:771–775.

68. Said ME, Goldstein H, Korra A, et al. Blindness prevalence rates in Egypt. Health Serv Rep 1973; 88:89–96.

69. Said ME, Goldstein H, Korra A, et al. Prevalence and causes of blindness in urban and rural areas in Egypt. Publ Health Rep 1970; 85:587–599.

70. Tabbara KF, Ross-Degnan D. Blindness in Saudi Arabia. JAMA 1986; 255:3378–3384.

71. El-Ashry MF, AbdEl-Aziz MM, Bhattacharya SS. A clinical and molecular genetic study of Egyptian and Saudi Arabian patients with primary congenital glaucoma (PCG). J Glaucoma 2007; 16:104–111.

72. Al-Hazmi A, Awad A, Zwaan J, et al. Correlation between surgical success rate and severity of congenital glaucoma. Br J Ophthalmol 2005; 89:449–453.

73. Eid TM, El-Hawary I, El-Manawy W. Frequency distribution of various types of glaucoma in newly diagnosed patients in the western region in Saudi Arabia: a hospital-based study. Paper submitted for presentation in the World Glaucoma Congress in Singapore, July 2007.

74. Egbert P. Glaucoma in West Africa: a neglected problem. Br J Ophthalmol 2002; 86:131–132.

75. Quigley HA. Number of people with glaucoma worldwide. Br J Ophthalmol 1996; 80:389–393.

76. Quigley HA, Buhrman RR, West SK, et al. Long term results of glaucoma surgery among participants in an African population survey. Br J Ophthalmol 2000; 84:860–864.

77. Verrey JD, Foster A, Wormald R, et al. Chronic glaucoma in northern Ghana – a retrospective study of 397 patients. Eye 1990; 4(Pt 1):115–120.

78. Bowman JC, Kirupananthan S. Glaucoma management in Africa: how to manage a patient with glaucoma in Africa. Community Eye Health J 2006; 19:59.

79. Anand N, Mielke C, Dawdar K. Trabulectomy outcomes in advanced glaucoma in Nigeria. Eye 2001; 15:274–278.

80. Lewallen S, Courtright P. Blindness in Africa: present situation and future needs. Br J Ophthalmol 2001; 85:897–903.

81. Thylefors BA. Global initiative for the education of avoidable blindness. Am J Ophthalmol 1999; 125:90–93.

82. Kocur I, Resnikoff S. Visual impairment and blindness in Europe and their prevention. Br J Ophthalmol 2002; 86:716–722.

83. Tuck MW, Crick RP. The projected increase in glaucoma due to an ageing population. Ophthalmic Physiol Opt 2003; 23:175–179.

84. Quigley HA, Broman AT. The number of people with glaucoma worldwide in 2010 and 2020. Br J Ophthalmol 2006; 90:262–267.

85. Taylor HR, Keeffe JE. World blindness: a 21st century perspective. Br J Ophthalmol 2001; 85:261–266.

86. Traverso CE, Walt JG, Kelly SP, et al. Direct costs of glaucoma and severity of the disease: a multinational long term study of resource utilisation in Europe. Br J Ophthalmol 2005; 89:1245–1249.

87. Rouland JF, Berdeaux G, Lafuma A. The economic burden of glaucoma and ocular hypertension. Drugs Aging 2005; 22:315–321.

88. Macleod SM, Clark R, Forrest J, et al. A review of glaucoma treatment in Scotland 1994–2004. Eye 2008; 22: 251–255.

89. Coyle D, Drummond M. The economic burden of glaucoma in the UK: the need for a far-sighted policy. Pharmacoeconomics 2005; 7:484–489.

90. Lafuma A, Brezin A, Lopatriello S, et al. Evaluation of non-medical costs associated with visual impairment in four European countries, France, Italy, Germany and the UK. Pharmacoeconomics 2006; 24:193–205.

91. Aspinall PA, Hill AR, Nelson P, et al. Quality of life in patients with glaucoma: a conjoint analysis approach. Vis Impair Res 2005; 7:13–26.

92. Hoevenaars JGMM, Schouten JSAG, van der Borne B, et al. Socioeconomic differences in glaucoma patients' knowledge, need for information and expectations of treatments. Acta Ophthalmol Scand 2006; 84:84–91.

93. Mvroforou A, Michalodimitrakis E. Physicians' liability in ophthalmology practice. Acta Ophthalmol Scand 2003; 81:321–325.

94. Chen PP. Blindness among patients with treated open angle glaucoma. Ophthalmology 2003; 110:723–733.

95. Fraser S, Bunce C, Wormald R, et al. Deprivation and late presentation of glaucoma. A case-control study. Br Med J 2001; 322:639–643.

96. Iwase A, Suzuki Y, Araie M, et al. The prevalence of primary open angle glaucoma in Japanese – the Tajimi Study. Ophthalmology 2004; 111:1641–1648.

97. Kunimatsu S, Tomidokoro A, Mishima K, et al. Prevalence of appositional angle closure determined by ultrasonic biomicroscopy in eyes with shallow anterior chamber. Ophthalmology 2005; 112:407–412.

98. Yamamoto T, Iwase A, Araie M, et al. Prevalence of primary angle closure and secondary glaucoma in a Japanese population. Ophthalmology 2005; 12:1661–1669.

99. Tsukahara S, Hosoda M, Asaka A, et al. Health economics study of glaucoma treatment. Chibret Int J Ophthalmol 1994; 10:20–28.

100. Heijl A, Leske MC, Bengtsson B, et al. for the Early Manifest Glaucoma Trial Group. Reduction of intraocular pressure and glaucoma progression. Arch Ophthalmol 2002; 120:1268–1279.

101. Sarfarazi M. Recent advances in molecular genetics of glaucomas. Hum Mol Genet 1997; 6:1667–1677.

102. Polansky JR, Juster RP, Spaeth GL. Association of the myocilin mt. 1 promoter variant with the worsening of glaucomatous disease over time. Clin Genet 2003; 64:18–27.

CHAPTER 25

Ocular Hypertension

Thad Labbe and Michael A Kass

INTRODUCTION

Glaucoma is the world's second most common cause of blindness.[1] Approximately 7 million people worldwide are blind from glaucoma.[2] In the United States alone, the direct medical cost associated with primary open-angle glaucoma (POAG) is estimated at US$2.86 billion per year.[3] Glaucomatous visual loss is irreversible, but early detection and appropriate treatment offer the opportunity to preserve vision. Ocular hypertension (OHT) is a leading risk factor for the development of POAG and is the one modifiable factor at present. The detection and proper management of ocular hypertension represents an opportunity to prevent or slow the development of POAG.

DEFINITION

Ocular hypertension is defined as an elevated intraocular pressure (IOP) without evidence of structural or functional damage by standard clinical tests. The patient with OHT must have open angles and no evidence of an ocular or systemic cause of the elevated IOP. Many different thresholds have been used to define OHT. The authors will use an IOP of greater than or equal to 21 mmHg as the definition of OHT in this chapter.

PREVALENCE

The prevalence of OHT varies in different ethnic groups. In the Blue Mountains Eye Study, the prevalence of OHT in Australian patients older than age 49 was 3.7%.[4] Similarly, the prevalence of OHT in Mexican-Americans older than age 40 was 3.56%.[5] In patients older than age 40, the prevalence of OHT was 1.1% in southern India[6] and 0.9% in Japan.[7] In contrast, the Afro-Caribbean population in the Barbados Eye Study had a prevalence of OHT of 12.6%.[8] The prevalence of OHT increases substantially with age. In the Framingham Eye Study, 6.2% of Caucasians under 65 had an IOP greater than 21 mmHg, while 8.7% over the age of 75 had an IOP greater than 21 mmHg.[9]

PATIENT ASSESSMENT

CLINICAL HISTORY

When a patient presents with OHT, a thorough medical and ocular history must be obtained. The clinician must have a good idea of the patient's general health and life expectancy in order to reach a proper diagnosis, plan future visits, and decide whether treatment is indicated. If a patient cannot provide a detailed history, family members or the patient's general physician can be contacted for additional information. It is important to determine if the patient has a history of previous elevations of eye pressure and if the patient has been treated before. Potential secondary causes of elevated IOP, such as trauma or uveitis, must be ruled out. The clinician must know what topical and systemic medications the patient is using because medications can raise or lower IOP. In this regard, it is especially important to determine if the patient is using corticosteroids, including inhaled or topical skin preparations, which can raise IOP. The patient should also be questioned about medications that can lower eye pressure, such as systemic β-adrenergic blockers.

The clinician should ask the patient about hypertension, hypotension, cardiac disease, and anemia, as all of these factors may influence the health of the optic nerve. Knowledge about cardiovascular disease may also be important in choosing ocular hypotensive medications for a patient. The patient should be asked about history of previous ocular trauma, which can cause eye pressure to rise months or years after an accident. In addition, patients with post-traumatic glaucoma in one eye often develop OHT in the fellow eye years later. A family history of POAG is also important in assessing a patient's risk of progressing from OHT to glaucoma.

INITIAL CLINICAL EXAMINATION

A complete ophthalmic examination must be performed to look for causes of elevated IOP and to determine if glaucoma is already present. A careful refraction and best-corrected visual acuity must be determined in

307

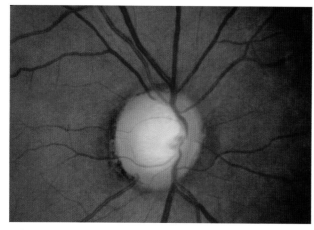

FIGURE 25.1 Focal thinning of neuroretinal rim. This optic nerve notching is a sign of glaucomatous damage. (Courtesy of Rhonda Curtis, CRA, COT.)

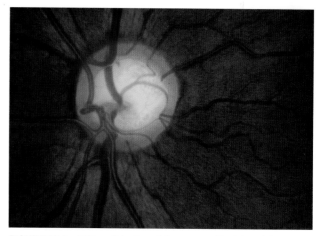

FIGURE 25.2 Diffuse thinning of the neuroretinal rim of the optic disc. Progressive thinning of the optic nerve rim is a sign of progression to glaucoma. (Courtesy of Rhonda Curtis, CRA, COT.)

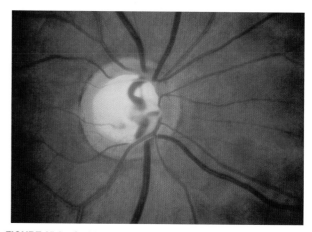

FIGURE 25.3 Sudden change in the direction of blood vessels in a patient who has glaucoma. (Courtesy of Rhonda Curtis, CRA, COT.)

order to perform and interpret visual fields. In addition, keratometry readings are useful for certain types of optic nerve imaging. An afferent pupillary defect may indicate subtle optic nerve damage due to early glaucoma or other disorders. A slit lamp examination can reveal signs of pigment dispersion, pseudoexfoliation, iritis, or trauma. Patients with these signs or conditions have a different pathogenesis of their elevated IOP and a different prognosis. Examination of the lens is also important because lens opacification can affect visual fields. Gonioscopy should always be performed to rule out angle closure or other causes of elevated IOP. The clinician must look for angle recession, increased pigmentation of the trabecular meshwork, peripheral anterior synechiae, or a narrow angle. Central corneal thickness should also be measured on all ocular hypertensive patients as this helps gauge risk of progression and may influence IOP readings.

When initially evaluating a patient with elevated IOP, the optic nerve and retinal nerve fiber layer should be carefully examined to determine baseline status and to rule out existing glaucomatous damage. Possible early signs of glaucomatous optic neuropathy include focal (Fig. 25.1) or generalized thinning of the optic disc rim (Fig. 25.2), a sudden change in the direction of a blood vessel on the surface of the disc[10] (Fig. 25.3), asymmetry of the optic discs, a disc hemorrhage, and focal or diffuse loss of the nerve fiber layer. It is also important to obtain initial stereoscopic optic disc photographs so optic nerve progression can be assessed during future examinations. Stereoscopic photographs also help in drawing optic disc nerve borders for imaging examinations such as Heidelberg retinal tomography (HRT). Many clinicians also do baseline HRT, GDx imaging, or optical coherence tomography (OCT) at the first or second visits. Many experts believe these modalities are useful because they can detect subtle glaucomatous progression; however, a number of studies have shown that careful comparison of optic disc photographs has comparable sensitivity and specificity in detecting progressive optic disc cupping.[11,12]

Measurement of cup-to-disc ratio helps determine the risk of progression, as patients with larger cup-to-disc ratios are at greater risk of developing POAG. Optic nerve evaluation is subjective, and studies have shown that glaucoma specialists often disagree in their assessments of cup-to-disc ratios.[13] On the other hand, when criteria for cup-to-disc measurement are clearly defined, glaucoma specialists and technicians are able to reproducibly grade cup-to-disc ratios. In fact, in the Ocular Hypertension Treatment Study (OHTS), only 1% of readings differed by greater than 0.2 disc diameters (DD).[14] It must be noted that reproducibility of cup-to-disc measurements decline as the cup-to-disc ratio enlarges. The most reproducible cup-to-disc measurements occur between 0.1 DD and 0.6 DD.[14]

Some studies suggest that neuroretinal rim area may be a better predictor of development of glaucoma than cup-to-disc ratio. While it is possible to calculate rim area from stereoscopic disc photographs, computerized measurements make this determination much quicker and perhaps more reproducible.[15] Thus, OCT and HRT can be very helpful in following ocular hypertensive patients.

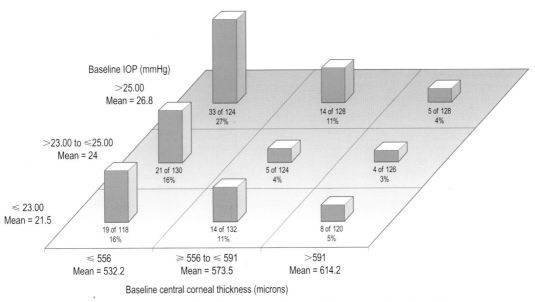

Baseline IOP (mmHg)

>25.00
Mean = 26.8

>23.00 to ≤25.00
Mean = 24

≤ 23.00
Mean = 21.5

33 of 124
27%

14 of 128
11%

5 of 128
4%

21 of 130
16%

5 of 124
4%

4 of 126
3%

19 of 118
16%

14 of 132
11%

8 of 120
5%

≤ 556
Mean = 532.2

≥ 556 to ≤ 591
Mean = 573.5

>591
Mean = 614.2

Baseline central corneal thickness (microns)

FIGURE 25.4 This graph demonstrates the cumulative effect of central corneal thickness and baseline IOP on progression to glaucoma in OHT patients. These results were derived from analysis of pooled data from OHTS and EGPS. (Reproduced from data presented in Ocular Hypertension Treatment Study Group, European Glaucoma Prevention Study Group. Validated prediction model for the development of primary open-angle glaucoma in individuals with ocular hypertension. Ophthalmology 2007; 114:10–19. Copyright 2007, with permission from American Academy of Ophthalmology. Copyright (2007), American Medical Association. All Rights reserved.)

A baseline visual field should be performed on every ocular hypertensive or glaucoma patient. Many patients demonstrate a learning effect with visual fields; therefore, more than one visual field is usually needed to establish a good baseline. Frequency doubling technology (FDT) perimetry has been shown to detect glaucomatous progression up to 4 years before changes in white-on-white perimetry occur.[16] The changes in FDT occur in the same regions as future changes in standard automated perimetry (SAP). Short-wavelength automated perimetry (SWAP) utilizes blue light presented on a yellow background. SWAP also can detect visual field changes earlier than SAP.[17] Although FDT has a shorter testing time than SWAP, the new SITA SWAP reduces the time differential between the tests.

RISK OF PROGRESSION TO GLAUCOMA

It is generally accepted that 1–2% of ocular hypertensive patients develop POAG per year. The incidence depends on the risk characteristics of the patients included in the study, the methods of examination, and the definitions of open-angle glaucoma. It is important to understand why some people with OHT develop POAG and others do not. Although part of the difference may be due to the indirect way we measure IOP, as well as the narrow timeframe of the measurement, different clinical responses to IOP are likely due to intrinsic factors that vary from patient to patient. Intrinsic neuroprotective factors, microstructural anatomy of the optic disc, immune responses, or differences in optic nerve blood flow may be part of the answer; however, there is no way to measure these factors clinically at this time. We must rely on clinical history and examination to estimate a patient's risk for progressing to glaucoma.

A patient's risk of progressing to glaucoma can be estimated from clinical and demographic variables. The OHTS and the European Glaucoma Prevention Study (EGPS) are both longitudinal randomized clinical trials that examined risk factors for progressing to glaucoma. Both trials found that older age, thinner central corneal thickness, increased cup-to-disc ratio, greater IOP, and greater pattern standard deviation were independent risk factors for progression to glaucoma. By definition, patients with OHT have no visual field changes indicative of glaucoma; however, a higher pattern standard deviation on the initial visual field tests increases a patient's risk of progressing to glaucoma.[18,19] The OHTS reported that IOP asymmetry between the eyes may also increase the risk of progression to glaucoma.[20] In OHTS, although African-American heritage increased the risk of progression, this increased risk could be attributed to thinner corneas and larger cup-to-disc ratios in African-Americans. Other studies suggest that a smaller neuroretinal rim area and a larger zone beta of peripapillary atrophy may increase the risk of progression to glaucoma.[21]

Factors can be combined to estimate risk of progressing to glaucoma. For example, a patient with thick corneas (greater than 588 μm) and an IOP of 22 mmHg has only a 2% risk of progression over 5 years without therapy. Patients with the same IOP but with thin corneas (less than 555 μm) have a 17% risk of progression over 5 years. If the patient has two risk factors, IOP greater than 26 mmHg and corneas thinner than 555 μm, the risk increases to 36% over 5 years.[18] Figure 25.4 demonstrates how the risk of progression to glaucoma in the OHTS increased as the IOP increased and as the central corneal thickness (CCT) decreased. Figure 25.5 shows

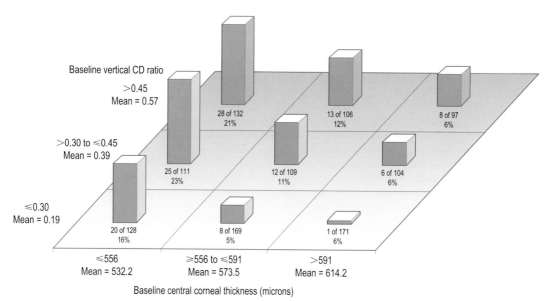

FIGURE 25.5 This graph demonstrates the cumulative effect of central corneal thickness and cup-to-disc ratio on progression to glaucoma in OHT patients. These results were derived from analysis of pooled data from OHTS and EGPS. (Reproduced from data presented in Ocular Hypertension Treatment Study Group, European Glaucoma Prevention Study Group. Validated prediction model for the development of primary open-angle glaucoma in individuals with ocular hypertension. Ophthalmology 2007; 114:10–19. Copyright 2007, with permission from American Academy of Ophthalmology. Copyright (2007), American Medical Association. All Rights reserved.)

TABLE 25.1 **Risk of progression from ocular hypertension to glaucoma**

	POINTS FOR BASELINE PREDICTOR				
BASELINE PREDICTOR	**0**	**1**	**2**	**3**	**4**
Age (years)	<45	45–<55	55–<65	65–<75	≥75
Mean IOP (mmHg)	<22	22–<24	24–<26	26–<28	≥28
Mean CCT (μm)	≥600	576–600	551–575	526–550	≤525
Vertical C/D ratio	<0.3	0.3–<0.4	0.4–<0.5	0.5–<0.6	≥0.6
Mean PSD (db)	<1.8	1.8–<2.0	2.0–<2.4	2.4–<2.8	≥2.8
Sum of points	0–6	7–8	9–10	11–12	>12
Estimated 5-year risk	≤4.0%	10%	15%	20%	≥33%

This table allows a clinician to predict the risk that a patient will progress from OHT to glaucoma over 5 years. Each risk factor increases the total number of points a patients receives. The sum of points allows the calculation of the estimated 5-year risk of progression.
Reproduced from data presented in Ocular Hypertension Treatment Study Group, European Glaucoma Prevention Study Group. Validated prediction model for the development of primary open-angle glaucoma in individuals with ocular hypertension. Ophthalmology 2007; 114:10–19. Copyright 2007, with permission from American Academy of Ophthalmology. Copyright (2007), American Medical Association. All Rights reserved.

how the rate of progression to glaucoma depends on baseline vertical cup-to disc ratio and CCT.

Mansberger[22] and Medeiros et al.[23] developed point systems for baseline predictive factors to help estimate the 5-year risk of progression to glaucoma. A more recent point system using data from the OHTS and EGPS also allows the estimation of the 5-year risk of progression from OHT to glaucoma (Table 25.1).[24]

DETECTING PROGRESSION

When following an ocular hypertensive patient, the optic nerve and the visual field must be assessed periodically to determine if early glaucomatous damage is present. The OHTS demonstrated that the earliest signs of progression to glaucoma are more likely to be detected by changes in the stereoscopic appearance of the optic nerve than by changes in the visual field.[25] In some patients, however, changes can be detected first in the visual field; in other patients, changes can occur simultaneously. The sequence by which early damage is detected is very dependent on the methods of assessment and the thresholds for damage. Because progression to glaucoma can occur either on or off ocular hypotensive medication, close observation is essential, even in patients who are being treated.

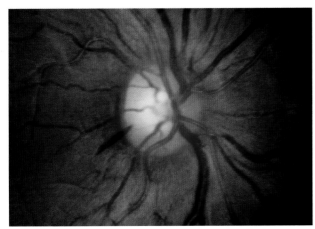

FIGURE 25.6 Disc hemorrhage seen on an optic nerve. (Courtesy of Rhonda Curtis, CRA, COT.)

DETECTING STRUCTURAL EVIDENCE OF PROGRESSION

A common way to assess optic disc change is with optic disc photographs. Side-by-side comparison of stereoscopic photographs with magnification is a very effective way to detect early thinning of the rim. HRT, GDX, and OCT are all capable of measuring structural optic disc parameters, such as rim area and nerve fiber layer thickness. These parameters can be followed to help identify progression. The clinician must look for changes larger than expected from chance variation. It is important to repeat tests so that deterioration can be confirmed. It is also important to determine if changes in the disc or nerve fiber layer correlate with changes in the visual field. A lack of correlation may suggest alternative causes of visual field loss.

Careful examination of the optic disc for a disc hemorrhage may be helpful for monitoring signs of progression. A disc hemorrhage is associated with a 125% increased risk of visual field deterioration in ocular hypertensive patients (Fig. 25.6).[26]

At least 25% of ganglion cells are lost before a significant change is seen on white-on-white perimetry;[27] therefore, many clinicians have sought more sensitive indicators of glaucomatous damage. Nerve fiber layer damage can be found clinically in 60% of OHT patients up to 6 years before changes are seen in perimetry (Fig. 25.7).[28] Although the nerve fiber layer was originally examined either through ophthalmoscopy with red-free light or with special nerve fiber layer photographs, new technology such as OCT, GDX, or HRT can now measure the nerve fiber layer and can help quantify nerve fiber layer loss.

DETECTING PROGRESSION ON VISUAL FIELDS

The earliest changes on visual field testing are more likely to affect the superior hemifield and most commonly present as a nasal step or a partial arcuate defect. The next most common initial visual field defect is a Bjerrum's scotoma.[29]

The type of testing chosen to assess visual function also may influence the ability of the clinician to detect progression. New visual field technology is more sensitive in detecting early visual field deterioration.[30] Standard white-on-white automated perimetry is much more sensitive to early glaucomatous functional changes than Goldmann visual fields. The OHTS showed that changes in standard automated perimetry can occur in some cases even before any apparent change is seen in the optic disc. SITA SWAP and FDT were shown to detect progression earlier than standard automated perimetry in some studies;[16,17] however, it is not clear yet if FDT or SWAP should be recommended for all patients with ocular hypertension. Regardless of the technology, if changes are seen on a visual field, it is important to repeat the field to confirm the change is reproducible. In OHTS, after one abnormal and reliable visual field, the next field is normal 86% of the time. After two abnormal and reliable fields, the next field is normal 40% of the time. Three abnormal fields and correlation of visual field change with the appearance of the optic nerve is helpful in confirming progression of OHT to glaucoma.

TREATMENT

Many issues must be taken into consideration when determining whether to treat a patient with ocular hypertension, including a patient's risk of progressing to glaucoma, a patient's preference for treatment, and the patient's age, health, and life expectancy. Patients should be educated on the risk of progression and the potential risks and benefits of treatment. For some patients with elevated IOP, anxiety linked to glaucoma may sway the decision for treatment. Some patients with ocular hypertension may prefer to remain on an ocular hypotensive medication previously prescribed, despite relatively low risk of progression. Some clinicians believe that a patient is more likely to return for follow-up visits if treatment is prescribed.

The decision to withhold treatment is based upon the assumption that treatment can be started at the earliest sign of glaucomatous damage. This implies that careful visual field studies and optic disc assessment can be performed. Some patients may have a condition, such as nystagmus, which makes examination difficult. In such cases it may be best to begin medical treatment because it would be difficult to diagnose glaucoma before substantial damage occurs. Furthermore, some patients may have other medical conditions, such as a history of a vascular occlusion in one eye, which makes treatment reasonable despite few risk factors for progression to glaucoma. Similarly, medical treatment may be initiated in a monocular patient or a young patient at relatively low risk. On the other hand, a patient with a short life expectancy may be better served by watchful waiting. It is important to follow such a patient

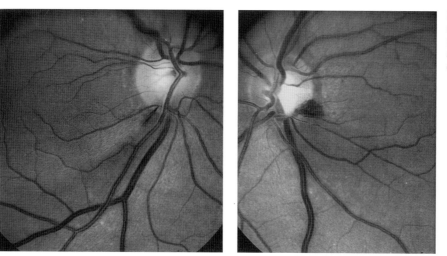

FIGURE 25.7 Nerve fiber layer dropout seen on a red-free photograph. A disc hemorrhage is also seen on the optic disc. (Courtesy of Rhonda Curtis, CRA, COT.)

with serial imaging and visual fields to assure that the goal of maintaining useful vision for the entirety of the patient's life is achieved.

In one cost–utility analysis, treating patients with greater than 2% yearly risk of progressing to glaucoma was cost-effective.[31] A panel of glaucoma experts recommended treating patients with ocular hypertension if the 5-year risk of converting to glaucoma was greater than 15%. The same panel recommended following patients without treatment if the 5-year risk of progression was less than 5%. Between these two values, clinical judgment and patient preference were recommended.[32] The authors' recommendation is to form judgments on treatment by considering the patient's health, life expectancy, preferences, and risk of progressing to glaucoma. Risk calculators are not a replacement for clinical judgment.

The usual treatment for OHT is medical. In rare situations, argon laser trabeculoplasty or selective laser trabeculoplasty may be considered. A variety of classes of topical medications can be used to treat OHT. Topical prostaglandin analogues or β-adrenergic antagonists are the most commonly used medications at this time. The variety of medications now available usually allows the clinician to find a topical medication that is safe and effective for the patient.

The medical treatment of OHT comes with a substantial cost. Medications to lower IOP by 20–25% cost on average US$465 per year in the United States in 2005.[31] Medical treatment also involves patient time and additional examinations, which add further to the cost of therapy. On the other hand, visual impairment that can occur from glaucoma has a major impact on patients and creates a great financial burden on society.

TREATMENT GOALS

Once the decision to treat has been made, a target IOP range or a percentage reduction should be chosen. In OHTS, a 20% reduction of IOP reduced the incidence of glaucoma more than 50%.[25] A 20–25% reduction of IOP is a goal achievable in most OHT patients with current medications. This pressure goal is often reached with the daily use of a prostaglandin analogue, but additional ocular medications may be needed. It is important to realize that a considerable number of patients will still progress to glaucoma, even with a 20% IOP reduction; therefore, it may be prudent to choose a more rigorous goal in a patient at very high risk. As patients are followed, signs of impending progression, such as disc hemorrhage, need to be detected. If a patient develops POAG despite treatment, his or her target IOP should be lowered, and compliance with therapy should be reinforced.

FREQUENCY OF FOLLOW-UP

The OHTS and EGPS showed that initial glaucomatous changes can be detected first in either the visual field or the optic nerve. It is therefore essential to follow both structural and functional parameters. The OHTS protocol included visual fields performed every 6 months. If a patient has few risk factors and is at low risk of progression, a visual field once a year may be appropriate. On the other hand, a patient with multiple risk factors with high risk of progression should be monitored more frequently. Visual fields every 4–6 months may be reasonable in certain very high-risk patients.

At each visit, the optic disc and nerve fiber layer should be examined. A careful search for changes in optic nerve appearance, disc hemorrhages, and nerve fiber layer thinning must be made. An initial stereoscopic optic disc photograph is crucial to allow assessment of optic nerve change over time. Yearly optic disc and nerve fiber layer imaging and computerized analysis with instruments such as OCT, HRT, or GDX can help in detection of subtle optic nerve changes. If early changes are suspected during clinical examination, repeat photographs or disc imaging should be performed to confirm or deny the suspicion.

Summary

Glaucoma is a major cause of blindness worldwide. Detecting OHT provides the clinician with an opportunity to prevent or slow the progress of glaucoma. A thorough examination must be performed to rule out secondary causes of OHT. Risk factors should be determined and assessed to estimate each patient's risk of progression to glaucoma. Follow-up and the decision to treat should be based on the patient's risk profile, as well as his or her age, medical status, life expectancy, and preferences. Treating OHT reduces the risk of progressing to glaucoma by over 50%.[25] The cost and potential side effects of treating OHT are outweighed by the benefits of treatment in patients with moderate to high risk of developing glaucoma.

Treatment should initially decrease IOP by 20–25%. Patients need to be followed for changes such as disc hemorrhages, which suggest an increased risk of progression. Both treated and untreated patients should be followed for structural or functional damage suggestive of glaucoma. If these changes are seen, treatment should be initiated or accelerated.

ACKNOWLEDGEMENTS

Special thanks to Mae Gordon, PhD, for her advice and help in preparation of this chapter.

REFERENCES

1. Resnikoff S, Pascolini D, Etya'ale D, et al. Global data on visual impairment in the year 2002. Bull World Health Organ 2004; 82:844–851.

2. Quigley HA. Number of people with glaucoma worldwide. Br J Ophthalmol 1996; 80:389–893.

3. Rein DB, Zhang P, Wirth KE, et al. The economic burden of major adult visual disorders in the United States. Arch Ophthalmol 2006; 124:1754–1760.

4. Mitchell P, Smith W, Attebo K, et al. Prevalence of open-angle glaucoma in Australia. The Blue Mountains Eye Study. Ophthalmology 1996; 103:1661–1669.

5. Varma R, Ying-Lai M, Francis BA, et al. Prevalence of open-angle glaucoma and ocular hypertension in Latinos: the Los Angeles Latino Eye Study. Ophthalmology 2004; 111:1439–1448.

6. Ramakrishnan R, Nirmalan PK, Krisnadas R, et al. Glaucoma in a rural population of southern India. The Aravind Comprehensive Eye Survey. Ophthalmology 2003; 110: 1484–1490.

7. Iwase A, Suzaki Y, Araie M, et al. The prevalence of primary open-angle glaucoma in Japanese: the Tajimi Study. Ophthalmology 2004; 111:1641–1648.

8. Nemesure B, Wu SY, Hennis A, et al. Factors related to the 4-year risk of high intraocular pressure: the Barbados Eye Studies. Arch Ophthalmol 2003; 121:856–862.

9. Leibowitz HM, Krueger DE, Maunder LR, et al. The Framingham Eye Study monograph: an ophthalmological and epidemiological study of cataract, glaucoma, diabetic retinopathy, macular degeneration, and visual acuity in a general population of 2631 adults, 1973–1975. Surv Ophthalmol 1980; 24(suppl):335–610.

10. Hitchings RA, Anderton S. Identification of glaucomatous visual field defects from examination of monocular photographs of the optic disc. Br J Ophthalmol 1983; 67:822–825.

11. Medeiros FA, Zangwill LM, Bowd C, et al. Use of progressive glaucomatous optic disk change as the reference standard for evaluation of diagnostic tests in glaucoma. Am J Ophthalmol 2005; 139:1010–1018.

12. Arthur SN, Aldridge AJ, Leon-Ortega J, et al. Agreement in assessing cup-to-disc ratio measurements among stereoscopic optic nerve head photographs, HRT II, and Stratus OCT. J Glaucoma 2006; 15:183–189.

13. Tielsch JM, Katz J, Quigley HA, et al. Intraobserver and interobserver agreement in measurement of optic disc characteristics. Ophthalmology 1988; 95:350–356.

14. Feuer WJ, Parrish RK, Schiffman JC, et al. The Ocular Hypertension Treatment Study: reproducibility of cup/disk ratio measurements over time at an optic disc reading center. Am J Ophthalmol 2002; 133:19–28.

15. Balazsi AG, Drance SM, Schulzer M, et al. Neuroretinal rim area in suspected glaucoma and early chronic open-angle glaucoma. Correlation with parameters of visual function. Arch Ophthalmol 1984; 102:1011–1014.

16. Medeiros FA, Sample PA, Weinreb RN. Frequency doubling technology perimetry abnormalities as predictors of glaucomatous visual field loss. Am J Ophthalmol 2004; 137:863–871.

17. Landers JA, Goldberg I, Graham SL. Detection of early visual field loss in glaucoma using frequency-doubling perimetry and short-wavelength automated perimetry. Arch Ophthalmol 2003; 121:1705–1710.

18. Gordon MO, Beiser JA, Brandt JD, et al. for the Ocular Hypertension Treatment Study Group. The Ocular Hypertension Treatment Study. Baseline factors that predict the onset of primary open-angle glaucoma. Arch Ophthalmol 2002; 120:714–720.

19. European Glaucoma Prevention Study Group. Predictive factors for open-angle glaucoma among patients with ocular hypertension in the European Glaucoma Prevention Study. Ophthalmology 2007; 114:3–9.

20. Levine RA, Demire S, Fan J, et al. Asymmetries and visual field summaries as predictors of glaucoma in the Ocular Hypertension Treatment Study. Invest Ophthalmol Vis Sci 2006; 47:3896–3903.

21. Jonas JB, Martus P, Budde WM, et al. Small neuroretinal rim and large parapapillary atrophy as predictive factors for progression of glaucomatous optic neuropathy. Ophthalmology 2002; 109:1561–1567.

22. Mansberger SL. A risk calculator to determine the probability of glaucoma. J Glaucoma 2004; 13:345–347.

23. Medeiros FA, Weinreb RN, Sample PA, et al. Validation of a predictive model to estimate the risk of conversion from ocular hypertension to glaucoma. Arch Ophthalmol 2005; 123: 1351–1360.

24. Ocular Hypertension Treatment Study Group, European Glaucoma Prevention Study Group. Validated prediction model for the development of primary open-angle glaucoma in individuals with ocular hypertension. Ophthalmology 2007; 114:10–19.

25. Kass MA, Heuer DK, Higginbotham EJ, et al. for the Ocular Hypertension Treatment Study. The Ocular Hypertension Treatment Study. A randomized trial determines that topical ocular hypotensive medication delays or prevents the onset of primary open-angle glaucoma. Arch Ophthalmol 2002; 120:701–713.

26. Keltner JL, Johnson CA, Anderson DR, et al. The association between glaucomatous visual fields and optic nerve head features in the Ocular Hypertension Treatment Study. Ophthalmology 2006; 113:1603–1612.

27. Kerrigan-Baumrind LA, Quigley HA, Pease ME, et al. Number of ganglion cells in glaucoma eyes compared with threshold visual field tests in the same persons. Invest Ophthalmol Vis Sci 2000; 41:741–748.

28. Sommer A, Katz J, Quigley HA, et al. Clinically detectable nerve fiber atrophy precedes the onset of glaucomatous field loss. Arch Ophthalmol 1991; 109:77–83.

29. Hart WM Jr, Becker. The onset and evolution of glaucomatous visual field defects. Ophthalmology 1982; 89:268–279.

30. Portnoy GL, Krohn MA. The limitations of kinetic perimetry in early scotoma detection. Ophthalmology 1978; 85: 287–293.

31. Kymes SM, Kass MA, Anderson DR, et al. Management of ocular hypertension: a cost-effectiveness approach from the Ocular Hypertension Treatment Study. Am J Ophthalmol 2006; 141:997–1008.

32. Weinreb RN, Friedman DS, Fechtner RD, et al. Risk assessment in the management of patients with ocular hypertension. Am J Ophthalmol 2004; 138:458–467.

CHAPTER 26

Primary Open-Angle Glaucoma

Albert S Khouri and Robert D Fechtner

INTRODUCTION

Glaucoma is a leading cause of irreversible visual loss. This potentially blinding disease is a progressive optic neuropathy associated with elevated intraocular pressure. The diagnosis of primary open-angle glaucoma is often made too late, after permanent visual damage has occurred. Preserving vision is best achieved with diagnosis prior to perceived functional damage by the patient. Often the diagnosis is presumptive, based on abnormal optic nerve findings, or loss on psychophysical testing. The diagnosis becomes definitive once progression of disease is detected over time. With the evolution of global risk assessment, and the refinement of diagnostic tools and technologies, our ability to detect early disease continues to improve. This allows clinicians to identify patients earlier for the institution of treatment. Recent clinical trials such as the Early Manifest Glaucoma Trial, Collaborative Initial Glaucoma Treatment Study, and Advanced Glaucoma Intervention Study have provided pivotal data on natural history, risk factors, and outcomes of treatment. The outcomes of clinical trials are discussed in a later section.

PREVALENCE

A recent review of published data from population-based studies of age-specific prevalence of primary open-angle glaucoma (POAG) combined with United Nations world population projections for 2010 and 2020 were analyzed to derive the estimated number of subjects with glaucoma. It was estimated that by 2010 around 45 million people will have POAG, increasing to 59 million by 2020. Bilateral blindness will be present in 4.5 million people with POAG, rising to 5.9 million in 2020, making glaucoma the second leading cause of blindness worldwide.[1]

In the 2002 World Health Organization report on the magnitude and causes of visual impairment, more than 161 million people were visually impaired, of whom 124 million people had low vision and 37 million were blind. In this report published in 2004, glaucoma contributed to blindness in about 4.5 million individuals. These figures represented the first global estimates since the early 1990s. Country and regional variations were notable, with more than 90% of the world's visually impaired living in developing countries. Although cataract remained the leading cause of blindness associated with aging in all regions of the world (except for the most developed countries), glaucoma was reported as the second leading cause of blindness globally as well as in most regions, with age-related macular degeneration (AMD) ranking third on the global scale.[2,3]

The prevalence of glaucoma is influenced by many variables, particularly age and race. Several population-based studies found the prevalence increased with age.[4–7] These showed that glaucoma prevalence increases with age by as much as five- to tenfold from the fifth to the eighth decade. However, individuals older than 75 years are poorly represented in population-based studies of glaucoma prevalence. Typically, younger individuals are included, as older individuals are the most difficult to bring in for screening and scheduled eye examinations.[8]

It is also well known that age-adjusted prevalence rates for POAG are higher in blacks compared with whites.[4] Rates among blacks in the Baltimore Eye Survey ranged from 1.23% (in those aged 40–49 years) to 11.26% (in those older than 80 years), whereas rates for whites ranged from 0.92% to 2.16%, respectively. In the more recent Salisbury Eye Evaluation Glaucoma Study a total of 1233 individuals were screened with eye examination.[8] The prevalence of POAG was 3.4% for white individuals aged 73 and 74 years, increasing to 9.4% for those older than 75 years. Among black persons, the prevalence was 5.7% in those aged 73 and 74 years and increased tremendously to 23.2% in those 75 years and older. Thus, black persons older than 75 years had substantially higher rates than whites the same age. These findings have important implications for public health initiatives and screening programs. This may also reflect a different racial genetic basis or susceptibility to the disease.

RISK FACTORS

Identifying risk factors for the development of glaucoma has been highlighted by the evolving understanding of risk assessment, and the way it has affected management options for glaucoma patients. The goal of identifying risk factors for glaucoma is to recognize patients at greatest risk for progression leading to symptomatic vision loss that may have a detrimental effect on their quality of life. In that sense, glaucoma presents an unusual situation where some of the putative risk factors for the disease are actually early pathologic signs, such as optic nerve cupping for example.

The ophthalmologist treating patients with early glaucoma is frequently faced with the clinical dilemma of how vigorous treatment goals should be. Not all patients with glaucoma will progress to symptomatic visual loss during their expected life span. Some with glaucoma will maintain useful vision for their entire lifetime. Simply put, risk assessment should allow us to identify those at greatest risk for developing glaucoma and for suffering symptomatic vision loss. Applying what we have learned from longitudinal studies of patients will help in making individualized risk assessment plans.

The literature has often described 'risk factors for glaucoma' without specifying whether it is a risk for developing the disease or a risk for it progressing. To better understand this issue, it is helpful to think of glaucoma as a spectrum ranging from a healthy appearance to the optic nerve with pre-detectable damage by current technologies, to early detectable damage with none to early asymptomatic vision loss, to more advanced degrees of damage and blindness. We should also not assume that all the risk factors remain the same or carry the same weight at all stages of the disease. Risk assessment in patients with ocular hypertension and glaucoma has been the subject of several reviews.[9–11]

Some risk factors can be identified by patient history, such as age, race, and family history, while others can be detected by clinical examination and testing, such as intraocular pressure and optic nerve cup-to-disc ratio. The strength of evidence supporting risk factors varies from strong to weak (Table 26.1). Several risk factors have been identified for progression from ocular hypertension to glaucoma. Those are discussed in detail in

Chapter 25. The authors have focused the discussion below on risk factors mostly associated with POAG and its progression.

OPTIC NERVE HEAD

The optic nerve head appearance is perhaps the most significant risk factor and diagnostic sign as its alteration basically defines glaucoma in most patients. With current limitations in imaging technologies as well as biologic variability it remains challenging to isolate well-defined optic nerve head parameters as risk factors. However, there exists strong evidence that a large cup-to-disc ratio in itself represents a risk factor for progression of glaucoma.[12,13] Whether an elevated cup-to-disc ratio represents a risk factor or undetected existing glaucoma damage has been debated.[14] Limitations in early detection of structural damage make it difficult to completely resolve this issue. Optic disc hemorrhages were associated with a faster rate of glaucoma progression in the Collaborative Normal Tension Glaucoma Study,[15] and with a sixfold increase (95% confidence interval [CI], 3.6–10.1; $p < 0.001$) in risk of developing POAG in the Ocular Hypertension Treatment Study participants.[16]

INTRAOCULAR PRESSURE

Intraocular pressure (IOP) is one of the strongest risk factors for glaucoma progression.[12,17–20] At high enough levels, IOP can be causative. Higher IOP levels are associated with glaucoma progression. Variability in diurnal IOP and large IOP differences between fellow eyes were found to be more common in patients with POAG (36%) than in normal subjects (6%).[21] The diurnal IOP range and the IOP range over multiple days were found to be significant risk factors for progression, even after adjusting for age, race, and visual field damage (relative hazards and 95% CI were 5.69 [1.86–17.35] and 5.76 [2.21–14.98]).[22] In the recent analysis of the Early Manifest Glaucoma Trial with a median follow-up of 8 years the results confirmed the earlier findings that elevated IOP is a strong factor for glaucoma progression, with a hazard ratio increasing by 11% for every 1mmHg of higher IOP (95% CI, 1.06–1.17; $p < 0.0001$).[23]

AGE

There is strong evidence that prevalence of primary open-angle glaucoma (POAG) increases with the age of the population being studied.[20,24,25] This was also confirmed in other population-based studies such as the visual impairment project[26] and the Barbados Family Study.[27]

RACE

Primary open-angle glaucoma was found to be four to six times more frequent among individuals of African-American origin compared to Caucasian.[4,28] On

TABLE 26.1 Risk factors for glaucoma by strength of evidence	
RISK FACTOR	**STRENGTH OF EVIDENCE**
Optic nerve head alteration	Strong
Elevated intraocular pressure	Strong
Older age	Strong
African origin	Strong
Confirmed family history	Moderate
Diabetes mellitus	Modest
Hypertension	Modest

average, POAG also began at an earlier age in African-Americans than Caucasians. Other studies have also reported a notably higher prevalence of glaucoma in individuals of black race when compared with other racial groups.[8,29]

FAMILY HISTORY

Family history of glaucoma increases the risk of an individual developing the disease. Although the exact inheritance pattern is still unknown, POAG would appear to be a multifactorial polygenetic disease. Several studies examined family history as a risk factor for glaucoma. The Glaucoma Inheritance Study in Tasmania compared the distribution of patients with genealogically confirmed familial POAG and those with sporadic POAG. The familial group was significantly younger at diagnosis and had more severe disease than the sporadic group.[30] This finding is in support of the value of tailored screening, particularly of family members of individuals with a positive family history.

Self-reporting can be unreliable, but in the Rotterdam Study family history was ascertained by direct examination of relatives and not by patient self-report.[31] The lifetime absolute risk of glaucoma at age 80 years was found to be almost 10 times higher for individuals having relatives with glaucoma than for patients with negative family history (22.0% vs 2.4%). The Barbados Family Study of Open-Angle Glaucoma investigated inheritance of POAG among families of black race and also found family history to be a major risk factor for glaucoma confirmed by direct examination of the relatives.[27] Still, family history alone cannot account for the observed prevalence of the disease, suggesting that nongenetic factors play a significant role in the overall occurrence of glaucoma.[17]

DIABETES

Several studies investigated the possible relationship between POAG and diabetes. Prevalence of POAG was higher in diabetic individuals compared to nondiabetics (4.2% vs 2.0%; $p = 0.004$).[32] In the Blue Mountains Eye Study, glaucoma prevalence and ocular hypertension (OHT) were more common in people with diabetes (odds ratio, 2.12; 95% CI, 1.18–3.79, and 1.86; 95% CI, 1.09–3.20, respectively).[33] Other prospective studies of glaucoma management reported a greater likelihood of progression in patients with diabetes.[34,35]

In the Baltimore Eye Survey, the association between glaucoma and diabetes was found to be weak (age-race-adjusted odds ratio, 1.03; 95% CI, 0.85–1.25).

Persons whose POAG had been diagnosed before they enrolled in the study showed a positive association with diabetes (odds ratio, 1.7; 95% CI, 1.03–2.86), indicating that selection bias into the healthcare system may have influenced the positive results of associations between diabetes and POAG in some studies.[36] The Ocular Hypertension Treatment Study suggested that diabetes actually protected against progression to

POAG (hazard ratio of 0.37 in the multivariate analysis with $p < 0.05$).[17,18] However, diabetes was not selected as a predictive factor in the analysis of pooled Ocular Hypertension Treatment Study and European Glaucoma Prevention Study datasets. The effect of diabetes on the development of POAG remains controversial.[37]

HYPERTENSION

In the Blue Mountains Eye Study, participants with glaucoma were more likely to have systemic hypertension than participants without glaucoma (65.7%; 95% CI, 56.6–74.8 vs 45.4%; 95% CI, 43.8–47.1).[38] Although a positive association between elevated blood pressure and POAG was reported,[39] larger population-based studies such as the Framingham Eye Study[40] and the Baltimore Eye Survey failed to confirm the association. However, systolic and diastolic blood pressure showed modest, positive association with POAG. Age-adjusted data indicated that individuals with a systolic blood pressure >130 mmHg had a higher prevalence of POAG. Lower perfusion pressure (blood pressure–intraocular pressure) was strongly associated with an increased prevalence of POAG, with a sixfold excess for those in the lowest category of perfusion pressure.[41]

OTHER RISK FACTORS

Various factors such as myopia, pseudoexfoliation, and migraine have been reported in the literature as risk factors. There seems to be an increased frequency of myopia among patients with OHT or POAG. In one study, 60% of eyes progressing from OHT to glaucoma were myopic.[42] In the Beijing Eye Study, subjects with myopic refractive error exceeding −6 diopters had a significantly higher glaucoma frequency than groups with low myopia (−0.5 to −3) or emmetropia.[43] There is evidence for pseudoexfoliation as a risk factor for glaucoma progression.[34] Migraine has also been reported as a risk factor for glaucoma progression.[44]

PATHOGENESIS

Despite the fact that POAG is the most commonly studied type of glaucoma, its pathogenesis remains unclear. Accordingly, POAG is by definition a primary disease with no identifiable cause. With the current definition, any time a cause is identified for glaucoma, it is labeled a secondary glaucoma rather than POAG. Several theories of mechanism have been suggested and remain a subject of debate.[45] Among those are the vascular and mechanical theories for optic nerve damage.

Abnormal resistance to aqueous outflow and alterations at various levels of the trabecular meshwork have been described. Among those were histologic abnormalities in collagen structure, intertrabecular spaces, juxtacanalicular connective tissue, and endothelial cell function in glaucoma eyes.[46,47] Collapse in Schlemm's canal has been proposed as a contributing factor to the increased resistance to outflow in POAG.[48] Interpretation of the various histologic findings and their implications on outflow resistance and IOP is difficult. The role of different components of the outflow system in regulating IOP, and the segmental variability of the system, makes simple interpretations elusive.[49] The understanding of complex mechano-transduction mechanisms of aqueous outflow continue to evolve, with new models proposed for outflow control and regulatory feedback of IOP.[50]

GENETICS

The advances in DNA-related technologies have led to significant leaps in our knowledge of the genetics of ophthalmic diseases. This progress has accelerated with the completion of the Human Genome Project in 2003 (aimed to identify all of the approximately 25 000 genes in human DNA, and to determine the sequences of approximately 3 billion base pairs that make up human DNA), and the International HapMap Project in 2005.[51–53] Perhaps a reason why it has been challenging to discover the genes for POAG relates to the fact that POAG (although thought of as a single disease) does not consist of a single 'phenotypic' variant. For example, some patients with POAG suffer optic nerve damage at IOP in the statistically normal range, while others produce damage with higher levels of IOP.[54]

Genetic factors have long been implicated in the pathophysiology of POAG. Myocilin, for example, was associated with both juvenile open-angle glaucoma and POAG. Although more than 40 different myocilin mutations have been described in POAG patients, as a group these mutations are associated with only 3–4% of POAG patient worldwide.[55] Other genetic sequence variations for POAG have been described but in general they still are responsible for only a small minority of all POAG.[56,57] In a recent study a genome-wide scan of IOP was performed using 486 pedigrees of a population-based cohort from the Beaver Dam Eye Study. Linkage analysis was performed using regression models and seven loci of interest were identified on chromosomes 2, 5, 6, 7, 12, 15, and 19. Two of the regions (chromosomes 2 and 19) were especially interesting since each has been identified as a potential linkage region for blood pressure.[58] Replicating these initial findings in other populations will assist in identifying genes that may control IOP.

DIAGNOSIS

PRESUMPTIVE VERSUS DEFINITIVE

Detecting glaucomatous optic neuropathy or the corresponding characteristic visual field loss is the basis of diagnosis. Structural and functional tests are useful for detection of glaucoma, and in its follow-up and management over time. Detection of change on either modality may not only indicate progression of disease but also may indicate with certainty the presence of POAG. Classic optic nerve head findings such as a large cup-to-disc ratio may show considerable overlap among POAG and normal subjects. Visual field sensitivity and performance fluctuate over time, and pathologic findings frequently disappear or decrease in intensity upon retesting. Frequently, the diagnosis of glaucoma is 'presumptive,' based on pathologic optic nerve or visual field findings. Having the ability to detect the most subtle signs of progression of disease once they occur constitutes the 'definitive' diagnosis for most subjects.

SIGNS OF PRIMARY OPEN-ANGLE GLAUCOMA

Clinical assessment of the optic nerve head to diagnose or exclude glaucoma is challenging because of the overlap in appearance and extent of cup-to-disc ratio between pathologic and normal subjects. Changes in the observations made with follow-up of subjects over time are a more sensitive indicator of progression of disease. Certain findings on examination are very suggestive of POAG and their presence, even on a single observation, can imply the presumptive diagnosis of glaucoma. Among these observations are nerve fiber layer (NFL) defects, optic nerve rim hemorrhages, and neuroretinal rim notching or relative thinning (Figs 26.1–26.3). The ISNT rule can be used to aid in the differentiation between normal and glaucomatous optic nerves. In normal eyes the neuroretinal rim follows a characteristic configuration whereby the inferior (I) rim is thickest, followed by the superior (S), then nasal (N), then temporal (T) rim, hence the ISNT rule. In many patients glaucomatous optic neuropathy may be advanced (Fig. 26.4) by the time visual impairment is noted.

STRUCTURAL ABNORMALITIES

It has been demonstrated that significant optic nerve damage may occur prior to the appearance of visual field loss.[59] In one study, nerve fiber layer defects were present

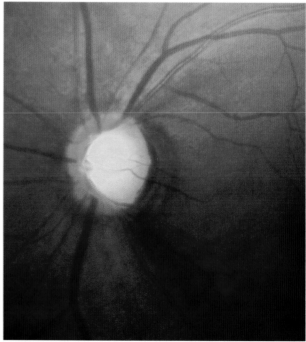

FIGURE 26.1 Inferior and superior nerve fiber layer defects.

in 88% of optic nerve photographs at the time field loss was first detected, with 60% of eyes showing nerve fiber layer defects 6 years before field loss.[60] Clinically, the evaluation of the optic nerve is done with biomicroscopy using a handheld lens (typically 78 D or 90 D), or through evaluation of stereoscopic optic nerve images.

The essential pathologic process in glaucoma is loss of ganglion cell axons. The appearance of the neural rim

and configuration of the optic cup reflect the amount of axon loss. The five rules described for optic nerve evaluation are: optic disc size, neuroretinal rim shape, retinal nerve fiber layer, presence of peripapillary atrophy, and presence of retinal or optic disc hemorrhages.[61] A large number of clinical features have been characterized (Table 26.2). None, however, seems to be universally present or absent. Thus, it remains essential to

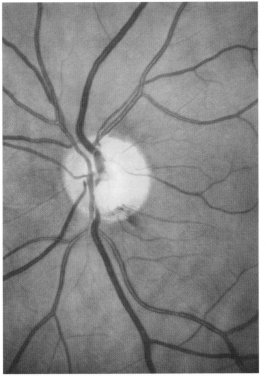

FIGURE 26.2 Inferior splinter hemorrhage with neural rim thinning and a corresponding nerve fiber layer defect.

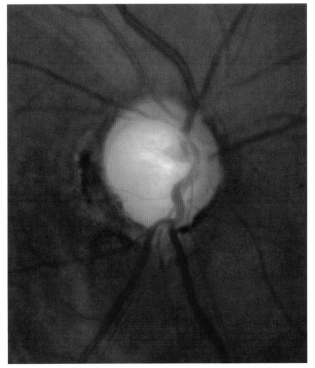

FIGURE 26.4 Advanced glaucomatous optic neuropathy.

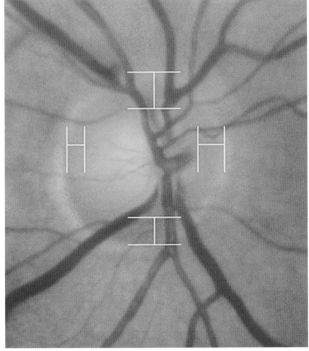

FIGURE 26.3 Relative thickness of the neuroretinal rim is outlined at the four poles of the disc in a patient with early POAG. Note the inferior rim is thin, violating the ISNT rule.

TABLE 26.2 Common optic disc and nerve fiber layer signs of glaucoma

SIGN	DESCRIPTION
Cup-to-disc ratio	Increased, usually >0.6
	Asymmetry between eyes, usually >0.2
	Vertical elongation, usually denoting loss of rim inferiorly or superiorly
Neuroretinal rim	Notching or focal loss
	Pallor
	Sloped rim is common temporally and is not a specific sign
Nerve fiber layer	Localized wedge defects
	Can be diffuse in advanced disease
	Often in relation with splinter hemorrhage
Vascular	Disc splinter hemorrhages
	Overpass with loss of rim underneath
	Bayonetting
	Narrowing, can be diffuse or focal
	Nasalization mostly with advanced cupping
Peripapillary atrophy	Common but not specific to glaucoma

correlate optic nerve findings with functional changes in vision, and to follow these alterations over time.

FUNCTIONAL DEFECTS

Visual field testing is mainstay for the diagnosis and management of POAG. Reproducible visual field defects confirm a presumptive diagnosis of glaucoma. Certain visual field patterns of loss have been classically associated with glaucoma such as arcuate and nasal step defects (Figs 26.5 and 26.6). Progression of visual field loss is probably the most commonly recognized indicator of disease worsening. However, perimetric testing generally is not sensitive to very small changes, and

true progression usually reflects significant loss of nerve tissue. It is important to realize that not all defects detected on sensitive perimetric testing persist on retesting and imply a pathologic glaucomatous process.

It is less common for glaucoma to be diagnosed before the appearance of visual field loss. The exception would be in patients with recurrent optic disc hemorrhages prior to manifesting visual field loss.[62,63] Standard automated perimetry (SAP) with static techniques has almost completely replaced kinetic manual perimetry, in large part because of the convenience of testing and quantitative measures provided by automated testing. In addition to white-on-white SAP, several other automated perimetry tests and algorithms exist for the

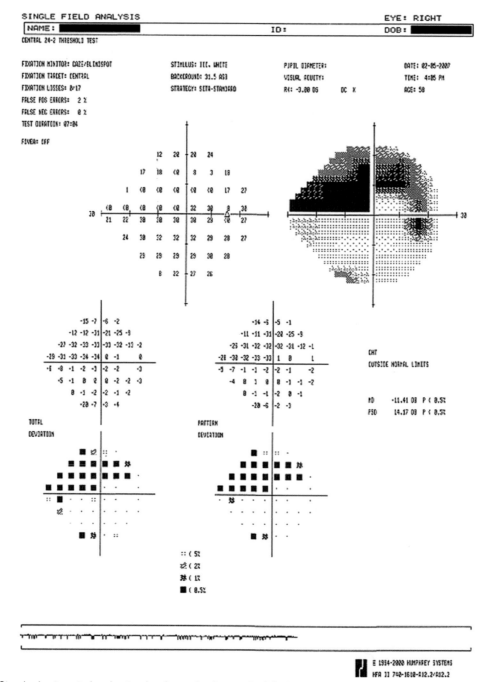

FIGURE 26.5 Standard automated perimetry showing a classic arcuate defect.

diagnosis and detection of glaucoma progression. Among those technologies are short-wavelength automated perimetry (SWAP) and frequency doubling technology (FDT) perimetry.

In brief, there is evidence that SWAP can detect visual field loss earlier than SAP, with a sensitivity and specificity of about 88% and 92%, respectively. However, SWAP testing can be lengthy when performed under a standard algorithm speed. It is also sensitive to media opacities such as nuclear sclerosis. In addition, SWAP showed greater long-term fluctuation compared with SAP, making it difficult to use in assessing accurate disease progression. Testing with FDT perimetry showed sensitivity and specificity more than 97% for detecting moderate and advanced glaucoma, and sensitivity of 85% and specificity of 90% for early glaucoma when compared to SAP. As FDT perimetry has a short testing time and is resistant to blur and pupil size, it may be a useful screening tool.[64]

ANCILLARY TESTS

Functional and structural testing is covered in detail in other sections. Below is an overview of tests commonly used in glaucoma diagnosis and follow-up.

Stereophotography Optic nerve head stereophotography allows the objective documentation of optic nerve

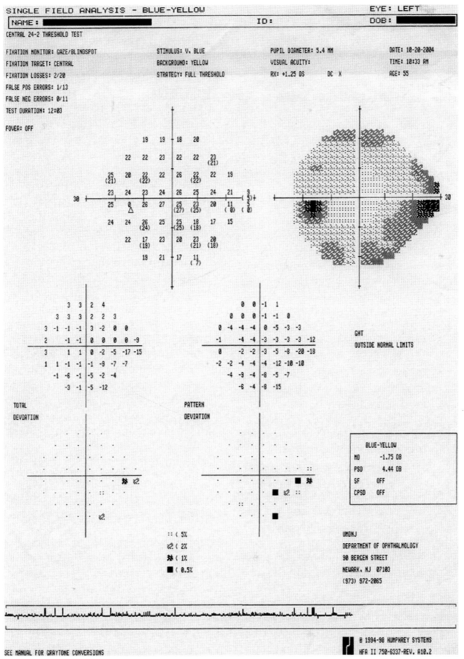

FIGURE 26.6 Short-wavelength automated perimetry showing an early inferior nasal step defect.

findings,[65] and is a strong comparative tool when used for serial comparison of photos over time.[66] The use of digital imaging is becoming common in ophthalmology, and has been a standard in recent major clinical trials. It allows immediate feedback on the quality of obtained images. Film and digital imaging seem comparable in the assessment of glaucomatous optic neuropathy.[67] Digital images can be transmitted to reading centers as is done in clinical trials and teleophthalmology without effects on clinical interpretation or image quality.[68] Digital images can also be analyzed with software-driven digital filters to expedite archiving and clinical assessment of images.[69,70]

Scanning laser polarimetry This technique measures the peripapillary NFL thickness by shining a laser beam onto the retina and assessing the change in polarization or retardation of the reflected beam. Laser retardation is due to the birefringent properties of the neurotubules in ganglion cell axons. Individualized compensation for corneal birefringence is performed. The GDx (Carl Zeiss Meditec, Inc., Dublin, CA) utilizes scanning laser polarimetry to generate a high-resolution image of the peripapillary retina. The NFL thickness is measured along a circle located 3.2 mm in diameter around the disc. The superior and inferior poles have the greatest NFL thickness, and when thickness is plotted graphically this typically manifests in a 'double hump' pattern in normal eyes. Measurements with this technology correlate well with glaucoma damage and visual field defects.[71,72]

Confocal scanning laser topography The principle of confocal scanning laser polarimetry is to illuminate the optic nerve and retina through a single pinhole and to allow light that returns from the point of interest to pass through the pinhole and be detected. To image a plane, rather than a point, an array of points in that plane must be scanned point by point, yielding an optical plane or section. The Heidelberg Retina Tomograph (HRT; Heidelberg Engineering GmbH, Heidelberg, Germany) creates a topographic image by a reconstruction of up to 64 scanned image planes. A contour line is placed by an operator and a series of topographic analyses are performed on the image. The latest HRT 3 software performs automated analyses based on the three-dimensional modeling of the entire topographical image. The constructed three-dimensional models of the optical nerve head (ONH) shape do not require placement of a contour line manually, and do not require a reference plane for analysis.[73] Many HRT parameters were found to be associated with the development of POAG, including large cup-to-disc area ratio, mean cup depth, cup volume, and neuroretinal rim area and volume.[74]

Optical coherence tomography The physical principles of this technology are similar those of ultrasound, yet provide a higher resolution. The Optical Coherence Tomograph (OCT; Carl Zeiss Meditec, Inc., Dublin, CA, USA) provides an axial cross-sectional image of tissues based on the optical backscatter of low-coherence laser light as it goes through the retinal layers including the NFL. The glaucoma algorithm measures NFL thickness along a circle 3.4 mm in diameter around the disc, and provides a reconstruction of the ONH. Optic nerve head parameters like cup-to-disc ratio and rim area, together with NFL measurement, can improve diagnostic accuracy for glaucoma detection using this instrument.[75] New spectral domain instruments are currently available, providing faster scans at a higher resolution.

Each of the above technologies has its merits and limitations in the diagnosis and detection of progression of POAG. The clinician should never rely solely on imaging devices to diagnose or follow up patients. Interpretation of test results is most accurate when made in light of the clinical assessment of individual patients.

TREATMENT OPTIONS AND SEQUENCING OF THERAPY

The selection of POAG treatment is usually determined by the stage of disease, the levels of IOP at which damage occurred or continues to progress, and the estimated lifetime risk of visual disability for patients. Although estimating lifetime risk remains challenging, our understanding of global risk assessment continues to evolve. The reality remains that IOP is the only risk factor currently modifiable by treatment. The IOP can be lowered by medical treatment, and laser or incisional surgery. The choice of initial therapy depends on numerous considerations that vary depending on the severity of the disease, ocular and systemic factors, as well as patient economic and lifestyle considerations. All these factors go into the decision-making process in formulating the best therapeutic strategy for an individual patient. In the USA, the majority of patients are treated with topical medications first or occasionally laser, followed by incisional treatments if therapeutic goals are unmet. The concept of maximal medical therapy continues to evolve.[76] For some patients it may represent a single, fixed combination therapy with or without a prostaglandin analogue. A full discussion of the therapeutics of glaucoma are beyond the scope of this chapter and are discussed in detail elsewhere in the book.

TARGET INTRAOCULAR PRESSURE

Establishing an upper limit of a range of IOP at which it is judged likely to retard further optic nerve damage is known as a 'target IOP.'[77] There exists no algorithm by which physicians can estimate this 'range target' below which further optic nerve damage will be prevented in any particular patient. Target IOP is usually determined based on the clinician's experience and on the knowledge of outcome data from clinical trials. It remains a largely individual, subjective process. If glaucoma progression occurs at the preset 'within target range,' then target IOP should be lowered further. Patients may progress despite achieving a very low target IOP. We must recognize there may be an IOP-independent contribution to damage in some patients.

It is helpful while choosing a target pressure to judge the severity of glaucoma on a simplified scale of mild, moderate or severe. According to the American Academy of Ophthalmology preferred practice patterns published in 2006 the severity of glaucoma can be classified as follows:

- *Mild*: characteristic optic nerve abnormalities and a normal visual field as tested with SAP.
- *Moderate*: characteristic optic nerve abnormalities and visual field abnormalities in one hemifield and not within 5 degrees of fixation.
- *Severe*: characteristic optic nerve abnormalities and visual field abnormalities in both hemifields and loss within 5 degrees of fixation in at least one hemifield.

There exists a large body of evidence supporting an initial target pressure selected at least 20% lower than the pretreatment IOP.[18,78,79] Additional reductions of the target IOP are recommended in patients with advanced disease or with rapid progression.[80]

MEDICAL TREATMENT

Topical prostaglandin analogs and β-adrenergic antagonists are the most frequently used eyedrops for initial lowering IOP in patients with glaucoma. Other agents include α_2-adrenergic agonists, topical and oral carbonic anhydrase inhibitors, and parasympathomimetics. If a drug fails to reduce IOP, it can be switched to another agent within the same pharmacologic class. Simplifying therapy helps patients avoid the burdens of complex therapeutic regimens. If a single medication is effective in lowering IOP but target pressure is not reached, combination therapy, or switching to an alternate therapy may be appropriate. Adequate medical treatment of glaucoma requires a high level of adherence to therapy.

Adherence with medical therapy Adherence is the consistent use of prescribed medications over time, while persistence is the continued use of prescribed medications over time. Adherence and persistence to treatment are vital in preventing visual loss, and subsequent loss of functioning, and quality of life.[81] Compliance is often defined as how well patients follow physicians' recommendations. In recent medical literature, less judgmental words such as 'adherence' and 'persistency' have been substituted for 'compliance' with glaucoma therapy.[82,83] Reducing the complexity of an eyedrop regimen helps to improve the compliance, adherence, and persistence with glaucoma treatment. This relationship, however, is by no means direct.

Levels of patient adherence to chronic medications are known to be variable and challenging to measure across areas of medicine.[84] Adherence studies are difficult to conduct, and are riddled with potential bias. Evidence of how different drug regimens may influence adherence is mixed. Increasing complexity of eyedrop regimens has been linked to worsening of [85,86] or no difference in adherence.[87] A review of nonadherence with glaucoma treatment found only 29 original studies and concluded that few clinically relevant guidelines could be discerned.[88] It is, however, generally accepted that simpler therapeutic regimens with less frequent dosing may be preferred by patients and could promote adherence.[49] In that sense, fixed-combination medications offer patients better convenience. If a single eyedrop from a single bottle can deliver the same efficacy as two separate drops from two separate bottles the benefit to the patient is obvious.

LASER AND INCISIONAL SURGERY

Laser may be considered as a first-line intervention in patients unable or unwilling to use medications, or in certain conditions such as pseudoexfoliation or pigmentary glaucoma where it can be very effective. Laser trabeculoplasty is often performed for additional IOP lowering. At times, it can serve as a temporizing procedure for control of IOP in eyes awaiting filtering surgery. As compared to eyes initially treated with medication, eyes initially treated with argon laser trabeculoplasty had 1.2 mmHg greater reduction in intraocular pressure.[89] Selective laser trabeculoplasty (532 nm Nd: YAG laser) appears to be as effective as argon trabeculoplasty techniques in lowering IOP.[90]

Trabeculectomy with antimetabolites is the most commonly performed incisional filtering procedure. Other surgical techniques to lower IOP include nonpenetrating glaucoma surgery and use of glaucoma drainage devices. Several sections of this textbook are dedicated to the full discussion of medical and surgical treatments of glaucoma.

SELECTED MAJOR CLINICAL TRIALS

A great deal of the current understanding of risk of progression and outcomes of treatment in POAG comes from the large prospective clinical trials supported by the National Eye Institute (http://www.nei.nih.gov). The Ocular Hypertension Treatment Study (OHTS) mainly focused on quantifying risk factors for developing POAG among ocular hypertensive subjects. Other clinical trials such as the Early Manifest Glaucoma Trial (EMGT) and the Collaborative Initial Glaucoma Treatment Study (CIGTS) studied long-term effects of treating newly diagnosed POAG patients. The Advanced Glaucoma Intervention Study (AGIS) enrolled POAG patients that were unsuccessfully controlled with medications, and assessed the long-term outcomes of different sequences of interventions involving trabeculectomy and argon laser trabeculoplasty. A summary is included in Table 26.3.

TABLE 26.3 Selected major POAG clinical trials

STUDY	GOAL	INTERVENTION	FOLLOW-UP	OUTCOME
OHTS[18]	20% IOP reduction	Medications	5 years	Probability of POAG: Treated 4.4% Untreated 9.5%
CNTGS[94]	30% IOP reduction	Medications and surgery	7 years	Glaucoma progression: Treated 12% Untreated 35%
EGMT[34]	Protocol driven	Trabeculoplasty (360°) + Betaxolol b.i.d.	5 years	POAG progression: Treated 45% Untreated 62%
CIGTS[91]	Protocol driven	Medications and surgery	4+ years	No significant difference in visual field loss between the medically and surgically treated patients
AGIS[79]	Protocol driven	Argon laser trabeculoplasty (A) and trabeculectomy (T) sequences: ATT and TAT	10 years (ongoing)	Visual function outcomes better in ATT sequence in blacks and better in TAT sequence in whites

EARLY MANIFEST GLAUCOMA TRIAL

The main purpose was to compare the effect of medical therapy to late or no treatment on the progression of newly detected POAG, and to measure the extent of IOP reduction and explore factors that may influence glaucoma progression. The EMGT was conducted in collaboration with the University of Lund in Sweden. The study was initiated with support from the Swedish Medical Research Council. Two hundred and fifty-five open-angle glaucoma patients were randomized to argon laser trabeculoplasty plus topical betaxolol or no immediate treatment (129 treated; 126 controls) and followed up every 3 months. After 6 years, 53% of patients progressed. Relative risk of progression decreased by about 10% with each millimeter of mercury of IOP reduction from baseline to the first follow-up visit (hazard ratio, 0.90 per 1 mmHg decrease; 95% CI, 0.86–0.94).[34] In a more recent analysis with a median follow-up time was 8 years (range, 0.1–11.1), 68% of the patients had progressed. Similar to the earlier findings that elevated IOP is a strong factor for glaucoma progression, the hazard ratio increased by 11% for every 1 mmHg of higher IOP (hazard ratio, 1.11; 95% CI, 1.06–1.17; $p < 0.0001$). Intraocular pressure fluctuation, however, was not related to progression (hazard ratio, 1.00; 95% CI, 0.81–1.24; $p = 0.999$).[23]

Summary

Primary open-angle glaucoma is the most prevalent of the open-angle glaucomas and a leading cause of worldwide blindness. Risk factors for the development or progression of POAG have been identified. A better understanding of risk factors may allow more targeted aggressive therapy for those patients at greatest risk of suffering visual disability. The treatment of POAG remains limited to lowering of IOP by medical, laser surgery, or incisional surgery approaches. Major clinical trials have demonstrated the benefit of IOP lowering.

The causes of primary open-angle glaucoma remain obscure. When elevated IOP is present, it seems due to increased resistance to aqueous outflow at the trabecular meshwork. Yet glaucomatous damage can occur at statistically normal IOPs and patients can tolerate elevated IOPs without glaucomatous damage. We have little understanding of the differential susceptibilities to glaucoma.

Primary open-angle glaucoma remains a challenge because the early disease is asymptomatic. Once symptoms are noticeable to the patient, the disease is usually fairly advanced. No adequate simple screening method exists. The best detection method remains the comprehensive eye evaluation. Since the damage of POAG is irreversible, eye treatment should be directed at preserving sufficient visual function to maintain quality of life.

REFERENCES

1. Quigley HA, Broman AT. The number of people with glaucoma worldwide in 2010 and 2020. Br J Ophthalmol 2006; 90:262–267.

2. World Health Organization. Magnitude and causes of visual impairment, Fact Sheet Number 282, Nov. 2004.

3. Resnikoff S, Pascolini D, Etya'ale D, et al. Global data on visual impairment in the year 2002. Bull World Health Organ 2004; 82:844–851.

4. Tielsch JM, Sommer A, Katz J, et al. Racial variations in the prevalence of primary open-angle glaucoma. The Baltimore Eye Survey. JAMA 1991; 266:369–374.

5. Mitchell P, Smith W, Attebo K, et al. Prevalence of open-angle glaucoma in Australia. The Blue Mountains Eye Study. Ophthalmology 1996; 103:1661–1669.

6. Klein BE, Klein R, Sponsel WE, et al. Prevalence of glaucoma. The Beaver Dam Eye Study. Ophthalmology 1992; 99:1499–1504.

7. Dielemans I, Vingerling JR, Wolfs RC, et al. The prevalence of primary open-angle glaucoma in a population-based study in The Netherlands. The Rotterdam Study. Ophthalmology 1994; 101:1851–1855.

8. Friedman DS, Jampel HD, Munoz B, et al. The prevalence of open-angle glaucoma among blacks and whites 73 years and older: The Salisbury Eye Evaluation Glaucoma Study. Arch Ophthalmol 2006; 124:1625–1630.

9. Fechtner RD, Khouri AS. Evolving global risk assessment of ocular hypertension to glaucoma. Curr Opin Ophthalmol 2007; 18:104–109.

10. Weinreb RN, Friedman DS, Fechtner RD, et al. Risk assessment in the management of patients with ocular hypertension. Am J Ophthalmol 2004; 138:458–467.

11. Chen PP. Risk and risk factors for blindness from glaucoma. Curr Opin Ophthalmol 2004; 15:107–111.

12. Schulzer M, Drance SM, Douglas GR. A comparison of treated and untreated glaucoma suspects. Ophthalmology 1991; 98:301–307.

13. Epstein DL, Krug JH Jr, Hertzmark E, et al. A long-term clinical trial of timolol therapy versus no treatment in the management of glaucoma suspects. Ophthalmology 1989; 96:1460–1467.

14. Cioffi GA, Liebmann JM. Translating the OHTS results into clinical practice. J Glaucoma 2002; 11:375–377.

15. Anderson DR. Collaborative Normal Tension Glaucoma Study. Curr Opin Ophthalmol 2003; 14:86–90.

16. Budenz DL, Anderson DR, Feuer WJ, et al. Detection and prognostic significance of optic disc hemorrhages during the Ocular Hypertension Treatment Study. Ophthalmology 2006; 113:2137–2143.

17. Gordon MO, Beiser JA, Brandt JD, et al. The Ocular Hypertension Treatment Study: baseline factors that predict the onset of primary open-angle glaucoma. Arch Ophthalmol 2002; 120:714–720; discussion 829–830.

18. Kass MA, Heuer DK, Higginbotham EJ, et al. The Ocular Hypertension Treatment Study: a randomized trial determines that topical ocular hypotensive medication delays or prevents the onset of primary open-angle glaucoma. Arch Ophthalmol 2002; 120:701–713; discussion 829–830.

19. Kass MA, Gordon MO, Hoff MR, et al. Topical timolol administration reduces the incidence of glaucomatous damage in ocular hypertensive individuals. A randomized, double-masked, long-term clinical trial. Arch Ophthalmol 1989; 107:1590–1598.

20. Quigley HA, Enger C, Katz J, et al. Risk factors for the development of glaucomatous visual field loss in ocular hypertension. Arch Ophthalmol 1994; 112:644–649.

21. Wilensky JT, Gieser DK, Dietsche ML, et al. Individual variability in the diurnal intraocular pressure curve. Ophthalmology 1993; 100:940–944.

22. Asrani S, Zeimer R, Wilensky J, et al. Large diurnal fluctuations in intraocular pressure are an independent risk factor in patients with glaucoma. J Glaucoma 2000; 9:134–142.

23. Bengtsson B, Leske MC, Hyman L, et al. Fluctuation of intraocular pressure and glaucoma progression in the Early Manifest Glaucoma Trial. Ophthalmology 2007; 114:205–209.

24. Martinez GS, Campbell AJ, Reinken J, et al. Prevalence of ocular disease in a population study of subjects 65 years old and older. Am J Ophthalmol 1982; 94:181–189.

25. Leske MC, Connell AM, Wu SY, et al. Risk factors for open-angle glaucoma. The Barbados Eye Study. Arch Ophthalmol 1995; 113:918–924.

26. Mukesh BN, McCarty CA, Rait JL, et al. Five-year incidence of open-angle glaucoma: the visual impairment project. Ophthalmology 2002; 109:1047–1051.

27. Leske MC, Nemesure B, He Q, et al. Patterns of open-angle glaucoma in the Barbados Family Study. Ophthalmology 2001; 108:1015–1022.

28. Sommer A, Tielsch JM, Katz J, et al. Racial differences in the cause-specific prevalence of blindness in east Baltimore. N Engl J Med 1991; 325:1412–1417.

29. Lichter PR, Musch DC, Gillespie BW, et al. Interim clinical outcomes in the Collaborative Initial Glaucoma Treatment Study comparing initial treatment randomized to medications or surgery. Ophthalmology 2001; 108:1943–1953.

30. Wu J, Hewitt AW, Green CM, et al. Disease severity of familial glaucoma compared with sporadic glaucoma. Arch Ophthalmol 2006; 124:950–954.

31. Wolfs RC, Klaver CC, Ramrattan RS, et al. Genetic risk of primary open-angle glaucoma. Population-based familial aggregation study. Arch Ophthalmol 1998; 116:1640–1645.

32. Klein BE, Klein R, Jensen SC. Open-angle glaucoma and older-onset diabetes. The Beaver Dam Eye Study. Ophthalmology 1994; 101:1173–1177.

33. Mitchell P, Smith W, Chey T, et al. Open-angle glaucoma and diabetes: the Blue Mountains Eye Study, Australia. Ophthalmology 1997; 104:712–718.

34. Leske MC, Heijl A, Hussein M, et al. Factors for glaucoma progression and the effect of treatment: the Early Manifest Glaucoma Trial. Arch Ophthalmol 2003; 121:48–56.

35. The Advanced Glaucoma Intervention Study (AGIS): 12. Baseline risk factors for sustained loss of visual field and visual acuity in patients with advanced glaucoma. Am J Ophthalmol 2002; 134:499–512.

36. Tielsch JM, Katz J, Quigley HA, et al. Diabetes, intraocular pressure, and primary open-angle glaucoma in the Baltimore Eye Survey. Ophthalmology 1995; 102:48–53.

37. Gordon MO, Torri V, Miglior S, et al. Validated prediction model for the development of primary open-angle glaucoma in individuals with ocular hypertension. Ophthalmology 2007; 114:10–19.

38. Lee AJ, Wang JJ, Kifley A, et al. Open-angle glaucoma and cardiovascular mortality: the Blue Mountains Eye Study. Ophthalmology 2006; 113:1069–1076.

39. Leighton DA, Phillips CI. Systemic blood pressure in open-angle glaucoma, low tension glaucoma, and the normal eye. Br J Ophthalmol 1972; 56:447–453.

40. Kahn HA, Leibowitz HM, Ganley JP, et al. The Framingham Eye Study. II. Association of ophthalmic pathology with single variables previously measured in the Framingham Heart Study. Am J Epidemiol 1977; 106:33–41.

41. Tielsch JM, Katz J, Sommer A, et al. Hypertension, perfusion pressure, and primary open-angle glaucoma. A population-based assessment. Arch Ophthalmol 1995; 113:216–221.

42. Perkins ES, Phelps CD. Open angle glaucoma, ocular hypertension, low-tension glaucoma, and refraction. Arch Ophthalmol 1982; 100:1464–1467.

43. Xu L, Wang Y, Wang S, et al. High myopia and glaucoma susceptibility. The Beijing Eye Study. Ophthalmology 2007; 114:216–220.

44. Drance S, Anderson DR, Schulzer M. Risk factors for progression of visual field abnormalities in normal-tension glaucoma. Am J Ophthalmol 2001; 131:699–708.

45. Fechtner RD, Weinreb RN. Mechanisms of optic nerve damage in primary open angle glaucoma. Surv Ophthalmol 1994; 39:23–42.

46. Finkelstein I, Trope GE, Basu PK, et al. Quantitative analysis of collagen content and amino acids in trabecular meshwork. Br J Ophthalmol 1990; 74:280–282.

47. Rohen JW, Lutjen-Drecoll E, Flugel C, et al. Ultrastructure of the trabecular meshwork in untreated cases of primary open-angle glaucoma (POAG). Exp Eye Res 1993; 56:683–692.

48. Moses RA, Grodzki WJ Jr, Etheridge EL, et al. Schlemm's canal: the effect of intraocular pressure. Invest Ophthalmol Vis Sci 1981; 20:61–68.

49. Buller C, Johnson D. Segmental variability of the trabecular meshwork in normal and glaucomatous eyes. Invest Ophthalmol Vis Sci 1994; 35:3841–3851.

50. Johnstone MA. The aqueous outflow system as a mechanical pump: evidence from examination of tissue and aqueous movement in human and non-human primates. J Glaucoma 2004; 13:421–438.

51. Lander ES, Linton LM, Birren B, et al. Initial sequencing and analysis of the human genome. Nature 2001; 409:860–921.

52. Venter JC, Adams MD, Myers EW, et al. The sequence of the human genome. Science 2001; 291:1304–1351.

53. Hyman L, Klein B, Nemesure B, et al. Ophthalmic genetics: at the dawn of discovery. Arch Ophthalmol 2007; 125:9–10.

54. Pasquale LR. Genes involved in the pathogenesis of primary open-angle glaucoma: in search of the Holy Grail. JAMA 2007; 297:306–307.

55. Fingert JH, Stone EM, Sheffield VC, et al. Myocilin glaucoma. Surv Ophthalmol 2002; 47:547–561.

56. Alward WL, Kwon YH, Kawase K, et al. Evaluation of optineurin sequence variations in 1,048 patients with open-angle glaucoma. Am J Ophthalmol 2003; 136:904–910.

57. Alward WL, Kwon YH, Khanna CL, et al. Variations in the myocilin gene in patients with open-angle glaucoma. Arch Ophthalmol 2002; 120:1189–1197.

58. Duggal P, Klein AP, Lee KE, et al. Identification of novel genetic loci for intraocular pressure: a genomewide scan of the Beaver Dam Eye Study. Arch Ophthalmol 2007; 125:74–79.

59. Quigley HA, Addicks EM, Green WR. Optic nerve damage in human glaucoma. III. Quantitative correlation of nerve fiber loss and visual field defect in glaucoma, ischemic neuropathy, papilledema, and toxic neuropathy. Arch Ophthalmol 1982; 100:135–146.

60. Sommer A, Katz J, Quigley HA, et al. Clinically detectable nerve fiber atrophy precedes the onset of glaucomatous field loss. Arch Ophthalmol 1991; 109:77–83.

61. Fingeret M, Medeiros FA, Susanna R Jr, et al. Five rules to evaluate the optic disc and retinal nerve fiber layer for glaucoma. Optometry 2005; 76:661–668.

62. Bengtsson B. Optic disc haemorrhages preceding manifest glaucoma. Acta Ophthalmol (Copenh) 1990; 68:450–454.

63. Drance SM. Disc hemorrhages in the glaucomas. Surv Ophthalmol 1989; 33:331–337.

64. Delgado MF, Nguyen NT, Cox TA, et al. Automated perimetry: a report by the American Academy of Ophthalmology. Ophthalmology 2002; 109:2362–2374.

65. Lichter PR. Variability of expert observers in evaluating the optic disc. Trans Am Ophthalmol Soc 1976; 74:532–572.

66. Zeyen T, Miglior S, Pfeiffer N, et al. Reproducibility of evaluation of optic disc change for glaucoma with stereo optic disc photographs. Ophthalmology 2003; 110:340–344.

67. Khouri AS, Szirth B, Realini T, et al. Comparison of digital and film stereo photography of the optic nerve in the evaluation of patients with glaucoma. Telemed J E Health 2006; 12:632–638.

68. Khouri A, Szirth B, Salti H, et al. DICOM transmission of simultaneous stereoscopic images of the optic nerve in patient with glaucoma. J Telemed Telecare 2007; 13:337–340.

69. B. Szirth, A. Khouri, K. Shahid, et al. New concepts in screening for vision threatening disease, ARVO abstract #1578, 2007.

70. Khouri A, Szirth B, Shahid K, et al. Software assisted optic nerve assessment for glaucoma screening. ARVO abstract #2767, 2007.

71. Medeiros FA, Zangwill LM, Bowd C, et al. Comparison of scanning laser polarimetry using variable corneal compensation and retinal nerve fiber layer photography for detection of glaucoma. Arch Ophthalmol 2004; 122:698–704.

72. Reus NJ, Lemij HG. The relationship between standard automated perimetry and GDx VCC measurements. Invest Ophthalmol Vis Sci 2004; 45:840–845.

73. Khouri AS, Fechtner RD, Murray F. Heidelberg retina tomography.In: Tasman W, Jaeger E, eds. Duane's ophthalmology solution. New York: Lippincott Williams & Wilkins; 2008 (www.duanessolution.com).

74. Zangwill LM, Weinreb RN, Beiser JA, et al. Baseline topographic optic disc measurements are associated with the development of primary open-angle glaucoma: the Confocal Scanning Laser Ophthalmoscopy Ancillary Study to the Ocular Hypertension Treatment Study. Arch Ophthalmol 2005; 123:1188–1197.

75. Medeiros FA, Zangwill LM, Bowd C, et al. Evaluation of retinal nerve fiber layer, optic nerve head, and macular thickness measurements for glaucoma detection using optical coherence tomography. Am J Ophthalmol 2005; 139:44–55.

76. Fechtner RD, Singh K. Maximal glaucoma therapy. J Glaucoma 2001; 10:S73–S75.

77. Jampel HD. Target pressure in glaucoma therapy. J Glaucoma 1997; 6:133–138.

78. The Advanced Glaucoma Intervention Study (AGIS): 7. The relationship between control of intraocular pressure and visual field deterioration. The AGIS Investigators. Am J Ophthalmol 2000; 130:429–440.

79. Ederer F, Gaasterland DA, Dally LG, et al. The Advanced Glaucoma Intervention Study (AGIS): 13. Comparison of treatment outcomes within race: 10-year results. Ophthalmology 2004; 111:651–664.

80. Leskea MC, Heijl A, Hyman L, et al. Factors for progression and glaucoma treatment: the Early Manifest Glaucoma Trial. Curr Opin Ophthalmol 2004; 15:102–106.

81. Lee PP. Patient perspectives in glaucoma care: introduction to the American Journal of Ophthalmology Supplement. Am J Ophthalmol 2006; 141:S1–S2.

82. Tilson HH. Adherence or compliance? Changes in terminology. Ann Pharmacother 2004; 38:161–162.

83. Schwartz GF. Compliance and persistency in glaucoma follow-up treatment. Curr Opin Ophthalmol 2005; 16:114–121.

84. McDonald HP, Garg AX, Haynes RB. Interventions to enhance patient adherence to medication prescriptions: scientific review. JAMA 2002; 288:2868–2879.

85. Konstas AG, Maskaleris G, Gratsonidis S, et al. Compliance and viewpoint of glaucoma patients in Greece. Eye 2000; 14(Pt 5):752–756.

86. Patel KH, Javitt JC, Tielsch JM, et al. Incidence of acute angle-closure glaucoma after pharmacologic mydriasis. Am J Ophthalmol 1995; 120:709–717.

87. Kass MA, Gordon M, Morley RE Jr, et al. Compliance with topical timolol treatment. Am J Ophthalmol 1987; 103:188–193.

88. Olthoff CM, Schouten JS, van de Borne BW, et al. Noncompliance with ocular hypotensive treatment in patients with glaucoma or ocular hypertension: an evidence-based review. Ophthalmology 2005; 112:953–961.

89. The Glaucoma Laser Trial (GLT) and glaucoma laser trial follow-up study: 7. Results. Glaucoma Laser Trial Research Group. Am J Ophthalmol 2000; 130:429–440.

90. Damji KF, Shah KC, Rock WJ, et al. Selective laser trabeculoplasty v argon laser trabeculoplasty: a prospective randomised clinical trial. Br J Ophthalmol 1999; 83:718–722.

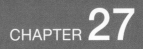

Primary Angle-Closure Glaucoma

Paul Foster and Sancy Low

INTRODUCTION

Glaucomatous optic neuropathy is the world's leading cause of irreversible blindness. Half of all cases blinded by glaucoma are affected by primary angle closure. The numerical importance of the condition has not been matched by proportionate clinical or research attention until recently. Efforts to understand the etiology and natural history and to develop effective management strategies have been hindered by the widespread use of a classification system that places great emphasis on the presence or absence of symptoms caused by dramatic fluctuations in intraocular pressure (IOP). Over the last decade, growing research interest in this condition has prompted a careful reexamination of the purposes that a classification system should serve, and whether these purposes had been well served by the traditional classification system. A key recognition, resulting directly from population-based research in South Africa, Taiwan, and Mongolia, has been that the majority of cases of angle-closure glaucoma suffer severe loss of vision without an 'acute' attack. This fact is vital to understanding how the disease should be detected and managed. However, there is undue emphasis on 'acute' symptomatic attacks, and the continuing propagation in textbooks of the message that acute angle closure is the most important manifestation of the disease. While acute attacks are an extremely unpleasant (but transient) manifestation of a sudden rise in IOP, and they do cause permanent loss of vision in some people (particularly if appropriate medical care is not immediately available), it is becoming apparent that the majority of people who suffer severe loss of vision from angle-closure glaucoma never experience acute symptoms.

Primary angle-closure glaucoma (PACG) is actually a secondary glaucoma. The glaucomatous optic neuropathy occurs as a direct consequence of elevated IOP caused by physical obstruction of aqueous outflow, or degenerative changes in the trabecular meshwork, resulting from iridotrabecular contact (ITC). It is this ITC which is the primary event, occurring as the result of anatomical disproportion of the anterior segment, whereas secondary angle closure most often occurs as a consequence of uveitis, iris neovascularization or iatrogenic misadventure. The most widely recognized anatomical characteristic associated with a PACG is a shallow anterior chamber. Other biometric characteristics of a crowded anterior segment are typically present. Iridotrabecular contact is a physical, anatomical phenomenon that directly affects ocular physiology. The anatomical characteristics of PACG have led many to believe that it is possible to screen either whole populations, or high-risk demographic subgroup populations, for those with an anatomical predisposition toward severe, sight-threatening disease, and to offer preventive treatment. Research is underway in Mongolia, Singapore, and China to examine the viability of this strategy.

Surgical iridectomy is the oldest surgical intervention targeted at glaucoma. It has been credited to von Graefe in 1857. The advent of argon and (later) YAG lasers has transformed an effective invasive procedure into a noninvasive, 'office' technique with minimal side effects. Iridectomy and iridotomy are highly effective techniques for treating pupil-block angle closure prior to the onset of irreversible trabecular meshwork damage. Pupil block is a major component responsible for angle closure in around 75% of cases. In others, anterior nonpupil-block mechanisms such as plateau iris and peripheral iris crowding play the predominant role. In these cases, laser iridoplasty or topical pilocarpine can be helpful in managing the condition. Lens-induced and ciliolenticular block are less common mechanisms. In both, pharmacological dilation of the pupil and lens extraction are appropriate initial treatments. Ultimately, in all cases, IOP control is the primary goal, with the aim of safeguarding visual function from glaucomatous optic neuropathy. Medical therapy of the types in widespread use for management of primary open-angle glaucoma (prostaglandin analogues, β-blockers, α-agonists, and carbonic anhydrase inhibitors) should be considered, once all practical steps to open the drainage angle have been taken. However, surgical intervention is often required in more advanced cases, by trabeculectomy, tube implant (in eyes rendered aphakic or pseudophakic) or cyclodestruction. Anecdotally, trabeculectomy in angle closure is prone to higher complication rates than in open-angle glaucoma cases. Of particular concern is the possibility of aqueous misdirection. However, modern surgical techniques, employing antimetabolites and an initially water-tight closure with releasable or adjustable sutures, have helped make this an unlikely event in the majority of cases.

The number of people affected in nonindustrialized nations, without access to sophisticated healthcare resources necessary for curative treatment, raises the issue of preventive management in the form of opportunistic or structured screening. This offers probably the greatest opportunity of making a significant reduction in blindness worldwide in the foreseeable future. However, it is important that hospital and clinic staff and services are developed in parallel. Gonioscopy is a key diagnostic skill in detection and management of PACG, and its mastery is something that all ophthalmologists should aspire to.

DEFINITION AND CLASSIFICATION

Approaches to classification of glaucoma vary according to the intended purpose. The most widely employed system identifies both etiology and mechanism, identifying adult glaucoma as either occurring secondary to another ocular or systemic pathology, or being primary, and whether closure of the drainage angle is present or not. This system is both logical and appropriate for clinical and research purposes. However, a solid evidence base for determining the division between angle-closure and open-angle mechanisms has been lacking. If gonioscopy reveals a narrow but open angle, the default approach is to assume an asymptomatic patient has an open-angle mechanism. As primary open-angle glaucoma is a diagnosis of exclusion, this is a mistake. It has been shown that the epidemiological threshold used to allocate a diagnosis of angle closure (an 'occludable' angle defined as one in which the posterior trabecular meshwork is hidden from view for three-quarters or more of the angle circumference) is heavily biased away from allocating a diagnosis of angle closure.[1]

There are several different approaches to the classification of angle closure, including the use of mechanisms, symptoms, or a staging approach. Of these, the most widely emphasized in educational media (and the most widely used in clinical practice) is that addressing the presence or absence of symptoms. Termed 'acute' and 'chronic', respectively, these cardinal forms of angle closure are often combined with subacute or intermittent to indicate self-aborting or remitting symptoms. Cases in which gonioscopic evidence (i.e. synechiae) or inducible pressure rises (a positive provocative test) is present are termed latent angle closure. Many have seen these forms of disease as analogous to a diagnosis of glaucoma, regardless of the presence or absence of an optic neuropathy. In fact, there is no evidence to link one of these subtypes with a particular prognosis or a significant risk of visual dysfunction. What is known is that once an individual has had an acute episode in one eye, the contralateral fellow is at high risk of a similar

TABLE 27.1 Conceptual stages in the natural history of primary angle-closure glaucoma

STAGE	DEFINITION
Primary angle-closure suspect	Iridotrabecular contact (ITC) with normal optic disc and visual field. IOP is normal and PAS are absent. Symptoms are absent
Primary angle closure	ITC + either raised IOP, PAS, or typical symptoms
Primary angle-closure glaucoma	ITC + structural glaucomatous changes in the optic nerve + visual field loss

episode. This observation, together with the fact that 'acute' angle closure causes transient but florid symptoms, is often subconsciously taken as justification for assuming that symptomatic forms of the disease are more serious than chronic, asymptomatic presentations. It is now emerging that the reverse may be true, with acute cases presenting in a relatively timely fashion for treatment, while asymptomatic angle closure typically presents later, with advanced loss of vision in at least one eye.[2] These facts have led to the suggestion that a symptom-based classification system is inappropriate, as it does not help to indicate prognosis or determine an appropriate strategy for management.

An alternative approach, based on the natural history of angle closure, identifies three conceptual stages of the disease. This is outlined in Table 27.1.

PREVALENCE, INCIDENCE, AND GEOGRAPHICAL VARIATION

INCIDENCE

Incidence is the rate of occurrence of new disease, and is a good index of the burden of transient manifestations of disease, where symptoms are short-lived, such as the acute form of angle closure. In this context it is expressed as cases/100 000 people/year, and is usually given for the population aged 30 years and older. Prevalence denotes the proportion of people affected at a specific point in time, and is a more appropriate measure of chronic, incurable disease, such as glaucomatous optic neuropathy. The incidence of symptomatic ('acute') angle closure has been studied in several countries: Finland,[3] Croatia,[4] Japan,[5] Israel,[6] Thailand,[5] Singapore,[7,8] and Hong Kong.[9] Age and gender standardized incidence ranges from 4.7 in Finland to 15.5 among Chinese Singaporeans. This is illustrated graphically in Figure 27.1, showing East Asian people (Japanese and Chinese from Singapore and Hong Kong) having the highest rates. Indian, Thai, and Malay people suffer less symptomatic angle closure.[5,8] European people have the lowest recorded rate of disease.[3,4] It is a recurring theme in these studies that older age and female gender are risk factors for 'acute' angle closure.

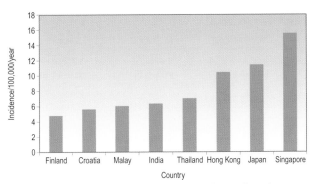

FIGURE 27.1 The incidence of symptomatic ('acute') angle closure in Finland,[3] Croatia,[4] Japan,[5] Israel,[6] Thailand,[5] Singapore,[7,8] and Hong Kong,[9] expressed as age and gender standardized incidence ranges from 4.7 in Finland to 15.5/100 000 people/year among Chinese Singaporeans. Figures relate to the population aged 40 years and older.

Data on the rate of progression from one category of disease to another (e.g. incidence of glaucomatous optic neuropathy in angle-closure cases) are scarce. One study in Greenland Inuits identified a 16% incidence of angle closure over a decade in high-risk suspects. Of the 12 incident cases, 10 were women.[10] Another study in southern India followed subjects enrolled in a population-based prevalence study 5 years after the original survey. This has provided important data on the natural history of angle closure. Among the people with narrow drainage angles, 22% had developed synechial or appositional angle closure (in a ratio of 2:1, respectively).[11] People with established angle closure when initially examined were advised to undergo laser iridotomy. Eight of 28 people examined had developed glaucomatous optic neuropathy over the 5-year follow-up period. One of 9 (11%) who underwent LPI progressed, compared to 7 of 19 (37%) who refused LPI.[12]

SYMPTOMS OF ANGLE CLOSURE

When interpreting the incidence data above, it is important to recognize that the majority are identified following a symptomatic episode. Symptoms of a sudden pressure rise are assumed to be so dramatic that the affected individual will immediately seek a medical opinion. However, in Singapore the median time to presentation was found to be 3 days, with some people waiting over 3 months.[7] This, coupled with the fact that in Asian populations only 25–40% of all cases of angle closure ever recall symptoms that accompany acute pressure spikes,[13–15] means that the figures from incidence studies probably represent less than a quarter of the incidence of primary angle closure. It is probable, but as yet unproven, that the same situation exists among European people.

The received wisdom is that symptomatic 'acute' angle closure is rapidly blinding. However, accounts of visual prognosis in those suffering a symptomatic episode of PACG suggest that 60–75% recover without any optic disc or visual field damage.[16–18] One retrospective study of IOP control following symptomatic angle closure in Singaporeans showed that 42% were successfully treated by laser iridotomy alone. The remaining 58% required additional treatment; 33% underwent trabeculectomy.[19] This may indicate that the prognosis may be less optimistic when measured in years instead of months. However, in a study of European people living in Rochester, Minnesota, the probability of becoming blind in one eye from PACG was 4% after 5 years among patients not blind at diagnosis.[20] What is becoming clear is that with prompt, appropriate management, the symptomatic phase of the disease will not necessarily result in catastrophic visual loss. The real challenge to preventing blindness lies in identifying and effectively managing the asymptomatic 'chronic' form of angle closure.

PREVALENCE

As with incidence data, angle closure (with or without glaucomatous optic neuropathy) is not commonly recognized as a major problem in European people. Studies suggest a prevalence of around 0.1% in people aged 40 years and older.[21–23] Although not published, the Baltimore Eye Study found a prevalence of 0.4% among white residents aged 40 years and older (Tielsch, personal communication). A population-based study in northern Italy has recently found a somewhat higher prevalence of 0.6%.[24] However, this study in a rather isolated Italian village may not be wholly representative of the general population of Italy. Similarly in Africa, angle closure is regarded as uncommon.[25] However, the heterogeneity of the continent's population means that sweeping generalizations about patterns of disease will be incorrect. In the Republic of South Africa, for instance, angle closure is rare in Zulus, whereas in the black population of the Temba region a prevalence of angle closure with glaucoma of 0.5% was found.[26] Among the Cape-Malay people, a group with mixed Southeast Asian, European, and African origins, angle closure (±glaucoma) was found in 2.3% of people over the age of 40.[27] Angle closure among African people is asymptomatic in more than 68% of cases.[28]

Among Asian people prevalence rates of primary angle closure (PAC) are relatively high. Table 27.2 gives prevalence of occludable drainage angles, PAC, and PACG for populations of Singapore, Mongolia, Japan, and China. In Mongolia, 91% of glaucoma cases were previously undiagnosed, whereas in Guangzhou, China, and Singapore, 57% and 79%, respectively, of cases of PACG had been diagnosed before.

Implications for China China seems to suffer a large burden of disease. With a population currently in excess of 1 billion people, this means the numbers affected will inevitably be large. However, until recently, population-based prevalence data for glaucoma in China was limited and of variable quality.[29,30] Using data from Mongolia and Singapore to make a cautious extrapolation to China, it has been estimated that 9.4 million people aged 40 years and older have glaucomatous optic neuropathy. The same study suggested that

TABLE 27.2 Primary angle-closure glaucoma prevalence in East Asian nations

	JAPAN	SINGAPORE	MONGOLIA	CHINA**
Occludable angles	*	6.3% (4.9–7.6)	6.4% (4.3–8.5)	10.2% (8.6–11.8)
PAC	1.3% (0.9–1.7)	2.2% (1.4–3.1)	2.0% (1.3–3.1)	2.4% (1.6–3.1)
PACG	0.6% (0.4–0.9)	0.8% (0.4–1.2)	0.8% (0.4–1.7)	1.5% (0.9–2.1)
% glaucoma cases blind in at least 1 eye	5%	50%	75%	43%

95% confidence intervals given in brackets. Figures for occludable angles includes PAC and PACG. Figures for PAC includes those with PACG.
*Gonioscopy was not performed on all subjects.
**Subjects aged 50 years and older. All other figures relate to people aged ≥40 years.

approximately 5.2 million people (55%) would be blind in at least one eye, and around 1.7 million (18.1%) would be blind in both eyes.[30] It is likely that PACG is responsible for the vast majority (91%) of bilateral glaucoma blindness in China. Around 28 million people have the anatomical trait predisposing to PACG (a narrow drainage angle), and of these 9 million have significant angle closure, indicated by peripheral anterior synechiae or raised intraocular pressure.[31]

Prevalence in India While PACG is acknowledged as a major cause of ocular morbidity in Chinese populations, the situation for people living on the Indian subcontinent is less clear. It has been widely believed that PACG is more common than in European people.[32] However, two recent population surveys have provided conflicting data. In Vellore, southern India, the prevalence of PACG was 4.3% among people aged 30 to 60 years. All the PACG cases detected were of the chronic type, making PACG about five times as common as POAG.[33] However, in neighboring Hyderabad, PACG and occludable angles without glaucoma were found with prevalence of 0.7% and 1.4%, respectively, in participants 30 years of age or older. The prevalence of these two conditions considered together increased significantly with age. Only 33% of PACG had been previously diagnosed, and only one of 12 (8%) had a peripheral iridotomy. PACG had caused blindness in at least one eye of 42%. Most (83%) of those with PACG had the chronic form of the disease.[34] The difference in prevalence of PACG between the people for Hyderabad and Vellore may, in part, be explicable on the grounds of differing definitions, although it seems unlikely that this is the sole reason. What can be gleaned from these studies is that PACG is probably more common in India than in European people and, as in the rest of Asia, has a tendency to be asymptomatic. Further data from India, using standardized definitions, would be helpful in verifying the results of these two projects.

ETIOLOGY AND MECHANISM

Primary angle closure is the result of physical crowding of the anterior segment, and the resultant contact between iris and trabecular meshwork (TM) may eventually cause an elevation in intraocular pressure (IOP) by various mechanisms. There are probably at least three conceptual routes to elevated IOP. First total physical obstruction of the trabecular meshwork by the iris will rapidly cause the IOP to rise. This is probably the precipitating event in symptomatic (acute) angle closure. In this context, iridotrabecular contact (ITC) has not occurred acutely; it will doubtless have been present for many years beforehand. The number of people with ITC in a population far exceeds the number suffering 'acute' episodes, or developing glaucomatous optic neuropathy. Hence the terms 'total' or 'symptomatic' angle closure are more accurate.

Secondly, prolonged appositional ITC, or an episode of anterior segment inflammation (such as may occur with a symptomatic episode of angle closure), may cause the formation of synechial scars between iris and trabecular meshwork, in turn physically obstructing aqueous outflow. From longitudinal studies in India, it appears that both appositional closure (probably causing intermittent pressure spikes) and permanent synechial closure are capable of impairing aqueous outflow sufficient to cause glaucomatous optic neuropathy.[12]

A third possible mechanism exists by which ITC may reduce aqueous outflow. Intermittent frictional contact between iris and TM over prolonged periods probably degrades TM architecture and, eventually, function. A hint that this may be the case is given by another study from India in which histological specimens of trabecular meshwork were harvested during trabeculectomy surgery. Not surprisingly, in cases that had suffered an acute, symptomatic attack, the trabecular meshwork was distorted, with free blood and pigment in the meshwork. However, more surprisingly, in cases of asymptomatic disease, similarly gross changes in TM architecture were seen. These were present in areas where peripheral anterior synechiae (PAS) had formed, but crucially, they also existed in areas without PAS. These observations point toward low-grade ITC being sufficient to cause TM functional degradation.[35]

The mechanisms which cause ITC to occur can be visualized as being of four different categories, each one acting at a progressively more posterior location than the previous. Undoubtedly, the major mechanism acting in primary angle closure is pupil block. Although the microanatomical basis of pupil block is debated, it is widely regarded that it is the result of simultaneous activation of the dilator and sphincter pupillae muscles. This produces a resultant force whose vector lies more or less perpendicular to the lens surface when the pupil is in the mid-dilated position. This theory is the anatomical basis for the pharmacological provocation test proposed by Mapstone, using topical pilocarpine and phenylephrine to induce pressure rises in angle-closure suspects.[36] The other mechanisms, in anatomical order, are anterior non-pupil block (also called plateau iris), lens induced and retrolenticular forces. The latter two are generally seen as secondary processes occurring as the result of changes in size or position of the lens, or as the result of a posterior segment mass effect caused by a large vitreous hemorrhage or iatrogenic causes such as a gas tamponade. The most widely misunderstood mechanism is that of the anterior non-pupil block, which includes the plateau iris form of angle closure. Publications based on ultrasound biomicroscopy imaging of the iridociliary and the lens equatorial sulcii suggest that the plateau iris phenomenon is caused by anteriorly positioned ciliary processes that result in an angulated profile in the peripheral iris and a narrow angle that fails to open after an iridotomy has been performed (Fig. 27.2).[37] However, this is an oversimplication. More detailed analysis of cases of ITC which did not have an increase in angle width after laser iridotomy reveal multiple characteristics of the iridotrabecular angle that are associated with a poor response to PI, including an especially narrow angle, a thicker iris with a more anterior insertion of iris into ciliary body, as well as more anteriorly positioned ciliary processes.[38] These latter findings may offer a means of predicting which cases will benefit from laser iridotomy, and which will not.

In the context of symptomatic angle closure, it is not uncommon for there to be an external precipitating event which triggers total closure of an anatomically narrow angle, and a subsequent pressure rise. The most commonly recognized scenario in which this might occur is pharmacological mydriasis for diagnostic or therapeutic purposes. Incidence of symptomatic PAC shows significant seasonal variation, and is highest at times of extremes of temperature.[3,6,7,39,40] It has been suggested that periods of unpleasant weather encourage people to stay indoors, and results in a 'city-wide darkroom provocation test.'

An association between incidence of symptomatic PAC and the number of sunspots over the preceding month has been described.[7,41] There is an acknowledged connection between number of sunspots and terrestrial weather conditions. Sunspots are related to variations in the amount of electromagnetic and charged-particle radiation emitted by the sun, which drives the earth's 'climatic engine' in the upper atmosphere. Temperatures in tropical regions correlate positively with sunspot numbers.

Oral and nebulized medication is linked with the onset of symptomatic angle closure. These agents tend to exert their effects by acting with sympathetic or parasympathetic arms of the autonomic system, either locally or systemically. Such agents include nebulized ipratropium bromide and salbutamol.[42] Tricyclic antidepressants (such as amitriptyline and imipramine) are associated with angle closure largely through mydriasis of susceptible patients' pupils, mediated by an antimuscarinic effect.[43] Paroxetine is a selective serotonin reuptake inhibitor (SSRI) with a weak antimuscarinic effect, and is also linked with angle closure.[44] Bilateral angle closure has also been reported after use of citalopram (an SSRI with antimuscarinic and serotonergic action).[45] Anticholinergics in the treatment of bladder instability can cause angle closure,[46] as can proprietary cold and flu remedies.[9] However, pharmacological mydriasis for diagnostic or therapeutic purpose is probably the most commonly recognized precipitating event.

RISK FACTORS

DEMOGRAPHIC FACTORS

Older age, female sex, and Asian parentage are well recognized as risk factors for angle closure. The Singapore Island-wide incidence study quantified these risks: female sex (relative risk [RR] = 2.4), Chinese ethnic origin (RR = 2.8), and age of 60 years or over (RR = 9.1).[7] All these factors can be explained by trends in ocular biometry.

Ocular biometry
Axial length of the globe Using ultrasound biometry, Lowe confirmed that people suffering angle closure had shorter axial lengths than did unaffected people.[47] In a study of Chinese people, those suffering 'acute' angle closure were found to have shorter axial lengths than those affected by asymptomatic angle closure. Both groups had shorter axial lengths than people judged normal.[48] Similarly, in India, a study of the ocular dimensions in groups of people with acute, subacute, and chronic angle closure found that all groups of people with angle closure had shorter axial lengths than age- and gender-matched controls.[49]

Anterior chamber depth A shallow anterior chamber is the major risk factor for development of angle closure. The demographic risk factors (increasing age, female gender, and Chinese ethnicity) are all associated with shallower anterior chambers. Women have shallower anterior chambers than men. One study in Inuits (M > F by 0.16 mm) found this difference to be highly significant.[50] In Mongolian people, a significantly shallower anterior chamber depth (ACD) in women was also identified, although the magnitude of the difference varied with age.[51] In all populations studied to date, people who have angle closure tend to have shallower anterior chambers than those who are not

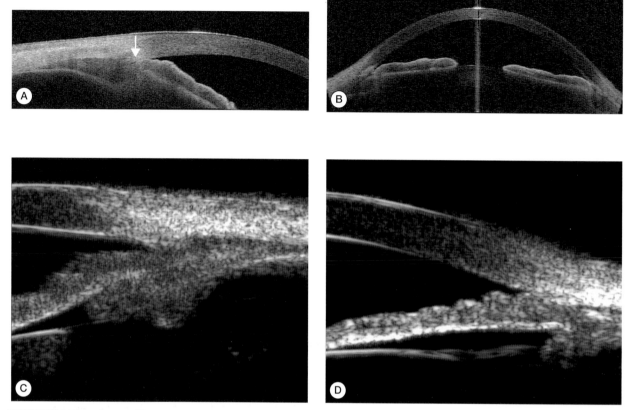

FIGURE 27.2 These images illustrate eyes with plateau iris configuration and angle closure. For an eye with plateau iris configuration to have clinically significant angle closure, manifest iridotrabecular contact (ITC) needs to be present, or judged to be occurring intermittently. **(A)** This high-resolution anterior segment optical coherence tomography (AS-OCT) image taken on eccentric fixation shows iridotrabecular contact anterior to the scleral spur (*arrow*). Note the angulation in the peripheral third of the iris, just proximal to its insertion. The plane of the iris, best assessed using the more reflective white line of the iris pigment epithelium, is flat, indicating an absence of pupil block. **(B)** This AS-OCT image shows a cross-section of the anterior chamber in the horizontal meridian of the same eye as shown in **(A)**. There is a slight prominence of the last iris roll, which is a sign frequently observed on gonioscopy in patients with residual ITC after a laser iridotomy. **(C)** Ultrasound biomicroscopy (UBM) image shows an eye in which a laser iridotomy has alleviated pupil block and produced an open angle. However, a very bulky ciliary process can be seen in contact with the posterior surface of the iris. Closure of the iridociliary sulcus is the anatomical hallmark of plateau iris, and is a common cause of failure of a laser iridotomy to open an appositionally closed angle. **(D)** This UBM image shows an example in which laser iridotomy fails to open the drainage angle. The flat contour of the iris pigment epithelium shows that there is no longer any element of pupil block. However, the iris lying immediately adjacent to the trabecular meshwork is almost twice as thick as the more axial iris. In addition, the iris inserts into the anterior scleral surface of the ciliary body. The very thick iris and very anterior insertion are the cause of residual ITC in this case, as the iridociliary sulcus is open. This is a variant of nonpupil-block angle closure which has a different mechanism from 'typical' plateau iris in which the iridociliary sulcus is closed.

affected.[50,51] As a generalization, racial groups that suffer high rates of angle closure tend to have shallower mean ACDs than those which are less severely affected.[51] However, this view is not universally accepted, and it is suggested that other ocular biometric parameters should be sought to explain the excess of PACG in Chinese people.[52] This discrepancy may be explained by the fact that the studies comparing risk of angle closure in different populations studied axial (central) anterior chamber depth only. The depth of the anterior chamber at the limbus is probably a stronger indicator of risk of angle closure than axial ACD. The limbal ACD is most often assessed using the van Herick technique (Fig. 27.3), in which a narrow beam of light is directed perpendicularly at the temporal limbus, and the depth of the most peripheral part of the anterior chamber graded as a fraction of the adjacent corneal thickness.[53] A narrower van Herick grade is a reliable indicator of the width of the angle on gonioscopy.[54]

Lens position and thickness The position and thickness of the lens determines the depth of the anterior chamber. Therefore, these factors are important in determining the risk of angle closure. Lowe developed an index of relative lens position (RLP), calculated as follows:

Relative lens position = anterior chamber depth + 1/2 (lens thickness) axial length.

He found ACD was 1.0 mm shallower in the group with angle closure compared with normal subjects. It was calculated that 66% of this difference was explained by a more anterior position of the lens, and

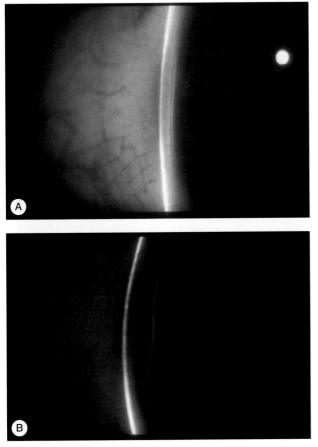

FIGURE 27.3 These color photographs illustrate the van Herick technique of estimating limbal anterior chamber depth at the temporal limbus. A very narrow beam of light is directed perpendicular to the surface of the eye at the temporal limbus. **(A)** A very shallow anterior chamber, approximately 5% of the adjacent peripheral cornea. This eye had a very narrow angle with some iridotrabecular contact. **(B)** An eye with a very deep anterior chamber, nearly twice that of corneal thickness. This eye had a very wide open drainage angle.

33% was attributable to the lens being thicker than normal. Among the same group of patients, eyes with PAC had a significantly shorter axial length than normal eyes. Furthermore, normal eyes showed an inverse relationship between axial length and lens thickness. This finding was not reproduced in eyes with PAC. It was concluded that less coordinated development of the intraocular anatomy was a feature of eyes with PAC.[55] Another anatomic trait thought to be associated with PAC is curvature of the anterior lens surface. In Europeans, there is a close correlation between thickness of the lens and anterior curvature of the lens, and an inverse correlation between axial length of the globe and lens curvature. The lens became more steeply curved with advancing age.[56]

REFRACTIVE ERROR AND ANGLE CLOSURE

While PACG shows a predilection for hypermetropic eyes, this is not an invariable association.[57] Current data on Singaporean people with occludable drainage angles shows that 41 had a hypermetropic refraction in their right eye, 15 were myopic, and 9 emmetropic. When considering people with PAS, the figures were 24 hypermetropes, 16 myopes, and 8 emmetropes. In Australia, Lowe found that 7/127 eyes with PACG had a myopic refraction (5.5%), 42 were emmetropic (33%), and 78 were hypermetropic (61.4%).[57] The data from Singapore suggest 23% of people graded as having an occludable angle, and 33% of those with PAS had a myopic refraction.

DIAGNOSIS, DIFFERENTIAL, AND TESTING

In making the diagnosis and planning management, the key questions are, firstly, deciding whether pathological angle closure is present, has previously occurred, or could occur in the future. Secondly, if any of these situations are present, it is important to determine why the angle is anatomically narrow, whether this has damaged any ocular tissues, and whether this damage constitutes a threat to vision.

The 'reference standard' diagnostic procedure for angle closure remains gonioscopy to identify iridotrabecular contact (ITC). Pathological angle closure is identified by elevated intraocular pressure, or by peripheral anterior synechiae (PAS). PAS do not have to be present for the pressure to be raised. Dynamic gonioscopy is essential to identify PAS. Most often, a four-mirror gonioscope is used to perform dynamic examinations, although, in most cases, with practice, it is possible to use the rim of a Goldmann gonioscope to indent the central cornea, and achieve the same results.

In assessing why the angle has closed, or is at high risk of closure, the underlying mechanism must be determined (see Etiology and mechanism, above). It is important to identify secondary pathology which may cause abrupt pressure rises, or ITC. The important differential diagnoses for an abrupt rise in IOP, where assessment of the angle is made difficult because of corneal edema, is hypertensive uveitis. Occasional neovascular angle closure (typically the result of a central retinal vein occlusion) may present in this way. ITC may result from:

- iris and ciliary body cysts
- iatrogenic – vitreoretinal surgery (early or late)
- posterior segment mass effect (hemorrhage, tumor)
- uveitis
- neovascularization (diabetes, CRVO)
- Marfan syndrome
- Axenfeld-Rieger syndrome
- trauma (usually with an unstable lens)
- tumors.

The use of pharmacological agents,[36] or exposure to darkness, or a face-down posture to provoke angle closure has been suggested as a method of identifying those at high risk of angle closure, by detecting dramatic rises in intraocular pressure. However, they have been denounced as time-consuming, misleading, and in some cases dangerous.[58]

Anterior segment imaging has evolved from an important research tool to a technique that is an important adjunct to clinical examination. Ultrasound biomicroscopy provides high-resolution images of cornea, iris, and anterior lens, and was instrumental in giving an insight into the mechanism responsible for plateau iris configuration.[37] Crucially, this technique gives good resolution of the relationship between iris, ciliary body, and anterior lens. However, it requires coupling fluid, and is messy and uncomfortable. The advent of anterior segment OCT has provided a noncontact method of obtaining similar quality images of the cornea and drainage angle. The important advantage of both UBM and OCT over gonioscopy is that both imaging techniques do not rely on visible light, and can be conducted in low light, or even dark conditions. This is very important as, in high illumination levels, the angle may appear open, whereas in the dark, it may be closed (Fig. 27.4). Studies suggest that this gives AS-OCT an advantage over gonioscopy in identifying angle closure.[59] The use of AS-OCT to image patients in light and dark provides a more physiological alternative to pharmacological provocative tests.

CLINICAL FEATURES, SIGNS, AND SYMPTOMS

Raised intraocular pressure in primary angle closure can cause glaucomatous optic neuropathy (GON). It has been shown that there is a significantly closer relationship between IOP and the development of GON in PACG than in POAG.[60] The pattern of visual field loss differs somewhat between the two forms of glaucoma, with the superior hemifield more severely affected than the inferior in POAG. This pattern is less pronounced in people with PACG.[61]

Following an acute episode of raised IOP, the thickness of the peripapillary retinal nerve fiber layer decreases significantly in the first 4 months.[62] Other ocular tissues may be damaged in angle-closure glaucoma. The development of anterior subcapsular lens opacities ('glaukomfleken') after high IOPs during acute episodes is well recognized. In addition, eyes that have suffered a previous symptomatic episode of primary angle closure have a significantly lower corneal endothelial cell count than their unaffected fellows.[63–65] One study noted that 33% of cases of unilateral acute angle closure had corneal endothelial guttata bilaterally.[63] Specular microscopy in eyes with primary angle-closure glaucoma showed a significant loss of endothelial cells in eyes that had visual field loss, a CDR >0.5, a previous acute attack of angle closure, or surgery in addition to peripheral iridectomy.[66] Part of this effect is probably related to either raised IOP or toxicity from medications or preservatives, as modest reductions in endothelial cell count have been reported in both POAG and PACG.[67]

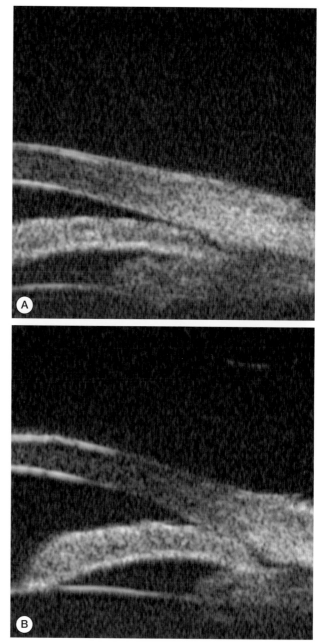

FIGURE 27.4 These images show ultrasound biomicroscope images of an eye with very narrow drainage angles. In the light **(A)** the angle is very narrow but open. In the dark **(B)** there is contact between iris and anterior trabecular meshwork as well as peripheral cornea. There is a small aqueous-filled space adjacent to the very peripheral iris and the posterior part of the trabecular meshwork. This eye has pupil block, manifesting as an anterior convexity of the iris (i.e. toward the cornea).

TREATMENT OPTIONS, OUTCOMES, AND PROGNOSIS

If a patient with angle closure has a visually significant cataract, this should be removed as the first intervention, effectively eradicating angle closure. If the lens is clear, pupillary block is the predominant mechanism in angle closure, and therefore iridotomy or iridectomy remain the cornerstones of management. Iridotomy results in a widening of the iridotrabecular angle, although 20–25% of those treated still have residual appositional angle closure afterwards.[68,69] Iridotomy is not effective in reversing synechial angle closure. Laser iridoplasty is effective for managing acute, symptomatic angle closure, and also for patients with asymptomatic disease, resulting in a reduction in IOP and an increase in drainage angle width, respectively.[70,71] Again, this technique is ineffective, and probably detrimental, if used when there is synechial angle closure. The association between lens thickness and position suggested that lens extraction should be similarly effective in managing the early to moderate angle closure. Both extracapsular and phacoemulsification surgery have been studied and found to be effective at increasing angle width and reducing IOP.[72,73] The combined use of lens extraction and mechanical synechialysis has been advocated within 6 months of an acute episode.[74] Pilocarpine remains an effective agent for mechanically opening drainage angles that are appositionally closed.[75]

Once a closed angle has been opened, any residual pressure elevation that needs to be treated can be tackled in the same manner as a secondary open-angle glaucoma case. Medical agents are similarly effective in PACG, with prostaglandins having been shown to outperform topical β-blockers for IOP control.[76] Trabeculectomy is appropriate for most cases of primary angle-closure glaucoma, with the exception of nanophthalmic eyes, or those with very anteriorly positioned lenses, in whom the risk of aqueous misdirection is high. If aqueous misdirection is considered more likely, lens extraction (prior or combined), localized ciliary body ablation, and intensive pharmacological mydriasis are all options.

The prognosis of angle-closure glaucoma varies according to the stage the disease has reached in its natural history. Untreated, angle-closure glaucoma causes blindness in at least one eye of 33–75% of those affected, versus 11–27% of eyes with open-angle glaucoma. However, in the earlier stages of disease, the majority of people (75–80%) with anatomically narrow angles can be effectively treated by laser iridotomy. In primary angle-closure glaucoma, laser iridotomy is not usually effective in achieving satisfactory long-term IOP control, with topical medication being needed in almost all cases, and trabeculectomy required in over half. The prognosis appears worse in people who have suffered an acute attack of angle closure.[77] Contralateral fellow eyes of those who have suffered an acute attack are at high risk of suffering a similar fate.[78,79] Laser iridotomy appears effective in preventing long-term IOP rises in around 90% of these eyes.[80]

Summary

- Primary angle-closure glaucoma is responsible for half of all glaucoma blindness worldwide.
- PACG is a more visually destructive form of disease than primary open-angle glaucoma.
- Older people, women, and Asians are high-risk demographic groups.
- Ocular biometric risk factors are a thicker lens, a more anteriorly positioned lens, a shorter axial length, all acting to form a shallower anterior chamber.
- Most angle closure is asymptomatic.
- Classification should identify the mechanism responsible for angle closure, and the stage of disease in terms of its natural history.
- Laser iridotomy and laser iridoplasty are very effective in the early stages of disease.

REFERENCES

1. Foster PJ, Nolan WP, Aung T, et al. Defining 'occludable' angles in population surveys: drainage angle width, peripheral anterior synechiae and glaucomatous optic neuropathy in East Asian people. Br J Ophthalmol 2004; 88:486–490.

2. Ang LP, Aung T, Chua WH, et al. Visual field loss from primary angle-closure glaucoma: a comparative study of symptomatic and asymptomatic disease. Ophthalmology 2004; 111: 1636–1640.

3. Teikari J, Raivio I, Nurminen M. Incidence of acute glaucoma in Finland from 1973 to 1982. Graefe's Arch Clin Exp Ophthalmol 1987; 225:357–360.

4. Ivanisevic M, Erceg M, Smoljanovic A, et al. The incidence and seasonal variations of acute primary angle-closure glaucoma. Coll Antropol 2002; 26:41–45.

5. Fujita K, Negishi K, Fujiki K, et al. Epidemiology of acute angle-closure glaucoma. Jpn J Clin Ophthalmol 1996; 37:625–629.

6. David R, Tessler Z, Yassur Y. Epidemiology of acute angle-closure glaucoma: incidence and seasonal variations. Ophthalmologica 1985; 191:4–7.

7. Seah SKL, Foster PJ, Chew PT, et al. Incidence of acute primary angle-closure glaucoma in Singapore. An island-wide survey. Arch Ophthalmol 1997; 115:1436–1440.

8. Wong TY, Foster PJ, Seah SKL, et al. Rates of hospital admissions for primary angle closure glaucoma among Chinese, Malays. and Indians in Singapore, Br J Ophthalmol 2000; 84:990–992.

9. Lai JS, Liu DT, Tham CC, et al. Epidemiology of acute primary angle-closure glaucoma in the Hong Kong Chinese population: prospective study. Hong Kong Med J 2001; 7:118–123.

10. Alsbirk PH. Anatomical risk factors in primary angle-closure glaucoma. A ten year follow up survey based on limbal and axial anterior chamber depths in a high risk population. Int Ophthalmol 1992; 16:265–272.

11. Thomas R, George R, Parikh R, et al. Five year risk of progression of primary angle closure suspects to primary angle closure: a population based study. Br J Ophthalmol 2003; 87:450–454.

12. Thomas R, Parikh R, Muliyil J, et al. Five-year risk of progression of primary angle closure to primary angle closure glaucoma: a population-based study. Acta Ophthalmol Scand 2003; 81:480–485.

13. Congdon N, Quigley HA, Hung PT, et al. Screening techniques for angle-closure glaucoma in rural Taiwan. Acta Ophthalmol Scand 1996; 74:113–119.

14. Foster PJ, Baasanhu J, Alsbirk PH, et al. Glaucoma in Mongolia – a population-based survey in Hövsgöl Province, Northern Mongolia. Arch Ophthalmol 1996; 114:1235–1241.

15. Foster PJ, Oen FT, Machin DS, et al. The prevalence of glaucoma in Chinese residents of Singapore. A cross-sectional population survey in Tanjong Pagar district. Arch Ophthalmol 2000; 118:1105–1111.

16. Douglas GR, Drance SM, Schulzer M. The visual field and nerve head in angle-closure glaucoma. A comparison of the effects of acute and chronic angle closure. Arch Ophthalmol 1975; 93:409–411.

17. Dhillon B, Chew PT, Lim ASM. Field loss in primary angle-closure glaucoma. Asia-Pac J Ophthalmol 1990; 2:85–87.

18. Aung T, Looi AL, Chew PT. The visual field following acute primary angle closure. Acta Ophthalmol Scand 2001; 79: 298–300.

19. Aung T, Ang LP, Chan SP, et al. Acute primary angle-closure: long-term intraocular pressure outcome in Asian eyes. Am J Ophthalmol 2001; 131:7–12.

20. Erie JC, Hodge DO, Gray DT. The incidence of primary angle-closure glaucoma in Olmstead County, Minnesota. Arch Ophthalmol 1997; 115:177–181.

21. Wensor MD, McCarty CA, Stanislavsky YL, et al. The prevalence of glaucoma in the Melbourne Visual Impairment Project. Ophthalmology 1998; 105:733–739.

22. Hollows FC, Graham PA. Intraocular pressure, glaucoma and glaucoma suspects in a defined population. Br J Ophthalmol 1966; 50:570–586.

23. Coffey M, Reidy A, Wormald R, et al. Prevalence of glaucoma in the west of Ireland. Br J Ophthalmol 1993; 77:17–21.

24. Bonomi L, Marchini G, Marrafa M, et al. Epidemiology of angle-closure glaucoma: prevalence, clinical types, and association with peripheral anterior chamber depth in the Egna-Neumarkt Glaucoma Study. Ophthalmology 2000; 107:998–1003.

25. Rotchford AP, Johnson GJ. Glaucoma in Zulus: a population-based cross-sectional survey in a rural district in South Africa. Arch Ophthalmol 2002; 120:471–478.

26. Rotchford AP, Kirwan JF, Muller MA, et al. Temba glaucoma study: a population-based cross-sectional survey in urban South Africa. Ophthalmology 2003; 110:376–382.

27. Salmon JF, Mermoud A, Ivey A, et al. The prevalence of primary angle-closure glaucoma and open-angle glaucoma in Mamre, Western Cape, South Africa. Arch Ophthalmol 1993; 111:1263–1269.

28. Luntz MH. Primary angle-closure glaucoma in urbanized South African caucasoid and negroid communities. Br J Ophthalmol 1973; 57:445–456.

29. Hu Z, Zhao ZL, Dong FT. [An epidemiological investigation of glaucoma in Beijing and Shun-yi county]. [Chinese]. Zhong-Hua Yen Ke Za Zhi [Chinese J Ophthalmol] 1989; 25:115–118.

30. Zhao JL. [An epidemiological survey of primary angle-closure glaucoma (PACG) in Tibet]. [Chinese]. Zhong-Hua Yen Ke Za Zhi [Chinese J Ophthalmol] 1990; 26:47–50.

31. Foster PJ, Johnson GJ. Glaucoma in China: how big is the problem? Br J Ophthalmol 2001; 85:1277–1282.

32. Congdon N, Wang F, Tielsch JM. Issues in the epidemiology and population-based screening of primary angle-closure glaucoma. Surv Ophthalmol 1992; 36:411–423.

33. Jacob A, Thomas R, Koshi SP, et al. Prevalence of primary glaucoma in an urban south Indian population. Ind J Ophthalmol 1998; 46:81–86.

34. Dandona L, Dandona R, Mandal P, et al. Angle-closure glaucoma in an urban population in southern India. The Andhra Pradesh eye disease study. Ophthalmology 2000; 107:1710–1716.

35. Sihota R, Lakshimaiah NC, Walia KB, et al. The trabecular meshwork in acute and chronic angle closure glaucoma. Ind J Ophthalmol 2001; 49:255–259.

36. Mapstone R. Provocative tests in closed-angle glaucoma. Br J Ophthalmol 1976; 60:115–119.

37. Pavlin CJ, Ritch R, Foster FS. Ultrasound biomicroscopy in plateau iris syndrome. Am J Ophthalmol 1992; 113:390–395.

38. He MG, Friedman DS, Ge J, et al. Laser peripheral iridotomy in eyes with narrow drainage angles: ultrasound biomicroscopy outcomes: The Liwan Eye Study. Ophthalmology 2007; 114:1513–1519.

39. Tupling MR, Junet EJ. Meteorological triggering of acute glaucoma attacks. Trans Ophthalmol Soc UK 1977; 97:185–188.

40. Gao F, Seah SKL, Foster PJ, et al. Angular regression and the detection of seasonal onset of disease. J Cancer Epidemiol Prevention 2002; 7:29–35.

41. Hillman JS, Turner JDC. Association between acute glaucoma and the weather and sunspot activity. Br J Ophthalmol 1977; 61:512–516.

42. Shah P, Dhurjon L, Metcalfe T, et al. Acute angle closure glaucoma associated with nebulised ipratropium bromide and salbutamol. Br Med J 1992; 304:40–41.

43. Epstein NE, Goldbloom DS. Oral imipramine and acute angle-closure glaucoma [letter; comment]. Arch Ophthalmol 1995; 113:698–699.

44. Eke T, Bates AK, Carr S. Acute angle-closure glaucoma associated with paroxetine. Br Med J 1997; 314:1387.

45. Croos R, Thirumalai S, Hassan S, et al. Citalopram associated with acute angle-closure glaucoma: case report. BMC Ophthalmol 2005; 4:23.

46. Kato K, Yoshida K, Suzuki K, et al. Managing patients with an overactive bladder and glaucoma: a questionnaire survey of Japanese urologists on the use of anticholinergics. BJU Int 2005; 95:98–101.

47. Lowe RF. Primary angle-closure glaucoma. A review of ocular biometry. Aust J Ophthalmol 1977; 5:9–17.

48. Sun X, Ji X, Zheng Y, et al. Primary chronic angle-closure glaucoma in Chinese – a clinical exploration of its pathogenesis and natural course. Yen Ke Xue Bao [Eye Science] 1994; 10:176–185.

49. Sihota R, Lakshimaiah NC, Agrawal HC, et al. Ocular parameters in the subgroups of angle closure glaucoma. Clin Exp Ophthalmol 2000; 28:253–258.

50. Alsbirk PH. Anterior chamber depth in Greenland Eskimos. I. A population study of variation with age and sex. Acta Ophthalmol 1974; 52:551–564.

51. Foster PJ, Alsbirk PH, Baasanhu J, et al. Anterior chamber depth in Mongolians. Variation with age, sex and method of measurement. Am J Ophthalmol 1997; 124:53–60.

52. Congdon NG, Qi Y, Quigley HA, et al. Biometry and primary angle-closure glaucoma among Chinese, white and black populations. Ophthalmology 1997; 104:1489–1495.

53. Becker B, Shaffer RN. Diagnosis and therapy of the glaucomas. St Louis: CV Mosby; 1965:42–53.

54. Foster PJ, Devereux JG, Alsbirk PH, et al. Detection of gonioscopically occludable angles and primary angle closure glaucoma by estimation of limbal chamber depth in Asians: modified grading scheme. Br J Ophthalmol 2000; 84:186–192.

55. Lowe RF. Causes of shallow anterior chamber in primary angle closure glaucoma. Ultrasonic biometry of normal and angle-closure eyes. Am J Ophthalmol 1969; 67:87–93.

56. Lowe RF, Clark BA. Radius of curvature of the anterior lens surface. Correlations in normal eyes and in eyes involved with primary angle-closure glaucoma. Br J Ophthalmol 1973; 57:471–474.

57. Lowe RF. Aetiology of the anatomical basis for primary angle-closure glaucoma. Biometrical comparisons between normal eyes and eyes with primary angle-closure glaucoma. Br J Ophthalmol 1970; 54:161–169.

58. Lowe RF. Primary angle-closure glaucoma. A review of provocative tests. Br J Ophthalmol 1967; 51:727–732.

59. Nolan WP, See J, Chew PT, et al. Detection of primary angle closure using anterior segment optical coherence tomography in Asian eyes. Ophthalmology 2007; 114:33–39.

60. Gazzard G, Foster PJ, Devereux JG, et al. Intraocular pressure and visual field loss in primary angle closure and primary open angle glaucomas. Br J Ophthalmol 2003; 87:720–725.

61. Gazzard G, Foster PJ, Viswanathan AC, et al. The severity and spatial distribution of visual field defects in primary glaucoma: a comparison of primary open-angle glaucoma and primary angle-closure glaucoma. Arch Ophthalmol 2002; 120: 1636–1643.

62. Aung T, Husain R, Gazzard G, et al. Changes in retinal nerve fiber layer thickness after acute primary angle closure. Ophthalmology 2004; 111:1475–1479.

63. Bigar F, Witmer R. Corneal endothelial changes in primary acute angle-closure glaucoma. Ophthalmology 1982; 89: 596–599.

64. Tham CC, Kwong YY, Lai JS, et al. Effect of a previous acute angle closure attack on the corneal endothelial cell density in chronic angle closure glaucoma patients. J Glaucoma 2006; 15:482–485.

65. Sihota R, Lakshimaiah NC, Titiyal JS, et al. Corneal endothelial status in the subtypes of primary angle closure glaucoma. Clin Exp Ophthalmol 2003; 31:492–495.

66. Markowitz SN, Morin JD. The endothelium in primary angle-closure glaucoma. Am J Ophthalmol 1984; 98:103–104.

67. Gagnon MM, Boisjoly HM, Brunette I, et al. Corneal endothelial cell density in glaucoma. Cornea 1997; 16:314–318.

68. He MG, Friedman DS, Ge J, et al. Laser peripheral iridotomy in primary angle-closure suspects: biometric and gonioscopic outcomes: the Liwan Eye Study. Ophthalmology 2007; 114:494–500.

69. Gazzard G, Friedman DS, Devereux JG, et al. A prospective ultrasound biomicroscopy evaluation of changes in anterior segment morphology after laser iridotomy in Asian eyes. Ophthalmology 2003; 110:630–638.

70. Lam DS, Lai JS, Tham CC, et al. Argon laser peripheral iridoplasty versus conventional systemic medical therapy in treatment of acute primary angle-closure glaucoma: a prospective, randomized, controlled trial. Ophthalmology 2002; 109:1591–1596.

71. Ritch R, Tham CC, Lam DS. Long-term success of argon laser peripheral iridoplasty in the management of plateau iris syndrome. Ophthalmology 2004; 111:104–108.

72. Greve EL. Primary angle-closure glaucoma: extracapsular cataract extraction or filtering procedure? Int Ophthalmol 1988; 12:157–1562.

73. Jacobi PC, Dietlein TS, Luke C, et al. Primary phacoemulsification and intraocular lens implantation for acute angle-closure glaucoma. Ophthalmology 2002; 109:1579–1603.

74. Teekhasaenee C, Ritch R. Combined phacoemulsification and goniosynechialysis for uncontrolled chronic angle-closure glaucoma after acute angle-closure glaucoma. Ophthalmology 1999; 106:669–674.

75. Kobayashi H, Kobayashi K, Kiryu J, et al. Pilocarpine induces an increase in the anterior chamber angular width in eyes with narrow angles. Br J Ophthalmol 1999; 83:553–558.

76. Chew PTK, Hung PT, Aung T. Efficacy of latanoprost in reducing intraocular pressure in patients with primary angle-closure glaucoma. Surv Ophthalmol 2002; 47:S125–S128.

77. Alsagoff Z, Aung T, Ang LP, et al. Long-term clinical course of primary angle-closure glaucoma in an Asian population. Ophthalmology 2000; 107:2300–2304.

78. Snow JT. Value of prophylactic peripheral iridectomy on the second eye in angle-closure glaucoma. Trans Ophthalmol Soc UK 1977; 97:189–191.

79. Lowe RF. Acute angle-closure glaucoma. The second eye: an analysis of 200 cases. Br J Ophthalmol 1962; 46:641–650.

80. Ang LP, Aung T, Chew PT. Acute primary angle closure in an Asian population: long-term outcome of the fellow eye after prophylactic laser peripheral iridotomy. Ophthalmology 2003; 107:2092–2096.

Exfoliation Syndrome and Exfoliative Glaucoma

Robert Ritch, Anastasios GP Konstas, and Ursula Schlötzer-Schrehardt

INTRODUCTION

Exfoliation syndrome (XFS), first described nearly a century ago, is the most common identifiable cause of open-angle glaucoma worldwide, comprising the majority of glaucoma in some countries.[1] Its incidence increases progressively with age, while its widespread distribution, its frequency, and its potential association with other diseases is only beginning to be realized. The subtlety of clinical signs results in the diagnosis of exfoliative glaucoma (XFG) being often overlooked, resulting in less than ideal management. Etiologically related ocular manifestations include angle closure, cataract, dry eye, and central retinal vein occlusion. Systemic associations are primarily related to vasculopathy and include transient ischemic attacks, stroke, myocardial infarction, cerebrovascular insufficiency, Alzheimer's disease, and hearing loss.

There are important differences in the clinical appearance, course, and prognosis of XFG versus primary open-angle glaucoma (POAG). Its prognosis is more severe than that of POAG, with greater 24-hour intraocular pressure (IOP) fluctuation, greater visual field loss and optic disc damage at the time of detection, more rapid progression, and greater need for surgical intervention. The ideal laser and medical treatment approaches differ from those of POAG. The hypotensive efficacy of the various treatment modalities may differ in XFG from their efficacy in POAG.

At the cellular and biochemical levels, XFS is a distinct entity, with a unique mechanism of development that is still being elucidated. It is characterized by the production and progressive accumulation of a fibrillar extracellular material in many ocular tissues. Innovative approaches may slow the progression, or even prevent the development of, XFS and XFG and potentially lead to a future cure. The epidemiology, etiology, clinical findings, mechanisms of glaucoma, associations, and treatment have been the subject of recent major reviews and the reader is referred to these for comprehensive information.[2–4]

DISEASE PREVALENCE AND INFLUENCE

Although long thought to be a disease peculiar to Scandinavia, XFS comprises over half the open-angle glaucoma in such diverse countries as Norway, Ireland, Greece, and Saudi Arabia, and has recently been found to be common in South African Zulus, Ethiopia, and Nepal. It has been estimated that between 60 and 70 million people are affected worldwide and it appears to account for about 20–25% of open-angle glaucoma.

The prevalence of XFS increases steadily with age in all populations. About two-thirds of patients have clinically unilateral involvement, but XFS can be diagnosed prior to the clinically visible appearance of classic exfoliation material on the lens surface by conjunctival biopsy, showing that the disease is present microscopically before it is detected clinically in the fellow eye. The reasons for this presentation remain unknown, but it is analogous to that of uveitis, which is also often clinically unilateral or markedly asymmetric.

RACIAL AND ETHNIC VARIATION

The reported prevalence of XFS in the United States is generally similar to that in Western Europe. It is much more common in Caucasians than in persons of African ancestry. However, whereas it was thought to be rare in Africa, recent reports suggest that it is common in Ethiopia and South Africa, and the Gambia in West Africa, a large area in which it was previously said not to exist. It is also common in Navajo Indians in the United States and in Australian Aborigines. In New Mexico, Spanish-American men are nearly six times as likely to develop XFS than are non-Spanish-Americans.[5] Although common in Japan and Mongolia, it is rare in southern China. Further epidemiological studies are necessary.

Ethnic and local variations exist also. In France, XFS is much more common in Brittany, the population of which has Celtic origins, than in southeastern France. It accounts for about 60% of the open-angle glaucoma in Ireland and in the Isle of Man, but only 10% in neighboring England. In central Norway, the prevalence in two adjacent towns (20%) was twice that in a third adjacent town. Interestingly, the prevalence of XFS in both members of 343 married couples (3.2%) was significantly higher ($p = 0.022$) than would be expected, suggesting the possibility of an infectious origin.[6] In Nepal, XFS was found in 12% of members of one ethnic group, the Gurung, and only 0.24% of non-Gurung of similar ages.[7] Other examples exist and why this is so has yet to be explained.

GEOGRAPHICAL VARIATION

In addition to the above, persons living at lower latitudes (Greece, Saudi Arabia, Iran) appear to develop XFS at younger ages. Exposure to sunlight (ultraviolet radiation) may or may not be implicated, as may dietary factors. Forsius and Luukka[8] found no XFS in Eskimos versus 20% of Lapps living at the same latitude. Persons living at higher altitude had a greater prevalence in two series[9,10] but not in a third.[11] In one series, eyes with blue irides were significantly more detected to have XFS than those with brown irides.[12]

RISK FACTORS AND PROGNOSIS

The risk of developing glaucoma is cumulative over time and it occurs 5 to 10 times as frequently in eyes with XFS than in those without it. About 25% of patients with XFS develop elevated IOP and one-third of these develop glaucoma. Patients with XFS are twice as likely to convert from ocular hypertension to glaucoma and, when glaucoma is present, to progress.[13,14]

Exfoliative glaucoma has a more serious clinical course and worse prognosis than POAG. The mean IOP is greater in normotensive patients with XFS than in the general population and greater in XFG patients at presentation than in POAG patients. At any specific IOP level, eyes with XFS are more likely to have glaucomatous damage than are eyes without XFS. There is a greater rate of conversion of ocular hypertensive patients to XFG than to POAG and damage progresses more rapidly in patients with XFG than in patients with POAG. There is a higher frequency and severity of optic nerve damage at the time of diagnosis, worse visual field damage, poorer response to medications, and more frequent necessity for surgical intervention. Greater fluctuation of the IOP is present in patients with XFS on diurnal measurement compared with POAG.[15] Glaucoma in XFS is more resistant to medical therapy than is POAG, responds for a shorter period of time, and fails more often.

ETIOLOGY AND PATHOGENESIS

ETIOLOGY

Besides geographical clustering, lines of evidence that support a genetic basis for XFS include familial aggregation, transmission in two-generation families, higher concordance rates in monozygous twins, an increased risk of XFS in relatives of affected patients, loss of heterozygosity, and HLA studies.[16,17] The disease appears to be inherited as an autosomal dominant trait, the late onset and incomplete penetrance of which pose considerable problems to genetic analyses. Most of the two-generation pedigrees published in the literature showed matrilineal inheritance, but additional evidence of paternal transmission has been provided recently.

Several chromosomal regions have been tentatively associated with XFS to date. Most recently, sequence variants in the LOXL1 gene, which catalyzes the formation of elastin fibers, have been implicated in the causation of exfoliative glaucoma in two separate groups of patients, one from Iceland and one from Sweden.[18]

However, a number of nongenetic factors, including dietary factors, autoimmunity, infectious agents, and trauma, have also been hypothesized to be involved in pathogenesis, but have not been proven. Interestingly, the exceptional diagnosis of XFS in patients under age 40 has often been preceded by prior intraocular surgery or anterior segment trauma, particularly to the iris, or to occur after corneal transplantation with grafts from elderly donors. These events may serve as a trigger for the premature development of XFS in a predisposed individual or even point to the possibility of a transmissible etiology. Altogether, it appears that XFS represents a complex, multifactorial, late-onset disease, involving both genetic and nongenetic factors in its pathogenesis.

PATHOGENESIS

The specific pathogenesis of XFS and the exact chemical composition of exfoliation material (XFM) are still not known. However, the pathologic process is characterized by the chronic accumulation of an abnormal fibrillar matrix product, which is either the result of an excessive production or insufficient breakdown or both, and which is regarded as pathognomonic for the disease, based on its unique light microscopic and ultrastructural criteria.[19]

Previous immunohistochemical studies have shown XFM to represent a complex glycoprotein/proteoglycan structure bearing epitopes of the basement membrane and elastic fiber system. The characteristic fibrils, composed of microfibrillar subunits surrounded by an amorphous matrix comprising various glycoconjugates, contain predominantly epitopes of elastic fibers, such as elastin, tropoelastin, amyloid P, vitronectin, and components of elastic microfibrils, such as fibrillin-1, microfibril-associated glycoprotein (MAGP-1), and latent transforming growth factor ($TGF-\beta_1$) binding proteins (LTBP-1 and LTBP-2) by immunohistochemistry. Recently, a direct analytical approach by using liquid chromatography coupled with tandem mass spectrometry (LC-MS/MS) has been accomplished and showed XFM to consist of the elastic microfibril components fibrillin-1, fibulin-2, and vitronectin, the proteoglycans syndecan and versican, the extracellular chaperone clusterin, the cross-linking enzyme lysyl oxidase, and other proteins, confirming many of the previously reported immunohistochemical data.[20]

A set of genes primarily involved in extracellular matrix metabolism and in cellular stress was found to be differentially expressed in anterior segment tissues of XFS eyes,[21,22] suggesting that the underlying pathophysiology of XFS is associated with excess production of elastic microfibril components, enzymatic cross-linking processes, overexpression of TGF-β_1, a proteolytic imbalance between matrix metalloproteinases (MMPs) and their tissue inhibitors (TIMPs), increased cellular and oxidative stress, and an impaired cellular stress response.

PATHOGENETIC CONCEPT

Immunohistochemical, biochemical, and molecular biologic data give strong support to the elastic microfibril theory of pathogenesis, which was first proposed by Streeten et al.[23] on the basis of histochemical similarities between XFM and zonular fibers and which explains XFS as a type of elastosis affecting elastic microfibrils. The currently proposed pathogenetic concept of XFS describes the condition as a specific type of stress-induced elastosis, an elastic microfibrillopathy, associated with the excessive production of elastic microfibrils and their aggregation into typical mature fibrils by a variety of potentially elastogenic cells.[4] Growth factors, particularly TGF-β_1, increased cellular and oxidative stress, an impaired cellular protection system, and the stable aggregation of misfolded stressed proteins appear to be involved in this fibrotic process. Due to an imbalance between MMPs and TIMPs and extensive cross-linking processes involved in fiber formation, the pathologic material is not properly degraded but progressively accumulates within the tissues over time (Fig. 28.1).

MECHANISMS OF GLAUCOMA

Chronic pressure elevation in XFS eyes is caused by increased outflow resistance in the trabecular meshwork, most probably due to blockage of the outflow channels by XFM. Although there may be deposits of XFM throughout the trabecular meshwork, the focus of accumulation and pathological alterations is the juxtacanalicular tissue beneath the inner wall of Schlemm's canal, the site of greatest resistance to aqueous outflow.[24] This critical area becomes thickened through gradual deposition of XFM, which appears to be locally produced by the endothelial cells lining Schlemm's canal. The gradual build-up of XFM in the juxtacanalicular tissue correlates with the IOP level and with the presence and severity of glaucomatous optic nerve damage,[25] and may be associated with progressive degenerative changes of Schlemm's canal, including narrowing, fragmentation, and obstruction in more advanced cases. These findings indicate a direct causative relationship between the build-up of XFM in the meshwork and glaucoma development and progression, and suggest that therapeutic efforts to improve outflow need to address the alterations in the juxtacanalicular area to obtain lasting intraocular pressure reduction. Partly, clumps of XFM may be also passively washed in with the aqueous flow after abrasion from the lens and pupillary margin and may become trapped in the uveal pores of the meshwork.

Apart from the obstruction of the trabecular outflow channels by XFM, contributions of pigment dispersion and increased aqueous protein concentrations to increased outflow resistance have also been proposed. Increased pigmentation is a prominent sign of XFS and may be an early diagnostic finding preceding the appearance of exfoliation deposits on the pupillary margin or anterior lens capsule.[26] In patients with clinically unilateral XFG, trabecular pigment is usually denser in the involved eye. Eyes with POAG or eyes without glaucoma tend to have less pigmentation than eyes with XFG. Glaucomatous damage is usually more advanced in the eye with greater trabecular pigmentation.

Although XFG is characteristically a high-pressure disease, pressure-independent risk factors, such as an impaired ocular and retrobulbar perfusion and abnormalities of elastic tissue of the lamina cribrosa, may be present and further increase the individual risk for glaucomatous damage. In a prospective study, Puska et al.[27] found that in normotensive XFS patients with clinically unilateral involvement, in whom IOP was equal throughout the follow-up period, disc changes took place only in the involved eye, suggesting that the exfoliation process itself may be a risk factor for optic disc changes.

Clinically, XFS often appears to be unilateral, although why this is so remains unknown. Although conjunctival XFM and iris abnormalities can almost always be found in fellow eyes on electron microscopy, clinically visible involvement of the fellow eye often does not occur. A protective mechanism, perhaps mediated through the immune system, may exist for the second eye. In addition, not all eyes with XFS develop elevated IOP, and extensive deposits of XFM may be found in the meshwork in normotensive eyes. Perhaps

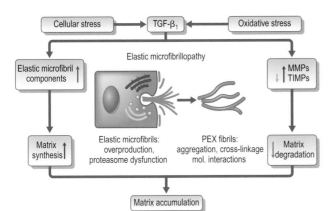

FIGURE 28.1 Current concept of the pathogenesis of exfoliation syndrome.

other factors, such as differences in managing the metabolic disturbance, genetic factors, and duration of the disease, may influence the progression from XFS to ocular hypertension and then XFG.

DIAGNOSIS AND ANCILLARY TESTING, AND DIFFERENTIAL DIAGNOSIS

The diagnosis is made by finding typical XFM on the anterior lens surface or pupillary border. The diagnosis should be suspected in the absence of XFM when ancillary pigment-related signs are present, which define patients as 'exfoliation suspects.'

OCULAR SIGNS

All anterior segment structures are involved in XFS. Deposits of white material on the anterior lens surface are the most consistent and important diagnostic feature. The classic pattern consists of three distinct zones that become visible when the pupil is fully dilated: a central disc, intermediate clear zone created by the iris rubbing exfoliation material from the lens surface during its physiologic excursions, and a granular peripheral zone (Figs 28.2 and 28.3). Exfoliation material is often found at the pupillary border (Fig. 28.4).

It leads not only to severe, chronic open-angle glaucoma but also to lens subluxation, angle closure, blood–aqueous barrier impairment, and serious complications at the time of cataract extraction, such as zonular dialysis, capsular rupture, and vitreous loss.

Pigment loss from the pupillary ruff and iris sphincter region and its deposition on anterior chamber structures is a hallmark of XFS. Just as the iris scrapes exfoliation material from the lens surface, the exfoliation material on the lens causes rupture of iris pigment epithelial cells with concomitant pigment dispersion into the anterior chamber. This leads to iris sphincter transillumination, loss of the ruff, increased trabecular pigmentation, and pigment deposition on the iris surface (Figs 28.5 and 28.6). Pigment dispersion in the

anterior chamber is common after pupillary dilation and may be profuse (Fig. 28.7). Marked IOP rises can occur after pharmacologic dilation and IOP should be measured routinely in all patients after dilation.

Exfoliation 'suspects' were initially defined as patients in whom one or both eyes exhibited one or more signs

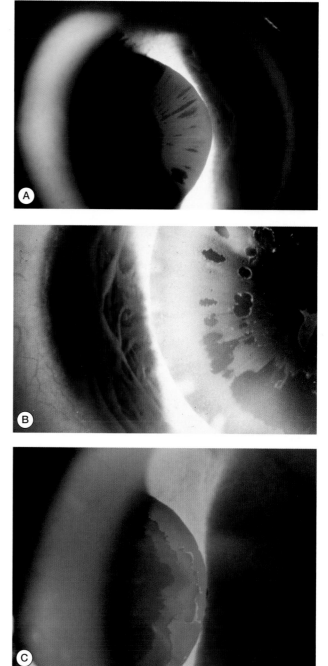

FIGURE 28.3 (A) An earlier stage than Figure 28.1, showing the future intermediate clear zone beginning to form as the iris excursions create clefts in the exfoliation material. **(B)** There is a relatively homogeneous central disc and the clear intermediate zone is partially complete. Alternating bridges and clefts demarcate the residual exfoliation material remaining in this zone. **(C)** The peripheral zone is granular and has a layered appearance resulting from the undisturbed build-up of exfoliation material on the lens surface.

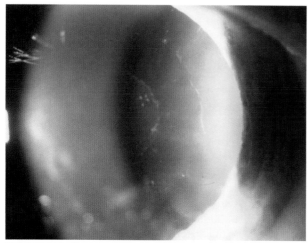

FIGURE 28.2 Classic appearance of XFS.

related to pigment dispersion in the absence of clinically identifiable XFM on the anterior lens capsule or pupillary margin in either eye.[26] Transmission electron microscopy of conjunctival biopsy specimens from patients previously diagnosed to have either POAG or

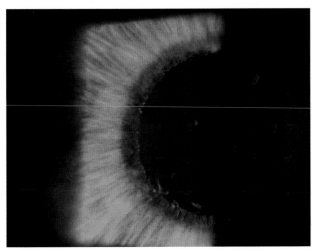

FIGURE 28.4 Exfoliation material on the pupillary border.

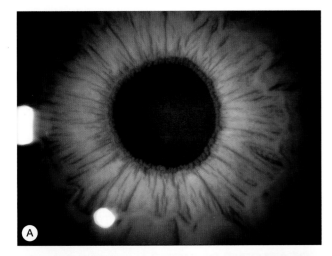

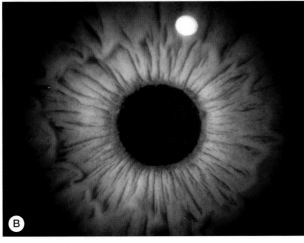

FIGURE 28.5 Intact pupillary ruff in the uninvolved eye **(A)** and virtually totally absent ruff in the involved eye in a patient with clinically unilateral XFS **(B)**.

ocular hypertension revealed exfoliation fibers in 8/23 suspect eyes. These pigment-related signs also correlated with the presence of extraocular exfoliation fibrils in 7 of 12 eyelid skin specimens in the absence of any clinically visible intraocular XFM.[28]

Exfoliation material may be detected earliest on the ciliary processes and zonules, which are often frayed and broken (Fig. 28.8). Phacodonesis is common, and spontaneous subluxation or dislocation of the lens can occur. Patients with XFS are much more prone to have complications at the time of cataract extraction. Zonular fragility increases the risk of lens dislocation, zonular dialysis, or vitreous loss up to 10 times during extracapsular extraction, while eyes with XFS dilate poorly and are prone to posterior synechia formation. Complications are fewer with phacoemulsification. Late postoperative decentration of intraocular lenses and capsular bags, capsular contraction syndrome, and posterior capsular opacification are more common in XFS.

OCULAR ASSOCIATIONS

There is an etiological association between XFS and cataract. Significantly reduced levels of ascorbic acid, an important free radical scavenger in the eye, have been reported in the aqueous humor of XFS patients,[29]

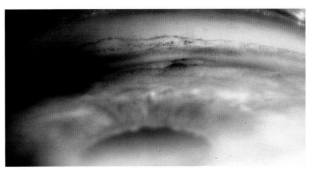

FIGURE 28.6 Typical iridocorneal angle appearance in an eye with XFS.

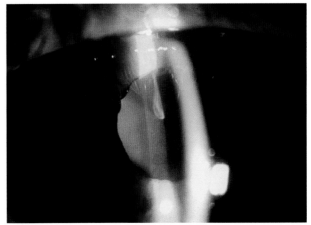

FIGURE 28.7 Pigment dispersion into the anterior chamber with pupillary dilation.

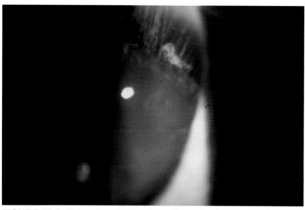

FIGURE 28.8 Extensive destruction of zonules in an eye with a spontaneously dislocated lens.

suggesting a faulty antioxidant defense system. Also, 8-iso-prostaglandin $F_{2\alpha}$ was significantly increased in the aqueous of patients with XFS, providing evidence of a role for free radical-induced oxidative damage in the pathobiology of XFS.[30] Serum ascorbate concentrations were much lower and malondialdehyde concentrations were much higher in XFS patients than controls, reflecting free radical damage to lipid peroxides.[31] Mean hydroxyproline levels are greater in the aqueous humor of XFS patients.

Exfoliation syndrome is associated with ocular ischemia and systemic vascular abnormalities. Iris ischemia is the rule and can be detected both on iris angiography[32] and histopathologically[33] in fellow eyes of patients with clinically unilateral involvement. Vessel lumens are often narrowed and may become obliterated, with marked alteration of the iris vasculature in advanced cases. Vessel dropout with collateral formation and iris hypoperfusion lead to anterior chamber hypoxia and patchy iris microneovascularization. There is chronic breakdown of the blood–aqueous barrier and greater protein levels in the anterior chamber.

Retinal vein occlusion has been associated with XFS at variable frequencies and based upon retrospective studies, which employed either slit lamp examination or histopathology. In a series of consecutive eyes with branch retinal vein occlusion (BRVO) (73 eyes of 70 patients) or central retinal vein occlusion (CRVO) (53 eyes of 49 patients), XFS was present in 6 of 73 eyes with BRVO (8.2%), 11 of 53 eyes with CRVO (20.8%), and 20 of 384 age-matched control eyes (5.2%).[34] Elevated IOP and glaucoma have been suggested as a cause for the association of XFS with CRVO. It is possible that a common pathophysiologic mechanism may predispose to XFS and CRVO. Abnormal homocysteine metabolism could be a candidate, as patients with XFS have significantly elevated plasma,[35] aqueous,[36] and tear fluid[37] homocysteine levels.

SYSTEMIC

Exfoliation syndrome is a generalized disorder of the extracellular matrix. Deposits of XFM have been identified in the walls of posterior ciliary arteries, vortex veins, and central retinal vessels as they exit the optic nerve. Electron microscopy reveals aggregates in heart, lung, liver, kidney, gall bladder, and cerebral meninges in patients with ocular XFS.[38,39] No clear-cut association of XFS with a systemic disease has yet been shown in the sense of the disease having conclusive evidence of a functional deficit in association with the presence of XFS. However, in addition to the vascular abnormalities described above, an increasing number of associations with specific systemic disorders are being reported, including transient ischemic attacks, hypertension, angina, myocardial infarction, stroke, asymptomatic myocardial dysfunction, Alzheimer's disease, and hearing loss. Some of these associations have been disputed and no clear evidence of increased mortality in patients with XFS, which one might expect with these associations, has been reported.

Ocular, retrobulbar, and cerebral blood flow are reduced in patients with XFS both with and without glaucoma. In clinically unilateral cases, ipsilateral pulsatile ocular blood flow and carotid blood flow have been reported to be reduced. Patients with XFS had greater decreases in blood flow velocities of the ophthalmic artery, the central retinal artery, and the short posterior ciliary arteries determined by color Doppler imaging than those without XFS. Blood flow of the lamina cribrosa and neural rim decreased with increasing glaucomatous damage. Patients with XFG have lower baseline fingertip cutaneous capillary perfusion than those with POAG or controls, longer time to maximal cold-induced flow reduction, and longer recovery time. Elevated levels of endothelin-1, a powerful vasoconstrictor, have been reported in the aqueous humor of patients with XFS. Recently, pathological carotid artery function, as well as altered parasympathetic vascular control, in XFS/XFG which increases with age and with higher homocysteine concentration, was reported. These findings have been nicely summarized in a well-referenced recent editorial.[40]

TREATMENT OPTIONS

The sole focus of therapy in XFG should not be the reduction of IOP. Understanding the mechanisms leading to elevated IOP in XFS could allow us to develop new, more logical approaches to therapy.

The initial approach to medical therapy of XFG has been similar to that for POAG. It includes topical prostaglandin analogues (bimatoprost, latanoprost, and travoprost), and aqueous suppressants. However, this approach has not been refined specifically for XFG by taking into account the response of this glaucoma to the various drugs. There is still limited information regarding the success of the newer medications in XFG. In a recent crossover trial comparing latanoprost to bimatoprost in XFG, bimatoprost provided a statistically greater IOP reduction for all time points and for the mean diurnal curve after 3 months of therapy (35% reduction with bimatoprost versus 31% reduction for latanoprost).[41] Another 24-hour study showed that both latanoprost and travoprost reduced IOP at each time point and for the 24-hour curve from untreated baseline.[42] However, travoprost provided a slightly greater hypotensive effect for the 24-hour curve (mean difference between groups was 0.5 mmHg).

Konstas et al.[43] demonstrated the benefit of IOP reduction and suggested a target IOP of 17 mmHg and lower to prevent or slow progressive damage. Latanoprost provided a narrower range of diurnal IOP fluctuation compared to timolol. Aqueous suppressants may lower IOP in eyes with XFS but do not interfere with the mechanism of the cause of progression of trabecular damage, i.e. iridolenticular friction and disruption of the iris pigment epithelial cells. Cholinergic agents have multiple beneficial actions in eyes with XFS. Not only do they lower IOP but, by increasing aqueous outflow, they should enable the trabecular meshwork to clear more rapidly and, by limiting pupillary movement, should slow the progression of the disease. Aqueous suppressants, on the other hand, by decreasing aqueous secretion, result in decreased aqueous flow through the trabecular meshwork. Becker[44] has presented suggestive evidence that treatment with aqueous suppressants leads to worsening of trabecular function.

Theoretically, miotics should be the first line of treatment. However, many patients have nuclear sclerosis, and miotics may reduce visual acuity or dim vision sufficiently to create difficulty. The long-term use of miotics may lead to the development of posterior synechiae. The authors have found that 2% pilocarpine q.h.s. can provide sufficient limitation of pupillary mobility without causing these side effects. An international, multi-institutional prospective trial (ICEST) is currently underway comparing latanoprost and 2% pilocarpine q.h.s. versus timolol/Cosopt for patients with XFS and ocular hypertension or glaucoma.

Because of the strong association with elevated homocysteine levels, one must also consider the possibility that patients with XFS may benefit from lowering of plasma homocysteine levels by supplemental vitamins B_6, B_{12}, and folic acid.

LASER THERAPY

Argon laser trabeculoplasty (ALT) is particularly effective, at least early on, in eyes with XFS. The baseline IOP is usually higher in XFG than in eyes with POAG undergoing ALT and thus the initial drop in IOP is greater in XFG. Primary ALT can delay the use of medical

therapy for up to 8 years in a significant proportion of these patients.[45] There is a gradual reduction in success over time, with long-term rates dropping to approximately 35–55% at 3–6 years.

Approximately 20% of patients develop sudden, late rises of IOP within the first 2 years after treatment.[46] Continued pigment liberation may overwhelm the restored functional capacity of the trabecular meshwork, and maintenance miotic therapy to minimize pupillary movement after ALT might counteract this. The authors have found empirically that 2% pilocarpine q.h.s. is sufficient to provide this protection. Selective laser trabeculoplasty (SLT) needs to be further evaluated as an effective and safe alternative to ALT in the treatment of XFG.

SURGICAL THERAPY

The results of trabeculectomy are comparable to those in POAG. In a recent study, trabeculectomy with mitomycin C obtained better 24-hour IOP control than successful maximal medical therapy in patients with advanced XFG or POAG.[47] However, surgical complications are more common in patients with XFG. In some cases, high preoperative IOP may predispose to choroidal hemorrhage, or effusion. Weakened zonular support may allow intraoperative lens movement or even subluxation in extreme cases. This could lead to inadvertent lens damage during iridectomy, vitreous loss, or late incarceration of vitreous into the internal ostium. Hyphema from the surgical iridectomy could be the result of undetected iris fine neovascularization, which occurs in XFG. After trabeculectomy there is an increased possibility of cataract progression in patients with XFG. The more advanced the disease and the longer its duration, the higher the likelihood for complications to occur.

Trabeculotomy, performed with the rationale that it may bypass mechanical blockage of the trabecular meshwork, has been reported successful.[48] Along similar lines of reasoning, Jacobi et al.[49] described a procedure termed trabecular aspiration, designed to improve outflow facility.

Deep sclerectomy and similar procedures including a deroofing of Schlemm's canal are becoming popular choices in some centers owing to the reduced risk profile of nonpenetrating surgery. More recently, XFG patients were reported to have significantly better success than POAG patients following deep sclerectomy with an implant.[50] Moreover, phacoemulsification combined with penetrating and nonpenetrating procedures does not seem to adversely influence success rate.

REFERENCES

1. Ritch R. Exfoliation syndrome: the most common identifiable cause of open-angle glaucoma. J Glaucoma 1994; 3:176–178.

2. Ritch R, Schlötzer-Schrehardt U, Konstas AGP. Why is glaucoma associated with exfoliation syndrome? Prog Retin Eye Res 2003; 22:253–275.

3. Ritch R, Schlötzer-Schrehardt U. Exfoliation syndrome. Surv Ophthalmol 2001; 45:265–315.

4. Schlötzer-Schrehardt U, Naumann GOH. Ocular and systemic pseudoexfoliation syndrome. Am J Ophthalmol 2006; 141:921–937.

5. Jones W, White RE, Magnus DE. Increased occurrence of exfoliation in the male, Spanish American population of New Mexico. J Am Optom Assoc 1992; 63:643–648.

6. Ringvold A, Blika S, Elsås T, et al. The Middle-Norway eye-screening study. I. Epidemiology of the pseudo-exfoliation syndrome. Acta Ophthalmol 1988; 66:652–657.

7. Shakya S, Koirala S, Karmacharya PCD. Pseudoexfoliation syndrome in Nepal: a hospital-based retrospective study. Asia-Pacific J Ophthalmol 2004; 16:13–16.

8. Forsius H, Luukka H. Pseudoexfoliation of the anterior capsule of the lens in Lapps and Eskimos. Can J Ophthalmol 1973; 8:274–277.

9. Mohammed S, Kazmi N. Subluxation of the lens and ocular hypertension in exfoliation syndrome. Pak J Ophthalmol 1986; 2:77–78.

10. Kozobolis VP, Papatzanaki M, Vlachonikolis IG, et al. Epidemiology of pseudoexfoliation in the island of Crete (Greece). Acta Ophthalmol 1997; 75:726–729.

11. Forsius H. Prevalence of pseudoexfoliation of the lens in Finns, Lapps, Icelanders, Eskimos, and Russians. Trans Ophthalmol Soc UK 1979; 99:296–298.

12. Konstas AGP, Dimitrakoulias N, Kourtzidou O, et al. Frequency of exfoliation syndrome in Greek cataract patients. Acta Ophthalmol 1996; 74:478–482.

13. Bengtsson B, Heijl A. A long-term prospective study of risk factors for glaucomatous visual field loss in patients with ocular hypertension. J Glaucoma 2005; 14:135–138.

14. Leske MC, Heijl A, Hussein M, et al. Factors for glaucoma progression and the effect of treatment. The Early Manifest Glaucoma Trial. Arch Ophthalmol 2003; 121:48–56.

15. Konstas AGP, Mantziris DA, Stewart WC. Diurnal intraocular pressure in untreated exfoliation and primary open-angle glaucoma. Arch Ophthalmol 1997; 115:182–185.

16. Damji KF. Is pseudoexfoliation syndrome inherited? A review of genetic and nongenetic factors and a new observation. Ophthalmic Genet 1998; 19:175–185.

17. Orr AC, Robitaille JM, Price PA, et al. Exfoliation syndrome: clinical and genetic features. Ophthalmic Genet 2001; 22:171–185.

18. Thorliefsson G, Magnusson KP, Sulem P, et al. Common sequence variants in the LOXL1 gene confer susceptibility to exfoliation glaucoma. Sciencexpress 2007. Online. Available: www.sciencexpress.org

19. Naumann GOH, Schlötzer-Schrehardt U, Küchle M. Pseudoexfoliation syndrome for the comprehensive ophthalmologist: intraocular and systemic manifestations. Ophthalmology 1998; 105:951–968.

20. Ovodenko B, Rostagno A, Neubert TA, et al. Proteomic analysis of lenticular exfoliation deposits. Invest Ophthalmol Vis Sci 2007; 48:1447–1457.

21. Zenkel M, Pöschl E, von der Mark K, et al. Differential gene expression in pseudoexfoliation syndrome. Invest Ophthalmol Vis Sci 2005; 46:3742–3752.

22. Zenkel M, Kruse FE, Jünemann AG, et al. Clusterin deficiency in eyes with pseudoexfoliation syndrome may be implicated in the aggregation and deposition of pseudoexfoliative material. Invest Ophthalmol Vis Sci 2006; 47:1982–1990.

23. Streeten BW, Gibson SA, Dark AJ. Pseudoexfoliative material contains an elastic microfibrillar-associated glycoprotein. Trans Am Ophthalmol Soc 1986; 84:304–320.

24. Schlötzer-Schrehardt U, Naumann GOH. Trabecular meshwork in pseudoexfoliation syndrome with and without open-angle glaucoma. A morphometric, ultrastructural study. Invest Ophthalmol Vis Sci 1995; 36:1750–1764.

25. Gottanka J, Flügel-Koch C, Martus P, et al. Correlation of pseudoexfoliation material and optic nerve damage in pseudoexfoliation syndrome. Invest Ophthalmol Vis Sci 1997; 38:2435–2446.

26. Prince AM, Streeten BW, Ritch R, et al. Preclinical diagnosis of pseudoexfoliation syndrome. Arch Ophthalmol 1987; 105:1076–1082.

27. Puska P, Vesti E, Tomita G, et al. Optic disc changes in normotensive persons with unilateral exfoliation syndrome: a 3-year follow-up study. Graefe's Arch Clin Exp Ophthalmol 1999; 237:457–462.

28. Schlötzer-Schrehardt U, Küchle M, Dorfler S, Naumann GOH. Pseudoexfoliative material in the eyelid skin of pseudoexfoliation-suspect patients: a clinico-histopathological correlation. German J Ophthalmol 1993; 2:51–60.

29. Koliakos GG, Konstas AGP, Schlötzer-Schrehardt U, et al. Ascorbic acid concentration is reduced in the aqueous humor of patients with exfoliation syndrome. Am J Ophthalmol 2002; 134:879–883.

30. Koliakos GG, Konstas AGP, Schlötzer-Schrehardt U, et al. 8-Isoprostaglandin F2a and ascorbic acid concentration in the aqueous humour of patients with exfoliation syndrome. Br J Ophthalmol 2003; 87:353–356.

31. Yilmaz A, Adiguzel U, Tamer L, et al. Serum oxidant/antioxidant balance in exfoliation syndrome. Clin Exp Ophthalmol 2005; 33:63–66.

32. Laatikainen L. Fluorescein angiographic studies of the peripapillary and perilimbal regions in simple, capsular and low-tension glaucoma. Acta Ophthalmol 1971; 111(Suppl):3–83.

33. Hammer T, Schlötzer-Schrehardt U, Naumann GOH. Unilateral or asymmetric pseudoexfoliation syndrome? An ultrastructural study. Arch Ophthalmol 2001; 119:1023–1031.

34. Saatci OA, Ferliel ST, Ferliel M, et al. Pseudoexfoliation and glaucoma in eyes with retinal vein occlusion. Int Ophthalmol 1999; 23:75–78.

35. Vessani RM, Liebmann JM, Jofe M, et al. Plasma homocysteine is elevated in patients with exfoliation syndrome. Am J Ophthalmol 2003; 136:41–46.

36. Bleich S, Roedl J, Von Ahsen N, et al. Elevated homocysteine levels in aqueous humor of patients with pseudoexfoliation glaucoma. Am J Ophthalmol 2004; 138:162–164.

37. Roedl JB, Bleich S, Reulbach U, et al. Homocysteine in tear fluid of patients with pseudoexfoliation glaucoma. J Glaucoma 2007; 16:234–239.

38. Schlötzer-Schrehardt U, Koca MR, Naumann GOH, et al. Pseudoexfoliation syndrome. Ocular manifestation of a systemic disorder? Arch Ophthalmol 1992; 110:1752–1756.

39. Streeten BW, Li ZY, Wallace RN, et al. Pseudoexfoliative fibrillopathy in visceral organs of a patient with pseudoexfoliation syndrome. Arch Ophthalmol 1992; 110:1757–1762.

40. Irkec M. Exfoliation and carotid stiffness (editorial). Br J Ophthalmol 2006; 90:529–530.

41. Konstas AGP, Holló G, Irkec M, et al. Diurnal IOP control with bimatoprost vs latanoprost in exfoliative glaucoma: a crossover observer-masked 3-center study. Br J Ophthalmol 2007; 91:757–760.

42. Konstas AGP, Kozobolis VP, Katsimpris IE, et al. Efficacy and safety of latanoprost versus travoprost in exfoliative glaucoma patients. Ophthalmology 2007; 114:653–657.

43. Konstas AGP, Holló G, Astakhov YS, et al. Factors associated with long-term progression or stability in exfoliation glaucoma. Arch Ophthalmol 2004; 122:29–33.

44. Becker B. Does hyposecretion of aqueous humor damage the trabecular meshwork? (editorial). J Glaucoma 1995; 4:303–305.

45. Odberg T, Sandvik L. The medium and long-term efficacy of primary argon laser trabeculoplasty in avoiding topical medication in open-angle glaucoma. Acta Ophthalmol 1999; 77:176–181.

46. Ritch R, Podos SM. Laser trabeculoplasty in exfoliation syndrome. Bull NY Acad Med 1983; 59:339–344.

47. Konstas AGP, Topouzis F, Leliopoulou O, et al. 24-hour intraocular pressure control with maximum medical therapy compared with surgery in patients with advanced open-angle glaucoma. Ophthalmology 2006; 113:761–765.

48. Tanihara H, Negi A, Akimoto M, et al. Surgical effect of trabeculotomy ab externo on adult eyes with primary open angle glaucoma and pseudoexfoliation syndrome. Arch Ophthalmol 1993; 111:1653–1661.

49. Jacobi PC, Dietlein TS. G.K. Krieglstein. Bimanual trabecular aspiration in pseudoexfoliation glaucoma – an alternative in nonfiltering glaucoma surgery,. Ophthalmology 1998; 105:886–894.

50. Drolsum L. Deep sclerectomy in patients with capsular glaucoma. Acta Ophthalmol Scand 2003; 81:567–572.

CHAPTER 29

Pigmentary Glaucoma

Stefano A Gandolfi, Nicola Ungaro, Paolo Mora, and Chiara Sangermani

INTRODUCTION

In 1949, Sugar and Barbour[1] described a novel clinical form of glaucoma with marked dispersion of pigment onto several structures in the anterior and posterior chamber. They named this entity as 'pigmentary glaucoma' (PG). The diagnostic triad consisted of: (1) slit-like midperipheral iris transillumination defects, (2) diffuse and dense brownish pigmentation of the anterior chamber angle, and (3) pigment granules on the corneal endothelium (the 'Krukenberg spindle'). When the triad was not paralleled by glaucoma, the clinical picture was named as 'pigment dispersion syndrome' (PDS).

Nowadays, PG is considered a 'secondary open angle glaucoma,' mainly triggered by a progressive loading of pigment in the trabecular meshwork. Eyes bearing a PDS are considered at risk for a future development of PG.

DISEASE PREVALENCE

The dispersion of pigment (PDS) was detected in as many as 2.5% of a Caucasian population screened for glaucoma (average age 41.5 years old in males, 35.9 years old in females).[2] There is no general agreement about the prevalence of PDS among genders: some studies reported that PDS is more common among males, while females were predominant in other series. In fact, no population-based studies have been performed so far. It is generally agreed that the conversion to pigmentary glaucoma occurs more often in males, the final male-to-female ratio being 3:1. Some authors speculated that a 15% greater anterior chamber depth, reported in males, could offer a possible explanation for the reported sex-linked incidence of pigmentary glaucoma.[3]

PDS, as well as PG, is claimed to occur almost exclusively in Caucasians, although the reported low prevalence among blacks could be explained by possible misdiagnosis: in fact, the thicker and dark iris makes the detection of pigment loss more difficult in blacks. Besides, the trabecular meshwork pigmentation can be easily interpreted as normal in the eyes of black people. The detection of pigment deposition onto the zonular structures (Fig. 29.1), explored in full mydriasis, has been claimed as a possible tool to identify those eyes, belonging to black people, that are actively dispersing pigment.[4] Therefore, the actual prevalence of pigment dispersion in black people is far from being ascertained.

There are no definite data on the age of onset of pigment dispersion. Based on the reported peak prevalence of pigmentary glaucoma (i.e. between the third and fourth decades) and on the measured average conversion rate from PDS to PG (10–15 years), one could speculate that pigment dispersion can start as early as in the mid-teens. Again, there are no population data consistent with this hypothesis.

The vast majority of eyes affected by pigment dispersion are also affected by mild-to-moderate myopia. There are no data linking the degree of myopia with the prevalence of PDS. However, it appears that eyes with pigmentary glaucoma are more myopic than those with

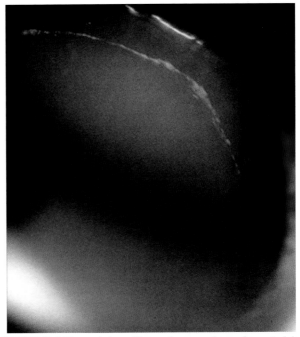

FIGURE 29.1 Pigment deposition on lens zonules and equatorial region. The deposits are clearly visible in full mydriasis.

the pigment dispersion syndrome. In particular, the higher the degree of refractive myopic error, the earlier seems to be the onset of the disease.[5]

In conclusion, as stated by Shields, 'the typical patient affected by PG is young, myopic, and male.'[6]

NATURAL HISTORY AND RISK FACTORS

The clinical course of the disease can be divided into three phases:

1. *The 'active' pigment dispersion phase*: This phase can start as early as in the mid-teens. During this phase, pigment is actively liberated and starts to accumulate in the anterior segment of the eye. This phase is mostly asymptomatic. During the whole phase, the intraocular pressure (IOP) remains normal. However, in some patients the dispersion of pigment can be accelerated by such environmental factors as (1) physical exercise, (2) emotional stress, and (3) naturally occurring and/or drug-induced mydriasis. In particular, phenylephrine-induced mydriasis has been associated with huge flush of pigment in the anterior chamber in some PDS. However provoked, an active dispersion of pigment is not always paralleled by a measurable IOP increase.[7]

2. *The 'conversion' to glaucoma*: In a recent population-based, retrospective study, it was estimated that 10% of PDS will eventually develop PG in 5 years, the incidence increasing to 15% after 15 years.[8] However, a PDS–PG conversion rate as high as 35% in a 5–35-year time span was also reported.[9] Conversely, in a case series, only 2 of 43 eyes showing a PDS developed an unquestionable glaucomatous field defect after 6 years of follow-up.[10] It appears that the apparent discrepancy between the individual surveys can be explained (at least in part) by the criteria adopted for the 'definition' of pigmentary glaucoma, ranging from a pure IOP elevation to a consistent visual field defect on Goldmann manual perimetry. Most studies agree on the 'active dispersion' of pigment being a remarkable risk factor for the future conversion from PDS to PG.[11] Moreover, high myopia has been claimed as a risk factor for conversion.[11]

3. *The possible 'self-healing' (regression) phase*: An interesting phenomenon was repeatedly described in individuals, affected by pigmentary glaucoma, upon aging: pigment starts clearing from the trabecular meshwork, the iris defects slowly disappears, and, in some patients, IOP recovers within the 'normal' range. This phase is called 'regression phase.'[12] The resulting phenotype can be clinically misleading: in fact, the eye still shows an unquestionable glaucomatous optic neuropathy (with or without a concurrent visual field defect), but the IOP is low and the patient can be labeled as having low-tension glaucoma. In these individuals, gonioscopy can be particularly useful: the pigment will appear more dense and dark in the upper than in the lower quadrants

of the angle. This sign (named 'pigment reversal sign') is by far not specific for a regressed PG and can be detected whenever the pigment spontaneously clears from the trabecular meshwork.

ETIOLOGY AND PATHOGENESIS

Mechanical, genetic, and environmental factors contribute to the pathogenesis of the dispersion of pigment.

MECHANICAL

In 1976, Rodrigues and co-workers, while analyzing iris specimens from eyes affected by PDS, found areas of focal atrophy of the pigment epithelium together with a hypertropic dilator muscle.[13] An epithelial abnormality was then supposed to be the primary lesion leading to the PDS phenotype. In 1979, Campbell, after having observed a consistency between the iris transillumination defects and the location of the zonular fibers, set a new theory: he hypothesized that a posterior bowing of the peripheral iris could induce a recurrent contact between the iris pigment epithelium and the lens zonular diaphragm, thus leading to a dispersion of pigment.[14] To bow posteriorly, the iris should have had some peculiar anatomical features: (1) a more posterior insertion to the sclera, (2) a concave profile paralleled by a deeper than normal peripheral anterior chamber, and (3) a floppier stroma, leading to a lower resistance to vectorial dynamic forces from the environment. Each of the required features was confirmed by ultrasound biomicroscopy (UBM) analysis: the distance between the base of the trabecular meshwork and the iris insertion proved greater in PDS than in control eyes;[15] a concave iris profile with a deeper anterior chamber (Fig. 29.2) was repeatedly described in PDS and PG eyes;[16] and the radial width of the iris proved longer than normal in PDS eyes,[17] thus leading to a potential flattening of the midperipheral iris against the lens–zonular complex

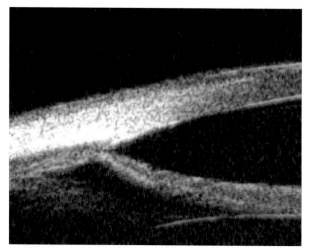

FIGURE 29.2 A concave profile of the midperipheral iris. The UBM image is showing a naturally occurring posterior bowing of the iris with a visible iris–lens contact in an eye affected by PDS.

(Fig. 29.3). The anatomical features, however, do not explain by themselves the occurrence of posterior bowing. A posteriorly directed pressure gradient must occur to trigger the phenomenon. For example, this can occur during blinking. In fact, during blinking, aqueous is moved into the anterior chamber against the normal pressure gradient. The pressure wave, thus created, will act on the iris and push it posteriorly towards the lens–zonular complex.[18] An abnormally great iris–lens contact will prevent equilibration of aqueous between the two chambers, anterior and posterior. Therefore, the iris will assume an even more pronounced concave profile and the rubbing against the zonules will be facilitated. This has been named as 'reverse pupillary block'.[19] Accommodation and bicycle exercise will also increase lens concavity and create a reverse block.[20,21] In particular, accommodation seems to act by displacing the lens forward, thus increasing the pressure in the anterior chamber (Fig. 29.4). As well as the anteriorly directed block, observed in narrow angles, the reverse block too is relieved by a YAG laser iridotomy. The iris profile then loses its concavity to assume a planar configuration (Fig. 29.5).[22] Pilocarpine has been shown to reduce the lens concavity observed after blinking and accommodation. Pilocarpine also prevents the anterior flush of pigment observed in PDS eyes upon physical exercise.[23] In fact, the iris profile after instillation of pilocarpine is convex rather than planar (Fig. 29.6). The mechanical theory has been extensively validated by UBM studies performed on affected subjects. However, a posterior bowing of the iris per se is not sufficient to explain the loss of pigment. In fact, normal eyes can exhibit transient concave iris configurations without visible dispersion of pigment.[21] Therefore, concurrent abnormalities of the iris, as well as comorbidities, must play a role in facilitating the loss of pigment from the posterior iris surface, leading eventually to glaucoma. Interestingly, long anterior zonules, inserted onto the central lens capsule, may also cause mechanical disruption of the pigment epithelium at the pupillary ruff and central iris, leading to pigment dispersion.

GENETIC

In humans, PDS/PG exhibits strong hereditary associations. In some families, linkage was initially reported between the disease phenotype and markers on 7q35-q36[24] and 18q.[25] However, causative mutations at this

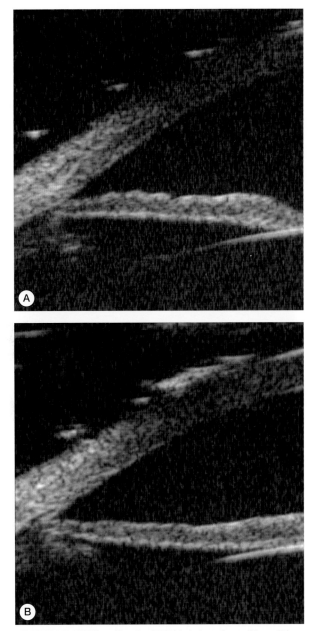

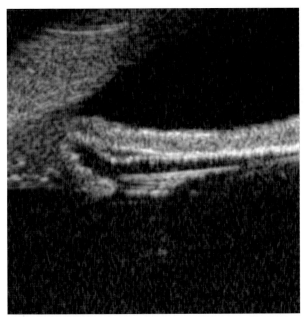

FIGURE 29.3 UBM profile of a 'longer-than-normal' iris in a PG. The iris is flattening onto the anterior lens surface. The lens zonules are clearly visible because of the increased echographic signal due to the deposition of pigment.

FIGURE 29.4 UBM profile of a PDS iris in basal conditions **(A)** and upon soliciting accommodation in the fellow eye **(B)**. An initial reverse pupillary block with a greater iris–lens contact is visible in the accommodative state.

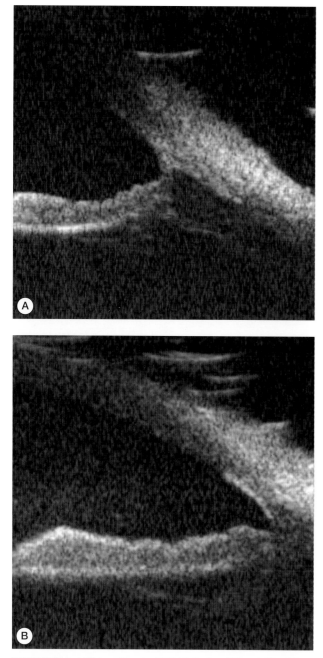

FIGURE 29.5 UBM profile of a PDS iris before **(A)** and after **(B)** iridotomy. The iris root becomes less concave and more planar after the iridotomy. A dense hyperechogenous band, due to accumulation of pigment, is visible on the trabecular meshwork. Gonioscopic view of the same eye is shown in Figure 29.12.

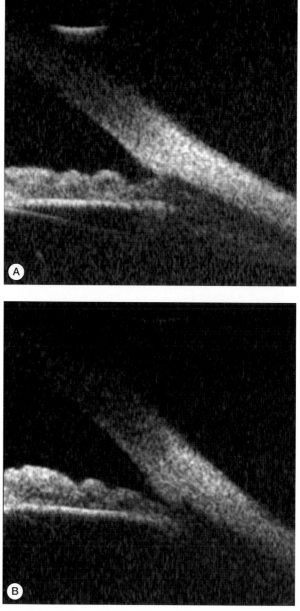

FIGURE 29.6 UBM profile of the iris of a PG eye showing a posterior bowing with concave iris configuration before **(A)** and after **(B)** instillation of 2% pilocarpine. The iris becomes less flat, assuming a very moderate convexity.

locus have thus far not been found. Interestingly, mice carrying a mutation in the DBA/2J (D2) gene complex will develop a glaucoma phenotype consistent with human pigmentary glaucoma.[26] These loci (*TYRP1* and *GPNMB*) are coding for melanosomal membrane glycoproteins, both involved in the tyrosinase activity: in particular *TYRP1* encodes a membrane-bound melanosomal protein with enzymatic activity involved in melanin synthesis.[27] A key function of melanosomes is to sequester the cytotoxic intermediates produced during melanin production. GPNMB and TYRP1 are both transmembrane melanosomal proteins and their mutation appears to promote iris disease by allowing leakage of toxic intermediates from the melanosomes. In fact, the melanosomes of DBA/2J mice are structurally abnormal, as are melanosomes in some human PDS/PG patients. Unfortunately, an analysis of the candidate genes suggested by experiments with D2 mice has so far failed to identify any clear mutations in families carrying the pigmentary glaucoma phenotype.[28] However, the lack of identified mutations in *GPNMB* and *TYRP1* in these families does not preclude the involvement of these genes (or genes of similar function) in patients of other families. Interestingly,

Mo and co-workers showed recently some evidence for immune aberrations and sustained, mild inflammation in eyes of D2-mutant mice.[29] They further proposed that a similar, and previously unsuspected, set of abnormalities may occur in human PDS/PG, thus tracing a role for bone marrow-derived cells and ocular immune privilege in the pathogenesis of PG. Another example of PDS/PG-like phenotype observed upon knocking down of selected genes is the collagen XVIII-endostatin deficient mouse (ColA8a1[−/−]). The absence of this collagen alters the properties of iris basal membranes and leads to severe defects in the iris. In addition, loss of collagen XVIII creates changes that allow clump cells to migrate out of the iris.[30] These cells are macrophage-like cells and are able to penetrate the inner limiting membrane, thus affecting the inner layers of the mouse retina. This phenomenon may disclose a totally new mechanism, leading directly to ganglion cell dysfunction in this model and (possibly) in human PG.

ENVIRONMENTAL

Mild subclinical inflammation and abnormal ocular immunity may contribute to human PDS. In fact, the IL-18, NF-κB, MAPK, MMP-2, TIMP-1, and apoptotic signaling components were altered in the D2-mutant mouse. In particular, elevated expression of IL-18 was correlated with the increased IOP and the death of retinal ganglion cells.[31] It is then possible that at least

some PDS represents the mild end of a spectrum of inflammatory diseases that attack the iris and cause glaucoma (including anterior uveitis). Although there is currently scant evidence for an inflammatory component in PDS, the issue has not been extensively studied. Indeed, pigment-containing macrophages are reported in histologic studies of eyes from human PDS patients and may not be simply involved in pigment cleaning. If immune genotype and inflammatory components are important in PDS susceptibility, factors affecting iris configuration and rubbing could cause the initial damage that primes the disease (either alone or by exacerbating the effects of melanosomal toxicity). Alternatively, but not exclusively, viral or other trauma could have the same effect.[32]

Once the pigment is liberated in the anterior chamber, its deposition onto the angle structure will trigger the mechanisms leading to outflow obstruction. In detail, the trabecular endothelial cells will take up the melanin carried by the pigmented granules. The overload of melanin will lead to cell death and denudation of the collagen beams within the trabecular meshwork. The structure will then collapse and fuse, leading to closure of the aqueous channels, increased resistance to flow, and elevated IOP (Fig. 29.7).[33] Therefore, those eyes whose trabecular meshwork has not yet collapsed (thus leading to an increased IOP) will mostly benefit from preventing further pigment dispersion. In fact, once the outflow system is knocked out, a spontaneous

1. Posterior bowing of mid-peripheral iris leading to iris-zonular contact

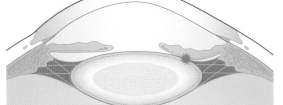

2. Co-morbidities capable of triggering pigment dispersion upon iris-zonular contact

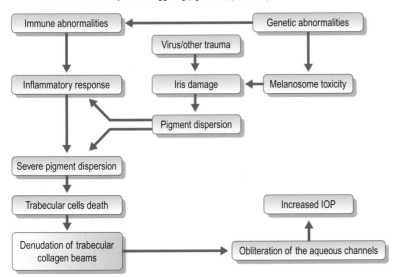

FIGURE 29.7 Schematic representation of the mechanisms leading to pigment liberation from the iris and to an eventual obstruction of trabecular flow and increase of IOP. The mechanical rubbing, between lens zonules and posterior iris, represents the initial triggering step. Liberation of pigment will then occur as a function of several possible comorbidities directly damaging the iris and weakening the epithelial cells of the posterior surface.

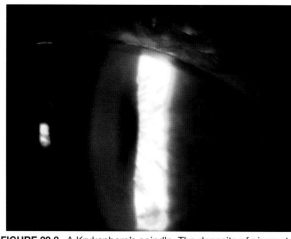

FIGURE 29.8 A Krukenberg's spindle. The deposits of pigment on the endothelium are vertically arranged to assume a tentlike configuration.

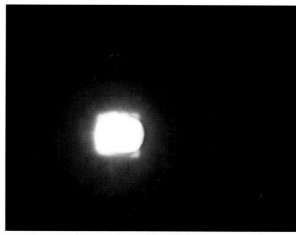

FIGURE 29.9 Slitlike midperipheral iris defects. Pupillary transillumination reveals the defects through the entire circumference of the iris.

self-healing, up to a complete recovery of basal normal steady state, will be more difficult, even upon stopping the pigment liberation from the iris.

SIGNS AND SYMPTOMS

Open-angle glaucomas are mostly asymptomatic until the disease reaches the advanced-to-end stages. Individuals with pigmentary glaucoma are somewhat different. Conditions triggering an acute dispersion of pigment (i.e. physical exercise, prolonged permanence in the dark, prolonged near work, night driving, etc.) can be paralleled by acute and intense rise of IOP. This may generate symptoms like (1) haloes surrounding light sources and, more generally, (2) blurred vision due to corneal edema. Conversely, patients with the pigment dispersion syndrome, having by definition a normal IOP, do not report symptoms related to their condition; the diagnosis is often made within the course of a routine ophthalmological examination, mostly requested because of the concurrent myopia.

ANTERIOR SEGMENT

Pigment can be theoretically detected on every structure of the anterior segment. A careful slit lamp examination will reveal deposits of pigment on the posterior cornea. Typically, the pigment granules are aligned in a vertically shaped fashion to create a spindlelike pattern on the central corneal endothelium (the so-called 'Krukenberg spindle') (Fig. 29.8). This occurs due to convection movements of aqueous humor in the anterior chamber: the pigment accumulates centrally to be eventually phagocyted by the endothelial cells that change their shape to create both polymorphisms and polymegathism. In spite of this phenomenon, no abnormalities in both endothelial cell count and central corneal thickness have been reported in eyes with PG.[34] Pigment deposits can be seen also on the lens zonules once the patient is put on mydriasis. Conversely of what is reported in pseudoexfoliation, accumulation of pigment does not seem to induce weakness of the zonular structures. Loss of iris pigment creates typical midperipheral, radial, slitlike defects (Fig. 29.9) detectable upon either retrollumination or transillumination, the latter technique showing a higher sensitivity than the former. In 1990, Alward and co-workers described a videographic technique that, so far, has proven to be the most sensitive method to detect iris transillumination defects in eyes where a slit lamp examination was negative.[35] Typically, the pigment particles can accumulate on the anterior iris surface, leading to a unique blend of hyperpigmented and thinner areas. Heterochromia can frequently occur in asymmetric cases. Eyes showing particularly profound transillumination defects will show a slightly more dilated pupil in basal conditions. If the disease is asymmetric, the clinician will diagnose anisocoria that, together with the possible heterochromia, will offer a 'Horner-like' picture.[36]

ANTERIOR CHAMBER ANGLE

The anterior chamber of both a PDS and a PG-affected eye is deeper than normal (Fig. 29.10). In particular, Strasser and Hauf, while examining patients with unilateral PDS, reported a deeper anterior chamber and a flatter lens in the affected eye.[37] The anterior chamber angle is wide open. The iris is inserted more posteriorly. The distance between the iris insertion and the scleral spur can range between 0.42 mm and 0.40 mm, while in control subjects the distance is 0.28–0.29 mm.[38] The iris root can be concave on gonioscopy both in basal conditions and upon soliciting accommodation in the contralateral eye. Typically, the concavity affects the midperipheral part of the iris. A band of dark-brown pigment on the trabecular meshwork is visible (Fig. 29.11). In some subjects, the pigment will cover the entire angle structures up to the Schwalbe line (Fig. 29.12). The pigmented band can be either thin or broad. Prominent ciliary processes in some phenotypes of PG were also described, thus leading to the hypothesis of concurrent malformations of the angle structures.

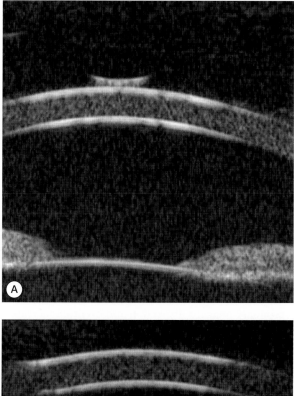

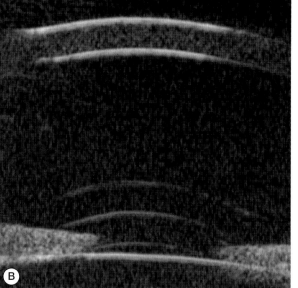

FIGURE 29.10 A UBM profile of the anterior chamber depth in a control eye **(A)** and in an eye affected by PG **(B)**. The depth is significantly increased in PG.

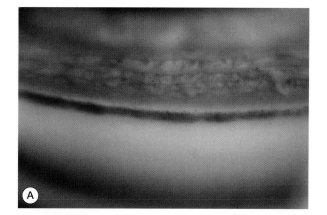

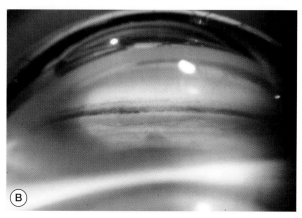

FIGURE 29.11 Gonioscopic view of an eye affected by PG. A band of dense brownish-like pigment is visible in both the upper **(A)** and the lower **(B)** quadrants. Pigment on the Schwalbe's line is clearly visible in the lower quadrants. (Courtesy of Tarek Shaarawy, MD.)

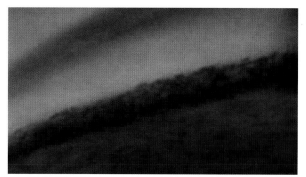

FIGURE 29.12 Gonioscopic view of an eye with PDS. A broad band of pigment covers most of the angle structures. A UBM profile of this eye is visible in Figure 29.5.

POSTERIOR SEGMENT

The peripheral retina is often abnormal in both PDS and PG eyes. A retinal detachment can occur in as many as 6–7% of affected eyes, irrespective of the degree of myopia.[39] Degeneration of the peripheral retina is common. Wesley and co-workers, while examining the fundi of 60 patients with PDS and PG, detected rhegmatogenous degenerations in 20% and a full-thickness retinal hole in 11% of the enrolled eyes.[40] This feature stresses the need for periodic retinal examination (in full mydriasis) for patients affected by PDS and PG. Recently, a bilateral retinal vein occlusion has been described in a 32-year-old male affected by PG with an untreated IOP >30 mmHg.[41]

DIFFERENTIAL DIAGNOSIS

See Table 29.1 for a summary of the diagnostic features of pigment dispersion syndrome and pigmentary glaucoma.

The occurrence of elevated intraocular pressure and dispersion of pigment granules in the anterior segment

TABLE 29.1 Diagnostic features of pigment dispersion syndrome and pigmentary glaucoma

Cornea	Krukenberg spindle Endothelial cells polymorphism on microscopy
Anterior chamber	Free-floating pigmented particles Increased depth
Iris	Slitlike midperipheral defects 'Patchy' deposits of pigment onto the anterior surface Heterochromia Anisocoria
Lens zonule	Deposits of pigment on anterior and posterior lens capsule AND on lens zonules
Anterior chamber angle	Heavily pigmented trabecular meshwork Deposits of pigment on Schwalbe's line Wide open Posterior insertion of the iris Concave iris profile (often but not always)
Posterior segment	Rhegmatogenous peripheral retina degenerations (i.e. lattice, etc.)

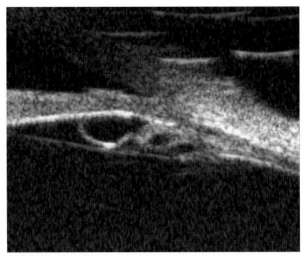

FIGURE 29.13 A UBM analysis of an eye bearing iris cysts. The cysts are pushing on the posterior surface of the iris, leading to an anterior convexity.

is by far not unique to PG. Pigment dispersion and iris transillumination defects can be detected in *pseudoexfoliation* (PEX). In fact, rubbing of the anterior lens capsule against the peripupillary border can induce the liberation of pigment in the anterior chamber. The deposits of pseudoexfoliative material on the anterior lens and on the pupillary border, together with the older age of the affected patients and the typical gonioscopic features such as the Sampaolesi line, will help in differentiating PEX from PG. However, both situations can occur in the same subject/eye.[42] A careful evaluation of the lens (in full mydriasis) as well as an accurate gonioscopy are then always needed.

Pigment dispersion can occur as a consequence of a disease of the posterior iris. *Cysts of the iris and ciliary body* can induce a loss of pigment, but an accurate gonioscopy with a complimentary UBM study (Fig. 29.13) will help in making a correct diagnosis. *Neoplasms of the iris–ciliary body complex* (i.e. melanomas) can induce liberation of pigmented granules in the anterior chamber. However, a careful examination will reveal neither a Krukenberg spindle nor the typical midperipheral transillumination defects. Conversely, the angle will appear narrow/closed in the segment affected by the body of the neoplasm.

A secondary pigmentary glaucoma can be provoked by an *incorrect implantation of posterior chamber intraocular lenses*, leading to displacement of the haptics and rubbing against the posterior iris (the so-called 'iris-chafing' syndrome).[43] The surgical history, as well as the unilaterality of the disease, will help in making a proper differential diagnosis with primary PDS or PG. Again, (1) implantation of *posterior chamber refractive IOLs* in phakic patients[44] and (2) *piggyback implantation of IOLs* in aphakic eyes[45] have been associated with

a secondary pigment dispersion and eventual increase of IOP. In every post-IOL case, the UBM can prove pivotal in directing the clinician to the diagnosis. In any case, reintervention with explantation of the IOLs is advised.

Pigment deposition onto the anterior chamber structures and elevated IOP can occur in recurrent *uveitis* as well as after a *trauma*. Again, the medical history and the absence of the typical features of the PDS/PG will help in making the correct diagnosis.

Recently, an asymmetric form of pigmentary glaucoma has been described in an individual affected by *Marfan's* syndrome.[46] A superiorly subluxated lens as well as an extreme zonular weakness has been considered as a possible mechanism responsible for the secondary glaucoma in this case.

As described above, the UBM is pivotal in studying cases of abnormal pigment liberation in the anterior segment. The recent availability of noncontact devices to study the anterior segment, such as the Pentacam® and the OCT Visante®, can potentially help the clinician in making the diagnosis. However, while the accuracy of UBM in studying the iris root insertion and conformation as well as the relationship with the other anatomical structures of the iridolenticular area has been extensively proven, more clinical studies are needed to trace the role of noncontact devices in the evaluation of PDS and PG patients.

TREATMENT OPTIONS

The treatment algorithm of pigmentary glaucoma is traditionally considered as comparable to what is applicable in primary open-angle glaucoma. Briefly, medical treatment is usually offered as a first-line approach. A more aggressive approach is considered when medications fail to keep IOP under a proper control. However, eyes affected by pigmentary glaucoma have some phenotypic characteristics that may affect both (1) the choice of the agent and (2) the timing of further nonmedical therapeutic strategies.

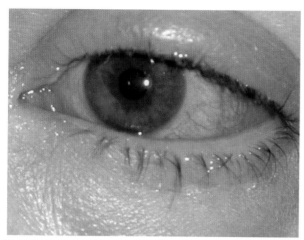

FIGURE 29.14 A PDS eye, with a 'hazel' iris, showing a toxic/allergic-like reaction to a prolonged use of an α_1-antagonist. The conjunctiva is diffusely inflamed. The anterior iris is showing the peripheral deposits of brownish pigment in areas of less dark stroma.

MEDICAL THERAPY

Drugs capable of reducing (if not eliminating) the contact between the posterior iris and the lens zonule should theoretically be considered as a first choice in pigmentary glaucoma. For example, *cholinergic agonists*, such as pilocarpine, have been extensively used in the past. Pilocarpine can, in fact, both reduce the liberation of pigment, by blocking the pupil in miosis, and decrease the IOP by increasing the trabecular outflow of aqueous. Interestingly, a prolonged use of pilocarpine was associated with *both* a decrease in the amount of pigment, detectable onto anterior segment, *and*, in some, reversal of the iris transillumination defects.[12] Unfortunately, (1) the relatively young age and (2) the concurrent myopia make pilocarpine poorly tolerated by the patients, who experience pain, a transient worsening of the myopic refractive error, and poor night vision. Besides, due to the higher incidence of rhegmatogenous lesions in PDS/PG eyes, a prolonged use of miotics could represent a further risk factor for retinal tears and detachment. *Alpha$_1$-receptor antagonists*, like dapiprazole and thymoxamine, have been offered as a therapeutic option to avoid physiological mydriasis in the affected eyes. These agents offer the therapeutic advantage of sparing the ciliary muscle and acting by relaxation of the dilator muscle.[47] The refraction is then unaffected. However, their long-term efficacy on both IOP control and pigment liberation is still controversial, and topical adverse events, such as burning and intolerable hyperemia, have been reported upon their prolonged use (Fig. 29.14). Due to the nature of the disease, aqueous outflow enhancers should be preferentially considered with respect to aqueous suppressants. In fact, *prostaglandin analogues* have been reported as greatly effective in decreasing IOP in eyes affected by pigmentary glaucoma. In a 12-month prospective, randomized, controlled trial, latanoprost was more effective than timolol in eyes affected by pigmentary

glaucoma.[48] However, it is necessary to stress that drugs that increase the uveoscleral outflow will not ameliorate either the trabecular function or the mechanism of continued pigment liberation from the posterior iris. Therefore, their mechanism of action can be considered as a medical 'bypass' of the trabecular meshwork, leaving the diseased tissue unaffected by therapy.

LASER TRABECULOPLASTY

If the anterior chamber angle is wide open, laser trabeculoplasty (both argon and selective) could be a reasonable option. Conversely to what is observed in primary open-angle glaucoma, laser trabeculoplasty seems more effective in young individuals affected by PG. Moreover, the longer the duration of the disease, the poorer the response to laser trabeculoplasty.[49] This is consistent with histologic data, showing that the majority of pigment is recovered far away from the trabecular meshwork in young patients and in the earlier stages of the disease. Technically speaking, PG patients do require a minimal laser energy, as low as 300 mW/spot (argon) or 0.4 mJ/spot (selective). In particular, the greater is the amount of pigment in the angle structures (as, for example, in older individuals), the lower is the amount of energy to be delivered, thus minimizing the risk of postoperative IOP increase due to excess absorption of energy and subsequent scarring of the meshwork anlage. In a recent prospective, randomized clinical trial comparing argon versus selective trabeculoplasty, the IOP decreased by 3.4 mmHg in the ALT ($n = 3$) and by 5.6 mmHg in the SLT ($n = 5$) groups on average at 12 months.[50]

LASER IRIDOTOMY

Laser iridotomy has been shown to reduce the chance of a reverse pupillary block. After a successful iridotomy, a concave iris root will flatten, thus producing a narrowing of the angle with decreased likelihood of iris-to-lens contact (Fig. 29.15).[16] Besides, Nd:YAG laser iridotomy results in significant (65%) decrease of aqueous melanin granules in eyes with primary pigment dispersion syndrome.[51] However, performing a laser iridotomy will liberate a huge amount of pigment in the anterior chamber. Therefore, the potential benefit of the procedure must be weighed against a theoretical increased morbidity. In a randomized, prospective, controlled clinical trial, laser iridotomy significantly reduced the 10-year incidence of increase in IOP in a series of PDS eyes showing a concave iris root and pigment granules in the anterior chamber upon medical dilation.[52,53] The effect was greater below the age of 40 years: this is consistent with the well-known exacerbation of a reverse pupillary block induced by accommodation. If iridotomy proved effective in PDS eyes, the results on IOP in PG eyes are still controversial. In a recent retrospective chart review, performed on 46 patients treated medically for PG and observed for 2 years or more, the mean intraocular pressure in the lasered eyes decreased

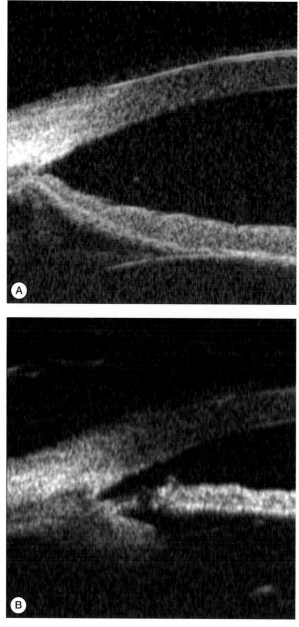

FIGURE 29.15 UBM profile of a PDS eye on reverse pupillary block before **(A)** and after **(B)** a YAG laser iridotomy. The iris root is moved forward and the posterior chamber is greater after the iridotomy. Interestingly, the post-laser dynamics are a mirror image of those observed in post-laser narrow angles with 'anteriorly directed' pupillary block.

the IOP is increased, the benefit of no further pigment overload in the tissue can be questionable and is by no means supported by the presently available scientific evidence.

SURGERY

Surgery is indicated when both medications and laser fail to control IOP. The peculiarity of the disease, a 'trabecular aspiration,' was recently investigated as a possible indication in both PDS and PG. In spite of an initial better success rate for PDS, the midterm data were somehow disappointing.[55] Therefore, trabecular aspiration is presently not indicated either in PDS or in PG. Since there are no specific data on the efficacy of nonpenetrating surgery in PG, proper filtration surgery still remains the first choice. Patients with PG are, on average, younger than patients with both POAG and PACG. When performing the trabeculectomy, the surgeon must consider the possible adjunctive use on antifibrotic agents. While performing surgery with mitomycin C (MMC), one should be aware of the higher risk of postoperative hypotony in young myopic eyes. Besides, minimizing the risk of intraoperative shallowing of the anterior chamber is pivotal to avoid tractions of the vitreous base on the peripheral retina. In fact, one should remember that eyes affected by PG have a higher prevalence of peripheral retinal degenerations and dystrophies, thus leading to a higher risk of retinal tears formation and rhegmatogenous retinal detachment. A careful postoperative monitoring of the peripheral retina is then advised.

TREATMENT OUTCOME AND PROGNOSIS

The risk for conversion from PDS to PG has been discussed above.

Long-term data on visual prognosis and treatment outcomes in pigmentary glaucoma are scanty. In a retrospective study, visual field progression was noted in 44% of 23 pigmentary glaucoma cases over a follow-up period of up to 15 years. During follow-up, the probability of surgical intervention for patients with pigmentary glaucoma was 18% for laser trabeculoplasty and 10% for filtration surgery by 10 years. For all patients with pigmentary glaucoma, the IOP on treatment at the last examination was 18.0 + 4.0 mmHg. Two of 23 patients developed legal blindness in at least one eye during the follow-up period.[8]

A worse glaucoma damage and a poorly controlled IOP were observed in those PG patients who, on therapy, showed a greater amount of pigment granules in the anterior chamber. Such a measure could (at least theoretically) offer some help in dissecting those PG eyes bearing a worse prognosis.[56]

No data are available on the relative risk of environmental and comportamental situations, inducing pigment dispersion, on long-term visual prognosis. Therefore, the impact of (1) intense physical exercise, (2) prolonged accommodative effort, and (3) spending

4.0 + 5.4 mmHg, compared with 1.9 + 3.8 mmHg in the fellow nonlasered eyes ($p = 0.005$), but the difference proved not significant when the data were subjected to rigid statistical analysis.[54] Therefore, in dissecting out eyes which might benefit from a peripheral iridotomy, one should treat eyes of individuals aged less than 45 years showing (1) a well-documented concave iris root, (2) a clinically detectable pigment flush in the anterior chamber upon medical dilation, and (3) a functioning trabecular meshwork, as documented by an IOP still reasonably controlled without treatment. In fact, once the trabecular meshwork is damaged and hours in a dark environment on visual field deterioration in PG eyes is far from being quantified.[57] Caution must thus be taken in counseling patients.

As a rule of thumb, the IOP should be also measured upon dilation and/or after a prolonged accommodation in every patient on treatment. In case either condition may induce a significant IOP rise, a more aggressive therapy should be considered as one usually does in other glaucoma phenotypes once spontaneous IOP fluctuations are detected.

Summary

- Pigment dispersion syndrome (PDS) and pigmentary glaucoma (PG) are not rare clinical entities. Siblings of affected individuals are at high risk for developing the pathological phenotype.
- PDS and PG are mostly diagnosed in individuals of a younger age than those diagnosed with either primary open-angle or primary angle-closure glaucoma.
- In PDS eyes, an active dispersion of pigment is a strong risk factor for conversion to PG.
- Pigment is liberated from the posterior iris due to two mechanisms: (1) mechanical rubbing against the lens zonules with a reverse pupillary block due to either a concave iris root or to a spontaneous flattening of a floppier and longer iris on the anterior lens surface, and (2) conditions (both genetic and environmental) leading to a weakness of the iris pigmented epithelium.
- Gonioscopy and evaluation of the anterior lens surface in full mydriasis are needed to perform a correct diagnosis. UBM can greatly help by offering pivotal information on the iris profile.
- PDS and PG are mostly bilateral. In case of an asymmetrical involvement, an accurate investigation on concurrent diseases leading to a secondary dispersion of pigment is needed.
- The treatment algorithm of PG is similar to that applicable in primary open-angle glaucoma. Miotics are still (at least theoretically) the drug of choice to cure the disease. Care must be taken in performing laser trabeculoplasty not to deliver too much energy to the trabecular meshwork.
- YAG laser iridotomy can be beneficial in individuals older than 45 years whose PDS eyes show a concave iris root and a high risk for conversion to PG as defined by an active dispersion of pigment. The potential benefit of an iridotomy in PG is still a matter of debate.
- PDS and PG eyes can develop serious retinal problems. While planning a follow-up, a routine examination of the retina in full mydriasis is mandatory.

REFERENCES

1. Sugar HS, Barbour FA. Pigmentary glaucoma: a rare clinical entity. Am J Ophthalmol 1949; 32:90–96.
2. Ritch R, Steinberger D, Liebmann JM. Prevalence of pigment dispersion syndrome in a population undergoing glaucoma screening. Am J Ophthalmol 1993; 115:707–710.
3. Orgul S, Hendrickson P, Flammer J. Anterior chamber depth and pigment dispersion syndrome. Am J Ophthalmol 1994; 117:575–583.
4. Roberts DK, Chaglasian MA, Metz RE. Clinical signs of the pigment dispersion syndrome in blacks. Optom Vis Sci 1997; 74:993–998.
5. Gramer E, Thiele H, Ritch R. Family history of glaucoma and risk factors in pigmentary glaucoma. A new clinical study. Klin Monatsbl Augenheilkd 1998; 212:454–464.
6. Pigmentary glaucomas and other glaucomas associated with disorders of the iris and ciliary body. In: Allingham RR, Damji K, Freedman S, et al., eds. Shields' textbook of glaucoma. Philadephia: Lippincott Williams & Wilkins; 2005:303.
7. Epstein DL, Boger WP, Grant WM. Phenylephrine provocative testing in the pigmentary dispersion syndrome. Am J Ophthalmol 1978; 85:43–51.
8. Siddiqui Y, Hulzen RDT, Cameron D, et al. What is the risk of developing pigmentary glaucoma from pigment dispersion syndrome? Am J Ophthalmol 2003; 135:794–799.
9. Migliazzo CV, Shaffer RN, Nykin R, et al. Long-term analysis of pigmentary dispersion syndrome and pigmentary glaucoma. Ophthalmology 1986; 93:528–536.
10. Wilensky JT, Buerk KM, Podos SM. Krukenberg's spindles. Am J Ophthalmol 1975; 79:220–225.
11. Farrar SM, Shields MB, Miller KN, et al. Risk factors for the development and severity of glaucoma in the pigment dispersion syndrome. Am J Ophthalmol 1989; 108:223–229.
12. Campbell DG. Improvement of pigmentary glaucoma and healing of transillumination defects with miotic therapy. Inv Ophthalmol Vis Sci (ARVO Suppl) 1983; 23:173.

13. Rodrigues MM, Spaeth GL, Weinreb S, et al. Spectrum of trabecular pigmentation in open-angle glaucoma: a clinico-pathologic study. Trans Sect Ophthalmol Am Acad Ophthalmol Otolaryngol 1976; 81:258–276.
14. Campbell DG. Pigmentary dispersion and glaucoma: a new theory. Arch Ophthalmol 1979; 97:1667–1672.
15. Sokol J, Stegman Z, Liebmann JM, et al. Location of the iris insertion in pigment dispersion syndrome. Ophthalmology 1996; 103:289–293.
16. Carassa RG, Bettin P, Fiori M, et al. Nd:YAG laser iridotomy in pigment dispersion syndrome: an ultrasound biomicroscopic study. Br J Ophthalmol 1998; 82:150–153.
17. Ritch R. A unification hypothesis of pigmentary dispersion syndrome. Trans Am Ophthalmol Soc 1996; 94:381–388.
18. McWhae JA, Piamontesi RL. Crichton ACS. Blinking and iris configuration in PDS. Ophthalmology 1996; 103:197–199.
19. Karickhoff JR. Pigment dispersion syndrome and pigmentary glaucoma: a new mechanism concept. A new treatment and a new technique. Ophthalm Surg 1992; 23:269–277.
20. Pavlin CJ, Harasiewicz K, Foster FS. Posterior iris bowing in pigmentary dispersion syndrome caused by accommodation. Am J Ophthalmol 1994; 118:114–116.
21. Haargard B, Jensen PK, Kessing SV, et al. Exercise and iris concavity in healthy eyes. Acta Ophthalmol Scand 2001; 79:277–282.
22. Pavlin CJ, Macken P, Trope GE, et al. Accommodation and iridotomy in the pigment dispersion syndrome. Ophthalmic Surg Lasers 1996; 27:113–120.
23. Haynes WL, Johnson AT, Alward WLM. Inhibition of exercise-induced pigment dispersion in a patient with the pigment dispersion syndrome. Am J Ophthalmol 1990; 109:599–601.
24. Andersen JS, Pralea AM, DelBono EA, et al. A gene responsible for the pigment dispersion syndrome maps to chromosome 7q35-q36. Arch Ophthalmol 1997; 115:384–388.

25. Andersen JS, DelBono EA, Haines JL, et al. Identification and genetic analysis of pigmentary glaucoma loci on 7q36 and 18q. Invest Ophthalmol Vis Sci (ARVO Suppl) 1999; 40:S596.

26. John SW, Smith RS, Savinova OV, et al. Essential iris atrophy, pigment dispersion, and glaucoma in DBA/2 J mice. Invest Ophthalmol Vis Sci 1998; 39:951–962.

27. Kobayashi T, Urabe K, Winder A, et al. DHICA oxidase activity of TRP1 and interactions with other melanogenic enzymes. Pigment Cell Res 1994; 7:227–234.

28. Lynch S, Yanagi G, DelBono E, et al. DNA sequence variants in the tyrosinase-related protein 1 (TYRP1) gene are not associated with human pigmentary glaucoma. Mol Vis 2002; 8:127–129.

29. Mo JS, Anderson MG, Gregory M, et al. By altering ocular immune privilege, bone marrow derived cells pathogenically contribute to DBA/2 J pigmentary glaucoma. J Exp Med 2003; 197:1335–1344.

30. Marneros AG, Olsen BR. Age-dependent iris abnormalities in collagen XVIII/endostatin deficient mice with similarities to human pigment dispersion syndrome. Inv Ophthalmol Vis Sci 2003; 44:2367–2372.

31. Zhou X, Li F, Kong L, et al. Involvement of inflammation degradation and apoptosis in a mouse model of glaucoma. J Biol Chem 2005; 280:31240–31248.

32. Libby R, Gould D, Anderson MG, et al. Complex genetics of glaucoma susceptibility. Annu Rev Genomics Hum Genet 2005; 6:15–44.

33. Alvarado JA, Murphy CG. Outflow obstruction in pigmentary and primary open angle glaucoma. Arch Ophthalmol 1992; 110:1769–1778.

34. Lehto I, Rousuvaara P, Setala K. Corneal endothelium in pigmentary glaucoma and pigment dispersion syndrome. Acta Ophthalmol Scand 1990; 68:703–710.

35. Alward WLM, Munden PM, Vedick RE, et al. Use of infrared videography to detect and record iris transillumination defects. Arch Ophthalmol 1990; 108:748–750.

36. Haynes WL, Thompson HS, Kardon RH, et al. Asymmetric pigment dispersion syndrome mimicking Horner's syndrome. Am J Ophthalmol 1991; 112:463–464.

37. Strasser G, Hauff E. Pigmentary dispersion syndrome. A biometric study. Acta Ophthalmol (Copenh) 1985; 63:721–722.

38. Kanadani FN, Dorairaj S, Langlieb AM, et al. Ultrasound biomicroscopy in asymmetric pigment dispersion syndrome and pigmentary glaucoma. Arch Ophthalmol 2006; 124:1573–1576.

39. Scheie HG, Cameron JD. Pigment dispersion syndrome: a clinical study. Br J Ophthalmol 1981; 65:264–269.

40. Wesley P, Liebmann JM, Walsh JB, et al. Lattice degeneration of the retina and the pigment dispersion syndrome. Am J Ophthalmol 1992; 114:539–545.

41. Gupta V, Sony P, Sihota R. Bilateral retinal venous occlusion in pigmentary glaucoma. Graefe's Arch Clin Exp Ophthalmol 2005; 243:731–733.

42. Ritch R, Mudumbai R, Liebmann JM. Combined exfoliation and pigment dispersion: an overlap syndrome. Ophthalmology 2000; 107:1004–1008.

43. Masket S. Pseudophakic posterior iris chafing syndrome. J Cat Refract Surg 1986; 12:252–256.

44. Chun YS, Park IK, Lee HI, et al. Iris and trabecular meshwork pigment changes after posterior chamber phakic intraocular lens implantation. J Cat Refract Surg 2006; 32:1452–1458.

45. Chang SHL, Lim G. Secondary pigmentary glaucoma associated with piggyback intraocular lens implantation. J Cat Refract Surg 2004; 30:2219–2222.

46. Doyle A, Hamard P, Puech M, et al. Asymmetric pigmentary glaucoma in a patient with Marfan's syndrome. Graefe's Arch Clin Exp Ophthalmol 2005; 243:955–957.

47. Mastropasqua L, Carpineto P, Ciancaglini M, et al. The usefulness of dapiprazole an alpha-adrenergic blocking agent in pigmentary glaucoma. Ophthalmic Surg Lasers 1996; 27:806–811.

48. Mastropasqua L, Carpineto P, Ciancaglini M, et al. A 12-month randomised, double masked study comparing latanoprost with timolol in pigmentary glaucoma. Ophthalmology 1999; 106:550–555.

49. Ritch R, Liebmann JM, Robin A, et al. Argon laser trabeculoplasty in pigmentary glaucoma. Ophthalmology 1993; 100:909–913.

50. Damji KF, Bovell AM, Hodge WG, et al. Selective laser trabeculoplasty versus argon laser trabeculoplasty: results from a 1-year randomised clinical trial. Br J Ophthalmol 2006; 90:1490–1494.

51. Kuchle MK, Nguyen NX, Mardin CY, et al. Effect of neodymium:YAG laser iridotomy on number of aqueous melanin granules in primary pigment dispersion syndrome. Graefe's Arch Clin Exp Ophthalmol 2001; 239:411–415.

52. Gandolfi SA, Vecchi M. Effect of a YAG-laser iridotomy on intraocular pressure in pigment dispersion syndrome. Ophthalmology 1996; 103:1693–1696.

53. Ungaro N, Sangermani C, Vecchi M, et al. YAG-laser iridotomy in pigment dispersion syndrome: 10 years later. Invest Ophthalmol Vis Sci (ARVO Suppl) 2003:P4293.

54. Reistad CE, Shields MB, Campbell DG, et al. The influence of peripheral iridotomy on the IOP course in patients with pigmentary glaucoma. J Glaucoma 2005; 14:255–259.

55. Jacobi PC, Dietlein TS, Krieglstein GK. Effect of trabecular aspiration on intraocular pressure in pigment dispersion syndrome and pigmentary glaucoma. Ophthalmology 2000; 107:417–421.

56. Mardin CY, Kuchle M, Nguyen NX, et al. Quantification of aqueous melanin granules IOP and glaucomatous damage in primary pigment dispersion syndrome. Ophthalmology 2000; 107:435–440.

57. Ritch R. Pigment dispersion syndrome – update 2003. In: Grehn F, Stamper R, eds. Glaucoma. Essentials in ophthalmology,. Berlin: Springer; 2004:177–191.

CHAPTER 30

Normal-Tension Glaucoma

Angelo P Tanna and Theodore Krupin

INTRODUCTION

The concept of glaucomatous optic neuropathy occurring in patients with normal intraocular pressure (IOP) has been an area of controversy since it was first described by von Graefe in 1857.[1] It is now well accepted that typical glaucomatous optic neuropathy occurs in some eyes despite normal IOP. We define normal-tension glaucoma (NTG) as an optic neuropathy characterized by optic disc excavation and corresponding visual field loss in the setting of an open anterior chamber angle and statistically normal IOP. Based upon the findings of population-based surveys,[2–4] we consider NTG part of the spectrum of primary open-angle glaucoma (POAG) and recognize that any separation based on normal or elevated IOP is intrinsically arbitrary. For the purposes of clarity and ease of discussion, we refer to POAG with IOP ≤21 mmHg as NTG and open-angle glaucoma (OAG) without secondary features and IOP >21 mmHg as POAG.

THE SCIENTIFIC BASIS FOR THE CONCEPT OF NORMAL INTRAOCULAR PRESSURE

The prevalence of OAG increases in a continuous fashion as a function of increasing IOP (Fig. 30.1). In a particular population, preferably subclassified according to ethnicity, age, race, and gender, one could theoretically determine the range of normal IOP by performing a large survey, and then defining the upper limit of normal as the mean plus two standard deviations. Such an approach using Schiøtz tonometry, without an attempt to subclassify the study population, led to the widely accepted definition of the upper limit of normal IOP: 21 mmHg. This is flawed because IOP measurements are not normally distributed, but are skewed toward higher pressures. The authors believe that any attempt to define an upper normal limit of IOP is strictly arbitrary. There is an advantage to classifying POAG patients separately from those with NTG. The hallmark of glaucomatous optic neuropathy is optic disc excavation. However, it is simplistic to believe that

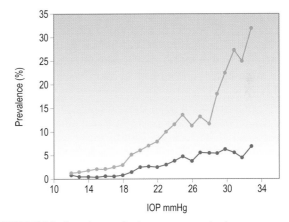

FIGURE 30.1 Prevalence of primary open-angle glaucoma (POAG) in black (orange circles) and white (blue circles) Americans in the Baltimore Eye Survey. The prevalence of POAG increases as a function of intraocular pressure (IOP) in both groups. (Reproduced with permission from Sommer et al.[2] Arch Ophthalmol 1991; 109: 1090–1095)

because optic disc excavation has a similar appearance in most eyes with glaucoma that this process represents a single disease. The phenotypic response of the optic nerve to injury is limited to a small number of morphological changes: the development of edema, excavation, and pallor. The authors propose that, on a molecular and cellular level, POAG and NTG are a group of many different diseases: there are a variety of molecular abnormalities that result in POAG or NTG. It seems likely that some particular molecular abnormalities are more prevalent in NTG and others more prevalent in POAG. For the purposes of research focused on pathogenesis and treatment, separately categorizing cases of NTG from POAG is meaningful.

DISEASE PREVALENCE

The prevalence of NTG varies among populations that have been studied. In the Baltimore Eye Survey, a population-based survey of 5308 black and white Americans aged ≥40 years, the prevalence of glaucoma was 2.4%. Among those with glaucoma, 24% had NTG.[2] The Beaver Dam Eye Study (4926 subjects) reported an

TABLE 30.1 Findings that suggest the possibility of a nonglaucomatous disease process
Optic disc pallor
Bitemporal or homonymous visual field defect
Vertically aligned visual field defects
Visual field defect out of proportion to the severity of optic disc excavation
Unexplained loss of visual acuity[1]
Dyschromatopsia[1]
Relative afferent pupillary defect[2]
These findings may occur in the setting of severe[1] or highly asymmetric[2] glaucoma damage.

overall 2.1% prevalence of OAG; 32% of cases had IOP <22 mmHg.[3] Population-based studies in Wales,[5] England,[6] Sweden,[7] the West Indies,[8] the Netherlands,[9] and Australia[10] show that 20–39% of OAG patients are classified as having NTG. In the Early Manifest Glaucoma Trial (EMGT) that recruited patients from a population-based screening in Sweden, baseline IOP was <21 mmHg in 52% ($n = 255$) of patients with OAG.[11]

The prevalence of glaucoma among Japanese was recently reported in a population-based survey of 3021 subjects age ≥40 years in Tajimi, Japan.[12] The prevalence of OAG was found to be 3.9%. IOP in 92% of these subjects was ≤21 mmHg, resulting in an overall prevalence of NTG of 3.6%. Unfortunately, the validity of utilizing the same arbitrary cutoff as has been used for Caucasian populations for the upper limit of normal IOP in a Japanese population is flawed. The mean IOP among Japanese without glaucoma in this study was 14.5 ± 2.7 mmHg, approximately 1 mmHg lower than in Caucasians.

DIFFERENTIAL DIAGNOSIS

The features, except for IOP, and differential diagnosis of NTG are identical to those for POAG (Table 30.1). Any optic neuropathy or retinal pathology that can mimic POAG can also mimic NTG. Historically it had been argued that patients with NTG actually have episodic IOP spikes or had previous episodes of IOP elevation. The authors believe this is an uncommon occurrence among patients diagnosed with NTG. Burnt-out pigmentary glaucoma, the phase of the disease in which IOP is no longer elevated and the classic signs of pigment dispersion may not be present, can mimic NTG.[13] The differential diagnosis between POAG and NTG can be blurred in eyes that have thin corneas, either inherently or following laser refractive surgery. Obviously, one must also rule out intermittent angle closure by performing careful dark-room gonioscopy (see Ch. 13).

Nonglaucomatous optic neuropathies, including those with compressive, infiltrative, or ischemic etiologies, can mimic glaucoma. A relative afferent pupillary defect can occur in the setting of asymmetric glaucoma damage; however, the presence of this finding necessitates extra attention to the possibility of a nonglaucomatous optic

nerve or retinal vascular disorder (such as a branch retinal artery occlusion). Acquired dyschromatopsia is highly suggestive of nonglaucomatous optic nerve disease. However, abnormal color vision can occur with glaucoma, particularly in the setting of severe damage. Central acuity is generally spared until fairly late in the glaucomatous disease process. Therefore, otherwise unexplained loss of acuity in the absence of very severe glaucoma damage should raise the consideration of a nonglaucomatous process. The location and degree of optic disc excavation should correspond with the visual field damage. If the degree of visual field loss is out of proportion to the extent of excavation or is vertically aligned, the possibility of a nonglaucomatous process should be considered.[14]

Just as optic disc excavation is the hallmark of glaucoma, pallor of the neuroretinal rim is the hallmark of a nonglaucomatous optic neuropathy. Subtle optic disc excavation can also occur in a variety of nonglaucomatous optic neuropathies including those with compressive, toxic, metabolic, hereditary, and ischemic etiologies; however, they are nearly always accompanied by neuroretinal rim pallor.

NTG patients with typical features of glaucomatous optic neuropathy do not require neuroimaging. Patients with the atypical characteristics described above should undergo directed diagnostic evaluation.

Branch retinal vascular occlusions can cause glaucomatous-appearing visual field and retinal nerve fiber layer defects as well as shallow optic disc excavation (Fig. 30.2). If the retinal embolus is no longer present, one could incorrectly arrive at a diagnosis of glaucoma.

Nonarteritic anterior ischemic optic neuropathy (NAION) typically results in the development of nerve fiber bundle visual field defects that mimic glaucomatous visual field defects. While optic disc excavation is rare in NAION, it is very common in arteritic anterior ischemic optic neuropathy.[15]

Moderate to highly myopic eyes with tilted optic discs and peripapillary atrophy can have nonprogressive, glaucomatous-appearing visual field defects. Also, these optic discs may have an excavated appearance or be difficult to interpret with respect to the degree of excavation.[16,17]

In myopic eyes the mean deviation on standard automated perimetry (SAP) decreases as a function of the axial length.[16] Myopic tilted discs may manifest focal visual field defects on SAP that have the appearance of a wedge-shaped defect above the physiologic blind spot, mimicking an arcuate defect. These field defects are due to the need for a different refractive correction in the region of the retina corresponding to the visual field defect due to the presence of a subtle staphyloma-like bulging of the eye wall in the region of the optic disc.[18] The use of an appropriate correction (for example, 4 D more myopic) reduces the severity of this defect.

In some myopic eyes, it may be unclear if the visual field and structural findings represent nonprogressive anomalies or NTG. It may be reasonable to carefully observe such eyes for evidence of progression prior to initiation of therapy. However, the myopic optic disc,

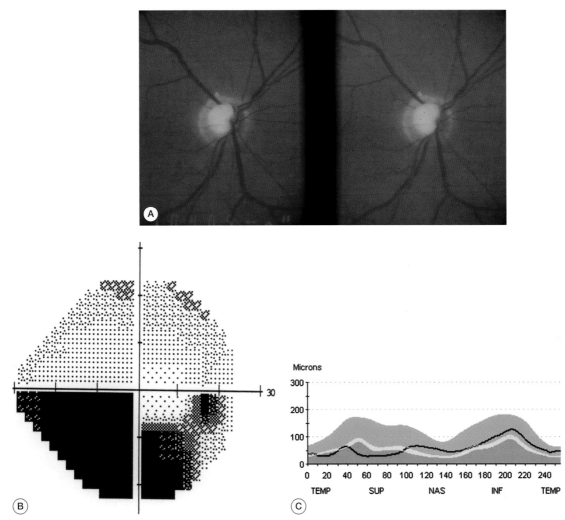

FIGURE 30.2 **(A)** Branch retinal artery occlusion with an embolus occluding the superior temporal retinal arteriole at the optic disc margin. **(B)** Visual field of the same eye disclosing the corresponding dense, inferior arcuate scotoma. **(C)** Time-domain optical coherence tomography of the peripapillary retinal nerve fiber layer, demonstrating severe thinning of the superior nerve fiber bundle. (TEMP = temporal; SUP = superior; NAS = nasal; INF = inferior)

retinal nerve fiber layer, and visual field are often very difficult to monitor for progression. Therefore, in eyes with visual field abnormalities, initiation of IOP-lowering therapy in the absence of evidence of progression should be considered. Non-glaucomatous causes of optic disc hemorrhages include diabetes, systemic hypertension, and acute posterior vitreous detachment.

PATHOGENESIS AND SYSTEMIC EVALUATION

The clinical appearance observed in patients with NTG is indistinguishable from that observed in POAG. The pathophysiology and etiology of NTG, as is also the case for POAG, are poorly understood. The fact that pharmacologic or surgical IOP reduction reduces the risk of progressive glaucoma damage in patients with NTG by two-thirds is taken as evidence that IOP likely plays a role in the pathogenesis of this disease. NTG and POAG are both multifactorial disease processes, however, in which IOP-dependent and IOP-independent

processes are thought to play a role. It seems likely that in most eyes with NTG, the IOP-independent causative factors play a relatively larger role.[4]

In NTG, other unique associations have been identified and suggested to represent pathogenic risk factors. However, ascertainment, referral, and recall bias may result in the incorrect identification of some of these associated characteristics.

SLEEP APNEA SYNDROME

In this condition, repetitive closure of the upper airway during sleep results in hypoxia, hypercapnia, and fragmented sleep. It has been postulated that abnormal autoregulation of blood flow to the optic nerve may occur as a result of the blood gas abnormalities.[19] The prevalence of NTG among patients with obstructive sleep apnea syndrome may be significantly increased compared to that seen in control cohorts.[19,20] However, this is controversial, with other investigators having found no association.[21,22] In NTG patients with a history of a sleep disturbance disorder, it may be prudent to obtain polysomnography.

BLOOD PRESSURE

An association between systemic blood pressure and NTG has been postulated. In addition, abnormalities in ocular blood flow are thought to play a role in POAG and NTG. In the Baltimore Eye Survey, low diastolic perfusion pressure (diastolic blood pressure – IOP) was found to be strongly associated with the prevalence of glaucoma.[23]

In the Low-pressure Glaucoma Treatment Study (LoGTS), concurrent systemic hypertension, as defined by the need for hypertensive treatment, occurred in 44.2% (n = 190) subjects,[24] similar to other studies.[25–27] NTG subjects have been reported to have a lower systemic blood pressure than POAG patients.[28] In LoGTS patients without systemic hypertension (n = 106), 17% were found to have a systolic pressure <110 mmHg and 21.7% a diastolic pressure <70 mmHg.[24] This may be an important association considering studies describing postural[29] and nocturnal hypotension[30,31] in NTG. A high prevalence of hypotensive episodes[25,32] and functional vasospasm with optic nerve hypoperfusion[28,32] has also been reported in NTG. In the LoGTS,[24] only two (2.1%) patients provided a history of a hypotensive episode and 16 (8.4%) patients provided a history of Raynaud's phenomenon.

MIGRAINE AND VASOSPASM

Phelps and Corbett[33] performed a case-control study in 1985 on the occurrence migraine in NTG. They found a positive migraine history in 37% of NTG patients. That was higher than that found in normal or POAG patients (approximately 22%). Subsequent studies by Lewis et al.[34] and the Beaver Dam Study[35] could not confirm this finding. This was also the situation in the LoGTS, with only 9 of 190 (4.7%) subjects providing a migraine history.[24]

The possible association of migraine and Raynaud's phenomenon with NTG is circumstantial evidence that abnormalities in blood flow, possibly caused by vasospasm or abnormal autoregulation, may play a role in NTG. Endothelin-1 (ET-1) is a vascular endothelium-derived vasoconstricting peptide that is thought to be involved in several vasospastic disorders. With exposure to cold, plasma ET-1 levels significantly rise in patients with glaucoma compared to healthy controls, and there is an associated decline in visual function among glaucoma patients with cold-induced vasospasm.[36] In another study, cold exposure resulted in a decline in ocular blood flow in glaucoma patients, but not in controls.[37]

DISC HEMORRHAGE

Optic disc hemorrhages occur in patients with all types of glaucoma; however, they are most commonly observed in eyes with NTG (Fig. 30.3). Furthermore, an optic disc hemorrhage is an independent risk factor for visual field deterioration.[38] Disc hemorrhages are likely the result of mechanical damage to the optic disc, particularly the lamina cribrosa, resulting in mechanical

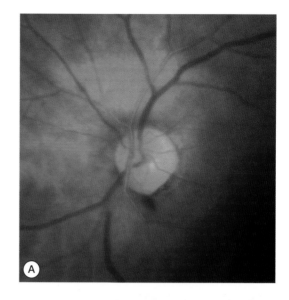

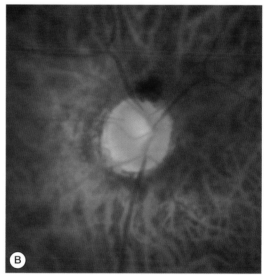

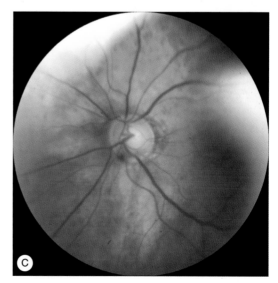

FIGURE 30.3 (A–C) Three examples of optic disc hemorrhages in eyes with normal-tension glaucoma. The presence of an optic disc hemorrhage may represent actively progressive disease. Disc hemorrhages are more common in eyes with normal-tension glaucoma compared to eyes with primary open-angle glaucoma.

trauma to capillaries that supply the optic disc. The authors hypothesize that when the IOP is normal, a sufficient volume of blood is able to extravasate from the ruptured blood vessel, resulting in a visible optic disc hemorrhage. In eyes with markedly elevated IOP, the ruptured vessel is tamponaded, resulting in the extravasation of too small a volume of blood to be detectable clinically.

AUTOIMMUNITY

There have been several reports indicating that autoimmunity may play a role in glaucoma. Autoantibodies to various antigens are present in the sera of glaucoma patients in higher concentrations than found in healthy controls. Antibodies to heat shock proteins, phosphatidylserine, α-fodrin, and several other antigens have been found in NTG patients.[39–41] The presence of these autoantibodies may be a marker of injury to the optic nerve in glaucoma rather than being causative. The case of α-fodrin is compelling in this regard, because antibodies to it have been found in other neurodegenerative diseases, such as Alzheimer's disease, and because anti-α-fodrin titers in patients with NTG are significantly higher than those found in POAG.[41] If the presence of this autoantibody were simply a result of optic nerve injury, similar titers would be expected in NTG and POAG.

TREATMENT

The only treatment approach proven to slow the progression of POAG and NTG is IOP reduction, with the means to accomplish this similar for both conditions. The strongest evidence that IOP reduction reduces the risk of subsequent glaucomatous visual field and optic disc deterioration in NTG is from the Collaborative Normal-Tension Glaucoma Study (CNTGS) that was initially designed in 1984.[42,43] This prospective, randomized, controlled clinical trial studied the effect of IOP reduction in NTG patients without a history of an IOP >24 mmHg in either eye. The basic strategy was to observe patients until progressive visual field or disc damage (progressive excavation or occurrence of a disc hemorrhage) was demonstrated. Randomization occurred at the outset if recent progressive field damage could reliably be demonstrated or if fixation was threatened. Two hundred and thirty eyes were enrolled, with 145 eyes randomized to one of two study arms: (1) observation without treatment or (2) treatment to achieve a 30% reduction in IOP. Eyes enrolled in the IOP reduction arm were treated with topical pilocarpine, systemic carbonic anhydrase inhibitors, argon laser trabeculoplasty, and/or incisional surgery. Eyes that underwent trabeculectomy were only required to achieve a 20% reduction in IOP.

Eyes were closely monitored for progressive visual field damage or optic disc excavation (the occurrence of a disc hemorrhage was not considered to represent a progression end point). The initial criteria for visual field progression were deemed non-specific early in the course of the study. Specifically, sensitivity loss, partly due to the development of cataract rather than to progressive glaucoma damage, led to false-positive progression end points. Accordingly, the investigators developed a new set of criteria that increased the magnitude of change required as evidence of progression, and required repeated testing to confirm the evidence of progression, thereby increasing the specificity for the detection of progressive glaucoma damage.

The intent-to-treat analysis of the CNTGS demonstrated no significant difference in the risk of progression between groups.[43] However, the frequency of cataract progression was significantly greater in the treated group, resulting in a high frequency of visual field deterioration that was not due to progressive glaucoma damage. Additionally, many eyes in the treatment arm required a prolonged period of time to achieve a 30% reduction in IOP. Accordingly, the data were reanalyzed such that visual fields in eyes with cataract were censored and the baseline visual field was defined as the one obtained after the IOP reduction goal was achieved. This alternative analysis demonstrated a 66% reduction in the risk of progression in the treatment arm. Sixty percent of untreated eyes in the CNTGS did not progress over a 3-year period and 40% did not progress over a 5-year period.

The EMGT enrolled 255 subjects with OAG (POAG, NTG, and exfoliation glaucoma), regardless of baseline IOP. About half of these patients had NTG. Subjects were randomized to treatment with betaxolol plus argon laser trabeculoplasty or observation without treatment. Patients with baseline IOP <21 mmHg had a significantly lower risk of progressing during the course of the study than did subjects with IOP ≥21 mmHg.[44] Furthermore, after a median 6-year follow-up period, in all eyes studied, including those with normal IOP at baseline, treatment was associated with a significant reduction in the risk of progression.[11]

GENERAL PRINCIPLES OF INTRAOCULAR PRESSURE-LOWERING TREATMENT

Because a large proportion of eyes with untreated NTG do not progress over a 5-year period, it is reasonable to closely observe patients with mild visual field loss prior to initiation of treatment. It is important to document the untreated IOPs to establish a target pressure. The IOP should be measured on at least three separate occasions, preferably including a diurnal curve. A 30% reduction below the mean of the untreated IOPs is a reasonable initial target. In patients in whom there is no contraindication, the authors usually use a prostaglandin analogue first, with laser trabeculoplasty a reasonable alternative. Topical carbonic anhydrase inhibitors, β-adrenergic antagonists, and α₂-adrenergic agonists can be used as primary or adjunctive agents.

At the time that the CNTGS was initially designed, it was expected that in order to achieve low IOP levels, a large proportion of eyes would require filtering surgery. However, a preliminary report[45] demonstrated that medical treatment (pilocarpine and oral carbonic anhydrase inhibitor) and laser trabeculoplasty effectively reduced IOP. Among 30 eyes that achieved a stable 30% reduction in IOP, only 43% required filtering surgery.

Adrenergic agents The use of nonselective α-adrenergic agonists is not recommended, given a lack of data regarding their potential benefit for NTG, because of their side-effect profile, and because of theoretical considerations surrounding their vasoconstrictive properties.

The α_2-selective adrenergic agonist brimonidine is in widespread use for the treatment of glaucoma and ocular hypertension. Experimental evidence in rodents strongly suggests that brimonidine may have neuroprotective properties beyond its ability to lower IOP.[46] However, neuroprotection has not been demonstrated in humans. The possible neuroprotective effect of brimonidine is under investigation in the LoGTS.[24] Other potential neuroprotective agents are discussed in Chapter 52.

Beta-adrenergic antagonists effectively lower IOP. Topical delivery of these agents may lower heart rate and blood pressure, thereby potentially reducing ocular perfusion pressure in NTG patients.[47] Additionally, a prospective study that included 131 NTG patients reported that topical β-adrenergic antagonist administration was associated with nocturnal arterial hypotension and was an independent risk factor for visual field progression.[48]

It has been shown that topical β-blockers have no impact on aqueous flow or IOP during the nocturnal period in eyes with POAG.[49] If β-blockers are to be used in patients with NTG, the authors recommend that they only be administered once-daily, in the morning.

Prostaglandin analogues Prostaglandin analogues have the potent IOP-lowering efficacy during the diurnal and nocturnal periods. It has been demonstrated in NTG and POAG that the highest IOPs occur during the nocturnal period when IOP is measured in the habitual position (sitting during the diurnal period and supine during the nocturnal period).[49] The prostaglandin analogues have been shown to lower IOP during the nocturnal period.[50]

Neuroprotection Although IOP reduction is the only therapeutic approach that has been proven to be effective in reducing the risk of progression in POAG and NTG, many other approaches have been or are under active investigation, including the use of N-methyl-D-aspartate (NMDA) receptor antagonists (e.g. menantine) and brimonidine. These are discussed in detail in Chapter 52.

Surgical therapy In a retrospective study of 61 eyes with NTG that underwent trabeculectomy, IOP was reduced significantly more in eyes treated with adjunctive mitomycin C (MMC) than in eyes treated with adjunctive 5-fluorouracil or no antifibrotic agent. In the subsequent 6 months, however, the incidence of visual field deterioration was significantly higher in the MMC group, possibly due to the higher incidence of hypotony observed in the MMC group.[51]

TREATMENT OUTCOMES AND PROGNOSIS

Data from the CNTGS and EMGT provide valuable information regarding the natural history of NTG as well as the prognosis in eyes that are treated. In the EMGT, after a median of 6 years, 40% of untreated eyes with NTG did not progress.[11] The risk of progression among eyes with baseline IOP <21 mmHg was significantly lower in the EMGT than among eyes with IOP ≥21 mmHg.[44]

In the CNTGS, the rate of progression was highly variable, with some untreated patients demonstrating progression a few months after enrollment, but about 40% showing no progression over a median of 5 years of observation.[52] The presence of disc hemorrhages and a history of migraine headache were independent risk factor for progression in CNTGS.[38] The importance of disc hemorrhages as risk factors for progression was verified in the EMGT.[44]

Overall, although historically a dreaded disease because it was felt to inexorably result in blindness, modern clinical trials have taught us that a large proportion of NTG patients do not progress over several years and that when progression does occur, it is often slow. Furthermore, and most importantly, these clinical trials have demonstrated the benefit of IOP-lowering therapy in reducing the risk of progression. Future advances in therapy such as the development of neuroprotective strategies will likely further improve the prognosis for patients with this vision-threatening disease.

REFERENCES

1. Werner EB. Normal-tension glaucoma. In: Ritch R, Shields MB, Krupin T, eds. The glaucomas. St. Louis: Mosby Year Book; 1996:769–797.

2. Sommer A, Tielsch JM, Katz J, et al. Relationship between intraocular pressure and primary open angle glaucoma among white and black Americans. The Baltimore Eye Survey. Arch Ophthalmol 1991; 109:1090–1095.

3. Klein BE, Klein R, Sponsel WE, et al. Prevalence of glaucoma. The Beaver Dam Eye Study, Ophthalmology 1992; 99:1499–1504.

4. Sommer A, Tielsch JM. Primary open-angle glaucoma: a clinical-epidemiologic perspective. In: Shields MB, Van Buskirk M, eds. 100 years of progress in glaucoma. Philadelphia: Lippincott-Raven; 1997:100–107.

5. Hollows FC, Graham PA. Intra-ocular pressure, glaucoma, and glaucoma suspects in a defined population. Br J Ophthalmol 1966; 50:570–586.

6. Perkins ES. The Bedford Glaucoma Survey. II. Rescreening of normal population. Br J Ophthalmol 1973; 57:186–192.

7. Bengtsson B. Further follow-up of the Dalby population. In: Krieglstein GK, ed. Glaucoma update III. Berlin: Springer-Verlag; 1987:112–114.

8. Mason RP, Kosoko O, Wilson MR, et al. National survey of the prevalence and risk factors of glaucoma in St. Lucia, West

Indies. I. Prevalence findings. Ophthalmology 1989; 96: 1363–1368.

9. Dielemans I, Vingerling JR, Wolfs RC, et al. The prevalence of primary open-angle glaucoma in a population-based study in the Netherlands. The Rotterdam Study. Ophthalmology 1994; 101:1851–1855.

10. Mitchell P, Smith W, Attebo K, et al. Prevalence of open-angle glaucoma in Australia. The Blue Mountains Eye Study. Ophthalmology 1996; 103:1661–1669.

11. Heijl A, Leske MC, Bengtsson B, et al. Reduction of intraocular pressure and glaucoma progression: results from the Early Manifest Glaucoma Trial. Arch Ophthalmol 2002; 120:1268–1279.

12. Iwase A, Suzuki Y, Araie M, et al. The prevalence of primary open-angle glaucoma in Japanese: The Tajimi Study. Ophthalmology 2004; 111:1641–1648.

13. Ritch R. Nonprogressive low-tension glaucoma with pigmentary glaucoma. Am J Ophthalmol 1992; 94:190–196.

14. Greenfield DS, Siatkowski RM, Glaser JS, et al. The cupped disc. Who needs neuroimaging? Ophthalmology 1998; 105:1866–1874.

15. Danesh-Meyer HV, Savino PJ, Sergott RC. The prevalence of cupping in end-stage arteritic and nonarteritic anterior ischemic optic neuropathy. Ophthalmology 2001; 108:593–598.

16. Aung T, Foster PF, Seah SK, et al. Automated static perimetry: the influence of myopia and its method of correction. Ophthalmology 2001; 108:290–295.

17. Doshi A, Kreidl KO, Lombardi L, et al. Nonprogressive glaucomatous cupping and visual field abnormalities in young Chinese males. Ophthalmology 2007; 114:472–479.

18. Anderson DR, Patella MV. Automated static perimetry. 2nd edn. St. Louis: Mosby; 1999:173–174.

19. Mojon DS, Hess CW, Goldblum D, et al. High prevalence of glaucoma in patients with sleep apnea syndrome. Ophthalmology 1999; 106:1009–1012.

20. Sergi M, Salerno DE, Rizzi M, et al. Prevalence of normal tension glaucoma in obstructive sleep apnea syndrome patients. J Glaucoma 2007; 16:42–46.

21. Geyer O, Cohen N, Segev E, et al. The prevalence of glaucoma in patients with sleep apnea syndrome: same as in the general population. Am J Ophthalmol 2003; 136:1093–1096.

22. Girkin CA, McGwin G Jr, McNeal SF, et al. Is there an association between pre-existing sleep apnoea and the development of glaucoma? Br J Ophthalmol 2006; 90: 679–681.

23. Tielsch JM, Katz J, Sommer A, et al. Hypertension, perfusion pressure, and primary open-angle glaucoma. A population-based assessment. Arch Ophthalmol 1995; 113:216–221.

24. Krupin T, Liebmann JM, Greenfield DS, et al. The Low-pressure Glaucoma Treatment Study (LoGTS): study design and baseline characteristics of enrolled patients. Ophthalmology 2005; 112:376–385.

25. Geijssen HC. Studies on normal-pressure glaucoma. Amstelveen: Kugler; 1991.

26. Goldberg I, Hollows FC, Kass MA, et al. Systemic factors in patients with low-tension glaucoma. Br J Ophthalmol 1981; 65:56–62.

27. Levene RZ. Low tension glaucoma: a critical review and new material. Surv Ophthalmol 1980; 24:621–664.

28. Drance SM, Sweeney VP, Morgan RW, et al. Studies of factors involved in the production of low tension glaucoma. Arch Ophthalmol 1973; 89:457–465.

29. Demailly P, Cambien F, Plouin PF, et al. Do patients with low tension glaucoma have particular cardiovascular characteristics? Ophthalmologica 1984; 188:65–75.

30. Hayreh SS, Zimmerman MB, Podhajsky P, et al. Nocturnal arterial hypotension and its role in optic nerve head and ocular ischaemic disorders. Am J Ophthalmol 1994; 117:603–624.

31. Meyer HJ, Brandi-Dohrn J, Funk J. Twenty-four-hour blood pressure monitoring in normal tension glaucoma. Br J Ophthalmol 1996; 80:864–867.

32. Gasser P, Flammer J. Influences of vasospasm on visual function. Doc Ophthalmol 1987; 66:3–18.

33. Phelps CD, Corbett JJ. Migraine and low-tension glaucoma. A case control study. Invest Ophthalmol Vis Sci 1985; 26: 1105–1108.

34. Lewis RA, Vijayan N, Watson C, et al. Visual field loss in migraine. Ophthalmology 1989; 96:321–326.

35. Klein BE, Klein R, Meuer SM, et al. Migraine headache and its association with open-angle glaucoma: the Beaver Dam Eye Study. Invest Ophthalmol Vis Sci 1993; 34:3024–3027.

36. Nicolela MT, Ferriers SN, Morrison CA, et al. Effects of cold-induced vasospasm in glaucoma: the role of endothelin-1. Invest Ophthalmol Vis Sci 2003; 44:2565–2572.

37. Gherghel D, Hosking SL, Cunliffe IA. Abnormal systemic and ocular vascular response to temperature provocation in primary open-angle glaucoma patients: a case for autonomic failure? Invest Ophthalmol Vis Sci 2004; 45:3546–3554.

38. Drance SM, Schulxer M. Collaborative Normal-Tension Study Group. Risk factors for progression of visual field abnormalities in normal-tension glaucoma. Am J Ophthalmol 2001; 131:699–708.

39. Wax WB, Tezel G, Saito I, et al. Anti-Ro/SS-A positivity and heat shock protein antibodies in patients with normal-pressure glaucoma. Am J Ophthalmol 1998; 125:145–157.

40. Kremmer S, Kreuzfelder E, Klein R, et al. Antiphosphatidylserine antibodies are elevated in normal tension glaucoma. Clin Exp Immunol 2001; 125:211–215.

41. Grus FH, Joachim SC, Bruns K, et al. Serum autoantibodies to alpha-fodrin are present in glaucoma patients from Germany and the United States. Invest Ophthalmol Vis Sci 2006; 47:968–976.

42. Collaborative Normal-Tension Study Group. Comparison of glaucomatous progression between untreated patients with normal-tension glaucoma and patients with therapeutically reduced intraocular pressures. Am J Ophthalmol 1998; 126:487–497.

43. Collaborative Normal-Tension Study Group. The effectiveness of intraocular pressure reduction in the treatment of normal-tension glaucoma. Am J Ophthalmol 1998; 126: 498–505.

44. Leske MC, Heijl A, Hussein M, et al. Factors for glaucoma progression and the effect of treatment: the Early Manifest Glaucoma Trial. Arch Ophthalmol 2003; 121:48–56.

45. Schulzer M. Intraocular pressure reduction in normal-tension glaucoma patients. The Normal Tension Glaucoma Study Group. Ophthalmology 1992; 99:1468–1470.

46. Wheeler L, Wolde Mussie E, Lai R. Role of alpha-2 agonists in neuroprotection. Surv Ophthalmol 2003; 48(Suppl 1): S47–S51.

47. Drance SM, Crichton A, Mills RP. Comparison of the effect of latanoprost 0.005% and timolol 0.5% on the calculated ocular perfusion pressure in patients with normal-tension glaucoma. Am J Ophthalmol 1998; 125:585–592.

48. Hayreh SS, Podhajsky P, Zimmerman MB. Beta-blocker eyedrops and nocturnal arterial hypotension. Am J Ophthalmol 1999; 128:301–309.

49. Liu JH, Kripke DF, Weinreb RN. Comparison of the nocturnal effects of once-daily timolol and latanoprost on intraocular pressure. Am J Ophthalmol 2004; 138:389–395.

50. Sit AJ, Weinreb RN, Crowston JG, et al. Sustained effect of travoprost on diurnal and nocturnal intraocular pressure. Am J Ophthalmol 2006; 141:1131–1133.

51. Membrey WL, Bunce C, Poinoosawmy DP, et al. Glaucoma surgery with or without adjunctive antiproliferatives in normal tension glaucoma: 2 Visual field progression. Br J Ophthalmol 2001; 85:696–701.

52. Anderson DR, Drance SM, Schulzer M. Collaborative Normal-Tension Glaucoma Study Group. Natural history of normal tension glaucoma. Ophthalmology 2001; 108:247–253.

Congenital Glaucoma and other Childhood Glaucomas

Camille Hylton and Allen Beck

INTRODUCTION

The evaluation and management of pediatric glaucoma differs greatly from the evaluation and management of adult forms of glaucoma. It is essential for the treating ophthalmologist to recognize the signs and symptoms of the various forms of glaucoma that occur in children. Because examination of children in an office setting can be challenging, examinations under anesthesia are often necessary for adequate assessment.

EVALUATION OF CHILDREN WITH GLAUCOMA

The examination of a child with glaucoma or suspected glaucoma generally begins with some determination of visual acuity. In general, prior to age 3, this will consist of assessing the child's ability to fixate and/or follow objects. The presence of nystagmus should also be noted in children as it can provide some indication of the chronicity and prognosis of disease. After age 3, visual acuity testing can be attempted with Allen picture, tumbling E, HOTV, or Snellen acuity charts.

A detailed external examination is another important step in the evaluation for childhood glaucomas. Since many of the childhood glaucomas can have associated facial and systemic features (e.g. nevus flammeus in Sturge-Weber syndrome [Fig. 31.1], eyelid neurofibroma in neurofibromatosis type 1 [Fig. 31.2]), it is important to carefully examine the eyelids, facial features, skin, and general appearance of the child. A careful history and examination can help determine whether associated systemic anomalies are present.

Tonometry in children in an office setting can be challenging. The intraocular pressure can be measured best in a cooperative child after applying topical anesthesia. In infants less than 1 year of age, this can often only be achieved if the child is feeding or otherwise distracted. Accurate measurements can be obtained with the Perkins or Kowa hand-held tonometer, pneumotonometry, or Tonopen. In older children, the standard slit lamp Goldmann tonometer can be used. If the child is crying or squeezing its eyelids,

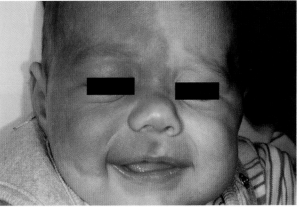

FIGURE 31.1 Nevus flammeus in Sturge-Weber syndrome. (Reproduced with permission from Paller AS, Mancini AJ, eds. Hurwitz clinical pediatric dermatology. 3rd edn. Philadelphia: Elsevier Saunders; 2006.)

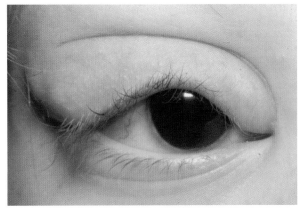

FIGURE 31.2 Plexiform neurofibroma in neurofibromatosis type 1.

falsely elevated pressures can occur, especially with the Tonopen. In these situations, it is best to measure the pressure under anesthesia immediately after sedation has been achieved. Most anesthetics, with the exception of ketamine, will lower the intraocular pressure. Thus, tonometry should be the initial step of an examination under anesthesia. Of note, applanation tonometry has

369

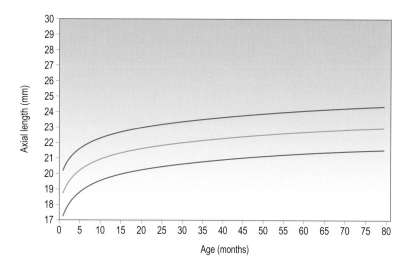

FIGURE 31.3 Axial length in millimeters (y-axis) versus age in months (x-axis). The area within the upper and lower parabolic curves represents the normal range of axial length, with the middle curve representing the mean axial length of normal eyes. (Adapted from Sampaolesi R, Caruso R. Ocular echometry in the diagnosis of congenital glaucoma. Arch Ophthalmol 1982; 100:574–577.[5]

been shown to underestimate the intraocular pressure in children under anesthesia.[1–4] Pneumotonometry seems to correlate best with true manometric pressure under general anesthesia.[4] The Tonopen tonometer has also been shown to reliably assess intraocular pressure in pediatric patients.[1]

Evaluation of the anterior segment, by penlight, portable slit lamp, or standard slit lamp, must also be performed. The cornea should be carefully assessed for corneal edema, breaks in Descemet's membrane (Haab's striae), and other anomalies. The corneal diameter ought to be measured. The most accurate measurements of corneal diameter are generally obtained during examination under anesthesia. Abnormalities of the iris, pupil, anterior chamber, and/or lens should be noted.

Gonioscopy can be performed successfully under anesthesia or at the slit lamp in cooperative children. The identification of the angle structures and gonioscopic appearance of the angle is important for the determination of the appropriate surgical procedure (see Ch. 107). Goniosurgery, such as goniotomy and trabeculotomy, is generally less successful in angles with significant peripheral anterior synechiae. Either direct (e.g. Koeppe lens) or indirect forms of gonioscopy (e.g. Zeiss or Posner goniolens) can be used to identify the appropriate anatomical landmarks. High iris insertions are typical of patients with primary congenital glaucoma; thus, the angle of insertion of the peripheral iris is important to note. Because corneal edema may be present, a clear view of the angle structures may not be possible. If goniotomy surgery is planned, it may be necessary to remove the corneal epithelium or give acetazolamide to maximize the view.

Ultrasonography is extremely useful in the evaluation of patients with childhood glaucoma. Axial length measurements are invaluable to the diagnosis and management of childhood glaucoma in patients under 3 years of age. After this age, the axial length tends to stabilize as the globe ceases to expand in response to increased intraocular pressure. The normal ocular axial growth curve is based on data published by Sampaolesi

and Caruso[5] in 1982 (Fig. 31.3). Prior to age 3, the axial length in glaucomatous eyes tends to increase at a rate well above that of normal eyes. If the glaucoma is subsequently controlled, the axial length can stabilize (and may even decrease) to follow the normal growth curve.[5,6] B-scan ultrasonography is also extremely useful in evaluating the posterior segment of eyes with hazy media due to corneal clouding, opacification, or cataract.

Fundoscopy is also essential in evaluating and following children with glaucoma. The fundoscopic evaluation begins with the assessment of the optic nerve. Children with normal eyes tend to have a cup-to-disc ratio <0.3. On the other hand, children with glaucoma can exhibit significant cupping (>0.3) and may also show evidence of cup-to-disc asymmetry. Fortunately, control of the glaucoma in many children can lead to reversal of the cupping phenomenon. If the intraocular pressure is lowered sufficiently the posterior bowing of the lamina cribrosa may resolve.[7] Fundoscopy is also useful for ruling out posterior pole pathology (e.g. retinoblastoma or diffuse choroidal hemangioma) which could indicate other types of glaucoma.

Cycloplegic refraction is helpful in the evaluation and management of children with glaucoma. If axial length increases significantly, these children will become progressively more myopic. Increasing axial length and myopia can be an indication of glaucomatous progression in children. Conversely, control of the glaucoma can result in stabilization of the myopia. Furthermore, loss of hyperopia can also indicate the presence of glaucoma.[8]

Visual field testing is useful once the child becomes old enough to perform a reliable test. Typically, visual field testing is attempted in children of normal development at 7–8 years of age.[9] If 'Humphrey fields' are not reliable, 'Goldmann visual fields' can often be obtained with good results.

Ancillary tests such as optic nerve head imaging and measurement of central corneal thickness may prove valuable once normative data for children have been attained and the utility of these tests has become more established.

CLASSIFICATION OF CHILDHOOD GLAUCOMAS

The terminology for pediatric glaucoma can be somewhat confusing. Both primary and secondary forms of glaucoma can occur in childhood and may or may not be associated with systemic features or syndromes.

Primary congenital glaucoma is the term generally applied to children who present with classic features (such as cloudy and/or enlarged corneas with Haab's striae). Newborn or birth-onset congenital glaucoma presents at birth or prior to 1 month of age. The most common age of presentation, after 1 month until 2 years of age, is known as infantile-onset primary congenital glaucoma. The terms late-onset or late-recognized primary infantile glaucoma are typically used to refer to patients who develop those same features after 2 years of age.[10] Juvenile open-angle glaucoma is an autosomal dominant form of glaucoma that occurs in patients who develop open-angle glaucoma in late childhood or early adulthood without signs of ocular enlargement. Other primary childhood glaucomas can be associated with specific ocular anomalies or systemic syndromes (Table 31.1).[11]

Secondary forms of glaucoma can also affect the pediatric population. Unlike primary forms of glaucoma, secondary glaucomas do not result from a primary developmental anomaly of the angle. Table 31.2 is an extensive list of possible mechanisms of secondary glaucoma in children.[11] One of the most common forms of secondary glaucoma results after surgery for congenital cataracts.

PRIMARY CONGENITAL GLAUCOMA

DISEASE PREVALENCE

Primary congenital glaucoma, whether presenting at birth or in the early infantile or childhood years, occurs in approximately 1 in 10 000 births.[12] Roughly 80% of all cases occur within the first year of life. About 25% of those cases present at or shortly after birth, and more than 60% present by age 6 months.[13,14] Congenital glaucoma occurs worldwide with a slightly higher incidence in males versus females. There does not appear to be any specific racial predilection. Approximately 65–80% of cases are bilateral. In some instances, there may be significant asymmetry in intraocular pressure at the initial presentation. However, the unsuspected eye may present with findings suggestive of glaucoma at a later stage.

RISK FACTORS

There are no known identifiable risk factors for congenital glaucoma. Most cases appear to occur sporadically with no known family history.[15] Approximately 10% of cases are familial and are inherited as an autosomal recessive trait with high penetrance.[16] At least two genetic loci, GLC3A (mapped to the 2p21 region) and GLC3B (mapped to the 1p36 region), have been

TABLE 31.1 Primary childhood glaucomas
A. Congenital open-angle glaucoma
1. Congenital
2. Infantile
3. Late-recognized
B. Juvenile open-angle glaucoma
C. Primary angle-closure glaucoma
D. Associated with systemic abnormalities (with or without ocular abnormalities)
1. Sturge-Weber syndrome
2. Axenfeld-Rieger syndrome
3. Neurofibromatosis type 1 (NF-1)
4. Lowe (oculocerebrorenal) syndrome
5. Stickler syndrome
6. Hepatorenal syndrome
7. Marfan syndrome
8. Rubenstein-Taybi syndrome
9. Infantile glaucoma associated with mental retardation and paralysis
10. Oculodentodigital dysplasia
11. Open-angle glaucoma associated with microcornea and absence of frontal sinuses
12. Mucopolysaccharidosis
13. Trisomy 13
14. Cutis marmorata telangiectatica congenita
15. Warburg syndrome
16. Kniest syndrome (skeletal dysplasia)
17. Michel syndrome
18. Nonprogressive hemiatrophy
E. Associated with ocular abnormalities
1. Aniridia
a. Congenital glaucoma
b. Acquired glaucoma
2. Peter's anomaly
3. Congenital ocular melanosis
4. Congenital glaucoma with iris and pupillary abnormalities
5. Iridotrabecular dysgenesis
6. Sclerocornea
7. Posterior polymorphous dystrophy
8. Iridotrabecular dysgenesis and ectropion uveae
9. Idiopathic or familial elevated episcleral venous pressure
10. Anterior corneal staphyloma
11. Congenital microcornea with myopia
12. Congenital hereditary iris stromal hypoplasia
13. Congenital hereditary endothelial dystrophy

Adapted from Walton DS. Glaucoma in infants and children. In: Nelson L, ed. Harley's pediatric ophthalmology. Philadelphia: WB Saunders; 1998.[11]

identified. Mutations in the gene for the 2p21 locus, CYP1B1 gene (cytochrome P4501B1) have been documented in patients with congenital glaucoma worldwide, with higher familial rates in cultures where consanguineous marriage is common.[16–24]

PATHOGENESIS

The pathogenesis of congenital glaucoma is not well understood. Initially, Barkan proposed that an impermeable membrane crossing the anterior chamber angle

TABLE 31.2 Secondary childhood glaucomas

A. Secondary to surgery for congenital cataract
  1. Lens material blockage of the trabecular meshwork (acute or subacute)
  2. Chronic open-angle glaucoma associated with angle defects
  3. Pupillary block

B. Secondary to uveitis
  1. Open-angle glaucoma
  2. Angle-closure glaucoma
    a. Synechial angle closure
    b. Iris bombe with pupillary block

C. Traumatic glaucoma
  1. Acute glaucoma
    a. Angle concussion
    b. Hyphema
    c. Ghost cell glaucoma
  2. Late-onset glaucoma with angle recession
  3. Arteriovenous fistula

D. Steroid-induced glaucoma

E. Secondary to intraocular neoplasm
  1. Retinoblastoma
  2. Juvenile xanthogranuloma
  3. Leukemia
  4. Melanoma
  5. Melanocytoma
  6. Iris rhabdomyosarcoma
  7. Aggressive nevi of the iris

F. Lens-induced glaucoma
  1. Subluxation-dislocation and pupillary block
    a. Marfan syndrome
    b. Homocystinuria
  2. Spherophakia and pupillary block
  3. Phacolytic glaucoma

G. Secondary angle-closure glaucoma
  1. Retinopathy of prematurity
  2. Microphthalmos
  3. Nanophthalmos
  4. Retinoblastoma
  5. Persistent hyperplastic primary vitreous
  6. Congenital papillary iris–lens membrane

H. Secondary to rubeosis
  1. Retinoblastoma
  2. Coats disease
  3. Medulloepithelioma
  4. Familial exudative vitreoretinopathy

I. Glaucoma associated with increased episcleral venous pressure
  1. Carotid or dural-venous fistula
  2. Orbital disease

J. Secondary to maternal rubella

K. Secondary to intraocular infection
  1. Acute recurrent toxoplasmosis
  2. Acute herpetic iritis

Adapted from Walton DS. Glaucoma in infants and children. In: Nelson L, ed. Harley's pediatric ophthalmology. Philadelphia: WB Saunders; 1998.[11]

was responsible for the impaired aqueous outflow in children.[25] However, subsequent histopathologic studies found no evidence for this membrane. More recent studies support the concept that congenital glaucoma results from the developmental arrest of the anterior chamber angle tissue (derived from neural crest cells). This arrest leads to a higher, more anterior insertion of the iris and ciliary body. This high insertion of the iris and ciliary body onto the posterior trabecular meshwork may result in the compression of the trabecular beams.[26–28]

SIGNS AND SYMPTOMS

Primary congenital glaucoma may present with one or more components of the classic clinical triad of epiphora, photophobia, and blepharospasm. Some parents may report that their child is tearing excessively or 'squinting' their eyes in response to light. Other parents might actually note that the cornea appears enlarged or cloudy, or that eye itself appears enlarged. Buphthalmos (ox eye) is the term applied to the enlargement of the globe that occurs in response to increased intraocular pressure. The immature collagen in infantile sclera tends to stretch in response to increased intraocular pressure until about 3 years of age.

On examination, corneal edema associated with Haab's striae (curvilinear breaks in Descemet's membrane, Fig. 31.4) is often present. The Haab's striae may not be readily visible if the corneal edema is extensive.

Corneal enlargement, suggested by a corneal diameter greater than 11.5 mm in a newborn, or greater than 12.5–13 mm in any infant or child, is highly suspicious for glaucoma.

Gonioscopic findings include a high, anterior iris insertion associated with a rather indistinct, translucent-appearing ciliary band, scleral spur, and trabecular meshwork (Fig. 31.5).

Intraocular pressure (IOP) measurements in children with congenital glaucoma show a range of elevation, with some studies noting a worse prognosis for cases with higher initial IOP.[29]

DIFFERENTIAL DIAGNOSIS

Congenital glaucoma should not be confused with other disorders in the differential diagnosis for infants with tearing, enlarged or opacified cornea, or pseudo-optic nerve cupping (Table 31.3). Causes of tearing, such as congenital lacrimal duct obstruction, conjunctivitis, or corneal irregularity, should be excluded. Similarly, other causes of corneal opacification, such as sclerocornea, choristomas, and corneal dystrophies, should also be excluded. Disorders associated with enlarged corneas should similarly be excluded. For example, megalocornea is a bilateral disorder of autosomal dominant or sporadic inheritance which presents with enlarged, clear corneas of normal thickness and no evidence of glaucoma. Furthermore, conditions associated with apparent optic disc cupping, such as physiologic cupping, optic nerve coloboma, and morning glory disc anomaly, should not be confused with congenital glaucoma.

TREATMENT OPTIONS

Surgical therapy is generally necessary for the treatment of primary congenital glaucoma. Medical therapy alone is rarely effective in the long term. Angle surgery (goniotomy

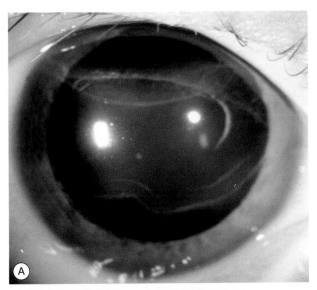

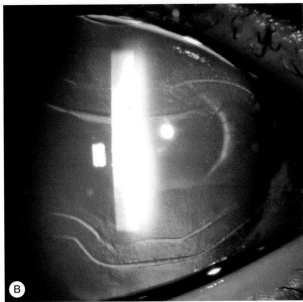

FIGURE 31.4 (A and B) Haab's striae. (Reproduced with permission from Krachmer JH, Palay DA. Cornea atlas. 2nd edn. St. Louis: Mosby; 2006.)

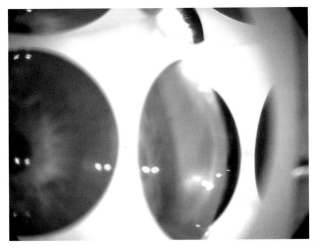

FIGURE 31.5 Surgical image of a patient with congenital glaucoma and high iris insertion with a blue Prolene suture delineating Schlemm's canal.

TABLE 31.3 Differential diagnosis of primary congenital glaucoma[31]
Conditions associated with enlarged corneas
Megalocornea
Conditions associated with epiphora
Congenital nasolacrimal duct obstruction
Keratitis
Corneal epithelial defect or abrasion
Conjunctivitis
Ocular inflammation (uveitis, trauma)
Conditions associated with corneal edema or opacification
Corneal dystrophy
Congenital hereditary endothelial dystrophy
Posterior polymorphous dystrophy
Forceps-related birth trauma with Descemet's tears
Storage diseases
Mucopolysaccharidoses
Mucolipidoses
Cystinosis
Congenital corneal anomalies
Sclerocornea
Peter's anomaly
Keratitis
Rubella
Herpetic
Phlyctenular
Conditions associated with apparent optic nerve cupping
Physiologically large optic cup
Optic nerve coloboma
Optic nerve pit
Optic atrophy
Morning glory disc anomaly
Optic nerve hypoplasia
Other optic nerve malformations

or trabeculotomy) is typically chosen as the initial surgical intervention. Goniotomy is a procedure in which a goniotomy knife is used to directly incise the trabecular meshwork under direct visualization with a gonioscopic lens. Trabeculotomy, on the other hand, is an external dissection of Schlemm's canal, which is less dependent on angle visualization than goniotomy. This dissection can be performed using two metal probes (trabeculotomes) inserted beneath a scleral flap to treat 120 to 180 degrees of the angle. It may also be performed by passing a 6-0 polypropylene suture beneath a scleral flap to treat the entire angle at once.[30,31] The major advantage of trabeculotomy over goniotomy is that trabeculotomy is less dependent on corneal clarity and can be performed successfully in eyes with cloudy corneas. The major advantage of goniotomy over trabeculotomy is that the conjunctiva is spared for future trabeculectomy if necessary. These procedures are discussed in detail in Chapter 107 of this text.

If one or more angle procedures are not successful in controlling childhood glaucoma, most surgeons will proceed to either trabeculectomy with antifibrotic agents or glaucoma implant surgery. Trabeculectomy with mitomycin has variable success rates in children. The major disadvantage of this procedure is the long-term risk of bleb leaks and endophthalmitis. Glaucoma drainage implant surgery (generally with

Molteno, Ahmed, or Baerveldt implants) can effectively reduce the intraocular pressure in children. However, many of these patients require adjunctive topical medical therapy postoperatively to achieve ultimate pressure control. Finally, if these procedures are not successful, cyclodestructive procedures may be helpful in controlling the intraocular pressure. These procedures are discussed in more detail in Chapter 108 of this text.

Medical therapy alone is rarely successful in the treatment of primary congenital glaucoma. However, medical therapy does play an important adjunctive role in the management of congenital glaucoma pre- and post-surgical intervention. Medications may also cause a modest reduction in intraocular pressure, which can be useful temporarily until surgery can be scheduled. For childhood glaucomas associated with a relatively poor surgical outcome, such as secondary glaucoma associated with aphakia, a medication trial is frequently warranted prior to surgical treatment. Medical therapy is also valuable postoperatively in controlling glaucoma in children in whom surgery is only moderately successful.

Medical treatment, when indicated, could include oral and topical carbonic anhydrase inhibitors, adrenergic agents, prostaglandins, and miotics. Frequently, oral carbonic anhydrase inhibitors are used to lower intraocular pressure in an attempt to clear the cornea for goniotomy surgery. The typical dose of oral acetazolamide (Diamox) is 5–15 mg/kg/day. Physicians must be aware of the potential side effects which include metabolic acidosis, diarrhea, lethargy, and decreased appetite. On the other hand, topical carbonic anhydrase inhibitors are both effective and safe adjunctive agents in the treatment of pediatric glaucoma. There are minimal systemic side effects, especially when compared to oral carbonic anhydrase inhibitors.[32] The most common difficulty with these drops is that that they burn or sting, making it more difficult for parental administration.

Topical β-blockers can also be used as first- or second-line auxiliary agents in the treatment of pediatric glaucoma. However, physicians need to be wary of their use in the early neonatal period and in premature or very small infants. There is a definite risk of bronchospasm and bradycardia. Parents should be adequately informed of these risks. Beta-blockers should not be used in infants or children with a history of reactive airway disease. Physicians may want to consider beginning treatment with the 0.25% formulation prior to prescribing the 0.50% formulation during infancy due to the potential for systemic β-blockade.[33] Consultation with the patient's pediatrician and/or pulmonologist or cardiologist may be worthwhile if surgical or other medical options are limited. The combination medication timolol 0.5% and dorzolamide 2% (Cosopt, Merck) is frequently helpful for parents due to the ability to dose two medications with two daily eyedrops.

Alpha2-agonists (brimonidine and apraclonidine) have limited utility in the treatment of young children with glaucoma. Apraclonidine may be more systemically safe than brimonidine in smaller children; however, it tends to be less effective and is associated with conjunctival hyperemia and allergy. *Brimonidine must not be used in infants or small children!* Brimonidine is associated with severe systemic side effects in infants, including apnea, bradycardia, hypotension, somnolence, severe lethargy, hypotonia, and hypothermia.[34–36] Its use should be limited to older, larger children greater than 20 kg or 6 years of age or older.[36] When used, parents should be adequately informed of the side effects and should be instructed to look for any unusual behavior in their children.

Prostaglandin analogues may be useful in lowering intraocular pressure in pediatric patients. Latanoprost (Xalatan) has been shown to successfully lower pressure in some patients, albeit with a nonresponse rate greater than that seen in adult patients. Latanoprost seems to be most effective in the juvenile open-angle glaucoma subtype of childhood glaucomas.[37,38]

Miotics tend to have limited value in the reduction of intraocular pressure in pediatric glaucomas. Most commonly, they are employed for the purpose of attaining miosis in the preoperative and postoperative settings when angle surgery has been planned. Miosis in the perioperative period may prevent the formation of peripheral anterior synechiae after angle surgery. Long-term use of miotics should be avoided in phakic and pseudophakic children because of the risk of posterior synechiae formation. However, miotics may be valuable in the treatment of glaucoma associated with aphakia.[3,39]

TREATMENT OUTCOMES AND PROGNOSIS

The initial surgical intervention for primary congenital glaucoma is typically angle surgery, namely, goniotomy or trabeculotomy. There is no clear evidence that one procedure is more effective than the other in terms of long-term surgical and visual outcomes. Poor visual outcomes are associated with high myopia, axial striae that lead to amblyopia, corneal decompensation, cataract, and progressive optic nerve damage or field loss. Visual outcomes are also affected by the age of diagnosis, the degree of corneal compensation prior to surgery, failure of the angle surgery, and poor compliance with follow-up and amblyopia therapy.[31] Newborn or birth-onset congenital glaucoma tends to have worse surgical outcomes, likely due to the fact that the corneal edema and nerve damage began in utero, and this presentation represents the most severe expression of the disease.[10] Infantile-onset primary congenital glaucoma demonstrates the best prognosis for successful angle surgery and the best visual outcomes. The outcomes and comparisons between goniotomy and trabeculotomy are discussed in more detail in Chapter 107 of this text.

Several studies on outcomes of trabeculectomy, aqueous shunt devices, nonpenetrating surgical techniques, and cyclodestructive procedures for congenital glaucoma and other childhood glaucomas have been performed. The outcomes and comparisons among the various procedures are discussed in more detail in Chapter 108 of this text.

JUVENILE OPEN-ANGLE GLAUCOMA

DISEASE PREVALENCE AND INFLUENCE

Juvenile open-angle glaucoma is a relatively rare form of childhood glaucoma. It typically presents after 4 years of age.

RISK FACTORS

Juvenile open-angle glaucoma is inherited as an autosomal dominant trait. The gene for the disease has been identified as a trabecular meshwork glucocorticoid response gene, otherwise known as the TIGR or myocilin gene.

PATHOGENESIS

It is not well understood how mutations in the myocilin gene cause glaucoma. However, it appears to do so by affecting trabecular outflow.

SIGNS AND SYMPTOMS

This form of glaucoma is typically asymptomatic and is often discovered incidentally on routine eye examination. Although the disease is generally bilateral, there can be marked asymmetry between the two eyes. The major signs of this disorder are increased intraocular pressure and optic nerve excavation. On gonioscopy, the angle appears normal. Features typical of primary infantile glaucoma, such as corneal edema and Haab's striae, are not present. Systemic features are not typically associated with juvenile open-angle glaucoma. Typical glaucomatous visual field defects can be documented.

DIFFERENTIAL DIAGNOSIS

The differential diagnosis of juvenile open-angle glaucoma includes other forms of open-angle glaucoma that can occur at any age. Late-recognized infantile glaucoma, steroid-induced glaucoma, traumatic glaucoma, and inflammatory glaucoma should be excluded prior to making this diagnosis.

TREATMENT OPTIONS, OUTCOMES, AND PROGNOSIS

Medical therapy is often useful in the treatment of juvenile open-angle glaucoma. When not successful, angle surgery, filtration surgery, and/or aqueous shunt devices can be considered. These procedures are discussed in more detail in Chapter 108 of this text.

PRIMARY CHILDHOOD GLAUCOMAS ASSOCIATED WITH SYSTEMIC SYNDROMES

Primary childhood glaucomas may occur in association with systemic syndromes. Some of the more common conditions in this category include Sturge-Weber syndrome, Axenfeld-Rieger syndrome, neurofibromatosis, and Lowe syndrome.

STURGE-WEBER SYNDROME

Disease prevalence and influence Sturge-Weber syndrome (encephalotrigeminal angiomatosis), one of the phakomatoses, is a syndrome associated with a facial nevus (nevus flammeus or port-wine stain) and ipsilateral leptomeningeal angiomatous lesions. Glaucoma occurs in about 50% of cases where an ipsilateral nevus flammeus is present in the first or second division of the trigeminal nerve. The disorder is typically unilateral, although several bilateral cases have been reported. No gender or racial predilection has been observed.

Risk factors There are no known risk factors for this disorder. No obvious hereditary pattern has been observed.

Pathogenesis Glaucoma in this disorder is caused by increased episcleral venous pressure due to abnormal episcleral vasculature.

Signs and symptoms Ocular signs include facial nevus flammeus in the ophthalmic and maxillary distribution of the trigeminal nerve (see Fig. 31.1), dilated episcleral vessels, and diffuse choroidal hemangioma on fundus examination. The angle generally appears normal, although blood in Schlemm's canal may be present. Increased intraocular pressure may cause corneal edema, corneal enlargement, or buphthalmos in infants with this disorder. These signs may be associated with symptoms of tearing, photophobia, or blepharospasm.

Systemic features of Sturge-Weber syndrome include the nevus flammeus, which may be associated with ipsilateral facial hemihypertrophy, as well as intracranial vascular angiomas. These intracranial lesions are likely responsible for the occurrence of seizures and epilepsy in these patients. Characteristic calcifications, known as 'railroad tracks,' can be identified in the cerebral cortex radiographically.

Differential diagnosis The differential diagnosis of Sturge-Weber syndrome includes other facial hemangiomas (e.g. capillary hemangioma), oculodermal melanocytosis, Klippel-Trenaunay-Weber syndrome, and other forms of infantile glaucoma.

Treatment options, outcomes, and prognosis Medical treatment is often the first line of therapy for patients with Sturge-Weber syndrome. If and when medical therapy fails, filtration surgery or aqueous shunt devices can be attempted. Angle surgery has shown limited success in patients in this category.[11]

AXENFELD-RIEGER SYNDROME

Disease prevalence and influence Axenfeld-Rieger syndrome is a spectrum of disease which was initially delineated by the presence of either Axenfeld anomaly (posterior embryotoxon associated with high peripheral iridocorneal adhesions), Rieger anomaly (Axenfeld anomaly with iris stromal thinning, iris holes, and/or corectopia), or Rieger syndrome (Rieger anomaly plus systemic developmental anomalies). The term Axenfeld-Rieger syndrome is now accepted as a spectrum of diseases which includes all clinical variations. The disease is bilateral. Glaucoma is reported to occur in greater than 50% of patients with the disorder.[40]

Risk factors The main risk factor for this disease is family history. The disease is inherited as an autosomal dominant trait. Several genes, including those at loci 4q25 (PITX2), 6p25 (FOXC1), and 13q14 (REIG2), have been identified.

Pathogenesis The pathogenesis of glaucoma due to Axenfeld-Rieger syndrome is thought to be related to an underlying trabeculodysgenesis, rather than to the degree of peripheral anterior synechiae or angle changes. The prevailing theory is that the mechanism of glaucoma is a developmental arrest of anterior segment tissue derived from neural crest cells.[40]

Signs and symptoms Ocular signs include the posterior embryotoxon (anteriorly displaced Schwalbe's line), high peripheral iris strands (adherent to the anteriorly displaced Schwalbe's line), ectropion uveae, iris stromal thinning, and hole formation. Abnormally shaped pupils or decentered pupils (corectopia), and/or the appearance of multiple pupils (polycoria), can occur as a result of these iris changes (Fig. 31.6).

Systemic developmental defects include dental anomalies (namely oligodontia and anodontia), craniofacial anomalies (especially maxillary hypoplasia with midface flattening), skeletal anomalies (e.g. growth hormone deficiency and short stature), umbilical anomalies (e.g. redundant umbilical skin), cardiac anomalies, deafness, and mental retardation.

Differential diagnosis The differential diagnosis of Axenfeld-Rieger syndrome includes iridocorneal endothelial syndrome, Peter's anomaly, aniridia, posterior polymorphous dystrophy, iridogoniodysgenesis,

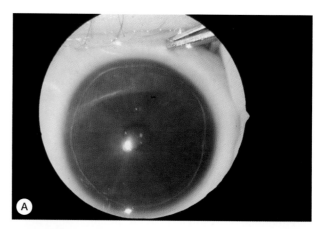

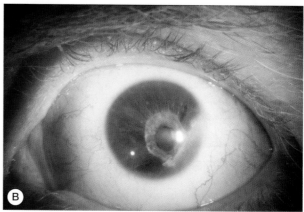

FIGURE 31.6 **(A)** Posterior embryotoxon. **(B)** Iris hypoplasia, stretch holes, iridocorneal adhesions, and correctopia. **((B).** Reproduced from Beck AD. Diagnosis and management of pediatric glaucoma. Ophthalmol Clin North Am 2001; 14: 501–512.)[3]

oculodentodigital dysplasia, ectopia lentis et pupillae, ectropion uveae, uveitic glaucoma, iris coloboma, iridodialysis, and iridoschisis.

Treatment options, outcomes, and prognosis The management of glaucoma associated with Axenfeld-Rieger syndrome begins with medical therapy. If this is ineffective, angle surgery can be attempted but has limited success rates. Trabeculectomy and aqueous shunt surgery are better surgical options for the management of glaucoma in these patients.

NEUROFIBROMATOSIS (TYPE 1)

Disease prevalence and influence Neurofibromatosis type 1, also known as von Recklinghausen's disease, is another one of the phakomatoses. It is associated with a 50% chance of congenital glaucoma when ipsilateral eyelid plexiform neurofibroma is present.[3]

Risk factors The main risk factor is family history. It is inherited as an autosomal dominant trait due to a mutation near the centromere on chromosome 17.[41]

Pathogenesis The pathogenesis of glaucoma due to neurofibromatosis is not well understood, but theories include an underlying trabecular dysgenesis and altered filtration due the observation of neurofibromatous tissue covering the angle.

Signs and symptoms Ocular signs of neurofibromatosis type 1 include S-shaped deformity of the upper eyelid (plexiform neurofibroma, see Fig. 31.2), hamartomatous lesions of the iris stroma (Lisch nodules), ectropion uveae, and ipsilateral hyperpigmentation of the fundus. The Lisch nodules and ectropion uveae may not appear until well after the first year of life. Chorioretinal hamartomas and optic nerve gliomas are occasionally present. Marked buphthalmos associated with corneal enlargement and edema can occur in infants with associated glaucoma.

The primary systemic feature is the presence of flat, hyperpigmented, well-circumscribed skin lesions known as café au lait spots (Fig. 31.7). Café au lait spots may not be present until after the first year of life. Nodular or subcutaneous neurofibromas may also occur.

Differential diagnosis The differential diagnosis includes congenital ectropion uveae and other forms of congenital glaucoma presenting with buphthalmos and corneal edema. Other disorders associated with upper eyelid swelling or masses should be excluded. Radiographic imaging of the orbit should be considered for confirmation of the diagnosis.

Treatment options, outcomes, and prognosis Treatment for glaucoma associated with neurofibromatosis can be difficult. Options include medical management, angle surgery (not often effective), filtration surgery, aqueous shunt devices, and cyclodestructive procedures in refractory cases.

LOWE SYNDROME

Disease prevalence and influence Lowe syndrome, also known as oculocerebrorenal syndrome, is characterized by a high incidence of bilateral cataract and glaucoma.

Risk factors The disease is X-linked recessive and has been linked to the locus Xq26.[42]

Pathogenesis The mechanism of the glaucoma is believed to be secondary to an underlying trabeculo-dysgenesis.

Signs and symptoms The most prominent ocular signs are the presence of glaucoma and cataract (Fig. 31.8). The corneal enlargement and edema may be somewhat mild despite the existence of elevated intraocular pressure. Pinpoint pupils that dilate poorly are another feature of this disorder. The appearance of the angle closely resembles that of primary congenital glaucoma. Other features which may occur include microphthalmia, strabismus, nystagmus, and iris atrophy.

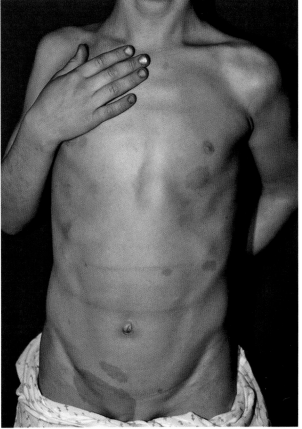

FIGURE 31.7 Café au lait spots in neurofibromatosis type 1 (NF-1). The presence of six or more café au lait spots greater than 0.5 cm in diameter in children and 1.5 cm in adolescents suggests the possibility of NF-1 (Reproduced with permission from Paller AS, Mancini AJ, eds. Hurwitz clinical pediatric dermatology. 3rd edn. Philadelphia: Elsevier Saunders; 2006.)

The systemic features include mental retardation, renal rickets, aminoaciduria, hypotonia, acidemia, and irritability.

Differential diagnosis The differential diagnosis includes other causes of congenital cataract and glaucoma.

Treatment options, outcomes, and prognosis Medications and angle surgery can be attempted. Drainage devices and cycloablative procedures may be necessary for refractory cases.

PRIMARY CHILDHOOD GLAUCOMAS ASSOCIATED WITH OCULAR ANOMALIES

Primary childhood glaucomas are often associated with ocular anomalies in the absence of systemic syndromes. The two most common conditions in this category are aniridia and Peter's anomaly.

ANIRIDIA

Disease prevalence and influence Aniridia is a bilateral condition characterized by the congenital absence

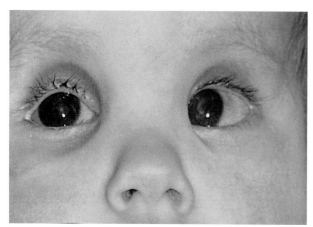

FIGURE 31.8 Glaucoma and cataract in Lowe syndrome. (Reproduced with permission from Albert DM, Jakobiec FA, eds. Principles and practice of ophthalmology. 2nd edn. Philadelphia: Saunders; 1999.)

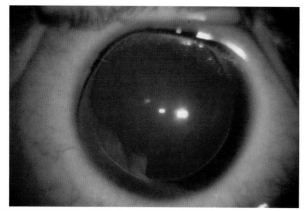

FIGURE 31.9 Absence of normal iris with rudimentary stump of peripheral iris tissue in aniridia.

of a normal iris and a variably sized rudimentary stump of peripheral iris tissue (Fig. 31.9). The disease is associated with glaucoma in approximately 50–70% of cases. However, the glaucoma may not present until later in childhood or adult life.

Risk factors Aniridia can be inherited as an autosomal dominant trait associated with mutations in the PAX6 gene, located at chromosome 11p13. It can also be inherited sporadically in approximately one-third of cases. Sporadic inheritance is associated with an increased risk of Wilms' tumor.

Pathogenesis The development of glaucoma in these eyes appears to relate to the gonioscopic appearance of the angle. The trabecular meshwork likely becomes progressively occluded by the movement of the rudimentary iris over the trabecula.

Signs and symptoms The most common ocular signs of aniridia include the appearance of only rudimentary

iris, corneal pannus, cataracts, foveal hypoplasia, and nystagmus. Visual acuity is typically poor due to foveal hypoplasia.

The most important systemic feature is that associated with sporadic forms of aniridia. Careful family history and screening for Wilms' tumor is essential in these patients.

Differential diagnosis The differential diagnosis includes iris coloboma and other forms of congenital glaucoma associated with iris anomalies.

Treatment options, outcomes, and prognosis Medical management can be attempted in patients with aniridia. Consideration should be given to the performance of prophylactic goniosurgery to prevent occlusion of the trabecular meshwork by iris tissue in patients with apparent progression of angle abnormalities.[43] Filtration surgery, aqueous shunt devices, and cyclodestructive procedures can be considered for more refractory cases.

PETER'S ANOMALY

Disease prevalence and influence Peter's anomaly is present at birth. The condition is typically bilateral, although marked asymmetry and unilateral cases can occur. Approximately 50% of patients present with associated congenital glaucoma.

Risk factors Most cases of Peter's anomaly are sporadic, although autosomal dominant and recessive forms have been reported. The anomaly can be caused by mutations in the PAX6, PITX2, CYPIB1, or FOXC1 genes.

Pathogenesis The mechanism of glaucoma is unclear, but is likely related to an underlying trabeculodysgenesis. In some cases, where marked peripheral anterior synechiae are present, angle closure may contribute to the mechanism.

Signs and symptoms The characteristic sign of Peter's anomaly is a central corneal leukoma (Fig. 31.10) due to a defect in Descemet's membrane. Iris adhesions may extend to the peripheral borders of the leukoma. Keratolenticular cataract and microphthalmia are present in some forms of the disorder. In rare cases, Peter's anomaly can be present in combination with Axenfeld-Rieger syndrome. Glaucoma, when present, may be severe.

Systemic associations with Peter's anomaly are rare. However, an association with lethal cardiac arrhythmias with bilateral forms of Peter's anomaly has been reported.

Differential diagnosis The differential diagnosis of Peter's anomaly includes other causes of corneal opacities

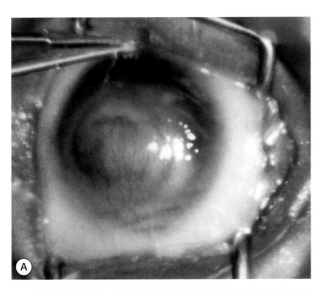

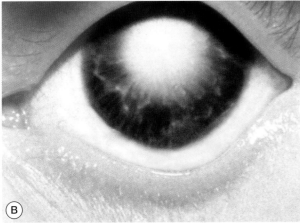

FIGURE 31.10 Central corneal leukomas with (A) and without (B) extensive superficial corneal pannus in Peter's anomaly. (Reproduced with permission from Krachmer JH, Palay DA. Cornea atlas. 2nd edn. St. Louis: Mosby; 2006.)

in infants (see Table 31.3). Congenital anterior staphyloma, which may represent one end of the spectrum of Peter's anomaly, is also in the differential, particularly in unilateral cases.

Treatment options, outcomes, and prognosis
Penetrating keratoplasty is frequently necessary for the prevention of amblyopia. Unfortunately, corneal graft failure occurs at high rates in these patients. Medical therapy and angle surgery can be attempted in milder cases. Frequently, aqueous shunt devices and cyclodestructive procedures are necessary to control the intraocular pressure. The visual prognosis in these patients is uniformly poor.

SECONDARY CHILDHOOD GLAUCOMAS

The most common condition in this category is glaucoma related to surgery for congenital cataract.

GLAUCOMA AFTER SURGERY FOR CONGENITAL CATARACT

Disease prevalence and influence The incidence of glaucoma after cataract surgery for congenital cataract has been reported to be as high as 75.9% (in patients who received follow-up for longer than 6 years after cataract surgery) with a mean onset of glaucoma at 4.0 ± 4.6 years status post cataract extraction.[44] There does not appear to be any racial or gender predilection.

Risk factors Several risk factors for the development of glaucoma after cataract surgery have been proposed including undergoing lensectomy in the first year of life, microcornea (specifically, corneal diameters <10 mm), microphthalmos, persistent fetal vasculature, and the complete and nuclear subtypes of congenital cataract.[44]

Pathogenesis The exact etiology of this type of glaucoma is still unclear. Open-angle mechanisms seem to be responsible for the majority of cases (93.9% according to one study).[34] Angle-closure glaucoma with pupillary block is less common with modern lensectomy techniques.

Signs and symptoms A history of congenital cataract and subsequent cataract extraction with increased intraocular pressure is the predominant feature of this disorder. Because the glaucoma often presents at a later age, buphthalmos and the characteristic corneal stigmata of primary congenital glaucoma do not typically occur. Since these eyes are frequently smaller than normal, a relative buphthalmos may occur.[8] Although gonioscopy generally reveals open angles, some degree of peripheral anterior synechiae may be present.[34]

Differential diagnosis The differential diagnosis includes other secondary glaucomas such as steroid-response glaucoma, inflammatory glaucoma, and traumatic glaucoma. In cases where angle closure is present, the glaucoma may be secondary to other coexisting disorders such as microphthalmos, nanophthalmos, retinopathy of prematurity, or persistent fetal vasculature.

Treatment options, outcomes, and prognosis Medical management can be attempted in these cases, but will not likely be successful in the long term. Unfortunately, the prognosis is guarded for this type of glaucoma.[34] Trabeculectomy can be performed, but has limited success. Aqueous shunt devices and cyclodestructive procedures may be necessary for long-term pressure control.

Summary

Primary congenital glaucoma and other childhood glaucomas are evaluated and managed differently from most adult forms of glaucoma. Most often, childhood glaucomas are managed best surgically, rather than medically. In primary congenital glaucoma, angle surgery is typically the initial surgical intervention. Other surgical options including trabeculectomy, drainage valves, and cyclodestructive procedures have proved valuable in the management of the various forms of childhood glaucoma. Medical treatment is often useful as adjunctive therapy or as an initial treatment in childhood glaucoma. However, the use of brimonidine is contraindicated in infants and small children.

Visual loss secondary to amblyopia in pediatric glaucoma is not uncommon.[45] Amblyopia must be treated aggressively in these patients. Management of childhood glaucomas in conjunction with a pediatric ophthalmologist should be considered by glaucoma specialists with limited experience in this field. Visual loss secondary to corneal decompensation, cataract, and progressive optic nerve or field loss can occur at any time. Primary congenital glaucoma has the best visual prognosis, with primary glaucomas associated with systemic/ocular anomalies and secondary childhood glaucomas demonstrating worse visual outcomes.[44,46] Lifelong follow-up for children with glaucoma is essential.

REFERENCES

1. Bordon AF, Katsumi O, Hirose T. Tonometry in pediatric patients: a comparative study among Tonopen, Perkins, and Schiotz tonometers. J Pediatr Ophthalmol Strabismus 1995; 32:373–377.

2. Jaafar MS, Kazi GA. Normal intraocular pressure in children: a comparative study of the Perkins applanation tonometer and the pneumotonometer. J Pediatr Ophthalmol Strabismus 1993; 30:284–287.

3. Beck AD. Diagnosis and management of pediatric glaucoma. Ophthalmol Clin North Am 2001; 14(3):501–512.

4. Eisenberg DL, Sherman BG, McKeown CA, et al. Tonometry in adults and children. A manometric evaluation of pneumotonometry, applanation, and Tonopen in vitro and in vivo. Ophthalmology 1998; 105:1173–1181.

5. Sampaolesi R, Caruso R. Ocular echometry in the diagnosis of congenital glaucoma. Arch Ophthalmol 1982; 100:574–577.

6. Law SK, Bui D, Caprioli J. Serial axial length measurements in congenital glaucoma. Am J Ophthalmol 2001; 132(6):926–928.

7. Quigley HA. The pathogenesis of reversible cupping in congenital glaucoma. Am J Ophthalmol 1977; 84:358–370.

8. Egbert JE, Kushner BJ. Excessive loss of hyperopia. A presenting sign of juvenile aphakic glaucoma. Arch Ophthalmol 1990; 108(9):1257–1259.

9. Morales J, Brown SM. The feasibility of short automated static perimetry in children. Ophthalmology 2001; 108:157–162.

10. Walton DS, Katsavounidou G. Newborn primary congenital glaucoma: 2005 Update. J Pediatr Ophthalmol Strabismus 2005; 42:1–8.

11. Walton DS. Glaucoma in infants and children. In: Nelson L, ed. Harley's pediatric ophthalmology. Philadelphia: WB Saunders; 1998.

12. Miller SJH. Genetic aspects of glaucoma. Trans Ophthalmol Soc UK 1962; 81:425.

13. Kolker AE, Hetherington JJ, eds. Becker-Shaffer's diagnosis and therapy of the glaucomas. 4th edn. St Louis: CV Mosby; 1976.

14. Chandler PA, Grant WM. Lectures in glaucoma. Philadelphia: Lea & Febiger; 1965.

15. Mattox C, Walton DS. Hereditary primary childhood glaucomas. Int Ophthalmol Clin 1993; 33:121–134.

16. Sarfarazi M, Akarsu AN, Hossain A, et al. Assignment of a locus (GLC3A) for congenital glaucoma (buphthalmos) to 2p21 and evidence for genetic heterogeneity. Genomics 1995; 30:171.

17. Sarfarazi M. Recent advances in molecular genetics of glaucomas. Hum Mol Genet 1997; 6:1677.

18. Kakiuchi-Matsumoto T, Isashiki Y, Ohba N, et al. Cytochrome P4501B1 gene mutations in Japanese patients with primary congenital glaucoma (1). Am J Ophthalmol 2001; 131:345.

19. Akarsu AN, Turacli ME, Aktan SG, et al. A second locus (GLC3B) for primary congenital glaucoma (Buphthalomos) maps to the 1p36 region. Hum Mol Genet 1996; 5:1199–1203.

20. Martin SN, Sutherland J, Levin AV, et al. Molecular characterization of congenital glaucoma in a consanguineous Canadian community: a step towards preventing glaucoma related blindness. J Med Genet 2000; 37:422.

21. Mashima Y, Suzuki Y, Sergeev Y, et al. Novel cytochrome P4501B1 (CYB1B1) gene mutations in Japanese patients with primary congenital glaucoma. Invest Ophthalmol Vis Sci 2001; 42:2211.

22. Pannicker SG, Reddy AB, Mandal AK, et al. Identification of novel mutations causing familial primary congenital glaucomas in Indian pedigrees. Invest Ophthalmol Vis Sci 2002; 43:1358.

23. Stoilov IR, Costa VP, Vasconellos JP, et al. Molecular genetics of primary congenital glaucoma in Brazil. Invest Ophthalmol Vis Sci 2002; 43:1820.

24. Vincent AL, Billingsley G, Buys Y, et al. Digenic inheritance of early-onset glaucoma: CYP1B1, a potential modifier gene. Am J Hum Genet 2002; 70:448.

25. Barkan O. Pathogenesis of congenital glaucoma: gonioscopic and anatomic observation of the angle of the anterior chamber in the normal eye and in congenital glaucoma. Am J Ophthalmol 1955; 40:1.

26. DeLuise VP, Anderson DR. Primary infantile glaucoma (congenital glaucoma). Surv Ophthalmol 1983; 28:1–19.

27. Maumenee AE. Further observations on the pathogenesis of congenital glaucoma. Trans Am Ophthalmol Soc 1963; 55:1163–1176.

28. Tawara A, Inomata H. Developmental immaturity of the trabecular meshwork in congenital glaucoma. Am J Ophthalmol 1981; 92:508–525.

29. Al-Hazmi A, Awad A, Zwaan A, et al. Correlation between surgical success and severity of congenital glaucoma. Br J Ophthalmol 2005; 89:449–453.

30. Shields MB, et al. Congenital glaucoma. Shields' textbook of glaucoma.. New York: Lippincott Williams & Wilkins; 2005.

31. Medicino ME, Lynch MG, Drack A, et al. Long-term surgical and visual outcomes in primary congenial glaucoma: 360° trabeculotomy versus goniotomy. J AAPOS 2000; 4(4):205–210.

32. Portellos M, Buckley EG, Freedman SF. Topical versus oral carbonic anhydrase inhibitor therapy for pediatric glaucoma. J AAPOS 1998; 2(1):43–47.

33. Passo MS, Palmer EA, Van Buskirk EM. Plasma timolol in glaucoma patients. Ophthalmology 1984; 91(11):1361–1363.

34. Carlson J, Zabriskie N, et al. Apparent central nervous system depression in infants after the use of topical brimonidine. Am J Ophthalmol 1999; 128:255.

35. Korsch E, Grote A, et al. Systemic adverse effects of topical treatment with brimonidine in an infant with secondary glaucoma. Eur J Pediatr 1999; 158:685.

36. Enyedi LB, Freedman SF. Safety and efficacy of brimonidine in children with glaucoma. J AAPOS 2001; 5:281.

37. Enyedi LB, Freedman SF, Buckley EG. The effectiveness of latanoprost for the treatment of pediatric glaucoma. J AAPOS 1999; 3:33.

38. Enyedi LB, Freedman SF. Latanoprost for the treatment of pediatric glaucoma. Surv Ophthalmol 2002; 47:S129.

39. Kwitko ML. Glaucoma in infants and children. New York: Appleton-Century-Crofts; 1973; 483-603.

40. Shields MB. Axenfeld-Rieger syndrome: a theory of mechanism and distinctions from the iridocorneal endothelial syndrome. Trans Am Ophthalmol Soc 1983; 81:736–784.

41. Barker D, Wright E, Nguyen K, et al. Gene for von Recklinghausen neurofibromatosis is in the pericentromeric region of chromosome 17. Science 1987; 236:1100–1102.

42. Mueller OT, Hartsfield JK Jr, Gallardo LA, et al. Lowe oculocerebrorenal syndrome in a female with a balanced X;20 translocation: mapping of the X chromosome breakpoint. Am J Hum Genet 1991; 49:804.

43. Chen TC, Walton DS. Goniosurgery for the prevention of aniridic glaucoma. Arch Ophthalmol 1999; 117(9):1144–1148.

44. Chen TC, Walton DS, Bhatia LS. Aphakic glaucoma after congenital cataract surgery. Arch Ophthalmol 2004; 122(12):1819–1825.

45. Robin AL, Quigley HA, Pollack IP, et al. An analysis of visual acuity, visual fields, and disk cupping in childhood glaucoma. Am J Ophthalmol 1979; 88(5):847–858.

46. Taylor RH, Ainsworth JR, Evans AR, et al. The epidemiology of pediatric glaucoma: the Toronto experience. J AAPOS 1999; 3(5):308–315.

CHAPTER 32

Secondary Angle-Closure Glaucoma

Syril Dorairaj, Jeffrey M Liebmann, and Robert Ritch

INTRODUCTION

ANGLE CLOSURE

Angle closure can be caused by a number of abnormalities in the absolute or relative sizes or positions of anterior segment structures or by abnormal forces in the posterior segment pushing forward and altering the anatomy of the anterior segment.[1] Angle-closure glaucoma can be classified as a primary or a secondary phenomenon. The term 'narrow-angle glaucoma' should not be used, as 'narrowing' of the anterior chamber angle in the absence of iridotrabecular contact does not cause elevated intraocular pressure (IOP) or glaucoma.

Primary angle closure Primary angle closure is attributable to relative pupillary block, where the flow of aqueous from the posterior chamber to the anterior chamber is limited by resistance in the region of iridolenticular contact. The limitation of aqueous flow creates a relative pressure gradient between the anterior and posterior chambers, causing the iris to bow anteriorly, thereby narrowing the angle.

Secondary angle closure Secondary angle closure refers to a wide variety of mechanisms other than relative pupillary block that can cause angle closure. In clinical practice, the presence of persistent iridotrabecular apposition following laser iridotomy suggests that a secondary mechanism is present.[2,3] Mechanisms of secondary angle closure include disorders of the ciliary body, lens-related angle closure (also known as phacomorphic glaucoma), or vectors acting posterior to the lens (e.g. malignant glaucoma). Each of these mechanisms presents with specific clinical signs, the identification of which allows for directed treatment of the underlying pathophysiology.

CLASSIFICATION

Angle closure is most reliably classified by using the *Ritch Four-point System*.[4] Diagnosis of the level of block permits specific treatment directed at the underlying disease mechanism.

I. Angle closure originating at the level of iris
   a. Relative pupillary block
   b. Iris thickness and architecture
II. Angle closure originating at the level of the ciliary body
   a. Plateau iris
      i. Plateau iris configuration
      ii. Plateau iris syndrome
      iii. Pseudoplateau iris
         • Iridociliary cysts
         • Solid lesions of the ciliary body
III. Angle closure originating at the level of the lens
   a. Enlargement or intumescence
   b. Dislocation or subluxation
IV. Angle closure originating posterior to the lens
   a. Malignant glaucoma
      i. Ciliary body detachment (supraciliary fluid)
      ii. Aqueous misdirection
   b. Choroidal effusion/swelling and ciliary body rotation/detachment
   c. Angle closure after scleral buckling procedure
   d. Angle closure after panretinal photocoagulation
   e. Angle closure after retinal vein occlusion
   f. Posterior segment tumors

DISEASE PREVALENCE AND INFLUENCE

Relative pupillary block, or primary angle closure, accounts for more than 90% of cases of angle closure. Secondary mechanisms account for the remainder.

RISK FACTORS, ETIOLOGY, AND DISEASE MECHANISMS

A number of different disease mechanisms may result in secondary angle closure, but all culminate in the common final pathway of iris apposition to the trabecular meshwork, elevated intraocular pressure, glaucomatous optic neuropathy, and visual field loss.

ANATOMY AND PATHOPHYSIOLOGY

Understanding of the anatomic and pathophysiologic mechanisms involved in the etiology of angle-closure glaucoma assists in diagnosis and optimizing the treatment course. Anatomic considerations, such as smaller corneal diameter, smaller radius of anterior corneal curvature (steeper corneal curvature), smaller radius of posterior corneal curvature, shallower anterior chamber, thicker lens, smaller radius of anterior lens curvature (steeper lens surface), more anterior lens position, and shorter axial length are all known to play a role in the angle-closure process.[5] However, a complete understanding of these parameters is still lacking since many eyes that have these anatomic findings do not go on to develop any form of angle closure.

Iris texture and thickness may have some influence on angle closure, although in persons of European ancestry there are no differences in the susceptibilities of blue, hazel, or brown irides.[6] Iris texture seems to be involved because a flaccid iris can likely assume a more convex configuration than a rigid iris, thus narrowing the angle further. Thickness and rigidity of the irides may contribute to a tendency towards angle closure.

SPECIFIC SECONDARY FORMS OF ANGLE CLOSURE

ANGLE CLOSURE ORIGINATING AT THE LEVEL OF THE CILIARY BODY

Plateau iris configuration As already mentioned, secondary angle closure refers to any mechanism other than relative pupillary block that causes angle closure. Plateau iris syndrome often presents as primary angle closure, and as such, some authors prefer to classify it as a form of primary angle closure. In plateau iris configuration and syndrome, anatomic variations to the iris anatomy predispose to angle closure, prompting others to classify the condition as a secondary form of angle closure.

In plateau iris configuration, the iris root angulates forward and then centrally due to an anteriorly positioned pars plicata, which mechanically holds the ciliary body against the trabecular meshwork (Fig. 32.1). Shallowing and narrowing of the angle may result from the anterior insertion of the iris and there is a sharp drop-off of the peripheral iris at the inner aspect of the angle.[7] On indentation gonioscopy, the 'double-hump' sign is seen, as the iris follows the convexity of the anterior lens capsule, dips posteriorly into the posterior chamber, and rises over the anteriorly positioned ciliary processes. It is important to note that more force is needed during indentation gonioscopy to open the angle in plateau iris than in pupillary block, as the pars plicata must be displaced posteriorly.

Plateau iris syndrome Plateau iris syndrome occurs when plateau configuration is present along with angle closure. The diagnosis of plateau iris should only be

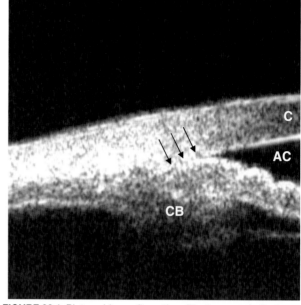

FIGURE 32.1 Plateau iris configuration. Black arrows indicate iridotrabecular apposition. C, cornea; AC, anterior chamber; I, iris; CB, ciliary body forcing the peripheral iris causing iridotrabecular apposition.

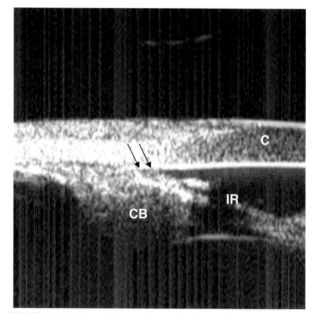

FIGURE 32.2 Plateau iris syndrome. In plateau iris syndrome, an anterior position of the ciliary body forces the peripheral iris to cause iridotrabecular apposition. Black arrows indicate iridotrabecular apposition. C, cornea; CB, ciliary body; IR, patent iridotomy.

made in the presence of a patent iridotomy (Fig. 32.2). On ultrasound biomicroscopy (UBM), anteriorly positioned ciliary processes and the absence of a ciliary sulcus are seen.[8] The syndrome can be complete or incomplete, with increased IOP primarily dependent on the level of iridotrabecular contact and trabecular damage.[9] In the complete syndrome, the iris occludes the trabecular meshwork up to Schwalbe's line, with subsequent angle closure and increase in IOP. In incomplete

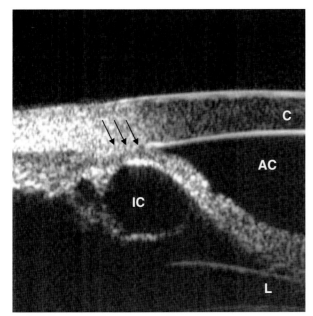

FIGURE 32.3 Iridociliary cyst. Iridociliary cysts are thin-walled echolucent lesions that may cause progressive focal iridotrabecular apposition. Black arrows indicate iridotrabecular apposition. C, cornea; AC, anterior chamber; IC, iridociliary cyst; L, lens.

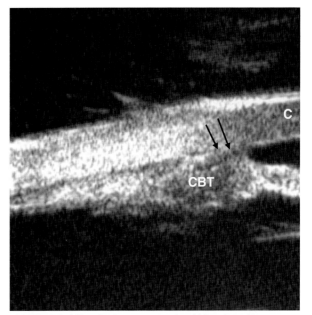

FIGURE 32.4 Ciliary body tumor causing iridotrabecular apposition. Black arrows indicate iridotrabecular apposition. C, cornea; I, iris; CBT, ciliary body tumor causing iridotrabecular apposition.

syndrome, the iris occludes the angle only to the level of midmeshwork. At this lower level of iridotrabecular contact no increase in IOP occurs. Incomplete plateau iris syndrome is more common and can result in peripheral anterior synechiae (PAS) years after a successful iridotomy.

Compared to those with relative pupillary block, patients with plateau iris tend to be younger, less hyperopic, and are more likely to be female. Many also have a family history of angle-closure glaucoma.

Secondary (pseudo-) plateau iris In secondary plateau iris, also known as pseudoplateau iris, cysts of the iris or ciliary body neuroepithelium cause anterior displacement of the peripheral iris (Fig. 32.3). The clinical appearance of the anterior chamber angle is similar to that seen in plateau iris syndrome and may occur with or without angle closure. Most cysts are thin-walled echolucent lesions on UBM. Iris and ciliary body cysts may potentially cause either acute or chronic angle-closure glaucoma. In a study of 67 young patients with angle closure, iridociliary cysts were reported as the cause in eight patients. The cysts were multiple and extended around the circumference of the angle, and all patients required iridotomy in at least one eye.[8] Solitary iridociliary cysts may cause focal iridotrabecular apposition but rarely cause elevated intraocular pressure.

Solid lesions of the ciliary body, although much more rare than iridociliary cysts, may also cause a secondary plateau iris, resulting in angle closure (Fig. 32.4).[10,11] A tumor in the posterior segment should be suspected, particularly if the fellow eye has a wide-open angle and the two eyes have a similar refraction. Ultrasound imaging should follow if the posterior segment cannot be visualized.

LENS-INDUCED GLAUCOMA

Phacomorphic glaucoma Phacomorphic glaucoma refers to glaucoma, the pathophysiology of which originates at the level of the lens. Marked swelling of the lens, known as intumescence, may convert an anterior chamber of medium depth into a shallow chamber, which subsequently precipitates acute angle closure (Fig. 32.5). As in any secondary angle-closure glaucoma, there may be some element of pupillary block present as well. Miotic-induced ciliary muscle contraction relaxes the zonules, which produces anterior lens movement, and increases lens thickness and curvature. Together, these actions augment pupillary block.

Following laser iridotomy in eyes with phacomorphic glaucoma, gonioscopy reveals iris contact with the anterior lens capsule. Considerable force may be required to move the lens posteriorly, and it may be difficult to open the angle with indentation.

Lens subluxation or dislocation is also a frequent cause of lens-induced angle closure. The most common cause of lens subluxation worldwide is exfoliation syndrome, in which zonular laxity or disintegration permits anterior lens movement, which can result in either increased pupillary block or angle closure related to the anterior lens position itself.

Younger patients with anterior lens movement often have underlying causes, such as ciliary block or Weill-Marchesani syndrome (WMS). WMS may cause secondary angle closure glaucoma in several ways, one of which is attributed to ectopia lentis. In WMS, abnormalities of the lens zonules and the ciliary body structure cause forward movement of the lens, and result in either angle-closure glaucoma or pupillary block glaucoma.[12] Microspherophakia, another feature of WMS,

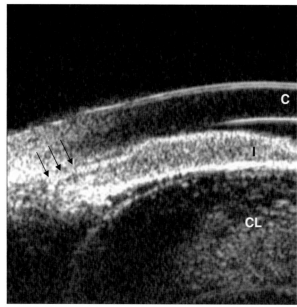

FIGURE 32.5 Lens-induced angle closure. Black arrows indicate iridotrabecular apposition. C, cornea; I, iris; CL, subluxated cataractous lens causing mechanical compression of the iris and ciliary body causing iridotrabecular apposition.

leads to a lens with a small diameter and a spherical shape, and thus, lens displacement.[13,14] Marfan's syndrome is the most common cause of hereditary ectopia lentis. Bilateral, early lens dislocation occurs in about 80% of patients and can occur in any direction, although it usually occurs in a superior or superotemporal direction.[15] In these cases, about 8% proceed to glaucoma. Ciliary block may also result if the lens moves further anteriorly.[16]

MALIGNANT GLAUCOMA

Malignant glaucoma is a multifactorial condition that involves a combination of some or all of the following: previous acute or chronic angle-closure glaucoma, a shallow anterior chamber, forward displacement of the lens, relaxation of the zonules, anterior rotation or swelling of the ciliary body, thickening of the anterior vitreous, and posterior aqueous displacement into or behind the vitreous.

Although malignant glaucoma was classically thought to be a postoperative condition occurring after any type of incisional procedure,[17] the term ciliary block glaucoma was suggested by Weiss and Shaffer to call attention to the region of the ciliary body.[18] Whereas in pupillary block the angle is occluded by the iris because of pressure differential between the posterior and anterior chambers, in malignant glaucoma, a pressure differential is created between the posterior and anterior segment compartments by aqueous misdirection into the vitreous, forcing the anterior segment structures to move forward.[19] This secondary angle-closure glaucoma is characterized by elevated IOP, shallow anterior chamber, patent iridectomy, and normal posterior segment anatomy by ophthalmoscopy or B-scan ultrasonography.

In eyes with malignant glaucoma, several anatomic features have been consistently observed in the region of the ciliary processes, lens equator, and anterior vitreous face. When viewed through a peripheral iridotomy, the tips of the ciliary processes may touch the lens. The ciliary processes are often rotated anteriorly. Phakic eyes with malignant glaucoma may have an anterior vitreous face that is abnormally forward behind the ciliary processes. In aphakic eyes, the anterior vitreous face may even touch or adhere to the ciliary processes.[17]

When the ciliary body swells or rotates anteriorly with forward rotation of the lens–iris diaphragm, relaxation of the zonular apparatus can contribute to anterior lens displacement, pushing the iris against the trabecular meshwork, and leading to angle closure. This also can be exacerbated by treatment with miotics. Physical findings that may suggest malignant glaucoma include unequal anterior chamber depths, progressively increasing myopia, and progressive shallowing of the anterior chamber.

UBM imaging of eyes with malignant glaucoma reveals two subtypes. In some eyes, a shallow supraciliary detachment, which is not evident on routine B-scan examination, is responsible for anterior rotation of the ciliary body (Fig. 32.6A). In eyes without supraciliary fluid, aqueous misdirection alone likely accounts for the aberrant anatomy (Fig. 32.6B).

The postoperative development of malignant glaucoma is highest in eyes with preexisting angle closure.[20] Intraocular pressure at the time of surgery is not a good indicator of the likelihood of developing malignant glaucoma postsurgically, as tension may be low preoperatively in some cases. There have also been cases in which IOP is normal due to the low rate of aqueous humor formation that occurs as a result of a spontaneous reaction to a previous acute attack of angle closure or secondary to medication use.[17]

Posterior chamber intraocular lens implantation following cataract surgery may also evolve into malignant glaucoma. In this circumstance, the differential diagnosis may include pupillary block, choroidal hemorrhage, or ciliochoroidal effusion with anterior rotation of the ciliary body. These pseudophakic patients tend to have shallowing of the central anterior chamber, unlike patients with pupillary block.

ANGLE CLOSURE DUE TO CHOROIDAL EFFUSION/SWELLING AND CILIARY BODY ROTATION/DETACHMENT

Idiosyncratic drug reactions have been shown to be a cause of secondary angle closure, although the exact pathophysiology of the reaction is unknown. Specifically, angle closure has been seen in patients after use of topiramate, venlafaxine, and fluvoxamine.[21–23] Sankar et al. reported two cases of uveal effusion thought to be associated with topiramate use. In one case the patient had been using fluvoxamine maleate for 2 days and had documented uveal effusion and forward shift of the ciliary body.[24] Rhee et al.

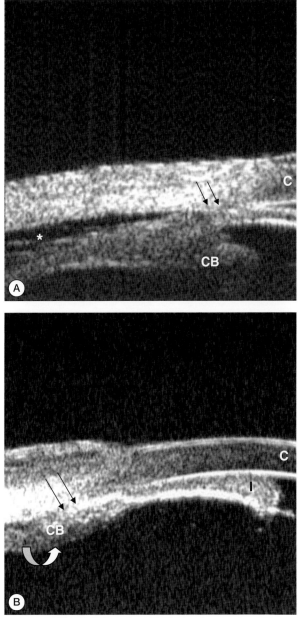

FIGURE 32.6 Malignant glaucoma. **(A)** Malignant glaucoma caused by ciliary body detachment and anterior rotation. Black arrows indicate iridotrabecular apposition. C, cornea; CB, ciliary body; LC, lens capsule; I, iris; S, sclera; asterisk points to the supraciliary effusion. **(B)** Malignant glaucoma caused by aqueous misdirection with absence of ciliary body detachment. Black arrows indicate iridotrabecular apposition. C, cornea; CB, ciliary body; I, iris; curved arrow indicates anterior rotation of the ciliary body.

described a case of bilateral angle closure in a patient using topiramate, which they attributed to ciliary body edema and forward displacement of the lens.[25]

SYSTEMIC INFLAMMATORY DISEASES AND NEOVASCULAR GLAUCOMA

Angle-closure glaucoma can also be part of systemic inflammatory diseases, for example, systemic lupus erythematosus (SLE) and Vogt-Koyanagi-Harada (VKH)

syndrome. Wisotsky et al. described a case of acute angle-closure glaucoma as the initial presentation of a patient with SLE.[26] On dilated funduscopy the patient revealed bilateral four-quadrant, annular, choroidal effusions with no overlying subretinal fluid. Due to failure of medical therapy and laser iridotomy to manage the glaucoma, the patient underwent partial-thickness sclerectomies with linear sclerostomies, which resulted in stabilization of IOP, resolution of choroidal effusions, and deepening of the anterior chamber. Although very rare, Rathinam et al. described three patients with VKH syndrome who presented with angle-closure glaucoma and poor response to laser iridotomy.[27]

Neovascular glaucoma is a severe type of secondary angle-closure glaucoma characterized by retinal or ocular ischemia or ocular inflammation. It is caused by a variety of disorders, including central retinal vein occlusion, diabetes mellitus, carotid artery occlusive disease, and intraocular tumor, among many others. Neovascularization begins as endothelial budding from capillaries at the pupil and progresses to glomerulus-like vascular tufts that lack a muscular layer or any supportive tissue.[28] These fine arborizing blood vessels on the surface of the iris and trabecular meshwork are accompanied by the creation of a fibrous membrane made up of proliferating myofibroblasts. The fibrous portion of this membrane causes a flattening of the iris surface. Contraction of this fibrous membrane also results in formation of peripheral anterior synechiae, which eventually coalesce and lead to the development of secondary angle-closure glaucoma (see also Ch. 34, Neovascular Glaucoma).

DIAGNOSTIC OPTIONS

GONIOSCOPY

On examination, angle closure, with or without ocular hypertension or glaucoma, is best recognized and diagnosed in clinical practice by anterior chamber gonioscopy. Accurate diagnosis of the specific type of angle closure relies on two modalities. The first is darkroom indentation gonioscopy. Using a four-mirror gonioscopy lens with a diameter smaller than that of the cornea, pressure is applied on the central cornea, displacing aqueous towards the peripheral anterior chamber. If reversible iridocorneal apposition is present, aqueous is forced into the angle and results in discernable angle widening and viewing of previously hidden angle landmarks. In addition, the behavior of the iris during indentation gonioscopy is specific to the level at which angle closure originates, as detailed below. In order to correctly discern a narrow, but open, angle from a closed one, it is of the utmost importance that gonioscopy be performed in a completely darkened room, as any light shone through the pupil will result in miosis and may prevent detection of iridotrabecular apposition. For this reason, the smallest square of light should be used for a slit beam, ensuring that it does not project into the pupil. The quadrant to be assessed

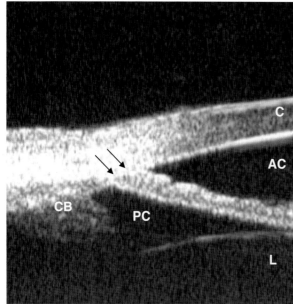

FIGURE 32.7 Peripheral anterior synechiae. Black arrows indicate iridotrabecular apposition. C, cornea; AC, anterior chamber; CB, ciliary body; PC, posterior chamber; L, lens.

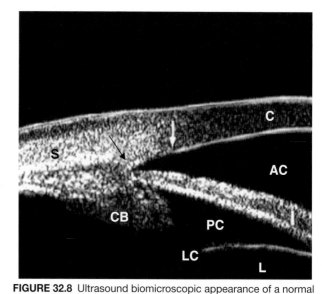

FIGURE 32.8 Ultrasound biomicroscopic appearance of a normal eye. Black arrow indicates scleral spur, white arrow indicates Schwalbe's line. C, cornea; AC, anterior chamber; CB, ciliary body; S, sclera; PC, posterior chamber; LC, lens capsule; L, lens.

is first examined without pressure on the cornea and with the patient looking toward the mirror, allowing the examiner to see as deeply into the angle as possible. The widest quadrant is usually, but not always, the inferior angle (superior mirror), so it is logical to begin the examination at this location. Corneal indentation is subsequently performed and any changes in angle and iris configuration are noted. Pressure on the cornea during gonioscopy forces aqueous humor into the angle, thus making it wide enough to permit viewing over the iris convexity. The presence and extent of synechial closure consequent to PAS (Fig. 32.7), as well as the depth of the angle, can be determined by this method. Information gathered by gonioscopy provides the key to clinical decisions regarding treatment (see also Ch. 13, Gonioscopy).

ULTRASOUND BIOMICROSCOPY

High-frequency, high-resolution ultrasound biomicroscopy (UBM) allows for imaging of the structures surrounding the posterior chamber and the anterior segment that cannot normally be seen during slit lamp biomicroscopy or gonioscopy. In vivo cross-sectional or transverse images can be obtained detailing the cornea, iris, ciliary body, anterior chamber angle, and peripheral sclera, and are similar to those seen on a low-power microscope (Fig. 32.8). This technology allows for better differentiation and diagnosis of causes of angle closure, which in turn leads to more informed decision-making and directed treatment. UBM augments gonioscopy in the qualitative and quantitative evaluation of pathologic changes leading to angle closure (see also Ch. 14, Ultrasound Biomicroscopy).

ANTERIOR SEGMENT OPTICAL COHERENCE TOMOGRAPHY

Anterior segment optical coherence tomography (AS-OCT) is a new imaging method that allows for objective and quantitative imaging of the anterior segment. AS-OCT is similar to UBM in its ability to quantitatively determine angle parameters, and has the benefit of being easier to use and does not require a coupling agent.[29,30] Due to its dependence on light rather than sound waves, AS-OCT has limited use in conditions that require imaging of structures posterior to the pigment epithelium of the iris and ciliary body, including plateau iris syndrome and tumors of the ciliary body. In these conditions, UBM is more suitable.

SIGNS AND SYMPTOMS OF SECONDARY ANGLE CLOSURE

Acute clinical presentations of secondary angle-closure glaucomas are identical to primary angle closure. Signs and symptoms include pain, blurred vision, nausea, and ocular injection. Their frequency is often described as acute, subacute, intermittent, or chronic. The specific presentation depends on what percentage of the filtering meshwork is occluded by the iris, the rapidity with which the occlusion occurs, and the ability to reverse the iridotrabecular blockage.

Elevation of intraocular pressure can result in severe corneal edema with blurred vision, intense pain, and possibly lacrimation and lid edema. Systemic vagal symptoms can include nausea and bradycardia, diaphoresis, nausea, and emesis. Relevant clinical signs of angle closure are markedly elevated IOP, and decreased visual acuity. Eyelids are swollen, and there is conjunctival

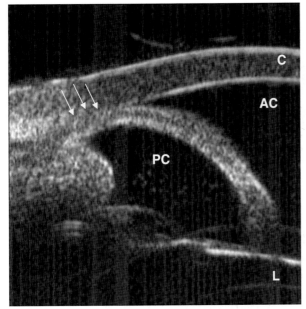

FIGURE 32.9 Iris bombe. White arrows indicate iridotrabecular apposition. C, cornea; AC, anterior chamber; PC, posterior chamber; CB, ciliary body; L, lens.

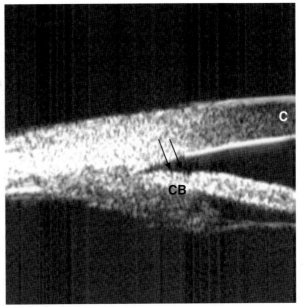

FIGURE 32.10 Plateau iris following argon laser peripheral iridoplasty. Black arrows indicate the site of iridoplasty. C, cornea; CB, ciliary body; asterisk points to the scleral spur indicating relief of iridotrabecular apposition following laser iridoplasty.

hyperemia and circumlimbal injection. Because of iris sphincter ischemia, the pupil is usually mid-dilated and/ or vertically oval, and the cornea may be edematous. The midperipheral iris is bowed anteriorly and may contact the cornea peripherally (Fig. 32.9); the anterior chamber may be shallow with evidence of an inflammatory reaction. With severe corneal damage, there may be chronic edema, lipid deposits, and fibrosis and vascularization of the cornea. When intraocular pressure is very high, glaukomflecken may form.

TREATMENT OPTIONS, OUTCOMES, AND PROGNOSIS

GENERAL TREATMENT OF ANGLE-CLOSURE GLAUCOMA

The mainstay of therapy for acute and chronic angle closure is reduction of intraocular pressure and appropriate laser surgery.

MEDICAL THERAPY

Pharmaceutical treatments for angle closure have several different mechanisms of action.

Aqueous suppression Suppression of aqueous humor formation is the mainstay of therapy. Therapeutic options include topical therapy with β-adrenergic antagonist, carbonic anhydrase inhibitors, or α-adrenergic agonists. Systemic carbonic anhydrase inhibition can be very effective, particularly in eyes with acute angle closure.

Miotics Miotic therapy with agents such as pilocarpine may be used to constrict the pupil and draw the

peripheral iris away from the trabecular meshwork. Eyes in which angle closure has some component of pupillary block are often improved by miotics; however, for eyes in which angle closure is caused by forward lens movement, ciliary block, or an intumescent lens, excessive miotic therapy may cause contraction of the ciliary ring, anterior lens movement, and paradoxical worsening of the angle-closure process.

LASER THERAPIES

The primary goal of treatment in angle-closure glaucoma, regardless of cause, is to eliminate the cause of angle closure, to reopen the filtration angle, and to prevent further damage to the optic nerve by lowering IOP.

LASER PERIPHERAL IRIDOTOMY AND IRIDOPLASTY

Virtually all individuals with angle closure have some component of relative pupillary block and therefore almost all eyes with angle closure require laser iridotomy. This disease process and treatment is described in detail elsewhere (see also Ch. 66, Laser Iridoplasty).

Eyes with secondary angle closure typically have continued appositional angle closure in the presence of a patent iridotomy. Residual appositional closure in these eyes can often be eliminated by argon laser peripheral iridoplasty. Peripheral iridoplasty is a procedure in which a ring of contraction burns is placed circumferentially on the peripheral iris, contracting the iris stroma between the burn site and angle, and thereby widening the angle (Fig. 32.10). The short-term effect of the peripheral iridoplasty procedure is related to heat shrinkage of collagen, and the long-term effect is secondary to contraction of a fibroblastic membrane in the region of the laser application.

Peripheral iridoplasty is effective in breaking attacks of angle closure due to plateau iris configuration and lens-induced angle closure. In these patients, the eye is often quite inflamed as a result of unsuccessful previous treatments, and breaking the attack with iridoplasty allows the inflammation to disappear and the corneal edema to ameliorate (see also Ch. 65, Peripheral Iridectomy).

GONIOSYNECHIALYSIS

Goniosynechialysis is a surgical procedure that removes PAS from the angle wall in eyes with synechial closure, leading to opening of the angle and variable restoration of trabecular meshwork function. Under viscoelastic cover, the angle is visualized with gonioscopy, and the iris is mechanically separated from the trabecular meshwork. This procedure is successful only if synechiae have been typically present for less than 1 year. Complications include bleeding, iridodialysis, and marked inflammation.

PLATEAU IRIS SYNDROME AND CONFIGURATION

Treatment of plateau iris syndrome requires differentiation of the condition from the more common configuration, as the latter requires only follow-up. In eyes with plateau iris syndrome, if the angle closes completely to the upper trabecular meshwork or Schwalbe's line, the IOP will rise. In patients with plateau iris syndrome for whom the angle only closes partially, leaving the upper portion of the filtering meshwork open, IOP will not rise; however, these patients may develop peripheral anterior synechiae (PAS) years after a successful iridotomy.[9]

The main objective of treatment in eyes with plateau iris syndrome is to prevent the development of PAS, chronic angle closure, and less commonly acute angle closure, and also to prevent the development of elevated IOP in the dark, as occurs with some patients. Iridotomy should be the first intervention to counteract an element of pupillary block, if present. If angle closure persists, argon laser peripheral iridoplasty (ALPI) is indicated, which, by compacting and contracting the peripheral iris stroma, physically opens the angle (see Fig. 32.10).[31,32]

Studies have documented the long-term success of argon laser peripheral iridoplasty in the treatment of plateau iris syndrome.[33] Ritch et al. showed that in 23 eyes treated with ALPI, 20 remained open throughout the entire follow-up period after only one treatment. Gradual reclosure occurred in the remaining three eyes 5–9 years after the initial ALPI. These eyes

were reopened and maintained open by a single repeat treatment.

Pilocarpine can widen the angle in plateau iris syndrome and works by thinning the iris. Its effect may not be long term, making a treatment of ALPI more preferable. Pilocarpine also has side effects, particularly in younger patients, making a single treatment with ALPI more preferable as it produces a more stable angle. Pilocarpine should be used at the lowest effective concentration and should be used only at night.

If the patient is diagnosed with plateau iris configuration, periodic gonioscopy is warranted to search for signs of possible angle closure. Treatment of plateau-like iris configuration as a result of ciliary body cysts using argon laser iridoplasty, with opening of drainage angle in both eyes, has been reported.[34]

LENS-INDUCED GLAUCOMA

Phacomorphic glaucoma is often unresponsive to medical therapy and paradoxical reactions to treatment with pilocarpine are common. Laser iridoplasty may be necessary to eliminate continued appositional closure and widen the angle if posterior lens position and open angle cannot be properly maintained with cycloplegics after iridotomy. PICP is shown to cause lasting widening of the angle; however, it can only be used if no visually significant lens opacification is present.[35] If cataract is present, lens extraction can lead to widening of the angle and lowering of IOP.[36,37] In eyes with complete or near-complete synechial angle closure, PICP or lens extraction will most likely not be beneficial in terms of angle widening and IOP lowering. If medication fails to lower IOP, trabeculectomy, with or without cataract extraction, is indicated.

Patients who develop slight lens subluxation with age have a generally good prognosis. In these cases, laser iridotomy usually eliminates the pupillary block and angle-closure components. However, younger patients with anterior lens movements may often require iridoplasty following iridotomy to eliminate apposition if cycloplegics cannot maintain a more posterior lens position and open angle. Rarely, cataract extraction may be required to relieve the angle closure.

MALIGNANT GLAUCOMA

Medical therapy for malignant glaucoma includes the concurrent use of mydriatic-cycloplegic drops, β-adrenergic blocking agents, carbonic anhydrase inhibitors, and hyperosmotics. This regimen should be continued until the anterior chamber is formed and pressure improves, or until 4–5 days. The regimen is gradually tapered after the condition is improved; however, the cycloplegic drops are continued indefinitely. Using this regimen, approximately 50% of malignant glaucoma cases are relieved within 4–5 days.[17]

In malignant glaucoma, laser iridotomy for angle closure is often only temporarily successful. In those cases where it is initially successful, lens enlargement from natural aging can cause return of appositional closure. In these cases, iridoplasty is often used, in addition to iridotomy, to flatten the peripheral iris and control angle closure.

In malignant glaucoma that results from surgery, there is often a need for reoperation, and the long-term prognosis for visual improvement is often poor. There exists a spectrum of disease severity. Approximately 50% of all cases of malignant glaucoma remit with intensive cycloplegia, aqueous suppression, and topical steroids. Malignant glaucoma caused primarily by aqueous misdirection may require surgical intervention. Therapy is best directed towards the anatomic cause of the disease, but malignant glaucoma is often a recalcitrant process with a poor prognosis.

Summary

In summary, the secondary causes of angle-closure glaucoma require careful examination, as interventions and prognosis are directly dependent on the correct identification of the mechanism involved. Although predominantly the result of pupillary block, angle-closure glaucoma can result from a variety of forces acting on the angle. These forces may either be intrinsic to the eye, or may be the ocular manifestation of a more widespread, systemic problem, affecting the entire body. The success of medical and surgical intervention for secondary angle-closure glaucoma is a direct reflection of the underlying mechanism. In some cases, medical intervention or simple iridotomy may rectify the angle closure. In other cases, for which more than one mechanism may be precipitating the angle closure, more complicated interventions may be required. Examination by experienced clinicians, with attention to new diagnostic modalities, is allowing for treatment of the secondary causes of angle closure with more successful outcomes than previously achieved.

REFERENCES

1. Ritch R, Liebmann JM. Role of ultrasound biomicroscopy in the differentiation of block glaucomas. Curr Opin Ophthalmol 1998; 9:39–45.

2. Ritch R. Argon laser treatment for medically unresponsive attacks of angle-closure glaucoma. Am J Ophthalmol 1982; 94:197.

3. Pavlin CJ, Ritch R, Foster FS. Ultrasound biomicroscopy in plateau iris syndrome. Am J Ophthalmol 1992; 113:390–395.

4. Ritch R, Liebmann JM, Tello C. A construct for understanding angle-closure glaucoma: the role of ultrasound biomicroscopy. Ophthalmol Clin North Am 1995; 8:281–293.

5. Dorairaj SK, Tello C, Liebmann JM, Ritch R. Why is the superior angle narrower than the inferior angle in patients with narrow angles? Archives 2007; 6; (in press).

6. Ritch R, Lowe RF. Angle-closure glaucoma; mechanisms and epidemiology. In: Ritch R, Shields MB, Krupin T, eds. The glaucomas. St Louis, MO: Mosby; 1996:807–808.

7. Ritch R. Plateau iris is caused by abnormally positioned ciliary processes. J Glaucoma 1992; 1:23–26.

8. Ritch R, Chang BM, Liebmann JM. Angle closure in younger patients. Ophthalmology 2003; 110:1880–1889.

9. Ritch R, Lowe RF. Angle-closure glaucoma; clinical types. In: Ritch R, Shields MB, Krupin T, eds. The glaucomas. St Louis, MO: Mosby; 1996:829–853.

10. Al-Torbak A, Karcioglu ZA, Abboud E, et al. Phacomorphic glaucoma associated with choroidal melanoma. Ophthalmic Surg Lasers 1998; 29:510–513.

11. Escalona-Benz E, Benz MS, Briggs JW, et al. Uveal melanoma presenting as acute angle-closure glaucoma: report of two cases. Am J Ophthalmol 2003; 136:756–758.

12. Chu BS. Weill-Marchesani syndrome and secondary glaucoma associated with ectopia lentis. Clin Exp Optom 2006; 89:95–99.

13. Chang BM, Liebmann JM, Ritch R. Angle closure in younger patients. Trans Am Ophthalmol Soc 2002; 10:201–214.

14. el Kettani A, Hamdani M, Rais L, et al. Weill-Marchesani syndrome. Report of a case. J Fr Ophtalmol 2001; 24:944–948.

15. Liebmann JM, Ritch R. Glaucoma associated with lens intumescence and dislocation. In: Ritch R, Shields MV, Krupin T, eds. The glaucomas. St Louis, MO: Mosby; 1996:1044.

16. Ritch R. Exfoliation syndrome. In: Ritch R, Shields MV, Krupin T, eds. The glaucomas. St Louis, MO: Mosby; 1996:1005.

17. Simmons RJ, Maestre FA. Malignant glaucoma. In: Ritch R, Shields MV, Krupin T, eds. The glaucomas. St Louis, MO: Mosby; 1996:841–847.

18. Weiss DI, Shaffer RN. Ciliary block (malignant) glaucoma. Trans Am Acad Ophthalmol Otolaryngol 1972; 76:450.

19. Shaffer RN. The role of vitreous detachment in aphakic and malignant glaucoma. Trans Am Acad Ophthalmol Otolaryngol 1954; 58:217–234.

20. Simmons RJ. Malignant glaucoma. In: Epstein D, ed. Chandler and Grant's glaucoma. Philadelphia: Lea & Febiger; 1986.

21. Medeiros FA, Zhang XY, Bernd AS, et al. Angle-closure glaucoma associated with ciliary body detachment in patients using topiramate. Arch Ophthalmol 2003; 121:282–285.

22. Jimenez-Jimenez FJ, Orti-Pareja M, Zurdo JM. Aggravation of glaucoma with fluvoxamine. Ann Pharmacother 2001; 35:1565–1566.

23. Aragona M, Inghilleri M. Increased ocular pressure in two patients with narrow angle glaucoma treated with venlafaxine. Clin Neuropharmacol 1998; 21:130–131.

24. Sankar PS, Pasquale LR, Grosskreutz CL. Uveal effusion and secondary angle-closure glaucoma associated with topiramate use. Arch Ophthalmol 2001; 119:1210–1211.

25. Rhee DJ, Goldberg MJ, Parrish RK. Bilateral angle-closure glaucoma and ciliary body swelling from topiramate. Arch Ophthalmol 2001; 119:1721–1723.

26. Wisotsky BJ, Mugat-Gordon CB, Puklin JE. Angle closure glaucoma as an initial presentation of systemic lupus erythematosus. Ophthalmology 1998; 105:1170–1172.

27. Rathinam SR, Namperumalsamy P, Nozik RA, et al. Angle closure glaucoma as a presenting sign of Vogt-Koyanagi-Harada syndrome. Br J Ophthalmol 1997; 81:608–609.

28. Wand M. Neovascular glaucoma. In: Ritch R, Shields MV, Krupin T, eds. The glaucomas. St Louis, MO: Mosby; 1996:1081.

29. Hoerauf H, Scholz C, Koch P, et al. Transscleral optical coherence tomography: a new imaging method for the anterior segment of the eye. Arch Ophthalmol 2002; 12:816–819.

30. Radhakrishnan S, Goldsmith J, Huang D, et al. Comparison of optical coherence tomography and ultrasound biomicroscopy for detection of narrow anterior chamber angles. Arch Ophthalmol 2005; 123:1053–1059.

31. Ritch R. Techniques of argon laser iridectomy and iridoplasty. Palo Alto: Coherent Medical Press; 1983.

32. Ritch R. Argon laser peripheral iridoplasty: an overview. J Glaucoma 1992; 1:206–213.

33. Ritch R, Tham CC, Lam DS. Long-term success of argon laser peripheral iridoplasty in the management of plateau iris syndrome. Ophthalmology 2004; 111:104–108.

34. Crowston JG, Medeiros FA, Mosaed S, et al. Argon laser iridoplasty in the treatment of plateau-like iris configuration as result of numerous ciliary body cysts. Am J Ophthalmol 2005; 139:381–383.

35. Ritch R. Argon laser treatment for medically unresponsive attacks of angle-closure glaucoma. Am J Ophthalmol 1982; 94:197–204.

36. Wishart PK, Atkinson PL. Extracapsular cataract extraction and posterior chamber lens implantation in patients with primary chronic angle-closure glaucoma: effect on intraocular pressure control. Eye 1989; 3:706–712.

37. Greve EL. Primary angle closure glaucoma: extracapsular cataract extraction or filtering procedure? Int Ophthalmol 1988; 12:157–162.

CHAPTER 33

Uveitic Glaucoma

Avinash Kulkarni and Keith Barton

INTRODUCTION

Glaucoma was noted to be a common complication of uveitis with a significant risk of visual loss as early as 1813.[1] In 1857, von Graefe published a series of 20 patients with uveitic glaucoma successfully treated by peripheral iridectomy.[2] In 1918, Elliot attributed inflammatory cases to infective causes and postulated that glaucoma developed as a result of changes in the aqueous humor and increased resistance in the outflow pathway induced by inflammatory cells and debris.[3] Interestingly, Elliot also remarked that treatment by trephination frequently failed due to closure of the fistula.

Infective causes are much less common today and the majority of uveitis is idiopathic. Nevertheless, the term *uveitic glaucoma* encompasses a number of diverse clinical entities with differing prognoses. A careful evaluation of the individual patient is therefore essential for the accurate diagnosis of the type of uveitis and an understanding of the mechanism of glaucoma.

EPIDEMIOLOGY

The prevalence of glaucoma in uveitis appears to range from 10% to 20%.[4–6] The accuracy of this estimate is uncertain because in most studies the criteria used to diagnose glaucoma have not been reported. Most have also used hospital ophthalmology clinics, rather than the primary care or community setting as a source of subjects. Finally, there has been little standardization for the type of uveitis, length of disease duration, and level of corticosteroid treatment that has been used. The effect of disease duration is especially important in a condition that is long-lasting. This has been illustrated by one retrospective uveitis clinic study. Neri et al. reported that, in 337 patients with chronic uveitis, the incidence of glaucoma at 1 and 5 years was 6.5% and 11.1%, respectively, but after 10 years this had increased to 22.7%.[7]

The reported prevalence of secondary glaucoma in patients with juvenile idiopathic arthritis has been particularly high, but one study to examine all those newly diagnosed cases in a rheumatology clinic found a lower prevalence of uveitis and secondary glaucoma than was reported in the past. Shorter follow-up accounts for some of this discrepancy, but it is likely that the prospective study methodology and the use of a rheumatology clinic as a source of subjects uses a more accurate denominator than traditional retrospective ophthalmology clinic-based reports.[8]

The prevalence of secondary glaucoma is related to age at presentation as well as the anatomical type, course, and severity of the uveitis. Although uveitis less commonly affects the very young and elderly, these groups are more prone to intraocular pressure (IOP) elevation. Children have a higher risk of corticosteroid-induced IOP elevation, and childhood uveitis is more likely to result in glaucoma. Again, using the example of juvenile idiopathic arthritis (JIA), a high risk of blindness was originally observed by Kanski and Shunshin, who reported that 35% of JIA eyes with secondary glaucoma lost all vision.[9] It is disconcerting that similarly poor outcomes have been reported by de Boer et al. in a more recent study in which 44% (11/25) of children with JIA developed glaucoma, and after 3 years 27% (3/11) had visual acuity worse than 20/200 as a consequence of glaucoma.[10] However, in that study, recalcitrant glaucoma was managed largely with carbonic anhydrase inhibitors in preference to surgery, a conservative strategy by modern standards.

The poor prognosis of glaucoma in JIA may be due to late presentation or the high level of topical corticosteroids required to control the disease in children. The risk of complications such as elevated IOP in JIA-associated uveitis has been reported by Edelsten et al. in a pediatric rheumatology clinic-based study to be higher in those with greater severity of uveitis at presentation and those whose treatment regimen varied from that particular clinic's standard practice.[11] Children seem to be particularly susceptible to the effect of topical steroids on IOP, but the relative effects of uveitis severity and treatment intensity on IOP are difficult to disentangle. More than 50% of nonuveitic children under 10 years old demonstrate a significant IOP response to topical corticosteroids.[12] It is worth noting that in children the IOP response to rimexolone, a drug with a lower propensity to increase the IOP in adults than either dexamethasone or prednisolone, may still be quite significant and has been reported to approximate to the response observed to dexamethasone in adults.[13]

Though uveitis is less common in the elderly, this group is more vulnerable to IOP elevation. In one study, of patients over 60 years of age presenting de novo with anterior uveitis, one-third had raised IOP.[14]

Other factors such as the chronicity of uveitis and involvement of predominantly the anterior rather than posterior segment increase the risk of IOP elevation.[7,15] The presence of posterior synechiae and the possession of the HLA-B27 antigen are also associated with a higher risk of secondary glaucoma, possibly because they are associated with more severe intraocular inflammation.[16,17]

ETIOLOGY AND PATHOGENESIS

Intraocular pressure elevation in association with uveitis is due to obstruction of aqueous outflow, either macroscopically with iris (secluded pupil and secondary pupil block, chronic synechial angle closure) or microscopically (chronic secondary open-angle glaucoma and corticosteroid-induced IOP elevation) (Table 33.1). In open-angle glaucoma secondary to uveitis, compromised outflow results from trabecular meshwork (TM) exposure to filtered inflammatory cells, cytokines, iris pigment, and corticosteroids.

ALTERATIONS IN AQUEOUS DYNAMICS AND COMPOSITION

In acute uveitis, the IOP often drops, and the reason is thought to be a combination of reduced aqueous production when the ciliary body is inflamed[18] and elevated uveoscleral outflow due to prostaglandin release. It is conceivable that these might lead to TM hypoperfusion and elevated conventional outflow resistance.

TABLE 33.1 Factors influencing IOP in uveitics

IOP-lowering influences:

Cyclitis reducing aqueous production

Prostaglandin release increasing uveoscleral outflow

IOP-elevating influences:

Influence of cytokines on trabeculocytes (IL-1, TGF-β)

Increased aqueous viscosity when protein levels are elevated

Increased trabecular resistance following TM hypoperfusion in severe cyclitis

Trabeculitis

Corticosteroid-induced TM dysfunction

Angle closure (pupil block, forward movement of the iris–lens diaphragm, PAS or neovascularization)

Pigment deposition/cells/debris/inflammatory nodules in the rido-trabecular angle

---

In theory, a paradoxical IOP elevation would then occur after the episode of uveitis has resolved. Trabecular meshwork culture studies suggest that TM perfusion of less than $1\,\mu L/min$ may have a detrimental effect on trabeculocyte survival[19] and hence TM function. An indirect clinical observation that supports this is the observation of a disproportionate elevation in IOP that often occurs following closure of a cyclodialysis cleft.[20] As cleft-induced hypotony is generally more extreme and much more prolonged than that observed in acute uveitis, and as the above effect is believed to be largely reversible, it is unlikely that hypoperfusion accounts solely for the IOP elevation in uveitis. However, it is possible that this mechanism may play a role in some cases of glaucoma after severe acute anterior uveitis.

Variability in aqueous protein binding has so far precluded the accurate measurement of aqueous dynamics in human uveitis, though generally laser flare photometry may be used to estimate aqueous protein content relative to normal.[21,22] Persistently increased vascular permeability after resolution of inflammation in uveitis results in chronic elevation of aqueous protein evident as anterior chamber flare on biomicroscopy. Aqueous composition, especially viscosity, influences outflow facility. Aqueous protein originates from ciliary body capillaries in normal eyes,[23] but does not cross the ciliary epithelium. Instead, protein diffuses into the anterior chamber aqueous via the iris stroma and anterior iris surface. It is likely that in acute uveitis, aqueous protein also comes from dilated iris vessels. Normal aqueous protein concentration is approximately 1% of that in serum, but increases in uveitis and may reach levels similar to undiluted serum.[24] Elliot originally hypothesized that elevated aqueous protein concentration in uveitis reduces outflow.[3] Cadaver studies in which trabecular meshwork was perfused with human serum demonstrated a 42% decrease in facility of outflow.[25] Interestingly, a persistent reduction was observed after irrigation with balanced salt solution, suggesting that protein might be sequestered in trabecular tissue.

THE ROLE OF INFLAMMATORY MEDIATORS

The role of inflammatory mediators in IOP elevation is uncertain. The predominance of CD4[+] T lymphocytes in human intraocular infiltrates,[26–32] animal models of uveitis,[33,34] and their role in adoptive transfer studies[35] imply an important role in the development of uveitis. Despite this, anterior chamber infiltrates are mostly composed of polymorphs and macrophages. Endotoxin-induced uveitis has been used as a model of anterior uveitis because the induced anterior chamber infiltrates are similar to those in human anterior uveitis, where polymorphs and macrophages predominate.[36,37] An imbalance in individual responsiveness to lipopolysaccharide (endotoxin), may also be involved in human anterior uveitis.[38]

Cytokines such as interleukin-1 (IL-1), IL-6, and tumor necrosis factor-α (TNF-α) are expressed in a variety of ocular tissues in experimental uveitis.[39] IL-1 activity in the trabecular meshwork has also been implicated in IOP elevation in primary open-angle glaucoma.[40] Whether this occurs as a result of IOP-related stress to the trabeculocytes, or alternatively represents part of the pathogenic mechanism, is unclear.

Transforming growth factor-β_2 (TGF-β_2) is present in unusually high concentrations in the aqueous of POAG patients,[41] and has been implicated in increased outflow resistance in POAG and in the aging eye. The role of TGF-β in uveitis has not been fully elucidated but, as an immunosuppressive cytokine that seems to have a suppressive role in uveitis,[42] it is perhaps not surprising that low aqueous humor TGF-β_2 levels have been reported in uveitics.[43,44]

Finally, certain cytokines are chemoattractant to trabeculocytes and it is possible that TM depopulation might result from chronic cytokine exposure,[45] with a consequent reduction in conventional outflow.

CHANGES IN TRABECULAR MESHWORK TISSUE ARCHITECTURE

There is little direct evidence of the effect of intraocular inflammation on TM structure, but indirect evidence from other secondary glaucomas suggests that outflow obstruction is more likely to be due to trabeculocyte loss than blockage with pigment, debris, etc. An example is pigmentary glaucoma, where chronic pigment dispersion results in chronic trabeculocyte depletion.[46] Loss of juxtacanalicular TM cells is associated with loss of trabecular surface area.

TRABECULITIS

It is hypothesized that, in Posner-Schlossman syndrome and herpetic keratouveitis, inflammation of the TM may be responsible for the marked increases in IOP that are observed, on the basis that these are disproportionate to the degree of visible anterior segment inflammation. To date, this has not been supported by histological evidence.

CORTICOSTEROID-INDUCED TRABECULAR MESHWORK DYSFUNCTION

Topical corticosteroids are the mainstay of treatment for most patients with uveitis. Although an IOP elevation of 6–15 mmHg occurs in one-third of normal subjects treated with topical corticosteroids, with a small proportion (4–5%) developing a greater elevation,[47,48] the likelihood of inducing an elevation in IOP increases if the aqueous outflow pathway is compromised. Fifty percent of POAG patients exhibit an IOP elevation of 15 mmHg or more with corticosteroids,[49] and in uveitis, where corticosteroid use may be prolonged, responsiveness is more frequent and may even be the predominant cause of secondary glaucoma. Periocular, inhaled, and systemic administration of corticosteroids may also cause ocular hypertension, but less commonly.[50–53] The influence of corticosteroids on outflow is more marked in those in whom outflow is already compromised. For instance, a significant IOP rise will take several weeks in a normal subject but in POAG patients may occur within hours.[50]

Corticosteroids have a number of effects on the TM that have been observed in perfused human anterior segments treated with dexamethasone. These include thickening of trabecular beams, decreased intertrabecular spaces, thickened juxtacanalicular tissue, activated trabecular meshwork cells, and increased amounts of extracellular material. These changes were observed in cultures from steroid responders but not nonresponders.[54]

The increased extracellular material observed in corticosteroid-induced glaucoma has been reported to differ in histological appearance from that described in POAG.[55]

The role of myocilin in corticosteroid-induced glaucoma is still unclear. Although mutations in the TIGR/MYOC gene are probably not involved in steroid-induced glaucoma,[56] myocilin was first described in connection with its appearance in the supernatant of cultured trabecular cells when exposed to corticosteroids.[57] It seems likely that extracellular myocilin protein is linked to aqueous outflow resistance.[58,59]

MACROSCOPIC CHANGES IN ANTERIOR CHAMBER ANGLE ANATOMY

The angle configuration in patients with uveitic glaucoma depends on the natural anatomical configuration of the angle, previous cataract surgery, the severity and chronicity of anterior segment inflammation, and the effect, if any, of inflammation on the morphology of the ciliary body. Most cases of uveitis associated with IOP elevation have an open angle but some degree of pigment deposition in the angle from previous inflammation. A significant proportion develops peripheral anterior synechiae (PAS) or angle closure that may be partly or wholly responsible for a rise in IOP. The extent of closure will have a significant bearing on the severity of secondary ocular hypertension, the likelihood of developing glaucoma, and the responsiveness to therapy.

ANGLE CLOSURE IN UVEITIS

Angle closure as a consequence of uveitis falls into two broad groups according to the mechanism: pupillary block and nonpupillary block. In the latter group iridotrabecular contact results from forward movement of the iris–lens diaphragm, anterior rotation of the ciliary processes, or iris neovascularization. If iridotrabecular contact persists for a sufficient period of time, permanent adhesions (PAS) also develop.

A proportion of eyes with uveitis will have an anatomical predisposition to primary angle closure (PAC), coincidental to their uveitis, as do nonuveitic eyes. In such cases a uveitic episode or mydriatic use may precipitate an episode of angle closure. As acute episodes of PAC are often associated with anterior segment inflammation, it can occasionally be unclear as to the nature of the initial process.

Pupillary block Seclusio pupillae or absolute pupillary block is a potent mechanism of angle closure that typically results from complete obstruction of aqueous flow through the pupil caused by the presence of 360° posterior synechiae, when it occurs in uveitis. *Seclusio pupillae* differs from pupillary block in primary angle closure (PAC) in that adhesions between pupil margin and lens result in absolute rather than relative obstruction of aqueous flow. The degree of forward ballooning of peripheral iris (iris bombe) is therefore greater than with PAC and the appearance can be dramatic. The central anterior chamber usually remains deep (Fig. 33.1AA). Laser iridotomies (PI) are surprisingly ineffective as they close very quickly even when more than one is performed. As a result, surgical iridectomies, synechiolysis, or lens extraction are almost inevitably required.

Angle closure in the absence of pupillary block

While there is often an element of pupillary block in other types of angle closure, posterior segment inflammatory disease may result in angle closure from forward movement of the iris–lens diaphragm or anterior rotation of the ciliary processes. These mechanisms must be differentiated from situations in which pupillary block is the predominant mechanism of angle closure (Fig. 33.1AB).

Forward movement of the iris–lens diaphragm

Angle closure secondary to forward movement of the iris–lens diaphragm occurs when expansion of posterior segment structures displace ciliary processes, zonules, lens, and iris forward, usually with marked shallowing of the anterior chamber and direct obstruction of the trabecular meshwork with iris (see Fig. 33.1AC). Typically, secondary angle closure due to this mechanism is not responsive to iridectomy either by laser or surgery because pupillary block is not the principle mechanism.

While the typical features of angle closure secondary to pupillary block are a relatively deep central anterior chamber and convex peripheral iris surface, the cardinal feature that distinguishes pupillary block from forward movement of the iris–lens diaphragm is the very marked shallowing of the central anterior chamber in the latter (see Fig. 33.1AC and AD). Phacomorphic angle closure is sometimes an exception to this rule. Cataract is common in uveitis and a swollen lens may result in pupillary block and secondary angle closure. In contrast to other forms of pupillary block, the central anterior chamber may be very shallow in phacomorphic glaucoma. It may be necessary to use imaging techniques such as ultrasound biomicroscopy in such cases to confirm the position of the ciliary processes and to measure the lens thickness to help differentiate phacomorphic angle closure from forward movement of the iris–lens diaphragm.

Typical causes of secondary angle closure due to forward movement of the iris–lens diaphragm are aqueous misdirection, posterior scleritis, retinal vein occlusion, or occasionally after extensive retinal photocoagulation.

Anterior rotation of the ciliary processes

Anterior rotation of the ciliary body is an alternative mechanism of angle closure secondary to posterior segment disease. This may be due to ciliary body edema, and if it were to occur in isolation, the clinical appearance would be similar to a plateau configuration of the peripheral iris, with a typical peripheral iris roll, without central anterior chamber shallowing. However, in the authors' experience, anterior rotation of the ciliary processes in uveitis is more often associated with severe episodes of anterior uveitis and concurrent hypotony than closed angle and IOP elevation.

Peripheral anterior synechiae

Prolonged iridotrabecular contact under normal circumstances eventually results in iridotrabecular adhesions (peripheral anterior synechiae, PAS). In inflamed anterior segments, a shorter duration of contact is believed to be required before adhesions become permanent. For this reason, PAS development is probably more common in uveitis than in eyes with intermittent PAC. Uveitis patients with preexisting narrow angles are probably at higher risk of PAS development by virtue of close tissue proximity. *Bridging* PAS, although less common, are particularly dramatic and are characteristically seen in the presence of an apparently wide-open angle (Fig. 33.1BA). These may be narrow and traverse a wide angle from anterior iris surface to Schwalbe's line and appear similar to those seen in Axenfeld's anomaly but are typically fewer in number than in the latter. Bridging synechiae develop when an acute attack of fibrinous anterior uveitis results in short-lived angle narrowing, either because of a temporary pupil block and iris bombe or anterior movement of the ciliary processes secondary to edema of the inflamed ciliary body. Either of these mechanisms may resolve with successful treatment of the acute inflammation and restoration of the original angle width, but leaving bridging synechiae as a persistent sequela.

More commonly, PAS are seen as broad-based adhesions to anterior TM or scleral spur (see Fig. 33.1BA). Some patients show signs of patchy PAS with seemingly open intervals of angle or areas of pigment smudging in between. The development of IOP elevation is probably dependent not only on the extent of PAS but also on whether or not the open portions that have been subjected to pigment deposition or smudging are functioning at full capacity. It is likely that occlusion of some areas of TM may be a visible marker indicating the TM

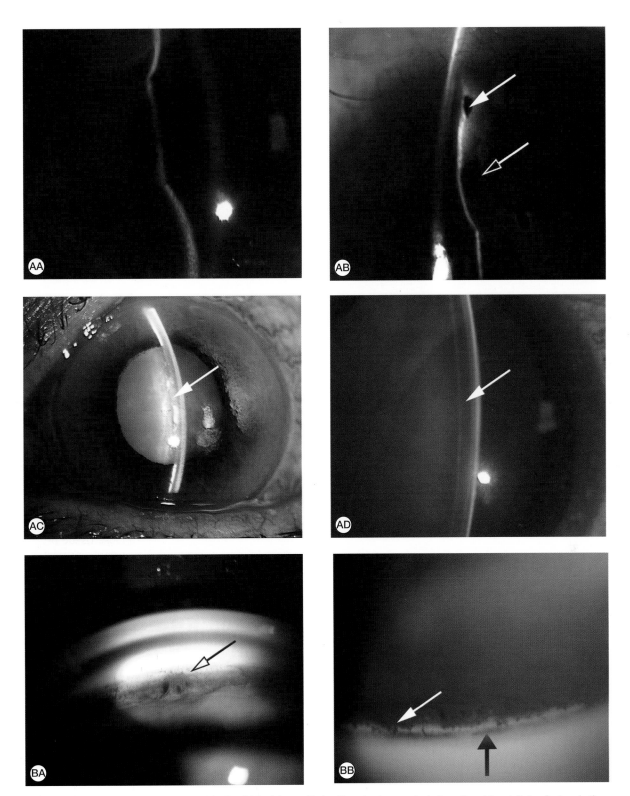

FIGURE 33.1 (A) Acute angle closure in uveitis. Pupil block in uveitis is often due to a secluded pupil and the defining feature is the deep central anterior chamber and often dramatic surrounding iris bombe **(AA)**. Laser iridotomy is usually ineffective in correcting uveitic pupil block due to rapid closure or loculation of aqueous behind the iris. In **(AB)** a patent iridotomy is present (solid arrow) yet there is persistent bombe of the iris and pupil block (transparent arrow). Pupil block must be distinguished from other causes of angle closure in uveitis such as phacomorphic glaucoma **(AC)** or forward movement of the iris–lens diaphragm **(AD)**, in this case due to vitreous hemorrhage. In both cases the shallow central anterior chamber is highlighted by the solid arrow.
(B) Peripheral anterior synechiae in uveitis. Peripheral anterior synechiae (PAS) are common in uveitis. Bridging synechiae from anterior iris surface to Schwalbe's line **(BA)** (transparent arrow) are relatively uncommon but particularly characteristic of uveitis. These are rarely seen in other types of angle closure, though they may occasionally be confused with Axenfeld's anomaly (reproduced from Spalton DJ, Hitchings RA, Hunter PA, et al (eds) Atlas of Clinical Ophthalmology (3rd edn). Harcourt, London. 2008 Reproduced with permission of Moorfields Eye Hospital NHS Foundation Trust). Small PAS **(BB)** (white arrow) are common in uveitis, but are often seen in the presence of other angle abnormalities such as pigment deposition (dark arrow).

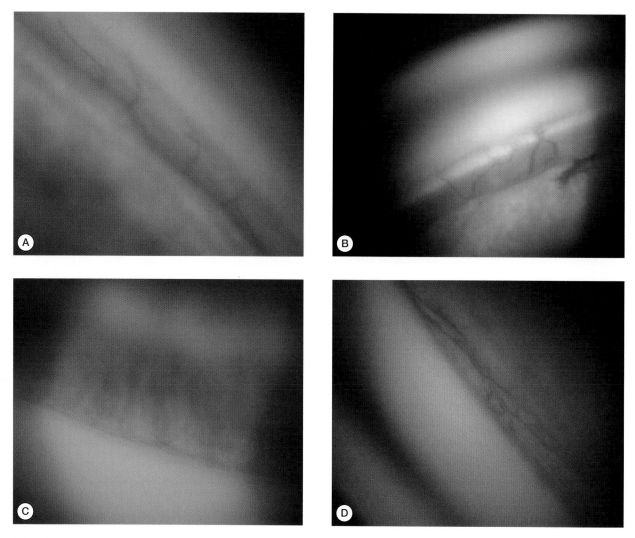

FIGURE 33.2 Angle neovascularization in uveitis. Angle neovascularization is not uncommon in uveitis. It is seen frequently in Fuchs' heterochromic cyclitis as fine vessels crossing the angle radially from iris root to peripheral cornea **(A)**. These are only of clinical significance because of their propensity to bleed on surgical decompression of the eye. Inflammatory neovascularization of the angle is often more aggressive and may also cross the iridocorneal angle **(B)**. This appearance contrasts with that seen in ischemic neovascular glaucoma, where the angle may be completely closed **(C)**, but without visible evidence of vessels in the angle other than on the peripheral iris surface **(D)**.

as a whole has suffered significantly from the effects of inflammation.

Neovascularization Neovascularization of the angle may also occur in some forms of uveitis such as Vogt-Koyanagi-Harada syndrome, sympathetic ophthalmia, and retinal vasculitis. By far the commonest association with neovascularization of the angle is Fuchs' heterochromic cyclitis which, in contrast to other types of uveitic neovascularization, does not result in synechiae or angle closure and is only of clinical significance due a tendency to cause hyphema during intraocular surgery (Amsler's sign) (Fig. 33.2A).

Clinically, it can be difficult to distinguish neovascularization in uveitis from inflammatory dilation of the iris vessels. In the angle, vessels that cross the scleral spur, especially if there is a circumferential component, are more likely neovascular (see Fig. 33.2B).

DIAGNOSIS AND CLASSIFICATION

The lack of consistent diagnostic criteria for uveitic glaucoma has confounded estimates of the prevalence of uveitic glaucoma. Foster et al.[60] proposed a classification of glaucomas based on the presence or absence of optic neuropathy. This has not generally been applied to secondary glaucomas.

In this chapter, the authors propose that it would be appropriate to adapt Foster's classification for use in uveitic glaucoma, i.e. that for cross-sectional epidemiological research the term *glaucoma* should be reserved for people with significant target organ damage.

The authors would propose that in IOP elevation secondary to uveitis, the term *glaucoma* should be reserved for those with evidence of optic nerve damage, and that uveitic or steroid-induced *ocular hypertension* be used in other cases of IOP elevation.

The difficulties in differentiating normal from abnormal that are encountered when attempting to diagnose other types of glaucoma also exist, perhaps to an even greater degree in uveitic eyes. The higher IOP levels encountered, often in younger patients, may cause apparent structural damage detected by optic disc imaging that disappears when the IOP level is corrected to normal. Foster proposed that the diagnosis of secondary glaucoma only be reserved for optic neuropathy in the presence of second ocular pathology. However, in cases of uncertainty, if the optic disc cannot be examined because of media opacity, a situation not uncommon in patients with uveitis, then an IOP exceeding 99.5th centile of the normal population, or evidence of previous filtration surgery should be taken as evidence of glaucoma. This exception applies to a great many patients with uveitis. Clearly untreated, the development of optic nerve damage would be inevitable, and after surgery it would seem appropriate to label these patients as suffering from *secondary glaucoma* rather than *ocular hypertension*, even though the optic nerves and intraocular pressures after surgery are normal.

While Foster's classification was intended for cross-sectional research, it would also be useful in clinical practice.

CLINICAL FEATURES AND INVESTIGATION

Late presentation of glaucoma secondary to uveitis is relatively uncommon because uveitis is usually sufficiently symptomatic to ensure early presentation to an ophthalmologist. For that reason, optic disc or visual field damage from glaucoma is often mild at presentation. An exception to this generalization is JIA-related uveitis. Before slit lamp examination of all JIA patients became routine, uveitis, and hence secondary glaucoma, often remained undiagnosed in children and presented eventually at a relatively late stage.

A number of syndromes commonly present with IOP elevation and in such patients accurate diagnosis depends partly on pattern recognition. However, careful clinical observation is also essential as there is considerable overlap in the presentation of conditions such as Fuchs' heterochromic cyclitis, herpetic keratouveitis, and Posner-Schlossman syndrome. A detailed gonioscopy and dilated fundus examination are essential in all patients in the diagnosis and management of IOP elevation in uveitis. The purpose of the examination is not only to identify specific syndromes such as those listed above but also to document both the type of uveitis and the mechanism of IOP elevation.

IOP elevation in association with uveitis differs from that in other conditions in that it may be short lived in some and chronic in others. In some eyes, IOP elevation may only be a problem during an episode of active uveitis, either due to the inflammation or the corticosteroid treatment. In others, a glaucomatous optic neuropathy develops either because of chronic IOP elevation or a high frequency of repeated short-lived episodes.

While the likely longevity of an episode of IOP elevation cannot be predicted with certainty, it is helpful to estimate into which group the patient falls, as the predicted longevity of the IOP elevation will influence the level of aggression with which it is to be treated.

A history of chronic or recurring IOP elevation and the presence of optic nerve damage or early optic disc asymmetry are obvious indicators. It is worth noting that in young uveitic patients, optic disc asymmetry in the presence of a very high IOP does not necessarily indicate damage, as a proportion of the optic disc cupping will reverse when the IOP is controlled. In an eye with a high IOP and a healthy optic nerve, the appearance of the drainage angle is a helpful indicator as to the likelihood of a long-term IOP problem.

Evidence of angle compromise such as PAS, smudging, or angle pigment increases the likelihood that the IOP elevation will be chronic rather than short lived. Absence of the above and a wide-open, pigment-free angle favors a more short-lived effect (Fig. 33.3).

Apart from the typical features of intraocular inflammation such as flare, cells, fibrin, and keratic precipitates that will not be described in detail, evidence of chronicity of the uveitis should also be sought. This includes the presence of iris nodules, angle neovascularization, and posterior segment disease. Abnormal nodules visible on the anterior iris surface are most common in Fuchs' heterochromic cyclitis but are also a typical feature of granulomatous disease and may be seen on the iris and in the drainage angle in uveitis associated with granulomatous conditions such as sarcoidosis.

In certain types of uveitis, specific signs may also be evident. It is important to note that in isolation none of these is pathognomonic. Examples of findings that point to specific syndromes associated with elevated IOP include corneal epithelial ulceration, with stromal edema and underlying keratic precipitates in herpetic keratouveitis. Stellate keratic precipitates, heterochromia, depigmentation, and stromal atrophy of the iris may be seen in Fuchs' heterochromic cyclitis.[61] Often, a careful comparison of iris stromal appearance with the other eye will help distinguish Fuchs' heterochromic cyclitis from other types of uveitis. In blue-eyed individuals, a typical moth-eaten appearance of iris depigmentation is seen on iris transillumination, whereas in brown eyes a difference in iris surface texture may be seen with accompanying nodules around the pupil margin (Fig. 33.4).

A history of sudden onset of symptoms in combination with few anterior segment cells plus one or

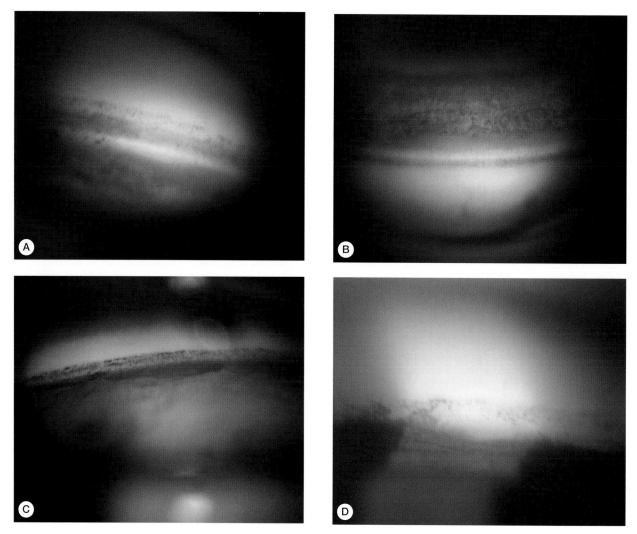

FIGURE 33.3. Angle pigmentation in uveitis. Pigmentation of the angle is common in uveitis, more often seen inferiorly than superiorly, as shown in two views of the same angle (**A** and **B**). In eyes with severe chronic inflammation, significant pigment deposition may be seen in the inferior angle (**C**). The mechanism of pigment deposition in the angle is different from that of pigment smudging (**D**), which results from intermittent iridotrabecular contact. It is not unusual to see a mixture of these as well as PAS in an eye with chronic uveitis.

two 'sentinel' keratic precipitates point to Posner-Schlossman syndrome.[62] These three conditions are virtually always unilateral.

A comprehensive examination should also reveal associated nonocular abnormalities, such as poliosis and vitiligo in Vogt-Koyanagi-Harada syndrome and lacrimal gland swelling in sarcoidosis.

The visual acuity may be affected to a variable degree. Dilated fundus examination with careful attention to the retinal periphery is important to exclude pars planitis. The vitreous may show few signs, as in anterior uveitis. The fundi should be examined for signs of choroidal and retinal inflammation, which often complicate many systemic inflammatory and infective disorders. Finally, the optic discs should be assessed for signs of glaucomatous optic neuropathy even if the recorded IOP is normal.

The ancillary investigation of uveitis is outside the remit of this chapter. Anterior segment imaging may be required to clarify the exact mechanism in a case of angle closure and occasionally in cases where the angle is open but obscured, e.g. by heavy pigment deposition. Both anterior segment optical coherence tomography (AS-OCT) and high-frequency ultrasound biomicroscopy (UBM) offer high-resolution images of the anterior segment angle.

When used in conjunction with gonioscopy, these imaging techniques are valuable in identifying angles at risk of closure. While AS-OCT offers a convenient, noncontact method of angle assessment, it is also a highly sensitive and reproducible technique. One particular advantage of AS-OCT over gonioscopy is its ability to image the angle in the dark.[63] UBM, on the other hand, is able to image ciliary body and lens. Changes in angle configuration can then be examined in the wider context of variations in ciliary body and lens anatomy.[64] It is important to note that these imaging techniques aid diagnosis but do not replace the role of gonioscopy in angle assessment.

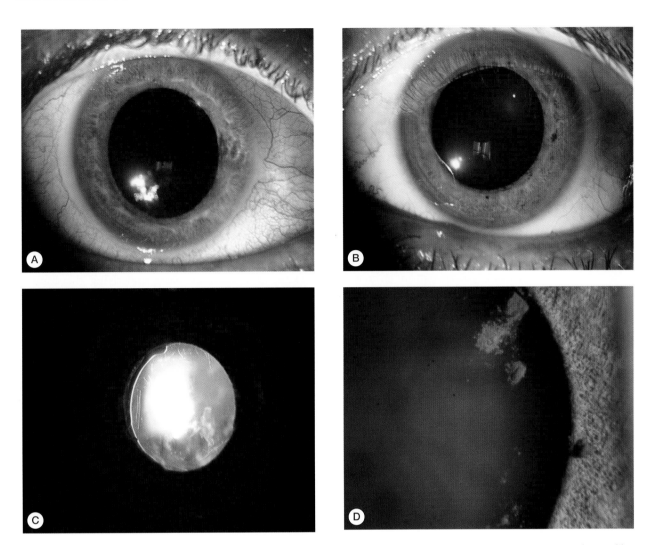

FIGURE 33.4 Fuchs' heterochromic cyclitis: diagnostic features. Although it is important to stand back and compare eyes when making the diagnosis of Fuchs' heterochromic cyclitis (FHC) (**A** and **B**), it is important to take other factors into consideration, such as the presence of diffuse iris transillumination in blue-eyed FHC (**C**), the presence of vitreous floaters (**C**), unilateral cataract or pseudophakia (**C**). It is also important to examine closely the texture of the iris stroma, which will usually differ significantly from the fellow eye. Brown-eyed FHC does not demonstrate iris transillumination, but occasionally iris nodules may be seen (**D**) and the iris stromal texture will also differ significantly from the fellow eye.

MANAGEMENT

MANAGEMENT OF UVEITIS

Successful management of uveitic glaucoma requires adequate, simultaneous treatment of both uveitis and IOP elevation. As a rule, suppression of inflammation should be the primary objective. Undertreatment of uveitis in order to avoid a corticosteroid-induced IOP rise is often a false economy that may result in further TM damage from ongoing inflammation.

Corticosteroid-induced IOP elevation may be especially resistant to ocular hypotensive therapy. For cases of uveitis where elevated IOP occurs only during periods of active disease, topical medical therapy will usually suffice. However, in other cases, the uveitis may be difficult to control without very high levels of corticosteroids and joint management with a uveitis specialist is essential. A uveitis specialist may be able to offer immunosuppression with drugs such as ciclosporin, mycophenolate mofetil, tacrolimus, azathioprine, methotrexate, or even anti-TNF-α antibody therapy (infliximab or etanercept) that will control inflammation and permit the use of lower doses of corticosteroids.

In eyes with a predominantly steroid-driven IOP elevation, topical corticosteroids such as rimexolone may also achieve control of inflammation with a lower degree of IOP elevation.

Depot steroid preparations, such as orbital floor methylprednisolone, triamcinolone, and intraocular steroid-containing implants should be used with caution in this particular subgroup of patients as the intraocular pressure effect may be long lasting. Nevertheless, it is often better to use these where necessary to achieve adequate control of inflammation. Surgical control of IOP elevation, when necessary, is generally more successful if performed in the setting of well-controlled inflammation.

In patients in whom IOP elevation is only a problem during intermittent courses of corticosteroid treatment, a careful judgment is required about the likelihood of further uveitis episodes and the future necessity for continued corticosteroid therapy. In contrast, in certain cases where IOP elevation is driven by ongoing inflammation, topical corticosteroids, by suppressing inflammation, may aid IOP control. Examples include herpetic keratouveitis and some cases of Posner-Schlossman syndrome.

OCULAR HYPOTENSIVE THERAPY

When prescribing ocular hypotensive treatment for uveitic glaucoma, some specific considerations should be borne in mind. Commonly used agents may demonstrate variable efficacy in the presence of inflammation or when administered with steroid treatment. There are no data comparing the efficacy of ocular hypotensive agents in uveitic glaucoma; however, there are relative contraindications to the use of some commonly prescribed glaucoma medications.

Beta-adrenergic antagonists In uveitis-associated IOP elevation, nonselective topical β-adrenergic antagonists remain the first-line agents of choice in patients without contraindications such as asthma or bradycardia. A number of reports of granulomatous anterior uveitis were reported as an adverse effect of higher concentrations (largely 0.6% and sometimes 0.3%) of metipranolol in the 1990s, initially in the United Kingdom but later in Europe and the United States.[65–68] This has also been reported in the unpreserved preparation[69] and seems to be an effect of the drug itself, which should therefore be avoided in uveitis unless there is no acceptable alternative.

Prostaglandin analogues Although prostaglandin analogues (PGAs) are generally believed to be effective in uveitic glaucoma, published efficacy data are sparse. In one study, the IOP response was measured after a single drop of latanoprost.[70] In that particular study a poor IOP reduction was observed. It is also worth noting that in patients using nonsteroidal antiinflammatory drugs, the IOP-lowering response to PGA may also be blunted,[71,72] an effect that has also been reported with nonsteroidals and α-agonists.[73]

The wider use of PGAs in uveitic glaucoma has been tempered by the expectation that they would induce or exacerbate uveitis, aqueous flare, and cystoid macular edema (CMO). Despite initial fears, it seems that anterior uveitis rarely arises de novo after PGA treatment in eyes with no other risk factors.[74] Although uncommon, a number of cases have been reported in which uveitis, apparently induced by a PGA, has recurred on rechallenge. In one report of four cases, all of which developed recurrent anterior uveitis when rechallenged with latanoprost, three eyes had previously undergone some form of intraocular surgery, and the fourth had traumatic glaucoma with a subluxed lens and a history of iritis in the fellow eye.[75]

The likelihood of reactivating quiescent preexisting uveitis by topical PGA treatment is also uncertain. In one retrospective study that attempted to examine this risk, 527 patients were studied, but only 13 had a history of uveitis and three of these were observed to reactivate on treatment with latanoprost (23%). Interestingly, none of nine patients with active uveitis treated with latanoprost was observed to worsen.[76]

The risk of increased aqueous flare or CMO with PGA treatment seems to mirror that of anterior uveitis, in that pseudophakes, aphakes, and others with certain predisposing factors are at higher risk,[77] whereas phakic eyes with no history of CMO are at a low risk.[74] At present, the level of risk of CMO in a patient with preexisting uveitis but no history of previous intraocular surgery or CMO is uncertain.

There is a scientific basis underlying the concern that PGA might result in reactivation or worsening of herpetic keratouveitis,. There is also some evidence in rabbit studies that this is the case.[78] However, despite anecdotal reports of epithelial herpetic keratitis recurring on rechallenge with latanoprost,[79,80] there does not seem to be an increase in prevalence in those treated with topical PGA.[81] In eyes with a history of herpetic keratitis or keratouveitis, PGAs are best avoided where possible.

Carbonic anhydrase inhibitors and hyperosmotic agents Topical carbonic anhydrase inhibitors are widely used in uveitic glaucoma and often as part of a dorzolamide-timolol fixed combination. In some uveitics, largely those with a chronic history and probable severe ciliary body damage, drugs such as dorzolamide and brinzolamide may profoundly reduce IOP. Although this is not necessarily a contraindication, lower doses than normal may be required.

Acetazolamide is frequently used to manage acute rises in IOP in uveitis patients if topical therapy proves inadequate. It is especially helpful in combination with topical therapy for treatment of refractory cases pending definitive surgery. Hyperosmotic drugs such as mannitol and glycerol are rarely indicated.

Alpha₂-adrenergic agonists Currently, the selective α₂-agonists apraclonidine and brimonidine are useful second-line drugs for the treatment of IOP elevation. Again, the efficacy of these drugs in uveitis has not been specifically studied. However, there is some evidence that α₂-adrenergic agonists act by prostaglandin release and that this may be inhibited if cyclooxygenase inhibitors (most nonsteroidal antiinflammatory drugs) are concurrently used.

Miotics Cholinergic agonists, such as pilocarpine, are best avoided in uveitic eyes because of their tendency to compromise the blood–aqueous barrier and aggravate inflammation. In addition, immobilization of the pupil in the uveitic eye promotes the development of posterior synechiae.

Mydriatics Mydriatics are used frequently in uveitis to prevent formation of posterior synechiae, and potent mydriatics such as atropine or homatropine may be helpful in glaucoma induced by anterior displacement of the iris–lens diaphragm or anterior rotation of the ciliary body. However, care must be taken as they may also exacerbate angle closure.

SURGICAL MANAGEMENT

Secondary angle-closure glaucoma with pupil block
Laser iridotomy is much less effective in controlling uveitic pupillary block than in PAC. Laser iridotomies in uveitics frequently close within a few days with recurrent pupillary block. Eyes with uveitic pupillary block often behave as if the aqueous is loculated behind the iris so that one laser iridotomy may decompress iris bombe in one area only, with pupillary block remaining in other quadrants. Finally, peripheral anterior synechiae develop quickly in uveitis and by the time laser iridotomy is performed, angle closure may be irreversible.

While laser iridotomy may be performed in an emergency attempt to break the block while awaiting surgery, the treatment of choice for uveitic pupillary block remains surgical iridectomy with synechiolysis. For phakic patients, lens extraction might be considered. However, phacoemulsification in uveitis is most successful when the uveitis is well controlled. Uveitic pupillary block is a relative emergency, and while an attempt should be made to control inflammation adequately, iridectomy and synechiolysis should be carried out as soon as possible, rather than waiting to control the inflammation sufficiently for phacoemulsification.

After iridotomy or iridectomy, intensive postoperative topical corticosteroids should be used with adjunctive intravitreal, periocular, or systemic corticosteroids as required.

In cases of pupil block caused by fibrin occlusion of the pupil, the block may sometimes be rapidly reversed by intracameral tissue plasminogen activator injection (12.5 µg).

Secondary angle closure without pupillary block
The management of secondary angle-closure due to anterior displacement of the iris–lens diaphragm depends on the underlying cause and many of these, such as aqueous misdirection, are dealt with in other chapters. In chronic, secondary angle-closure glaucoma due to creeping PAS formation, laser iridotomy has been advocated in PAC, in an attempt to prevent further PAS formation. There is no evidence that this is beneficial in uveitics and the short-lived effect of laser iridotomies would limit any long-term benefit. In a patient where PAC and uveitis coincide, laser iridotomy might be appropriate if the uveitis is mild and well controlled.

In chronic angle closure, IOP control may be achieved with medical therapy, but a significant proportion ultimately requires surgery because of refractory glaucoma caused by progressive synechial angle closure. In the hypermetropic uveitic eye with a narrow angle, lens extraction may be indicated in preference to trabeculectomy if the narrow angle is the predominant problem rather than the uveitis.

Secondary open angle glaucoma
In uveitic glaucoma with an open angle, the decision to operate is based on the degree of IOP elevation, tolerability and response to medication, and the extent of glaucomatous optic neuropathy. Tolerability is an important issue in uveitic glaucoma in which high, unsustainable levels of medication, including systemic carbonic anhydrase inhibitors, may control the IOP in the short term, but do not offer a realistic long-term solution.

Ideally, intraocular inflammation should be well controlled for at least 3 months before surgery is contemplated. In practice this is not often achievable, because surgery for uveitic glaucoma is typically planned on a semiurgent basis. Preoperative administration of topical steroids helps to reduce the severity of the postoperative inflammatory response, which may be a result of suppression of the preoperative conjunctival inflammatory cell population.[82,83]

In particularly labile inflammatory disease, a short course of perioperative systemic steroids is often useful (0.5–1.0 mg/kg oral prednisolone). Alternatively, 40 mg of infraorbital methylprednisolone or intravitreal triamcinolone may be given as a depot preparation in the absence of a history of steroid-induced elevated IOP.

Prior to surgical or laser intervention in uveitic eyes, inflammation should be minimized with topical and, in severe uveitis or systemic disease, systemic corticosteroids for 1–2 weeks.

Filtration surgery
In refractory cases of uveitic glaucoma, unresponsive to maximal, tolerated medical therapy, surgery is indicated to limit further progression. Trabeculectomy is the procedure of choice except in aphakic uveitics, cases with coincidental anterior segment neovascularization, and patients with poor visual function or prognosis in the affected eye.

Trabeculectomy without antiproliferative agents has been reported to be poorly successful in uveitic eyes.[84] Better long-term results, with 53% achieving IOP control without adjunctive medication, and 78% with medication at 5 years, have been reported in one study.[85] However, despite a paucity of studies reporting follow-up of more than 2 years, and an absence of randomized controlled trials, antiproliferative trabeculectomy and specifically the use of adjunctive mitomycin C (MMC) is, at the time of writing, the standard of care in most international tertiary referral centers.[86,87] At present, this standard is more likely to be replaced by primary aqueous shunt implantation for uveitic glaucoma than a return to non-antiproliferative trabeculectomy. The reason for this potential replacement is that in a number of the shorter-term studies that have been published, even MMC-enhanced trabeculectomy has not produced success rates that are noticeably better than those reported with 5-fluorouracil (5-FU).[88–91]

Yet, case selection has a profound influence on success rates in surgical studies, and uveitis is no exception. It is conceivable that in a tertiary referral uveitis clinic, where patients are treated aggressively with corticosteroids and have relatively short-term exposure to glaucoma medications, the success rate of trabeculectomy without antiproliferatives might prove higher than expected, whereas in centers where use of corticosteroids is more conservative the opposite might be true.

Nevertheless, the long-term function of a trabeculectomy in uveitis is likely to be challenged by recurrent inflammation and it seems likely that adjunctive use of MMC by providing lower initial IOP, indicating greater functional reserve in the trabeculectomy, might help the bleb weather this long-term attrition better than the use of 5-FU or no antiproliferative agent.

Cataract and the uveitic trabeculectomy Cataract surgery compromises the outcome of trabeculectomy[92] and this is a major confounding influence on judging the success of uveitic trabeculectomy because cataract is very common in uveitis, and trabeculectomy accelerates the rate of cataract formation.[93]

Given that isolated trabeculectomy induces less postoperative anterior chamber flare[94] and is more successful than phacotrabeculectomy,[95] the logical sequence for optimal long-term IOP control should be cataract surgery followed later by trabeculectomy. In practice, this is not something that can usually be planned as the order of precedence of the two procedures is more often dictated by the degree of IOP elevation. Under these circumstances, the use of antiproliferatives at the time of filtering surgery may help to offset any detrimental effect from subsequent cataract surgery. Furthermore, the use of a temporal clear corneal incision in sequential cataract surgery may minimize the risk to a functioning trabeculectomy.[96]

Meticulous technique is essential for successful filtration surgery in uveitic glaucoma. Younger patients, labile aqueous production, and the use of MMC predispose to early hypotony, necessitating tight scleral suturing at the time of surgery to minimize early drainage. With aggressive postoperative suture manipulation, removal of releasables or laser suture lysis, as required, the IOP level can be brought into the desired range. Following surgery, attention should be paid to the degree of intraocular inflammation and conjunctival bleb morphology with appropriate titration of topical and systemic steroid therapy, typically over several months for topical steroids and much sooner for systemic steroids, if there is no ongoing indication for treatment of uveitis. Occasionally in the early postoperative period, steroid therapy is tapered more rapidly than usual if persistent hypotony results from overdrainage.

Aqueous shunt implantation and other surgical procedures Aqueous shunt implantation is often performed as a primary surgical procedure in uveitic patients. Some specialists would classify uveitic glaucoma requiring IOP-lowering surgery as an indication in itself for shunt implantation, but many agree that in eyes with other risk factors in addition to uveitis, the success rate of a shunt is likely to be better than a trabeculectomy. These include uveitis secondary to JIA, previous failed trabeculectomy, aphakic eyes, eyes with prior silicone oil injection, and eyes that have had neovascularization (other than that commonly seen in Fuchs' heterochromic cyclitis).

IOP control after aqueous shunt implantation in uveitics has been reported to be better than that after shunt implantation for other types of glaucoma. In a prospective series of 41 implants in 40 eyes of 35 patients, Molteno reported the mean IOP fell from 30.86 mmHg preoperatively to 14.51 mmHg after 5 years, at which point 87% of operated eyes were controlled (IOP < 21 mmHg) on an average of 0.44 medications. At 10 years, follow-up data were available on 14 eyes, of which 93% maintained IOP control (<21 mmHg) on an average of 0.32 medications.[97] The success of IOP control with the Baerveldt glaucoma implant[98] appears to be good in the short term. Likewise, the Ahmed glaucoma valve seems successful in uveitics at 1 year [99] although in one reported study, success was considerably lower in the second year of follow-up. Longer-term data are not yet available.

Nonpenetrating filtration surgery An alternative to trabeculectomy is nonpenetrating surgery and for patients with steroid-induced IOP elevation, minimal optic disc cupping, and a high intraocular pressure, nonpenetrating filtration surgery is an attractive option, avoiding anterior chamber entry and hypotony in eyes in which a very low target IOP is probably not required. Uveitic eyes have a higher risk of hypotony after penetrating filtration surgery than others, and uveitic patients who tend to be younger with more elastic sclera are more prone to maculopathy and astigmatism should hypotony develop.

The potential disadvantage is uncertainty over long-term IOP control in uveitics after nonpenetrating surgery.

Goniotomy Goniotomy has been reported to be a useful primary procedure for uveitic glaucoma in children.[100] However, goniotomy is a procedure that requires considerable skill and experience and is best avoided by specialists who do not perform it on a regular basis.

Cyclophotocoagulation Cyclophotocoagulation is best avoided in uveitics as this treatment can act as a 'double blow' to a ciliary body that has already been compromised by cyclitis, resulting in a higher rate of hypotony than is seen in other types of glaucoma[101] and potentially tipping the eye into chronic ciliary insufficiency.

Laser trabeculoplasty Laser trabeculoplasty has no role in the management of uveitic glaucoma.

Summary

Uveitic glaucoma is an umbrella term for a range of disorders whose common end result is glaucomatous optic neuropathy. Glaucoma in uveitis is distinguished from other glaucomas by its episodic, partly iatrogenic nature and very high intraocular pressures that untreated may result in much more rapid glaucoma progression than is commonly seen in POAG.

Most patients are young and of working age and may be greatly debilitated by their glaucoma. Rapid diagnosis and high-quality care are required to safeguard their vision in the long term and keep these patients in employment.

Management of uveitic glaucoma requires careful diagnosis and management of both uveitis and glaucoma. It is essential to identify the mechanisms of IOP elevation so the correct treatment can be instituted. Management of the patient in a multidisciplinary fashion with the involvement of both uveitis and glaucoma specialists offers the best chance of a successful outcome.

It is not unusual for patients to require both IOP-lowering surgery and cataract surgery. It is therefore imperative that the first procedure is performed optimally to afford the best chance of long-term IOP control. Finally, uveitic glaucoma patients require lifelong care and supervision, which should be undertaken in dedicated, specialized centers which are appropriately staffed and equipped.

REFERENCES

1. Beer J. Die Lehre v. d. Augenkrankheiten. Vienna, 1813; 1:633.

2. von Graefe A. Ueber die Iridectomie bei Glaucom und über den glaocomatösen Process. Arch Für Ophthalmologie 1857; 3:456–560.

3. Elliot RH. A treatise on glaucoma. London: Oxford Medical Publications; 1918.

4. Merayo-Lloves J, Power WJ, Rodriguez A, et al. Secondary glaucoma in patients with uveitis. Ophthalmologica 1999; 213:300–304.

5. Takahashi T, Ohtani S, Miyata K, et al. A clinical evaluation of uveitis-associated secondary glaucoma. Jpn J Ophthalmol 2002; 46:556–562.

6. Herbert HM, Viswanathan A, Jackson H, et al. Risk factors for elevated intraocular pressure in uveitis. J Glaucoma 2004; 13:96–99.

7. Neri P, Azuara-Blanco A, Forrester JV. Incidence of glaucoma in patients with uveitis. J Glaucoma 2004; 13:461–465.

8. Kotaniemi K, Kautiainen H, Karma A, et al. Occurrence of uveitis in recently diagnosed juvenile chronic arthritis: a prospective study. Ophthalmology 2001; 108:2071–2075.

9. Kanski JJ, Shun-Shin GA. Systemic uveitis syndromes in childhood: an analysis of 340 cases. Ophthalmology 1984; 91:1247–1252.

10. de Boer J, Wulffraat N, Rothova A. Visual loss in uveitis of childhood. Br J Ophthalmol 2003; 87:879–884.

11. Edelsten C, Lee V, Bentley CR, et al. An evaluation of baseline risk factors predicting severity in juvenile idiopathic arthritis associated uveitis and other chronic anterior uveitis in early childhood. Br J Ophthalmol 2002; 86:51–56.

12. Kwok AK, Lam DS, Ng JS, et al. Ocular-hypertensive response to topical steroids in children. Ophthalmology 1997; 104:2112–2116.

13. Fan DS, Yu CB, Chiu TY, et al. Ocular-hypertensive and anti-inflammatory response to rimexolone therapy in children. Arch Ophthalmol 2003; 121:1716–1721.

14. Barton K, Pavesio CE, Towler HMA, et al. Uveitis presenting de novo in the elderly. Eye 1994; 8:288–291.

15. Panek WC, Holland GN, Lee DA, et al. Glaucoma in patients with uveitis. Br J Ophthalmol 1990; 74:223–227.

16. Wolf MD, Lichter PR, Ragsdale CG. Prognostic factors in the uveitis of juvenile rheumatoid arthritis. Ophthalmology 1987; 94:1242–1248.

17. Rothova A, van Veenendaal WG, Linssen A, et al. Clinical features of acute anterior uveitis. Am J Ophthalmol 1987; 103:137–145.

18. Toris CB, Pederson JE. Aqueous humor dynamics in experimental iridocyclitis. Invest Ophthalmol Vis Sci 1987; 28:477–481.

19. Johnson DH. Human trabecular meshwork cell survival is dependent on perfusion rate. Invest Ophthalmol Vis Sci 1996; 37:1204–1208.

20. Epstein DL. Cyclodialysis. In: Epstein DL, Allingham RR, Schuman JS, eds. Chandler and Grant's glaucoma. 4th edn. Baltimore: Williams & Wilkins; 1997:573–579.

21. McLaren JW, Trocme SD, Relf S, et al. Rate of flow of aqueous humor determined from measurements of aqueous flare. Invest Ophthalmol Vis Sci 1990; 31:339–346.

22. Ladas JG, Yu F, Loo R, et al. Relationship between aqueous humor protein level and outflow facility in patients with uveitis. Invest Ophthalmol Vis Sci 2001; 42:2584–2588.

23. Barsotti MF, Bartels SP, Freddo TF, et al. The source of protein in the aqueous humor of the normal monkey eye. Invest Ophthalmol Vis Sci 1992; 33:581–595.

24. Peretz WL, Tomasi TB. Aqueous humor proteins in uveitis. Immunoelectrophoretic and gel diffusion studies on normal and pathological human aqueous humor. Arch Ophthalmol 1961; 65:20–23.

25. Epstein DL, Hashimoto JM, Grant WM. Serum obstruction of aqueous outflow in enucleated eyes. Am J Ophthalmol 1978; 86:101–105.

26. Chan C-C, BenEzra D, Hsu SM, et al. Granulomas in sympathetic ophthalmia and sarcoidosis. Arch Ophthalmol 1985; 103:198–202.

27. Wakefield D, Lloyd A. The role of cytokines in the pathogenesis of inflammatory eye disease. Cytokine 1992; 4:1–5.

28. Chan C-C, Palestine AG, Kuwabara T, et al. Immunopathologic study of Vogt-Koyanagi-Harada syndrome. Am J Ophthalmol 1988; 105:607–611.

29. Charteris DG, Barton K, McCartney ACE, et al. CD4[+] lymphocyte involvement in ocular Behçet's disease. Autoimmunity 1992; 12:201–206.

30. Modlin RL, Hofman FM, Meyer PR, et al. In situ demonstration of T lymphocyte subsets in granulomatous inflammation: leprosy, rhinoscleroma and sarcoidosis. Clin Exp Immunol 1983; 51:430–438.

31. Shah DN, Piacentini MA, Burnier MN Jr, et al. Inflammatory cellular kinetics in sympathetic ophthalmia. Ocular Immunol Inflamm 1993; 1:255–262.

32. Wetzig RP, Chan C-C, Nussenblatt RB, et al. Clinical and immunopathological studies of pars planitis in a family. Br J Ophthalmol 1988; 72:5–10.

33. Barton K, Calder VL, Lightman S. Isolation of lymphocytes from the retina in experimental autoimmune uveoretinitis: phenotypic and functional characterisation. Immunology 1993; 78:393–398.

34. Barton K, McLauchlan M, Calder VL, et al. The kinetics of cytokine mRNA expression in the retina during experimental autoimmune uveoretinitis. Cell Immunol 1995; 164: 133–140.

35. Caspi RR, Chan C-C, Fujino Y, et al. Recruitment of antigen-nonspecific cells plays a pivotal role in the pathogenesis of a T cell-mediated organ-specific autoimmune disease, experimental

autoimmune uveoretinitis. J Neuroimmunol 1993; 47:177–188.

36. Bhattacherjee P, Williams RN, Eakins KE. An evaluation of ocular inflammation following the injection of bacterial endotoxin into the rat foot pad. Invest Ophthalmol Vis Sci 1983; 24:196–202.

37. Okumura A, Mochizuki M. Endotoxin-induced uveitis in rats: morphological and biochemical study. Invest Ophthalmol Vis Sci 1988; 32:457–465.

38. Chang JH, Hampartzoumian T, Everett B, et al. Changes in Toll-like receptor (TLR)-2 and TLR4 expression and function but not polymorphisms are associated with acute anterior uveitis. Invest Ophthalmol Vis Sci 2007; 48:1711–1717.

39. Planck SR, Huang X-N, Robertson JE, et al. Cytokine mRNA levels in rat ocular tissues after systemic endotoxin treatment. Invest Ophthalmol Vis Sci 1994; 35:924–930.

40. Wang N, Chintala SK, Fini ME, et al. Activation of a tissue-specific stress response in the aqueous outflow pathway of the eye defines the glaucoma disease phenotype. Nat Med 2001; 7:304–309.

41. Tripathi RC, Chan WF, Li J, et al. Trabecular cells express the TGF-beta 2 gene and secrete the cytokine. Exp Eye Res 1994; 58:523–528.

42. Xu H, Silver PB, Tarrant TK, et al. TGF-beta inhibits activation and uveitogenicity of primary but not of fully polarized retinal antigen-specific memory-effector T cells. Invest Ophthalmol Vis Sci 2003; 44:4805–4812.

43. Min SH, Lee TI, Chung YS, et al. Transforming growth factor-beta levels in human aqueous humor of glaucomatous, diabetic and uveitic eyes. Korean J Ophthalmol 2006; 20: 162–165.

44. de Boer JH, Limpens J, Orengo-Nania S, et al. Low mature TGF-beta 2 levels in aqueous humor during uveitis. Invest Ophthalmol Vis Sci 1994; 35:3702–3710.

45. Hogg P, Calthorpe M, Batterbury M, et al. Aqueous humor stimulates the migration of human trabecular meshwork cells in vitro. Invest Ophthalmol Vis Sci 2000; 41:1091–1098.

46. Alvarado JA, Murphy CG. Outflow obstruction in pigmentary and primary open angle glaucoma. Arch Ophthalmol 1992; 110:1769–1778.

47. Armaly MF. Statistical attributes of the steroid hypertensive response in the clinically normal eye. I. The demonstration of three levels of response. Invest Ophthalmol 1965; 4:187–197.

48. Armaly MF. The heritable nature of dexamethasone-induced ocular hypertension. Arch Ophthalmol 1966; 75:32–35.

49. Becker B. Intraocular pressure response to topical steroids. Invest Ophthalmol 1965; 4:198–205.

50. Weinreb RN, Polansky JR, Kramer SG, et al. Acute effects of dexamethasone on intraocular pressure in glaucoma. Invest Ophthalmol Vis Sci 1985; 26:170–175.

51. Dreyer EB. Inhaled steroid use and glaucoma. N Engl J Med 1993; 329:1822.

52. Mitchell P, Cumming RG, Mackey DA. Inhaled corticosteroids, family history, and risk of glaucoma. Ophthalmology 1999; 106:2301–2306.

53. Levin DS, Han DP, Dev S, et al. Subtenon's depot corticosteroid injections in patients with a history of corticosteroid-induced intraocular pressure elevation. Am J Ophthalmol 2002; 133:196–202.

54. Clark AF, Wilson K, de Kater AW, et al. Dexamethasone-induced ocular hypertension in perfusion-cultured human eyes. Invest Ophthalmol Vis Sci 1995; 36:478–489.

55. Johnson D, Gottanka J, Flugel C, et al. Ultrastructural changes in the trabecular meshwork of human eyes treated with corticosteroids. Arch Ophthalmol 1997; 115:375–383.

56. Fingert JH, Clark AF, Craig JE, et al. Evaluation of the myocilin (MYOC) glaucoma gene in monkey and human steroid-induced ocular hypertension. Invest Ophthalmol Vis Sci 2001; 42:145–152.

57. Nguyen TD, Chen P, Huang WD, et al. Gene structure and properties of TIGR, an olfactomedin-related glycoprotein cloned from glucocorticoid-induced trabecular meshwork cells. J Biol Chem 1998; 273:6341–6350.

58. Clark AF, Steely HT, Dickerson JE Jr, et al. Glucocorticoid induction of the glaucoma gene MYOC in human and monkey trabecular meshwork cells and tissues. Invest Ophthalmol Vis Sci 2001; 42:1769–1780.

59. Fautsch MP, Bahler CK, Vrabel AM, et al. Perfusion of his-tagged eukaryotic myocilin increases outflow resistance in human anterior segments in the presence of aqueous humor. Invest Ophthalmol Vis Sci 2006; 47:213–221.

60. Foster PJ, Buhrmann R, Quigley HA, et al. The definition and classification of glaucoma in prevalence surveys. Br J Ophthalmol 2002; 86:238–242.

61. Franceschetti A. Heterochromic cyclitis. Am J Ophthalmol 1955; 39:50–58.

62. Posner A, Schlossman A. Syndrome of recurrent attacks of glaucoma with cyclitic symptoms. Arch Ophthalmol 1948; 39:517–533.

63. Nolan WP, See JL, Chew PT, et al. Detection of primary angle closure using anterior segment optical coherence tomography in Asian eyes. Ophthalmology 2006; 114:33–39.

64. Dorairaj SK, Tello C, Liebmann JM, et al. Narrow angles and angle closure: anatomic reasons for earlier closure of the superior portion of the iridocorneal angle. Arch Ophthalmol 2007; 125:734–739.

65. Akingbehin T, Villada JR. Metipranolol-associated granulomatous anterior uveitis. Br J Ophthalmol 1991; 75:519–523.

66. KeBler C. Possible bilateral anterior uveitis secondary to metipranolol (OptiPranolol) therapy. Arch Ophthalmol 1994; 112:1277.

67. Patel NP, Patel KH, Moster MR, et al. Metipranolol-associated nongranulomatous anterior uveitis. Am J Ophthalmol 1997; 123:843–844.

68. Watanabe TM, Hodes BL. Bilateral anterior uveitis associated with a brand of metipranolol. Arch Ophthalmol 1997; 115:421–422.

69. Kamalarajah S, Johnston PB. Bilateral anterior uveitis associated with 0.3% minims metipranolol. Eye 1999; 13(Pt 3a):380–381.

70. Kiuchi Y, Okada K, Ito N, et al. Effect of a single drop of latanoprost on intraocular pressure and blood–aqueous barrier permeability in patients with uveitis. Kobe J Med Sci 2002; 48:153–159.

71. Kashiwagi K, Tsukahara S. Effect of non-steroidal anti-inflammatory ophthalmic solution on intraocular pressure reduction by latanoprost. Br J Ophthalmol 2003; 87:297–301.

72. Chiba T, Kashiwagi K, Chiba N, et al. Effect of non-steroidal anti-inflammatory ophthalmic solution on intraocular pressure reduction by latanoprost in patients with primary open angle glaucoma or ocular hypertension. Br J Ophthalmol 2006; 90:314–317.

73. Sponsel WE, Paris G, Trigo Y, et al. Latanoprost and brimonidine: therapeutic and physiologic assessment before and after oral nonsteroidal anti-inflammatory therapy. Am J Ophthalmol 2002; 133:11–18.

74. Schumer RA, Camras CB, Mandahl AK. Putative side effects of prostaglandin analogs. Surv Ophthalmol 2002; 47(Suppl 1):S219.

75. Fechtner RD, Khouri AS, Zimmerman TJ, et al. Anterior uveitis associated with latanoprost. Am J Ophthalmol 1998; 126:37–41.

76. Smith SL, Pruitt CA, Sine CS, et al. Latanoprost 0.005% and anterior segment uveitis. Acta Ophthalmol Scand 1999; 77:668–672.

77. Arcieri ES, Santana A, Rocha FN, et al. Blood–aqueous barrier changes after the use of prostaglandin analogues in patients

with pseudophakia and aphakia: a 6-month randomized trial. Arch Ophthalmol 2005; 123:186–192.

78. Kaufman HE, Varnell ED, Toshida H, et al. Effects of topical unoprostone and latanoprost on acute and recurrent herpetic keratitis in the rabbit. Am J Ophthalmol 2001; 131:643–646.

79. Wand M, Gilbert CM, Liesegang TJ. Latanoprost and herpes simplex keratitis. Am J Ophthalmol 1999; 127:602–604.

80. Ekatomatis P. Herpes simplex dendritic keratitis after treatment with latanoprost for primary open angle glaucoma. Br J Ophthalmol 2001; 85:1008–1009.

81. Bean G, Reardon G, Zimmerman TJ. Association between ocular herpes simplex virus and topical ocular hypotensive therapy. J Glaucoma 2004; 13:361–364.

82. Broadway DC, Bates AK, Lightman SL, et al. The importance of cellular changes in the conjunctiva of patients with uveitic glaucoma undergoing trabeculectomy. Eye 1993; 7(Pt 4): 495–501.

83. Broadway DC, Grierson I, Stürmer J, et al. Reversal of topical antiglaucoma medication effects on the conjunctiva. Arch Ophthalmol 1996; 114:262–267.

84. Towler HM, Bates AK, Broadway DC, et al. Primary trabeculectomy with 5-fluorouracil for glaucoma secondary to uveitis. Ocular Immunol Inflamm 1995; 3:163–170.

85. Stavrou P, Murray PI. Long-term follow-up of trabeculectomy without antimetabolites in patients with uveitis. Am J Ophthalmol 1999; 128:434–439.

86. Towler HM, McCluskey P, Shaer B, et al. Long-term follow-up of trabeculectomy with intraoperative 5-fluorouracil for uveitis-related glaucoma. Ophthalmology 2000; 107:1822–1828.

87. Yalvac IS, Sungur G, Turhan E, et al. Trabeculectomy with mitomycin-C in uveitic glaucoma associated with Behçet disease. J Glaucoma 2004; 13:450–453.

88. Ceballos EM, Beck AD, Lynn MJ. Trabeculectomy with antiproliferative agents in uveitic glaucoma. J Glaucoma 2002; 11:189–196.

89. Wright MM, McGehee RF, Pederson JE. Intraoperative mitomycin-C for glaucoma associated with ocular inflammation. Ophthalmic Surg Lasers 1997; 28:370–376.

90. Prata JA Jr, Neves RA, Minckler DS, et al. Trabeculectomy with mitomycin C in glaucoma associated with uveitis. Ophthalmic Surg 1994; 25:616–620.

91. Elgin U, Berker N, Batman A, et al. Trabeculectomy with mitomycin C in secondary glaucoma associated with Behçet disease. J Glaucoma 2007; 16:68–72.

92. Chen PP, Weaver YK, Budenz DL, et al. Trabeculectomy function after cataract extraction. Ophthalmology 1998; 105:1928–1935.

93. Lichter PR, Musch DC, Gillespie BW, et al. Interim clinical outcomes in the Collaborative Initial Glaucoma Treatment Study comparing initial treatment randomized to medications or surgery. Ophthalmology 2001; 108:1943–1953.

94. Siriwardena D, Kotecha A, Minassian D, et al. Anterior chamber flare after trabeculectomy and after phacoemulsification. Br J Ophthalmol 2000; 84:1056–1057.

95. Park H-J, Weitzman M, Caprioli J. Temporal corneal phacoemulsification combined with superior trabeculectomy. Arch Ophthalmol 1997; 115:318–323.

96. Park HJ, Kwon YH, Weitzman M, et al. Temporal corneal phacoemulsification in patients with filtered glaucoma. Arch Ophthalmol 1997; 115:1375–1380.

97. Molteno AC, Sayawat N, Herbison P. Otago Glaucoma Surgery Outcome Study: long-term results of uveitis with secondary glaucoma drained by Molteno implants. Ophthalmology 2001; 108:605–613.

98. Ceballos EM, Parrish RK, Schiffman JC. Outcome of Baerveldt glaucoma drainage implants for the treatment of uveitic glaucoma. Ophthalmology 2002; 109:2256–2260.

99. Da Mata A, Burk SE, Netland PA, et al. Management of uveitic glaucoma with Ahmed glaucoma valve implantation. Ophthalmology 1999; 106:2168–2172.

100. Ho CL, Wong EY, Walton DS. Goniosurgery for glaucoma complicating chronic childhood uveitis. Arch Ophthalmol 2004; 122:838–844.

101. Murphy CC, Burnett CA, Spry PG, et al. A two centre study of the dose-response relation for transscleral diode laser cyclophotocoagulation in refractory glaucoma. Br J Ophthalmol 2003; 87:1252–1257.

CHAPTER 34

Neovascular Glaucoma

Danny Kim, Arun D Singh, and Annapurna Singh

INTRODUCTION

Neovascular glaucoma (NVG) was first described in the late nineteenth century as a condition in which the eye developed progressive neovascularization of the iris (NVI) and angle (NVA). Though widely described as congestive glaucoma, rubeotic glaucoma, thrombotic glaucoma, and hemorrhagic glaucoma, the current preferred terminology is *neovascular glaucoma* as proposed by Weiss et al.[1] It has since been discovered that there are numerous systemic diseases and secondary ocular conditions that share one common underlying etiology: retinal ischemia and hypoxia. Under conditions of retinal ischemia, a pro-angiogenic cascade is triggered that promotes the development of new, fragile, leaky blood vessels on the surface of the iris and the angle. NVG progresses through the growth of a fibrovascular membrane over the trabecular meshwork in the anterior chamber angle that can contract and cause secondary closed-angle glaucoma. Left untreated, NVG causes advanced glaucomatous optic neuropathy and irreversible visual loss. Both early diagnosis and aggressive treatment are necessary to prevent these serious complications.

DISEASE PREVALENCE AND INFLUENCE

Although the overall incidence and prevalence of NVG has not been accurately reported, a retrospective study has shown a prevalence rate of 3.9%.[2] The most common conditions associated with NVG are central retinal vein occlusion (CRVO), proliferative diabetic retinopathy (PDR), and other conditions such as ocular ischemic syndrome and tumors. Approximately 36% of NVG occurs after CRVO, 32% with PDR, and 13% occurs after carotid artery obstruction.[3] Given that the underlying etiology of developing NVG is some form of retinal ischemia, it is more prevalent in elderly patients who have significant cardiovascular risk factors such as hypertension, diabetes, dyslipidemia, and a history of smoking. In addition, there are numerous retinal diseases and ocular/extraocular disorders that predispose to NVG (Table 34.1).

RISK FACTORS FOR DEVELOPING NEOVASCULAR GLAUCOMA

Regardless of the systemic or ocular condition that is associated with the development of NVG, the underlying process of retinal ischemia is the initiating factor for the angiogenic cascade. The most common conditions associated with NVG are CRVO, PDR, and ocular ischemic syndrome.[4]

CENTRAL RETINAL VEIN OCCLUSION

The predominant risk factor for the development of neovascular complications following central retinal vein occlusion (CRVO) is the extent, location, and duration of retinal ischemia (ischemic drive).[5] Whereas anterior segment neovascularization is rare in nonischemic CRVO, the incidence of iris neovascularization is as high as 60% in ischemic eyes, usually occurring at a mean 3–5 months after the CRVO.[6]

The importance of closely following patients with CRVO was demonstrated by the landmark Central Vein Occlusion Study (CVOS). The CVOS showed that 15% of nonischemic CRVO could proceed to ischemic CRVO in the first 4 months.[7] During the next 32 months an additional 19% of eyes were found to have converted to the ischemic form for a total of 34% after 3 years. The development of nonperfusion or ischemia was most rapid in the first 4 months and progressed continuously throughout the entire duration of follow-up. Iris neovascularization of at least two clock hours, and/or NVA developed in 16% of eyes. The CVOS also found that the most important risk factor predictive of rubeosis iridis was poor visual acuity.

In a prospective clinical and fluorescein angiographic study of patients with CRVO, 20% developed NVG.[8] The eyes were classified as having either an ischemic or a hyperpermeable type of CRVO according to the extent of retinal capillary nonperfusion demonstrated by the initial fluorescein angiogram. The risk of developing NVG was approximately 60% in those eyes with extensive retinal ischemia. The tendency for rapid progression

TABLE 34.1 Predisposing factors for neovascular glaucoma			
RETINAL ISCHEMIA	Diabetic retinopathy	Central retinal vein occlusion	Central retinal artery occlusion
	Branch retinal vein occlusion	Branch retinal artery occlusion	Retinal detachment
	Coats' exudative retinopathy	Eales disease	Retinopathy of prematurity
	Sickle cell retinopathy	Retinal vasculitis	Persistent hyperplastic primary vitreous
INFLAMMATORY DISEASES	Behçet disease	Chronic iridocyclitis	Vogt-Koyanagi-Harada syndrome
	Sympathetic ophthalmia	Sarcoidosis	Crohn's disease
TUMORS	Iris melanoma	Ciliary body melanoma	Choroidal melanoma
	Retinoblastoma	Metastasis	Medulloepithelioma
EXTRAOCULAR DISORDERS	Carotid-cavernous fistula	Sequelae of dural shunt embolization	Carotid artery obstructive disease
	Takayasu's syndrome	Wyburn-Mason syndrome	Temporal arteritis
IRRADIATION	External beam radiation	Proton beam radiation	Plaques radiation
SURGICAL	Cataract extraction	Pars plana vitrectomy or lensectomy	Scleral buckling

of early NVI to NVG makes early recognition of eyes at high risk to develop NVG essential.

DIABETIC RETINOPATHY

In most cases of diabetic retinopathy, many years elapse before rubeosis becomes evident. Approximately one-third of patients with rubeosis iridis have diabetic retinopathy.[9,10] The Diabetes Control and Complications Trial (DCCT) demonstrated that tight control of blood glucose levels delayed the onset of diabetic retinopathy and slowed progression to proliferative retinopathy.[11] The overall prevalence of NVG in diabetes mellitus is about 2%, but increases to over 21% in PDR, where the frequency of rubeosis iridis can be as high as 65%. If a diabetic patient develops NVG in one eye, the fellow eye is also at higher risk of developing NVG if prophylactic panretinal photocoagulation (PRP) treatment is not performed. About 80% of eyes with a detached retina, as compared with 4% of eyes with an attached retina, develop NVG following pars plana vitrectomy for complications of diabetic retinopathy.[12]

OCULAR ISCHEMIC SYNDROME

Ocular ischemic syndrome occurs when there is chronic, severe, carotid artery obstruction. Ocular ischemic syndrome is often misdiagnosed and treated as primary open-angle glaucoma, or later on as neovascular glaucoma. Typically, a 90% or greater ipsilateral obstruction is necessary to cause ocular ischemic syndrome. Anterior segment signs include rubeosis iridis in up to 66% of patients.[13] Although the prevalence of rubeosis iridis is very high in these patients, the intraocular pressure (IOP) is typically low or normal, presumably due to impaired ciliary body perfusion. In cases of iris neovascularization or midperipheral hemorrhages, Doppler sonography of carotid arteries should be performed. A combined effort between the ophthalmologist, radiologist, and vascular surgeon following carotid endarterectomy can be effective in slowing the progression of ocular ischemic syndrome.[14]

CENTRAL RETINAL ARTERY OCCLUSION

Ischemia/reperfusion injury of the retina after central retinal artery occlusion (CRAO) predisposes to rubeosis iridis in 18% of cases within 3 months, although rubeosis iridis can develop much later.[15] In one prospective study of 33 patients, rubeosis iridis appeared as early as 12 days to as late as 15 weeks following CRAO, with an overall incidence of 18%.[16] Five of the six patients (15% of the total) later developed NVG. Another patient in this series developed neovascularization of the optic disc without neovascularization of the iris, an incidence of 3%. Only two of the seven patients with ocular neovascularization had ipsilateral hemodynamically significant carotid artery disease as determined by noninvasive carotid artery testing. This study confirms results of previous retrospective studies that the incidence of ocular neovascularization after CRAO is higher than commonly thought. It also shows that, in the majority of cases, carotid artery disease is not responsible for the neovascularization seen after CRAO. Although not as common, NVG has been reported to occur after branch retinal artery occlusion.[17]

OTHER CONDITIONS ASSOCIATED WITH NEOVASCULAR GLAUCOMA

As listed in Table 34.1, there are numerous other ocular and extraocular diseases that are associated with NVG. Ocular tumors such as choroidal melanoma, uveal melanoma, and retinoblastoma have been described to increase the risk of developing NVG.[18–20] Lymphoma that has metastasized to the iris and ciliary body causing

NVG highlights the importance of ultrasound biomicroscopy in detecting ciliary body tumors.[21] A rare case of ocular neovascularization in a patient with Fanconi anemia has been described in which NVG, vitreous hemorrhage, optic disc neovascularization, and peripheral ischemic retinopathy were evident.[22] NVG in a young patient with X-linked juvenile retinoschisis was recently reported.[23] Systemic cryoglobulinemia may be associated with anterior segment ischemia and neovascularization, and should be considered in the differential diagnosis of iris neovascularization in the absence of apparent retinal ischemia.[24] The association of sarcoidosis with rubeosis iridis and NVG has also been described.[25]

ETIOLOGY AND PATHOGENESIS

In ischemic retinal disease, hypoxia induces production of vascular endothelial growth factor (VEGF), a vasoproliferative substance, which acts upon healthy endothelial cells of viable capillaries to stimulate the formation of fragile new vessels (neovascularization). In cases of extreme retinal hypoxia, there are essentially very few viable retinal capillaries available. In that instance, VEGF is theorized to diffuse forward to the nearest area of viable capillaries, namely the posterior iris. Neovascularization buds off from the capillaries of the posterior iris, grows along the posterior iris, through the pupil, along the anterior surface of the iris, and then into the angle. Once in the angle, the neovascularization, along with its fibrovascular support membrane, acts to both physically block the angle as well as bridge the angle and pull the iris and cornea into apposition, thus blocking the trabecular meshwork. Scanning electron microscopy revealed extensive peripheral anterior synechiae formation and flattening and effacement of the anterior iridic surface by a confluent fibrovascular membrane.[26] New vessels on the anterior iris uniformly were hidden beneath a clinically invisible layer of myofibroblasts. Myofibroblasts provide the motive force for synechial closure and ectropion iridis in NVG. The result is a secondary angle closure without pupillary block.

DIAGNOSIS AND ANCILLARY TESTING

In patients who have ocular conditions that predispose them to developing NVG, clinicians should perform a comprehensive ophthalmologic exam with particular attention to the pupillary margin (Fig. 34.1).[27] An undilated slit lamp examination and gonioscopy are essential for the detection of NVI and NVA. Although NVI usually precedes NVA, new vessels may occasionally be found in the angle without evidence of iris neovascularization. Fluorescein angiography of the anterior segment and fluorescein gonio-angiography may be contributive to the diagnosis of early rubeosis iridis (Fig. 34.2).

DIFFERENTIAL DIAGNOSIS

It is important to distinguish NVG in the open-angle stage from other types of glaucoma such as inflammatory

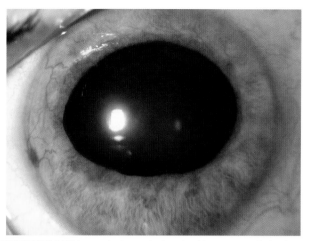

FIGURE 34.1 Slit lamp photograph showing iris neovascularization.

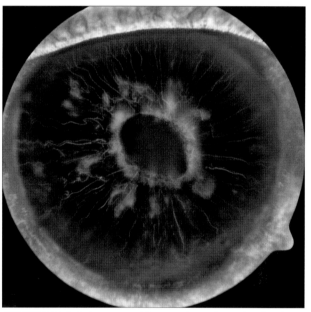

FIGURE 34.2 Anterior segment fluorescein angiography showing leakage from iris neovascularization.

glaucoma associated with anterior uveitis or angle-closure glaucoma. This differentiation can typically be made on the basis of detecting neovascularization on the surface of the iris and in the angle in NVG. Fuchs heterochromic iridocyclitis also can present with new vessels in the anterior chamber angle. In the angle-closure glaucoma stage, the differential diagnosis must also include other causes of iris distortion and peripheral anterior synechiae, such as prior ocular trauma and iridocorneal endothelial syndromes.

SIGNS AND SYMPTOMS

Depending on the severity of intraocular pressure elevation, intraocular inflammation, and glaucomatous optic neuropathy, patients can present with various signs and symptoms of NVG that include decreased vision, photophobia, corneal edema, conjunctival injection, rubeosis, elevated intraocular pressure, inflammation, hyphema, and vitreous hemorrhage. If the inflammation

TABLE 34.2 Stages of neovascular glaucoma		
Stage 1	Rubeosis iridis	Mild iris and/or angle neovascularization. Tufts of rubeosis can be found at the pupillary margin and/or angle. IOP is normal (unless preexisting open-angle glaucoma is present)
Stage 2	Open-angle glaucoma	Mild–moderate rubeosis iridis and/or angle neovascularization. Growth of fibrovascular tissue over trabecular meshwork, decreases aqueous outflow and increases IOP in an aberrantly open angle. IOP is elevated, but can also rise suddenly. Some level of inflammation can be present. Hyphema can also develop
Stage 3	Angle-closure glaucoma	Moderate–severe iris and angle neovascularization. Fibrovascular membrane proliferates and contracts, causing progressive angle closure and ectropion uveae. Possible hyphema with inflammation. IOP can be as high as 60–70 mmHg

is severe, or the elevation in IOP is acute, the patient may exhibit severe pain, headache, nausea, and/or vomiting.

STAGES OF NEOVASCULAR GLAUCOMA

The typical clinical presentation can be divided into the following three stages: (1) rubeosis iridis, (2) open-angle glaucoma stage, and (3) angle-closure glaucoma stage. These stages generally follow each other in progression. The relevant clinical signs and symptoms are included in this section and summarized in Table 34.2.

STAGE 1: RUBEOSIS IRIDIS

At this stage tufts of rubeosis can be found at the pupillary margin and/or rubeotic vessels may be found in the angle (Fig. 34.3). Although slit lamp biomicroscopy can detect iris neovascularization, iris fluorescein angiography has been shown to be more reliable in detecting very early iris neovascularization.[28] In one study of 200 randomly selected fluorescein angiograms of the iris, rubeosis iridis was detected in 97.2% with a false-positive rate of only 1%.[29] Furthermore, iris angiography detects rubeosis prior to it becoming clinically evident on slit lamp biomicroscopy in approximately 33% of the eyes. Although neovascularization is usually seen first at the peripupillary iris, a thorough gonioscopic examination should be performed since NVA can sometimes precede rubeosis.[30] Intraocular pressure is typically normal, but can be elevated if a preexisting open-angle glaucoma is present. Patients are typically asymptomatic at this stage unless a complication of an underlying condition such as vitreous hemorrhage from underlying diabetic retinopathy or visual field loss from CRVO develops.

STAGE 2: OPEN-ANGLE GLAUCOMA

At this stage, the IOP begins to rise and stays elevated. The elevated IOP can also rise suddenly, causing acute-onset glaucoma. Due to the fragile nature of the new vessels, a hyphema can also present at this stage. The degree of rubeosis iridis is usually more prominent and the anterior chamber can show some level of inflammation. Gonioscopy typically shows an open angle, but NVA can be significant. The NVI can be continuous

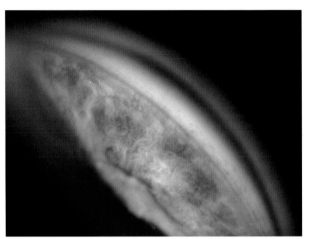

FIGURE 34.3 Slit lamp goniophotograph of iris and angle neovascularization.

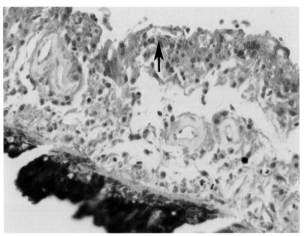

FIGURE 34.4 Iris neovascularization appears as fine vascular channels (*arrow*) on the anterior surface of the iris. (Hematoxylin and eosin; original magnification 40×.)

with the new vessels in the angle. Histopathologically, the hallmark of this stage is growth of a fibrovascular membrane, including rubeotic vessels on the iris surface that extend over the trabecular meshwork, decreasing aqueous outflow and increasing IOP in an aberrantly open angle (Fig. 34.4).[31] Both inflammation in the anterior chamber and possible hyphema can exacerbate the disease process.

STAGE 3: ANGLE-CLOSURE GLAUCOMA

The contraction of the fibrovascular membrane causes progressive angle closure, ectropion uveae, peripheral anterior synechiae formation, and a flat, glistening appearance to the iris. Patients will often complain of photophobia, reduced visual acuity, acute severe pain, headache, nausea, and/or vomiting. Rubeosis is usually severe, with possible hyphema, moderate inflammation, and IOP as high as 60–70 mmHg. Conjunctival injection and corneal edema are frequently present. Fundoscopic examination may reveal optic nerve cupping. The glaucoma at this stage is severe and usually requires some form of surgical intervention.

TREATMENT OPTIONS

The treatment of NVG varies depending on the stage of the disease and the clarity of the media.

TREATMENT OF NEOVASCULARIZATION

Once rubeosis iridis has begun, the primary goal of treatment is to reduce the ischemic drive of neovascularization. This is best accomplished with panretinal photocoagulation (PRP) to destroy ischemic retina, minimize oxygen demand of the eye, and reduce the amount of VEGF being released. PRP tends to be effective in causing regression and involution of anterior segment neovascularization.

If the patient has NVI or NVA, with normal IOP, the clarity of the media usually dictates what form of treatment can be initiated. If the media is clear, PRP is recommended. The ablation of the peripheral retina is considered to be first-line therapy to counter the angiogenic cascade. It is important to understand that adequate PRP treatment must be performed. In one study that reported using 1200 to 1600 laser spots, there was a regression of rubeosis in nearly 71% of diabetic patients, whereas using 400 to 650 spots produced a regression of only 36%.[32] Another study involved 256 patients with PDR and 21 patients with retinal vascular occlusions with ischemic involvement that were all treated with prophylactic PRP; only three patients from the entire treated group developed NVG.[33]

However, in patients with CRVO, the benefits of prophylactic PRP in a 10-year prospective study of eyes with no evidence of neovascularization showed no significant difference in the incidence of NVG compared to eyes without PRP.[32] The CVOS essentially recommended performing PRP only when two clock hours of NVI and/or NVA was observed. Therefore, for patients with CRVO, the standard practice is to monitor them closely with slit lamp biomicroscopy and gonioscopy, and to treat with PRP at the earliest sign of NVI and/or NVA.

If the media is cloudy because of vitreous hemorrhage, a pars plana vitrectomy and endolaser treatment,

which can be combined with direct laser coagulation of the ciliary processes, are likely to be most effective.[34] In conjunction with vitrectomy, the use of silicone oil infusion in severe PDR was found to be beneficial in treating rubeosis iridis, presumably by acting as a barrier for the flow of pro-angiogenic factors between the anterior and posterior segments.[35] If the media is cloudy because of a visually significant cataract, cataract extraction and immediate PRP should be considered to prevent further worsening of the neovascularization, which can progress rapidly after cataract extraction. In one study, patients with PDR who underwent prophylactic PRP were less likely to develop rubeosis iridis after cataract extraction than those not receiving PRP.[36]

Other treatment modalities when the media is not clear include diode laser retinopexy (peripheral transscleral retinal diode laser photocoagulation)[37] and panretinal cryotherapy. Diode laser retinopexy may be combined with transscleral cyclophotocoagulation therapy to manage concurrent high intraocular pressure in rubeotic glaucoma, but this involves a risk of postoperative hypotony.

TREATMENT OF NEOVASCULAR GLAUCOMA

Once a patient has progressed beyond the early stages of rubeosis iridis and has elevated IOP with an open- or closed-angle glaucoma, the primary goals of treatment are to regress any neovascularization as described above and control IOP.

Medical management of elevated intraocular pressure If the angle is open and the eye still has relatively useful vision, but IOP is above normal, initiate medical therapy to reduce aqueous production. Patients may require a combination of carbonic anhydrase inhibitors (topical or systemic), topical β-blockers, and/or α$_2$-agonists to control IOP. Prostaglandin analogues are generally not recommended since there is compromised access to the uveoscleral route. In addition, antiinflammatory agents such as topical steroid drops and cycloplegic agents may be indicated to control any inflammation and pain.

Surgical management of elevated intraocular pressure Occasionally, although the angle is open, it may not be possible to control IOP on medical management alone. Surgical glaucoma intervention involving filtering surgery, drainage implants, and/or cyclodestructive procedures may be necessary.

Filtering surgery Filtering surgery is relatively effective in controlling elevated IOP associated with NVG. Results from two recent studies involving early trabeculectomy with mitomycin C (MMC) have shown successful IOP control of 53% at 13 months[38] and 66.7% at 28 months.[39] Another study in which trabeculectomy with MMC was performed on eyes with active NVG secondary to PDR showed success rates of 67%

at 1 year and 61.8% after 2–3 years.[40] Trabeculectomy combined with implantation of a silicone rubber slice successfully lowered IOP at 18-month follow-up.[41] In a more recent study, 72 eyes of 72 patients with NVG who underwent primary trabeculectomy with MMC combined with direct cauterization of peripheral iris before iridectomy had successful IOP reduction at 6-month follow-up and decreased incidence of both intra-operative bleeding and early postoperative hyphema.[42] Another study of early trabeculectomy with MMC in the treatment of NVG with hazy ocular media showed a 52.7% success rate in controlling IOP at mean follow-up of 13 months.[38] Trabeculectomy with 5-fluorouracil had a higher risk of long-term failure, with success rates at the 1, 3, and 5 years of 71%, 61%, and 28%, respectively.[43]

The success rate has improved with performing adequate PRP prior to surgery.[44] When complete PRP was combined with pars plana vitrectomy and trabeculectomy with MMC in patients with NVG, IOP was effectively reduced in 81.2% after 3 years follow-up compared to only 18.5% after 2 years in patients without prior PRP.

Drainage implants Aqueous tube shunt implants have some success in the treatment of refractory NVG, especially in situations where conventional filtering surgery has failed.[45,46] Although the initial response to Ahmed valve and Molteno implants is relatively good, the long-term outcome is poor. In one study, the cumulative success was 63.2% at 1 year, 56.2% at 2 years, 43.2% at 3 years, 37.8% at 4 years, and 25.2% at 5 years in the Ahmed valve group, whereas the cumulative probabilities of success were 37.0% at 1 year, 29.6% at 2 years, 29.6% at 3 years, 29.6% at 4 years, and 29.6% at 5 years with the Molteno implant.[47] Baerveldt implantation is also effective in controlling IOP elevation associated with neovascular glaucoma, with success rates of 79% and 56% at the 12- and 18-month follow-up, respectively.[48] Young patients with poor preoperative visual acuity are at risk of surgical failure.

Improved success rates have been shown in patients with refractory NVG when the drainage tube is implanted via the pars plana and combined with pars plana vitrectomy.[49] Although these results are somewhat satisfactory in the treatment of refractory NVG, the visual outcomes are generally very poor, with no light perception developing in as high as 31%.

Cyclodestructive procedures Cyclodestruction to reduce production of aqueous humor can be achieved with photocoagulation or cryotherapy. Long-term results of noncontact neodymium:yttrium–aluminum–garnet cyclophoto-coagulation in neovascular glaucoma showed success rates of 65%, 49.8%, and 34.8% at 1-, 3-, and 6-year follow-up, respectively.[50] Contact transscleral diode cyclophotocoagulation is effective in lowering IOP in eyes with neovascular glaucoma.[51] Currently, a standardized cyclophotocoagulation protocol in NVG has not yet been established. Although the IOP can often be controlled,

visual outcomes are typically very poor, with the rate of long-term visual loss in patients who have NVG approaching nearly 50%.[52]

TREATMENT OF LATE STAGES OF NEOVASCULAR GLAUCOMA

If the eye no longer has visual potential, it is recommended to initiate medical therapy to control IOP, including cycloplegic agents, steroid drops for comfort, and PRP if the media is clear. If the media is cloudy, then panretinal cryotherapy and cyclodestructive surgery to control IOP will likely be needed. In a study of 70 patients with NVG resistant to medical and surgical treatment that were treated with transconjunctival cyclocryocoagulation, there was a significant decrease in IOP and eye pain after 180 days.[53] However, if the eye has no vision and medical therapy is not controlling the pain and discomfort, more aggressive action may be needed such as performing retrobulbar alcohol injection, evisceration, or enucleation.

FUTURE TREATMENT OPTIONS

Several novel treatments for NVG in eyes with intractable glaucoma are under clinical investigation. Investigators have tried using photodynamic therapy with verteporfin to occlude new iris vessels without damaging the adjacent tissue or normal iris vessels, and some of the preliminary studies show promising results. In one study of 4 eyes with NVG, 100% showed complete obliteration of angle neovascularization, partial occlusion of iris neovascularization, and a reduction in IOP only 1 week after photodynamic therapy.[54] Long-term follow-up results of this novel approach have not yet been reported.

Intravitreal injection of crystalline triamcinolone has also been shown to cause a regression of iris neovascularization. In one study, 14 eyes of 14 patients with NVG due to PDR and CRVO had a significant reduction in rubeosis, IOP, and pain following intravitreal injection of triamcinolone (either alone or in combination with other surgical procedures), although visual acuity was not significantly improved postoperatively.[55] Again, long-term follow-up data have not yet been published.

Perhaps the most promising therapeutic approach involves the modulation of the angiogenic cascade by inhibiting vascular endothelial growth factor (VEGF). VEGF plays a critical role in the pathogenesis of retinal neovascularization in linking tissue ischemia to angiogenesis. Novel anti-VEGF compounds, which include bevacizumab (Avastin [Genentech, Inc.]), small interfering RNA (siRNA) directed against VEGF or VEGF receptor 1, and VEGF trap are being considered.[56–58] Intravitreal injection of bevacizumab (Avastin) has shown significant promise in treating NVG. One study reported rapid regression of iris and angle neovascularization in patients with NVG and refractory IOP elevation (Fig. 34.5).[59] More recent studies also show a similar response to intravitreal bevacizumab.[60]

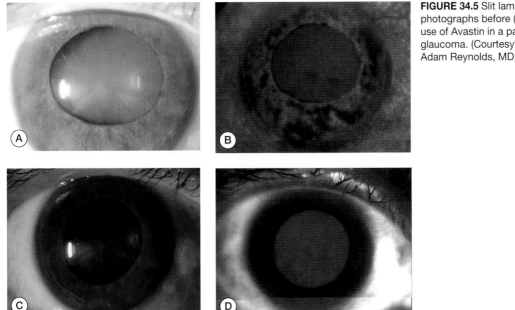

FIGURE 34.5 Slit lamp and fluorescein photographs before (**A, B**) and after (**C, D**) use of Avastin in a patient with neovascular glaucoma. (Courtesy of Eugene Eng, MD, and Adam Reynolds, MD.)

Pigment-epithelium-derived factor (PEDF), an endogenous angiogenesis inhibitor, shows promise in the treatment of rubeosis. PEDF acts broadly at the earliest stages of the angiogenic cascade. PEDF aims at balancing the levels of pro-angiogenic and angiostatic molecules.[61] It is secreted by the retinal pigment epithelium (RPE) and a select number of other cell types in the eye, as well as by other tissues in the body. PEDF was originally defined by its ability to induce differentiation in retinoblastoma cells. PEDF has tremendous specificity for causing the regression of new vessels with little harmful effect on mature vessels.[62] In a mouse model of ischemia-induced retinal neovascularization and on VEGF-induced migration and growth of cultured vascular endothelial cells, elevated concentrations of PEDF inhibit VEGF-induced retinal endothelial cell growth and migration and retinal neovascularization.[63] There are human clinical trials underway to evaluate the safety of PEDF in conditions such as neovascular age-related macular degeneration (AMD) that may someday be applicable to neovascular glaucoma. In one such phase I clinical trial, 28 patients with advanced neovascular AMD were given a single intravitreal injection of an adeno-viral vector-delivered PEDF and up 71% of patients showed improvement in lesion size from baseline at 6 months.[64]

Summary

Neovascular glaucoma is a devastating ocular disease often associated with poor visual prognosis. It is a relatively common complication of several retinal disorders, especially central retinal vein occlusion, proliferative diabetic retinopathy, and ocular ischemic syndrome. The pathophysiology of neovascular glaucoma involves the formation of new blood vessels on the surface of the iris and the angle of the anterior chamber, which initially impedes aqueous outflow, but later contracts to produce an angle-closure form of glaucoma. Currently used medical or surgical treatment has a low success rate. The most effective treatment involves retinal ablation, which reduces the level of retinal hypoxia and slows the subsequent angiogenic cascade. The best hope for preventing blindness associated with NVG is continued research into the angiogenesis pathway that has already produced many novel and promising therapeutic options for AMD.

REFERENCES

1. Weiss DI, Shaffer RN, Nehrenberg TR. Neovascular glaucoma complicating carotid-cavernous fistula. Arch Ophthalmol 1963; 69:304.

2. Mocanu C, Barascu D, Marinescu F. Neovascular glaucoma – retrospective study. Oftalmologia 2005;49:58–65.

3. Vancea PP, Abu-Taleb A. Current trends in neovascular glaucoma treatment. Rev Med Chir Soc Med Nat Iasi 2005; 109:264–268.

4. Brown GC, Magargal LE, Schachat A, et al. Neovascular glaucoma. Etiologic considerations. Ophthalmology 1984; 91:315–320.

5. Magargal LE, Donoso LA, Sanborn GE. Retinal ischemia and risk of neovascularization following central retinal vein occlusion. Ophthalmology 1982; 89:1241–1245.

6. Zegarra H, Gutman FA, Conforto J. The natural course of central retinal vein occlusion. Ophthalmology 1979; 6:1931–1942.

7. Central Vein Occlusion Study Group. Baseline and early natural history report. The Central Vein Occlusion Study. Arch Ophthalmol 1993; 11:1087–1095.

8. Magargal LE, Brown GC, Augsburger JJ, et al. Neovascular glaucoma following central retinal vein obstruction. Ophthalmology 1981; 8:1095–1101.

9. Hoskins HD Jr. Neovascular glaucoma: current concepts. Trans Am Acad Ophthalmol Otolaryngol 1994; 78:330–333.

10. Brown GC, Magargal LE, Schachat A, et al. Neovascular glaucoma: Etiologic considerations. Ophthalmology 1984; 91:315–320.

11. Diabetes Control and Complications Trial (DCCT) Research Group. The effect of intensive treatment of diabetes on the development and progression of long-term complications in insulin-dependent diabetes mellitus. N Engl J Med 1993; 329:977.

12. Wand M, Madigan JC, Gaudio AR, et al. Neovascular glaucoma following pars plana vitrectomy for complications of diabetic retinopathy. Ophthalmic Surg 1990; 21:113–118.

13. Brown GC. Ocular ishchemic syndrome. In: Ryan SJ, ed. Retina. 3rd edn. St. Louis: Mosby; 2001:1516–1529.

14. Pecold-Stepniewska H, Karokzak-Kulesza M, Wasilewłcz R, Krasiński Z, Kulesza J. Glaucoma and ocular ischemic syndrome–case report. Klin Oczna 2004; 106:258–260.

15. Schafer S, Lang GE. Iris neovascularization as a complication of central retinal artery occlusion. Klin Monatsbl Augeheilkd 2005; 222:343–345.

16. Duker JS, Sivalingam A, Brown GC, et al. A prospective study of acute central retinal artery obstruction. The incidence of secondary ocular neovascularization. Arch Ophthalmol 1991; 109:339–342.

17. Yamamoto K, Tsujikawa A, Hangai M, et al. Neovascular glaucoma after branch retinal artery occlusion. Jpn J Ophthalmol 2005; 49:388–390.

18. Hirasawa N, Triji H, Ishikawa H, et al. Risk factors for neovascular glaucoma after carbon ion radiotherapy of choroidal melanoma using dose-volume histogram analysis. Int J Radiat Oncol Biol Phys 2007; 67:538–543.

19. Detorakis ET, Engstrom RE Jr, Wallace R, et al. Iris and anterior chamber angle neovascularization after iodine 125 brachytherapy for uveal melanoma. Ophthalmology 2005; 112:505–510.

20. Egbert PR, Donaldson SS, Moazed K, et al. Visual results and ocular complications following radiotherapy for retinoblastoma. Arch Ophthalmol 1978; 96:1826–1830.

21. Matsui N, Kamao T, Azumi A. Case of metastatic intraocular malignant lymphoma with neovascular glaucoma. Nippon Ganka Gakkai Zasshi 2005; 109:434–439.

22. Yahia SB, Touffahi SA, Zeghidi H, et al. Ocular neovascularization in a patient with Fanconi anemia. Can J Ophthalmol 2006; 41:778–779.

23. Zuo C, Chen C, Xing Y, et al. Neovascular glaucoma in a patient with X-linked juvenile retinoschisis. Yan Ke Xue Bao 2005; 21:140–141.

24. Telander DG, Holland GN, Wax MB, et al. Rubeosis and anterior segment ischemia associated with systemic cryoglobulinemia. Am J Ophthalmol 2006; 142:689–690.

25. Mayer J, Brouillette G, Corriveau LA. Sarcoidosis and rubeosis iridis. Can J Ophthalmol 1983; 18:197–198.

26. John T, Sassani JW, Eagle RC Jr. The myofibroblastic component of rubeosis iridis. Ophthalmology 1983; 90:721–728.

27. Detry-Morel M. Neovascular glaucoma in the diabetic patient. Bull Soc Belge Ophthalmol 1995; 256:133–141.

28. Oya Y, Sugiyama W, Ando N. Anterior segment fluorescein angiography for evaluating the effect of vitrectomy for neovascular glaucoma. Nippon Ganka Gakkai Zasshi 2005; 109:741–747.

29. Sanborn GE, Symes DJ, Magargal LE. Fundu-iris fluorescein angiography: evaluation of its use in the diagnosis of rubeosis iridis. Ann Ophthalmol 1986; 18:52–58.

30. Browning DJ, Scott AQ, Peterson CB, et al. The risk of missing angle neovascularization by omitting screening gonioscopy in acute central retinal vein occlusion. Arch Ophthalmol 1998; 105:776.

31. Anderson DM, Morin JD, Hunter WS. Rubeosis iridis. Can J Ophthalmol 1971; 6:183.

32. Hayreh SS, Klugman MR, Podhajsky P, et al. Argon laser panretinal photocoagulation in ischemic central retinal vein occlusion. A 10-year prospective study. Graefe's Arch Clin Exp Ophthalmol 1990; 228:281–296.

33. Preda M, Davidescu L, Damian C, et al. Neovascular glaucoma – prevention. Oftalmologia 2006; 50:108–114.

34. Bartz-Schmidt KU, Thumann G, Psichias A, et al. Pars plana vitrectomy, endolaser coagulation of the retina and the ciliary body combined with silicone oil endotamponade in the treatment of uncontrolled neovascular glaucoma. Graefe's Arch Clin Exp Ophthalmol 1999; 237:969–975.

35. Castellarin A, Grigorian R, Bhagat N, et al. Vitrectomy with silicone oil infusion in severe diabetic retinopathy. Br J Ophthalmol 2003; 87:1303–1304.

36. Aiello LM, Wang M, Liang G. Neovascular glaucoma and vitreous hemorrhage after cataract surgery in patients with diabetes mellitus. Ophthalmology 1983; 90:814–820.

37. Flaxel CJ, Larkin GB, Broadway DB, et al. Peripheral transscleral retinal diode laser for rubeosis iridis. Retina 1998; 18:389.

38. Euswas A, Warrasak S. Long-term results of early trabeculectomy with mitomycin C and subsequent posterior segment intervention in the treatment of neovascular glaucoma with hazy ocular media. J Med Assoc Thai 2005; 88:1582–1590.

39. Mandal AK, Majji AB, Mandal SP, et al. Mitomycin-C augmented trabeculectomy for neovascular glaucoma. A preliminary report. Indian J Ophthalmol 2002; 50:287–293.

40. Kiuchi Y, Sugimoto R, Nakae K, et al. Trabeculectomy with mitomycin C for treatment of neovascular glaucoma in diabetic patients. Ophthalmologica 2006; 220:383–388.

41. Yang W, Deng F. Treatment of neovascular glaucoma using trabeculectomy combined with implantation of silicone rubber slice. Yan Ke Xue Bao 2001; 17:183–185.

42. Elgin U, Berker N, Batman A, et al. Trabeculectomy with mitomycin C combined with direct cauterization of peripheral iris in the management of neovascular glaucoma. J Glaucoma 2006; 15:466–470.

43. Tsai JC, Feuer WJ, Parrish RK 2nd, et al. 5-Fluorouracil filtering surgery and neovascular glaucoma. Long-term follow-up of the original pilot study. Ophthalmology 1995; 102:887–892.

44. Allen RC, Bellows AR, Hutchinson BT, et al. Filtration surgery in the treatment of neovascular glaucoma. Ophthalmology 1982; 89:1181–1187.

45. Mermoud A, Salmon JF, Alexander P, et al. Molteno tube implantation for neovascular glaucoma. Long-term results and factors influencing the outcome. Ophthalmology 1993; 100:897–902.

46. Tsai JC, Johnson CC, Dietrich MS. The Ahmed shunt versus the Baerveldt shunt for refractory glaucoma: a single-surgeon comparison of outcome. Ophthalmology 2003; 110:1814–1821.

47. Yalvac IS, Eksioglu U, Satana B, et al. Long-term results of Ahmed glaucoma valve and Molteno implant in neovascular glaucoma. Eye 2007; 21:65–70.

48. Sidoti PA, Dunphy TR, Baerveldt G, et al. Experience with the Baerveldt glaucoma implant in treating neovascular glaucoma. Ophthalmology 1995; 102:1107–1118.

49. Luttrull JK, Avery RL. Pars plana implant and vitrectomy for treatment of neovascular glaucoma. Retina 1995; 15:379–387.

50. Delgado MF, Dickens CJ, Iwach AG, et al. Long-term results of noncontact neodymium:yttrium–aluminum–garnet cyclophotocoagulation in neovascular glaucoma. Ophthalmology 2003; 110:895–899.

51. Threlkeld AB, Johnson MH. Contact transscleral diode cyclophotocoagulation for refractory glaucoma. J Glaucoma 1999; 8:3–7.

52. Shields MB, Shields SE. Noncontact transscleral Nd:YAG cyclophotocoagulation: a long-term follow-up of 500 patients.

Trans Am Ophthalmol Soc 1994; 92:271–283; discussion: 283–287.

53. Kovacic Z, Ivanisevic M, Rogosic V, et al. Cyclocryocoagulation in treatment of neovascular glaucoma. Lijec Vjesn 2004; 126:240–242.

54. Parodi MB, Iacono P. Photodynamic therapy with verteporfin for anterior segment neovascularizations in neovascular glaucoma. Am J Ophthalmol 2004; 138:157.

55. Jonas JB, Hayler JK, Sofker A, et al. Regression of neovascular iris vessels by intravitreal injection of crystalline cortisone. J Glaucoma 2001; 10:284.

56. Avery RL. Regression of retinal and iris neovascularization after intravitreal bevacizumab (Avastin) treatment. Retina 2006; 26:352–354.

57. Campochiaro PA. Potential applications for RNAi to probe pathogenesis and develop new treatments for ocular disorders. Gene Ther 2006; 13:559–562.

58. Lau SC, Rosa DD, Jayson G. Technology evaluation: VEGF Trap (cancer), Regeneron/sanofi-aventis. Curr Opin Mol Ther 2005; 7:493–501.

59. Iliev ME, Domig D, Wolf-Schnurrbursch U, et al. Intravitreal bevacizumab (Avastin) in the treatment of neovascular glaucoma. Am J Ophthalmol 2006; 142:1054–1056.

60. Mason JO 3rd, Albert MA Jr, Mays A, et al. Regression of neovascular iris vessels by intravitreal injection of bevacizumab. Retina 2006; 26:839–841.

61. Eichler W, Yafai Y, Wiedemann P, et al. Antineovascular agents in the treatment of eye diseases. Curr Pharm Des 2006; 12:2645–2660.

62. Dawson DW, Volpert OV, Gillis P, et al. Pigment epithelium-derived factor: a potent inhibitor of angiogenesis. Science 1999; 285:245–248.

63. Duh EJ, et al. Pigment epithelium derived factor suppresses ischemia-induced retinal neovascularization and VEGF-induced migration and growth. Invest Ophthalmol Vis Sci 2002; 43:821–829.

64. Campochiaro PA, Nguyen QD, Shah SM, et al. Adenoviral vector-delivered pigment epithelium-derived factor for neovascular age-related macular degeneration: results of a phase I clinical trial. Hum Gene Ther 2006; 17:167–176.

CHAPTER 35

Other Secondary Glaucomas

Jody Piltz-Seymour and Tara A Uhler

INTRODUCTION

Secondary glaucomas are the end result of a multitude of processes that ultimately impair trabecular outflow and cause elevated intraocular pressure (IOP). This chapter will cover those secondary glaucomas not otherwise addressed in prior chapters, including lens-induced open-angle glaucomas, glaucomas associated with disorders of the corneal endothelium, corticosteroid-induced glaucoma, as well as glaucomas associated with elevated episcleral venous pressure, vitreoretinal disorders, and epithelial and fibrous ingrowth.

LENS-INDUCED OPEN-ANGLE GLAUCOMAS

There are three main forms of lens-induced open angle glaucomas: phacolytic, phacoanaphylactic, and lens-particle glaucoma (Table 35.1). The mechanisms for the intraocular pressure elevation differs in these three diseases, but all ultimately result in obstruction of the trabecular meshwork with diminished outflow facility.

PHACOLYTIC GLAUCOMA

Etiology/pathogenesis Phacolytic glaucoma is an acute open-angle glaucoma that develops from leakage of lens proteins in an eye with a mature or hypermature cataract.[1] The lens capsule normally acts like a barrier against leakage of lenticular material. As lenses become mature, small microscopic defects can develop in the capsule, allowing release of high molecular weight proteins. These proteins impede outflow through the trabecular meshwork, causing an acute rise in intraocular pressure.[2] Outflow can be further compromised by obstruction of the trabecular meshwork by protein-laden macrophages.

Signs and symptoms While vision usually declines gradually as the cataract progresses, the intraocular pressure rise in phacolytic glaucoma typically develops acutely and is accompanied by pain and conjunctival injection. Examination reveals diffuse corneal edema, marked aqueous flare, and a mature white cataract or hypermature lens with small compact nucleus floating in liquefied cortex. Engorged macrophages may be visible as large cells in the anterior chamber and iridescent particles may also be visible in the aqueous. The clinical course may be indolent when the lens is dislocated into the vitreous.

Diagnosis The diagnosis of phacolytic glaucoma is based on the clinical presentation described above. A diagnostic paracentesis can be performed to demonstrate swollen macrophages, but frequently there is paucity of macrophages in the aspirate. Detection of macrophages may be enhanced by using a millipore filter and phase contrast microscopy.

Treatment Treatment of phacolytic glaucoma is aimed at lowering the pressure and quieting the eye with topical steroids in preparation for urgent cataract surgery. The use of a capsular stain such as Trypan blue can help facilitate capsulorrhexis in these mature cataracts. In most cases the glaucoma reverses rapidly after cataract removal.

TABLE 35.1 Lens-induced open-angle glaucomas	
TYPE	MECHANISM
Phacolytic glaucoma	Leakage of high molecular weight proteins through an intact lens capsule
Phacoanaphylactic glaucoma	Immune complex formation following sensitization to lens proteins resulting in a granulomatous uveitis
Lens-particle glaucoma	Trabecular obstruction from retained lens material and inflammatory cells

PHACOANAPHYLAXIS OR PHACOANTIGENIC UVEITIS

Etiology/pathogenesis Phacoanaphylactic or phacoantigenic uveitis is a rare severe granulomatous uveitis that develops after either traumatic or surgical lens disruption.[3,4] The term phacoanaphylaxis is a misnomer since this is not a true IgE-mediated anaphylactic response. Rather, phacoantigenic uveitis results from immune complex formation following sensitization to lens proteins and loss of normal tolerance to these lens proteins. Histopathology reveals a zonal granulomatous infiltrate surrounding the damaged lens.

Signs and symptoms The clinical onset of the uveitis may occur days to years after the initial insult. Patients demonstrate conjunctival hyperemia and corneal edema. The degree of uveitis may vary from mild to severe and may involve the vitreous. Hypopyon and keratic precipitates may be present. Retained lens material is evident.[3]

Intraocular pressure is often normal but may become elevated from a variety of mechanisms. Trabecular outflow may become compromised by inflammatory cells and high molecular weight proteins, or synechiae may develop leading to chronic angle closure or pupil-block angle closure.

Treatment Without removal of the lens material, topical steroids have little effect on the uveitis and may lead to steroid-induced IOP elevation. Surgery is required to remove all residual lens material including the lens capsule and intraocular lens. Pathologic evaluation of these specimens is crucial in making the diagnosis.

LENS-PARTICLE GLAUCOMA (RETAINED LENS FRAGMENT)

Etiology/pathogenesis Disruption of the lens capsule can lead to release of cortical and capsular material into the aqueous, obstructing trabecular outflow and resulting in lens-particle glaucoma. The inciting event may be cataract surgery, penetrating ocular trauma or Nd: YAG laser capsulotomy (Fig. 35.1).

Signs and symptoms After injury, cortical material accumulates in the anterior chamber and can be visualized as white fluffy debris. An inflammatory response may ensue, resulting in cell and flare. Intraocular pressure may rise as the trabecular meshwork becomes clogged by the lens particles and inflammatory debris.[2] Glaucoma can also develop from synechial angle closure or pupil block. Eyes with impaired outflow facility are more likely to develop elevated intraocular pressure from retained lens material.

Treatment Medical treatment should be initiated with aqueous suppressant and corticosteroids. If there is substantial retained cortical material, surgical removal will lead to more rapid control of the glaucoma and inflammation.

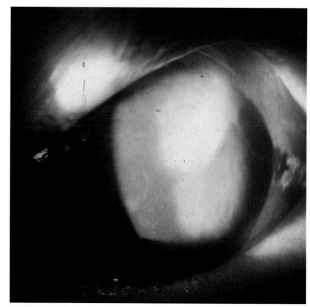

FIGURE 35.1 Retained lens fragment. The retained lens fragment causes an inflammatory response and obstruction of trabecular outflow.

GLAUCOMAS ASSOCIATED WITH DISORDERS OF THE CORNEAL ENDOTHELIUM

IRIDOCORNEAL ENDOTHELIAL SYNDROME

The iridocorneal endothelial syndrome (ICE) is a group of disorders characterized by abnormal physiology of the corneal endothelium, leading to varying degrees of progressive iris atrophy, corneal edema, and/or synechial angle closure.[5,6] ICE syndrome is more common in females, is clinically unilateral, and usually presents in the fourth to fifth decades of life. There is no consistent inheritance pattern.

There are three main variations of this disorder: progressive iris atrophy, Chandler's syndrome, and Cogan-Reese syndrome (Table 35.2). Chandler's syndrome accounts for half the cases of ICE syndrome; the other two entities each account for a quarter of cases.

Etiology/pathogenesis The common feature in the three variants of ICE is a hammered, silver/gray appearance to the corneal endothelial layer which is clearly evident on slit lamp examination.[7] Pleomorphism and polymegathism of endothelial cells can be demonstrated on specular microscopy. The abnormal endothelial cells proliferate and migrate over the anterior chamber angle and onto the iris surface, leading to peripheral anterior synechiae formation. Confocal microscopy can visualize 'epithelium-like' changes in the corneal endothelium even in the presence of corneal edema.[8,9]

A viral etiology for ICE has been postulated. Epstein-Barr virus has been detected serologically in patients with ICE.[10] More compelling was the detection of herpes simplex virus DNA in the corneal endothelium

TABLE 35.2 Iridocorneal endothelial syndrome

SYNDROME TYPE	SIGNS AND SYMPTOMS
Progressive iris atrophy	Corectopia, iris atrophy, iris hole formation, ectropion uveae, peripheral anterior synechiae
Chandler's syndrome	Corneal edema, decreased vision, pain
Cogan-Reese syndrome	Pedunculated iris outcroppings, peripheral anterior synechiae

of 16 out of 25 corneal specimens using polymerase chain reaction (PCR) analysis.[11]

Signs and symptoms Essential iris atrophy is characterized by corectopia, iris atrophy, iris hole formation, and ectropion uveae. The abnormal endothelial layer proliferates to cover the angle and iris. Contracture of this membrane leads to peripheral anterior synechiae, pupil distortion, and iris hole formation opposite the area of the peripheral anterior synechiae (PAS). Iris hole formation may also develop without corectopia and may be related to iris ischemia (Figs 35.2–35.4).

Corneal edema is the most common prominent feature of Chandler's syndrome. Patients frequently present with decreased vision and pain. Iris abnormalities are not typical. Corneal edema and blurred vision are often worse upon awakening in the early stage of the disease. Later in the disease, the corneal edema, decreased vision, and pain may persist throughout the day.

In Cogan-Reese syndrome, contracture of the proliferating endothelial membrane on the iris face forms multiple pedunculated outcroppings of normal iris tissue.

Cogan Reese has been called iris nevis syndrome since these artcroppings resemble small nevi on the iris surface. This name is a misnomer since the artcroppings consist of normal iris tissue, and are histologically unrelated to nevi.

Patients may have manifestations of more than one of these clinical entities (Fig. 35.5 and see Fig. 35.4).

Glaucoma develops in most eyes with progressive iris atrophy and Cogan-Reese syndrome, but may be less common with Chandler's syndrome. Glaucoma results from the proliferation of the endothelial membrane over the anterior chamber angle and from the subsequent PAS development. Intraocular pressure elevation does not correlate with the extent of the PAS. Uncontrolled glaucoma may worsen corneal edema and cause increased pain.

Treatment Treatment may be required for corneal edema and/or glaucoma. Corneal edema can be treated initially with hypertonic saline, contact lens, and IOP lowering, but corneal surgery may eventually be required.

Aqueous suppressants are the first-line therapy for IOP elevation in ICE syndrome. The effect of prostaglandin analogues is variable and laser trabeculoplasty is not helpful. It is common for filtering blebs to fail as the membrane proliferates through the sclerostomy,

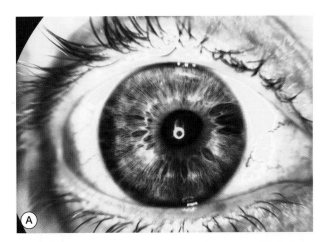

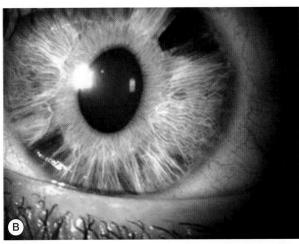

FIGURE 35.2 (A,B) Iridocorneal endothelial syndrome/essential iris atrophy. These two patients had early signs of essential iris atrophy with focal thinning of the iris stroma and minimal corectopia. (Fig. 35.2B courtesy of Stephen Orlin, MD.)

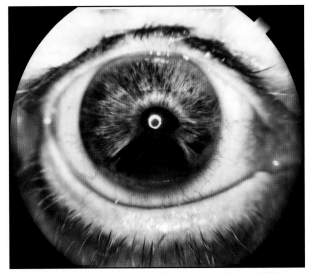

FIGURE 35.3 Iridocorneal endothelial syndrome/essential iris atrophy. The inferior iris has become stretched and thin, resulting in full-thickness atrophic holes (polycoria). Corectopia, which is often present at this stage, is absent in this eye.

421

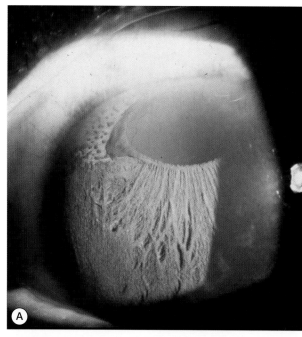

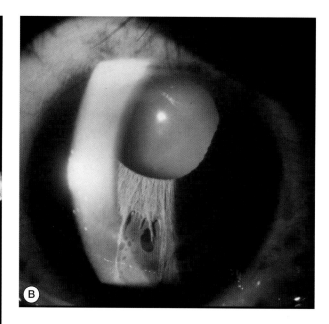

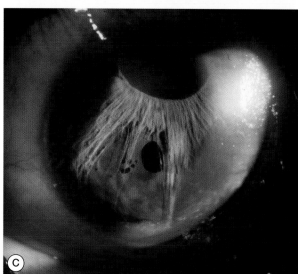

FIGURE 35.4 Iridocorneal endothelial syndrome. This eye demonstrates the classic features of progressive corectopia, polycoria, and ectropion uveae. Features of both essential iris atropy and Cogan-Reese syndrome are present. **(A)** 1983. Corectopia with iris nevi (*thin arrow*) and ectropion uveae (*short arrow*) seen superionasally. **(B)** 1985. Same eye 2 years later with progressive thinning of the iris stoma with iris hole formation (*arrow*). **(C)** 1992. Seven years later the iris has continued to thin (*short arrow*) with increased hole formation (*thin arrow*).

forming an impermeable layer on the inner bleb surface. Glaucoma drainage tubes can also be compromised by the membrane proliferation and some advocate using a longer tube in the anterior chamber or pars plana tube placement to minimize failure.

Differential diagnosis Iridocorneal endothelial syndrome is readily distinguished from Rieger's syndrome, which is a bilateral, dominantly inherited congenital disorder with nonprogressive iris findings.

POSTERIOR POLYMORPHOUS DYSTROPHY

Posterior polymorphous corneal dystrophy is a rare bilateral congenital progressive disorder in which the corneal endothelial layer takes on epithelial-like qualities with thickening of Descemet's membrane. It has an autosomal dominant mode of inheritance with variable expression.o

Signs and symptoms Slit lamp examination reveals small vesicular opacifications of the inner cornea that may form a band configuration or geographic lesions with posterior corneal haze. Visual acuity can be normal or compromised, depending on the extent of corneal involvement. Corneal involvement is bilateral but may be asymmetric. Occasionally, broad PAS, corectopia, and ectropion uveae may develop.[12]

Gonioscopy may reveal either an anterior iris insertion or frank PAS. Glaucoma develops in approximately 13% of patients with posterior polymorphous dystrophy as a result of membrane proliferation of the angle surface or angle closure from PAS.

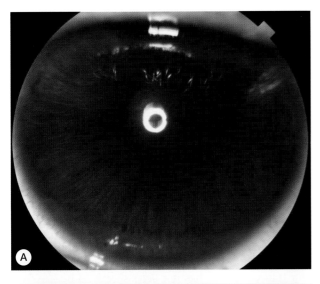

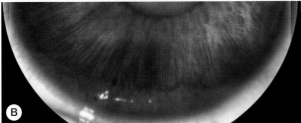

FIGURE 35.5 Iridocorneal endothelial syndrome/Cogan-Reese syndrome. **(A)** This patient presented with elevated pressure, a round central pupil, and a thickened, hammered silver appearance to the corneal endothelium. The glaucoma was unresponsive to medical therapy. Trabeculectomy failed, and the intraocular pressure was controlled with a glaucoma drainage tube. The iris became updrawn toward the tube and, over the next 8 years, iris changes consistent with Cogan-Reese (iris nevus syndrome) began to develop inferiorly. **(B)** Highlighted view of the inferior iris demonstrating the pedunculated iris outcropping. The name iris nevus syndrome is a misnomer, since the pedunculated areas are actually islands of normal iris formed by contracture of the proliferating endothelial-like membrane growing over the iris surface.

Treatment Treatment is similar to that of ICE syndrome with hypertonic saline and aqueous suppressants. Glaucoma and corneal surgery may be required.

CORTICOSTEROID-INDUCED OCULAR HYPERTENSION AND GLAUCOMA

Ocular hypertension secondary to systemic corticosteroids was first described over 50 years ago;[13] since then, it has been reported with topical, periocular, and inhaled corticosteroid therapy as well. Approximately one-third of patients treated with topical steroids exhibit an increase in IOP of 6–15 mmHg.[14] Understanding its prevalence, risk factors, and pathophysiology may help clinicians prevent, monitor, and treat any clinically significant rise in IOP and associated glaucoma.

TABLE 35.3 Risk factors for corticosteroid-induced ocular hypertension
POAG
Glaucoma suspect
First-degree relative with POAG
Previous steroid response
Age
Connective tissue disease
High myopia
Type 1 diabetes

RISK FACTORS

A number of predisposing risk factors for corticosteroid-induced ocular hypertension have been reported (Table 35.3). In particular, patients with primary open-angle glaucoma (POAG) or classified as glaucoma suspects are much more likely to exhibit a significant response to steroids.[15] Simply having a first-degree relative with POAG appears to increase a patient's risk.

Age is another significant risk factor. Older adults are more likely to demonstrate a steroid response than younger adults. However, as a class, children have been shown to be greater steroid responders than adults, with children 6 years of age or less exhibiting the greatest response.[16]

In addition, an increased risk of steroid response has been reported in patients, especially men, with connective tissue disease. Patients with type 1 diabetes and high myopia are also more likely to be steroid responders.

ETIOLOGY/PATHOGENESIS

Corticosteroid-induced ocular hypertension appears to be the result of increased resistance to aqueous outflow. The mechanism of this is not clearly understood but several studies have implicated glucocorticoid-induced changes in the trabecular meshwork and suggested a genetic predisposition.[17]

Glucocorticoid-induced changes Corticosteroids affect the trabecular meshwork by inducing microstructural changes, increasing deposition of extracellular material, and inhibiting protease and phagocytic activity. Morphological changes include thickened trabecular beams, decreased intertrabecular spaces, thickened juxtacanalicular tissues, and increased deposition of extracellular material such as glycosaminoglycan, elastin, and fibronectin. In addition, trabecular meshwork cultures treated with dexamethasone exhibit decreased levels of tissue plasminogen activator, stromelysin, and metalloproteinases as well as reduced arachidonic acid metabolism and phagocytic activity. These corticosteroid-induced changes may lead to both an increased accumulation and a decreased clearance of channel debris. The net effect is decreased facility of outflow, contributing to the observed ocular hypertensive response.

Genetics A genetic susceptibility to corticosteroid-induced ocular hypertension has been proposed and several genes have been shown to be upregulated in dexamethasone-treated trabecular meshwork cells. In particular, the myocilin gene (previously referred to as TIGR and identical to GCL1A) has generated interest because myocilin expression is induced by glucocorticoids in a manner which mirrors the timing and dosing of steroid administration required to raise IOP. However, the exact role of this gene is poorly understood, with experimental studies offering conflicting results. Further investigation of myocilin and other corticosteroid-induced gene products will be necessary to better understand the pathogenesis of and susceptibility to corticosteroid-induced hypertension.

INTRAOCULAR PRESSURE RESPONSE

The onset and magnitude of the ocular hypertensive effect are influenced by the type and potency of the corticosteroid, the frequency and mode of administration, and the susceptibility of the patient.

The greater the potency of the corticosteroid, the greater the risk of IOP elevation.[18] Some corticosteroid preparations, such as fluoromethalone, rimexolone, or loteprednol, are less likely to increase IOP than prednisolone or dexamethasone. However, weaker preparations or lower concentrations of stronger agents may still cause an increased IOP in susceptible individuals.

Increased IOP is more common with topical administration and typically occurs within 1 to 4 weeks. Although rare, a rapid rise in IOP has been described. Such acute responses appear to be more common in patients with a history of glaucoma or in children. Importantly, intravitreal injection of triamcinolone is becoming increasingly popular and has been associated with an acute elevation of IOP in approximately 50% of patients.[19,20] Elevated IOP is less common with systemic administration and typically occurs over weeks to years although a rapid response, particularly in children, has also been described.

After cessation of steroid therapy, resolution of steroid response typically mirrors the onset. Most commonly, the chronic steroid response resolves within 1 to 4 weeks after cessation of steroids. The rare, acute response may resolve in a few days.

TREATMENT

The management of clinically significant corticosteroid-induced IOP elevation and associated glaucoma is similar to that of primary open-angle glaucoma or ocular hypertension. Prevention and early detection are important. A glaucoma evaluation and baseline IOP measurement should be performed prior to the start of corticosteroid therapy. After initiating topical or periocular treatment, patients should have their pressure rechecked every 2 weeks for the first month, monthly for 2–3 months, and then every 3 to 6 months thereafter for long-term steroid therapy. Importantly, patients who receive a single dose of intravitreal triamcinolone should be monitored for several months since some patients have demonstrated significant increases in IOP more than 3 months after injection.[20,21] Patients taking systemic corticosteroids should have IOP measured at regular intervals.

Clinically significant ocular hypertension may be treated with topical ocular antihypertensives. Beta-blockers and carbonic anhydrase inhibitors are popular and effective choices. Use of prostaglandin analogues to control IOP increases have been shown to be as effective as cessation of corticosteroids. However, like α-agonists and miotics, prostaglandin analogues are relatively contraindicated in patients with uveitis or cystoid macular edema. Argon laser trabeculoplasty has not been shown to be effective. Trabeculectomy may be necessary in cases refractory to medical therapy.

If possible, once clinically significant corticosteroid-induced ocular hypertension or glaucoma is diagnosed, corticosteroid therapy should be discontinued. In patients who do not respond to medical therapy, surgical removal of depot steroids can be attempted. Cushing syndrome patients with corticosteroid-induced ocular hypertension generally demonstrate normalization of IOP after the corticosteroid-producing tumor or hyperplastic tissue is excised.

If topical antiinflammatory drugs are necessary, substituting less potent corticosteroid preparations or nonsteroidal antiinflammatory drugs may be helpful. Switching from a topical to systemic steroid may also diminish the ocular hypertensive effect.

For patients requiring systemic therapy, consultation with a physician who has experience with immunosuppressive agents may be useful.

In approximately 3% of cases, the elevation in IOP may not be reversible despite cessation of steroid use. This appears to be more likely in patients with a family history of glaucoma or chronic steroid use for several years. In these cases, management remains similar to that for chronic open-angle glaucoma.

SUMMARY

Although the mechanism of corticosteroid-induced ocular hypertension is incompletely understood, some risk factors and patterns of response have been identified. All patients receiving corticosteroid therapy should be monitored. Whenever possible, clinicians should prescribe the least potent steroid for the shortest period of time necessary to achieve therapeutic results. It may be prudent to avoid depot forms of steroid administration such as sub-Tenon's or intravitreal injections in high-risk individuals. If clinically significant corticosteroid-induced ocular hypertension occurs, used alternative antiinflammatory or immunosuppressive agents, IOP-lowering medications, and glaucoma surgery may be necessary.

ELEVATED EPISCLERAL VENOUS PRESSURE

There is little diurnal variation of episcleral venous pressure. Episcleral venous pressure has been shown to increase in the supine position and to be higher in older patients and in some patients with primary glaucoma, although the significance of this is unknown.[21,22] There are several conditions, however, in which episcleral venous pressure is pathologically elevated with a pronounced increase in IOP and the potential to cause secondary glaucomatous damage.

EFFECT ON INTRAOCULAR PRESSURE

To understand the effect of elevated episcleral venous pressure on IOP, it is useful to review the Goldmann equation: $P = (F/C) + Pe$. Intraocular pressure (P) depends upon: the rate of aqueous formation (F), which is normally 2–3 μL/min; the facility of outflow (C), which is normally 0.2–0.3 μL/min/mmHg; and the episcleral venous pressure (Pe), which is normally 8–10 mmHg. A commonly quoted rule of thumb is that for every millimeter rise in the episcleral venous pressure, there is approximately 1 mmHg rise in IOP. In reality, this relationship is not exactly one-to-one, but there is a direct effect of increased episcleral venous pressure on IOP.

Acutely, facility of outflow is not affected by increased episcleral venous pressure, and a normalization of episcleral venous pressure should result in normalization of IOP. However, with chronically increased episcleral venous pressure, outflow facility may be adversely affected and may not return to normal with normalization of episcleral venous pressure.

SIGNS AND SYMPTOMS

Although the clinical picture depends upon the cause, the most consistent features of elevated episcleral venous pressure are dilated and tortuous episcleral vessels and elevated intraocular pressure. Additional signs may include chemosis, proptosis, or orbital bruit. Increased ocular pulse amplitude may be observed during tonometry. Gonioscopy may reveal blood in Schlemm's canal.

ETIOLOGY/PATHOGENESIS

Causes of increased episcleral venous pressure can be divided into three categories: venous obstruction, arteriovenous abnormalities, and idiopathic.

Venous obstruction Causes of venous obstruction include: thyroid ophthalmopathy, superior vena cava syndrome, retrobulbar tumors, and cavernous sinus thrombosis.

Thyroid ophthalmopathy, or Graves disease, results from infiltration of the orbit, including extraocular muscles, by lymphocytes, mast cells, and plasma cells. Elevated episcleral venous pressure may occur in severe cases with marked proptosis and orbital congestion due to obstruction of venous flow.[23]

Superior vena cava syndrome occurs when lesions of the upper thorax obstruct venous return from the head. Associated signs includes exophthalmos, edema, cyanosis of the face and neck, and dilation of veins of the head, neck, chest, and upper extremities.

Other conditions which have been associated with obstruction of venous drainage and elevation of episcleral venous pressure include localized amyloidosis as well as retrobulbar tumors and cavernous sinus thrombosis.

Arteriovenous abnormalities Arteriovenous fistulas are the most common cause of ocular injection with increased IOP due to elevated episcleral venous pressure. Carotid–cavernous sinus fistulas may be divided into two types: traumatic and spontaneous.[24] Traumatic fistulas are the most common and are characterized by high flow through a communication between the internal carotid artery and surrounding cavernous sinus venous plexus. Shunting blood through this fistula increases blood flow and produces high orbital and episcleral venous pressure. In addition to dilated, tortuous episcleral veins, associated signs include pulsating exophthalmos, orbital bruit, restricted motility, and ocular ischemia.

The spontaneous type occurs more often in middle-aged to elderly females without a history of trauma. They are small and are typically characterized by a low flow indirect or dural communication low flow between small meningeal branches of the carotid arteries with the venous circulation of the cavernous sinus or an adjacent dural vein that connects with the cavernous sinus. Mixing of arterial and venous blood reduces arterial pressure and increases orbital and episcleral venous pressure. Signs and symptoms are similar but milder low flow fistulas cause than those associated with high-flow fistulas; prominent episcleral and conjunctival vessels but minimal proptosis and no pulsations or bruit. Many low flow fistulas resolve spontaneously without intervention (Fig. 35.6).[25]

Orbital varices may also cause increased episcleral venous pressure. Varices usually present with intermittent proptosis exacerbated by Valsalva maneuvers, and episcleral venous pressure is usually normal between episodes. As a result, glaucoma is uncommon and conservative management with medications, if necessary, is usually sufficient.[26]

Elevated episcleral venous pressure due to episcleral hemangiomas and arteriovenous fistulas is thought to be one mechanism of IOP elevation in Sturge-Weber syndrome. This syndrome is reviewed in more detail in Chapter 28.

Idiopathic Several cases of idiopathic dilated episcleral veins with open-angle glaucoma and without proptosis or a known cause of venous congestion have been described (Table 35.4).[27] The observed injection is less pronounced without arterialization of vessels described in arteriovenous fistulas. The condition has been reported in both younger and older patients and within a family. Proposed mechanisms have included localized venous obstruction

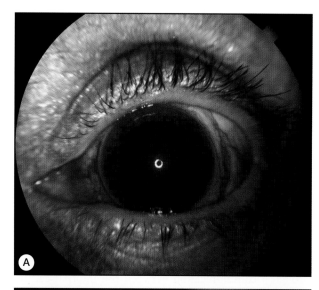

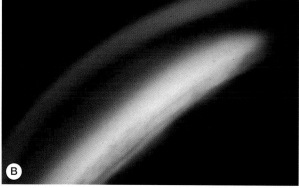

FIGURE 35.6 Elevated episcleral venous pressure resulting from a low-flow dural sinus fistula. **(A)** Note the prominent episcleral and conjunctival vessels without proptosis. **(B)** There is reflux of blood in Schlemm's canal viewed on gonioscopy.

TABLE 35.4 Causes of increased episcleral venous pressure
Venous obstruction
Thyroid ophthalmopathy
Superior vena cava syndrome
Retrobulbar tumors
Cavernous sinus thrombosis
Arteriovenous abnormalities
Carotid–cavernous sinus fistula
Orbital varix
Sturge-Weber syndrome
Idiopathic

at the region of the extraocular muscles, congenital anomaly of the vasculature, and a familial predisposition.

Orbital color Doppler imaging may be useful in distinguishing patients with idiopathic dilated episcleral veins from those with fistulas who may need invasive catheter angiography. In patients with fistulas, a characteristic reversal of blood flow in a dilated superior ophthalmic vein is observed; in a patient with idiopathic dilated episcleral veins, orbital color Doppler imaging demonstrated normal retrograde flow through a superior ophthalmic vein of normal caliber.[28]

MECHANISM

Elevated episcleral venous pressure may cause glaucoma through several mechanisms: direct effect on IOP, reduced outflow facility, angle closure, and neovascular glaucoma.

Acutely, elevated episcleral venous pressure causes glaucoma through a direct, though often nonlinear, effect on the Goldmann equation. Initially, outflow facility is typically normal; however, with chronic venous pressure elevation, outflow may decrease and fail to recover even after venous pressure is normalized. This explains why drugs which enhance outflow are not useful in cases of acute episcleral venous elevation, but may be beneficial in chronic cases when IOP fails to normalize after the episcleral venous pressure normalizes.

Both acute angle closure and neovascular glaucoma have been reported with elevated episcleral venous pressure in the setting of arteriovenous abnormalities. Angle closure is associated with venous stasis in the vortex veins with subsequent choroidal detachment and anterior displacement of the lens–iris diaphragm. Decreased arterial flow such as that observed with carotid–cavernous sinus fistulas may cause ocular ischemia and neovascularization. Neovascular glaucoma has also been reported as a complication of attempted superior ophthalmic vein embolization of a carotid–cavernous sinus fistula.[29]

TREATMENT

Ideally, management of ocular hypertension or glaucoma associated with elevated episcleral venous pressure should include treatment of the underlying cause such as thyroid ophthalmopathy, superior vena cava syndrome, retrobulbar tumors, or cavernous sinus thrombosis. Often only short-term control of IOP is required and achievable with medications. For example, low-flow carotid–cavernous fistulas may resolve spontaneously or close after diagnostic angiography. In other cases, however, treatment of the underlying cause may not be possible; for example, embolization of high-flow carotid–cavernous fistulas is risky and may be unsuccessful.

If medical therapy is attempted, aqueous suppressants including β-blockers, carbonic anhydrase inhibitors, and α-agonists are the most effective drugs. As predicted by the Goldmann equation, trabeculoplasty or drugs which affect the outflow pathway are not as effective. However, in chronic cases where outflow facility may be impaired, drugs which improve outflow may have a role.

If the underlying cause cannot be eliminated and IOP remains uncontrolled with medications, it may be necessary to consider glaucoma surgery or, if the eye has poor visual potential, a cyclodestructive procedure. The goal is often to simply normalize IOP and not achieve an extremely low pressure. Certain complications are more likely to occur in the setting of elevated episcleral venous pressure: hypotony, choroidal effusion, suprachoroidal hemorrhage, and flat anterior chamber. Consideration should be given to preoperative mannitol, prophylactic sclerotomies, and intracameral viscoelastic. With a guarded filtration surgery, scleral flap sutures may be preplaced before entering the anterior chamber. To further reduce the risk of hypotony, moderately tight flap sutures may be placed with the plan to pull releasable sutures or perform suture lysis later. Antifibrotic agents should be used judiciously to avoid extremely low IOP. If a tube shunt is placed, a valved device with an external ligation or a two-stage procedure may be considered.

SUMMARY

Elevated episcleral venous pressure is an important cause of ocular hypertension and associated glaucoma. It should be considered in the differential diagnosis of ocular injection with elevated IOP. Causes include venous obstruction, arteriovenous abnormalities, and idiopathic factors. Initial management should be directed at treating the underlying cause when possible and controlling IOP with aqueous suppressants. If glaucoma surgery is necessary, efforts to reduce the risk of hypotony, choroidal effusion, suprachoroidal hemorrhage, and flat anterior chamber should be maximized.

VITREORETINAL AND RETINAL DISORDERS

ANGLE-CLOSURE MECHANISMS

Retinal and vitreoretinal disorders can lead to both open-angle and angle-closure glaucoma. Angle closure in the pediatric population can be caused by retinopathy of prematurity, familial exudative vitreoretinopathy, Coats' disease and other congenital malformations and inflammatory conditions. Nanophthalmos can cause angle closure from pupil block or uveal effusion. Other causes of uveal expansion, such as Topamax sensitivity, AIDS, choroidal detachments, choroidal hemorrhage, or central retinal vein occlusion, can lead to angle closure by pushing the lens–iris diaphragm anteriorly. Retinal ischemia from diabetes, central retinal vein occlusion, carotid insufficiency, and other mechanisms can lead to neovascular glaucoma. These angle-closure entities are discussed elsewhere in this text (see Ch. 32).

OPEN-ANGLE MECHANISMS

Stickler's syndrome Stickler's syndrome, or hereditary arthro-ophthalmopathy, is an autosomal dominant connective tissue disease with ocular, aural, facial, and skeletal manifestations.[30] A genetic defect in collagen synthesis has been identified. The most prominent ocular findings in Stickler's syndrome are high myopia, vitreoretinal degeneration, and retinal detachment.[31] The myopia is congenital and progressive throughout childhood and usually exceeds 10 diopters. The majority of patients with Stickler's develop retinal detachments in one or both eyes. Other common ocular findings include presenile cataracts, open-angle glaucoma, strabismus, and amblyopia.

Glaucoma in patients with Stickler's syndrome may be difficult to monitor. Optic discs are often tilted and anomalous. Visual fields may be influenced by the high refractive error, amblyopia, lens changes, and retinal degenerations. Systemic findings include hyperextendible and lax joints, neurosensory hearing loss, and orofacial/dental anomalies. Progressive arthritis commonly develops. Miotic therapy should be avoided.

Ghost-cell glaucoma Degenerating red blood cells sequestered in the vitreous may form rigid 'ghost' cells. When released into the aqueous, these ghost cells occlude the trabecular meshwork and elevate the intraocular pressure. Ghost-cell glaucoma develops most commonly after vitreous hemorrhage (Fig. 35.7) (see Ch. 36).

Schwartz syndrome Rhegmatogenous retinal detachments typically produce a moderate reduction in

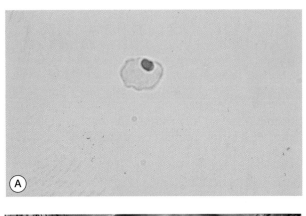

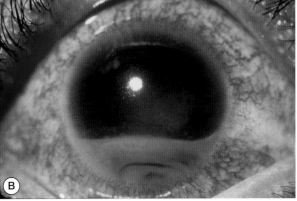

FIGURE 35.7 Ghost cell. **(A)** Light microscopy of degenerated red blood cell in aqueous aspirate of patient with ghost-cell glaucoma. **(B)** Classic khaki-colored hyphema in an eye with ghost-cell glaucoma. The hyphema is composed of the tan ghost cells.

intraocular pressure. Occasionally, patients with retinal detachment without underlying glaucoma develop a form of open-angle glaucoma called Schwartz syndrome.[32] In Schwartz syndrome, photoreceptor outer segments are released through a retinal break into the anterior chamber. These pigmented cells obstruct the trabecular meshwork and lead to increased intraocular pressure.[33] The glaucoma of Schwartz syndrome typically resolves after the retinal detachment is repaired.

GLAUCOMA ASSOCIATED WITH RETINAL SURGERY

Increased intraocular pressure is one of the most common postoperative complications of many vitreoretinal procedures. There are several mechanisms for these pressure elevations, including corticosteroid-induced ocular hypertension, secondary angle closure, and increased episcleral venous pressure.

As described previously, intravitreal injections of triamcinolone acetate may be associated with corticosteroid-induced ocular hypertension. As therapeutic indications for this procedure continue to expand, intravitreal triamcinolone will become increasingly more common. Almost half of patients experience a significant rise in IOP which may not manifest for several months after injection.[19,20]

Scleral buckling procedures, especially with encircling bands, may shallow the anterior chamber and cause angle closure. This is usually associated with congestion and swelling of the ciliary body due to a temporary interference by the scleral buckle with venous drainage.[34] Choroidal effusion and anterior rotation of the ciliary body usually resolves over days to weeks. Temporary medical management includes antiinflammatory agents, cycloplegics, and aqueous suppressants. If medical therapy is unsuccessful, drainage of suprachoroidal fluid or, possibly, adjustment of the buckle may be necessary.

Injection of air, expansile gases, or silicone oil may cause increased IOP and secondary angle closure. Following pneumatic retinopexy, an immediate, temporary increase in IOP is common and may collapse the central retinal artery; however, the IOP usually drops within 1 hour.

Significantly elevated IOP has been reported in approximately 50% of patients following pars plana vitrectomy with silicone oil injection. Silicone oil used in the treatment of complicated retinal detachments can cause both open- and closed-angle glaucoma. Tamponade of the pupil can result in papillary-block angle closure, which can be prevented or treated with inferior iridectomy (Fig. 35.8). If the silicone oil droplets become dispersed in the aqueous, the droplets can clog the trabecular meshwork outflow pathways and cause secondary open-angle glaucoma. If prophylactic placement of inferior iridotomies is not successful and IOP cannot be controlled medically, surgical management with glaucoma drainage devices, cyclodestructive procedures, or removal of silicone oil may be necessary.[35]

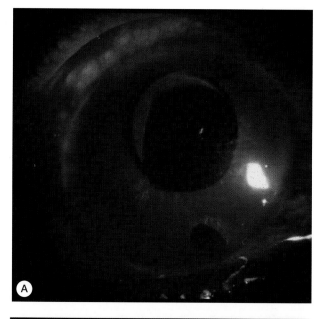

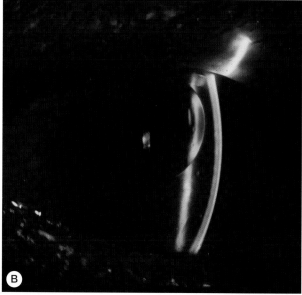

FIGURE 35.8 (A) Silicone oil causing pupillary block. Angle closure was prevented by a prophylactically placed inferior iridotomy. **(B)** Slit view of silicone oil prolapsed through the pupil.

The mechanism for increased IOP after panretinal photocoagulation is not clearly understood and has been observed even with an open angle. It has also been associated with development of both early and late angle closure secondary to thickening and anterior rotation of the ciliary body. This form of angle closure is generally self-limited, requiring temporary medical management with topical corticosteroids, cycloplegic agents, and aqueous suppressants.

EPITHELIAL AND FIBROUS INGROWTH

EPITHELIAL INGROWTH

Epithelial ingrowth is a rare but devastating complication of anterior segment surgery or trauma. It is more likely to develop after trauma, penetrating keratoplasty, or complicated surgery, particularly if there is suboptimal wound construction or incarceration of vitreous, lens material, iris, or conjunctiva in the operative wound.[36] With the introduction of microsurgical techniques and improved wound design, the incidence of epithelial ingrowth has markedly decreased. However, cases of epithelial ingrowth have been reported after sutureless cataract surgery, which may have unstable wounds in the immediate postoperative period.[37]

Most cases of epithelial ingrowth present within 1 year of surgery. Eyes are inflamed with conjunctival injection; wound gape and a positive Seidel test may be apparent. A posterior corneal membrane extending from the wound is demarcated by a gray line, which is the leading edge of the proliferating epithelial sheet. Corneal edema may overly the membrane and keratic precipitates are typically absent. There may be vascularization of the deep corneal stroma in 50% of cases. The epithelial sheet grows over the anterior chamber angle, resulting in PAS formation and necrosis of the trabecular meshwork. A fistula may cause hypotony, or glaucoma may develop from pupil block, inflammation, or steroid use. The membrane rarely extends more than halfway down the cornea, but it rapidly grows over the iris and ciliary body and structures of the posterior chamber (Fig. 35.9). The pupil may become distorted with ectropion uveae formation.[38]

Histology reveals a multilayered, nonkeratinized, stratified squamous epithelial membrane thickest at the leading edge. Argon laser photocoagulation can aid in the diagnosis of epithelial ingrowth. When the iris is treated with argon laser (100 mW, 500 μm for 0.1 seconds), a sharply demarcated burn forms on normal iris, while a fluffy white burn forms in the areas where the membrane covers the iris.[39]

Epithelium can also proliferate in the anterior chamber as an inclusion cyst connected to the operative or traumatic wound (Fig. 35.10). These cysts may have a relatively benign course or may grow rapidly, occluding the visual axis, or cause inflammation and glaucoma. Surgical intervention is avoided if possible, since the proliferation often recurs as the more aggressive sheet-like epithelial ingrowth. A case of successful treatment of an epithelial inclusion cyst with needle aspiration and intralesional mitomycin C injection has recently been reported.[40]

The prognosis for eyes with epithelial ingrowth is very poor. Surgical intervention includes delineating the extent of the iris membrane with argon laser, removal of involved ocular structures, an anterior vitrectomy, and fistula repair. Air is placed in the anterior segment and cryotherapy is applied. Success rates are variable and prognosis for good vision is guarded at best.

FIBROUS INGROWTH

The same factors that predispose to epithelial ingrowth can lead to fibrous ingrowth. Fibrous ingrowth occurs

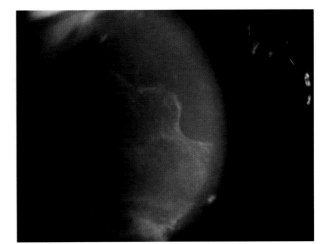

FIGURE 35.9 Epithelial ingrowth. An epithelial membrane is proliferating as a sheet growing over the corneal endothelium. The leading edge of the sheet is demarcated by a gray line. The membrane rarely grows more than halfway down the cornea, but grows rapidly over the iris and anterior chamber angle. (Courtesy of Stephen Orlin, MD.)

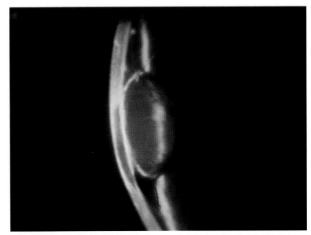

FIGURE 35.10 Epithelial inclusion cyst. This epithelial inclusion cyst remained stable long term and was followed without surgical intervention. (Courtesy of Stephen Orlin, MD.)

more commonly after penetrating keratoplasty than from cataract surgery.[41] Typically, a pale gray retrocorneal membrane extends down from the penetrating wound. The membrane may proliferate over the drainage angle and onto the iris surface.

The clinical course for fibrous ingrowth is more variable than for epithelial ingrowth. Some cases of fibrous ingrowth are self-limited and spontaneously regress, while others develop extensive anterior segment fibrosis with severe glaucoma. In mild cases, treatment is aimed at observation and medical therapy for glaucoma, corneal edema, and inflammation. Surgical intervention can be attempted for more severe cases but prognosis is poor.

REFERENCES

1. Flocks M, Littwin CS, Zimmerman LE. Phacolytic glaucoma: a clinicopathological study of one hundred thirty-eight cases of glaucoma associated with hypermature cataract. Arch Ophthalmol 1955; 54:37.

2. Epstein DL, Jedziniak JA, Grant WM. Obstruction of aqueous outflow by lens particles and by heavy molecular weight soluble lens proteins. Invest Ophthalmol Vis Sci 1978; 17:272.

3. Marak GE. Phacoanaphylactic endophthalmitis. Surv Ophthalmol 1992; 36:325.

4. Riise P. Endophthalmitis phacoanaphylactica. Am J Ophthalmol 1965; 60:911.

5. Campbell DG, Shields MB, Smith TR. The corneal endothelium and the spectrum of essential iris atrophy. Am J Ophthalmol 1978; 86:317.

6. Shields MB. Progressive essential iris atrophy, Chandler's syndrome, and the iris nevus (Cogan-Reese) syndrome: a spectrum of disease. Surv Ophthalmol 1979; 24:3.

7. Eagle RC Jr, Font RL, Yanoff M, et al. Proliferative endotheliopathy with iris abnormalities: the iridocorneal endothelial syndrome. Arch Ophthalmol 1979; 97:2104–2111.

8. Garibaldi DC, Schein OD, Jun A. Features of the iridocorneal endothelial syndrome on confocal microscopy. Cornea 2005; 24:349–351.

9. Sheppard JD, Lattanzio FA, Williams PB, et al. Confocal microscopy used as the definitive, early diagnostic method in Chandler syndrome. Cornea 2005; 24:227–229.

10. Tsai CS, Ritch R, Straus SE, Peny HD, Hscih FY. Antibodies to Epstein-Barr virus in iridocorneal endothelial syndrome. Arch Ophthalmol 1990; 108:1572–1576.

11. Alvarado JA, Underwood JL, Green WR, et al. Detection of herpes simplex viral DNA in the iridocorneal endothelial syndrome. Arch Ophthalmol 1994; 112:1601–1609.

12. Krachmer JH. Posterior polymorphous corneal dystrophy: a disease characterized by epithelial dystrophy. Am J Ophthalmol 1983; 95:143.

13. McLean JM. Use of ACTH and cortisone. Trans Am Ophthalmol Soc 1950; 48:293–296.

14. Becker B, Hahn KA. Topical corticosteroids and heredity in primary open-angle glaucoma. Am J Ophthalmol 1964; 57:543–551.

15. Armaly MF. Effect of corticosteroids on intraocular pressure and fluid dynamics: II. The effect of dexamethasone on the glaucomatous eye. Arch Ophthalmol 1963; 70:492–499.

16. Lam DSC, Fan DSP, Ng JSK, et al. Ocular hypertensive and anti-inflammatory responses to different dosages of topical dexamethasone in children: a randomized trial. Clin Exp Ophthalmol 2005; 33:252–258.

17. Kersey JP, Broadway DC. Corticosteroid-induced glaucoma: a review of the literature. Eye 2006; 20:407–416.

18. Cantrill HL, Palmberg P, Zink HA, et al. Comparison of in vitro potency of corticosteroids with ability to raise intraocular pressure. Am J Ophthalmol 1975; 79:1012–1017.

19. Jonas JB, Degenrigh RF, Kreissig I, et al. Intraocular pressure elevation after intravitreal triamcinolone acetonide injection. Ophthalmology 2005; 112:593–598.

20. Smithen LM, Ober MD, Marana L, et al. Intravitreal triamcinolone acetonide and intraocular pressure. Am J Ophthalmol 2004; 138:740–743.

21. Selbach JM, Posielek K, Steuhl KP, et al. Episcleral venous pressure in untreated primary open-angle and normal-tension glaucoma. Ophthalmologica 2005; 219(6):357–361.

22. Sultan M, Blondeau P. Episcleral venous pressure in younger and older subjects in the sitting and supine positions. J Glaucoma 2003; 12(4):370–373.

23. Dev S, Damji KF, DeBacker CM, et al. Decrease in intraocular pressure after orbital decompression for thyroid orbitopathy. Can J Ophthalmol 1998; 33(6):314–319.

24. Keltner JL, Satterfield D, Dublin AB, et al. Dural and carotid cavernous sinus fistulas. Diagnosis, management, and complications. Ophthalmology 1987; 94:1585–1600.

25. Goldberg RA, Goldey SH, Duckwiler G, et al. Management of cavernous sinus–dural fistulas. Indications and techniques for primary embolization via the superior ophthalmic vein. Arch Ophthalmol 1996; 114(6):707–714.

26. Kollarits CR, Gasterland D, Di Chiro G, et al. Management of a patient with orbital varices, visual loss, and ipsilateral glaucoma. Ophthalmic Surg 1977; 8:54–62.

27. Minas TF, Podos SM. Familial glaucoma associated with elevated episcleral venous pressure. Arch Ophthalmol 1968; 80:202–208.

28. Foroozan R, Buono LM, Savino PJ, et al. Idiopathic dilated episcleral veins and increased intraocular pressure. Br J Ophthalmol 2003; 87(5):652–654.

29. Gupta N, Kikkawa DO, Levi L, et al. Severe vision loss and neovascular glaucoma complicating superior ophthalmic vein approach to carotid–cavernous sinus fistula. Am J Ophthalmol 1997; 124(6):853–855.

30. Stickler GB, Belau PG, Forell FJ, et al. Hereditary progressive arthro-ophthalmology. Mayo Clinic Proc 1965; 40:433–455.

31. Blair NP, Albert DM, Liberfarb RM, Hirose T. Hereditary progressive arthro-ophthalmology of Stickler. Am J Ophthalmol 1979; 88:876–888.

32. Schwartz A. Chronic open angle glaucoma secondary to rhegmatogenous retinal detachment. Am J Ophthalmol 1973; 75:205.

33. Matsuo N, Takabatake M, Ueno H, Nakayama T, Matsuo T. Photoreceptor outer segments in the aqueous humor in rhegmatogenous retinal detachment. Am J Ophthalmol 1986; 101:673–679.

34. Perez RN, Phelps CD, Burton TC. Angle-closure glaucoma following scleral buckling operations. Trans Sect Ophthalmol Am Acad Ophthalmol Otolaryngol 1976; 81(2):247–252.

35. Nguyen QH, Lloyd MA, Huer DK, et al. Incidence and management of glaucoma after intravitreal silicone oil injection for complicated retinal detachments. Ophthamology 1992; 99:1520–1526.

36. Bangert A, Bialisiewicz AA, Endglemann K, et al. Intraocular epithelial downgrowth – report on 14 cases from 1986 to 2000. Klin Monatsbl Augenheilkd 2004; 221:197–203.

37. Holliday JN, Buller CR, Bourne WM. Specular microscopy and fluorophotometry in the diagnosis of epithelial downgrowth after a sutureless cataract operation. Am J Ophthalmol 1993; 116:238.

38. Weiner MJ, Trentawite J, Pon DM, Albert DM. Epithelial downgrowth: a 30 year clinicopathological review. Br J Ophthalmol 1989; 73:611.

39. Stark WJ, Michels RG, Maumenee AE, Cupples H. Surgical management of epithelial ingrowth. Am J Ophthalmol 1978; 85:772–780.

40. Yu CS, Chiu SI, Tse RK. Treatment of cystic epithelial downgrowth with intralesional administration of mitomycin C. Cornea 2005; 24:884–886.

41. Kurz GH, D'Amico RA. Histopathology of corneal graft failures. Am J Ophthalmol 1968; 66:184.

CHAPTER 36

Post-Traumatic Glaucoma

Sheila Bazzaz, L Jay Katz, and Jonathan S Myers

INTRODUCTION

Ocular trauma is a leading cause of ocular morbidity with early- and late-onset complications that may affect the final visual outcome. Trauma-related glaucoma is a potentially devastating complication that may present acutely or develop later on in an individual's lifetime. Thorough evaluation of the anterior segment as well as careful follow-up is necessary to detect the predilection for glaucoma and to initiate management. The complications from elevated intraocular pressure after trauma are usually preventable if management is initiated appropriately.

PREVALENCE AND INCIDENCE

Ocular trauma is not uncommon and frequently results in hospitalization. In a survey of hospital discharge data between 1984 and 1987 the average annual rate of principal diagnosis of ocular trauma was 13.2 per 100 000.[1] Of these patients 40% were diagnosed with primary contusion of the eyeball, adnexa or orbital fracture. Most ocular trauma patients are young, typically less than 30 years of age.[2–4] Children represent 27–48% of the total number of patients with ocular trauma.[3,4] Males are more likely to sustain an ocular injury than females: the male to female ratio ranges from 3.4:1 to 13.2:1.[1,3,5]

The circumstances that lead to ocular trauma vary considerably and are influenced by numerous factors. The age of the patient is associated with the environmental cause of injury, whether it is at play in children; versus sports or assault in young adults; versus occupational and domestic accidents being most prevalent in older adults.[6] Historically, most accidents occurred in the workplace, but there has been an increase in ocular injuries associated with leisure activities, motor vehicle accidents, and violent behavior. Geographic, socioeconomic, and cultural influences factor into the etiology of ocular trauma. In Great Britain,[4,7] assault accounts for only 1–21% of ocular injuries, whereas in Los Angeles County, California, it accounts for 41%.[6] Patients from lower socioeconomic groups have a higher incidence and severity of ocular trauma. Another cause of ocular trauma with a relatively recent increase in prevalence is air bag injury related to motor vehicle accidents.[8]

NONPENETRATING TRAUMA

Contusion trauma to the anterior segment results in physiologic alterations to various structures. Campbell[9] described the seven rings of anterior segment tissue that can become damaged by ocular contusion injury as the anterior–posterior forces are translated into an equatorial stretching: (1) sphincter pupillae, resulting in an irregular pupil with decreased light reaction or a traumatic mydriasis; (2) iris base, resulting in iridodialysis; (3) anterior ciliary body, resulting in a tear in the ciliary body muscles or angle recession; (4) attachment of the ciliary body muscle fibers to the scleral spur, resulting in a cyclodialysis cleft; (5) trabecular meshwork, tear in the anterior portion of the meshwork; (6) zonular attachments, resulting in subluxation or dislocation of the lens; and (7) attachment of the retina at the ora serrata, resulting in a retinal dialysis and detachment. All of these possible injuries present an acute or chronic cause of elevated intraocular pressure and glaucoma.

Blunt trauma initially indents and stretches the globe, resulting in a distortion of the normal anatomy. This compression of the eye elevates the pressure of the anterior chamber, which leads to a posterior displacement of the lens–iris diaphragm. The resultant posterior movement leads to tearing and distortion of the highly vascularized ciliary body and iris. Bleeding of the ciliary body vessels eventually stops, secondary to the elevated intraocular pressure, vasospasm of the ciliary body vessels, and clot formation. The clot reaches maximum organization in approximately 4 to 7 days. The clot is then removed from the anterior chamber via the fibrinolytic system. The blood and breakdown products are subsequently removed via the trabecular meshwork.

CLINICAL FINDINGS

Hyphema The anterior segment of the eye is the most commonly injured after ocular trauma, with hyphema being the most common complication (see also Ch. 51).

Clinically, hyphema is defined as red blood cells circulating in the anterior chamber (Fig. 36.1). The incidence of hyphema with blunt trauma varies from 6% reported in a pediatric population,[4] up to 55.2% in a survey of penetrating injuries caused by assault.[10] Sports-related injuries and assault account for the large majority of ocular trauma resulting in hyphema. Typically, this is seen in young male patients.

It is important to document the extent of hemorrhage within the anterior chamber. One useful technique for longitudinal monitoring is measurement of the height of the hyphema at the slit lamp. Another method is to grade the amount of blood within the anterior chamber. Grade I is less than one-third filling of the anterior chamber, grade II is one-third to one-half of the anterior chamber, and grade III is one-half to near total filling of the anterior chamber. A grade IV hyphema is a complete filling of the anterior chamber. It is important to distinguish between a total hyphema with bright red blood and an *eight-ball hyphema* which is characterized by dark red-black blood. The complete filling of the anterior chamber impairs the aqueous circulation, leading to a decreased oxygen concentration in the anterior chamber and the black appearance of the clot. An eight-ball hyphema is often associated with a dumbbell-shaped clot that leads to pupillary block and secondary angle-closure glaucoma.

Complications If the hyphema persists longer than 7 days there may be: (1) damage to the trabecular meshwork inhibiting outflow; (2) uveitis; (3) a vitreous hemorrhage with spillover of red blood cells into the anterior chamber; or (4) possible rebleeding into the anterior chamber. Rebleeding is one of the most common complications of hyphema (Fig. 36.2). The prevalence varies from 3.5% to 38%.[11] As the initial clot begins to retract and lyse from day 2 to day 5, the originally injured vessels may bleed again. Patients with an increased risk of rebleed include: those with ocular hypotony[12] or elevated intraocular pressure, a 50% or greater hyphema,[13] systemic hypertension,[14] use of aspirin,[15] black patients,[16] and those from urban populations. In general, the recurrent hemorrhage into the anterior chamber is more severe and often leads to glaucoma, corneal blood staining, and synechiae.

The visual prognosis varies in the literature regarding patients with a rebleed after a traumatic hyphema. The final visual acuity of 13 patients with rebleed was not worse compared to patients that did not rebleed in a retrospective review of 314 patients with hyphemas.[7] This finding was supported by another retrospective review where six of the 119 cases of traumatic hyphema developed rebleed without any adverse impact on visual prognosis.[11] All of these studies attributed the diminished visual acuity to retinal pathology. One prospective study of 238 patients with traumatic hyphema found a statistically significant decline in visual acuity after traumatic hyphema.[17]

Sickle cell anemia Special consideration should be given in patients who may be at risk for sickle cell anemia. This hereditary condition causes normal

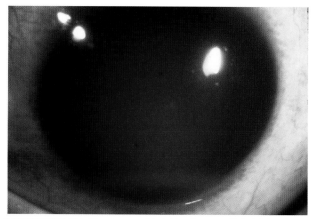

FIGURE 36.1 Total hyphema. A total hyphema with bright red blood filling the anterior chamber after blunt ocular trauma.

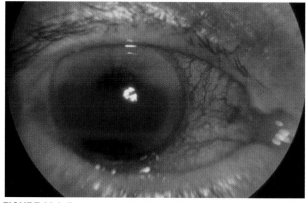

FIGURE 36.2 Recurrent hemorrhage. Recurrent hemorrhage into the anterior chamber demonstrated by fresh red blood layered above the darker clot.

red blood cells to become deformed and rigid, with a slightly decreased oxygen concentration. These sickled cells, when present in the anterior chamber, clog the trabecular meshwork and mechanically impede outflow of aqueous. As the intraocular pressure rises, further hypoxia develops and further sickling occurs. This condition is more common in the black population, but is also found in Hispanic patients or any patient with a positive family history of blood dyscrasias. Therefore, a careful history and sickle cell prep should be sent on all patients who may be at risk. It is important to note that patients with sickle cell disease and those with the trait are at risk for red blood cell sickling during hypoxia. Sickle cell trait affects approximately 10% of the black population. Nasrullah and Kerr[18] described 99 children with hyphema, 13 of whom had sickle cell trait. Eleven of the sickle cell patients had elevated intraocular pressure, with six of those patients requiring anterior chamber washout to control the intraocular pressure. Sickle cell disease patients are also at increased risk for vaso-occlusive events due to the sickling, which may compromise blood flow to the optic nerve at even mildly elevated intraocular pressures.

Angle recession Blunt ocular trauma imparts shearing forces upon the globe with the potential tearing of multiple structures within the anterior chamber. In many patients with a hyphema, once the hemorrhage has cleared, visualization of the angle reveals ruptures within various structures. The most common of these is angle recession, which is clinically diagnosed as an irregularly widened ciliary body band on gonioscopy (Fig. 36.3). Histologically, this represents a separation between the longitudinal and circular muscle fibers of the ciliary body (Fig. 36.4). Angle recession is reported to occur in 60–94% of eyes with a traumatic hyphema.[19–21] In one population-based glaucoma survey, angle recession was noted on gonioscopy in 14.8%, of which 5.5% of those individuals had glaucoma.[22] With angle recession the intraocular pressure may be elevated, but usually not in the immediate post-injury period. Additionally, patients with angle recession have a predisposition to chronic open-angle glaucoma and steroid-response glaucoma.[20] One study demonstrated that patients with glaucoma secondary to angle recession appear to have at least a 50% chance of developing open-angle glaucoma in the nontraumatized fellow eyes.[23]

Additional injuries to the angle include: iridodialysis, a tear in the root of the iris, and cyclodialysis, which is a separation of the ciliary body from its insertion at the scleral spur. Anatomically, a cyclodialysis creates a communication between the anterior chamber and the suprachorioidal space, which theoretically increases uveoscleral outflow. A very low pressure may be present in the initial post-injury period. Historically, it was thought that the cyclodialysis itself was the cause of the lower intraocular pressure, but studies have shown that the reduced aqueous humor flow in an eye with acute cyclodialysis is due to the concomitant inflammation rather than the cyclodialysis itself.[24] If the cyclodialysis cleft suddenly closes, the intraocular pressure may abruptly, transiently rise to extreme values.[25] Clefts may be closed by dilation, and reopened by miotics.

Inflammation The contusion injury to the anterior chamber incites a cascade of inflammatory mediators. The level of inflammation varies depending on the severity of injury, from a mild iritis to a severe inflammatory reaction with deposition of keratic precipitates in the anterior chamber angle. It is important to document and follow the degree of inflammation for proper management as well as prevention of potential chronic changes to the anterior chamber and angle. In the immediate post-injury setting, a mild trabeculitis may be noted with keratic precipitates in the angle and an elevated intraocular pressure. With chronic inflammation, synechiae may develop between either the pupillary margin or anterior lens capsule, with potential pupillary block and elevation of intraocular pressure. Additionally, peripheral anterior synechiae (PAS) may develop in the angle, leading to chronic angle-closure glaucoma.

Although the mechanism of injury may appear to be due to blunt trauma it is always important to be aware of possible penetrating injuries with a potential intraocular foreign body. Careful retroillumination of the iris may reveal a transillumination defect where a foreign body may have entered into the posterior chamber.

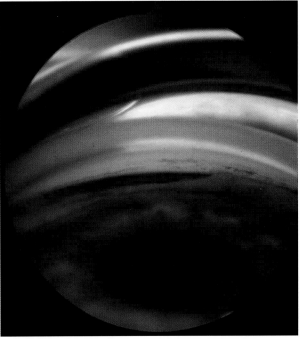

FIGURE 36.3 Angle recession. Gonioscopic view of angle recession, demonstrated by a widened ciliary body band.

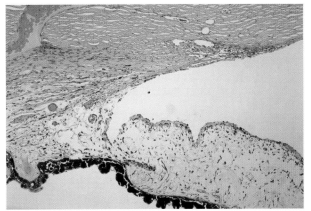

FIGURE 36.4 Angle recession. Contusion injury to the ciliary body. There is a disruption in the ciliary body between the external longitudinal muscle fibers and the internal oblique and circular muscle fibers.

Gonioscopy may also uncover an unsuspected foreign body in the angle that was not visible at slit lamp examination. The need for close questioning regarding the mechanism of injury, and thorough examination of the cornea, conjunctiva, and sclera cannot be overemphasized. Subconjunctival hemorrhages may mask entry wounds.

Blunt trauma may also cause disruption of the zonular fibers with a resultant lens subluxation or dislocation, posteriorly or anteriorly. It is important to carefully examine for disruption of the anterior lens capsule, which may lead to cataract formation and/or release of lens particles into the anterior chamber. Vitreous can also protrude through the ruptured zonules into the anterior chamber and cause pupillary block glaucoma.

MECHANISMS OF GLAUCOMA

Early post-traumatic period Patients in the early post-injury period may present with a slightly reduced intraocular pressure. This may be secondary to inflammation in the anterior chamber and subsequent reduction of aqueous humor production by the ciliary body or possibly an increase in outflow from a disruption in the angle structures, retinal tear, or occult rupture.

Conversely, other patients may have an elevated intraocular pressure in the acute post-injury phase. Intraocular pressure may be elevated without any obvious damage to the eye, but more often the pressure rises acutely as red blood cells, inflammatory cells, and debris obstructs the trabecular meshwork. Usually, this rise in intraocular pressure is transient and returns to baseline within several days.

Hyphema The prevalence of elevated intraocular pressure has been shown to be related to the amount of hyphema,[26] except in patients with sickle cell anemia or trait where a small amount of red blood cells in the anterior chamber may cause an elevation in intraocular pressure. Eight-ball hyphemas can cause a pupillary block secondary to the clot in the anterior chamber or mechanical blockage of the trabecular meshwork. In one study of 235 cases, glaucoma occurred in 13.5% of the eyes in which the hyphema filled less than 50% of the anterior chamber, 27% in eyes in which the hyphema was greater than 50%, and 52% of eyes developed glaucoma with a total hyphema.[27] Patients with a rebleed have a greater than 50% likelihood of developing glaucoma.

Management Conservative management of hyphemas is the first line of therapy. Historically, patients were admitted to the hospital for 5 days of bed rest with elevation of the head of the bed and monocular or binocular patching. Studies have shown that it is reasonable to follow those with hyphemas as outpatients and to allow limited ambulation, with a shield to protect the injured eye. Hospitalization is indicated in very large hyphemas, sickle cell disease or trait, or if the patient cannot be relied upon to maintain limited activity or to return for follow-up visits. Aspirin and nonsteroidal agents should be avoided.

Topical cycloplegics and steroids are given to decrease the amount of inflammation and prevent synechiae formation. Aminocaproic acid, an antifibrinolytic, was shown by Crouch and Frenkel[28] to significantly reduce the incidence of rebleeding when 100 mg/kg was given orally every 4 hours for 5 days. Aminocaproic acid may cause postural hypotension, nausea, and vomiting and should be avoided in pregnant patients and those with cardiac, hepatic, or renal disease. Topical aminocaproic acid has also been shown to be a safe and effective treatment to prevent secondary hemorrhage in traumatic hyphema.[29] Tranexamic acid also competitively inhibits activation of plasminogen to plasmin, but is more potent than aminocaproic acid and has fewer side effects.[30] A recent randomized study compared the use of tranexamic acid, oral prednisolone, and placebo in 238 patients.[23] The rate of rebleed was 10% in the tranexamic acid group, 18% in the oral steroid group, and 26% in the placebo group. Although there was a higher than expected rate of rebleed in the tranexamic group, there was a statistical difference between the tranexamic group and placebo.

If the intraocular pressure is elevated, it is advisable to protect the optic nerve head and enhance absorption of the hyphema. Pressure reduction is best accomplished with aqueous suppressants such as β-adrenergic antagonists, topical or oral carbonic anhydrase inhibitors, or α-adrenergic agonists. Due to the inflammatory response that is concurrent with the hyphema, miotics and prostaglandin analogues should be avoided. Hyperosmotic agents such as mannitol can also be utilized if topical medications do not adequately reduce intraocular pressure.

Surgical intervention becomes necessary if the intraocular pressure remains elevated despite medical management and threatens the optic nerve or is associated with corneal blood staining. Approximately 5% of patients with hyphemas require surgical intervention.[31] The exact timing of surgery depends on the status of the optic nerve. A patient with a healthy optic nerve may tolerate intraocular pressures of 40–50 mmHg for up to a week, but a patient with prior glaucomatous optic neuropathy may only tolerate a pressure in the high 30 range for 2 to 3 days.[32] A total or complete hyphema without resolution after 4 days is also an indication for surgical intervention.[33]

The precise surgical technique of anterior chamber washout varies depending on the surgeon and degree of hyphema. Manual irrigation and aspiration of the blood is a common technique. Using either a manual irrigation–aspiration system or just an irrigation cannula, a washout of the anterior chamber debris can be done through one or two corneal incisions. Occasionally, the clot is larger and denser than can be removed with an irrigation–aspiration handpiece. A vitrectomy instrument may be used through a larger corneal incision to remove the clot and debris. This may also facilitate debulking the clot without causing shearing in the angle associated with forcible removal of the entire clot. Care needs to be taken to protect the corneal endothelium, anterior lens capsule, and the iris during the procedure. Anterior chamber stability is very important throughout the procedure. The bottle height should be fairly high so as to keep the intraocular pressure from becoming too low and potentially causing a secondary hemorrhage. If a secondary hemorrhage occurs, the bottle height should be raised as high as possible to tamponade the bleeding. Viscoelastic can be placed into the anterior chamber after evacuation of the initial clot. If necessary, diathermy may be used if the site of bleeding can be localized and is accessible.[26] It is not necessary to remove the entire clot, but to decrease the anterior chamber inflammatory and hemorrhagic debris.

Limbal clot delivery has become less frequently used due to the large limbal wound, potential conjunctival scarring, and inadvertent prolapse of uveal tissue that may occur. Large eight-ball hyphemas may be more safely removed with this technique if visibility cannot be obtained with irrigation and viscoelastic use. If this method is used, it is best to wait until the clot has matured and retraction has occurred by approximately day 4. Vitrectomy instruments can also be helpful for eight-ball hyphemas, but care must be taken to avoid damage to anterior segment structures if visualization is not adequate.

Guarded filtration surgery in combination with an anterior chamber washout is another alternative. Patients with evidence of optic nerve damage and elevated intraocular pressure which has failed medical therapy may benefit from a filtering procedure. Sickle cell patients may also benefit from this approach as there is a reduced chance of postoperative spikes as compared to washout alone. This approach was first described by Weiss et al.[33] and has been used by others to control the intraocular pressure while the remaining blood is cleared. Although the amount of inflammation and debris that is present usually leads to early scarring and failure of the filtration site, it provides adequate time for the intraocular pressure to return to baseline.

It is important to be cautious in patients who may be at risk for sickle cell disease or trait, as carbonic anhydrase inhibitors increase the concentration of ascorbic acid in the aqueous humor, leading to more sickling in the anterior chamber.[34] Epinephrine may also increase intravascular and intracameral sickling by its vasoconstrictive and subsequent deoxygenating properties. There is a poor prognosis in patients with sickle cell trait if intraocular pressure is not aggressively controlled in the first 24 hours. Therefore, it is reasonable to hospitalize these patients for administration of topical, oral, and possibly intravenous medications, as well as close observation of the intraocular pressure. Sickle cell patients should have early surgical intervention if their pressures are not controlled within the first 24 hours.

Hemolytic glaucoma Hemolytic glaucoma is a form of open-angle glaucoma that develops days to weeks after a large intraocular hemorrhage. The elevated intraocular pressure is associated with hemolytic and inflammatory debris which mechanically obstructs the outflow through the trabecular meshwork. On gonioscopy, the angle is open with reddish-brown pigmented deposits on the trabecular meshwork, especially inferiorly.

Management Hemolytic glaucoma is usually a self-limited condition, which responds to medical management with β-adrenergic antagonists, carbonic anhydrase inhibitors, α2-agonists, and hyperosmotic agents. Rare cases that do not respond may require anterior chamber washout with possible vitrectomy. It is important to send an aqueous sample for cytology to ensure that the pigmented cells in the angle are due to old hemorrhage and not malignancy.[35]

Ghost-cell glaucoma A subset of patients with vitreous hemorrhage secondary to either ocular trauma, retinal

disease, or after intraocular surgery, develop a condition called 'ghost-cell glaucoma.' The erythrocytes in the vitreous cavity degenerate from their typical biconvex shape into spherical, khaki-colored cells. The degenerated erythrocytes migrate forward into the anterior chamber through a disrupted anterior hyaloid face. The term 'ghost cell' is used because the cells appear empty except for clumps of denatured hemoglobin seen on histopathology (Heinz bodies) (Fig. 36.5). These cells are more rigid and do not easily pass through the trabecular meshwork, resulting in obstruction of the outflow pathway. A pseudohypopyon may form in some situations where there is a large number of 'ghost cells.'

Management Ghost-cell glaucoma is often a transient problem, which may take months for resolution of the intraocular pressure back to baseline. It may last for months before all of the denatured cells clear from the anterior chamber angle. Most patients can be controlled with topical aqueous suppressants, including β-adrenergic antagonists, carbonic anhydrase inhibitors, and α2-agonists. In some situations the use of oral carbonic anhydrase inhibitors and intravenous hyperosmotic agents may become necessary. Refractory cases may require surgical intervention, such as an anterior chamber washout with pars plana vitrectomy, to remove all the remaining ghost cells.

Lens subluxation Blunt ocular trauma may cause disruption of zonular fibers with lens subluxation or even total lens dislocation into either the anterior chamber or vitreous cavity (Fig. 36.6). With lens subluxation, the forward rotation of the lens or protrusion of vitreous through the ruptured zonules may cause pupillary block with resultant secondary angle-closure glaucoma. Total lens dislocation into the anterior chamber may cause iris bombe with pupillary block, and angle-closure or open-angle glaucoma may occur from direct obstruction of the angle by the lens or lens fragments.

Management The definitive treatment for lens dislocation or subluxation is either extracapsular or

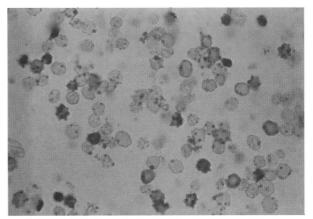

FIGURE 36.5 Ghost-cell glaucoma. Degenerating erythrocytes are spherical in shape and rigid, which makes outflow through the trabecular meshwork difficult.

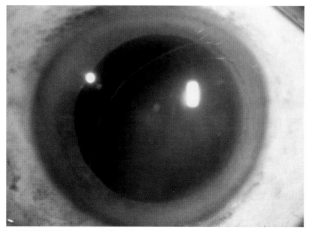

FIGURE 36.6 Lens subluxation. Inferior nasal subluxation of the lens with zonular dehiscence after blunt ocular trauma.

intracapsular cataract extraction, depending on the amount of zonular dehiscence. In the interim, dilation of the pupil while the patient is supine may allow the lens to fall back into the posterior chamber, decreasing the urgency of surgical intervention. If there is any lenticular corneal touch, corneal decompensation may occur, requiring immediate surgical intervention. If there is pupillary block, laser iridotomy is indicated to relieve the block, subsequently allowing for safer surgical removal of the lens.

Lens particle glaucoma Days to weeks after ocular trauma the intraocular pressure may potentially spike due to mechanical obstruction of the trabecular meshwork with lens particles. If the anterior or posterior lens capsule is torn, lenticular material can be seen in the anterior chamber. Chronic inflammation may lead to the formation of peripheral anterior and posterior synechiae. Anterior chamber aspirate shows lens cortical fibers and lens particles.

Management Initial treatment with topical steroids and cycloplegia in the acute phase is necessary to decrease the inflammatory reaction. Aqueous suppression with β-adrenergic antagonists, carbonic anhydrase inhibitors, and α₂-agonists will aid in control of the intraocular pressure, but the definitive treatment is cataract extraction with careful anterior chamber washout to ensure removal of all inflammatory mediators and lens particles.

Other reported causes of elevated intraocular pressure following blunt ocular trauma include: shallowing of the anterior chamber due to anterior rotation of the lens–iris diaphragm secondary to a uveal effusion,[36] vitreous prolapse into the anterior chamber,[37] and Schwartz-Matsuo syndrome, which may have fluctuant intraocular pressures in association with a retinal detachment and a tear in the nonpigmented epithelium of the ciliary body.[38] In this syndrome, photoreceptor outer segments clog the trabecular meshwork, and may be mistaken for uveitis in the anterior chamber.

Late post-traumatic period

Angle recession Although elevation in intraocular pressure is usually transient, it is important to follow all patients with a history of ocular trauma because a reported 4–9% of patients with angle recession greater than 180° develop a chronic glaucoma, often many years later.[39] Angle-recession glaucoma is not directly due to the tear in the ciliary body, but secondary to the degenerative changes in the trabecular meshwork tissue after the trauma and subsequent inflammation, which cause an obstruction to outflow. This theory was initially introduced by Wolff and Zimmerman[40] and later supported by clinical and animal studies by Herschler.[41] He demonstrated tears in the trabecular meshwork just posterior to Schwalbe's line during the early post-traumatic period. This tear produced a flap of trabecular tissue, which scarred with time, ultimately leading to chronic obstruction in the aqueous outflow pathway.

Management Glaucomas following ocular trauma usually do not respond adequately to medical management, but some patients can be controlled with β-adrenergic antagonists, carbonic anhydrase inhibitors, and α₂-agonists. Patients with angle recession respond poorly to laser trabeculoplasty. One series of 13 patients who had undergone laser trabeculoplasty for angle-recession glaucoma only had a 23% success rate with a mean 36-month follow-up.[42] Numerous other studies have shown similar results.

Glaucoma filtering surgery has also shown poor results in patients with angle recession. Studies have shown an increased failure rate of guarded filtration surgery and tube shunt in patients with angle recession when compared to patients with chronic open-angle glaucoma.[43,44] The failures of filtration in these studies were attributed to the increased fibrosis of the fistula or filtering bleb within the first 3 months postoperatively. Subsequent to ocular injury, patients have a heightened fibroblast proliferation after filtering surgery. The use of antimetabolite agents, such as mitomycin C, in filtration surgery has been demonstrated to statistically improve long-term success rates in patients with angle-recession glaucoma.[45]

PENETRATING TRAUMA

Penetrating injuries of the globe can result from blunt force, sharp lacerations, or missiles. As with blunt ocular trauma, young males are the most vulnerable to penetrating ocular injuries. The National Eye Trauma System (NETS) reported 6% of penetrating globe injuries secondary to assault and 35% due to occupational injuries involved an intraocular foreign body.[10] The median ages of patients collected by the NETS with assault-related and occupational penetrating injuries were 28 and 30 years, respectively, with males involved in 97% and 83% of the cases, respectively.[10]

The intraocular pressure after a penetrating ocular injury is usually low because of the open wound, but after surgical repair glaucoma may develop because of intraocular changes induced by the penetrating injury. During the early post-injury period the intraocular pressure may be elevated secondary to hyphema, inflammation, or angle closure due to lenticular trauma, as discussed previously. As these conditions subside, chronic changes may develop as a result of the inflammation.

Cyclitic membranes may form in the anterior chamber, pulling the lens–iris diaphragm forward with secondary angle closure or obstructing the pupil with subsequent iris bombe. Peripheral anterior synechiae may also develop, leading to angle closure due to chronic inflammation or a prolonged shallow/flat anterior chamber. Prompt administration of topical anti-inflammatory agents and cycloplegics may prevent synechiae formation and decrease the strong inflammatory response. Additionally, reformation of the anterior chamber early on is important to prevent peripheral anterior synechiae.

Additional causes of glaucoma are sympathetic ophthalmia and epithelial downgrowth after a penetrating ocular injury (Fig. 36.7). Epithelial tissue may migrate through the intraocular injury, leading to obstruction of the outflow through the trabecular meshwork. It should be suspected in patients with penetrating ocular trauma and chronic elevation of intraocular pressure but without other identifiable causes (see Ch. 32). White burns seen with argon laser application to the surface of the iris are indicative of epithelial downgrowth.

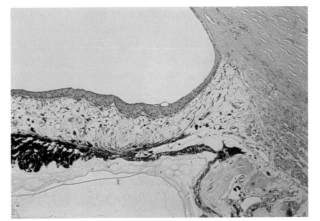

FIGURE 36.7 Epithelial downgrowth. Histological representation of multilayered epithelial cells on the anterior surface of the iris.

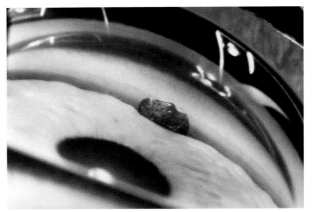

FIGURE 36.8 Retained intraocular foreign body. Penetrating ocular injury with occult metallic foreign body in the inferior angle.

RETAINED INTRAOCULAR FOREIGN BODY

Penetrating ocular trauma should always raise a high suspicion for a retained intraocular foreign body (Fig. 36.8). All patients with penetrating injuries should undergo radiographic imaging to evaluate for any potential metallic foreign bodies. Patients with a retained intraocular foreign body may develop elevated intraocular pressures through all the same mechanisms as described earlier for simple penetrating trauma, but may also develop glaucoma due to the late sequela of retained metallic foreign bodies. Iron released from a retained metallic foreign body is toxic to the trabecular meshwork, leading to a decreased outflow and elevated intraocular pressures (siderosis). Copper may be oxidized within the eye, causing similar trabecular changes as with iron, but with less frequency (chalcosis).

Management The management for all foreign bodies should be prompt removal to prevent the complications previously described. Once glaucoma is present, a foreign body may be so encapsulated that standard extraction techniques may be difficult. The visual prognosis is also limited due to the retinal toxicity associated with a retained metallic foreign body. Treatment with corticosteroids to avoid cyclitic membranes and antibiotics for endophthalmitis prophylaxis is important. Elevated intraocular pressure can be treated with β-adrenergic antagonists, carbonic anhydrase inhibitors, α_2-agonists, and hyperosmotic agents. Occasionally, patients may

require filtration surgery if medical therapy fails. In selected cases, serial electroretinograms (ERGs) may be helpful to watch for retinal pathology from retained metallic foreign bodies.

CHEMICAL BURNS

Alkali burns Alkaline chemicals may penetrate into the anterior chamber within seconds of contact, causing severe anterior segment damage. Alkali burns of the eye may produce characteristic intraocular pressure changes. There is an initial rapid rise in intraocular pressure, which has been attributed to anterior segment shrinkage[46] and increased uveal blood flow,[47] which may be prostaglandin mediated. If there is severe damage to the ciliary body, decreased aqueous production may produce early hypotony. Patients with severe alkali burns may not recover from this hypotonous phase. There is also a severe inflammatory reaction, which may lead to hypopyon formation in some patients.

Weeks to months after the injury the anterior segment undergoes repair, scarring, and further inflammation. There may be irreversible damage to the trabecular meshwork as a direct consequence of the original alkali injury or the sequela of peripheral anterior synechiae formation from inflammation or pupillary block. Patients may develop glaucoma in this phase secondary to pupillary block from synechiae to the lens capsule or cataract formation and forward rotation of the lens, or by a phacolytic mechanism when lens materials are released.

Management Measurement of intraocular pressure with applanation may be difficult in these patients due to the disorganized corneal tissue. Tonopen and pneumotonometry may provide a more accurate intraocular pressure reading. Elevated intraocular pressure in the early phase can be controlled with β-adrenergic antagonists, carbonic anhydrase inhibitors, α$_2$-agonists, and hyperosmotic agents. Topical medications may inhibit reepithelialization of the cornea; therefore, it may be preferential in these patients to use oral or intravenous agents.

The resultant damage from alkali burns is predominantly due to the aggressive inflammatory reaction. Topical corticosteroids have been shown to be safe in rabbits for use in the first week after an alkali burn, but are contraindicated because of the risk of stromal lysis after the first week.[48] Oral corticosteroids should be used to decrease the inflammatory reaction and potential scarring that will occur.

Chronic elevation of intraocular pressure is a result of direct damage to the outflow pathway and resultant synechiae formation and scarring of the anterior segment from the severe inflammation. If glaucoma develops due to pupillary block, medical management should be initiated, but if it fails laser iridotomy should be performed. Elevation of intraocular pressure due to the lens may not respond to medical therapy and the eye should undergo cataract extraction.

Acid burns Acidic chemicals cause coagulation of tissue proteins, which limits the penetration, resulting in more superficial injuries, unless the acid concentration is high or there is prolonged exposure. The intraocular pressure has been shown to become elevated after acid burns in rabbits. A spike in intraocular pressure occurs acutely, lasting up to 3 hours. Similar to alkali burns, the shrinkage of corneal and scleral tissues is thought to cause the initial rise in intraocular pressure. A sustained elevated intraocular pressure is thought to be mediated by prostaglandin release. Treatment of any resultant glaucoma is similar to alkali burns.

REFERENCES

1. Klopfer J, Tielsch JM, Vitale S, et al. Ocular trauma in the United States. Eye injuries resulting in hospitalization, 1984–1987. Arch Ophthalmol 1992; 110:838–842.

2. Blomdahl S, Norell S. Perforating eye injury in the Stockholm population. An epidemiological study. Acta Ophthalmol 1983; 62:378–390.

3. Canavan YM, Archer DB. Anterior segment consequences of blunt ocular injury. Br J Ophthalmol 1982; 66:549–555.

4. MacEwen CJ. Eye injuries: a prospective survey of 5671 cases. Br J Ophthalmol 1989; 73:888–894.

5. Moreira CA, Debert-Ribeiro M, Belfort R. Epidemiological study of eye injuries in Brazilian children. Arch Ophthalmol 1988; 106:781–788.

6. Liggett PE, Pince KJ, Barlow W, et al. Ocular trauma in an urban population. Review of 1131 cases. Ophthalmology 1990; 97:581–584.

7. Kearns P. Traumatic hyphaema: a retrospective study of 314 cases. Br J Ophthalmol 1991; 75:137–141.

8. Lesher MP, Durrie DA, Stiles MC. Corneal edema, hyphema, and angle recession after air bag inflation. Arch Ophthalmol 1993; 111:1320–1322.

9. Campbell D. Traumatic glaucoma. In: Shingleton B, Hersh P, Kenyon K, eds. Eye trauma. St. Louis: Mosby Year Book; 1991:117–125.

10. Dannenberg AL, Parver LM, Fowler CJ. Penetrating eye injuries related to assault. The National Eye Trauma System Registry. Arch Ophthalmol 1992; 110:849–852.

11. Volpe NJ, Larrison WI, Hersh PS, et al. Secondary hemorrhage in traumatic hyphema. Am J Ophthalmol 1991; 112:507–513.

12. Howard GM, Hutchinson BT, Frederick AR. Hyphema resulting from blunt trauma. Gonioscopic, tonographic, and ophthalmoscopic observations following resolution of the hemorrhage. Trans Am Acad Ophthalmol Otolaryngol 1965; 69:294–306.

13. Edwards WC, Layden WF. Traumatic hyphema. A report of 184 consecutive cases. Am J Ophthalmol 1973; 75:110–116.

14. Fong LP. Secondary hemorrhage in traumatic hyphema. Predictive factors for selective prophylaxis. Ophthalmology 1994; 101:1583–1588.

15. Ganley JP, Geiger JM, Clement JR, et al. Aspirin and recurrent hyphema after blunt ocular trauma. Am J Ophthalmol 1983; 96:797–801.

16. Spoor TC, Kwito GM, O'Grady JM, et al. Traumatic hyphema in an urban population. Am J Ophthalmol 1990; 109:23–27.

17. Rahmani B, Jahadi HR, Rajaeefard A. An analysis of risk for secondary hemorrhage in traumatic hyphema. Ophthalmology 1999; 106:380–85.

18. Nasrullah A, Kerr NC. Sickle cell as a risk factor for secondary hemorrhage in children with traumatic hyphema. Am J Ophthalmol 1997; 123:783–790.

19. Mooney D. Angle recession and secondary glaucoma. Br J Ophthalmol 1973; 57:608–612.

20. Spaeth GL. Traumatic hyphema, angle recession, dexamethasone hypertension, and glaucoma. Arch Ophthalmol 1967; 78:714–721.

21. Blanton FM. Anterior chamber angle recession and secondary glaucoma: a study of the after effects of traumatic hyphemas. Arch Ophthalmol 1964; 72:39–43.

22. Salmon JF, Mermoud A, Ivey A, et al. The detection of post-traumatic angle recession by gonioscopy in a population-based glaucoma survey. Ophthalmology 1994; 101:1844–1850.

23. Tesluk GC, Spaeth GL. The occurrence of primary open-angle glaucoma in the fellow eye of patients with unilateral angle-cleavage glaucoma. Ophthalmology 1985; 92:904–911.

24. Pederson JE. Ocular hypotony. Trans Ophthalmol Soc UK 1986; 105:220–226.

25. Kronfeld PC. The fluid exchange in the successfully cyclodialyzed eye. Trans Am Ophthalmol Soc 1954; 52:249–263.

26. Crouch ER Jr, Crouch ER. Management of traumatic hyphema: therapeutic options. J Pediatr Ophthalmol Strabismus 1999; 36:238–250.

27. Coles WH. Traumatic hyphema: an analysis of 235 cases. South Med J 1968; 61:813–816.

28. Crouch ER, Frenkel M. Aminocaproic acid in the treatment of hyphema. Am J Ophthalmol 1976; 81:355–360.

29. Crouch ER Jr, Williams PB, Gray KM, et al. Topical aminocaproic acid in the treatment of traumatic hyphema. Arch Ophthalmol 1997; 115:1106–1112.

30. Deans R, Noeel LP, Clarke WN. Oral administration of tranexamic acid in the management of traumatic hyphema in children. Can J Ophthalmol 1992; 27:181–183.

31. Rahmani B, Jahadi H. Comparison of tranexamic acid and prednisolone in the treatment of traumatic hyphema. Ophthalmology 1999; 106:375–379.

32. Wilson FM. Traumatic hyphema. Pathogenesis and management. Ophthalmology 1980; 87:910–919.

33. Weiss JS, Parrish RK, Anderson DR. Surgical therapy of traumatic hyphema. Ophthalmic Surg 1983; 14:343–345.

34. Goldberg MF. Sickled erythrocytes, hyphema, and secondary glaucoma: V. The effect of vitamin C on erythrocyte sickling in aqueous humor. Ophthalmic Surg 1979; 10:70–77.

35. Phelps CD, Watzke RC. Hemolytic glaucoma. Am J Ophthalmol 1975; 80:690–695.

36. Dotan S, Oliver M. Shallow anterior chamber and uveal effusion after nonperforating trauma to the eye. Am J Ophthalmol 1982; 94:782–784.

37. Samples JR, Van Buskirk EM. Open-angle glaucoma associated with vitreous humor filling the anterior chamber. Am J Ophthalmol 1986; 102:759–761.

38. Matsuo T, Muraoka N, Shiraga F, et al. Schwartz-Matsuo syndrome in retinal detachment with tears of the nonpigmented epithelium of the ciliary body. Acta Ophthalmol Scand 1998; 76:481–485.

39. Kaufman JH, Tolpin DW. Glaucoma after traumatic angle recession: a ten-year prospective study. Am J Ophthalmol 1974; 79:648–654.

40. Wolff SM, Zimmerman LE. Chronic secondary glaucoma: associated with retrodisplacement of iris root and deepening of the anterior chamber angle secondary to contusion. Am J Ophthalmol 1962; 54:547–563.

41. Herschler J. Trabecular damage due to blunt anterior segment injury and its relationship to traumatic glaucoma. Trans Am Acad Ophthalmol Otolaryngol 1977; 83:239–248.

42. Scharf B, Chi T, Grayson D, et al. Argon laser trabeculoplasty for angle recession glaucoma. Invest Ophthalmol Vis Sci 1992; 33(Suppl):1159.

43. Mermoud A, Salmon JF, Barron A, et al. Surgical management of post-traumatic angle recession glaucoma. Ophthalmology 1993; 100:634–642.

44. Mermoud A, Salmon JF, Straker C, et al. Post-traumatic angle recession glaucoma: a risk factor for bleb failure after trabeculectomy. Br J Ophthalmol 1993; 77:631–634.

45. Mermoud A, Salmon JF, Murray AD. Trabeculectomy with mitomycin-C for refractory glaucoma in blacks. Am J Ophthalmol 1993; 116:72–78.

46. Paterson CA, Pfister RR. Intraocular pressure changes after alkali burns. Arch Ophthalmol 1974; 91:211–218.

47. Green K, Paterson CA, Siddiqui A. Ocular blood flow after experimental alkali burns and prostaglandin administration. Arch Ophthalmol 1985; 103:569–571.

48. Donshik PC, Berman MB, Dohlman CH, et al. Effect of topical corticosteroids on ulceration in alkali-burned corneas. Arch Ophthalmol 1978; 96:2117–2120.

CHAPTER 37

Glaucoma and Intraocular Tumors

Kathryn Bollinger, Annapurna Singh, and Arun D Singh

INTRODUCTION

The prevalence of ocular hypertension and glaucoma in patients with intraocular tumors varies depending on the tumor type and location. For example, anterior segment melanomas of the iris or ciliary body cause raised intraocular pressure (IOP) more frequently than posterior segment tumors such as choroidal melanoma. Many estimates are skewed because they are based on ophthalmology referral services. One survey of 2597 patients with intraocular tumors found elevated IOP in 5% of tumor-containing eyes at the time of diagnosis.[1] Of the 2597 eyes with intraocular tumors, 2111 had uveal melanoma. Of these, secondary IOP elevation was present in 3%. This included 17% with ciliary body melanoma, 7% of eyes with iris melanoma, and 2% with choroidal melanoma. A study of 227 cases of carcinoma metastatic to the eye and orbit found that glaucoma was present in 7.5% of the total group.[2] In a second series of 256 eyes with uveal metastases, glaucoma occurred in 5% of these.[1]

Glaucoma is also a frequent complication of retinoblastoma. A combined histopathologic and clinical examination of 149 eyes revealed histologic evidence of glaucoma in 50% and clinically increased IOP in 23%.[3] Other intraocular tumors such as leukemia and lymphoma in adults and medulloepithelioma and juvenile xanthogranuloma in children may also cause glaucoma. Benign tumors including iris nevus, iris cyst, melanocytoma, melanocytosis, and adenoma may also increase IOP.

ETIOLOGY AND PATHOGENESIS

Intraocular tumors can increase IOP by multiple mechanisms.

OPEN-ANGLE GLAUCOMA

There are three main mechanisms by which tumors cause open-angle glaucoma. First, direct invasion of the anterior chamber angle may occur. All types of melanoma, and even nevi, can extend across the trabecular meshwork, leading to increased IOP.[1] When intraocular metastases cause glaucoma, the mechanism of increased IOP is generally direct infiltration of the trabecular meshwork by neoplastic tissue (Fig. 37.1).[1,4]

Secondly, tumor cells seeding the anterior chamber angle may cause open-angle glaucoma. This generally occurs in cases of intraocular melanoma when pigmented cells are dispersed into the anterior chamber and settle within the trabecular meshwork, thereby disrupting the outflow of aqueous (Fig. 37.2).[5] Intraocular metastasis from systemic melanoma can also cause glaucoma by this mechanism. In addition, leukemia and lymphoma can invade the anterior chamber, resulting in tumor cells that deposit within the angle as a pseudo-hypopyon and cause open-angle glaucoma.

The third mechanism is called melanomalytic glaucoma and is specific to melanotic tumors. This occurs when necrotic melanoma cells are engulfed by macrophages that occlude the trabecular meshwork and cause raised intraocular pressure.[5,6] This can occur in association with both anterior and posterior uveal melanomas.

ANGLE-CLOSURE GLAUCOMA

Closure of the anterior chamber angle is also a common cause of glaucoma in patients with intraocular tumors. Angle closure occurs through three main mechanisms. First, patients can present with angle closure secondary to forward movement of the lens–iris diaphragm. This is often associated with posterior segment tumors such as choroidal melanomas and is frequently accompanied by retinal detachment. Therefore, an underlying malignant melanoma should be considered in any patient with unilateral serous retinal detachment and glaucoma. In addition, anterior uveal tumors such as ciliary body melanoma can lead to angle closure by forward movement of the iris, causing occlusion of the trabecular meshwork and peripheral anterior synechiae (PAS) formation. Massive subretinal hemorrhage can occur in patients with leukemia or myelodysplastic syndrome and may cause angle closure.[7,8]

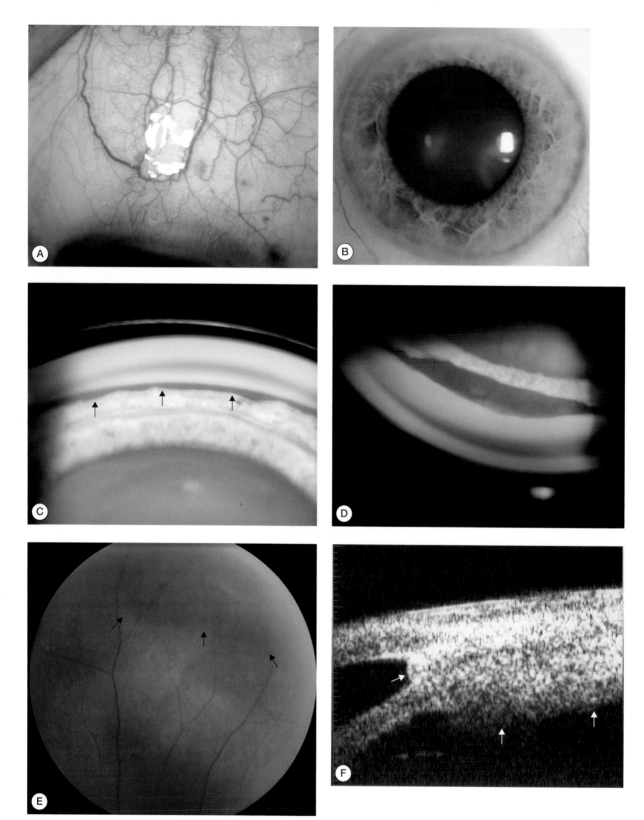

FIGURE 37.1 A 64-year-old woman was diagnosed with ocular hypertension OS (left eye). The IOP was 35 mmHg. On external examination prominent sentinel vessels with episcleral pigmentation were noted superiorly **(A)**. The anterior segment appeared normal **(B)**. On gonioscopy there was diffuse pigment seeding in the angle **(C,** *arrows***)** with area of tumor extension from 12 to 1 o'clock meridian **(D)**. Ophthalmoscopy revealed peripheral choroidal melanoma **(E,** *arrows***)**. Ciliary body and angle extension (*arrows*) was confirmed by ultrasound biomicroscopy **(F,** *arrows***)**.

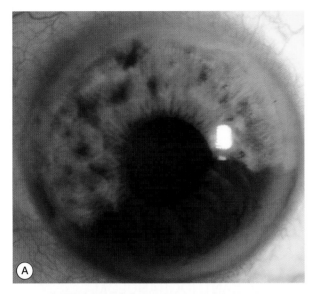

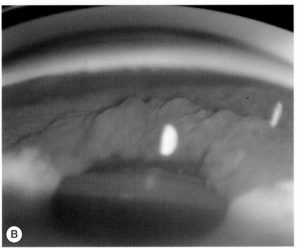

FIGURE 37.2 (A) Diffuse iris melanoma of the lower half of the iris causing secondary glaucoma (IOP = 26 mmHg). **(B)** Gonioscopy confirmed pigment seeding in the angle.

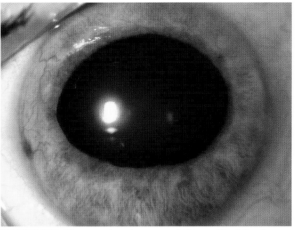

FIGURE 37.3 Neovascular glaucoma at 13 months following iodine 125 plaque radiotherapy for a medium-sized choroidal melanoma.

NEOVASCULAR GLAUCOMA

Neovascular glaucoma is a common cause of angle-closure glaucoma in intraocular melanomas.[1,5] This is also the mechanism for raised IOP in some cases of nonmelanotic intraocular metastasis and retinoblastoma. Medulloepithelioma has a specific tendency to induce iris neovascularization. Radiation, a common modality used for treating malignant intraocular tumors, is an important cause of neovascular glaucoma due to radiation-induced retinal ischemia (Fig. 37.3).

DIAGNOSTIC EVALUATION

An intraocular tumor should be considered in any patient who presents with unilateral glaucoma. A careful ophthalmic examination including slit lamp biomicroscopy, gonioscopy, transillumination of the globe, and posterior segment examination is critical. On slit lamp examination, several findings are indicative of an intraocular tumor. The iris may reveal a melanotic or nonmelanotic lesion. Pigmented cells may be present in the anterior chamber indicative of an anterior or posterior melanoma.[5,6] Also, the iris may be displaced or the lens subluxed or focally opacified. Neovascularization of the iris may also be identified on slit lamp examination.

Gonioscopy may reveal direct tumor invasion of the anterior chamber angle.[1,9] In addition, angle seeding by pigmented or nonpigmented neoplastic cells may be apparent inferiorly. Gonioscopic examination may also show neovascularization of the angle or angle closure in the setting of pupillary block secondary to intraocular tumor.[5]

Transillumination of the globe can aid in the diagnosis of intraocular melanoma. These tumors cast a shadow when transilluminated and ciliary body, ring, or choroidal melanomas may be apparent using this method.[1]

Posterior segment examination with direct and indirect ophthalmoscopy may reveal a choroidal tumor or retinal detachment associated with posterior segment malignancy. If the angle is occluded or occludable, dilation should be postponed until after peripheral iridotomy or iridectomy.

Definitive diagnosis may be difficult based on clinical examination alone. In particular, nevi of the iris may be clinically indistinguishable from melanoma. Ancillary studies such as fluorescein angiography of the iris can aid in differentiating between benign and malignant lesions.[10] Although ultrasound biomicroscopy can aid in the detection of ciliary body and choroidal tumors, this technique cannot reliably distinguish between a benign and a malignant neoplasm.[11,12] Cytopathologic or tissue analysis by fine needle aspiration may be helpful.[13] Depending on the clinical and histopathologic characteristics of the lesion, additional therapy may be needed.

DIFFERENTIAL DIAGNOSIS: CHILDHOOD GLAUCOMA

Childhood glaucoma is associated with a variety of congenital and developmental anomalies, most of which are easily distinguishable from secondary glaucoma due to intraocular tumors. When the mechanism of glaucoma is neovascular angle closure, a specific set of differential diagnoses must be considered. Neovascularization of the iris is the most common cause of glaucoma associated with retinoblastoma but it is not pathognomonic (Fig. 37.4). Iris neovascularization has been reported as the initial sign in 7% of cases.[14] Rubeosis iridis can easily be missed on examination and should be considered in any child with retinoblastoma. Conversely, any child with neovascular glaucoma must be evaluated for retinoblastoma. Other conditions such as retinopathy of prematurity, persistent hyperplastic primary vitreous, retinal dysplasia, Coats' disease, toxocariasis, and infantile retinal detachment can present with neovascular glaucoma.[15] Other specific entities in the differential diagnosis of childhood glaucoma include phakomatoses, juvenile xanthogranuloma, and medulloepithelioma.

PHAKOMATOSES

The phakomatoses are a group of congenital disorders characterized by systemic hamartosis with preferential neuro-oculo-cutaneous involvement. Glaucoma can occur in association with Sturge-Weber syndrome, neurofibromatosis, and von Hippel-Lindau disease.

Sturge-Weber syndrome Sturge-Weber syndrome is characterized by vascular hamartomas or hemangiomas within the skin along the distribution of the fifth cranial nerve. Patients generally present with the characteristic cutaneous hemangioma. The condition also involves the central nervous system, resulting in leptomeningeal angioma and cortical calcifications. Ocular examination may reveal dilated and tortuous episcleral veins and telangiectatic conjunctival vessels.[16] Glaucoma occurs in approximately half of patients and likely results either from a developmental defect within the anterior chamber or, more commonly, secondary to elevated episcleral venous pressure.[17]

Neurofibromatosis type 1 Neurofibromatosis type 1 is characterized by hyperpigmented lesions called café-au-lait spots and neurofibromas within the peripheral nervous system. Eye findings within the anterior segment include hamartomatous lesions of the iris and are called Lisch nodules. Elevated IOP can result from infiltration of the anterior chamber angle by neurofibromatous tissue, iris neovascularization, or developmental anomalies.[18] Glaucoma is more likely to occur in individuals who have neurofibromas of the upper eyelid.

Von Hippel-Lindau disease Von Hippel-Lindau disease is the third type of phakomatosis that may be associated with glaucoma. Patients are affected by retinal capillary hemangioma, which in neglected cases can cause neovascular glaucoma.

JUVENILE XANTHOGRANULOMA

Juvenile xanthogranuloma is generally diagnosed in infants and young children. Ocular manifestations of this condition include lightly pigmented iris lesions that are histologically composed of foamy histiocytes and Touton giant cells. These lesions can cause spontaneous hyphema. Glaucoma occurs secondary to hyphema or from direct invasion of the anterior chamber angle by histiocytes. Patients with this condition also have yellow papular skin lesions on the head and neck.[19]

MEDULLOEPITHELIOMA

Medulloepithelioma is a childhood tumor that arises most frequently from the nonpigmented epithelium of the ciliary body. Lesions can be benign or malignant and appear clinically as a whitish-gray mass of the ciliary body or iris. Glaucoma occurs secondary to neovascularization of the anterior chamber angle or because of forward displacement of the iris and PAS formation (Fig. 37.5).[20,21]

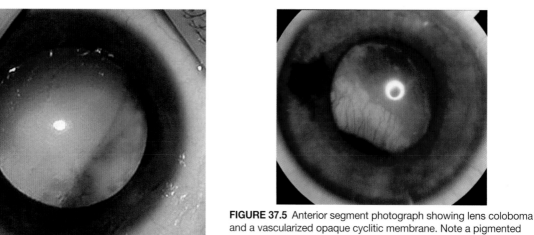

FIGURE 37.4 Neovascular glaucoma associated with stage E (international classification) retinoblastoma. Note ectropion iridis.

FIGURE 37.5 Anterior segment photograph showing lens coloboma and a vascularized opaque cyclitic membrane. Note a pigmented mass in the ciliary body region. (Reproduced with permission from Singh A, Singh AD, Shields CL, Shields JA. Iris neovascularization in children: a manifestation of underlying medulloepithelioma. J Pediatr Ophthalmol Strabismus 2001; 38:224–228.)

DIFFERENTIAL DIAGNOSIS: ADULT GLAUCOMA

IRIS CYSTS

Iris cysts arise primarily from the pigment epithelium of the iris or ciliary body. Stromal cysts may also occur secondarily following surgery or trauma. Both angle-closure and open-angle mechanisms may be involved.[22] Ultrasound biomicroscopy can be helpful in differentiating iris or ciliary body cysts from malignant lesions.[23]

MELANOCYTOMA

Melanocytomas are benign pigmented lesions that most frequently affect the optic nerve. Rarely, these occur within the anterior segment affecting the iris or ciliary body. Melanocytomas can cause glaucoma by extension into the trabecular meshwork or through obstruction by dispersed pigment or necrotic melanocytoma cells.[24]

FUCHS' ADENOMA

Fuchs' adenoma is a benign tumor of the ciliary body that can involve the iris primarily or secondarily. These lesions have been reported to cause glaucoma through a pigment dispersion mechanism.[25]

UVEAL MELANOMA

Iris melanoma is typically visible at the slit lamp as an elevated brown mass. When melanomas arise within the ciliary body, early detection can be more difficult. Typically, the mass presents as a dome-shaped elevation of the iris and may be visible between the iris and the lens on dilated gonioscopic examination. In some cases, a patient may present with unilateral glaucoma, and a mass extends circumferentially around the trabecular meshwork. This type of tumor is termed a ring melanoma and can arise from the iris, the ciliary body, or the trabecular meshwork.[9] Tapioca melanoma is a rare variant of anterior uveal melanoma with a pale, nodular appearance that resembles tapioca pudding.[26]

Choroidal melanoma that causes glaucoma is frequently a large mass that pushes the lens–iris diaphragm forward. Associated retinal detachment or vitreous hemorrhage may present with pigment dispersion into the vitreous and melanomalytic glaucoma. Neovascular glaucoma is a late sequelae.

METASTATIC TUMORS

Carcinomas of the lung and breast are the most common sources of intraocular metastases.[27] The choroid is the most frequent metastatic site. However, glaucoma is more commonly associated with anterior segment metastatic tumors.[4] Clinically, a metastasis to the iris or ciliary body is translucent and gelatinous in appearance and may be indistinguishable from an amelanotic melanoma. These intraocular tumors are frequently associated with iris neovascularization or hyphema (Fig. 37.6).

LEUKEMIA/LYMPHOMA

Choroidal infiltration can cause massive subretinal hemorrhage and induce acute angle-closure glaucoma.[7] Anterior segment involvement may lead to hypopyon or hyphema with resultant open-angle glaucoma.[28] Rarely, lymphoma can affect the anterior segment and present as iritis with elevated IOP.[29] A patient with iritis and a history of leukemia or lymphoma should be investigated for recurrence.

MYELODYSPLASTIC SYNDROME/ MULTIPLE MYELOMA

Cases of myelodysplastic syndrome have been reported in which patients presented with serous retinal detachment and angle-closure glaucoma.[8] Multiple myeloma has been shown to manifest as iritis, wherein cytologic analysis of the aqueous sample revealed neoplastic plasma cells.[30]

MANAGEMENT

The management of glaucoma associated with intraocular tumors is dependent on the mechanism of elevated intraocular pressure. In addition, with respect to malignancies such as uveal melanoma, metastatic carcinoma, and retinoblastoma, filtering surgery carries the risk of iatrogenic dissemination and should not be attempted.[31] Therefore, medical therapy should be the first line of management and a cyclodestructive procedure can be considered in some situations of uncontrolled IOP after the tumor has been treated. In many cases of ciliary body or choroidal melanoma associated with glaucoma, the treatment of choice is enucleation. This is also the case for many patients with retinoblastoma and glaucoma.

Management of glaucoma associated with Sturge-Weber syndrome requires special consideration. With respect to patients affected by the mechanism of elevated

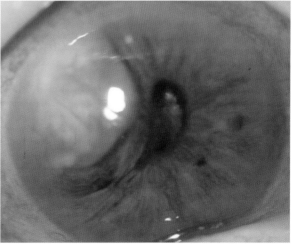

FIGURE 37.6 Iris metastasis from endometrial carcinoma causing neovascular glaucoma.

episcleral venous pressure, surgical therapy is frequently required. Patients who undergo trabeculectomy have an increased risk of intraoperative choroidal effusion and expulsive hemorrhage.[32] Goniotomy has been successful in some patients and carries a smaller risk of complications.[33] Glaucoma implant surgery with valved or nonvalved drainage devices has also been advocated.

PROGNOSIS

The prognosis for patients with intraocular tumors and glaucoma is particularly relevant in cases of malignancy. Histopathologic analyses of patients with ciliary body melanoma and glaucoma have revealed tumor cells within the aqueous outflow tract, and increased intraocular pressure may contribute to extraocular dissemination.[34] Patients with ring melanoma of the trabecular meshwork tend to also have a high rate of metastases.[9] In addition, patients with choroidal melanoma and glaucoma have a worse prognosis secondary to large tumor size at the time of presentation. With respect to retinoblastoma, glaucoma is generally associated with larger tumor size and these patients tend to have a worse prognosis.[35] Iris neovascularization is also indicative of poor prognosis irrespective of the presence of glaucoma.

Summary

Glaucoma is a manifestation of intraocular neoplasia that affects the health of the eye and may affect the patient's systemic prognosis. Intraocular tumors can cause elevated IOP through both open-angle and angle-closure mechanisms. It is important to consider intraocular tumors in the differential diagnosis of a patient with unilateral glaucoma.

REFERENCES

1. Shields CL, Shields JA, Shields MB, et al. Prevalence and mechanisms of secondary intraocular pressure elevation in eyes with intraocular tumors. Ophthalmology 1987; 94:839–846.

2. Ferry AP. Font RL. Carcinoma metastatic to the eye and orbit. I. A clinicopathologic study of 227 cases. Arch Ophthalmol 1974; 92:276–286.

3. Yoshizumi MO, Thomas JV, Smith TR. Glaucoma-inducing mechanisms in eyes with retinoblastoma. Arch Ophthalmol 1978; 96:105–110.

4. Ferry AP, Font RL. Carcinoma metastatic to the eye and orbit. II. A clinicopathological study of 26 patients with carcinoma metastatic to the anterior segment of the eye. Arch Ophthalmol 1975; 93:472–482.

5. Yanoff M. Glaucoma mechanisms in ocular malignant melanomas. Am J Ophthalmol 1970; 70:898–904.

6. Yanoff M, Scheie HG. Melanomalytic glaucoma. Report of a case. Arch Ophthalmol 1970; 84:471–473.

7. Kozlowski IM, Hirose T, Jalkh AE. Massive subretinal hemorrhage with acute angle-closure glaucoma in chronic myelocytic leukemia. Am J Ophthalmol 1987; 103:837–838.

8. Wohlrab TM, Pleyer U, Rohrbach JM, et al. Sudden increase in intraocular pressure as an initial manifestation of myelodysplastic syndrome. Am J Ophthalmol 1995; 119:370–372.

9. Demirci H, Shields CL, Shields JA, et al. Ring melanoma of the anterior chamber angle: a report of fourteen cases. Am J Ophthalmol 2001; 132:336–342.

10. Jakobiec FA, Depot MJ, Henkind P, et al. Fluorescein angiographic patterns of iris melanocytic tumors. Arch Ophthalmol 1982; 100:1288–1299.

11. Pavlin CJ, McWhae JA, McGowan HD, et al. Ultrasound biomicroscopy of anterior segment tumors. Ophthalmology 1992; 99:1220–1228.

12. Maberly DA, Pavlin CJ, McGowan HD, et al. Ultrasound biomicroscopic imaging of the anterior aspect of peripheral choroidal melanomas. Am J Ophthalmol 1997; 123:506–514.

13. Midena E, Segato T, Piermarocchi S, et al. Fine needle aspiration biopsy in ophthalmology. Surv Ophthalmol 1985; 29:410–422.

14. Ellsworth RM. The practical management of retinoblastoma. Trans Am Ophthalmol Soc 1969; 7:462–534.

15. Moazed K, Albert D, Smith TR. Rubeosis iridis in 'pseudogliomas.' Surv Ophthalmol 1980; 25:85–90.

16. Sullivan TJ, Clarke MP, Morin JD. The ocular manifestations of the Sturge-Weber syndrome. J Pediatr Ophthalmol Strabismus 1992; 29:349–356.

17. Cibis GW, Tripathi RC, Tripathi BJ. Glaucoma in Sturge-Weber syndrome. Ophthalmology 1984; 91:1061–1071.

18. Grant WM, Walton DS. Distinctive gonioscopic findings in glaucoma due to neurofibromatosis. Arch Ophthalmol 1968; 79:127–134.

19. Zimmerman LE. Ocular lesions of juvenile xanthogranuloma. Nevoxanthoedothelioma. Am J Ophthalmol 1965; 60:1011–1035.

20. Broughton WL, Zimmerman LE. A clinicopathologic study of 56 cases of intraocular medulloepitheliomas. Am J Ophthalmol 1978; 85:407–418.

21. Singh A, Singh AD, Shields CL, Shields JA. Iris neovascularization in children as a manifestation of underlying medulloepithelioma. J Pediatr Ophthalmol Strabismus 2001; 38:224–228.

22. Shields JA, Kline MW, Augsburger JJ. Primary iris cysts: a review of the literature and report of 62 cases. Br J Ophthalmol 1984; 68:152–166.

23. Marigo FA, Esaki K, Finger PT, et al. Differential diagnosis of anterior segment cysts by ultrasound biomicroscopy. Ophthalmology 1999; 106:2131–2135.

24. Nakazawa M, Tamai M. Iris melanocytoma with secondary glaucoma. Am J Ophthalmol 1984; 97:797–799.

25. Shields JA, Augsburger JJ, Sanborn GE, et al. Adenoma of the iris-pigment epithelium. Ophthalmology 1983; 90:735–739.

26. Reese AB, Mund ML, Iwamoto T. Tapioca melanoma of the iris. 1. Clinical and light microscopy studies. Am J Ophthalmol 1972; 74:840–850.

27. Bloch RS, Gartner S. The incidence of ocular metastatic carcinoma. Arch Ophthalmol 1971; 85:673–675.

28. Rosenthal AR. Ocular manifestations of leukemia. A review. Ophthalmology 1983; 90:899–905.

29. Saga T, Ohno S, Matsuda H, et al. Ocular involvement by a peripheral T-cell lymphoma. Arch Ophthalmol 1984; 102:399–402.

30. Shakin EP, Augsburger JJ, Eagle RC Jr, et al. Multiple myeloma involving the iris. Arch Ophthalmol 1988; 106:524–526.

31. Grossniklaus HE, Brown RH, Stulting RD, et al. Iris melanoma seeding through a trabeculectomy site. Arch Ophthalmol 1990; 108:1287–1290.

32. Christensen GR, Records RE. Glaucoma and expulsive hemorrhage mechanisms in the Sturge-Weber syndrome. Ophthalmology 1979; 86:1360–1366.

33. Iwach AG, Hoskins HD Jr, Hetherington J Jr, et al. Analysis of surgical and medical management of glaucoma in Sturge-Weber syndrome. Ophthalmology 1990; 97:904–909.

34. Shields MB, Klintworth GK. Anterior uveal melanomas and intraocular pressure. Ophthalmology 1980; 87:503–517.

35. Haik BG, Dunleavy SA, Cooke C, et al. Retinoblastoma with anterior chamber extension. Ophthalmology 1987; 94:367–370.

PRINCIPLES OF MANAGEMENT

Management of Ocular Hypertension and Primary Open-Angle Glaucoma

Roger A Hitchings

INTRODUCTION

This chapter sets out the principles of management of ocular hypertension and primary open-angle glaucoma. For the purpose of this chapter ocular hypertension (OHT) is defined as an eye having an intraocular pressure (IOP) lying two standard deviations or more above the mean IOP for the population, in the absence of any visible acquired change in the topography of the optic nerve head, or visual field defect characteristic for glaucoma (see Ch. 25, Ocular Hypertension). Usually this means an IOP consistently exceeding 21 mmHg, but for some populations this might be a higher or (as in the case of native Japanese) lower than 21 mmHg.

Primary open-angle glaucoma (POAG) is said to be present when there is a characteristic deformity of the optic nerve head, characterized as glaucomatous cupping, usually with a demonstrable reduction in visual function, shown as reduced retinal sensitivity in spatial location corresponding with the anatomic change (see Ch 26, Primary Open-Angle Glaucoma). The 'angle' of the anterior chamber is said to be 'open' and there is often an elevated IOP without visible cause. Some eyes may have an appearance of the optic nerve head or defects in visual function that could be misconstrued as glaucoma and in some cases the diagnosis of glaucoma may only be confirmed by disease progression.

Treatment for OHT and POAG is restricted to reducing intraocular pressure. Currently there is no proven 'non-IOP' antiglaucoma therapy available.

Management is based on the assessment of risk, the response to therapy, rate of progression, and the patient's needs. It requires initial assessment, target setting, and monitoring. This chapter will look at management from these three viewpoints and discuss each in turn (see also Ch. 40, Target Intraocular Pressure and Ch. 45, Benefit versus Risk). The same principles will apply for the management of glaucoma secondary to other (chronic) ocular conditions (especially pigment dispersion and pseudoexfoliation) and, apart from specific indications for the primary condition, the principles of management would be the same.

OCULAR HYPERTENSION

The case for treating ocular hypertension need to be balanced against the cost and the patient's perceived benefits. Although ocular hypertension is an established risk factor for developing POAG, it is not the only one, and does not inevitably lead to 'conversion' to POAG.

The cost of treating OHT may become a societal one, with pharmaceutical costs being a significant restricting factor in the widespread use of topical hypotensives.

BACKGROUND

The Ocular Hypertension Treatment Study (OHTS) demonstrated that sustained IOP reduction halved the conversion rate to POAG in a selected group of subjects.[1] A number of baseline factors were good predictors of 'conversion.'[2] The European Glaucoma Prevention Study (EGPS) did not demonstrate such protection, a fact attributable at least in part to differences in study design and a lower mean IOP difference between the two arms of the study.[3] However, a comparison of the untreated arms from the two studies showed that data from EGPS confirmed the predictive factors for 'conversion' shown in the OHTS.[4] These were baseline age, intraocular pressure, central corneal thickness, vertical cup-to-disc ratio, and Humphrey VF pattern standard deviation. A retrospective review of patients followed in the Diagnostic Interventions in Glaucoma Study (DIGS) agreed with the ability of such risk factors to predict which patients were most likely to 'convert' to glaucoma.[5]

Treatment by reducing (elevated) IOP offers protection from developing POAG within 5 years in higher-risk patients. Who should receive treatment? Kymes and colleagues looked at the outcomes from the OHTS and concluded that the treatment of those patients with IOP of ≥24 mmHg and a ≥2% annual risk of the development of glaucoma is likely to be cost-effective, identifying US$42 430 per quality-adjusted life year for this group[6] (see also Ch. 3, Economics of Glaucoma Care).

In contrast, Thomas and colleagues expressed concern that as ocular hypertension has an 'effective' PAR of 8.5%, this is a value not considered high enough to warrant public health intervention (*at least in 'developing countries'* – author's addition in italics) (see also Ch. 45, Benefit versus Risk).[7]

Public perception and national health budgets will inevitably play a role in the allocation of resources for the management of OHT.

ASSESSMENT

Identification of a patient with elevated IOP will lead to assessment, a decision on whether hypotensive therapy was needed from the outset and then formulation of plans for long-term monitoring.

Recognition of elevated IOP needs to be followed by an assessment of primary or secondary cause, consistent together with mean IOP level. Baseline risk factors as identified by OHTS/EGPS need to be looked for.

Identification of risk factors allows a prediction of 5-year risk; this will help the advice given to the patient.

In consultation with the patient about risk, an informed decision is taken on whether to initiate therapy. Influencing factors will include the absolute IOP level, the presence of a positive family history (particularly in siblings), cost, patient concern, and likely compliance.

MONITORING

Following initial assessment and therapeutic management decisions, a course for monitoring needs to be set. To do this, baseline values for visual function, optic nerve head and retinal nerve fiber layer imaging, and response to initial therapy need to be obtained.

Long-term follow-up needs to be at a frequency compatible with the patient's wishes and ability to attend, combined with the perceived likelihood of demonstrable change (suggesting 'conversion') between visits. For OHT without treatment (low risk), an annual visit usually suffices. With treatment, a biannual visit may be required. Image and functional assessment should be undertaken once a year to look for stability or change.

PRIMARY OPEN-ANGLE GLAUCOMA

The expectation is for elevated IOP to coexist with acquired change at the optic disc and in visual function. However, in many populations POAG may occur without elevated IOP. Whereas the management of OHT is relatively straightforward – a decision whether or not to lower the IOP – management in POAG becomes more complicated when the IOP lies in the normal range (see Ch. 30, Normal-Tension Glaucoma).

BACKGROUND

Two randomized treatment/no treatment trials have demonstrated a benefit from IOP reduction, the Collaborative Normal-Tension Glaucoma Study (CNTGS),[8] and the Early Manifest Glaucoma Trial (EMGT).[9] However, in both studies it was noted that for a significant subset of patients visual field progression in the untreated group might not be detected for 5 years or more. Risk factors for progression in CNTGS included disc hemorrhages, female gender, and migraine, but not age or baseline IOP.[10] The EMGT noted that risk factors for progression were a higher baseline IOP, exfoliation, bilateral disease, worse mean deviation, and older age, as well as frequent disc hemorrhages during follow-up.[11]

IOP reduction in POAG can slow if not halt progression. Even in developing countries, hypotensive treatment can be considered justifiable with a population attributable risk (PAR) of 16%.[7]

DIAGNOSIS

As for OHT, management for POAG starts with initial assessment, the defining of treatment (IOP reduction) goals, and then long-term monitoring. Successful management will be to prevent visual disability during the patient's lifetime, even if that means that some disease progression may have occurred. Clearly, the sooner the patient is diagnosed the better, even if the decision is made to defer treatment.

Management of glaucoma in any defined population has to be organized in such a way that early cases of glaucomatous cupping with visual field defects can be identified. This means the recognition that elevated IOP is not needed for the diagnosis of POAG. For presymptomatic glaucoma this means diagnosis in primary care, whether by other healthcare professionals, physicians, ophthalmologists, or glaucoma specialists. Two studies have demonstrated a cost increase for treating glaucoma in the later stages of disease.[12,13] Additionally, the response to hypotensive treatment would appear less marked with later stages of disease[14] while the risk of going blind despite good IOP control is increased.[15] Glaucoma management then can be summarized as the diagnosis of glaucoma at an early and certainly presymptomatic stage, followed by assessment, the setting of IOP targets, and adequate long-term monitoring.

COMPLIANCE AND ADHERENCE

A major issue for long-term management of chronic glaucoma is compliance[16] (see Ch. 43, Adherence and Persistence) and adherence with treatment.[17] It has been demonstrated that adherence may be improved by simplification of drop regimens, education, and self-reporting. All measures depend on patient cooperation and understanding, as well as a realization that failure to maintain IOP control can lead to significant disability. A recent study demonstrated that the main fear was disability such as loss of the driving license and blindness rather than the mode of treatment.[18]

ASSESSMENT

Initial assessment of the patient recently diagnosed with POAG involves looking at the risk of visual disability developing in the patient's lifetime. This will involve assessment of binocular function, age, likely compliance, as well as severity of disease in the two eyes, and any comorbidity, whether ocular (such as external eye inflammation, cataract or age-related macular degeneration), or systemic (such as diabetes).

It is important to identify the IOP level at which glaucomatous optic nerve damage occurred. This may require phasing over 24 hours if the initial readings are within the normal range.

The patient will require indefinite monitoring. Training is needed to obtain repeatable performances on visual field testing (see Ch. 10, Visual Fields). Two or three visual field tests may be needed for this. Baseline imaging of the optic nerve head and retinal nerve fiber layer is helpful, for the promise of software development that will identify change in the future. Baseline photographs of the optic disc (preferably stereophotographs) form a reasonable alternative at the present time (See Ch. 17, Optic Disc Photography in the Diagnosis of Glaucoma and Ch. 18, Optic Disc Imaging).

TREATMENT

The decision on whether to initiate medical treatment will depend upon the baseline IOP and the presence of other risk factors identified from the no-treatment studies. Additionally, the response to acceptable trials of therapy and the availability and affordability of hypotensive medications need to be considered. Many patients with normal-tension glaucoma are elderly and, if they have early visual field loss, may be safely watched as progression will be slow, if at all. Some patients with moderately elevated 'high tension glaucoma' respond little to therapy, or prove to be poor compliers. Other patients cannot obtain or instill medications (and may not be able to comply with the demands of monitoring). For this last group a decision needs be taken whether to offer laser or conventional surgery, or, again, just to monitor them. In conjunction with the patient, a decision to monitor without treatment may be the chosen option.

A 'target pressure' for the patient needs to be set, and an assessment made, if the 'target' is not met, whether to add therapy or switch medications (see Ch. 40, Target Intraocular Pressure). A trial of therapy should mean the application of hypotensive medication to one eye, the other remaining as a control (assuming that the response would be equal in the two eyes).[19]

MONITORING

Whatever the chosen target pressure, there is no guarantee that progression will have been halted. All patients with POAG, whether treated or not, should be closely monitored for the first 2 years. This gives the clinician an opportunity to identify the 'rapid progressors' and amend therapy appropriately. After the first 2 years, those eyes without apparent progression can have the recall intervals extended. Eventually, biannual or even less frequent intervals can be achieved.

Progression despite achieving a target IOP offers the physician three choices. First, to ask whether the IOPs measured at a clinic visit accurately reflect levels the rest of the time. Here, an investigation into compliance, adherence, and diurnal IOPs is warranted. Secondly, to further lower the IOP. This may be achieved medically by adding further medications or switching to an alternative. The former may be achieved by the use of combination therapy, although two drugs in combination do not always provide the expected IOP reduction from their actions when given alone. Thirdly, to switch to or add laser trabeculoplasty, or to offer filtration surgery. If the third choice is taken, it is necessary to recall that cataract- and bleb-related infections are a sequel of standard guarded filtration procedures ('trabeculectomy') and that the IOP level achieved after nonfiltration procedures may not be as low that for trabeculectomy.

REFERENCES

1. Kass MA, Heuer DK, Higginbotham EJ, et al. The Ocular Hypertension Treatment Study: a randomized trial determines that topical ocular hypotensive medication delays or prevents the onset of primary open-angle glaucoma. Arch Ophthalmol 2002; 120:701–713.

2. Gordon MO, Beiser JA, Brandt JD, et al. The Ocular Hypertension Treatment Study: baseline factors that predict the onset of primary open-angle glaucoma. Arch Ophthalmol 2002; 120:714–720.

3. Miglior S, Zeyen T, Pfeiffer N, et al. Results of the European Glaucoma Prevention Study. Ophthalmology 2005; 112: 366–375.

4. Ocular Hypertension Treatment Study Group; European Glaucoma Prevention Study Group, Gordon MD, Torri V, Miglior S, et al. Validated prediction model for the development of primary open-angle glaucoma in individuals with ocular hypertension. Ophthalmology 2007; 114:10–19.

5. Medeiros FA, Weinreb RN, Sample PA, et al. Validation of a predictive model to estimate the risk of conversion from ocular hypertension to glaucoma. Arch Ophthalmol 2005; 123:1351–1360.

6. Kymes SM, Kass MA, Anderson DR, et al. Management of ocular hypertension: a cost-effectiveness approach from the Ocular Hypertension Treatment Study. Am J Ophthalmol 2006; 141:997–1008.

7. Thomas R, Kumar RS, Chandrasekhar G, et al. Applying the recent clinical trials on primary open angle glaucoma: the developing world perspective. J Glaucoma 2005; 14:324–327.

8. The effectiveness of intraocular pressure reduction in the treatment of normal-tension glaucoma. Collaborative Normal-Tension Glaucoma Study Group. Am J Ophthalmol 1998; 126:498–505.

9. Heijl A, Leske MC, Bengtsson B, et al. Reduction of intraocular pressure and glaucoma progression: results from the Early

Manifest Glaucoma Trial. Arch Ophthalmol 2002; 120: 1268–1279.

10. Drance S, Anderson DR, Schulzer M, Collaborative Normal-Tension Glaucoma Study Group. Risk factors for progression of visual field abnormalities in normal-tension glaucoma. Am J Ophthalmol 2001; 131:699–708.

11. Leske MC, Heijl A, Hussein M, et al. Factors for glaucoma progression and the effect of treatment: the Early Manifest Glaucoma Trial. Arch Ophthalmol 2003; 121:48–56.

12. Lee PP, Walt JG, Doyle JJ, et al. A multicenter, retrospective pilot study of resource use and costs associated with severity of disease in glaucoma. Arch Ophthalmol 2006; 124:12–19.

13. Traverso CE, Walt JG, Kelly SP, et al. Direct costs of glaucoma and severity of the disease: a multinational long term study of resource utilisation in Europe. Br J Ophthalmol 2005; 89:1245–1249.

14. Oliver JE, Hattenhauer MG, Herman D, et al. Blindness and glaucoma: a comparison of patients progressing to blindness from glaucoma with patients maintaining vision. Am J Ophthalmol 2002; 133:764–772.

15. Forsman E, Kivela T, Vesti E. Lifetime visual disability in open-angle glaucoma and ocular hypertension. J Glaucoma 2007; 16:313–319.

16. Shaya FT. Compliance with medicine. Ophthalmol Clin North Am 2005; 18:611–617.

17. Tsai JC. Medication adherence in glaucoma: approaches for optimizing patient compliance. Curr Opin Ophthalmol 2006; 17:190–195.

18. Bhargava JS, Patel B, Foss AJ, et al. Views of glaucoma patients on aspects of their treatment: an assessment of patient preference by conjoint analysis. Invest Ophthalmol Vis Sci 2006; 47:2885–2888.

19. Realini T, Fechtner RD, Atreides SP, et al. The uniocular drug trial and second-eye response to glaucoma medications. Ophthalmology 2004; 111:421–426.

CHAPTER 39

An Overview of Angle-Closure Management

Chaiwat Teekhasaenee

INTRODUCTION

Angle closure is defined by iris obstruction of the anterior chamber angle resulting in an elevation of intraocular pressure (IOP). The obstruction may be due to a preexisting anatomical predisposition (primary) or a pathological process (secondary). The condition constitutes a number of different disorders with various pathogenic mechanisms that have iris apposition to the angle wall as a common finding. In general, the mechanisms of angle closure may be classified into 'pushing' or 'pulling' the iris forward with or without pupillary block. Multiple mechanisms may coexist in an eye. Proper management depends on the accurate diagnosis of the pathogenesis of angle closure. A thorough ocular history and comprehensive examination including dynamic gonioscopy, biometry, and imaging with ultrasonic biomicroscopy (UBM) or optical coherence tomography (OCT) are vital in identifying the underlying mechanisms.[1–5] (See Chapter 27, Primary Angle-Closure Glaucoma, for a more detailed discussion; also see Chapters 13, Gonioscopy, and 15, Angle Imaging.)

Primary angle closure (PAC) is the most common form of angle closure. Recent studies have shown that PAC is highly prevalent in East Asia, including China and India where almost half of the world's population lives.[6–9] The condition is highly destructive and causes ocular damage more than primary open-angle glaucoma (POAG). A study has shown that bilateral blindness in China from primary angle-closure glaucoma (PACG) exceeds that from POAG.[9] It is generally believed that PAC is uncommon in Caucasians. However, a recent study in northern Italy has shown that the prevalence of PAC in a white population is not as uncommon as previously thought.[10] Furthermore, a study comparing chronic PAC in Asians and North Americans has also found no difference in the clinical course of the disease among different racial populations.[11]

Recently, a new nomenclature of PAC based on end-organ damage or stage of the disease has been proposed. At the earliest stage of development, an eye that has a narrow or occludable angle as the only abnormal finding is termed primary angle-closure suspect (PACS).

When synechial formation and IOP elevation occur, the term primary angle closure (PAC) is applied. Finally, primary angle-closure glaucoma (PACG) is reserved for those with glaucomatous optic neuropathy and visual field loss.[12] (See Chapter 27, Primary Angle-Closure Glaucoma, for a more detailed discussion.)

PAC is a complex entity that can present in acute, subacute (intermittent), or chronic form. Although they behave differently, the three clinical manifestations overlap and may coexist in an eye. An acute attack superimposing on preexisting chronic PAC is not an uncommon finding. Chronic PAC is the most prevalent form of PAC and is responsible for worldwide blindness.[6–8] Chronic PAC may develop either after acute PAC with persistent peripheral anterior synechiae (PAS) (residual synechial angle closure) or more commonly following gradual asymptomatic closure of the angle. The lack of symptoms makes the latter frequently underdiagnosed in most populations.

IOP control in patients with PAC depends on the amount of trabecular meshwork damage and extent of PAS. There is a direct but nonlinear relationship between IOP and degrees of PAS.[13] The IOP is usually elevated when >180° of the angle is closed by the PAS.[14] Since the pathogenesis of glaucomatous damage in angle closure is primarily pressure dependent, lowering of the IOP should arrest the progression of the disease. In addition, since the trabecular meshwork is intrinsically normal, reopening of the angle prior to ultrastructural changes should restore the natural outflow pathway.

Therefore, the goals of the treatment for PAC consist of prompt reduction of IOP, reopening the anterior chamber angle and preventing recurrent angle closure and, finally, controlling residual IOP elevation if irreversible trabecular meshwork dysfunction has occurred.

REDUCTION OF INTRAOCULAR PRESSURE

ACUTE PRIMARY ANGLE CLOSURE

Acute PAC accounts for 15–45% of PAC and poses a severe threat to vision.[6–8] The extremely elevated IOP that occurs during the attack leads to rapid and permanent blindness if not properly treated. The longer the duration of an attack, the greater the damage to the ocular structures.[15] Recent imaging studies have found significant nerve fiber layer defects following an acute attack.[16,17] An acute attack should be considered as an ocular emergency requiring immediate treatment. Prompt reduction of the IOP provides a better final visual outcome than delayed treatment.

Acute PAC is initially treated with antiglaucoma medications including topical β-adrenergic blockers, systemic carbonic anhydrase inhibitors, and hyperosmotic agents. A miotic is frequently ineffective during the high IOP period and should be given when the IOP has been reduced. Copious administration of pilocarpine or the use of a strong miotic does not offer advantages over a low-dose regimen.[18–20] Topical carbonic anhydrase inhibitors can aggravate corneal edema and should be avoided. Recently, a prostaglandin analogue has been shown to be effective in reducing IOP in PAC patients whose angle is still partially open.[21] Another randomized clinical trial has shown latanoprost superior to timolol in reducing the IOP in patients who had undergone laser iridotomy.[22] Alpha$_2$-agonists have been shown to exert a neuroprotective effect in experimental models of optic nerve injury in addition to lowering of the IOP.[23,24] However, a study in patients with acute PAC failed to demonstrate superiority of the medication in protecting visual field when compared to timolol.[25]

Although effective in a majority of cases, medical treatment takes times to reduce the IOP to a safe level. Patients may have to suffer a prolonged period of severe pain. In addition, serious systemic side effects from the medications including metabolic acidosis and electrolyte disturbance can occur. Because of these problems with medical treatment, alternate approaches have been developed. The idea that initial treatment for the acute attack should be with medications has been challenged by an approach that used argon laser peripheral iridoplasty (LPI) and immediate paracentesis.[26–28] It was shown that LPI or paracentesis reduced IOP and relieved the symptoms much more rapidly than medications. Although the reported complications of paracentesis were minimal, the procedure is considered invasive and should be reserved for a competent ophthalmologist.

CHRONIC PRIMARY ANGLE CLOSURE

When the anterior chamber angle is closed >180°, chronic treatment with hypotensive medications is usually necessary. Medical treatment of chronic PAC resembles that of POAG. However, a miotic is ineffective in eyes with extensive PAS and may lead to a paradoxical rise of the IOP. Latanoprost decreases IOP in eyes with PAC more than timolol.[21,22,29,30] Travoprost is equally effective to latanoprost in treating patients with PAC.[31] Interestingly, the IOP-reducing efficacy of latanoprost did not correlate with the degree of angle narrowing or extent of PAS.[32] Since the pathogenesis of glaucomatous damage in PACG is primarily pressure dependent, the benefit of lowering IOP to a very low target level as in POAG is yet to be determined.

REOPENING OF THE ANTERIOR CHAMBER ANGLE

LASER IRIDOTOMY

See also Chapter 65, Peripheral Iridectomy.

Acute primary angle closure Laser iridotomy is currently considered the definitive treatment of acute PAC with pupillary block. Surgical iridectomy is indicated only when the laser treatment cannot be accomplished. The procedure provides an alternative route for aqueous trapped in the posterior chamber to enter the anterior chamber. When the pressure difference between the posterior and anterior chambers diminishes, the appositional iris may recede from the angle wall. Ultrasound biomicroscopy reveals a significant widening of the anterior chamber angle after laser iridotomy.[33–35]

However, laser iridotomy is not always effective. It is probably most beneficial for patients with early synechial development. Those eyes with chronic PAS and glaucomatous optic neuropathy (PACG) respond poorly to the laser procedure and frequently need further treatment.[36] A study in Asian eyes with acute PAC that had undergone laser iridotomy showed that 58.1% continued to have elevated IOP and 32.7% eventually required trabeculectomy.[36] A study comparing chronic PAC in Asians and North Americans reported similar results.[11] In addition, the procedure does not always provide a long-term efficacy.[36,37] Recurrent attacks and progressive PAS formation (creeping angle closure) can occur if nonpupillary block mechanisms are also present. A study showed that 32.2% of 59 eyes with acute PAC had progression of PAS following a successful laser iridotomy.[38] Repeat gonioscopy and constant monitoring of the IOP are essential when following these patients.

The fellow eye The fellow eye of a patient who develops an acute attack has a 40–80% chance of developing an acute attack within 5–10 years.[39–41] Biometric studies reveal that these eyes tend to be shorter and have more crowded anterior segments than those of healthy eyes.[42] Chronic administration of pilocarpine usually fails to prevent the attack. In contrast, both surgical iridectomy and laser iridotomy have been shown to be highly effective in preventing the attack in most cases.[43–45] A prompt prophylactic laser iridotomy is therefore recommended in the contralateral eye unless the angle is obviously nonoccludable.[46]

An occludable angle (primary angle-closure suspect, primary angle closure) Because of high patient acceptance and simplicity, laser iridotomy has gained widespread popularity since its introduction in the 1970s. The number of the procedures performed annually has increased considerably not only for PAC, PACG, and fellow eyes but also for PACS. One study showed that the number of laser iridotomies was more than four times the annual rate of surgical iridectomies performed before the laser was available.[47] With the increasing availability of laser instruments and relatively low risk of the procedure, prophylactic laser iridotomy has become widely popular not only in general eye clinics but also in mobile screening community campaigns. Since only a small number of PACS progresses to PAC,[48,49] performing prophylactic laser iridotomy routinely in all suspicious eyes without a comprehensive assessment of the angle configuration can result in overtreatment. Although laser iridotomy is considered relatively safe, the procedure also has potential risks. Postoperative transient focal lenticular and corneal endothelial burns are common. Progressive corneal edema requiring penetrating keratoplasty and subclinical cystoid macular edema after prophylactic argon laser iridotomy can occur.[50–52] Since laser iridotomy alters the natural passage of aqueous flow resulting in an increase in lens–iris contact and, theoretically, a possible disturbance of lens metabolism, the procedure can predispose to cataract formation.[53] It has shown that there is a significant rate of cataract progression (7.7%) requiring cataract surgery within 1 year following prophylactic laser iridotomy.[54] Unexpectedly, this simple prophylactic treatment can result in another cause of visual morbidity.

Although several studies have demonstrated the efficacy of prophylactic laser iridotomy in the fellow eye of a patient with monocular PAC, there is no long-term prospective study evaluating the risk-to-benefit ratio of the procedure in PACS. A recent population-based intervention study has shown that in spite of a significant increase in the angle width following laser iridotomy, one-fifth of the patients with PACS continue to have appositional angle closure.[35] Obviously, laser iridotomy is insufficient for PACS whose other pathogenic mechanisms, apart from pupillary block, do exist. Therefore, it would be unjustified to advocate prophylactic laser iridotomy as a universal treatment for all PACS. A decision to treat PACS should be based on a thorough assessment of the angle configuration by gonioscopy and clinical judgment. To help in this process, biometric and imaging studies with UBM and OCT can be valuable tools in evaluating the suspicious angle.[1–5]

Chronic primary angle closure Coexistence of PAS and appositional closure usually presents in an eye with chronic PAC. Laser iridotomy is indicated only in the presence of appositional closure. Eyes with extensive PAS respond poorly to the procedure. Like acute PACG, multiple disease mechanisms may coexist in chronic PACG. Those with nonpupillary block can develop progressive PAS in spite of a patent laser iridotomy.

LASER PERIPHERAL IRIDOPLASTY

See also Chapter 66, Laser Iridoplasty.

Acute primary angle closure Laser peripheral iridoplasty (LPI) has been shown to be effective in lowering IOP in patients with an acute attack that is unresponsive to medical therapy and laser iridotomy cannot be performed.[27,55–57] Tightening of the peripheral iris by applying a series of laser burns mechanically pulls open the appositionally closed angle. A rapid reduction of the IOP usually occurs within 1 hour following the laser treatment.

Recently, it has been shown that an acute attack may be broken by LPI alone without the use of topical antiglaucoma medications.[27,28,58] Another study has also shown that initial treatment of acute PAC with LPI is safe and even more effective than systemic antiglaucoma medications.[26] Patients who underwent LPI had a more rapid IOP reduction than those treated with hypotensive medications. Since LPI only temporarily breaks the attack and does not terminate pupillary block, laser iridotomy should be performed subsequently as the definitive treatment.

Chronic primary angle closure A mix of PAS and appositional angle closure may coexist in an eye with chronic PAC. Only eyes with appositional closure respond favorably to LPI. Although laser gonioplasty, a similar contraction laser procedure performed through a mirror of a gonioscopy lens, may separate recent synechiae, it is unlikely that LPI will break long-standing PAS.[59,60]

Plateau iris See also above and Chapter 32, Secondary Angle-Closure Glaucomas.

Plateau iris is another form of PAC. It is caused by anteriorly positioned or large ciliary processes. Since pupillary block always coexists with the condition, a laser iridotomy should be performed before making the diagnosis. The condition typically presents with persistent appositional closure despite a patent laser iridotomy. LPI effectively flattens the plateau iris configuration and opens the appositionally closed angle. Long-term effectiveness of laser iridoplasty in preventing the progression of PAS in plateau iris has been reported, although a small number of patients required additional treatment.[61]

LENS EXTRACTION

Primary angle closure (PAC) is an anatomical disorder of the eye with abnormal relationships of the anterior segment structures. The most remarkable biometric feature in an eye with PAC is a shallow anterior chamber. Although several anatomic predispositions are involved, the anterior chamber depth is primarily determined by the lens thickness and anterior position of the lens.[62,63] A thick and anteriorly positioned lens plays a pivotal role in the pathogenesis of both pupillary block and crowding of the anterior segment. Removal of the lens in eyes with PAC results in a significant increase in anterior chamber depth and angle width.[64–66] The narrower the preoperative anterior chamber angle, the greater the postoperative angle widening. Replacement of the natural lens with an intraocular lens (IOL) in

PAC patients can provide up to 4 mm more axial distance within the anterior chamber, or almost a threefold increase in the central anterior chamber depth and effectively eliminates both pupillary block and angle crowding.[67] In addition, anterior chamber deepening with a viscoelastic during the operation may break recently formed synechiae.

Several clinical studies have shown that lens extraction either by extracapsular cataract extraction (ECCE)[68–72] or phacoemulsification[73–76] is effective in opening the angle and decreasing IOP in patients who had developed an acute attack. Phacoemulsification has several advantages over ECCE. The small incision procedure offers a higher success rate in removing of the lens with less inflammation and fewer complications. In addition, the temporal clear corneal approach spares the superior conjunctiva for a possible filtering surgery. The procedure is highly effective in PAC patients with appositional closure or recently developed synechiae. Those with long-standing PAS and advanced glaucomatous optic neuropathy respond less favorably to the treatment.

Lens extraction has long been the definitive treatment for phacomorphic glaucoma. Currently, it is being considered for uncontrolled PAC as well. In the presence of a cataract, the procedure can be considered early in the course of the disease. However, the decision is more controversial when the lens is relatively clear. Early removal of a clear lens as a treatment for uncontrolled PAC has been debated for years. With the advancement of surgical techniques and instrumentation in lens extraction and several promising clinical evidences, removal of a clear lens as a treatment for PAC is gaining more popularity.[74,77] Furthermore, it has been shown that cataract formation develops rapidly following an acute attack.[78,79] The issue of trading a clear problematic lens for a possible control of the glaucoma is becoming more logically and ethically acceptable.

Lens removal in patients with acute PAC is not without risks. Performing a surgery in an inflamed eye with elevated IOP and a shallow anterior chamber requires a competent surgical skill. Inadvertent corneal damage, malignant glaucoma, and lens dislocation are potential intraoperative complications. Postoperative fibrinous anterior chamber reaction and transient pressure spike can occur.[67] Therefore, initial treatment of PAC patients should follow the standard protocols including medical and laser treatment. If the standard treatment fails to control the IOP and surgical intervention is necessary, lens extraction can be considered. Combined lens extraction with trabeculectomy or nonpenetrating deep sclerectomy has been reported as an effective surgical option for patients with chronic PACG who are unlikely to respond to lens extraction alone.[80,81]

GONIOSYNECHIALYSIS

Up to 60% of patients with acute PAC have persistent pressure elevation requiring glaucoma medications

following laser iridotomy.[36,73,78,82,83] Possible factors accounting for the development of residual synechial angle closure include delayed initial presentation, pre-existing chronic PAC prior to the acute attack, severity of the acute attack, and the coexistence of nonpupillary block mechanisms.[84–86] Postoperative IOP control depends on the amount of trabecular meshwork damage and extent of PAS. Irreversible damage to the trabecular meshwork will eventually occur if the PAS remain untreated. A logical approach is to eliminate the PAS and restore the trabecular function prior to the irreversible ultrastructural changes. Filtration through the natural pathway should be more physiologic and reliable than the artificial pathway of filtering surgery.

Surgical goniosynechialysis (GSL) is an effective procedure designed to strip the PAS from the angle wall and restore the trabecular outflow.[14,87] The procedure was successful in 80% of eyes with minimal complications if the PAS had been present for less than 1 year.[14] Later studies have confirmed the effectiveness of the procedure in reducing PAS and improving IOP control.[88–96] The success of the procedure depends not only on the preoperative duration but also on the recurrence of the PAS.

One of the major contributing factors in reformation of the PAS is the crystalline lens. A thickening lens would crowd the anterior chamber and force the iris back against the trabecular meshwork. GSL becomes more effective when performed after lens removal. An increase in the anterior chamber space provides ample room to perform the procedure and decreases the chance of synechial reformation. Combined phacoemulsification and GSL (phaco-GSL) has been shown to be safe and highly effective in controlling the IOP and decreased PAS in >90% of 52 eyes that developed acute angle closure within 6 months and had persistent IOP elevation following the laser treatment.[67,97,98] Recurrence of the PAS, although uncommon, might occur during the first 3 months. The success of phaco-GSL have been stable since the third postoperative month for up to 14 years of follow-up, providing a long-lasting or possibly permanent cure.[67] Phaco-GSL is best for PAC patients who have had a previously normal trabecular meshwork that has recently developed synechiae. Patients with long-standing PAS of more than 6 months are poor candidates. The shorter the duration of synechial closure, the better the prognosis. However, a postoperative fibrinous anterior chamber reaction commonly occurs if the operation is performed during the first 4 weeks after the acute attack. The optimal timing for the operation is suggested at week 6 after the acute attack when the inflammation subsides.[67]

CONTROLLING RESIDUAL INTRAOCULAR ELEVATION

FILTERING SURGERY

When >270° of the angle is closed, medical therapy is usually ineffective in controlling the IOP, and trabeculectomy is generally performed.[14] However, the surgical outcomes following trabeculectomy are far from ideal. The procedure is associated with several sight-threatening complications that tend to occur in eyes with PAC.[99] In a retrospective case series of patients with medically uncontrolled acute PAC who underwent urgent trabeculectomy only 56.2% had successful long-term IOP control without antiglaucoma medication during the mean follow-up of 22 months.[99] Approximately, one-third of them developed a shallow anterior chamber. Filtration through the artificial pathway is subjected to closure by healing process and the success rate decreases over time. The routine use of antifibrotic agents in trabeculectomy increases postoperative endophthalmitis and bleb leaks. Because of a low success rate and a high incidence of complications, trabeculectomy in PAC is becoming less popular and is considered inferior to lens extraction.[72]

Summary

Primary angle-closure glaucoma is a leading cause of glaucoma blindness worldwide and remains a major public health problem. Although severe and highly destructive in nature, treating PAC is challenging and rewarding. It is possible to prevent and permanently cure the condition if an appropriate treatment is instituted early enough before irreversible changes in the trabecular meshwork and glaucomatous damage have occurred. Since several pathogenic mechanisms may coexist in an eye, proper treatment depends on the accurate diagnosis of the underlying mechanisms. In addition to gonioscopy, biometry and imaging with UBM and OCT are becoming vital tools for assessing the angle. Laser iridotomy effectively eliminates pupillary block in PAC. Prophylactic laser iridotomy is routinely recommended for the fellow eye of monocular PAC but not for all PACS. Eyes with nonpupillary block mechanisms respond unfavorably to the laser treatment and can develop recurrent attacks or progressive PAS. Lens extraction is effective for both pupillary block and angle crowding. With the advancement of surgical techniques and instrumentation, early lens extraction with or without GSL is gaining more popularity. It is replacing trabeculectomy as the definitive treatment for refractory PAC.

REFERENCES

1. Marchini G, Pagliarusco A, Toscano A, et al. Ultrasound biomicroscopic and conventional ultrasonographic study of ocular dimension in primary angle closure glaucoma. Ophthalmology 1998; 105:2091–2098.

2. Leung CK, Yung W, et al. Novel approach for anterior chamber angle analysis. Arch Ophthalmol 2006; 124:1395–1401.

3. Radhakrishnan S, Goldsmith J, Huang D, et al. Comparison of optical coherence tomography and ultrasound biomicroscopy for detection of narrow anterior chamber angles. Arch Ophthalmol 2005; 123:1053–1059.

4. Leung CK, Chan WM, Ko CY, et al. Visualization of anterior chamber angle dynamics using optical coherence tomography. Ophthalmology 2005; 112:980–984.

5. Nolan WP, See JL, Chew PT, et al. Detection of primary angle closure using anterior segment optical coherence tomography in Asian eyes. Ophthalmology 2007; 114:33–39.

6. Foster PJ, Baasanhu J, Alsbirk PH, et al. Glaucoma in Mongolia – a population-based survey in Hovsgol Province, Northern Mongolia. Arch Ophthalmol 1996; 114:1235–1241.

7. Foster PJ, Oen FT, Machin D, et al. The prevalence of glaucoma in Chinese residents of Singapore: a cross-sectional population survey of the Tanjong Pagar district. Arch Ophthalmol 2000; 118:1105–1111.

8. Dandona L, Dandona R, Mandal P, et al. Angle closure glaucoma in an urban population in southern India. The Andhra Pradesh Eye Disease Study. Ophthalmology 2000; 107:1710–1716.

9. Foster PJ, Johnson GJ. Glaucoma in China: how big is the problem? Br J Ophthalmol 2001; 85:238–242.

10. Bonomi L, Marchini G, Marraffa M, et al. Epidemiology of angle-closure glaucoma, prevalence, clinical types, and association with peripheral anterior chamber depth in the Egna-Neumarket Glaucoma Study. Ophthalmology 2000; 107:998–1003.

11. Rosman M, Aung T, Ang LPK, et al. Chronic angle-closure with glaucomatous damage: long-term clinical course in a North American population and comparison with an Asian population. Ophthalmology 2002; 109:2227–2231.

12. Foster PJ, Buhrmann RR, Quigley HA, et al. The definition and classification of glaucoma in prevalence surveys. Br J Ophthalmol 2002; 86:238–242.

13. Chandler PA. Narrow-angle glaucoma. Arch Ophthalmol 1952; 47:695–716.

14. Campbell DG, Vela A. Modern goniosynechialysis for the treatment of synechial angle-closure glaucoma. Ophthalmology 1984; 91:1052–1060.

15. David R, Tessler Z, Yassur Y. Long-term outcome of primary acute angle-closure glaucoma. Br J Ophthalmol 1985; 69: 261–262.

16. Aung T, Husain R, Gazzard G, et al. Changes in retinal nerve fiber layer thickness after acute primary angle closure. Ophthalmology 2004; 88:1475–1479.

17. Fang A, Qu J, Ji B. Measurement of retinal nerve fiber layer in primary angle closure glaucoma by optical coherence tomography. J Glaucoma 2007; 16:178–184.

18. Ganias F, Mapstone R. Miotics in closed-angle glaucoma. Br J Ophthalmol 1975; 59:205–206.

19. Airaksinen PJ, Saari KM, Tiainen TJ, et al. Management of acute closed-angle glaucoma with miotics and timolol. Br J Ophthalmol 1979; 63:822–825.

20. Edwards RS. A comparative study of Ocusert Pilo 40, intensive pilocarpine and low-dose pilocarpine in the initial treatment of primary angle-closure glaucoma. Curr Med Res Opin 1997; 13:501–509.

21. Aung T, Wong HT, Yip CC, et al. Comparison of the intraocular pressure-lowering effect of latanoprost and timolol in patients with chronic angle closure glaucoma: a preliminary study. Ophthalmology 2000; 107:1178–1183.

22. Chew PT, Aung T, Aquino MV, et al. Intraocular pressure-reducing effects and safety of latanoprost versus timolol in subjects with chronic angle closure glaucoma. Ophthalmology 2004; 111:427–434.

23. Yoles E, Wheeler LA, Schwartz M. Alpha 2-adrenoreceptor agonists are neuroprotective in a rat model of optic nerve degeneration. Invest Ophthalmol Vis Sci 1999; 40:65–73.

24. Mussie Wolde E, Ruiz G, Wijono M, et al. Neuroprotection of retinal ganglion cells by brimonidine in rats with laser-induced chronic ocular hypertension. Invest Ophthalmol Vis Sci 2001; 42:2849–2855.

25. Aung T, Oen FTS, Wong HT, et al. Randomised controlled trial comparing the effect of brimonidine and timolol on visual field

loss after acute primary angle closure. Br J Ophthalmol 2004; 88:88–94.

26. Lam DSC, Chua JKH, Tham CCY, et al. Efficacy and safety of immediate anterior chamber paracentesis in the treatment of acute primary angle-closure glaucoma. A pilot study. Ophthalmology 2002; 109:64–70.

27. Agarwal HC, Kumar R, Kalra VK, et al. Argon laser iridoplasty: a primary mode of therapy in primary angle-closure glaucoma. Indian J Ophthalmol 1991; 39:87–90.

28. Lam DSC, Lai JSM, Tham CCY. Argon laser peripheral iridoplasty versus conventional systemic medical therapy in treatment of acute primary angle-closure glaucoma. A prospective, randomized, controlled trial. Ophthalmology 2002; 109:1591–1596.

29. Sihota R, Saxena R, Agarwal HC, et al. Crossover comparison of timolol and latanoprost in chronic primary angle-closure glaucoma. Arch Ophthalmol 2004; 122:185–189.

30. Hung PT, Hsieh JW, Chen YF, et al. Efficacy of latanoprost as an adjunct to medical therapy for residual angle-closure glaucoma after iridectomy. J Ocul Pharmacol Ther 2000; 16:43–47.

31. Chen MJ, Chen YC, Chou CK, et al. Comparison of the effects of latanoprost and travoprost on intraocular pressure in chronic angle-closure glaucoma. J Ocul Pharmacol Ther 2006; 22:449–454.

32. Aung T, Chan YH, Chew TK. Degree of angle closure and the intraocular pressure-lowering effect of latanoprost in subjects with chronic angle-closure glaucoma. Ophthalmology 2005; 112:267–271.

33. Gazzard G, Friedman D, Devereux JG, et al. A prospective ultrasound biomicroscopy evaluation of changes in anterior segment morphology after laser iridotomy in Asian eyes. Ophthalmology 2003; 110:630–638.

34. Lim LS, Aung T, Husain R, et al. Acute primary angle closure configuration of the drainage angle in the first year after laser peripheral iridotomy. Ophthalmology 2004; 111:1470–1474.

35. He M, Friedman DS, Ge J, et al. Laser peripheral iridotomy in primary angle-closure suspects: biometric and gonioscopic outcomes. Ophthalmology 2007; 114:494–500.

36. Aung T, Ang LP, Chan SP, et al. Acute primary angle closure: long-term intraocular pressure outcome in Asian eyes. Am J Ophthalmol 2001; 131:7–12.

37. Nolan WP, Foster PJ, Devereux JG, et al. YAG laser iridotomy treatment for primary angle closure in East Asian eyes. Br J Ophthalmol 2000; 84:1255–1259.

38. Choi JS, Kim YY. Progression of peripheral anterior synechiae after laser iridotomy. Am J Ophthalmol 2005; 140:1125–1127.

39. Lowe RF. The natural history and principles of treatment of primary angle-closure glaucoma. Am J Ophthalmol 1966; 61:642–651.

40. Edwards RS. Behaviour of the fellow eye in acute angle-closure glaucoma. Br J Ophthalmol 1982; 66:576–579.

41. Snow JT. Value of prophylactic peripheral iridectomy on the second eye in angle-closure glaucoma. Trans Ophthalmol Soc UK 1977; 97:189–191.

42. Friedman DS, Gazzard G, Foster P, et al. Ultrasonographic biomicroscopy, Scheimpflug photography, and novel provocative tests in contralateral eyes of Chinese patients initially seen with acute angle closure. Arch Ophthalmol 2003; 121:633–642.

43. Lowe RF. Acute angle-closure glaucoma: the second eye: an analysis of 200 cases. Br J Ophthalmol 1962; 46:641–650.

44. Fleck BW, Wright E, Fairley EA. A randomised prospective comparison of operative peripheral iridectomy and Nd:YAG laser iridotomy treatment of acute angle closure glaucoma: 3-year visual acuity and intraocular pressure control outcome. Br J Ophthalmol 1997; 81:884–888.

45. Ang LP, Aung T, Chew PT. Acute primary angle closure in an Asian population: long-term outcome of the fellow eye after prophylactic laser peripheral iridotomy. Ophthalmology 2000; 107:2092–2096.

46. Saw SM, Gazzard G, Friedman DS. Interventions for angle-closure glaucoma. An evidence-based update. Ophthalmology 2003; 110:1869–1879.

47. Rivera AH, Brown RH, Anderson DR. Laser iridotomy vs surgical iridectomy. Have the indications changed? Arch Ophthalmol 1985; 103:1350–1354.

48. Thomas R, Parikh R, Muliyil J, et al. Five-year risk of progression of primary angle closure to primary angle closure glaucoma; a population based study. Acta Ophthalmol Scand 2003; 81:480–485.

49. Thomas R, George R, Parikh R, et al. Five year risk of progression of primary angle closure suspects to primary angle closure; a population based study. Br J Ophthalmol 2003; 87:450–454.

50. Schwartz AL, Martin NF, Weber PA. Corneal decompensation after argon laser iridectomy. Arch Ophthalmol 1988; 106:1572–1574.

51. Lim LS, Ho CL, Ang LPK, et al. Inferior corneal decompensation following laser peripheral iridotomy in the superior iris. Am J Ophthalmol 2006; 142:166–168.

52. Sakai H, Ishikawa H, Shinzato M, et al. Prevalence of ciliochoroidal effusion after prophylactic laser iridotomy. Am J Ophthalmol 2003; 136:537–538.

53. Caronia RM, Liebmann JM, Stegman Z, et al. Increase in iris-lens contact after laser iridotomy for pupillary block angle closure. Am J Ophthalmol 1996; 122:53–57.

54. Lim L, Hussain R, Gazzard G, et al. Cataract progression after prophylactic laser peripheral iridotomy. Potential implications for the prevention of glaucoma blindness. Ophthalmology 2005; 112:1355–1359.

55. Ritch R. Argon laser treatment for medically unresponsive attacks of angle-closure glaucoma. Ophthalmology 1982; 111:197–204.

56. Matai A, Consul S. Argon laser iridoplasty. Indian J Ophthalmol 1987; 35:290–292.

57. Lim AS, Tan A, Chew P, et al. Laser iridoplasty in the treatment of severe acute angle closure glaucoma. Int Ophthalmol 1993; 17:33–36.

58. Lam DSC, Lai JSM, Tham CCY. Immediate argon laser peripheral iridoplasty as treatment for acute attack of primary angle-closure glaucoma: a preliminary study. Ophthalmology 1998; 105:2231–2236.

59. Weiss HS, Shingleton BJ, Goode SM, et al. Argon laser gonioplasty in the treatment of angle-closure glaucoma. Am J Ophthalmol 1992; 114:14–18.

60. Wand M. Argon laser gonioplasty for synechial angle closure. Arch Ophthalmol 1992; 110:353–367.

61. Ritch R, Tham CCY, Lam DSC. Long-term success of argon laser peripheral iridoplasty in the management of plateau iris syndrome. Ophthalmology 2004; 111:104–108.

62. Lowe RF. Aetiology of the anatomical basis for primary angle-closure glaucoma. Biometrical comparisons between normal eyes and eyes with primary angle-closure glaucoma. Br J Ophthalmol 1970; 54:161–169.

63. George R, Paul PG, Baskaran M, et al. Ocular biometry in occludable angles and angle closure glaucoma: a population based survey. Br J Ophthalmol 2003; 87:399–402.

64. Hayashi K, Hayashi H, Nakao F, et al. Changes in anterior chamber angle width and depth after intraocular lens implantation in eyes with glaucoma. Ophthalmology 2000; 107:698–703.

65. Kurimoto Y, Park M, Sakaue H, et al. Changes in the anterior chamber configuration after small-incision cataract surgery with posterior chamber intraocular lens implantation. Am J Ophthalmol 1997; 124:775–780.

66. Pereira FA, Cronemberger S. Ultrasound biomicroscopic study of anterior segment changes after phacoemulsification and foldable IOL implantation. Ophthalmology 2003; 110:1799–1806.

67. Teekhasaenee C, Ritch R. Combined phacoemulsification and goniosynechialysis for uncontrolled chronic angle-closure glaucoma after acute angle-closure glaucoma. Ophthalmology 1999; 106:669–675.

68. Gunning FP, Greve EL. Uncontrolled primary angle closure glaucoma: results of early intercapsular cataract extraction and posterior chamber lens implantation. Int Ophthalmol 1991; 15:237–247.

69. Gunning FP, Greve EL. Lens extraction for uncontrolled angle-closure glaucoma: long-term follow-up. J Cataract Refract Surg 1998; 24:1347–1356.

70. Acton J, Salmon JF, Scholtz R. Extracapsular cataract extraction with posterior chamber lens implantation in primary angle closure glaucoma. J Cataract Refract Surg 1997; 23:930–934.

71. Wishart PK, Atkinson PL. Extracapsular cataract extraction and posterior chamber lens implantation in patients with primary chronic angle-closure glaucoma: effect on intraocular pressure control. Eye 1989; 3:706–712.

72. Greve E. Primary angle closure glaucoma: extracapsular cataract extraction or filtering procedure? Int Ophthalmol 1988; 12:157–162.

73. Jacobi PC, Dietlein TS, Luke C, et al. Primary phacoemulsification and intraocular lens implantation for acute angle closure glaucoma. Ophthalmology 2002; 109: 1597–1603.

74. Roberts TV, Francis IC, Lertusumitkul S, et al. Primary phacoemulsification for uncontrolled angle-closure glaucoma. J Cataract Refract Surg 2000; 26:1012–1016.

75. Nonaka A, Kondo T, Kikuchi M, et al. Cataract surgery for residual angle closure after peripheral laser iridotomy. Ophthalmology 2005; 112:974–979.

76. Liu CJ, Cheng CY, Wu CW, et al. Factors predicting intraocular pressure control after phacoemulsification in angle-closure glaucoma. Arch Ophthalmol 2006; 124:1390–1394.

77. Zhi Ming Z, Lim AS, Yin Wong T. A pilot study of lens extraction in the management of acute primary angle-closure glaucoma. Am J Ophthalmol 2003; 135:534–536.

78. Buckley SA, Reeves B, Burdon M, et al. Acute angle closure glaucoma: relative failure of YAG iridotomy in affected eyes and factors influencing outcome. Br J Ophthalmol 1994; 78:529–533.

79. Aung T, Friedman DS, Chew PT, et al. Long-term outcomes in Asians after acute primary angle closure. Ophthalmology 2004; 111:464–469.

80. Lai JSM, Tham CCY, Chan JC, et al. Phacotrabeculectomy in treatment of primary angle-closure glaucoma and primary open-angle glaucoma. Jpn J Ophthalmol 2004; 48:408-4-11.

81. Yuen NS, Chan OC, Hui SP, et al. Combined phacoemulsification and nonpenetrating deep sclerectomy in the treatment of chronic angle-closure glaucoma with cataract. Eur J Ophthalmol 2007; 17:208–215.

82. Krupin T, Mitchell KB, Johnson MF, et al. The long term effects of iridectomy for primary acute angle-closure glaucoma. Am J Ophthalmol 1978; 86:506–509.

83. Murphy MB, Spaeth GL. Iridectomy in primary angle-closure glaucoma. Classification and differential diagnosis of glaucoma associated with narrowness of the angle. Arch Ophthalmol 1974; 91:114–119.

84. Del Priore LV, Robin AL, Pollack IP. Neodymium:YAG and argon laser iridotomy. Long-term follow-up in a prospective, randomized clinical trial. Ophthalmology 1988; 95:1207–1211.

85. Robin AL, Pollack IP. Argon laser peripheral iridotomies in the treatment of primary angle closure glaucoma: long-term follow-up. Arch Ophthalmol 1982; 100:919–923.

86. Seah SK, Foster PJ, Chew PT, et al. Incidence of acute primary angle closure glaucoma in Singapore. An island-wide survey. Arch Ophthalmol 1997; 115:1436–1440.

87. Shaffer RN. Operating room gonioscopy in angle closure glaucoma surgery. Trans Am Ophthalmol 1957; 55:59–66.

88. Shingleton BJ, Chang MA, Bellows AR, et al. Surgical goniosynechialysis for angle-closure glaucoma. Ophthalmology 1990; 97:551–556.

89. Tanihara H, Nishiwaki K, Nagata M. Surgical results and complications of goniosynechialysis. Graefe's Arch Clin Exp Ophthalmol 1992; 230:309–313.

90. Assalian A, Sebag M, Desjardins DC, et al. Successful goniosynechialysis for angle-closure glaucoma after vitreoretinal surgery. Am J Ophthalmol 2000; 130:834–836.

91. Canlas OAQ, Ishikawa H, Liebmann JM, et al. Ultrasound biomicroscopy before and after goniosynechialysis. Am J Ophthalmol 2001; 132:570–571.

92. Yoshimura N, Iwaki M. Goniosynechialysis for secondary angle-closure glaucoma after previously failed filtering procedures. Am J Ophthalmol 1988; 106:493.

93. Nagata M, Nezu N. Goniosynechialysis as a new treatment for chronic angle-closure glaucoma. Jpn J Clin Ophthalmol 1985; 349:707–710.

94. Ando H, Kitagawa K, Ogino N. Results of goniosynechialysis for synechial angle-closure glaucoma after pupillary block. Folia Ophthalmol Jpn 1990; 41:883–886.

95. Lai JSM, Tham CCY, Chua JKH, et al. Efficacy and safety of inferior 180° goniosynechialysis followed by diode laser peripheral iridoplasty in the treatment of chronic angle-closure glaucoma. J Glaucoma 2000; 9:388–391.

96. Tanihara H, Negi A, Akimoto M, et al. Long-term results of non-filtering surgery for the treatment of primary angle-closure glaucoma. Graefe's Arch Clin Exp Ophthalmol 1995; 223: 563–567.

97. Harasymowycz PJ, Papamatheakis DG, Ahmed I, et al. Phacoemulsification and goniosynechialysis in the management of unresponsive primary angle closure. J Glaucoma 2005; 14:186–189.

98. Kanamori A, Nakamura M, et al. Goniosynechialysis with lens aspiration and posterior intraocular lens implantation for glaucoma in spherophakia. J Cataract Refract Surg 2004; 30:513–516.

99. Aung T, Tow SL, Yap EY, et al. Trabeculectomy for acute primary angle closure. Ophthalmology 2000; 107:1298–1302.

CHAPTER 40

Target Intraocular Pressure

Nitin Anand

INTRODUCTION

The origin of the concept of 'target' intraocular pressure (IOP) is unclear. However, the idea that lowering the IOP in glaucoma might be helpful was first proposed more than a hundred years ago. By the 1950s, studies had established the mean IOP in the normal population to be 15–16 mmHg, with the statistical upper limit being 22 mmHg. IOP more than 22 mmHg became to be considered as glaucoma and vice versa. The aim of therapy became lowering IOP to less than 22 mmHg, the de facto target IOP for glaucoma therapy. This had unfortunate consequences. No treatment was offered to glaucoma patients with low pressures and some patients with low-risk ocular hypertension were unnecessarily exposed to the risks of medications or surgery. In the early 1960s, Chandler had observed the need for varying target IOPs according to the severity of glaucoma and said: 'Eyes with advanced glaucoma require a pressure below the average while eyes with limited cupping, confined to one pole of the disc, appear to withstand pressure better, and eyes with a normal disc appear to withstand pressure well over many years.'[1] Epidemiologic studies since then have contested the concept of raised IOP being glaucoma by showing that there were many people in the population with raised IOP without glaucoma and people with glaucoma and no raised IOP. The Baltimore Eye Survey confirmed that while IOP was a major risk factor, half the glaucoma patients had an IOP less than 21 mmHg on diagnosis and there was no correlation between IOP levels and the diagnoses of glaucoma.[2]

DEFINITION

The American Academy of Ophthalmology Preferred Practice Pattern Panel has defined target IOP as the upper limit of the range of measured intraocular pressures adequate to stop progressive pressure-induced injury of the optic nerve head.[3] The European Glaucoma Society Panel has defined target IOP as the estimate of the mean IOP obtained with treatment that is expected to prevent further glaucomatous damage.[4]

Another definition provided by Henry Jampel is that the target IOP is the highest IOP in a given eye which does not contribute to the development of *clinically apparent* glaucomatous optic nerve damage.[5] This definition takes into account the fact that glaucomatous damage of the optic nerve is not important as long as it is not apparent in visual function tests and to the patient.

The term IOP modulation has recently been suggested by Joseph Caprioli. This includes the concept of robust IOP reduction to the target IOP range and reduction of long-term IOP fluctuation.[6]

THE RATIONALE FOR TARGET INTRAOCULAR PRESSURE

Intraocular pressure is the only known risk factor which can be modified to arrest or slow progressive glaucomatous optic neuropathy. Once the assumption that lowering IOP is beneficial for glaucoma is made, a fundamental question that arises every time therapy is initiated is the degree to which the IOP should be lowered. The target IOP is hence the treatment goal for glaucoma along with periodic evaluation of optic nerve head and visual field parameter.

EVIDENCE JUSTIFYING THE SETTING OF A TARGET INTRAOCULAR PRESSURE

Results from large prospective, randomized, multicenter trials have provided evidence for the concept of target IOP and the basis for setting the level of target IOP for the individual patient.

OCULAR HYPERTENSION

Ocular Hypertension Treatment Study The multicenter, prospective Ocular Hypertension Treatment Study (OHTS) trial[7,8] was conducted in the USA on patients with a normal ocular examination, except for elevated IOP between 24 and 32 mmHg in one eye and between 21 and 32 mmHg in the other eye. In the treatment group of this study, the aim was to achieve a 20% reduction of IOP.

1. The risk of progression to glaucoma was significantly less in treated patients compared to controls. The cumulative risk of conversion was 4.4% in treated eyes and 9% in controls.
2. Progression was evidenced by optic nerve head changes in a majority of patients.
3. More than 90% of patients had not converted to glaucoma over 5 years.
4. The relative risk of progression increased 10% for every millimeter of mercury increase in average IOP.
5. Baseline age, vertical and horizontal cup-to-disc ratio, PSD, and IOP were good predictors for the conversion to primary open-angle glaucoma (POAG). The strongest association was with central corneal thickness (CCT). Once CCT was taken into account, race was not a significant risk factor for progression.
6. There was a weak but statistically significant inverse correlation between CCT and IOP lowering. Treatment eyes with thicker corneas had a lower measured IOP response compared to eyes with thinner corneas.[9]

European Glaucoma Prevention Study

In the European Glaucoma Prevention Study (EGPS),[10–12] patients were randomized to receive either topical dorzolamide or the vehicle for the commercially available solution without a specific target IOP.

1. The mean percentage reduction in IOP in the dorzolamide group was 15% after 6 months and 22% after 5 years. Mean IOP declined by 9% after 6 months and by 19% after 5 years in the placebo group. These differences were not statistically significant.
2. At 60 months, the cumulative probability of conversion was 13.4% in the dorzolamide group and 14.1% in the placebo group and this difference was not statistically significant.

The EGPS has been criticized for several reasons.[13] There was substantial loss to follow-up (60%) in both groups. Patients with high or fluctuating IOP were removed from the study, thus explaining the beneficial effect of placebo. There was no target IOP and dorzolamide has a modest IOP-lowering effect when used as monotherapy. In EGPS, the baseline IOP was calculated from two to three measurements per eye at the eligibility visit and one measurement per eye at the 6-month follow-up visit. In OHTS, the mean IOP for each eye was calculated using two to three IOP measurements from each of the two qualifying visits and the randomization visit. Therefore, it is possible that in EGPS a number of patients had their peak IOPs considered as baseline IOP and the subsequent IOPs were much lower, irrespective of group (regression to the mean). Two subsequent reports by the EGPS authors show that

the predictive factors for conversion in untreated ocular hypertension (OHT) were identical to that of OHTS, and the risk of progression was 10% for every millimeter of mercury rise in IOP, similar to that in OHTS.[11,12] A combined OHT risk calculation model has been developed. This model – available online at http://www.ohts.wustl.edu/risk – may assist in decisions about the frequency of tests and visits, as well as the possibility of early preventive treatment (see also Ch. 45, Benefit versus Risk).

Early Manifest Glaucoma Trial

In the Early Manifest Glaucoma Trial (EMGT),[14–17] patients with newly detected and untreated glaucoma, identified by population-based screening in Sweden, were studied. They were randomized to a treatment group and a control group which received no treatment. *Patients with advanced glaucoma were excluded.* The treatment group all received argon laser trabeculoplasty and betaxolol. No target IOPs were assigned.

1. The mean IOP on detection was 20.6 mmHg, and 82.3% of patients with newly detected glaucoma had IOP values of 30 mmHg or less.
2. Patients detected by population screening had less severe glaucoma (lower visual field mean deviation scores), lower IOPs (52.9% less than 21 mmHg in both eyes), and a lower frequency of pseudoexfoliation than self-selected patients from the same population.[17]
3. Progression by visual field criteria was significantly less in the treatment group (45%) compared to the control group (62%). Mean IOP reduction was 5.1 mmHg (25%) in the treatment group.
4. Multivariate analyses of the IOP outcomes illustrated the importance of lowering IOP in glaucoma therapy. Each millimeter of mercury of higher mean IOP at follow-up increased risk of progression by 13%. A 25% decrease of IOP from baseline and a maximum absolute level of 25 mmHg reduced the risk of progression by 50%.
5. The mean rates of progression of visual field loss were quite slow, being 6 dB of mean deviation (MD) per decade in the control group and 3.6 dB per decade in treated patients.
6. Pseudoexfoliation was a strong positive risk factor for progression to glaucoma.[16] Ocular hypertensives (IOP 24–32 mmHg) detected during screening were reviewed after a mean period of 8 years. The risk of conversion to glaucoma was twice that in patients with (55.1%) than in those without (27.6%) pseudoexfoliation.

Collaborative Normal Tension Glaucoma Study

A multicenter, prospective, randomized trial compared treatment versus no treatment in the Collaborative Normal Tension Glaucoma Study (CNTGS).[18–21] Eligible patients had to show signs of visual field progression or field defects threatening fixation or new optic disc hemorrhages. The baseline IOP was an average of 10 IOP measurements after washout and the median IOP had to be less than 20 mmHg and a maximum of 24 mmHg. Three baseline visual fields were done and the visual acuity had to be 6/9 or better. Progression was detected by visual field and optic disc photographs. The target was a 30% reduction from the baseline IOP. Treatment was escalated depending on response, i.e. medical, laser, and finally surgical. Trabeculectomy was performed in half the eyes to achieve the target IOP.

1. The probability of progression was 20% at 5 years in the treatment group and 60% in the control group. The treatment benefit in the survival analysis was evident only after exclusion (censoring) at time of cataract extraction. More eyes in the treatment group (35%) had cataract extraction than in the control group (14%).
2. The study showed that visual field progression was variable but slow in most untreated normal-tension glaucoma. Before randomization, 62 out of 109 untreated eyes did not show any progression and the remainder showed a decline of 0.2 dB to 2 dB per year. About half of the eventually untreated eyes showed some localized deterioration but no extension of the field defects over 7 years.[19]
3. A faster rate of progression was observed in women, in patients with migraine headaches, and in the presence of disc hemorrhages.[21]
4. Despite its many shortcomings this was the first major trial to show a benefit of lowering IOP by 30% in normal-pressure glaucoma.

The Collaborative Initial Glaucoma Treatment Study

The Collaborative Initial Glaucoma Treatment Study (CIGTS)[22,23] was a multicenter, randomized, controlled trial in the USA. Newly diagnosed patients were randomized into a medical therapy and trabeculectomy group. Individual target IOPs were calculated by a predetermined formula.

1. The trabeculectomy group had mean IOPs of 14–15 mmHg and the medical therapy group had mean IOPs of 17–18 mmHg. The rate of visual field loss was not significantly different between the two intervention groups 5 years into the study.
2. In CIGTS subjects with only mild baseline visual field loss (mean deviation, −2 dB or better), subsequent loss of MD was minimal for both the initial medication and initial surgery groups.
3. However, in those patients with more advanced visual field loss (−10 dB), subsequent visual field loss progression was more in the medication group compared to the surgery group.[23]

Advanced Glaucoma Intervention Study

The multicenter Advanced Glaucoma Intervention Study (AGIS)[24,25] comprised patients with glaucoma with higher initial presenting pressures and IOP that could not be controlled with medication alone. Patients were randomized into treatment sequences: argon laser trabeculoplasty, trabeculectomy, trabeculectomy (ATT), or trabeculectomy, argon laser trabeculoplasty and trabeculectomy (TAT). The target IOP was less than 18 mmHg. Progression was detected by visual field criteria. Patients were phakic at the outset and those with advanced field loss (MD more than 16 dB) were excluded. The relevant findings from this study were from the secondary analyses.

1. There was a clear relationship between the degree of IOP lowering and preservation of visual fields.
2. Eyes with average IOP greater than 17.5 mmHg over the first three 6-month visits showed significantly greater visual field deterioration compared to the eyes with IOP less than 14 mmHg in the same time period.
3. Eyes with IOP less than 18 mmHg at 100% of the visits over 6 years (mean IOP of 12.7 mmHg) were less likely to show an increase of their initial visual field defect compared to other eyes.
4. The beneficial effect of lowering the IOP was independent of baseline IOP, sex, race, and systemic disease.
5. Various multivariate regression models of AGIS data showed that the only consistent factor associated with worsening of field defects was long-term IOP fluctuation. Eyes with an IOP fluctuation (standard deviation of 6-monthly IOP measurements) of less than 3 mmHg were more likely to remain stable.[25]

'More Flow' (Moorfields/UK MRC) Study

The 'More Flow' (Moorfields/UK MRC) Study[26] was a randomized, multicenter trial designed to test the hypothesis that intraoperative 5-FU supplementation during trabeculectomy was more effective than placebo in lowering IOP over the long term.

1. At 5 years, visual field defect or optic disc damage progression increased relative to IOP, ranging from 0% of patients with less than 14 mmHg to 24% of patients greater than 21 mmHg.

Table 40.1 summarizes the characteristics of these randomized trials. These trials have confirmed that lowering IOP decreases the risk of progression from ocular hypertension to glaucoma and the progression of visual field loss in early and advanced glaucoma. The protective effect of IOP does appear to be dose dependent. To prevent progression, in eyes with significant field loss, IOP should be lowered below 14–15 mmHg with minimal visit-to-visit IOP fluctuation.

FACTORS INFLUENCING TARGET INTRAOCULAR PRESSURE

While the randomized trials have now shown a clear benefit of lowering the IOP on visual fields, the target IOP must be individualized (Fig. 40.1).

TABLE 40.1 Characteristics of the randomized trials				
	STUDY POPULATION	BASELINE IOP (mmHg)	TARGET IOP OR IOP REDUCTION	RESULTS
Ocular Hypertension Treatment Study (OHTS)	OHT	25	20%	Conversion to POAG 4.4% in treated and 9% in controls
European Glaucoma Prevention Study (EGPS)	OHT	23.5	None	Conversion to POAG 13.4% in dorzolamide and 14% in controls
Early Manifest Glaucoma Trial (EMGT)	POAG diagnosed by population screening	21	None	Progression 45% in treated, 60% in controls
Collaborative Normal Tension Glaucoma Study (CNTG)	NTG	16	30%	Progression 20% in treated, 60% in controls
Collaborative Initial Glaucoma Treatment Study (CIGTS)	Newly diagnosed POAG	28	40% (according to formula)	Mean IOP after surgery 14–15, with meds/laser 17–18 mmHg
Advanced Glaucoma Intervention Study (AGIS)	POAG not controlled by medication	24	18 mmHg	IOP <18 mmHg on all visits, no progression in 85%

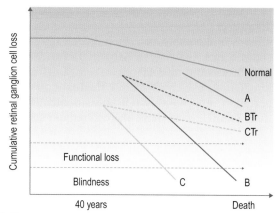

FIGURE 40.1 Schematic representation for tailoring therapy according to severity of glaucoma, age, and life expectancy. Deterioration is rarely linear as shown, often step-like. (A) Patient with early glaucoma/OHT diagnosed late in life or with limited life expectancy. No treatment required; observe. (B) Patient with moderate glaucoma diagnosed at age of 50+ at risk of developing functional visual impairment. Treatment with medications and/or laser to lower IOP by 30% may slow the rate of deterioration (*line Btr*) to the extent that the patient never experiences visual problems. (C) Patient with advanced glaucoma, significant risk for functional loss. Low target IOPs are required to slow rate of ganglion cell loss to that of the normal aging eyes. Treatment with medications, laser and/or surgery to decrease IOP to low teens may slow the rate of deterioration (line

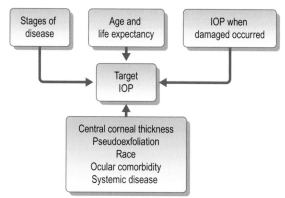

FIGURE 40.2 Factors that singly or combined identify the need for a low target IOP.

The most important factors to consider while setting target IOP level for a glaucoma patient are severity (measured either as visual field defect [MD] or glaucomatous cupping [CD]), baseline IOP, age, and life expectancy (Fig. 40.2).

1. *Stage of disease*: The severity of glaucomatous damage to the optic nerve head is one of the most important factors for setting the target IOP. Severity is assessed by optic disc evaluation and extent of visual field loss. Visual field loss encroaching on fixation should prompt the physician to set a low target IOP regardless of the baseline pressure.

2. *Age*: There is a gradual, steady decrease in the number of nerve fibers in the optic nerve head with age, with loss estimated to be 4–5% per decade after the age of 50.[27] In glaucoma, the rate of retinal ganglion cell death is accelerated above that of the normal aging process. However, the rate of progression is variable and slow in most patients. In the EMGT study, the average visual field loss progression in the untreated group was about 6 dB per year and 3.6 dB per year with protocol-directed treatment.[14] In the CNTGS, 56% of the untreated patients did not progress over a period of 3 years or while the rest showed a gradual decline, between 2 and 20 dB per decade.[19]

This implies that elderly patients with early glaucoma may not need to be treated aggressively unless central fixation is threatened. Younger patients are perhaps better monitored for disease progression by observing optic disc parameters. It may be reasonable to aim for lower target IOPs in young patients with advanced disc changes and no visual field loss. Life expectancy is a function of age of the patient and other systemic factors. For example a 60-year-old, obese, male smoker has a lower life expectancy than a healthy 80-year-old female nonsmoker.

3. *Baseline intraocular pressure*: It is essential to get an accurate estimate of the baseline IOP. Ideally, a 24-hour IOP curve should be obtained before starting treatment. This is rarely practical and the best compromise is the mean of 4–6 IOP readings at different times of the day over 2–3 visits. The incidence of glaucoma rises with increasing IOP in population studies.[2] The risk for conversion to glaucoma increases with rising IOP and finally the risk of progression increases significantly with increasing IOP. The target IOP is a function of the baseline IOP at which glaucomatous damage had occurred, though for glaucoma with significant field loss it may also be appropriate to aim to lower the IOP below a specified level. It should be set keeping this in mind, and the other factors such as life expectancy, severity, and CCT.

4. *Central corneal thickness*: The pooled results of the OHTS and the EGPS show that CCT was a significant predictor for conversion to glaucoma.[12] In the OHTS prediction model, the risk for developing glaucoma doubles for every 40 μm of CCT thinning.[7] In glaucoma, more advanced disease and a greater risk for progression may be seen in eyes with thin corneas.[28] The concern for clinicians has been that IOP measurements with the Goldmann tonometer may be under- or overestimated in eyes with thin and thick corneas, respectively, altering their clinical decision-making.[29] However, a study on manometric IOP measurements has shown the effect of CCT on applanation tonometry to be significantly less than suggested by older studies. An error of ±0.4 mmHg per 10 μm CCT increment was reported.[30] The effect of CCT on IOP measurements is probably not important except in the eyes with extremely thick or thin corneas. The biomechanical properties of the cornea probably have a more significant effect on IOP than CCT. It is more appropriate to think of CCT as an independent predictor for glaucoma and a marker for severity in glaucoma. It is more appropriate to stratify eyes on the basis of CCT: thick (>590 μm), average (540–590 μm), and thin corneas (<550 μm). Setting lower target IOPs in glaucoma on the basis of low CCT values only is, however, debatable. On current evidence, CCT measurements are crucial for the appropriate management of OHT.

5. *Associated ocular disease*: Pseudoexfoliation has been associated with an increased risk for conversion from OHT to POAG.[16] Ocular diseases which have already

compromised the vision must be kept in mind. For example, in advanced age-related macular degeneration aggressive lowering of the IOP is unlikely to benefit the patient's vision. Surgery in some instances may make the vision worse with no tangible benefit to the patient. Target IOP should be secondary to quality-of-life (QOL) issues in these patients.

6. *Race*: The Baltimore Eye Survey found that the overall prevalence of glaucoma was 4–5 times higher in African-Americans than Caucasians.[2] A finding of OHTS was that race was not a significant risk factor for conversion to glaucoma once CCT was included in the prediction model. However, it must be kept in mind that in people of West African origin the incidence of glaucoma is high, the onset is earlier, and it leads to blindness more often than in Caucasians.[31]

7. *Risks of treatment*: Glaucoma medications are not without risks. The Blue Mountains Eye Study showed a significant association between cardiovascular mortality and glaucoma, particularly in patients also treated with topical timolol.[32] The association between timolol and respiratory compromise is well documented in the literature. In older individuals or early glaucoma, it may be acceptable to leave the IOP higher than the target rather than prescribe topical β-blockers or perform glaucoma surgery.

8. *Systemic morbidity*: The role of systemic illnesses such as hypertension and diabetes is still not clearly elucidated. Studies are ongoing looking into non-IOP factors contributing to the disease. The practical impact of the presence of systemic diseases on the target IOP decision-making process is relatively minor other than that of its effect on the patient's life expectancy.

LIMITATIONS OF TARGET INTRAOCULAR PRESSURE

Rigorously pursuing the target IOP can be detrimental for the patient. The goal of glaucoma therapy is to slow or arrest retinal ganglion death (and blindness) and we have no way of knowing that achieving a particular target IOP does that. This can only be determined by serial, long-term assessment. On occasion, it may better to accept that the target IOP cannot be achieved and to withhold the next level of treatment, which may have serious effects on the patients' QOL.

1. *IOP measurements*: There are numerous reasons for inaccurate tonometry, but these are outside the scope of this chapter.[33] The effect on CCT has already been discussed above. It is important not to be obsessed with absolute numbers for target IOP. This implies that if the target IOP is set at 14 mmHg for an eye but the IOP is slightly higher, say 16 mmHg, the next step should be to repeat tonometry on a subsequent visit rather than modify therapy.

2. *IOP fluctuation*: IOP is measured infrequently. For most of the author's patients there is very little information on their diurnal IOP variation. The findings of a recent report suggest that the majority of patients with advanced glaucoma or disease which is disproportionate to IOP measurement have IOP peaks after office hours: at night or early morning.[34] Eyes with greater IOP fluctuation regardless of mean IOP tend to show more visual field loss.[25,35]

3. *Normal-pressure glaucoma*: Evidence for efficacy of treatment (and hence target IOP) of early normal-tension glaucoma (NTG) or the NTG suspect is not forthcoming from the recent large studies. A retrospective report showed very little progression over normal fellow eyes of patients with NTG and in eyes with field loss not encroaching fixation over a period of 5 years or more.[36]

4. *Very low target IOPs*: The benefit of setting the target IOPs to less than 10 mmHg is questionable. IOPs below 10 mmHg are usually attained by surgery with antimetabolites and there is a significant risk of postoperative hypotonic maculopathy and bleb-related infections.

SETTING THE TARGET INTRAOCULAR PRESSURE

To decide on the target IOP on an individual basis, it is essential to first establish the true baseline, peak, and trough IOP. One IOP reading is inadequate as the IOP in glaucoma patients has a wide diurnal fluctuation, with spikes in the night or early morning. Twenty-four-hour IOP monitoring may not be possible or indeed necessary in all cases. At the very least, four to six IOP measurements over two or more visits should be used to establish the baseline IOP. A measurement between 7:00 a.m. and 9:00 a.m. has a 75% likelihood of being close to the peak IOP.[37] Various methods have been described to derive a target IOP. The target IOP must be individualized according to factors previously mentioned. It must be emphasized that these are best-estimation techniques and that there is no certain, proven way of determining an IOP level below which no further damage occurs to the optic nerve.

Estimation methods The commonest and simplest method for setting the target IOP is to aim for a percentage drop from the baseline IOP of 30–50%. The drop should be at least 20% to account for the diurnal fluctuation and inaccuracies in current IOP measurement techniques. The recommendations of the American Academy of Ophthalmology Preferred Practice Panel are shown in Figure 40.3. However, this technique has its limitations. For example, in advanced glaucoma if the baseline is 40 mmHg a target of 50% would mean lowering the IOP to 20 mmHg, which may not be enough, as per AGIS Report 7. Therefore, specific arbitrary levels of target IOP based on severity of glaucoma may also be considered.[24] Commonly set levels are less than 19, 15, or 13 mmHg. The best

approach would be a combined approach of percentage IOP drop and absolute levels. Table 40.2 represents the consensus opinion of a Delphi Panel of 18 glaucoma specialists in the USA who reviewed all of the recent trials and made recommendations for initial target pressures.[38]

Formulas for calculating target intraocular pressure Complicated formulas have also been proposed that attempt to include various factors presumed to be relevant, such as race, age, refractive error, and degree of nerve damage and visual field loss. Although logical and reasonably inclusive of the risk factors that we have some basis for considering important, the practical applications of these concepts are quite limited and remain unproven by any study to be accurate or effective.

Jampel suggested the following formula for the target range:

$$\text{Target range} = [\text{initial IOP} \times (1 - \text{initial IOP}/100) - Z + Y \pm 1\,\text{mmHg}]$$

Z is an optic nerve damage severity factor and Y is a burden of therapy factor.[5] Table 40.3 explains the grading scale. Jampel's formula has been subsequently modified by other researchers. The Y factor (burden of therapy) was excluded as it is difficult to grade or quantify accurately.

Zeyen reported a simplified version:

$$\text{Target IOP} = \text{maximum IOP} - \text{maximum IOP\%} - Z$$

In this formula, the value of Z is the same as in Jampel's formula.[39]

The CGITS[22] formula for target IOP was calculated as follows:

$$\text{Target IOP} = [1 - (\text{reference IOP} + \text{VF score})/100] \times (\text{reference IOP})$$

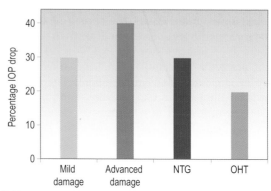

FIGURE 40.3 AAO recommendation for IOP-lowering in glaucoma and OHT. (Redrawn from American Academy of Ophthalmology. Primary open-angle glaucoma. Preferred practice pattern. 2006. American Academy of Ophthalmology, San Francisco, CA.)

TABLE 40.2 Delphi Panel recommendations for initial target pressures. (Data reproduced from Katz LJ.[38] with permission of Lippincott, Williams & Wilkins Visioncare Group.)

PATIENTS WITH HIGH IOP AT PRESENTATION	PREFERRED TARGET IOP (mmHg)	ACCEPTABLE IOP RANGE (mmHg)	RECOMMENDED MINIMUM PERCENTAGE IOP REDUCTION
Mild glaucoma	18	16–21	25%
Moderate glaucoma	16	14–18	30%
Severe glaucoma	12	18–24	20%
Glaucoma suspects	22	18–24	20%
Moderate normal-tension glaucoma	Not determined	Not determined	20%
Severe normal-tension glaucoma	Not determined	Not determined	30%

TABLE 40.3 Grading scale for Jampel's formula for calculating target IOP. (Reproduced from Jampel HD[5] J Glaucoma 1997; 6: 133–138.)

VALUE OF Z AND Y	Z, OPTIC NERVE DAMAGE	Y, BURDEN OF THERAPY
0	Normal disc and visual field	No effect on patients' QOL
1	Abnormal disc and normal visual field	Small effect
2	Visual field loss not threatening fixation	Moderate effect
3	Visual field loss threatening fixation	Larger effect

The reference IOP was the mean of six separate IOP measurements taken in the course of the two baseline visits. The reference visual field score was the mean of VF scores from at least two Humphrey 24–2 visual field tests taken during the two baseline visits.

Summary

Target IOP is the mean IOP obtained with treatment that is expected to prevent further damage to the glaucomatous eye. It is at best an estimate, and the evidence for it is derived from studies designed for other purposes. Besides target IOP, recent evidence suggests that the diurnal and long-term IOP fluctuation should also be minimized to preserve visual function in glaucoma. The management of glaucoma should include the concept of individualized target IOP. Prior to

setting a target IOP, the baseline parameters such as IOP and visual field status should be firmly established by multiple measurements. The steps taken to achieve this target should be in proportion to the disease severity and the probability of the patient losing vision due to glaucoma. There is no a priori way of deriving the target IOP or being certain that achieving target IOP will prevent disease progression in an individual. The target IOP should be flexible and modified as the ocular and physical condition of the patient changes. Achieving target IOP should not make the physician complacent, and constant monitoring of the optic nerve and visual fields in glaucoma is mandatory (Fig. 40.4).

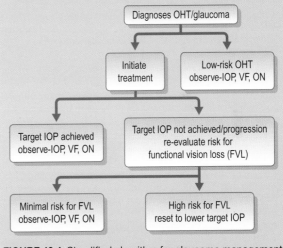

FIGURE 40.4 Simplified algorithm for glaucoma management by lowering IOP to target level. ON, optic nerve; FVL, functional vision loss; VF, visual fields.

REFERENCES

1. Chandler PA. Long-term results in glaucoma therapy. Am J Ophthalmol 1960; 49:221–246.

2. Sommer A, Tielsch JM, Katz J, et al. Relationship between intraocular pressure and primary open angle glaucoma among white and black Americans. The Baltimore Eye Survey. Arch Ophthalmol 1991; 109:1090–1095.

3. American Academy of Ophthalmology. Primary open-angle glaucoma. Preferred practice pattern. CA: San Francisco: American Academy of Ophthalmology; 2006.

4. European Glaucoma Society. Terminology and guidelines for glaucoma. 2nd edn. Savona, Italy: Dogma; 2003.

5. Jampel HD. Target pressure in glaucoma therapy. J Glaucoma 1997; 6:133–138.

6. Caprioli, J. Intraocular pressure revisited. Glaucoma Topics Trends 2006; 1:1–4. Ethis Communications, Inc. and the University of Florida School of Medicine.

7. Gordon MO, Beiser JA, Brandt JD, et al. The Ocular Hypertension Treatment Study: baseline factors that predict the onset of primary open-angle glaucoma. Arch Ophthalmol 2002; 120:714–720.

8. Kass MA, Heuer DK, Higginbotham EJ, et al. The Ocular Hypertension Treatment Study: a randomized trial determines that topical ocular hypotensive medication delays or prevents

the onset of primary open-angle glaucoma. Arch Ophthalmol 2002; 120:701–713.

9. Brandt JD, Beiser JA, Gordon MO, et al. Central corneal thickness and measured IOP response to topical ocular hypotensive medication in the Ocular Hypertension Treatment Study. Am J Ophthalmol 2004; 138:717–722.

10. Miglior S, Zeyen T, Pfeiffer N, et al. Results of the European Glaucoma Prevention Study. Ophthalmology 2005; 112:366–375.

11. European Glaucoma Prevention Study (EGPS) Group. Predictive factors for open-angle glaucoma among patients with ocular hypertension in the European Glaucoma Prevention Study. Ophthalmology 2007; 114:3–9.

12. Ocular Hypertension Treatment Study Group EGPSG. Validated prediction model for the development of primary open-angle glaucoma in individuals with ocular hypertension. Ophthalmology 2007; 114:10–19.

13. Quigley HA. European Glaucoma Prevention Study. Ophthalmology 2005; 112:1642–1643.

14. Heijl A, Leske MC, Bengtsson B, et al. Reduction of intraocular pressure and glaucoma progression: results from the Early Manifest Glaucoma Trial. Arch Ophthalmol 2002; 120:1268–1279.

15. Leske MC, Heijl A, Hussein M, et al. Factors for glaucoma progression and the effect of treatment: the Early Manifest Glaucoma Trial. Arch Ophthalmol 2003; 121:48–56.

16. Grodum K, Heijl A, Bengtsson B. Risk of glaucoma in ocular hypertension with and without pseudoexfoliation. Ophthalmology 2005; 112:386–390.

17. Grodum K, Heijl A, Bengtsson B. A comparison of glaucoma patients identified through mass screening and in routine clinical practice. Acta Ophthalmol Scand 2002; 80:627–631.

18. Collaborative Normal-Tension Glaucoma Study Group. The effectiveness of intraocular pressure reduction in the treatment of normal-tension glaucoma. Am J Ophthalmol 1998; 126:498–505.

19. Anderson DR, Drance SM, Schulzer M. Natural history of normal-tension glaucoma. Ophthalmology 2001; 108:247–253.

20. Anderson DR, Drance SM, Schulzer M. Factors that predict the benefit of lowering intraocular pressure in normal-tension glaucoma. Am J Ophthalmol 2003; 136:820–829.

21. Drance S, Anderson DR, Schulzer M. Risk factors for progression of visual field abnormalities in normal-tension glaucoma. Am J Ophthalmol 2001; 131:699–708.

22. Lichter PR, Musch DC, Gillespie BW, et al. Interim clinical outcomes in the Collaborative Initial Glaucoma Treatment Study comparing initial treatment randomized to medications or surgery. Ophthalmology 2001; 108:1943–1953.

23. Lichter P, Musch D. Initial surgery favorable for patients with advanced visual field loss in the Collaborative Initial Glaucoma Treatment Study (CIGTS). Paper presented at: annual meeting of the American Academy of Ophthalmology (AAO); November 14, 2006; Las Vegas, NV.

24. The Advanced Glaucoma Intervention Study (AGIS): 7. The relationship between control of intraocular pressure and visual field deterioration. The AGIS Investigators. Am J Ophthalmol 2000; 130:429–440.

25. Nouri-Mahdavi K, Hoffman D, Coleman AL, et al. Predictive factors for glaucomatous visual field progression in the Advanced Glaucoma Intervention Study. Ophthalmology 2004; 111:1627–1635.

26. Khaw PT, Minassian D, Farewell V, et al., and More Flow Study Group. The More Flow (Moorfields/UK MRC) Study: A prospective randomized trial of intraoperative 5-fluorouracil vs placebo: effect on long-term pressure control and glaucoma progression. American Academy of Ophthalmology and the European Society of Ophthalmology, Annual Meeting. 24-10-20.

27. Jonas JB, Schmidt AM, Muller-Bergh JA, et al. Human optic nerve fiber count and optic disc size. Invest Ophthalmol Vis Sci 1992; 33:2012–2018.

28. Congdon NG, Broman AT, Bandeen-Roche K, et al. Central corneal thickness and corneal hysteresis associated with glaucoma damage. Am J Ophthalmol 2006; 141:868–875.

29. Shih CY, Graff Zivin JS, Trokel SL, et al. Clinical significance of central corneal thickness in the management of glaucoma. Arch Ophthalmol 2004; 122:1270–1275.

30. Kohlhaas M, Boehm AG, Spoerl E, et al. Effect of central corneal thickness, corneal curvature, and axial length on applanation tonometry. Arch Ophthalmol 2006; 124:471–476.

31. Wilson MR, Kosoko O, Cowan CL, et al. Progression of visual field loss in untreated glaucoma patients and glaucoma suspects in St. Lucia, West Indies. Am J Ophthalmol 2002; 134:399–405.

32. Lee AJ, Wang JJ, Kifley A, et al. Open-angle glaucoma and cardiovascular mortality: the Blue Mountains Eye Study. Ophthalmology 2006; 113:1069–1076.

33. Whitacre MM, Stein R. Sources of error with use of Goldmann-type tonometers. Surv Ophthalmol 1993; 38:1–30.

34. Barkana Y, Gerber Y, Mora R, et al. Effect of eye testing order on automated perimetry results using the Swedish Interactive Threshold Algorithm standard 24–2. Arch Ophthalmol 2006; 124:781–784.

35. Bergea B, Bodin L, Svedbergh B. Impact of intraocular pressure regulation on visual fields in open-angle glaucoma. Ophthalmology 1999; 106:997–1004.

36. Membrey WL, Poinoosawmy DP, Bunce C, et al. Comparison of visual field progression in patients with normal pressure glaucoma between eyes with and without visual field loss that threatens fixation. Br J Ophthalmol 2000; 84:1154–1158.

37. Jonas JB, Budde W, Stroux A, et al. Single intraocular pressure measurements and diurnal intraocular pressure profiles. Am J Ophthalmol 2005; 139:1136–1137.

38. Katz LJ. Prostaglandin as first-line therapy. Ophthalmology management. Online. Available: http://www.ophmanagement. com/article.aspx?article = 865. Lippincott, Williams & Wilkins Visioncare Group; 2006.

39. Zeyen T. Target pressures in glaucoma. Bull Soc Belge Ophtalmol 1999; 274:61–65.

CHAPTER 41

Quality of Life

Alexander Spratt, Aachal Kotecha, and Ananth Viswanathan

INTRODUCTION

Just as beauty is in the eye of the beholder, so ophthalmic patients will always have the upper hand in their assessment of disease severity. Nevertheless, it is alarming just how wide this gulf of understanding between ophthalmologists and patients has been shown to be.

A sizeable and growing body of evidence clearly demonstrates that patients value their vision more highly than most ophthalmologists realize.[1] Closing this gap in knowledge between patients' experiences and ophthalmologists' perceptions remains an elusive but worthwhile goal; in failing to do so we risk doing less than our best for patients.

'Success' in glaucoma has always been a moving target. It has evolved from the hope that an intraocular pressure (IOP) of 21 mmHg or less would prevent visual loss to encompass the results of a complex battery of hospital-administered tests including assessment of IOP, visual field stability, optic nerve and nerve fiber layer status and, more recently, measures of optic nerve hemodynamics and corneal rigidity. Such parameters, with their logical foundations, have sparked countless exciting scientific publications and given rise to a new language of glaucoma.

Conspicuous by their absence are attempts to evaluate patients' ability to perform visually demanding tasks, to understand patients' satisfaction with their vision, and to tackle patients' fears. The initial aim of this chapter is to remind ophthalmologists that it is these factors, and how they impact on quality of life (QOL), that patients consider to be critically important. Redefining success as judged by these terms may be just what the patient ordered.

The main purpose of this chapter is to explain how the unfocused term 'quality of life' has been conceptualized and processed to yield quantitative measures, to review the literature on the QOL impacts of glaucoma, and to consider the assessment instruments used. Finally, the use of QOL measures in determining the effectiveness of treatments and the cost-efficiency of healthcare will be discussed. For additional discussion, see also Chapter 42, Optimizing QOL.

DEFINITION

Put simply, QOL is determined by an individual's own assessment of his or her physical, psychological, and social well-being. The right to drive and the freedom to live independently and enjoy life all contribute to a 'good' QOL and each of these has a sight-dependent component.

It is, of course, well recognized that patients with similar disease states, including those suffering glaucomatous visual loss, are likely to rate its impact on their QOL quite differently. Perceived QOL differs between individuals, with variability based on cultural beliefs, social circumstances, and personal expectations. It also varies within individuals over time, based on life experiences and changing personal expectations. However, even with this variable personal resilience, research studies with sufficiently large sample sizes do provide useful information about the QOL impact of glaucoma.

WHY IS QOL IMPORTANT?

1. 'Patient-centered care' demands that the needs and wants of patients are central to how healthcare is organized and provided. In the spirit of this, many health strategists advocate that the perspectives of patients be integrated with the preferences of doctors and healthcare funders in reaching important decisions. After all, it is the patient alone who lives with the consequences of treatment choices. Improving understanding of how glaucoma impacts on QOL should bring the perceptions of ophthalmologists and patients closer together and in doing so help simplify the process of shared decision-making.

2. Our psychophysical tests are not capable of describing the functional ability of patients in their own activities of daily living and our history taking is often too closely focused on glaucoma or, at best, sight in general. There is a real danger that in treating glaucoma according to the best guidelines of the finest landmark studies we neglect to fully treat our patients. Should not equal importance be attached to studies correlating loss of visual function in the

elderly with reduced cognitive and functional ability and increased mortality?[2,3] By more thoroughly understanding the effects of glaucoma on patients' QOL at different stages of the disease we can hope to plan more sensible treatment strategies, serve our patients better, and become more complete doctors. Examples of notable results from QOL research include the findings that more than 25% of glaucoma patients with relatively minor binocular field loss report a moderate to severe mobility restriction[4] and that patients with moderate and severe visual field loss both experience a similar level of disability from glare and reduced dark adaptation, suggesting a subjective plateau beyond which further disease progression does not increase this perceived disability.

3. Finally, a measurement of QOL in glaucoma is also needed to calculate and judge the cost-effectiveness of medical and surgical interventions. Such cost-utility analyses help those who allocate finite health resources to reach their difficult decisions and most successfully achieve 'ethical rationing'. Finding an acceptable way to deal with the competing financial demands of expensive medical interventions may be one of the greatest healthcare challenges of the twenty-first century. A value-based medical approach measuring costs expended against both quality and length of life yielded may be a part of the solution.

ASSESSMENT OF QOL IN GLAUCOMA

Although researchers now have a choice of techniques with which to measure QOL in glaucoma, this still remains a relatively new endeavor. It is only in the last decade that systematic efforts have been made to understand how glaucoma affects patients' lives.

This young science now incorporates self-reported visual ability by questionnaire, directly observed performance-based evidence, and utility analyses in its forms of assessment.

QUESTIONNAIRES

Historically, health-related QOL research has been carried out using interview-administered or self-reported questionnaires to present a subjective, patient-based assessment of the impact of a disease and its treatment on the patient's well-being. In vision research, questionnaires are used to assess patients' perceived visual functional abilities, with responses often compared with objective measures such as visual acuity and visual field to confirm a causal link and thereby 'validity'. Results are often then used to infer that patients with reduced visual abilities have a poorer vision-related QOL.

Health questionnaires can be broadly divided into those assessing general health, those which are system specific in their questioning, and those which are disease specific. Each of these types has been used to assess QOL in patients with glaucoma.

GENERAL HEALTH-RELATED QOL QUESTIONNAIRES

These were first developed to provide a patient-derived outcome measure of the overall impact of sickness or surgery and have since been used to assess the effects of ophthalmic interventions and visual loss on patients' QOL. Part of the value of providing a generic overview of health is that it allows for comparison of data across various disease states.

The Medical Outcomes Study Short-Form Health Survey (SF-36) is a general health-related QOL questionnaire for the assessment of chronically ill patients. It measures patients' perceptions in eight areas: general health, physical function, role limitations due to physical and mental disability, social function, vitality, mental health, and bodily pain. Studies using the SF-36 in glaucoma patients have found a weak or absent correlation with binocular visual field loss in glaucoma patients[5,6] and a mixed ability to discriminate between patients with and without glaucoma.[6,7]

The Collaborative Initial Glaucoma Treatment Study (CIGTS) is one of the largest randomized, controlled clinical trials to have collected longitudinal data on QOL in newly diagnosed glaucoma patients. Their QOL assessment used six questionnaires to assess disease-specific and general health aspects of impairment, functional status, and health perceptions. One questionnaire, the Sickness Impact Profile (SIP) – a modified general health QOL questionnaire – showed no association between reduced functional health status and newly diagnosed glaucoma.[7]

With such weak associations, general health questionnaires used in isolation play only a very limited role in the assessment of the QOL impact of glaucoma.

VISION-SPECIFIC QOL QUESTIONNAIRES

These were developed in the early 1990s with the initial aim of assessing the effect of cataract on patients' perceptions of visual ability. They are designed to assess ocular symptoms and specific difficulties with vision-dependent tasks. Questions investigating a similar theme are often grouped into 'subscales' to allow for subanalysis. Examples of such subscales include ocular pain, distance vision, driving, and role limitations and reflect the origins of these questionnaires in the investigation of visual impact of cataract. Vision-specific questionnaires are more discerning for ocular disease but do not allow for comparison with differing non-ocular disease states.

The Activities of Daily Vision Scale (ADVS) was the first vision-specific QOL questionnaire. It was designed to assess the visual ability of cataract patients and consists of 22 questions grouped into five subscales: near vision, distance vision, glare disability, daytime driving, and night driving. The questionnaire asks patients to rate the difficulty of each visual task on a five-point scale ranging from 'no difficulty at all' to 'stopped doing because of vision.' Studies have suggested that only the near vision and night driving subscales are statistically independent; the other three subscales show intercorrelations. All subscales, however, are significantly associated with clinical measures of visual function.[8] When applied to glaucoma, the ADVS was able to reliably differentiate glaucoma patients from normal controls, and poorer overall ADVS scores were shown to correlate well with the degree of field loss.[9]

The Visual Function Index (VF-14) was also developed to assess functional impairment in patients with cataract. Its questions were established by expert consensus to encompass a broad spectrum of vision-dependent activities including cooking, reading newsprint, seeing stairs, and night driving. As with the ADVS, it requires the patient to rate the difficulty of each task. The outcome, in the form of a single visual function score, was only moderately correlated in cataract patients with visual acuity in the better eye but was strongly correlated with self-reported overall visual trouble and overall satisfaction with vision. When used in the assessment of glaucoma, the difference between the VF-14 scores of glaucoma patients and normal controls did not reach statistical significance.[5] However, VF-14 scores did correlate with the extent of visual field loss, albeit to a lesser degree than that observed using the ADVS questionnaire.[5,9]

The Visual Activities Questionnaire (VAQ) was developed to assess difficulty with everyday visual tasks experienced by elderly patients. It consists of 33 questions grouped into 10 subscales encompassing visual abilities that are recognized to decline with age. As it has a subscale specifically assessing peripheral vision, it was selected for inclusion in the QOL assessments of the CIGTS which found overall VAQ scores to correlate with both visual acuity and visual field.[7] The peripheral vision subscale not only correlated highly with the presence of visual field impairment but also showed correlation with the degree of severity of visual field loss in the worse eye.[7]

The Impact of Vision Impairment (IVI) questionnaire was developed to measure the restrictive effects of impaired vision on common daily experiences, originally for the purposes of visual rehabilitation assessment. It asks 32 questions, covering a broad range of practical and psychosocial activities within five subscales. Used in the assessment of glaucoma, no correlation was demonstrated between visual field loss and the overall IVI score, although a correlation was found to responses in the mobility subscale. Notably, a quarter of glaucoma patients with relatively minor binocular field loss reported a moderate to severe mobility restriction[4] in keeping with previous observations of mobility performance in glaucoma.[10]

The National Eye Institute Visual Function Questionnaire (NEI-VFQ) was developed with the help of patient focus groups to measure the effects of a variety of ocular conditions on daily functioning and QOL. It was originally designed as a 51-point questionnaire and later redeveloped for convenience using 25 of the original questions (NEI-VFQ25). Both formats have been validated and widely used by researchers to assess ocular disease and, by comparison, used to authenticate the results of other questionnaires. When used in the assessment of glaucoma, the severity of visual field loss correlated with the overall NEI-VFQ25 score and the peripheral vision and vision-specific dependency subscales of the original NEI-VFQ.[5,11] Furthermore, the NEI-VFQ scores of glaucoma patients were lower across most subscales, including driving and vision-specific role difficulties, poorer scores correlating with more severe visual field defects of the better eye.[12]

GLAUCOMA-SPECIFIC QOL QUESTIONNAIRES

These were developed in response to the relative weaknesses of vision-specific questionnaires. By incorporating questions specific to the visual disabilities experienced by glaucoma patients, investigators hoped to find an alternative method of determining disease severity. Questions usually focus on straightforward visual ability, specific task performance, and the impact of reduced visual ability on patients. They aim to assess the hidden symptoms which patients often overcome by developing subconscious coping strategies. There are currently five glaucoma specific questionnaires in the literature.

The Glaucoma Symptom Scale (GSS) asks subjects to score 10 symptoms commonly experienced by glaucoma patients on a five-point rating scale (Fig. 41.1). Questions are divided into those assessing nonvisual symptoms, including stinging and foreign-body sensation, and those assessing visual symptoms, which include difficulty seeing in daylight and blurry vision; the GSS does not assess specific task performance. The GSS is able to effectively discriminate between glaucoma patients and normal controls,[13] but another study found no association between Esterman visual field scores and those of the GSS.[4] The GSS may therefore have a niche role in measuring the symptoms of medical and surgical treatments of glaucoma, rather than providing a rounded measure of quality of life.

The Viswanathan Questionnaire, as named by Iester and Zingirian,[14] also consists of 10 questions but asks subjects to make a binary 'yes' or 'no' response (Fig. 41.2).[15] It includes questions about bumping into things, finding dropped objects, and tripping/difficulty with stairs. This questionnaire evolved from Mills and Drance's earlier questionnaire designed to assess visual disability in patients with severe glaucoma.[16] Responses correlate well with visual field mean deviation and pattern standard deviation[14] and also with Esterman visual field score,[15] suggesting that this questionnaire effectively targets activities specific to glaucoma. Of note, this questionnaire has also demonstrated that even patients with only mild to moderate glaucomatous visual field loss have subjectively perceived visual disability.[15]

The Glaucoma Quality of Life (GQL-15) questionnaire asks 15 rating-scored questions to assess the degree of functional disability caused by glaucoma. The

		Yes, very bothersome	Yes, somewhat bothersome	Yes, a little bothersome	Yes, but not bothersome at all	No, absent
(1)	Burning, smarting, stinging					
(2)	Tearing					
(3)	Dryness					
(4)	Itching					
(5)	Soreness, tiredness					
(6)	Blurry or dim vision					
(7)	Feeling of something in the eye					
(8)	Hard to see in daylight					
(9)	Hard to see in dark places					
(10)	Halos around lights					

FIGURE 41.1 The Glaucoma Symptom Scale. (From Lee BL, Gutierrez P, Gordon M, et al. The Glaucoma Symptom Scale. A brief index of glaucoma-specific symptoms. Arch Ophthalmol 1998; 116:861–866.)

Please answer the questions below:	Yes	No
Do you ever notice that parts of your field of vision are missing?		
Have you noticed any deterioration in your sight over the last few years?		
Do you ever have trouble following a line of print or finding the next line when reading?		
Do you notice variation in colour intensity?		
Do you bump into things sometimes?		
Do you trip on things or have difficulty with stairs?		
Have you had to give up activities because of your sight?		
Do you have difficulty finding things that you have dropped?		
Are you troubled by glare or dazzled on sunny days or in bright lighting?		
Do you have particular difficulty seeing after moving from a light to a dark room?		

FIGURE 41.2 The Viswanathan Questionnaire. (From Viswanathan AC, McNaught AI, Poinoosawmy D, et al. Severity and stability of glaucoma: patient perception compared with objective measurement. Arch Ophthalmol 1999; 117:450–454.)

questions used were the 15 most significant predictors of visual field loss derived from an original 62–point questionnaire. They comprise six questions relating to actions demanding functional peripheral vision, six relating to dark adaptation and glare, two relating to central and near vision, and one relating to outdoor mobility (Table 41.1). None of the original questions relating to personal care or household tasks qualified for inclusion in the final GQL-15. A significant correlation exists between overall GQL-15 scores and a number of psychophysical tests, including contrast sensitivity, glare disability, dark adaptation, stereopsis, and Esterman visual field score.[17] The same study also found significantly greater perceived visual disability among glaucoma patients with mild visual field loss (defined

as unilateral visual field loss of less than a hemifield) compared with control subjects, suggesting that early glaucomatous loss is readily discernible to patients. This extends to the findings of Viswanathan and colleagues and further challenges the belief that glaucoma is an asymptomatic condition in its early stages.

The Symptom Impact Glaucoma (SIG) and *Glaucoma Health Perceptions Index* (GHPI) are glaucoma-specific questionnaires developed by the CIGTS group with the aim of providing a more complete understanding of the overall impact of glaucoma.[7] The SIG consists of 43 questions, including psychological and systemic inquiries, derived from discussions with patient focus groups and ophthalmologists. Patients were asked whether they had experienced a symptom and, if so, to what degree

---

TABLE 41.1 The Glaucoma Quality of Life (GQL-15) questionnaire

THE GLAUCOMA QUALITY OF LIFE-15 QUESTIONNAIRE

Patient instruction: Please circle the correct answer on the scale from 1 to 5 where [1] stands for no difficulty, [2] for a little bit of difficulty, [3] for some difficulty, [4] for quite a lot of difficulty, and [5] for severe difficulty. If you do not perform any of the activities for reasons other than vision, please circle [0].

Does your vision give you any difficulty, even with glasses with the following activities?

	NONE	A LITTLE BIT	SOME	QUITE A LOT	SEVERE	DO NOT PERFORM FOR NONVISUAL REASONS
Reading newspapers	1	2	3	4	5	0
Walking after dark	1	2	3	4	5	0
Seeing at night	1	2	3	4	5	0
Walking on uneven ground	1	2	3	4	5	0
Adjusting to bright lights	1	2	3	4	5	0
Adjusting to dim lights	1	2	3	4	5	0
Going from a light to a dark room or vice versa	1	2	3	4	5	0
Tripping over objects	1	2	3	4	5	0
Seeing objects coming from the side	1	2	3	4	5	0
Crossing the road	1	2	3	4	5	0
Walking on steps/stairs	1	2	3	4	5	0
Bumping into objects	1	2	3	4	5	0
Judging distance of foot to step/curb	1	2	3	4	5	0
Finding dropped objects	1	2	3	4	5	0
Recognizing faces	1	2	3	4	5	0

List of daily activities with the strongest relationship with visual field loss in glaucoma. (From Nelson P, Aspinall P, Papasouliotis O, et al. Quality of life in glaucoma and its relationship with visual function. J Glaucoma 2003; 12:139–150.)

---

they felt it was attributable to glaucoma or its treatment. The CIGTS group also developed the six-question GHPI, which assessed the impact of glaucoma on patients' emotional, physical, social, and cognitive well-being and assessed the stress caused by having glaucoma and the level of concern felt about blindness. The questionnaires were administered to newly diagnosed glaucoma patients with varying disease severity. Correlations with visual field test scores were weak for both questionnaires but showed some improvement when compared with simulated binocular visual field test scores.

QUESTIONNAIRE SCORING SYSTEMS: LIKERT AND RASCH ANALYSIS

Visual function questionnaires have taken their design from assessments commonly used in the fields of education and psychology. In such tests the scoring system is dichotomous, having either a 'correct' or 'incorrect' answer, with the questions in each subscale becoming progressively more difficult. Calculating the number of correct answers within each subscale reveals the relative aptitude of a student compared to his peers. This scoring system is representative of 'classical test theory' (CTT), where the total score is assumed to represent the strength of the trait being measured.

Similarly, visual function questionnaires are usually scored by summating the average score of each subscale to produce a final score of visual ability. However, many feel this approach is inadequate, as visual function questionnaires, unlike questions assessing aptitude, have no correct answer.[18] In addition, many questionnaires use a rating, or Likert, scale, in which the patients score the difficulty of each task. These scales represent an ordinal rather than interval scale, with the difference between each score varying subjectively between individuals. Summating such scores does not allow for this difference in patient subjectivity. An additional feature of aptitude tests is that questions testing a similar ability become progressively more difficult, such that higher scores indicate better ability. In visual function questionnaires, individual questions assess specific visual abilities and cannot be organized in such a way that levels of difficulty are ascribed. Further, averaging patient responses in each subscale may have the effect of masking very different QOL experiences. To use color vision as an example, two patients with equally reduced color vision may return similar questionnaire scores but if one is a painter this deficiency will have a greater impact on the QOL.

An alternative approach to scoring visual function questionnaires is the use of 'item response theory' (IRT). Using this method, responses to questions are mathematically modeled to take into account individuals' responses to other questions within the same questionnaire. This modeling re-scales questionnaire answers in an attempt to remove some of the unhelpful subjectivity of the test. An additional advantage of this method is that test scores are not dependent on specific questionnaires, allowing for inter-test comparisons to be made.

The Rasch scoring system is a form of IRT commonly used in questionnaires assessing QOL in other medical specialties. This system of scoring weighs the relative importance of subscales against each other for an individual. It takes into account an individual's perceived level of difficulty with each task compared with the actual level of difficulty, and so transforms raw ordinal scores into an interval scale. In vision research, Rasch scoring has been applied to the NEI-VFQ and IVI questionnaires but its use remains rare, perhaps because of its perceived mathematical complexity. It has not yet been used to score a glaucoma-specific questionnaire.

LIMITATIONS OF USING QUESTIONNAIRES TO MEASURE QOL

Visual function questionnaires have been developed to measure patients' perceptions of their abilities to perform the activities of daily living. They offer an interesting and valid measure of disease severity alongside clinical tests, reflected in the strong correlations between some questionnaire scores and clinical measures of disease severity. They are, however, a highly subjective form of self-evaluation and draw heavily upon a patient's own perception, expectations, and belief system. As such, their usefulness will perhaps always be limited. A superior method of assessing the impact of glaucoma on patients' visual abilities may be the direct observation of how well they perform visually demanding tasks.

PERFORMANCE-BASED ASSESSMENT OF VISUAL FUNCTION IN GLAUCOMA

Performance-based testing offers several distinct advantages over self-reported evaluation of visual ability. Self-reports are based on patients' understanding of what the presented task might involve, their assessment of the task's relative difficulty, and their own perceptions of their ability to perform that task. Performance-based testing removes this subjectivity and simply involves observing a patient's actual ability to perform a given task.

Performance-based testing is not new to medicine; it is familiar territory in the diagnosis and monitoring of stroke and other neurological conditions, and is used to assess other problems encountered by the elderly.[19] It has also been used in ophthalmology to assess

the effects of the aging process on visual abilities in the elderly and in studies assessing the functional abilities of low-vision patients. Studies have also looked more directly at the impact of glaucoma on mobility[10] and the ability to drive,[20,21] but none has fully assessed a patient's ability to carry out the activities of daily living. A recent addition to ophthalmological performance-based testing is the *Assessment of Function Related to Vision* (AFREV) test which aims to evaluate the effect of visual impairment from any cause on patients' functional ability.[22] The AFREV is unique in its use of Rasch analysis to determine a score of functional ability based on an individual patient's ability in each task. Although the test battery is not glaucoma specific, it has been used on glaucoma patients and has shown strong correlations between overall scores and Esterman visual field scores. However, many of the items on the AFREV are functional tests of central vision and, as this area is left intact until relatively late in glaucoma, the use of performance-based tests concentrating on central visual abilities may not fully describe the impairments of glaucoma patients with early disease. The challenge still remains to develop a performance-based test specific to the needs of glaucoma patients.

UTILITY MEASURES

Another common criticism made of the use of questionnaires to assess QOL is that they provide a measure of an individual's general health status but fall short of describing true quality of life.

Utility theory aims to overcome the composite approach of questionnaires, instead using preference-based choices to provide a single, patient-derived, numerical value representative of quality of life. In doing so, it reveals patients' perceptions of QOL related to a disease state. This technique has also been applied to medicine as a method to ascertain the cost-effectiveness of medical interventions.

Utility measures are rated on a scale of 0.0 to 1.0, zero representing death and 1.0 representing perfect health. A strength of this design is that it allows for effective comparison between various health states in a way not permitted by other disease-specific measures of QOL. An example of this is that severe angina and bilateral reduced visual acuity of 6/60 have both been associated with a utility value of 0.50, suggesting that these disparate conditions have a comparable impact on QOL.

Utility values can also be obtained from third parties, often with interesting results. In the case of age-related macular degeneration it has been demonstrated that the general public, non-ophthalmic clinicians, and ophthalmologists all significantly underestimate the QOL impact of this condition when compared with the patients who suffer from the disease.[23]

Several methods of assessing utility values exist. The two most commonly used measures are the time trade-off method and the standard gamble method.

Time trade-off (TTO) utility values are determined by asking patients how many years they expect to live and how many of those remaining years of life they would be willing to trade in return for perfect vision. The proportion of their future life expectancy traded is then subtracted from 1.0 to obtain the utility value.

The Standard Gamble (SG) method presents patients with an imaginary treatment that has two possible outcomes: either perfect health (or in the case of utility measures in ophthalmic disease, perfect sight in both eyes) with no side effects for the remainder of their life in cases where the treatment works, or immediate death (gamble 1) or blindness (gamble 2) when the treatment does not work. Patients are then asked what percentage chance of death (or blindness) they would be prepared to risk before refusing the treatment offered. This percentage is then subtracted from 1.0 to obtain the utility value.

The Linear Scale Thermometer is a less commonly used method of determining utility values.[24] Patients are presented with two 'thermometers.' The first is labeled 'perfect vision' at the top and 'blind' at the bottom and patients are asked to rate their current level of vision by placing a mark on this thermometer. The second thermometer is labeled 'perfect health' at the top and 'death' at the bottom. Patients are asked to make two marks on this thermometer, one rating their overall current level of health assuming they had perfect vision, and another rating their current health as if they were completely blind. Individuals' rating of vision on the first thermometer on a 'blind to perfect vision' scale can then be transferred onto the second 'life or death' thermometer to derive a vision-dependent QOL score (Fig. 41.3).

Utility values have been used to assess glaucoma patients. A study of 191 glaucoma patients and 46 glaucoma suspects found that only 22% of glaucoma and 11% of glaucoma suspect patients were willing to trade any life expectancy for perfect vision, giving modest average TTO utility values of 0.93 and 0.98, respectively.[6] These utility values showed poor correlation with Esterman visual fields. By comparison, 12 blind patients from the same study had an average TTO utility value of 0.67, meaning they were willing to trade a third of their remaining life expectancy for a permanent return to perfect vision. A study of 213 Chinese Singaporean glaucoma patients found that most were not willing to trade life expectancy or risk blindness for a glaucoma-free life; their mean TTO utility value was 0.88 and SG for death and blindness 0.94 and 0.95, respectively.[25] By contrast, a study of 105 Indian glaucoma patients found an average TTO utility value of 0.64 unrelated to the extent of visual field loss.[26] The authors suggest the marked difference in their utility value may reflect the severity of glaucoma in their patients and the differing impact of chronic disease and visual impairment in developing countries.[26]

QALYs AND DALYs

Utility values provide a snapshot measure of the QOL associated with a particular disease state. That they can

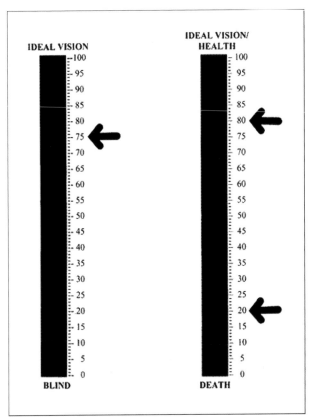

FIGURE 41.3 The Linear Scale Thermometer. In this example, the patient has rated his current level of vision as '75' (left thermometer). On the right thermometer he was asked to score his current overall health status imagining a scenario in which he has perfect vision (scored as '80') and another in which he is completely blind (scored as '20'). To yield his utility score, his perceived visual disability value is transposed onto the right thermometer. The adjusted linear rating is 75% of the distance between 20 and 80, yielding a utility score of 65. (Courtesy of Henry Jampel MD, Johns Hopkins University, Baltimore.)

change with disease progression or following successful medical intervention makes them suited to longitudinal use. Both the degree of improved health conferred by an intervention and the duration of that improvement can be considered together using the quality-adjusted life year (QALY). This is calculated by multiplying the utility value gain obtained by an intervention by the years of benefit gained. For example, if a surgical intervention such as cataract extraction results in an improved utility value from 0.5 preoperatively to 0.8 after surgery and that benefit is felt for the remaining 20 years of a patient's life, this translates into 6.0 QALYs gained (0.3 × 20) from that intervention.

When the number of QALYs gained and the costs associated with the intervention are both known, the cost per QALY can be calculated. Treatments costing less than US$20 000/QALY have been suggested to be cost-effective. Calculating cost-per-QALY for various treatments allows objective comparison of the cost-effectiveness of various treatments and permits a relative evaluation of the financial merits of competing interventions.

The disability-adjusted life year (DALY) is another construct by which to understand the impact of disease. Developed by the World Bank, DALYs assist health economists in planning service provision and setting health priorities, and can provide a measure of the usefulness of interventions. DALYs represent the sum of years of life lost to premature death (YLL), and the number of years spent living with disability (YLD):

$$DALYs = YLL + YLD$$

DALYs describe the mortality and morbidity burden of disease to societies and reflect the loss of productivity of patients and the time period over which that productivity is lost and can be used to calculate the cost-effectiveness of interventions.[27] One DALY can be considered a loss of 1 year of healthy life. As with QALYs, the cost-effectiveness of cataract extraction has been calculated in DALYs. This intervention is reported to cost between I\$730 and I\$2400 per DALY averted in the developed world and between I\$90 and I\$370 per DALY averted in developing countries. Costs are calculated in international dollars (I\$), a hypothetical unit of currency that has the same purchasing power as US\$1 had in the *United States* in the year 2000. DALYs have not yet been used to assess glaucoma and its treatments.

Summary

The value of quality of life research in glaucoma lies in our ability to better understand the impact of this disease on individuals and their ability to perform the activities of daily living. On a practical level, the results of questionnaire-based research have confirmed that the severity of patients' glaucomatous visual field loss is measurable by this method and therein subjectively, if subconsciously, discernible to them.

Specific difficulties with mobility and dark adaptation were highlighted by more than one study. Closed questioning in the clinic which puts this knowledge into practice may yield greater clinical insight than more general enquiries as to patients' visual status.

By contrast, the knowledge that questions regarding personal care and household task ability failed to qualify for inclusion on the short list of the GQL-15, from the originally piloted 62-point questionnaire, suggests that we need not regard them as significant or practical indicators of disease severity.

Finally, those parts of the GSS which were effective at measuring the symptoms and side-effects of medical and surgical glaucoma treatments should be of use to ophthalmologists seeking to monitor the iatrogenic morbidity associated with glaucoma.

Clearly much more research remains to be done, with increased use of utility analyses and performance-based testing likely to further the knowledge base in years to come. Only in achieving this can we hope to better understand our patients, comprehend what it is they want from us and at what personal cost, and begin to calculate the true worth of our treatments to patients and society.

REFERENCES

1. Stein JD. Disparities between ophthalmologists and their patients in estimating quality of life. Curr Opin Ophthalmol 2004; 15:238–243.

2. West SK, Rubin GS, Broman AT, et al. How does visual impairment affect performance on tasks of everyday life? The SEE Project. Salisbury Eye Evaluation. Arch Ophthalmol 2002; 120:774–780.

3. Lee DJ, Gomez-Marin O, Lam BL, et al. Visual impairment and unintentional injury mortality: the National Health Interview Survey 1986–1994. Am J Ophthalmol 2003; 136:1152–1154.

4. Noe G, Ferraro J, Lamoureux E, et al. Associations between glaucomatous visual field loss and participation in activities of daily living. Clin Experiment Ophthalmol 2003; 31:482–486.

5. Parrish RK 2nd, Gedde SJ, Scott IU, et al. Visual function and quality of life among patients with glaucoma. Arch Ophthalmol 1997; 115:1447–1455.

6. Jampel HD, Schwartz A, Pollack I, et al. Glaucoma patients' assessment of their visual function and quality of life. J Glaucoma 2002; 11:154–163.

7. Janz NK, Wren PA, Lichter PR, et al. Quality of life in newly diagnosed glaucoma patients: The Collaborative Initial Glaucoma Treatment Study. Ophthalmology 2001; 108:887–897; discussion 898.

8. Valbuena M, Bandeen-Roche K, Rubin GS, et al. Self-reported assessment of visual function in a population-based study: the SEE project. Salisbury Eye Evaluation. Invest Ophthalmol Vis Sci 1999; 40:280–288.

9. Sherwood MB, Garcia-Siekavizza A, Meltzer MI, et al. Glaucoma's impact on quality of life and its relation to clinical indicators: a pilot study. Ophthalmology 1998; 105:561–566.

10. Turano KA, Rubin GS, Quigley HA. Mobility performance in glaucoma. Invest Ophthalmol Vis Sci 1999; 40:2803–2809.

11. Jampel HD, Friedman DS, Quigley H, et al. Correlation of the binocular visual field with patient assessment of vision. Invest Ophthalmol Vis Sci 2002; 43:1059–1067.

12. Gutierrez P, Wilson MR, Johnson C, et al. Influence of glaucomatous visual field loss on health-related quality of life. Arch Ophthalmol 1997; 115:777–784.

13. Lee BL, Gutierrez P, Gordon M, et al. The Glaucoma Symptom Scale. A brief index of glaucoma-specific symptoms. Arch Ophthalmol 1998; 116:861–866.

14. Iester M, Zingirian M. Quality of life in patients with early, moderate and advanced glaucoma. Eye 2002; 16:44–49.

15. Viswanathan AC, McNaught AI, Poinoosawmy D, et al. Severity and stability of glaucoma: patient perception compared with objective measurement. Arch Ophthalmol 1999; 117:450–454.

16. Mills RP, Drance SM. Esterman disability rating in severe glaucoma. Ophthalmology 1986; 93:371–378.

17. Nelson P, Aspinall P, Papasouliotis O, et al. Quality of life in glaucoma and its relationship with visual function. J Glaucoma 2003; 12:139–150.

18. Massof RW, Rubin GS. Visual function assessment questionnaires. Surv Ophthalmol 2001; 45:531–548.

19. Rozzini R, Frisoni GB, Ferrucci L, et al. The effect of chronic diseases on physical function. Comparison between activities of daily living scales and the Physical Performance Test. Age Ageing 1997; 26:281–287.

20. McGwin G Jr, Mays A, Joiner W, et al. Is glaucoma associated with motor vehicle collision involvement and driving avoidance? Invest Ophthalmol Vis Sci 2004; 45:3934–3939.

21. Adler G, Bauer MJ, Rottunda S, et al. Driving habits and patterns in older men with glaucoma. Soc Work Health Care 2005; 40:75–87.

22. Altangerel U, Spaeth GL, Steinmann WC. Assessment of function related to vision (AFREV). Ophthalmic Epidemiol 2006; 13:67–80.

23. Brown GC, Brown MM, Sharma S. Difference between ophthalmologists' and patients' perceptions of quality of life associated with age-related macular degeneration. Can J Ophthalmol 2000; 35:127–133.

24. Jampel HD. Glaucoma patients' assessment of their visual function and quality of life. Trans Am Ophthalmol Soc 2001; 99:301–317.

25. Saw SM, Gazzard G, Eong KG, et al. Utility values in Singapore Chinese adults with primary open-angle and primary angle-closure glaucoma. J Glaucoma 2005; 14:455–462.

26. Gupta V, Srinivasan G, Mei SS, et al. Utility values among glaucoma patients: an impact on the quality of life. Br J Ophthalmol 2005; 89:1241–1244.

27. Barker C, Green A. Opening the debate on DALYs (disability-adjusted life years). Health Policy Plan 1996; 11:179–183.

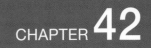

CHAPTER 42

Optimizing Quality of Life: Low-Vision Rehabilitation in Glaucoma

Jill E Keeffe

INTRODUCTION

People with glaucoma-related loss of vision, be it visual field or acuity, are likely to need and possibly benefit from referral for vision-related rehabilitation. This chapter will describe the visual, economic, and psychosocial consequences of impaired vision, discuss the needs of patients to be considered for referral for low-vision care, and the delivery of low-vision services (see also Ch. 41, Quality of Life).

Low vision is defined by the World Health Organization (WHO) in the ICD-10 as visual acuity of <6/18 (<20/60) to 3/60 (20/400) with <3/60 defined as blindness.[1] In meetings to discuss low-vision services a functional definition was adopted. This too uses <6/18 as the criterion for low vision but defines blindness from the functional point of view: that is, people with no perception of light.[2]

Visual acuity of <6/18 was used as a guide for referral to low-vision services although many people are not referred until vision is much worse that this.[3,4] Studies such as the Melbourne Visual Impairment Project[5] and the Blue Mountains Eye Study[6] demonstrated the link between impaired vision <6/12 and morbidity and the social consequences of vision loss. Data from these and other studies were combined using the criterion of <6/12 to report summary of prevalence data of vision impairment[7] and glaucoma.[8] A WHO Consultation discussed changing the definition to the criterion of <6/12 but concluded that further research was needed to establish the change in threshold.[9] Since then, there have been studies that indicate that the level of vision loss for referral to low-vision services should be <6/12.[4] While there has been research into the relationship between visual acuity and the need for low-vision care, the criterion to be used for loss of visual field is much less clear.

CONSEQUENCES OF LOW VISION

The consequences of vision loss from glaucoma on quality of life are a combination and interaction of a number of factors (Fig. 42.1). These include vision (glaucoma

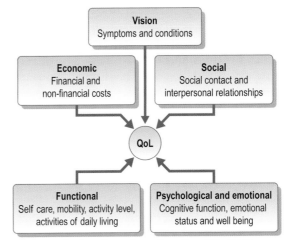

FIGURE 42.1 The key dimensions of quality of life (QOL).

diagnosis symptoms and visual functions), economic impact, the functional aspects of vision which relate to use of vision for activities of daily living, and the psychosocial factors of emotional well-being, social contact, and interpersonal relationships. For each person it is the unique interaction that determines the impact on quality of life and the possible need for low-vision services. For each of these factors involved there are many tools available to assess the impact and to then plan for possible intervention.

VISION

After the clinical diagnosis of glaucoma, the first of these factors measured is vision. This would normally include distance and near visual acuity, visual fields, color vision, dark and light adaptation, and stereoscopic vision. For people with low vision, a test of contrast sensitivity should also be included. For both high- and low-contrast visual acuity tests, a LogMAR chart is essential to obtain a measure of acuity, especially in people with profound impairment. A LogMAR chart based on the first one developed by Bailey and Lovie[10] is also necessary to measure vision for the prescription of low-vision devices. Near and distance LogMAR charts are available to test the vision of adults and children, with preschool children able to be tested by matching symbols.

A tool to measure glaucoma-specific symptoms is the Glaucoma Symptom Scale (GSS).[11] Items in the GSS cover nonvisual symptoms such as tearing, itching, burning/stinging, and dryness, and visual ones such as difficulty seeing in bright or dark light, blurry vision, or presence of halos.

A disturbing symptom for many people with vision loss from glaucoma is the presence of Charles Bonnet syndrome.[12] This has been documented in adults but little is known about the syndrome in children. The hallucinations experienced usually cause great concern to those who experience them as it is often not included in an examination to ask about or explain their possible presence. The visual hallucinations are 'well formed, vivid, elaborate, and often stereotyped.'[12] They can be flashes of light, patterns, or complex scenes involving animals or figures. The correct diagnosis of this distressing but not uncommon condition is of utmost importance, considering the serious implications of the alternative diagnoses.

ECONOMIC

The economic impact for both adults and children has been documented.[13-15] The alleviation of the financial impact for individuals is in the policy domain of governments with the availability of welfare and subsidies. For patients with glaucoma the out-of-pocket expenditure on medications depends on the availability of pharmaceutical benefit schemes as to whether the patient pays the whole or a subsidized cost. In a study of personal expenditure assessed using diaries, annual out-of-pocket expenditure was investigated.[13,14] The group of participants with glaucoma included people with minimal as well as those with significant vision loss. In comparison to other causes of vision loss, patients with glaucoma had greater expenditure on medications than people with other causes of vision loss who incurred greater expenditure on transport and community services. The latter groups also relied to a greater extent on carers for help with vision-related tasks. It is the vision loss rather than the diagnosis of glaucoma that has the greatest impact on independence and thus the need for carers and dependent mobility. Retaining the ability to hold a driver's licence is critical in this.

The costs of glaucoma treatment categorized by disease severity found an increase in costs with increasing severity of disease.[15] Lee and colleagues also found that the highest category of expenditure was the costs of medications. Direct costs for low-vision care were only recorded for the most severe of the five stages, the end stage of glaucoma.

FUNCTIONAL VISION

Until relatively recently, a decision for referral for low-vision care, similar to one for cataract surgery, relied mainly on a diagnosis of eye disease and some determined level of loss of visual acuity and fields. The use of questionnaires such as the VF-14 demonstrated that visual acuity alone did not predict the need for services.[16] There have been many questionnaires developed that assess functional vision: i.e., how vision is or can be used for activities of daily living. Examples of these are the Melbourne Low Vision ADL Index (MLVAI), which is a performance measure of disability,[17] and the Activities of Daily Vision Scale (ADVS), a self-report scale.[18] Some items in them are the same; in the MLVAI the person has to write a check on a form, while the ADVS asks the person to rate their difficulty in writing a check. Most scales of this type have items related to reading near and distant print and signs, threading needles, and preparing meals.

There are numerous checklists designed to assess children's use of vision in and out of the classroom: some are for specific purposes such as mobility and others are more general. Erin and Paul give a list of questionnaires and checklists with information about their application.[19]

While the checklists and questionnaires are useful guides to the restriction in activities (disability) imposed by impaired vision, the items do not necessarily reflect quality of life if the activities are not those a person needs to do.

SOCIAL, PSYCHOLOGICAL, AND EMOTIONAL FACTORS

These factors are often referred to as the psychosocial aspects that are assessed to gain a measure of quality of life. To determine the need for low-vision care it is essential to assess if vision restricts a person's participation in her or his desired or chosen way of life. The presence of vision impairment, be it visual acuity and/or visual fields alone, does not suggest the need for specialized low-vision care. Whilst there is a relationship between the degree of vision loss and restrictions in participation, some people with severe vision impairment rate the consequences of their vision impairment as having no or only little impact on their lives, thus not seeing the need for low-vision care.[20] The contextual factors (age, culture, profession, etc.) are most likely to account for these differences.

The International Classification of Functioning (ICF) provides a useful overview to examine and assess the interactions between vision, visual functions, activities, and participation of a person within his or her environment (Fig. 42.2).[21]

The ICF uses the terms 'activities' and 'participation' as opposed to those used in the ICD-10 of 'disability' and 'handicap.' It is not only a matter of language, as the concepts are important from a rehabilitation point of view, as the inclusion of the contextual factors. It is not only the person that is the focus of rehabilitation but also an understanding of the interaction of factors that causes a restriction in activities or limits participation. The ICF thus provides an overview of the comprehensive assessment needed to understand the effects

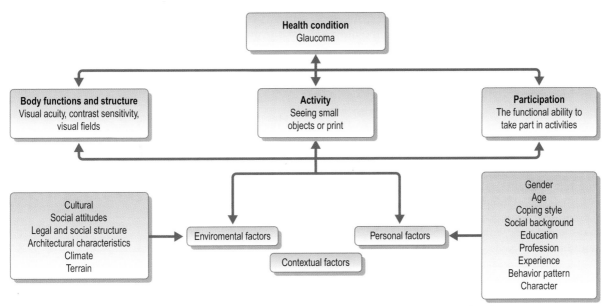

FIGURE 42.2 The World Health Organization's International Classification of Functioning with examples for glaucoma.

on quality of life which are the focus of rehabilitation interventions.

Questionnaires provide an understanding from patients' perspectives regarding consequences of the onset and progression of vision loss. As opposed to most of the items in the functional or activity scales, the content of questionnaires assessing participation is usually derived from focus groups of people with impaired vision, including those with glaucoma (Table 42.1). Examples of such questionnaires are the National Eye Institute Visual Function Questionnaire (NEI-VFQ)[22] and the Impact of Vision Impairment (IVI).[23] These vision-targeted questionnaires have been found to be more sensitive and relevant to glaucoma than generic quality of life instruments to measure differences in disease severity.[24] Some questionnaires such as the Veterans Affairs Low Vision Visual Functioning Questionnaire (VA LV VFQ-48) that was designed to assess change in rating of concern or difficulty with activities in patients that undergo vision-related rehabilitation are a combination of activities and participation.[25]

The rating of difficulty or concern of items that are important to people guide the content of a low-vision rehabilitation program. For example, if social isolation is important, the reasons for that can be assessed; they could be related to mobility, inability to read timetables for public transport, or read instructions. Similarly, difficulty with meal preparation can arise from a number of vision-related problems. The solutions can be related to equipment or training in vision and vision substitution techniques.

CONTEXTUAL FACTORS: CONSIDERATIONS FOR REHABILITATION

Most questionnaires have been developed in Western, developed countries which will make them unsuitable

TABLE 42.1 Quotes from focus groups of people with vision impairment on the consequences of their vision loss

Mobility:

'It's made me very slow and very careful and quite nervous.'

'The fact of not being able to see properly is very tiring because you have to concentrate whether you're in the house and doubly so when you are outside the house.'

'I miss the freedom of having a car.'

Emotional wellbeing:

'I think it is the frustration in the first place. It's total frustration and depression.'

'I was very angry that I couldn't see and do the things I wanted to do.'

'Frustrated because you can't get and keep a proper job so you are financially disadvantaged.'

Social:

'I withdrew from mixing with strangers.'

'I think it depends on your interaction with other people, with sighted people, how your day goes …'

'It's difficult to just pop over and visit someone and because you can't reciprocate you lose friends, they just drift away.'

for use in countries where cultures and values are different. The ICF demonstrates that the interaction of vision factors with personal and environmental ones are important considerations.

In many cultures, interdependence within the community and family support are of prime importance. This will have an impact on goals for rehabilitation: thus, the inclusion of traditional orientation and mobility skills for independent mobility. LaGrow illustrated this with reference to the Maori people in New Zealand whose goals are not for independence but for connection with the community.[26] Similarly, he speaks about young people in the Pacific Islands who travel around in groups, thus having different needs for rehabilitation, not necessarily including independent mobility.

The IVI was used as the basis for the development of a new quality of life instrument for use in the Pacific Islands. After translation, existing items were assessed for suitability and relevance of language, and areas not included were canvassed with health workers and patients. After administration of the IVI_M (Melanesian version) in Vanuatu, the structure of the IVI_M was analyzed.[27] While the IVI has three domains – reading and accessing information; mobility and independence; and emotional well-being[4] – the IVI_M has two domains – activities of daily living and emotional well-being.[27] Rehabilitation programs offered in different cultures need to reflect areas of need and importance.

All the research so far on QOL has been conducted with adults but almost none with children. While there are functional vision questionnaires and checklists of activities, there have been no quality of life tools. The Centre for Eye Research Australia has recently validated a new children's version of the IVI, IVI_C.[28] This is now available to study the impact of congenital and later-onset glaucoma in children. As the numbers of such children are relatively small, multicenter studies will be needed for either cross-sectional or longitudinal studies.

LOW-VISION SERVICES

Low-vision services consist of more than prescribing magnifiers! Ideally, comprehensive low-vision care is part of the continuum of care for people with impaired vision.

The methods of delivery of low-vision services vary across organizations and countries but the content is similar. The range of services includes:

- Clinical assessment of vision and prescription of low-vision devices (Figs 42.3 and 42.4)
- Advice on lighting, contrast, and modifications to the environment
- Advice or supply of nonoptical devices such as felt-tipped bold pens, kitchen equipment, 'talking' watches, scales, etc. (Figs 42.5–42.8)
- Orientation and mobility training
- Training for skills related to activities of daily living
- Employment and training
- Support for education
- Counseling for depression and Charles Bonnet syndrome
- Activity groups
- Self-management programs
- Peer support groups.

One thing that has come consistently from questionnaires is the impact of vision loss on emotional well-being. Many low-vision services do not provide specialist counselors as an integral part of their services but many organizations are now looking at ways to address the need for support. The introduction of self-management programs is one way of addressing the mental health of people with vision loss by incorporating ways to accept, understand, and cope with depression.[29]

LOW-VISION DEVICES

The main types of low-vision devices for near tasks are either spectacle-mounted, hand-held, or stand magnifiers. The type of magnifier prescribed depends on what it is to be used for. For prolonged use such as reading a newspaper, a stand magnifier might be preferred while 'spot reading' of instructions on food labels, prices, or timetables will be best with a hand-held device. The most common range of near magnifiers prescribed and/or taken are in the range of 3× to 7× magnification even though higher magnification allows smaller sizes of print to be seen.

Many older people prefer to have high plus segments as bifocals or as separate reading glasses. The advantage of spectacle-mounted magnifiers is that they leave hands free but the focal distance is relatively short depending on the power of the lens.

Distance devices such as telescopes are commonly used by children and young adults, but few older people choose to use telescopes for distance tasks (see Fig. 42.4).

An appreciation of the consequences of vision loss from glaucoma also provides the information needed to select services required. The personal factors listed in the ICF such as age, gender, employment, and place of residence will influence the types of service required. Most people who use low-vision services use the first three services listed.[30]

The focus groups conducted with children resulted in a very strong message about the importance of social skills and communication as part of low-vision and educational support.[28] Skills to enhance social interaction need to be included within the low-vision program for children and adolescents.

TECHNOLOGY

Advances in technology have made access to information and communication for people with impaired vision easier. Special equipment with enlarged, audio or tactile displays or output is available but regular computers can also be adapted to make screens more visible. Settings within the computer can increase the size of icons and menu bars. The polarity can also be changed to produce white print on a black background to ease the glare from the computer. Global positioning systems (GPS) can be linked to an audio or Braille display as a means to give instructions for orientation and independent mobility. Information and equipment and training are available on the websites listed below.

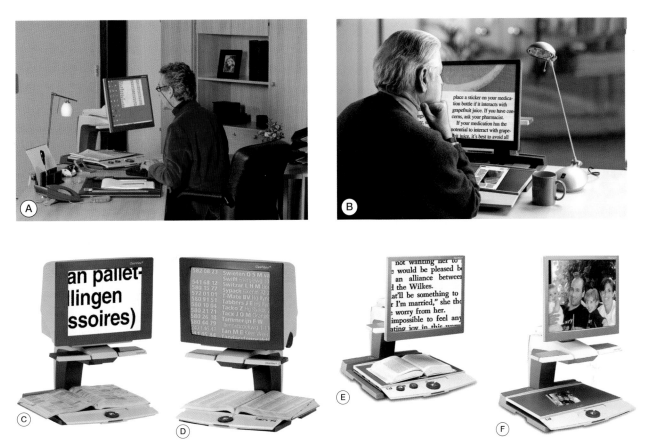

FIGURE 42.3 (A–F) When traditional magnifiers do not provide sufficient magnification, electronic devices provide high magnification for everyday needs such as print, pictures, and objects. Note the use of extra desk lighting and high-contrast objects on the desk and bookshelves in **(A)**. (Images courtesy of Tim Connell of Quantum Technology.)

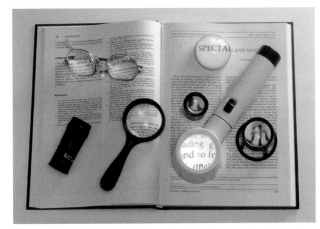

FIGURE 42.4 Magnifiers for near activities are available as spectacles and hand-held or stand magnifiers, with or without extra illumination. Telescopes assist in viewing of distant objects such as blackboards in a classroom or at outdoor activities to help with mobility of viewing a favorite sporting event.

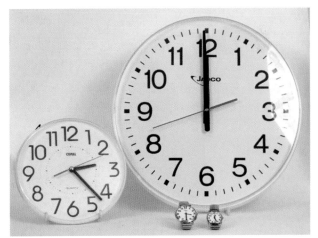

FIGURE 42.5 Both size and contrast are important for visibility. Many readily available items assist people with low vision.

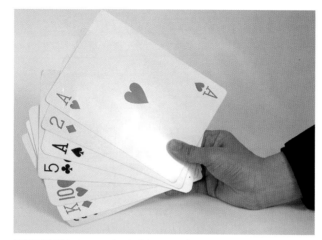

FIGURE 42.6 Large-sized objects such as these playing cards make it possible for people with low vision to join in everyday activities. These are usually available from agencies that provide support and equipment for people who are vision impaired.

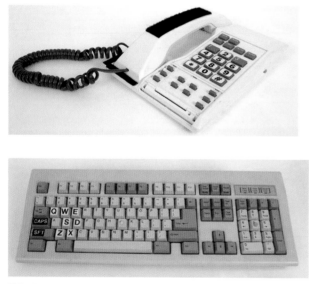

FIGURE 42.7 Large stick-on numbers or letters are readily available to make items more easy to identify.

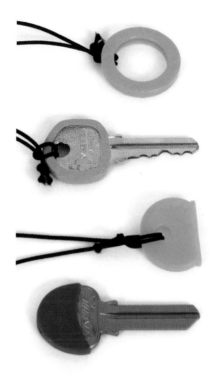

FIGURE 42.8 Had trouble finding your keys? Simple solutions such as brightly colored, high-contrast plastic can be added to items such as keys to make them easier to find.

Summary

- Visual acuity <6/12 is an indication to ask a patient about the effect that vision has on quality of life.
- Vision, economic, functional, and psychosocial factors interact to impact on quality of life of people with low vision.
- Consideration needs to be given to personal and environmental contextual factors as to how they influence perceptions and needs for service.
- Optical and nonoptical low-vision devices can enhance everyday visual functioning.
- Patients select services from the range offered by a comprehensive low-vision service according to their needs.
- Simple solutions are as good, or often better, than the 'high tech' solutions in improving functional vision.

REFERENCES

1. World Health Organization. International Classification of Diseases – 10th Revision (ICD-10). Geneva: World Health Organization; 1992.

2. World Health Organization. Management of low vision in children. World Health Organization, WHO/PBL/93.27.

3. Keeffe JE, Lovie-Kitchin JE, Taylor HR, et al. Referrals by ophthalmologists for low vision services. Aust NZ J Ophthalmol 1996; 24:207–214.

4. Lamoureux E, Pallant J, Pesudovs K, et al. The Impact of Vision Impairment questionnaire: an assessment of its domain structure using confirmatory factor analysis and Rasch analysis. Invest Ophthalmol Vis Sci 2007; 48:1001–1006.

5. Weih LM, McCarty CA, Taylor HR. Functional implications of vision impairment. Clin Exp Ophthalmol 2000; 28:153–155.

6. Wang JJ, Mitchell P, Smith W, et al. Factors associated with use of community support services in an older Australian population. Aust NZ J Public Health 1999; 23:146–153.

7. The Eye Diseases Prevalence Research Group. Causes and prevalence of visual impairment among adults in the United States. Arch Ophthalmol 2004; 122:477–485.

8. The Eye Diseases Prevalence Research Group. Prevalence of open-angle glaucoma among adults in the United States. Arch Ophthalmol 2004; 122:532–538.

9. World Health Organization. Consultation on development of standards for characterization of vision loss and visual functioning. Geneva: World Health Organization, Prevention of Blindness and Deafness; 2003; WHO/PBL/03.91..

10. Bailey IL. Lovie, JE. New design principles for visual acuity letter charts. Am J Optom Physiol Opt 1974; 53:740–745.

11. Lee B, Gutierrez P, Gordon M, et al. The Glaucoma Symptom Scale – a brief index of glaucoma-specific symptoms. Arch Ophthalmol 1998; 116:861–866.

12. Jacob A, Prasad S, Boggild M, et al. Charles Bonnet syndrome – elderly people and visual hallucinations. Br Med J 2004; 328:1552–1554.

13. Wong EYH, Chou SL, Lamoureux EL, et al. Personal costs of vision impairment for common eye diseases and severity of vision loss. Ophthal Epidemiol in press.

14. O'Connor PM, Chou SL, Lamoureux EL, et al. The cost of vision impairment in childhood and adolescence: case study reports from diary records, Optom Vis Sci in press.

15. Lee PP, Walt JG, Doyle JJ, et al. A multicenter, retrospective pilot study of resource use and costs associated with severity of disease in glaucoma. Arch Ophthalmol 2006; 124:12–19.

16. Steinberg EP, Javitt JC, Legro MW, et al. The VF-14. An index of functional impairment in patients with cataract. Arch Ophthalmol 1994; 112:630–638.

17. Haymes S, Johnston A, Heyes A. A weighted version of the Melbourne low-vision ADL index: a measure of disability impact. Optom Vis Sci 2001; 78:565–579.

18. Rubin G, Bandeen-Roche K, Huang G, et al. The association of multiple visual impairments with self-reported visual disability: SEE project. Invest Ophthalmol Vis Sci 2001; 42:64–72.

19. Erin JN, Paul B. Functional vision assessment and instruction of children and youths in academic programs. In: Corn AL, Koenig AJ, eds. Foundations of low vision: clinical and functional perspectives. New York: AFB Press; 1996.

20. World Health Organization. Asia Pacific Regional Low Vision Workshop. Geneva: World Health Organization; 2001; WHO/PBL/02.87.

21. World Health Organization. Towards a common language for functioning, disability, and health: ICF. Geneva: World Health Organization; 2002.

22. Mangione CM, Spritzer K, Berry S, et al. Development of the 25-item National Eye Institute Visual Function Questionnaire. Arch Ophthalmol 2001; 119:1050–1058.

23. Lamoureux E, Pallant J, Pesudovs K, et al. The Impact of Vision Impairment Questionnaire: an evaluation of its measurement properties using Rasch analysis. Invest Ophthalmol Vis Sci 2006; 47:4732–4741.

24. Gutierrez P, Wilson M, Johnson C, et al. Influence of glaucomatous visual field loss on health-related quality of life. Arch Ophthalmol 1997; 115:777–784.

25. Stelmack J, Szlyk J, Stelmack T, et al. Measuring outcomes of vision rehabilitation with the Veterans Affairs Low Vision Visual Functioning Questionnaire. Invest Ophthalmol Vis Sci 2006; 47:3253–3261.

26. LaGrow SJ. A cultural perspective on orientation and mobility. J Vis Impair Blindness 1998; 92:260–264.

27. Scarr BC. Vision-related quality of life in Melanesia. Bachelor of Medical Science thesis. The University of Melbourne. 2006.

28. Cochrane G, Lamoureux EL, Keeffe JE. Defining the content for a new quality of life questionnaire for students with low vision (the Impact of Vision Impairment on Children: IVI_C). Ophthalmic Epidemiol 2008; 15:114–120.

29. Rees G, Saw CL, Lamoureux S, et al. Self management programs for adults with low vision: needs and challenges. Patient Educ Couns 2007; 69:39–46.

30. Lamoureux EL, Pallant JF, Pesudovs K, et al. The effectiveness of low vision rehabilitation on participation in daily living and quality of life. Invest Ophthalmol Vis Sci 2007; 48:1476–1482.

SUGGESTED READING

O'Connor PM, Keeffe JE. Focus on low vision. The Centre for Eye Research Australia, Melbourne 2007. ISBN978-0-9757695-8-4. Online. Available: www.cera.org.au/publications

Fletcher D, ed. Low vision rehabilitation. San Francisco: American Academy of Ophthalmology; 2003.

USEFUL WEBSITES

. http//:www.rnib.org.
. http//:www.visionaustralia.org.
. http//:www.lighthouse.org.
. http//:www.visionaware.org.
. http//:www.lowvisiononline.org.

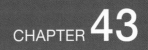

Adherence and Persistence

Gail F Schwartz

INTRODUCTION

'Drugs don't work for patients who don't take them.'[1] Those nine words encapsulate the problem that physicians face when their patients do not take their medications as prescribed over time. Failures in adherence (the extent to which patients' behaviors correspond with providers' recommendations) and persistence (the extent to which a recommended therapy is continued over time) are common, particularly among patients with chronic conditions who require lifelong medication and follow-up.[2] (The term 'adherence' is used herein as it more explicitly takes into account patient responsibility and involvement in care, although the alternate term, 'compliance,' is frequently used in the literature.)

Problems with medication adherence and persistence often begin before the patient even takes a medication home. Approximately 9% of prescriptions written are never filled,[3] and up to 20% of prescriptions that are filled remain unclaimed at pharmacies.[4] Even among patients who do fill and claim their prescriptions, it has been estimated that few completely follow providers' recommendations. Thus, approximately one-sixth of patients who claim their prescriptions will have perfect adherence over time, one-sixth will take nearly all doses with some timing irregularities, one-sixth will occasionally miss a dose, one-sixth will take a drug holiday three or four times a year, one-sixth will take a drug holiday at least monthly, and one-sixth will take few or no doses while giving the impression of good adherence.[5,6]

It is difficult for physicians to determine into which sixth of the adherence/persistence continuum a given patient falls, and even spot testing of drug levels cannot provide a complete picture. For example, a study using microelectronic pill monitors found that patients receiving antiepileptic medications for seizure control had a significant decline in adherence 1 month after their clinic visit (from 88% adherence in the 5 days previsit and 86% in the 5 days postvisit to 67% 1 month postvisit).[7] Estimates of a given patient's adherence would have varied substantially depending on when blood levels were monitored.

Adherence and persistence are problematic across therapeutic areas and impact health outcomes and costs.[8–11] Determining the magnitude of and minimizing the impact of these problems in patients with glaucoma is important given the prevalence of the condition. Worldwide, glaucoma affects more than 66 million individuals, and at least 6 to 8 million are bilaterally blind due to the condition.[12] The effect of glaucoma on healthcare systems is substantial, with more than 7 million glaucoma-related office visits occurring in the United States alone each year.[13,14]

This chapter discusses: (1) the scope of the problems with adherence and persistence in glaucoma therapy, (2) issues related to identifying patients with adherence or persistence problems, and (3) approaches to improving patient adherence and persistence.

SCOPE OF THE PROBLEMS

Estimates of rates of adherence with topical ocular hypotensive medication have been quite variable. For example, a 12-week, randomized, observer-masked, crossover study[15] of two formulations of a topical β-blocker conducted in 202 patients with primary open-angle glaucoma or ocular hypertension found that 98% and 96% of patients, respectively, reported never or rarely forgetting their medication. A 12-month, retrospective, population-based study[16] of more than 2400 glaucoma patients with a pharmacy claim for a prostaglandin analogue found that patients had medication available for use on 76.3% of days. In contrast, all 21 patients in a focus group of patients who had seen at least two ophthalmologists and were taking at least two topical medications for glaucoma reported some level of nonadherence.[17] Adherence also varies with patient diagnosis and medication prescribed. A retrospective cohort study[18] using health insurance claims data included 3623 patients with diagnosed glaucoma and 1677 with suspect glaucoma. As Figure 43.1[18] demonstrates, adherence (prevalence of use at various time points) was higher in patients with diagnosed than with suspect glaucoma (relative risk, 1.11; 95% confidence interval [CI], 1.05–1.18), and use of a prostaglandin was

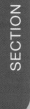
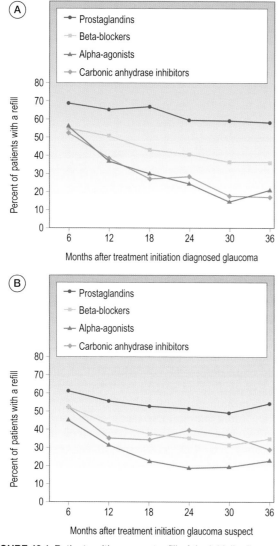

FIGURE 43.1 Patients with a current refill of the initially dispensed medication at each 6-month interval following treatment initiation for patients with diagnosed glaucoma **(A)** or suspect glaucoma **(B)**. (Reproduced with permission from Nordstrom BL, Friedman DS, Mozaffari E, et al. Persistance and adherence with topical glaucoma therapy. Am J Ophthalmol 2005; 140:598–606.)

associated with higher rates of adherence. Among those prescribed a prostaglandin, though, adherence may be negatively affected by a change from monotherapy to adjunctive therapy. An open-label, retrospective review[19] of nearly 5000 patient records found that the mean refill interval for latanoprost increased by 6.7 ± 25.6 days after the addition of a second drug, and the interval increased by >2 weeks for 22.9% of patients.

The wide range of medication adherence estimates reflects, in large part, heterogeneity in study methods, time frames, patient samples, and adherence measures. Methodologies have included, among others, retrospective cohort designs,[20,21] a cross-sectional patient survey and concomitant chart review,[22] a retrospective, population-based design,[16] and focus groups and in-depth interviews.[17] Time frames for adherence estimation have ranged from the unspecific ('Do you ever miss a dose?') to measurement of the prevalence of use at a variety of specified time points.[18] Study samples frequently

have been drawn from among patients treated in glaucoma subspecialty practices; however, some researchers included any patient seen in the practice[23–25] while others used a variety of inclusion and exclusion criteria.[17,19,22] Sample sizes have ranged from fewer than 50 participants[17,23] to more than 4000.[18,19] Although adherence most commonly has been measured by patient self-report either via self-administered questionnaire or structured interview by trained personnel,[23,25–28] other measures have included medication possession ratios (MPRs) and mean days without therapy.[16,20,21] In addition to variability in adherence estimates caused by the differences enumerated above, findings can be impacted by variation among studies in patient recall bias and in patient overestimation of adherence to meet what patients believe to be investigators' expectations.[29]

As with adherence, evaluating medication persistence across the population of patients prescribed ocular hypotensive therapies remains a significant challenge. A common approach has been the use of survival analysis to estimate time to discontinuation or change in therapy.[18,30–36] Although estimates have varied, persistence, which reflects not only the patient's satisfaction with an agent's tolerability but also the physician's satisfaction with the level of intraocular pressure control,[37] generally has been found to be poor. For example, among 28 741 patients dispensed any of seven ocular hypotensives, 33% of those receiving a prostaglandin and only 19% of those treated with any other therapy had not discontinued the initial agent after 12 months.[31] Among 1474 primary open-angle glaucoma suspects, 39% of those treated initially with a prostaglandin and 25% of patients treated first with a β-blocker had not discontinued treatment at month 12.[34] A study that included patients with either diagnosed or suspect glaucoma (n = 5300) found that nearly half of patients discontinued all ocular hypotensive therapy within 6 months, and only 37% recently had refilled the initial medication 3 years after the first dispensing date.[18] Persistence was marginally better in those with diagnosed glaucoma (hazard ratio, 0.92; 95% CI, 0.86–1.00) and was substantially higher with prostaglandins than with any other medication class. Variability in persistence has been seen within the prostaglandin class, though, with latanoprost-treated patients demonstrating greater persistence than those treated with bimatoprost or travoprost at 12 months.[33] Interestingly, discontinuation patterns for the three prostaglandins were similar between age cohorts (20 through 64 years vs ≥ 65 years) for the first 9 months, but younger patients demonstrated somewhat greater persistence for all agents at month 12 (Fig. 43.2).[38]

Physicians need to distinguish between lack of clinical response and lack of persistence, and including restarts of therapy is important to making such distinctions. A recent 6-month study[39] found that one-third of current users, defined as those who either persisted with the index prostaglandin or who restarted the index therapy after a discontinuation, had restarted the index drug. However, more than half of those who discontinued the index drug did not restart any topical ocular hypotensive

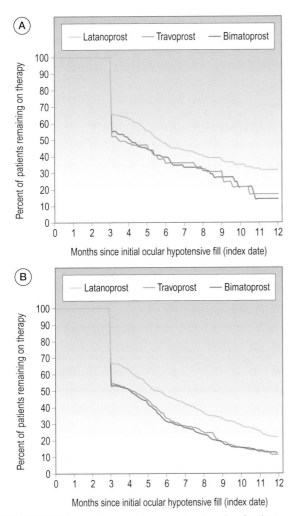

FIGURE 43.2 Kaplan–Meier plots of survival function for time to discontinuation of initial prostaglandin for patients ages 20 through 64 **(A)** and ⩾ 65 **(B)** years of age.[38]

both have been shown to decrease over time while patients treated with prostaglandins consistently have been found to be substantially more adherent and persistent than those receiving other agents.[18,30–32,34–36] More specifically, adherence has been found to be greater in patients with diagnosed than with suspect glaucoma, to be associated with increasing age in patients with diagnosed glaucoma, and to be lower among patients with suspect glaucoma in the Southeast than in the Midwest.[18] The greatest risk of therapy discontinuation was noted in patients between 40 and 49 years of age and in females (in diagnosed glaucoma patients) and in those living in the Southeast region (in diagnosed and suspect glaucoma patients).[18]

Although population-level data are informative, they do not help physicians identify individual patients who need to change behaviors. To make those identifications, physicians must obtain information concerning patients' medication-taking behavior outside the office, a task usually accomplished by asking patients directly. Still, the difficulty of relying on patient self-reports is demonstrated by results of a study on the reliability of blood glucose monitoring by patients with diabetes.[40] Nineteen patients with insulin-dependent diabetes mellitus were surreptitiously given standard reflectance meters modified with memory chips that stored glucose readings by date and time. Patients also continued to record meter readings in a logbook. After 2 weeks, mean reported glucose recordings were lower in the logbooks in three-quarters of patients, two-thirds obscured clinically significant hyperglycemia or hypoglycemia, and an average of 26% of logbook entries did not correspond completely to meter values. Similar disparities between observed and reported adherence have been noted in glaucoma patients. For example, the 30-day adherence rate measured by eyedrop monitor (76%) was lower than rates recorded by medication log (99%) or patient interview (97%); in addition, physicians could not accurately predict which patients would have ocular hypotensive medication adherence rates of <50% versus >90%.[41]

The Glaucoma Adherence and Persistency Study (GAPS) is the most recent series of publications evaluating pharmacy claims (n = 13 977), physicians charts (n = 301), physician interviews (n = 103), and patient interviews (n = 300).[42–44] This is a more complete view of actual medication usage as compared with reported use and provides greater insight into the drivers of adherence. The MPR was the main measure of adherence in GAPS.[43] Lower mean MPR values were noted among patients who heard all of what they know about glaucoma from the doctor (compared to some or no information) and among those who did not believe that reduced vision is a risk of not taking medication as recommended. Patients who reported having a problem paying for medications and those who stated that they had difficulty taking their medication while traveling or away from home also had lower mean MPRs. Lower mean MPR values were seen among patients who did not acknowledge stinging and burning, who were non-white, and who received samples. Finally, patients who

therapy. Most studies showing poor persistence with glaucoma therapy have not evaluated restarts, but analyses including restarts are critical to evaluating long-term glaucoma treatment.

It is important to recognize that analyses of persistence based on retrospective pharmacy claims have advantages and disadvantages. Although such studies often include large numbers of patients and their results can be used to compare agents within a drug class, they cannot identify reasons for differences in persistence among therapies or patient groups nor can the impact on health outcomes be estimated. Future research should combine patient interviews, routine clinical monitoring, and analyses of claims data in order to develop a more robust picture of medication persistence.

IDENTIFYING PATIENTS WITH ADHERENCE OR PERSISTENCE PROBLEMS

Identifying patients with adherence or persistence problems presents a substantial challenge for ophthalmologists. At the population level, adherence and persistence did not receive a phone call visit reminder had lower MPRs.[43] These findings may help tailor physician behavior to specific patient barriers with the goal of improving adherence.

IMPROVING ADHERENCE AND PERSISTENCE

Given the current state of the art, physicians might consider several approaches to optimizing adherence and persistence in patients receiving glaucoma therapy.

1. *Maximize patient motivation and knowledge by reinforcing the importance of adherence and persistence.* Glaucoma patients must be active, engaged, and knowledgeable participants in the management of their disease. Over the long term, adherence and persistence depend on the patient's understanding of his or her medication and follow-up regimens as well as the impact his or her own behavior has on controlling the disease. Conversations between the patient and the ophthalmologist will likely continue for many years. The ophthalmologist should use each interaction to reinforce the goals and benefits of medical therapy and ongoing follow-up, should stress the need for active patient participation, and should address patient concerns about treatment and barriers to adherence and persistence. The more patients know, the more adherent and persistent they will be.

2. *Give the patient literature to read at home.* Reinforce the information provided during office visits by providing written materials for the patient and his or her family to read at home.

3. *Assess the medication and follow-up regimen regularly, especially when initiating care.* In general, the simplest medication and follow-up regimen that meets the patient's needs should be considered. Questions concerning potential side effects that might interfere with medication adherence or persistence should be asked at each visit. Changes in the treatment regimen should be considered if problems arise, particularly if visible side effects, such as hyperemia, are present. When starting care, frequent follow-up visits provide an opportunity for the physician to address the patient's questions and concerns, to adjust the treatment regimen if needed, and to reinforce the importance of following instructions. Close early monitoring may circumvent later adherence and persistence problems.

4. *Ask the patient about adherence and persistence at every visit and be alert to 'white coat adherence.'* A technician should ask when the patient last filled a prescription, how much medication is left in the bottle at home, and how long a bottle of medication typically lasts. Patients also should be asked when they administered the last drop and to estimate how many doses they missed in the last month, 3 months, and since the last visit. These latter questions should be asked more than once during each visit since different answers may be given.

Technicians should be trained to make open-ended, nonjudgmental inquiries that reduce the stigma of nonadherence by normalizing and universalizing the behavior. Technicians also should be educated to identify cues of 'white coat adherence,' the tendency for patients to improve adherence around the time of a visit.[7,45] For example, Cramer et al.[7] found that patients were best at dosing 5 days prior to an office visit, with a sharp decline in adherence a month later.

5. *Assess the patient's ability to instill drops and minimize wastage.* Consider dispensing a practice bottle of artificial tears for the patient learning to instill drops. At each visit, have a technician watch while the patient instills drops to be sure skills are maintained and wastage is minimized. Don't assume that patients know how to use eyedrops: watch them and show them. Consider prescribing a device to aid in drop administration for patients having problems.

6. *Write down drop directions and consider an easy-to-read chart.* Be sure the patient understands the timing and spacing of drops by providing written drop directions and an easy-to-read chart that details the dosing schedule. Have the patient review the instructions in the office and recite them back; written instructions only work if the patient reads and understands them. Advise patients concerning what they should do if they miss a dose. A copy of all written materials provided to the patient should be kept in the medical record.

7. *Help patients integrate the treatment regimen into their lifestyles.* Help patients identify cues that will aid them in remembering to instill their eyedrops. For example, they might associate their drops with drinking their morning coffee, brushing their teeth, or taking other medications. Patients having problems with forgetfulness might be asked to keep a medication diary or calendar to be reviewed during office visits. Patients who work can be encouraged to keep an extra bottle at the work site.

8. *Use reminder phone calls rather than postcards and provide an office system for tracking patients who miss appointments.*

9. *Be sensitive to health system issues, including costs.* Patients may be embarrassed to admit they cannot afford their medication or follow-up visits. A referral to a medication assistance program sponsored by a pharmaceutical company might help offset the cost issue and improve adherence and persistence. Samples can be given to help patients become accustomed to taking medication and to encourage them to refill prescriptions. For patients with pharmacy benefits, physicians should know what is covered by the plan and provide refills with 90-day supplies whenever possible. Reliable patients should be given a generous number of refills.

10. *Make the office adherence and persistence friendly.* Implement systems for medication refill requests called in by patients. Provide mail and telephone

reminders of appointments and contact patients who miss appointments. Give phone numbers to patients that they can use for routine questions and in case of perceived emergencies.

11. *Encourage the pharmaceutical industry to continue working to improve patient adherence and persistence.* Pharmaceutical companies have a role to play in improving patient adherence and persistence. Support is needed for the development of innovative approaches to inform doctors and patients of missed refills at pharmacies. Industry-sponsored research can facilitate the development of effective patient education programs and materials targeted to changing patient behaviors. Research and development teams can bring to market long-acting ocular hypotensive medications that are simple to administer as well as medication monitors whose information can be easily downloaded into office databases.

Summary

As with other chronic and often asymptomatic conditions, patients with glaucoma frequently are nonadherent and poorly persistent with treatment regimens. The inability to distinguish between problems of efficacy versus those of adherence and persistence may result in suboptimal patient outcomes and unnecessary and costly changes in therapy. Physicians can take several approaches to identifying patients with suboptimal adherence or persistence and to working with patients to improve adherence and persistence.

REFERENCES

1. Cramer JA. Effect of partial compliance on cardiovascular medication effectiveness. Heart 2002; 88:203–206.
2. Osterberg L, Blaschke T. Adherence to medication. N Engl J Med 2005; 353:487–497.
3. Robbins J. Improving patient compliance: is there a pharmacist in the house? Schering Report XIV 1992; 6:1–16.
4. Farmer KC, Gumbhir AK. Unclaimed prescriptions: an overlooked opportunity. Am Pharm NS 1992; NS32:819–823.
5. Urquhart J. The electronic medication event monitor: lessons for pharmacotherapy. Clin Pharmacokinet 1997; 32:345–356.
6. Urquhart J. The odds of the three nons when an aptly prescribed medicine isn't working: non-compliance, non-absorption, non-response. Br J Clin Pharmacol 2002; 54:212–220.
7. Cramer JA, Scheyer RD, Mattson RH. Compliance declines between clinic visits. Arch Intern Med 1990; 150:1509–1510.
8. Caro JJ, Salas M, Speckman JL, et al. Persistence with treatment for hypertension in actual practice. CMAJ 1999; 160:31–37.
9. Degli Esposti L, Di Martino M, Saragoni S, et al. Pharmacoeconomics of antihypertensive drug treatment: an analysis of how long patients remain on various antihypertensive therapies. J Clin Hypertens (Greenwich) 2004; 6:76–82.
10. DiMatteo MR. Variations in patients' adherence to medical recommendations: a quantitative review of 50 years of research. Med Care 2004; 42:200–209.
11. McCombs JS, Nichol MB, Newman CM, et al. The costs of interrupting antihypertensive drug therapy in a Medicaid population. Med Care 1994; 32:214–226.
12. Quigley HA. Number of people with glaucoma worldwide. Br J Ophthalmol 1996; 80:389–393.
13. Javitt JC, Chiang YP. Preparing for managed competition: utilization of ophthalmologic services varies by state. Arch Ophthalmol 1993; 111:1469–1470.
14. Quigley HA, Vitale S. Models of open-angle glaucoma prevalence and incidence in the United States. Invest Ophthalmol Vis Sci 1997; 38:83–91.
15. Schenker H, Maloney S, Liss C, et al. Patient preference, efficacy, and compliance with timolol maleate ophthalmic gel-forming solution versus timolol maleate ophthalmic solution in patients with ocular hypertension or open-angle glaucoma. Clin Ther 1999; 21:138–147.
16. Wilensky J, Fiscella RG, Carlson AM, et al. Measurement of persistence and adherence to regimens of IOP-lowering glaucoma medications using pharmacy claims data. Am J Ophthalmol 2006; 141 (suppl):28–33.
17. Taylor SA, Galbraith SM, Mills RP. Causes of non-compliance with drug regimens in glaucoma patients: a qualitative study. J Ocul Pharmacol Ther 2002; 18:401–409.
18. Nordstrom BL, Friedman DS, Mozaffari E, et al. Persistence and adherence with topical glaucoma therapy. Am J Ophthalmol 2005; 140:598–606.
19. Robin AL, Covert D. Does adjunctive glaucoma therapy affect adherence to the initial primary therapy? Ophthalmology 2005; 112:863–868.
20. Gurwitz JH, Glynn RJ, Monane M, et al. Treatment for glaucoma: adherence by the elderly. Am J Public Health 1993; 83:711–716.
21. Gurwitz JH, Yeomans SM, Glynn RJ, et al. Patient noncompliance in the managed care setting. The case of medical therapy for glaucoma. Med Care 1998; 36:357–369.
22. Muir KW, Santiago-Turla C, Stinnett S, et al. Health literacy and adherence to glaucoma therapy. Am J Ophthalmol 2006; 142:223–226.
23. Tsai JC, McClure CA, Ramos SE, et al. Compliance barriers in glaucoma: a systematic classification. J Glaucoma 2003; 12:393–398.
24. Jampel HD, Schwartz GF, Robin AL, et al. Patient preferences for eye drop characteristics: a willingness-to-pay analysis. Arch Ophthalmol 2003; 121:540–546.
25. Patel SC, Spaeth GL. Compliance in patients prescribed eyedrops for glaucoma. Ophthalmic Surg 1995; 26:233–236.
26. Konstas AG, Maskaleris G, Gratsonidis S, et al. Compliance and viewpoint of glaucoma patients in Greece. Eye 2000; 14:752–756.
27. Kosoko O, Quigley HA, Vitale S, et al. Risk factors for noncompliance with glaucoma follow-up visits in a resident's eye clinic. Ophthalmology 1998; 105:2105–2111.
28. Rotchford AP, Murphy KM. Compliance with timolol treatment in glaucoma. Eye 1998; 12:234–236.
29. Krousel-Wood M, Thomas S, Muntner P, et al. Medication adherence: a key factor in achieving blood pressure control and good clinical outcomes in hypertensive patients. Curr Opin Cardiol 2004; 19:357–362.
30. Dasgupta S, Oates V, Bookhart BK, et al. Population-based persistency rates for topical glaucoma medications measured with pharmacy claims data. Am J Manag Care 2002; 8(suppl):S255–S261.
31. Reardon G, Schwartz GF, Mozaffari E. Patient persistency with topical ocular hypotensive therapy in a managed care population. Am J Ophthalmol 2004; 137(suppl):S3–S12.

32. Reardon G, Schwartz GF, Mozaffari E. Patient persistency with pharmacotherapy in the management of glaucoma. Eur J Ophthalmol 2003; 13(suppl):S44–S52.

33. Reardon G, Schwartz GF, Mozaffari E. Patient persistency with ocular prostaglandin therapy: a population-based, retrospective study. Clin Ther 2003; 25:1172–1185.

34. Schwartz GF, Reardon G, Mozaffari E. Persistency with latanoprost or timolol in primary open-angle glaucoma suspects. Am J Ophthalmol 2004; 137(suppl):S13–S16.

35. Spooner JJ, Bullano MF, Ikeda LI, et al. Rates of discontinuation and change of glaucoma therapy in a managed care setting. Am J Manag Care 2002; 8(suppl):S262–S270.

36. Zhou Z, Althin R, Sforzolini BS, et al. Persistence and treatment failure in newly diagnosed open angle glaucoma patients in the United Kingdom. Br J Ophthalmol 2004; 88:1391–1394.

37. Schwartz GF. Persistency and tolerability of ocular hypotensive agents: population-based evidence in the management of glaucoma. Am J Ophthalmol 2004; 137(suppl):S1–S2.

38. Schwartz GF, Reardon G, Shah SN. Persistence on ocular prostaglandin therapy: a comparison of Medicare-aged patients to the general glaucoma patient population. Invest Ophthalmol Vis Sci 2006; 47; E-Abstract 4395.

39. Schwartz GF, Platt R, Reardon G, et al. Accounting for restart rates in evaluating persistence with ocular hypertensives. Ophthalmology 2007; 114:648–652.

40. Mazze RS, Shamoon H, Pasmantier R, et al. Reliability of blood glucose monitoring by patients with diabetes mellitus. Am J Med 1984; 77:211–217.

41. Kass MA, Gordon M, Meltzer DW. Can ophthalmologists correctly identify patients defaulting from pilocarpine therapy? Am J Ophthalmol 1986; 101:524–530.

42. Quigley HA, Friedman DS, Hahn SR. Evaluation of practice patterns for the care of open-angle glaucoma compared with claims data: Glaucoma Adherence and Persistency Study. Ophthalmology 2007; 114:1599–1606.

43. Friedman DS, Hahn SR, Gelb L, et al. Doctor-patient communication, health-related beliefs, and adherence in glaucoma: results from the Glaucoma Adherence and Persistency Study (GAPS). Ophthalmology 2007; 114:1599–1606.

44. Friedman DS, Quigley HQ, Gelb L, et al. Using pharmacy claims data to study adherence to glaucoma medications: methodology of the Glaucoma Adherence and Persistency Study (GAPS). Invest Ophthalmol Vis Sci 2007; 48:5052–5057.

45. Feinstein AR. On white-coat effects and the electronic monitoring of compliance. Arch Intern Med 1990; 150:1377–1378.

CHAPTER 44

Outcomes

Ridia Lim and Ivan Goldberg

INTRODUCTION AND DEFINITION

Our ultimate goals for our patients are to preserve visual function, to avoid visual disability, and to minimize disruption to their quality of life (QOL). Outcomes are the achievements of healthcare delivery.

Historically, medicine has focused on clinical end points of healthcare delivery and has ignored this holistic approach: to improve the health of the whole person and to observe the Hippocratic Oath's 'First, do no harm.'

Outcomes focus clinicians onto ultimate goals, to encourage more appropriate application of the therapeutic index: the consideration of potential good versus possible harm from any clinical intervention. Outcomes research is important in all areas of medicine, especially glaucoma, as a chronic, incurable, progressive disease.

Depending on one's bias, scientists, clinicians, patients, and society as a whole view the disease glaucoma and glaucomatous progression very differently:[1] to the scientist, it is retinal ganglion cell death; to the clinician, disc and visual field changes and intraocular pressure (IOP) levels; to the patient, fear of visual loss and disability; to society, resources required to avoid dependency or to provide appropriate support if dependency occurs (Fig. 44.1). Delineating and harmonizing these various concepts and the desired outcomes that flow from them is crucial for effective understanding, communication, and planning.

Generally, chronic glaucoma is a slowly progressive disease. As final end points can take decades to eventuate, intermediate, surrogate end points have been used in most clinical studies. As clinicians, we need constantly to distinguish between final and surrogate end points: we are managing a whole person, not an IOP level, an optic disc appearance, or visual field sensitivity.

Historically, it has been the available technology that has driven concepts of glaucoma, as well as methods of diagnosis and measurement of outcomes. After Helmholtz invented the direct ophthalmoscope and von Graefe described glaucomatous optic neuropathy in the 1850s and 1860s, glaucoma was conceived as an optic nerve head excavation with pallor. When reasonably reliable tonometers became available in the 1890s, disease definitions and concepts focused on IOP levels. Perimetry emerged at the third feature in the classic, now-abandoned glaucoma 'triad' after Bjerrum advanced quantitative perimetry in 1898. With newer technologies precisely quantifying optic disc features, the emphasis has shifted back to glaucomatous optic neuropathy as the key. The disease itself has not changed! Unless we remain alert to this influence, true focus can be lost in the technology.

In bringing reliable tonometry and perimetry to clinical practice, Goldmann stressed, 'It is not pressure that frightens the glaucoma patient, but fear of blindness.'[2] As the ultimate goal of glaucoma management

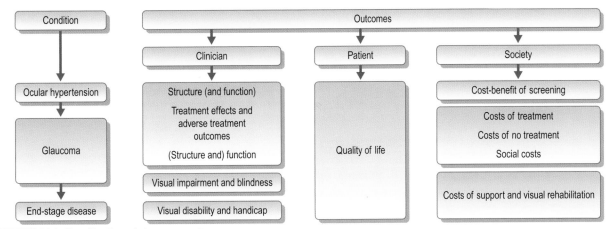

FIGURE 44.1 Classification of glaucoma outcomes.

is to preserve visual function and to maintain QOL, for the individual patient's lifetime, each individual's needs and life expectancy must be assessed; they may vary widely. From the patient's point of view, the main clinical outcome is preservation of visual function and independence (often linked with maintaining a driver's license): perimetry, optic disc evaluation, and IOP levels are intermediate outcomes. They are strategies to achieve the main outcome. QOL, too, is a high priority. Resources are limited and justification is required increasingly for any health expenditure. Glaucoma therapy needs to be shown to be cost-effective.

CLINICAL OUTCOMES: PHYSICIAN'S VIEW

Detection of disease (diagnosis) and subsequent detection of progressive damage are the main clinical glaucoma outcomes. Although there is general agreement on what glaucoma is, until recently[3] there has been no consensus on definitions for glaucoma diagnosis and glaucoma progression; study-specific definitions have been commonplace.

Glaucoma is an optic neuropathy with both characteristic architectural changes of the optic nerve head and matching visual field changes. IOP (whether or not it lies above the statistically derived upper limit of normal) is the biggest risk factor for incidence and progression of disease.

Sophisticated nerve head and nerve fiber layer measurement technologies have identified eyes with glaucomatous damage in which standard automated perimetric sensitivities lie within normal limits. As another example of the state of technology determining concepts, this has spawned the idea of 'pre-perimetric' glaucoma. The recent World Glaucoma Association consensus meeting on glaucoma diagnosis described glaucoma as 'progressive structural optic nerve damage' without reference to perimetry.[3]

In contrast, definition of disease progression remains controversial. Physicians are interested in changes in visual function: surrogate outcome measures are IOP, optic nerve head appearance and retinal nerve fiber layer thickness, visual field sensitivities, color vision, contrast sensitivity, and visual impairment. Patient day-to-day performance as determined by vision has been largely ignored in the past by studies of the various technologies.

GLAUCOMA DIAGNOSIS AND GLAUCOMA PROGRESSION: MEASURING STRUCTURE AND FUNCTION

Lack of consensus on glaucoma diagnosis and progression makes assessment of measurement tools difficult. What is the particular tool's validity (does it measure what it is trying to measure?), reliability, and reproducibility? What is its sensitivity, its specificity (Fig. 44.2)?

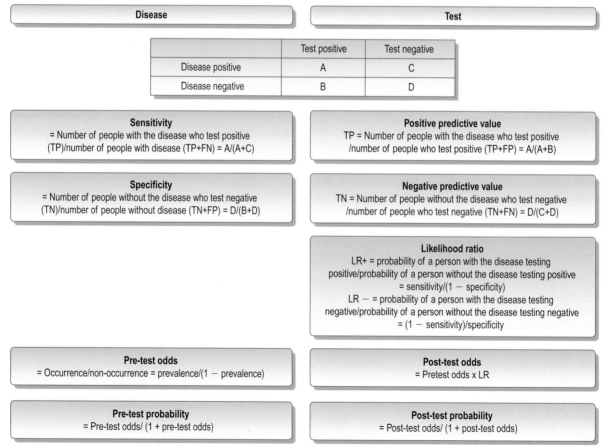

FIGURE 44.2 Understanding test outcomes. TP, true positive; TN, true negative; SpPin, a positive test with a high specificity rules in disease; SnNout, a negative test with a high sensitivity rules out disease.

What are its positive and negative predictive values? Probably, the most valuable indices for a measurement technology are the likelihood ratio and the post-test odds/probability (see Fig. 44.2). Calculation of the likelihood ratio requires sensitivity and specificity; post-test odds/probability needs disease prevalence in the tested population.

A gold standard test is the accepted best available test to measure an outcome. In glaucoma studies, there is no widely accepted gold standard. Standard automated perimetry (SAP), which is used frequently, does not diagnose early glaucoma and there are no widely accepted criteria for glaucoma progression. Even though optic disc change documented by stereophotography, where a panel of experts agree on disease or progression of disease, is the best candidate for the gold standard test, such changes are slow. A variety of different end points have been used in recent major glaucoma studies (Table 44.1).

To understand how good a reported test is, some criteria should be met during its critique. Reid et al. outline 7 methodological standards vital for evaluating how good diagnostic tests are:[4]

1. *Spectrum composition*: to understand what is the population tested, as sensitivities and specificities will vary with the tested population; the tested population are often individuals with significant disease whereas the population on whom the test will be used will not have a high prevalence of the disease. This also influences the ability to generalize the results of the test.

2. *Analysis of pertinent subgroups*: to yield indices for pertinent subgroups as subgroup results may vary widely.

3. *Avoidance of work-up bias*: to channel patients with a positive or negative gold standard test to be assessed by the new test.

4. *Avoidance of review bias*: to ensure that the reviewer of the new test is not aware of the results with the gold standard.

5. *Precision of results for test accuracy*: to present point estimates and confidence intervals.

6. *Presentation of indeterminate or equivocal test results*: most tests are given as positive or negative while, in practice, indeterminate and equivocal results occur frequently. Merit is awarded to a study if equivocal results are included.

7. *Test reproducibility*: any possible observer variation is recognized and measured.

Intraocular pressure While IOP elevated above the statistical 'usual' is no longer part of the diagnosis of glaucoma, IOP remains the most important modifiable risk factor. As it is a reliable and reproducible short-term clinical outcome for management strategies, it remains an end point in many studies. Success in these studies is frequently measured as an arbitrary IOP: in the past most frequently, 21 mmHg. The lack of true validity of this outcome measure has been recognized.[5] Mean IOP, diurnal and long-term fluctuations, and target IOP are important concepts in day-to-day glaucoma management. 'IOP' is not glaucoma, however; up to one-third of glaucoma patients do not have an elevated

TABLE 44.1 Definitions of the end points used in recent major clinical studies of ocular hypertension and glaucoma

STUDY	OUTCOMES
OHTS	'End-point committee'; either a disc change (generalized or localized thinning of the disc rim) or a visual field change (initial end point was a CPSD of $p < 0.05$ or GHT 'outside normal limits' in two consecutive tests but many reverted to normal; the revised end point required three consecutive abnormal results on visual field tests with the same type, location, and index of abnormality).[6]
EPGS	A reproducible disc change (photographic evidence of disc rim narrowing, either localized or diffuse, agreed on by masked graders) or visual field change (three adjacent points decreasing 5 dB from baseline, two adjacent points decreasing 10 dB from baseline or a difference of 10 or more in two or more points across the nasal horizontal meridian) or both; and a safety end point of IOP >35 mmHg.[7]
CNTGS	Either a disc change detected by the reading team or visual field change – a reproducible (at 4 weeks and two VFs at 3 months) new defect (three non-edge points that decrease 5 dB, one point by at least 10 dB), a deepening or expanding existing defect (two contiguous points within or adjacent to existing defect, decrease by 10 dB or three times SF) or a new or expanding defect at fixation.[8]
EMGT	Disc change as measured by a disc reading center (photographs were compared using flicker chronoscopy and judged to have progressed if the change was reproduced 6 months later) or visual field criteria – 'definite visual field progression' defined as three same points progressing ($p < 0.05$) in the EMGT pattern change probability maps in three consecutive 30-2 full threshold.[9]
AGIS	No disc outcome was used. Visual function outcome was either a decrease of visual field (DVF) or decrease of visual acuity (DVA) attributable to glaucoma – DVF was an increase in the AGIS score of 4 or more from baseline. AGIS score (0, no defect to 20, end stage) was calculated using grouped points from the total deviation plot. DVA was a doubling of the visual angle or more. Other outcome variables were time to intervention failure, time to cataract surgery, number of glaucoma medications, and IOP.[10,11]
CIGTS	No disc outcome was used. Visual field outcome used a modified AGIS technique; the CIGTS score (0–20) was calculated from the total deviation probability plot. An increase of three points denoted change. Health-related quality of life was performed using a specific instrument designed for this study incorporating other known instruments. Visual acuity, changes in IOP, and cataract extraction were secondary outcomes.[12]

IOP. It is not useful in diagnosis, but most often is the most identifiable risk factor for progressive disease (see also Ch. 40, Target Intraocular Pressure).

As with all numerical outcomes, a mean is only one way to represent the sample; a range of data leads to the formation of the mean.

Optic disc outcomes

Optic disc diagnosis In incident glaucoma, changes to the optic disc usually can be detected before a visual field defect. Optic disc morphology must be documented by the most objective method available, preferably by color stereophotography or computer-based image analysis. If these are not available, nonstereoscopic photography or a detailed drawing should be used.[13,14]

Once diagnosed, disease severity can be graded. Although patterns of past or ongoing disc damage do not necessarily follow any particular pattern, grading systems may be beneficial for patient care by staging disc change and possible progression (Table 44.2). While Armaly's vertical cup-to-disc ratio is the most popular disc parameter recorded, it needs to be placed in the context of disc size and cup location.[14]

No grading system accounts for descriptive qualities such as disc hemorrhages; presence, size, location, and type of peripapillary atrophy; and the state of retinal blood vessels. While grading systems are useful, other forms of documentation, diagrams or photographs, are also necessary.

The disc grading system proposed by Spaeth,[15] the Disc Damage Likelihood Scale (DDLS), offers a user-friendly system which takes into account disc size (Fig. 44.3). This 10–stage system assesses the narrowest rim width (rim/disc ratio) rather than cup-to-disc ratio. Where there is no rim, it assesses the circumferential extent of the total rim loss. The DDLS system has shown good correlation with Heidelberg retina tomography (HRT) parameters and correlates well with function.[16] An increase in DDLS stage indicates disease progression. Care needs to be used with the DDLS because of inter- and intraobserver variation and the effect these may have influencing interpretation.

Depending on the level of observer training and photograph quality, disc stereophotography is the best way to discriminate between normal and abnormal optic nerves. It remains the gold standard with which comparisons are made. Simultaneous stereophotographs perform better than sequential stereophotographs. While computerized imaging systems are not superior to assessment of stereophotographs by an expert panel, they should perform better than a nonexpert observer. Three commercially available imaging systems have been detailed in previous chapters: the HRT 3, Stratus OCT, and GDx VCC. In a recent comparison of glaucoma detection, the parameters with the best AUROC were HRT 2 linear discriminant function (AUC = 0.86), inferior Stratus OCT retinal nerve fiber layer (RNFL) inferior thickness (AUC = 0.92), and GDx VCC nerve fiber indicator (NFI) (AUC = 0.91).[17] When using the best predictive parameter of each quantitative

instrument, the ROC curves are almost equivalent for all three technologies (Fig. 44.4).[18]

Over time, all these technologies have evolved: hardware and/or software have changed at a rate faster than studies can be performed and published. Results from older studies may no longer be relevant. Although CSLO performed best in one study,[18] the general consensus is that no one technology is better than the others at diagnosing glaucoma at present.[3] As patients identified as having glaucoma with one technology or another do not completely correspond (but do overlap), for the individual patient, we cannot know which of these technologies is the most useful.

Optic disc progression Without technologies, detection of optic disc progression clinically is subjective and difficult to quantify. It may manifest as an increase in cup-to-disc ratio, a decrease in rim-to-disc ratio, a loss of the ISNT rule, and/or an increase in beta-peripapillary atrophy. Optic disc hemorrhages, not an outcome on their own, are significant risk factors for subsequent progression.[19] In the Ocular Hypertension Treatment Study (OHTS), 55% had a disc-only end point for glaucoma diagnosis,[20] while in Early Manifest Glaucoma Trial (EMGT) all the participants with progression met the visual field criteria except for one, who met the disc criteria only.[9] This may reflect their disc progression protocol, which was designed to be highly specific. In general, disc changes may be more sensitive earlier in the disease than visual field changes.

Studied most with respect to optic disc progression, the HRT 3 looks at trends using a point-by-point topographic change analysis (TCA), which incorporates a super-pixel strategy.[21] Furthermore, a trend-based analysis looks at and plots area and volume change over time within a cluster of significant pixels. For GDx and OCT to date, there is no consensus and no adequate studies. The GDx VCC currently presents some serial data: the Advanced Serial Analysis looks at the RNFL over time, with TSNIT graphs, a summary measure analysis of NFI over time and a topographical, point-by-point, color-coded RNFL thickness change from baseline. To date, no data have been published on the validity of these GDx measures.

Visual field outcomes Standard automated perimetry (SAP) remains the gold standard for visual field assessment. An abnormality of visual function is measured in terms of decreased visual field sensitivity. SAP abnormality remains a necessity for many glaucoma treatment paradigms, and an abnormal visual field is a criterion for glaucoma diagnosis in many studies. The main outcomes are presence of visual field abnormality and visual field progression.

Visual field diagnosis Standard automated perimetry (SAP) is a subjective test susceptible to both short- and long-term fluctuations, observer variability, and artifacts. Distinguishing fluctuations from true field change is the greatest challenge in interpreting perimetric

TABLE 44.2 Comparison between the different optic disc staging systems

SYSTEM	BASIS OF SYSTEM	NUMBER OF STAGES	USER FRIENDLY	DISC SIZE CORRECTION	REPRODUCIBILITY	VALIDITY	DETECTS EARLY-STAGE CHANGES	INCLUDES VARIOUS MODES OF DISC DETERIORATION	STUDIED FOR ABILITY TO MONITOR CHANGE	WIDELY USED
Armaly, 1969	Compares diameter of 'cup' to diameter of 'disc' in same axis (cup:disc ratio)	9	Yes	No	Varies	Moderate	Yes	No	Yes	Yes
Read & Spaeth, 1974	Cup:disc ratio combined with rim/disc ratio	6	Yes	No	Not tested	Not tested	Yes	Yes	No	Yes
Shiose, 1974	Rim width change related to different methods of cupping – 3 parallel tracks	6	No	No	Not tested	Not tested	No	Yes	No	No
Richardson, 1978	Many variables, including disc ratio, amount of disc pallor, and nature of visual field defect	5	Moderate	No	Not tested	Not tested	Yes	Yes	No	No
Nesterov, 1981	Combination of disc characteristics including cup:disc ratio and circumferential extent of rim loss	6	No	No	Not tested	Not tested	No	Yes	No	No
Jonas, 1988	Amount of rim notching	5	Yes	No	Not tested	Not tested	No	Yes	No	No
Spaeth, 2003	Width of narrowest rim or circumferential extent of rim absence	10	Yes	Yes	Yes	Yes	Yes	Yes	Yes	No

Reprinted from Spaeth et al.[15] with permission of Survey of Ophthalmology.

	DDLS stage	Narrowest rim width (rim/disc ratio) (average disc size: 1.50 - 2.00 mm)	Example
At risk	1	0.4 or more	
	2	0.3 to 0.39	
	3	0.2 to 0.29	
	4	0.1 to 0.19	
Glaucoma damage	5	less than 0.1	
	6	0 (extension: less than 45°)	
	7	0 (extension: 46° to 90°)	
Glaucoma disability	8	0 (extension: 91° to 180°)	
	9	0 (extension: 181° to 270°)	
	10	0 (extension: more than 270°)	

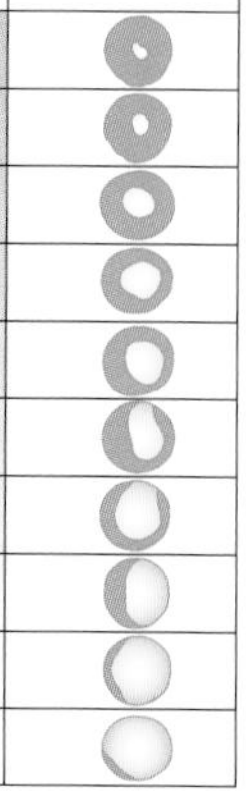

FIGURE 44.3 The Disc Damage Likelihood Scale (DDLS). For small discs (diameter < 1.5 mm) DDLS stage is increased by 1; for large discs (diameter > 2 mm) the DDLS stages should be decreased by 1. (Reprinted from Spaeth et al.[15] with permission of Survey of Ophthalmology.)

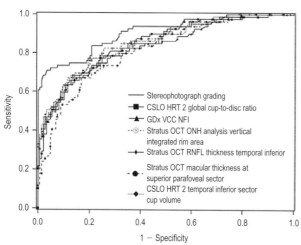

FIGURE 44.4 ROC curves comparing stereophotographs and the best parameter in each imaging technique. (Reprinted from Deleon-Ortega et al.[18] with permission of IOVS/Copyright.com.)

results. Eighty-six percent of an individual's initial visual field defects in OHTS were not reproducible.[22] When a defect was found in two VF tests, the third was normal in 66% whereas if three VF were abnormal, the fourth was normal in only 12%.[23]

The Anderson criteria remain classic to diagnose glaucomatous perimetric defects.[24] One of the following must be present on two consecutive occasions:

1. An abnormal glaucoma hemifield test (GHT).
2. Three contiguous non-edge points (allowing the two nasal step edge points) on a Humphrey program 30–2 or 24–2 visual field with $p < 5\%$ on the total deviation (TD) plot, with at least one point having $p < 1\%$
3. A $p < 5\%$ for corrected pattern standard deviation (CPSD) on full-threshold tests or pattern standard deviation (PSD) for SITA standard tests.

Sensitivity is greatest if any one criterion is used to diagnose glaucoma, while specificity increases with two or more criteria. Other definitions have been used (Table 44.3).

Once a glaucomatous visual field defect has been detected, we can use a system to grade the defect (judging its severity) (Table 44.4). Aulhorn and Karmeyer's descriptions remain classic.[28] Designed for research purposes, the AGIS and CIGTS systems[27] are too complex to use in everyday clinical practice. Based on the Bascom Palmer scale, the Glaucoma Staging System (GSS) can be used in everyday practice, but is time consuming (Table 44.5).[29]

Visual field progression The major clinical studies have used different criteria and various algorithms to detect and to quantify visual field progression (Table 44.6). This reflects the difficulty that clinicians experience in judging progression; it is a most complex task. Progression has to be differentiated from long-term fluctuation, which is higher in glaucomatous eyes and in damaged areas of the field, and increases with worsening disease.

TABLE 44.3 Definitions of a glaucomatous visual field defect in major glaucoma studies

STUDY	DEFINITION OF GLAUCOMATOUS VISUAL FIELD DEFECT
OHTS	GHT 'outside normal limits' and/or the CPSD $p < 5\%$.[23]
EPGS	(1) ≥3 horizontally or vertically adjacent points that differ ≥5 dB from baseline or (2) ≥2 horizontally or vertically adjacent points that differ ≥10 dB from baseline or (3) a difference >10 dB across the nasal horizontal meridian at ≥ two adjacent points.[7]
CNTGS	Confirmed localized defect with a cluster of three or more non-edge points depressed 5 dB from the average normal value for age and a nucleus of one point depressed 10 dB.[8]
EMGT	A classification of 'outside normal limits' affecting the same GHT sector (or sector 1 or 2) on two consecutive tests performed on different days or a classification of 'borderline' affecting the same GHT sector of the visual field on two consecutive tests performed on different days, and obvious localized glaucomatous changes of the optic disc in an area corresponding to the field defect.[25]
AGIS	Visual defect due to glaucoma, with the defect marked by an AGIS score of at least 1 (scores of no more than 16 at an initial pre-intervention test was admitted into the study). The score is based on the number and depth of adjacent depressed points in the nasal, superior, or inferior hemifield (0 no defect, 20 all test points depressed).[26,27]
CIGTS	Humphrey 24–2 visual field result that includes at least two or three contiguous points (depending on IOP) on the total deviation probability plot $p < 2\%$ and a GHT 'outside normal limits.'[12]

TABLE 44.4 Grading systems for perimetric defects in glaucoma

GRADING SYSTEMS	YEAR	DESCRIPTION
Aulhorn and Karmeyer	1977	Five descriptive stages based on extent and depth of the defect.[28]
Hodapp–Parrish–Anderson	1993	Three glaucoma stages: early, moderate, severe, based on MD and proximity to fixation.[30]
AGIS	1994	Score 1–20, uses the total deviation plot of 24–2, threshold values.[27]
CIGTS	1993 (enrolment started)	Score 1–20, uses the total deviation plot of 24–2, probability values.[27]
Brusini's Glaucoma Staging System (GSS) and GSS 2	1996, 2006	Based on MD and PSD, can be used on Humphrey and Octopus visual fields; is provided on the printout of the Oculus visual field.[31]
Glaucoma Staging System (GSS) and GSS 2	2006	Six-stage system based on MD, proximity to fixation, and number of points affected.[29]

TABLE 44.5 Glaucoma Staging System

STAGE	HUMPHREY MD SCORE		PROBABILITY PLOT/PATTERN DEVIATION		DB PLOT (STAGES 2–4) OR CPSD/PSD (STAGE 1)		DB PLOT (STAGES 2–4) OR HEMIFIELD TEST (STAGE 1)
Stage 0 – Ocular hypertension/ earliest glaucoma	>0.00	AND		OR	Does not meet any criteria for Stage 1	OR	
Stage 1 – Early glaucoma	−0.01 to −5.00 ($p < 0.05$)		Points below 5%: >3 contiguous AND >1 of the points below 1%		CPSD/PSD significant at $p < 0.05$		Glaucoma hemifield test 'outside normal limits'
Stage 2 – Moderate glaucoma	−5.01 to −12.00		Points below 5%: 19–36 AND Points below 1%: 12–18		Point(s) within the central 5° with sensitivity of <15 dB: >1 AND point(s) within the central 5° with sensitivity of <0 dB: None (0)		Point(s) with sensitivity <15 dB within 5° of fixation: only 1 hemifield (1 or 2)
Stage 3 – Advanced glaucoma	−12.01 to −20.00		Points below 5%: 37–55 AND Points below 1%: 19–36		Point(s) within the central 5° with sensitivity of <0 dB: 1 only		Point(s) with sensitivity <15 dB within 5° of fixation: both hemifields, at least 1 in each
Stage 4 – Severe glaucoma	−20.01 or worse		Points below 5%: 56–74 AND Points below 1%: 37–74		Point(s) within the central 5° with sensitivity of <0 dB: 2–4		Point(s) with sensitivity <15 dB within 5° of fixation: both hemifields, 2 in each (ALL)
Stage 5 – End-stage glaucoma/ blind	No HVF in 'worst eye'		HVF not possible attributable to central scotoma in 'worst eye' OR 'worst eye' acuity of 20/200 or worse attributable to glaucoma. Best eye may fall into any of above stages.				

CPSD/PSD, corrected pattern standard deviation/pattern standard deviation; dB, decibel; HVF, Humphrey visual field; <D, mean deviation. If a patient fits the MD criteria for a stage but does not fulfill one of the other criteria, they are classed in the preceding stage. If a patient fits the MD for a stage but fulfils one of the criteria for the following stage, they are classed in the following stage. If a patient fits the MD criteria for a stage but fulfils one of the criteria for the preceding stage and one for the following stage, they remain in the same stage. (Reprinted from Mills et al.[29] with permission of American Journal of Ophthalmology.)

While frequent repeated testing improves detection and reliability, in the clinical situation this has resource allocation implications and may prove impractical.

'Judgment' is still the method used by many clinicians; it is 'easy,' inexpensive, and not time consuming. Typically, a clinician uses all the information available on the visual field printout, assesses test reliability, and adds in other clinical information to make a judgment about disease progression. However, when clinical judgment is studied as a test of detecting progression, it has proved to be relatively unreliable, with poor interobserver agreement.[32] The Humphrey overview printout assists in the subjective evaluation of multiple visual fields. Arbitrary cutoff points can be added to define progression such as in the CNTGS; however, the authors found their first-choice criteria to be too sensitive with low specificity; the criteria had to be changed.[8]

TABLE 44.6 Definition of visual field progression in recent major clinical studies

STUDY	DEFINITION OF GLAUCOMATOUS VISUAL FIELD PROGRESSION
CNTGS	Changed during the study because too many reached end point and there was a high false-positive rate (57% vs 2% with second end point). The second end point (twice confirmed) was two contiguous points within or adjacent to a baseline visual field defect decreasing in sensitivity by at least 10 dB or three times their baseline SF (which ever is greater) or a new defect.[8]
EMGT	Forms the basis for the Humphrey glaucoma progression analysis (GPA). Tentative visual field progression is at least three test points that are flagged as significantly ($p < 5\%$) progressing at the same location in the EMGT pattern change probability maps of two consecutive tests. Definite visual field progression is at least three significantly progressing points at the same locations in three consecutive tests.[9]
AGIS	Decrease visual field (DVF) was an increase in AGIS score by 4 on two consecutive examinations from a single baseline test or a score of 19 or 20.[11,27]
CIGTS	Substantial visual field loss was an increase in CIGTS score by 3 or more from baseline (mean of two test results), and confirmed on two sequential examinations.[27]

Classification systems are useful to grade the severity of glaucoma; however, progression does not necessarily pass neatly from one defined stage to the next in every patient, and the steps from one stage to the next are not necessarily linear (see Table 44.5). By design, perimetric measurements are logarithmic. The AGIS and CIGTS scores are the most objective but when tested on the same population, identify different patients as 'progressors.'[33]

Trend analysis such as the PROGRESSOR software (Moorfields Eye Hospital, London, UK/Medisoft Ltd., Leeds, UK), looks at trends point-by-point and uses all the visual fields available. To detect progression, it may be more sensitive than Statpac 2 glaucoma change probability (GCP) analysis.[34] It assumes an age-related decline of 0.1 dB per year and picks up a rate 10 times that as abnormal. Peridata (Peridata Software GmbH, Huerth, Germany), which can be used with most perimeters, has a progression analysis with a box plot curve and a trend analysis with significance calculated for every point (see Ch. 10, Visual Fields).[35]

Event analysis looks for specified criteria to be fulfilled, comparing the current visual field to a baseline field. In the Statpac 2 program of the Humphrey Field Analyzer (Carl Zeiss Meditec, Dublin, CA), GCP compares the current visual field, point-for-point, from baseline using the total deviation plot. The Humphrey glaucoma progression analysis (GPA), derived from the analysis used in the EMGT study and now available for Humphrey Field Analyzers, uses the pattern deviation plot, point-by-point, to detect progression (see Ch. 15, Angle Imaging; Ch. 18, Optic Disc Imaging; Ch. 56, Ultrastructural Imaging).

Technologies for early detection such as short-wave automated perimetry (SWAP) and frequency doubling technology (FDT) and objective measures such as multifocal visual evoked potential (MFVEP) are covered in more detail in other chapters.

STRUCTURE AND FUNCTION RELATIONSHIP

Combining structure and function testing with clinical data increases the value of all tests significantly.[36]

Using data from combined tests, the sensitivity approaches the highest sensitivity of the component tests and the specificity, the lowest of the component tests.[37] Likelihood ratios (see Fig. 44.2) should be calculated and used to refine the pre-test odds to the post-test odds of glaucoma being present.

Glaucoma progression is measured by disc and/or field change, with disc change usually preceding field change, especially in early to moderate stages of the disease. Perhaps it is the functional reserve that accounts for this. Another theory is that if function is scaled linearly rather than logarithmically (as it is in all SAP), it has a linear relationship to structural change.[38] The apparent difference may simply reflect limits of current technology. There is no consensus on the true nature of the structure–function relationship.

Structure and function studies have focused on the relationship between optic disc and RNFL parameter with perimetry. A few recent studies have looked at the relationship between retinal ganglion cell (RGC) density and perimetry.[39] In studies by Quigley et al., 50% of RGC were lost before reproducible defects with manual quantitative kinetic perimetry;[40] however, with SAP, in eye bank eyes with documented glaucoma, a 5 dB reduction in the visual threshold on SAP was seen with a 25% local RGC loss and a generalized loss of about 10% of RGC population.[41]

VISUAL IMPAIRMENT, BLINDNESS, AND VISUAL DISABILITY

Patients' greatest fear is visual loss and disability (see also Ch. 41, Quality of Life). There are more than 65 definitions of visual impairment and blindness (Table 44.7).[42] The definition of legal blindness varies from country to country and many studies incorporate one of these definitions of blindness. Uniformity of definition would greatly enhance understanding of current existing data, preferably, the WHO ICD-9 definitions. West and Sommer[43] have suggested that at a level less than 6/18, functional capacity and employment ability is affected and that we should use this 'economic blindness' level as a benchmark of visual loss to prevent the economic and social burden that comes with dependency. Since this is essentially equivalent to the ICD-9 definition of

TABLE 44.7 Blindness and visual impairment from glaucoma

IMPAIRMENT		DEFINITION
Blindness:	WHO ICD-9	Best corrected visual acuity (BCVA) <3/60 (6/120 or 20/400) Visual field (VF) <10 degrees
	Legal blindness – USA	BCVA ≤ 6/60 VF < 20 degrees
	Legal blindness – Australia	BCVA ≤ 6/60 VF < 10 degrees
Visual impairment	Low vision ICD-9	BCVA < 6/18 in the better eye VF < 20 degrees
Visual disability		The loss of the ability to perform vision-related activities for daily living (reading, writing, driving, and occupation)
Vision handicap		The social consequence of visual disability

low vision, the authors recommend the use of the ICD-9 criteria for blindness and low vision as a uniform benchmark in future studies. In glaucoma, central acuity loss occurs very late in the disease; the patient can be 'visually disabled' from visual field loss long before this.

Several studies have looked at blindness rates from glaucoma. Hattenhauer et al.[44] conducted a retrospective, community-based, longitudinal study in Olmsted County, Minnesota, of 295 patients with open-angle glaucoma and treated ocular hypertension. They had a 9% cumulative probability of bilateral blindness (legal US) at 20 years, 8% on VF criteria, 5% by VA criteria. By extrapolation, there were 42% unilateral and 15% bilateral blindness from classical glaucoma at 15 years. Over this time, 4% of treated ocular hypertensive patients went blind and 22% of classical glaucoma patients went blind. There was a 27% cumulative probability of unilateral blindness at 20 years: 11% on VF criteria and 23% by VA criteria (14% of treated ocular hypertensives and 54% of classical glaucoma). Variability of IOP was a risk factor for blindness.

Chen reported his retrospective cohort study of 186 patients in a tertiary referral center in Washington State. Unilateral blindness (legal US) occurred in 14.6% in 15 years and bilateral blindness, 6.4%. Risk factors for blindness were noncompliance, worse initial visual field, and non-white race.[45] Wilson[46] looked at untreated African-derived people in the St. Lucia study and found the cumulative probability of visual field blindness (defined as an AGIS score = 18) was 16% unilateral and 9% bilateral at 10 years [bilateral figure extrapolated from the text].

Using the WHO ICD-9 definitions in a population-based study in Singapore, Foster et al.[47] reported 50% unilateral blindness, 36% bilateral blindness [5/14 extrapolated from the text] in angle-closure glaucoma, and 27% unilateral blindness in open-angle glaucoma. Glaucoma was the leading cause of blindness in this study.

Who goes blind from glaucoma? From the studies quoted above, the following circumstances are significant:
- developing countries with few resources
- African-derived populations
- undiagnosed or late-diagnosed glaucoma
- noncompliance
- worse visual field on presentation
- bilateral glaucoma.

ADVERSE TREATMENT OUTCOMES

At least in the early stages of glaucoma, treatment may cause more patient harm than good (Fig. 44.5) (see Section 6: Medical Therapy). In a study by Odberg et al., 4% experienced subjective problems from glaucoma and more than 25% had moderate side effects from treatment.[48] Of course, as disease progresses, this balance shifts, as the graph demonstrates.

A uniform reporting method for adverse outcomes would be useful. The COMTOL questionnaire (Comparison of Ophthalmic Medications for Tolerability) is one such tool.[49]

LIFE EXPECTANCY

Life expectancy calculation is useful in patient assessment; once the rate of visual field loss has been determined, a clinician can estimate whether or not the functional visual reserve is likely to be sufficient for the individual. Actuarial calculations of life expectancy are an integral part of life insurance premium and risk assessment.

Apart from medical history, other influencing factors include age, sex, family history, physical status, education and income, driving habits, and drug and alcohol history. In the USA, in 2003, life expectancies were: white males, 75.4 years; black males, 69.2 years; white females, 80.5 years; and black females, 76.1 years.[50] Using actuarial calculations from the average age of a glaucoma patient at diagnosis, Quigley and Vitale have estimated that a person diagnosed with glaucoma has an average life expectancy of 13 years.[51]

Do glaucoma patients have a reduced life expectancy? This question is based on potential comorbidities or the effects of medical therapy. Many of the earlier studies, which suggested this association, had methodological weaknesses. A recent large Swedish population-based

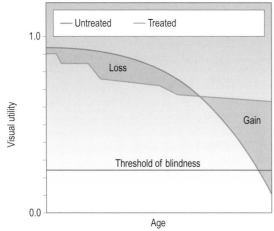

FIGURE 44.5 Effect of treatment on visual utility in a theoretical case of chronic glaucoma. (Reprinted from Brubaker[57] with permission of Ophthalmology.)

study did not show a difference in mortality between glaucoma patients and controls:[52] their 5–year mortalities were similar at 9.2% (glaucoma) and 11.9% (controls). Population-based studies have not demonstrated a significant link.[53,54] There is no good evidence for higher mortality in glaucoma patients.

OUTCOMES FOR THE PATIENT

Subjective symptoms from glaucoma vary widely between patients. In some, perhaps an observant young patient, a small relative scotoma may be symptomatic, while others with large areas of absolute scotoma will attest to no visual problems. This may be due partly to varying visual demands. It is also dependent on bilaterally overlapping scotomas.

Quality of life (QOL) is affected in glaucoma in many ways: any visual effects, impact of diagnosis, treatment side effects, and cost (see Ch. 41, Quality of Life).

There have been few studies of the feelings experienced by glaucoma patients. Patient satisfaction is the patient's emotional response to the disease and its treatment. Odberg et al.[48] found that 80% of patients report negative emotions on diagnosis and an immediate reduction in QOL. They recommend only informing patients of the diagnosis when it has been confirmed. One-third of participants were afraid of going blind, although half reported no visual problems at all. As many as 70% thought they would go blind without treatment, even though 44% had no visual field defect[55] and only 4% had extensive bilateral defects. Moderate to severe side effects from treatment affected 25%. The same study found that 90% were quite satisfied by the information their physician gave them, but their knowledge of glaucoma, particularly cause, treatment, and prognosis, was incomplete.

General, vision-specific, and glaucoma-specific tools have been used to assess the QOL in glaucoma patients. Utility values have more recently been used in the glaucoma population. Health-related quality-of-life instruments measure a patient's ability to function, while utility values measure a patient's perception of his/her own health status. Jampel first applied the concept of utility to glaucoma.[56] Various methods are used to calculate utilities: time trade, standard gamble, and category scaling.[57]

Bhargava et al.[58] studied patients' views of what is important in their own glaucoma management. In a conjoint analysis using 10 scenarios, the most important factors were risks of moderate visual loss, especially the ability to continue to drive (mean importance, 39%) and long-term blindness (mean importance, 27%). In contrast to what clinicians might believe, treatment methods, eyedrops, and complicated surgery were of much less importance. This study highlights the discrepancies between what patients regard as important outcomes and what clinicians assume.

Functional outcomes (the inability to perform tasks such as driving) are the hallmark of visual disability. One of an ophthalmologist's most difficult tasks is to inform a patient that driving is no longer permitted. As this is an ability no patient wishes to lose, this has a major impact on quality of life.[58] In a population screening study of 10 000 volunteers, patients with bilateral visual field defects were twice as likely to have traffic accidents and driving convictions as age- and sex-matched controls.[59] Rates for people with unilateral visual field defects did not vary significantly from normals.

There is no standardized method to assess what constitutes glaucomatous visual disability. As important as these concepts are, there has been a paucity of research and very few publications.[60,61] Visual disability is sometimes expressed as what percentage of the whole person is affected by the visual handicap. For example, total loss of vision in both eyes is a 100% disability of vision, but only an 85% disability of the whole person.[62]

Questionnaires have been developed to assess visual disability in glaucoma. The American Academy of Ophthalmology preferred practice guidelines[63] suggest that, to assess functional disabilities, the history should include general questions directed in four specific areas:
- problem areas and their significance to the patient (How has life changed? What do you miss most?)
- home-based near vision tasks (reading, paying bills, using magnifiers)
- distance vision skills (faces, traffic lights, driving)
- mobility and community skills (steps, bumping into objects, shopping, managing money, job performance).

A new performance-based outcome measure, the assessment of function related to vision (AFREV), has been validated and used on a glaucoma population.[64] This measures the observed performance of patients in an outpatient setting. The final model included:
- putting a stick into five holes of different sizes
- finding big objects: five boxes of different sizes, same color
- finding small objects: three coins (quarter, nickel, dime)
- reading small print
- reading in reduced illumination.

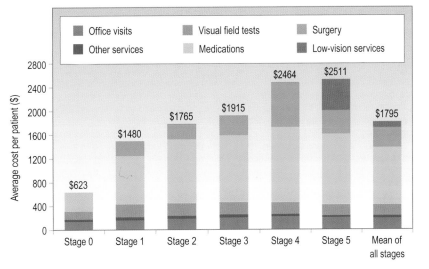

FIGURE 44.6 Total annual direct cost of glaucoma treatment per patient by stage. (Reprinted from Lee et al.,[66] with permission of

This recently validated, performance-based measure provides information that is currently not obtained from standard clinical measures of function such as visual acuity, visual field, or from self-reported quality-of-life measures.

OUTCOMES FOR SOCIETY

Provision of care for glaucoma comes at a cost to society. Besides direct costs of treatment to the individual or to society (depending on the system of eye care delivery), there are losses of work days and thus productivity, emotional costs, costs to the carer/family member, and costs to the employer and to the tax payer. Technology and treatments all come at a price. To make an economic evaluation of the impact from glaucoma, the cost of detection, management, and outcomes need to be considered. This is in its infancy. Economists face similar problems to the clinician: what is a useful outcome measure?[65] IOP, perimetric outcomes, and quality-adjusted life years (QALYs) are all surrogates.

Resource utilization has been estimated for patients with different severities of glaucoma. With increasing severity, resource utilization increased as did direct costs of care (Fig. 44.6; see also Fig. 3.4).[66,67] In the USA, the direct costs of glaucoma care have been estimated to be US$623 per patient per year for ocular hypertension; this increased as disease severity worsened to an estimated US$2511 per patient per year for stage 5 patients (Glaucoma Staging System, see above). Most of the costs arise from medications and office visits. In end-stage glaucoma, vision rehabilitation services contribute.

SPOTLIGHT: PRINCIPLES OF MANAGEMENT: OUTCOMES

Paul R Lichter

For chronic, nonfatal, diseases such as glaucoma, osteoarthritis, many dermatologic entities, and the like, quality of life (QOL) is the critical outcome measure. Functional status is closely tied to QOL and outcomes that include measurements of functional status are very important. Where function can be expected to be lost without proper treatment, the challenge comes in deciding when and how aggressively to treat a patient. In potentially fatal diseases such as heart disease, stroke, or cancer, physicians cannot wait to see how the disease behaves before deciding to treat. Yet, with chronic diseases such as open-angle glaucoma, there is only rarely an emergent treatment need. On the one hand, many patients with ocular hypertension or with suspicious optic discs, or even with early visual field loss, may not need treatment or, if treatment is needed, it may not need to be the most aggressive treatment to prevent a decrement in vision-related QOL. On the other hand, it is reasonable to overtreat some patients to be sure that none of them is allowed to lose significant vision so as to impair their QOL.

As the authors of this chapter so aptly state, the disease, glaucoma, has not changed, but there have been many changes in how we describe the disease and how we approach its diagnosis and treatment. In some ways, it is fair to say that we have learned most about glaucoma from epidemiologic studies and from randomized, controlled, clinical trials. That is to say, as this chapter's authors point out, we recognize that intraocular pressure (IOP) is a risk factor for glaucomatous damage, but that the disease is not defined by it. Rather, we have realized that glaucoma is an optic neuropathy, but one that is unique because of its relationship to IOP. The term 'IOP-sensitive optic neuropathy' can be used to distinguish glaucoma from all other optic neuropathies.

Thus, while there have been many new drugs to reduce IOP – for IOP is still the only treatable measure in patients with glaucoma – and new instruments to measure optic nerve parameters and retinal nerve fiber layer thickness, none of these drugs and instruments has proven magical in preservation of visual function any more than old drugs such as pilocarpine and epinephrine or tests such as tangent screen visual fields did years ago. There are more drugs today to lower IOP and drugs with less vision-related side effects than has pilocarpine. But in terms of vision-related QOL outcomes, there is no evidence that new pharmaceuticals and new-testing technology have, in themselves, led to glaucoma breakthroughs. Rather, the small breakthroughs we have seen in the past two decades have come from a better understanding of what glaucoma is and is not.

Unfortunately, all of the new drugs and devices have, to some extent, caused us to lose sight of the ball in glaucoma outcomes. We dwell on things such as glaucoma treatment formulas or how to detect the first loss of a ganglion cell. Because there is no need to show that an instrument has any real value in disease detection or management before it is brought to market, we become enamored with sophisticated analysis algorithms and colorful printouts before we have studies that show what the results of the tests mean. This approach is fueled, of course, by economic interests. Industry is motivated to create product and we provide the key opinion leaders to drive the use of what is developed. There is no economic advantage to physicians or to industry in promoting QOL outcomes in glaucoma. While it may be part of the dialogue in discussions about the disease, QOL is often given only lip-service and is lost amidst the pharmaceutical assault on IOP and the instrumentation assault on perimetric sophistication and imaging techniques. Cynical as it seems, these devices belong in the laboratory, including the clinical research laboratory, before they are marketed as being of value and before billing codes are established for their use that simply drive up the cost of care without making any impact whatsoever on the critical outcome in glaucoma – preservation of vision-related QOL.

We face a dilemma in a chronic, nonfatal disease such as glaucoma. On the one hand, we do not want to let a patient lose vision-related QOL, but we do not want to treat people who do not need treatment – because using eyedrops, having laser or incisional surgery, and coming for too-frequent testing all have a negative QOL impact, including on the patients' and society's pocketbooks. We know that some patients can have what any of us would call significant visual field loss in both eyes, yet have no impairment in vision-related QOL due to visual field overlap. That helps explain why so many of our glaucoma patients maintain their useful vision throughout their lives despite having had significant glaucomatous damage. That is not to say that we want to allow our patients to have

substantial damage. However, we should realize that we likely have a lot of leeway in terms of a good vision-related QOL outcome for patients with ocular hypertension (OHT) or early glaucoma if we take our time in deciding how aggressively to treat them. There are risk factors for which we are gaining a better understanding that may help us to pick out early those at great risk. Those are the people we need to worry about and who need to be treated aggressively. We do not need fancy visual field techniques and algorithms, clever treatment calculators, or sophisticated imaging devices to find these people. Rather, we need to keep at the top of our minds the question, 'Is this patient likely to lose vision-related QOL in their lifetime if I do not treat him/her now or if I do not treat that person aggressively now?' Regrettably, we do not have long-term, lifetime follow-up data on a controlled glaucoma cohort to help us make that judgment. We have to use what we do have – namely predicted long-term outcomes based only on relatively short-term clinical trial data and observational studies. Those studies need to be current, however. We can not get caught up in studies based on decades-old data and on long-outdated concepts of what glaucoma is and how it is best treated. We know very well that glaucoma patients can go blind without treatment or with inferior treatment. We do not need to invoke old studies that show that glaucoma patients can go blind with poor – old fashioned – management to justify treating everyone we see who has OHT or treating aggressively all of those with the earliest signs of glaucomatous damage. Those old studies tell us nothing about today's patients or about how to make judgments about vision-related QOL outcomes.

In potentially fatal diseases such as cancer and heart disease, we can have short-term outcome measures that serve as surrogates for ultimate QOL outcomes. That is because we know a lot about those diseases and what will likely happen without aggressive treatment. We wish we had that knowledge in glaucoma, but we do not. What we do have, though, is an ever-increasing understanding of what glaucoma is and which patients – e.g. those with advanced visual field loss at diagnosis – are at greatest risk for loss of vision-related QOL in their lifetime.

Clinical outcomes in glaucoma require our careful attention to keep our eyes on the lifetime vision-related QOL ball and not be distracted by relatively trivial end points, however intellectually interesting and stimulating they may be. And we need to think twice before being driven by industry – and their key opinion leaders – to embrace new technology before it is shown to have any value in helping to achieve the ultimate outcome goal.

Summary

To qualify as quality, management must be outcomes aware. In common with other chronic, progressive, incurable diseases, glaucoma management needs to incorporate the overall health of the patient and to avoid visual disability in the patient's lifetime. This requires effective communication with each patient: what is the attitude to the condition and its treatment, what expectations and understanding do they have? This becomes even more important in end-stage disease when structural and functional parameters offer less guidance. For all our management recommendations, we must consider the therapeutic index: potential benefits versus possible risks (see Ch. 45, Benefit versus Risk).

Which outcome measures are the most relevant? How can we standardize our outcome measures for comparison when basic uniform definitions are lacking? How do we justify what we do as clinicians to our communities, to payors, and to our patients? This field of study cries out for increased attention.

- Outcome measures depend on perspective; all points of view are valid.

- Consensus is needed on definitions of clinical outcomes for glaucoma diagnosis and progression.
- Optic disc stereophotography remains the gold standard for structural outcomes.
- No one type of optic disc and retinal nerve fiber layer imaging performs better than others for glaucoma diagnosis and only limited data are available on their ability to detect glaucoma progression.
- Study outcomes need to be viewed critically and to include clinically relevant measures such as likelihood ratios and post-test probability.
- Quality of life is affected immediately on glaucoma diagnosis.
- Cost of glaucoma increases with severity of damage.
- Be skeptical of 'fashions' in glaucoma outcome assessment, which are often technology driven.
- Manage the patient as a whole human being.

REFERENCES

1. Lee PP. Outcomes and endpoints in glaucoma. J Glaucoma 1996; 5:295–297.

2. Shaffer RN. The centennial history of glaucoma (1896–1996). American Academy of Ophthalmology. Ophthalmology 1996; 103:S40–S50.

3. Societies Aoig. Glaucoma diagnosis: structure and function. The Hague, The Netherlands: Kugler Publications; 2004.

4. Reid MC, Lachs MS, Feinstein AR. Use of methodological standards in diagnostic test research. Getting better but still not good. JAMA 1995; 274:551–645.

5. Spaeth GL. Proper outcome measurements regarding glaucoma: the inadequacy of using intraocular pressure alone. Eur J Ophthalmol 1996; 6:101–105.

6. Gordon MO, Kass MA. The Ocular Hypertension Treatment Study: design and baseline description of the participants. Arch Ophthalmol 1999; 117:573–583.

7. Miglior S, Zeyen T, Pfeiffer N, et al. The European Glaucoma Prevention Study design and baseline description of the participants. Ophthalmology 2002; 109:1612–1621.

8. Schulzer M. Errors in the diagnosis of visual field progression in normal-tension glaucoma. Ophthalmology 1994; 101: 1589–1594; discussion 1595.

9. Heijl A, Leske MC, Bengtsson B, et al. Reduction of intraocular pressure and glaucoma progression: results from the Early Manifest Glaucoma Trial. Arch Ophthalmol 2002; 120: 1268–1279.

10. The Advanced Glaucoma Intervention Study (AGIS): 4. Comparison of treatment outcomes within race. Seven-year results. Ophthalmology 1998; 105:1146–1164.

11. Ederer F, Gaasterland DA, Dally LG, et al. The Advanced Glaucoma Intervention Study (AGIS): 13. Comparison of treatment outcomes within race: 10-year results. Ophthalmology 2004; 111:651–664.

12. Musch DC, Lichter PR, Guire KE, et al. The Collaborative Initial Glaucoma Treatment Study: study design, methods, and baseline characteristics of enrolled patients. Ophthalmology 1999; 106:653–662.

13. Ophthalmology AAO. Primary Open-Angle Glaucoma, Preferred Practice Pattern. San Francisco: American Academy of Ophthalmology; 2005. Online. Available: http://www.aao.org/ppp

14. Group SEAGIG. South East Asia Glaucoma Interest Group. Asia Pacific Glaucoma Guidelines, 2003–4. Online. Available: http//:www.seagig.org

15. Spaeth GL, Lopes JF, Junk AK, et al. Systems for staging the amount of optic nerve damage in glaucoma: a critical review and new material. Surv Ophthalmol 2006; 51:293–315.

16. Danesh-Meyer HV, Gaskin BJ, Jayusundera T, et al. Comparison of disc damage likelihood scale, cup to disc ratio, and Heidelberg retina tomograph in the diagnosis of glaucoma. Br J Ophthalmol 2006; 90:437–441.

17. Medeiros FA, Zangwill LM, Bowd C, et al. Comparison of the GDx VCC scanning laser polarimeter, HRT II confocal scanning laser ophthalmoscope, and stratus OCT optical coherence tomograph for the detection of glaucoma. Arch Ophthalmol 2004; 122:827–837.

18. Deleon-Ortega JE, Arthur SN, McGwin G Jr, et al. Discrimination between glaucomatous and nonglaucomatous eyes using quantitative imaging devices and subjective optic nerve head assessment. Invest Ophthalmol Vis Sci 2006; 47:3374–3380.

19. Rasker MT, van den Enden A, Bakker D, et al. Deterioration of visual fields in patients with glaucoma with and without optic disc hemorrhages. Arch Ophthalmol 1997; 115:1257–1262.

20. Kass MA, Heuer DK, Higginbotham EJ, et al. The Ocular Hypertension Treatment Study: a randomized trial determines that topical ocular hypotensive medication delays or prevents the onset of primary open-angle glaucoma. Arch Ophthalmol 2002; 120:701–713; discussion 829–830.

21. Chauhan BC, Blanchard JW, Hamilton DC, et al. Technique for detecting serial topographic changes in the optic disc and peripapillary retina using scanning laser tomography. Invest Ophthalmol Vis Sci 2000; 41:775–782.

22. Keltner JL, Johnson CA, Quigg JM, et al. Confirmation of visual field abnormalities in the Ocular Hypertension Treatment Study. Ocular Hypertension Treatment Study Group. Arch Ophthalmol 2000; 118:1187–1194.

23. Keltner JL, Johnson CA, Levine RA, et al. Normal visual field test results following glaucomatous visual field end points in the Ocular Hypertension Treatment Study. Arch Ophthalmol 2005; 123:1201–1206.

24. Anderson DR. Automated static perimetry. St Louis: CV Mosby; 1992.

25. Leske MC, Heijl A, Hyman L, et al. Early Manifest Glaucoma Trial: design and baseline data. Ophthalmology 1999; 106:2144–2153.

26. Advanced Glaucoma Intervention Study. 2. Visual field test scoring and reliability. Ophthalmology 1994; 101:1445–1455.

27. Katz J. Scoring systems for measuring progression of visual field loss in clinical trials of glaucoma treatment. Ophthalmology 1999; 106:391–395.

28. Aulhorn E, Karmeyer H. Frequency distribution in early glaucomatous visual field defects. Doc Ophthalmol Proc Ser 1977; 14:75–83.

29. Mills RP, Budenz DL, Lee PP, et al. Categorizing the stage of glaucoma from pre-diagnosis to end-stage disease. Am J Ophthalmol 2006; 141:24–30.

30. Hodapp E, Parrish RI, Anderson D. Clinical decisions in glaucoma. St. Louis: CV Mosby; 1993; 52–61.

31. Brusini P, Filacorda S. Enhanced Glaucoma Staging System (GSS 2) for classifying functional damage in glaucoma. J Glaucoma 2006; 15:40–46.

32. Werner EB, Bishop KI, Koelle J, et al. A comparison of experienced clinical observers and statistical tests in detection of progressive visual field loss in glaucoma using automated perimetry. Arch Ophthalmol 1988; 106:619–623.

33. Katz J, Congdon N, Friedman DS. Methodological variations in estimating apparent progressive visual field loss in clinical trials of glaucoma treatment. Arch Ophthalmol 1999; 117:1137–1142.

34. Viswanathan AC, Fitzke FW, Hitchings RA. Early detection of visual field progression in glaucoma: a comparison of PROGRESSOR and STATPAC 2. Br J Ophthalmol 1997; 81:1037–1042.

35. Peridata. Online. Available: http://www.peridata.org (accessed February 5, 2007).

36. Shah NN, Bowd C, Medeiros FA, et al. Combining structural and functional testing for detection of glaucoma. Ophthalmology 2006; 113:1593–1602.

37. Garway-Heath DF, Friedman DS. How should results from clinical tests be integrated into the diagnostic process? Ophthalmology 2006; 113:1479–1480.

38. Garway-Heath DF, Holder GE, Fitzke FW, et al. Relationship between electrophysiological, psychophysical, and anatomical measurements in glaucoma. Invest Ophthalmol Vis Sci 2002; 43:2213–2220.

39. Harwerth RS, Quigley HA. Visual field defects and retinal ganglion cell losses in patients with glaucoma. Arch Ophthalmol 2006; 124:853–859.

40. Quigley HA, Addicks EM, Green WR. Optic nerve damage in human glaucoma. III. Quantitative correlation of nerve fiber loss and visual field defect in glaucoma, ischemic neuropathy, papilledema, and toxic neuropathy. Arch Ophthalmol 1982; 100:135–146.

41. Kerrigan-Baumrind LA, Quigley HA, Pease ME, et al. Number of ganglion cells in glaucoma eyes compared with threshold visual field tests in the same persons. Invest Ophthalmol Vis Sci 2000; 41:741–748.

42. World Health Organization. Blindness information collected from various sources. Epidemiol Vital Stat Rep 1966; 19:437–511.

43. West S, Sommer A. Prevention of blindness and priorities for the future. Bull World Health Organ 2001; 79:244–248.

44. Hattenhauer MG, Johnson DH, Ing HH, et al. The probability of blindness from open-angle glaucoma. Ophthalmology 1998; 105:2099–2104.

45. Chen PP. Blindness in patients with treated open-angle glaucoma. Ophthalmology 2003; 110:726–733.

46. Wilson MR. Progression of visual field loss in untreated glaucoma patients and suspects in St. Lucia, West Indies. Trans Am Ophthalmol Soc 2002; 100:365–410.

47. Foster PJ, Oen FT, Machin D, et al. The prevalence of glaucoma in Chinese residents of Singapore: a cross-sectional population survey of the Tanjong Pagar district. Arch Ophthalmol 2000; 118:1105–1111.

48. Odberg T, Jakobsen JE, Hultgren SJ, et al. The impact of glaucoma on the quality of life of patients in Norway. I. Results from a self-administered questionnaire. Acta Ophthalmol Scand 2001; 79:116–120.

49. Barber BL, Strahlman ER, Laibovitz R, et al. Validation of a questionnaire for comparing the tolerability of ophthalmic medications. Ophthalmology 1997; 104:334–342.

50. Online. Available: http://www.cdc.gov/nchs/pressroom/05facts/lifeexpectancy.htm (accessed 25 Jan 2007).

51. Quigley HA, Vitale S. Models of open-angle glaucoma prevalence and incidence in the United States. Invest Ophthalmol Vis Sci 1997; 38:83–91.

52. Grodum K, Heijl A, Bengtsson B. Glaucoma and mortality. Graefe's Arch Clin Exp Ophthalmol 2004; 242:397–401.

53. Knudtson MD, Klein BE, Klein R. Age-related eye disease, visual impairment, and survival: the Beaver Dam Eye Study. Arch Ophthalmol 2006; 124:243–249.

54. Borger PH, van Leeuwen R, Hulsman CA, et al. Is there a direct association between age-related eye diseases and mortality? The Rotterdam Study. Ophthalmology 2003; 110:1292–1296.

55. Odberg T, Jakobsen JE, Hultgren SJ, et al. The impact of glaucoma on the quality of life of patients in Norway. II. Patient response correlated to objective data. Acta Ophthalmol Scand 2001; 79:121–124.

56. Jampel HD. Glaucoma patients' assessment of their visual function and quality of life. Trans Am Ophthalmol Soc 2001; 99:301–317.

57. Brubaker RF. Decisions, decisions. Ophthalmology 1999; 106:165–168.

58. Bhargava JS, Patel B, Foss AJ, et al. Views of glaucoma patients on aspects of their treatment: an assessment of patient preference by conjoint analysis. Invest Ophthalmol Vis Sci 2006; 7:2885–2888.

59. Johnson CA, Keltner JL. Incidence of visual field loss in 20,000 eyes and its relationship to driving performance. Arch Ophthalmol 1983; 101:371–375.

60. Zimmerman TJ, Karunaratne N, Fechtner RD. Glaucoma: outcomeology (Part I). J Glaucoma 1996; 5:299.

61. Zimmerman TJ, Karunaratne N, Fechtner RD. Glaucoma: outcomeology (Part II). J Glaucoma 1996; 5:152–155.

62. American Academy of Ophthalmology fact sheet. Online. Available: https://secure3.aao.org/pdf/057135.pdf (accessed 14 Feb 2007).

63. Ophthalmology AAO. Vision rehabilitation for adults, preferred practice pattern. San Francisco: American Academy of Ophthalmology; 2001. Online. Available: http://www.aao.org/ppp

64. Altangerel U, Spaeth GL, Steinmann WC. Assessment of function related to vision (AFREV). Ophthalmic Epidemiol 2006; 13:67–80.

65. Kobelt G. Health economics, economic evaluation, and glaucoma. J Glaucoma 2002; 11:531–539.

66. Lee PP, Walt JG, Doyle JJ, et al. A multicenter, retrospective pilot study of resource use and costs associated with severity of disease in glaucoma. Arch Ophthalmol 2006; 124:12–19.

67. Traverso CE, Walt JG, Kelly SP, et al. Direct costs of glaucoma and severity of the disease: a multinational long term study of resource utilisation in Europe. Br J Ophthalmol 2005; 89: 1245–1249.

CHAPTER 45

Benefit versus Risk

Ravi Thomas and Rajul S Parikh

INTRODUCTION

This is an unusual, but important topic for a chapter. A consideration (and discussion) of benefit versus risk that should be the basis of any management decision is either superficially addressed or neglected in most books and articles. All of us intuitively consider the possible risks and benefits before we prescribe any treatment. We don't avoid a treatment just because it has serious side effects. Aspirin comes to mind. The side effects of this commonly prescribed drug would frighten any patient (and physician) but it is the most commonly prescribed drug. A single drop of a β-blocker can have significant side effects and yet for years it was the most commonly prescribed treatment for glaucoma. The issue is more serious with surgery. Even the successful and technologically superb modern cataract surgery can result in blindness or loss of the eye; yet it is the most commonly performed operation. The potential side effects of trabeculectomy are, unfortunately, far more serious and more frequent than those of cataract surgery. And even an 'extraocular' transscleral cyclophotocoagulation can lead to phthisis, or worse still, sympathetic ophthalmia.

Many decisions are straightforward. In days gone by, if penicillin was not prescribed for pneumonia, the patients died. There was no choice: the risk of a fatal anaphylactic reaction in this scenario had to be acceptable. If cataract surgery is not undertaken, the patients remain blind; the low risk (2%) of a poor outcome or disaster is acceptable.

While most patients accept such decisions unquestioningly, it is important to discuss the benefits and risks with them and consider their view. It is not only necessary from the medicolegal of view but, equally importantly, is the right thing to do. Alas, patients hear what they want to hear; cognitive dissonance is a real problem.

There are, of course, too many situations where evidence is lacking and where benefits and risks are not so straightforward. How do we make decisions in these situations? Some experienced physicians have the good clinical judgment to do this correctly each time. As Dr Arthur Jampolsky once asked, 'How do we develop good clinical judgment? From experience, of course! And how do we get experience? By making some very bad clinical judgments.' Some of our teachers had the intuition, experience, and judgment to practice the 'art of medicine.' Is there a science behind that 'art' that can be learned (and transmitted) to properly assess the benefits and risks, while minimizing the 'bad clinical judgments' phase? The authors believe there is.

The concepts practiced and taught to weigh up risks and benefits while making important decisions are the 'number needed to treat' (NNT) and the 'number needed to be treated to produce harm' (NNH). In most cases, weighing up these two numbers is all that is required to make a decision. In more complicated situations, the individual patient's values and risk-taking behavior can be blended into this assessment by using the 'likelihood of help versus harm' (LHH). The LHH allows one to quantify, from the patient's perspective, the probability of benefit or harm from an intervention. It allows one to 'individualize' the intervention.

To apply the concepts of NNT, NNH, and LHH, one needs to familiarize oneself with terms such as 'absolute risk' (AR) and 'absolute risk reduction' (ARR). Additionally, as terms such as 'relative risk' (RR) and 'relative risk reduction' (RRR) also crop up in the literature and can be misleading, they will briefly be discussed too.

NUMBER NEEDED TO TREAT AND NUMBER NEEDED TO BE TREATED TO PRODUCE HARM

The number needed to treat (NNT) tells us the number of patients we need to treat with the particular drug or procedure in order to achieve one good outcome (or prevent one complication) as compared to an alternative approach (which in some cases may be no treatment at all). It is calculated from the absolute risk and absolute risk reduction.[1–3]

Consider a situation where the patient is at risk for a particular complication. If one does not intervene, there is a chance (risk) that the patient will develop the complication – the absolute risk (AR) with no intervention. If one intervenes, there may be a reduced risk of encountering the complication – the AR of having the complication despite intervention. The difference between the risk of complication occurring without intervention and that of having it despite intervention gives the absolute risk reduction (ARR). For most ophthalmologists, this is a fraction that is a little difficult to understand and makes little sense. However, the inverse of the ARR yields a number that is more intuitive as well as clinically helpful – the number of patients needed to be treated with the intervention (for a defined duration) in order to achieve one benefit. That is the NNT.

In practice, when confronted with a statistically significant intervention, one examines the three elements that make NNT useful. First, one compares the risk of doing nothing at all with the benefits of the recommended procedure. Next, one examines the potential to cause harm – side effects, toxicity, complications, and so on, arising out of the intervention. Finally, one tries to identify high-risk or high-response subgroups of patients who have the most to gain from the intervention in question.

The calculation for the NNH is similar. If one intervenes, there is an AR of a complication, say expulsive hemorrhage. If one does not intervene, that particular AR is (almost) zero. The difference between the AR with intervention and no intervention is the 'absolute risk increase' (ARI). This fraction too is not intuitive and doesn't mean much. However, if one takes the inverse of the ARI, one gets the NNH: the number needed to be treated with the intervention to harm one patient, to produce one additional harmful effect, in this case, expulsive hemorrhage.

The calculation of NNT and NNH are easy enough and are briefly summarized and referenced in other texts.[1–3]

The Ocular Hypertension Treatment Study (OHTS) has been used to explain ARR, NNT, and NNH. Over a 5-year period the absolute risk of progression to glaucoma with no treatment in OHTS was 9.5%.[4,5] Treatment reduced this risk to 4.4%, an absolute risk reduction (ARR) of 5%. The inverse of this ARR (100/5 = 20), provides the NNT for the representative patient recruited in the OHTS study.[6] That means one needs to treat 20 'average' patients with ocular hypertension (of the type recruited in the OHTS trial) for 5 years in order to prevent one from progressing to early primary open-angle glaucoma (POAG).

This brings up the question of what is a 'good' NNT. Is an NNT of 20 for ocular hypertension a good NNT? That would depend on the seriousness of the outcome one is trying to prevent, and the opportunity cost of doing so. Whether an NNT of 20 is good for ocular hypertension would also depend on the answer to another question, one constantly asked by clinical epidemiologists, one that is relevant to most situations: 'Compared to what?'

The NNT for the treatment of systemic hypertension (diastolic 115–129 mmHg) with the objective of preventing death, stroke, or myocardial infarction over 1.5 years is 3. (That for a diastolic of 90–109 mmHg for a similar period is 470.[4]) The NNT for surgical treatment of symptomatic high-grade carotid stenosis with the objective of preventing major stroke or death over a period of 2 years is 10.[5]

Generally, 20 would be considered a good NNT, provided the outcome one is trying to prevent is something serious, such as blindness or a very high known probability of blindness. What one is preventing here is early glaucoma, disc changes in half the cases and very early field defect. Both are changes that may or may not eventually affect the patient's quality of life. Treating 20 patients effectively for 5 years with a modern intraocular pressure (IOP)-lowering drug is not inexpensive; and there are other interventions, including cataract surgery, competing for the same financial resources. As one is not really preventing blindness, these competing interventions, or 'opportunity' costs, are likely to win out.

The advantage of NNT is that it allows us to look for subgroups where the absolute risk is higher (and the NNT lower) and therefore costs of treatment (and its justification) are more acceptable. For ocular hypertension (OHT) one might want to treat those with a pressure of >25.75 mmHg. The risk of progression in these patients is three times higher and the NNT is three times lower: six patients.[6] This number might be more acceptable. However, as one is still not preventing changes in quality of life or blindness, for the developing world at least, perhaps we should treat only those OHT with such higher pressures *and* larger cup-to-disc ratios and/or thinner corneas. This would bring the NNT down to a lower, more acceptable (and justifiable) level.

Continuing with the OHTS example, the incidence of serious side effects with treatment was minimal (zero).[4] The ARI is therefore zero, and its inverse, the NNH, very, very large: infinite.

In another example, the Early Manifest Glaucoma Trial (EMGT), medical treatment was used in one group and the other group served as controls.[7] The side effect is cataract requiring surgery. Two of 126 patients in the control group developed cataracts that required surgery (AR, 1.6%). Cataract surgery was needed in 6 of 128 in the treatment group (AR, 4.7%). The ARI is therefore 3.1% (4.7–1.6). The NNH is 100/3.1 = 32.2. By convention, this is rounded to the next higher number: an NNH of 33. If this were a true side effect of medical treatment (OHTS didn't show this), most of physicians would be comfortable with one extra cataract surgery for every 33 patients treated with medical therapy and or laser. After all, the intended outcome is to prevent blindness from glaucoma, the treatment is known to work and, while the cataract surgical rate in this group is high, more importantly, such surgery usually has a good outcome. Accordingly, the decision to treat, even if made intuitively, is easy. And even with the use the NNT versus NNH, one is unlikely to discuss cataract surgery with the patient at this stage unless, of course, the patient asks.

On the other hand, consider the Collaborative Initial Glaucoma Treatment Study (CIGTS).[8] The rate of cataract formation in those undergoing medical therapy was 19/307 (6.1%). This rate following trabeculectomy was

51/300 (17.3%). The ARI is 11.2% and the NNH is 9 (100/11.2). If nine patients undergo trabeculectomy (as opposed to being put on medical treatment), there is likely to be one more cataract procedure to perform. This NNH is high enough to include a discussion of the possible need for cataract surgery in the future, if trabeculectomy is performed.

In most cases, as in the examples above, a comparison of NNT versus NNH will help make the decision. In other cases, especially when the evidence for benefit is marginal (or even if it is strong) but the risk of severe side effects is high, it may be necessary to (literally) incorporate the patient's values (perspective) on the risk versus benefit into the equation. This is done using the 'likelihood of help versus harm.'[9]

LIKELIHOOD OF HELP VERSUS HARM

In one case, a 60-year-old otherwise healthy monocular man had uncontrolled glaucoma. His left eye was enucleated following trauma in childhood; the visual acuity in the right eye was 20/60. The anterior segment examination was within normal limits for his age. The IOP on fixed combination timolol–dorzolamide, latanoprost 0.005%, and brimonidine 0.15% varied between 26 and 34 mmHg. The central corneal thickness was 536 μm. Gonioscopy in dim illumination showed open angles. The medium-sized optic nerve head showed 0.8:1 cup-to-disc ratio with a bipolar notch and a corresponding biarcuate scotoma; the latest field examination showed progression to a split fixation with a size V target on the macular program with white on white perimetry.

How does one decide the management of this one-eyed patient? This decision is not as straightforward as starting medical treatment or performing a trabeculectomy on a patient with early glaucoma. The potential for serious side effects and even loss of useful vision in this one-eyed patient (even if low) requires his understanding and consent. One can, of course, 'talk to him,' but despite all explanations, the patient may be averse to any surgical intervention. How does one communicate and agree on a management plan while incorporating all existing knowledge (benefits of therapy as well as accompanying risks) as well as the patient's views on the relative severity of the event prevented by treatment relative to the bad outcome caused by intervention. In other words, how does one combine the NNT and the NNH with the patient's risk-taking behavior?

In this situation, the management choice is probably best determined as a formal clinical decision analysis with the assistance of an experienced clinical epidemiologist. A rapid version of such an analysis that 'doesn't do too much violence to the truth' can also be used.[9] This depends on calculating a 'likelihood of help versus harm' (LHH).

One discusses the objectives of treatment and options with the patient. The goal is to preserve existing vision for the patient's lifetime. In this healthy 60-year-old whose parents died after the age of 80, one has to plan the treatment for at least another 20 years. If continued on medical treatment, the probability of loosing all useful vision with the relevant pressures over the next 5–10 years has to be close to 100% (AR = 100%). The planned procedure is a trabeculectomy, which has a success rate of 80% (AR of failure 20%). This is an ARR of 80 and an NNT of 2.

This is a good NNT, but, being one-eyed, the patient is naturally worried about loosing his vision as a result of surgery and wants more details of possible sight-threatening complications.

For an intervention in this kind of advanced disease, the chances of a wipe out of the visual field are about 1% (R Thomas, unpublished data on 100 eyes with advanced glaucoma as evidenced by split fixation with a size V target on the macular program). If one uses the higher end of the confidence interval for this risk of wipe out of the visual field, which is 3%, the number needed to harm (NNH) is therefore 33.

At this stage, the LHH is 1/NNT : 1/NNH or 1/2 : 1/33. That is, 17 in favor of treatment. The patient is then asked what value he puts on preserved vision for 5–10 years, relative to the risk of actually loosing his vision in the immediate postoperative period. There are graphical means of doing this.[9] (A scale and brief description of its use are provided in the Appendix.) If the patient's risk-taking behavior is in favor of the long term, and he feels that long-term visual preservation is 5 times more preferable, the LHH becomes 1/2 × 5: 1/33 = 83 times more likely to be helped versus harmed.

On the other hand, if, as is usual, the patient considers a small risk of immediate loss of vision to be worse, say 10 times worse, than the LHH for loosing vision over a period of 5–10 years is 1/2: 1/33 × 10. He is still twice as likely to be helped versus harmed.

One then does a sensitivity analysis. For example, what if the patient feels that 'immediate' loss of sight is 100 times worse than a slow loss? The LHH becomes 1/2: 1/33 × 100 = 7 times as likely to be harmed versus helped. What if patient considers 'immediate' loss to be 5 times worse than a slow loss? Here, the LHH is 1/2: 1/33 × 5 = 4 times likely to be helped versus harmed. The sensitivity analysis can be repeated for different, 'sensible' NNTs and NNHs, different relative severity of effects, and at different times to get a true feeling for the direction the patient really wants to go. If this is consistent, that is what does one do? The reader is referred to the authors' clinical bible for a more detailed explanation as well as alternative methods of such an analysis.[10]

This method can be extended to incorporate other serious adverse events to adjust the LHH. It can also be used to compare opposing treatments.

RELATIVE RISK, RELATIVE RISK REDUCTION, AND THEIR USE IN RISK–BENEFIT ASSESSMENT

Some actions are based on publications that report the terms referred to above. For example, one may be encouraged to decrease the IOP as much as possible, because every 1 mmHg decreases the risk of glaucoma by 10%. It is therefore important to understand these terms.

The relative risk (RR) tells us the risk of an outcome in one group with the risk factor (i.e. increased IOP) as compared to the risk of an outcome in a group without the risk factor (i.e. normal IOP). A derivation of the RR, the relative risk reduction (RRR) indicates the proportion of the baseline risk that can potentially be removed by treating the risk factor in question. Relative risk reduction and excess risk (explained later) are useful,[2,11] but may sometimes erroneously direct one toward intervention (especially useful when intervention effects are small).

Consider the EMGT. Over a 5–year period, 62% of untreated subjects (absolute risk in controls) progressed compared to 45% in the treated group (absolute risk in the treated group). The RR of progression in the EMGT was therefore 1.38 (62/45). How is this RR interpreted? Back to the earlier question: 'What is a "good" RR?' The authors' clinical bible says that RRs below 2 are rarely significant. According to this publication, depending on the type of study, RRs of 3–4 are likely significant, and 20 is probably high enough to attribute causality. As an example, an RR of 5.7, with confidence intervals of 1.9–17.1 ascribed to diurnal variation, is impressive on its own.[12] This sort of RR does not require any manipulation to make it look more impressive. The point estimate of RR is over 5, and even the lower end of the confidence interval is very close to 2, the value at which one's interest becomes aroused.

What if the relative risk is lower than what would usually be considered significant, such as 1.38 as in the EMGT? A good way to present a small RR, especially to decision-makers, is to use the 'relative risk reduction' (RRR):

((AR in the control group – AR in the treated group) ÷ AR in the control group) × 100

For the EMGT, $((62 - 45) ÷ 62) × 100 = 27.42\%$. (This is more easily calculated as RR–1/RR, which provides the same result.)

This RRR implies that if there is a cause-and-effect relationship between IOP and progression, one can potentially remove 27.4% of that risk by lowering the IOP. And this is very important. However, RRR does not provide much useful clinical information. A relative risk reduction (or relative risk) of 50% could mean an 'absolute' reduction from 100% to 50% or from 1% to 0.5%. These figures translate into an NNT of 2 for the first example versus 200 for the second. The RRR in the two examples is the same, but the clinical connotation and potential clinical decisions are totally different. All else being equal, one would probably always use the therapy that provides an NNT of 2 and rarely use one with an NNT of 200.

There is little doubt about the role of raised IOP in the causation and progression of glaucoma. However, results from some recent studies have been presented in an isolated manner that might encourage very aggressive lowering of the IOP with possibly detrimental effects.

Both the OHTS and the EMGT state that each 1 mmHg lowering of IOP is associated with a 10% lowering of risk. First, one must remember that in both these studies this conclusion was the result of post hoc analysis; such analyses are always interpreted with care. In the EMGT, this association was demonstrated using a Cox's hazard model and the hazard ratio was found to be 1.1. Hazard ratio is like RR and is interpreted in the same manner.

A relative risk of 1.1 is small (large numbers can make anything statistically significant). If the relative risk is small (like 1.1), one way to make it look attractive, as we learned, is the RRR. The RRR for a relative risk of 1.1 (RR–1/RR) is 9%. Another way to make this look more attractive is to use 'excess' risk. The formula for excess risk is RR–1 expressed as a percentage $(1.1 - 1 = 10\%)$. This derivation (with other assumptions) has probably led to the '10% reduction per 1 mmHg reduction' interpretation. While it is the true, the statement is perhaps best interpreted by keeping the overall picture in mind.

The authors personally feel that a combination of all the measures – absolute risk, relative risk, relative risk reduction, NNT, and NNH – provides far more useful and clinically useable information than the RR (or RRR) alone. As far as assessment of benefit versus risk is concerned, it is the NNT and NNH that the authors use.

Summary

Most clinicians intuitively assess benefit versus risk before making management decisions. In more difficult situations, a simple consideration of NNT versus NNH provides direction. In more complicated cases, especially where patient values may make a major difference, the calculation of LHH is a useful way to demonstrate to the patient how the patient's own preferences will direct the management. In really difficult situations, a formal decision analysis may be desirable.

APPENDIX

The authors provide patients with an explanation about the disease and discuss the benefits and risks of treatment, the hoped-for prevention of adverse outcomes, and the complications that may result as a consequence of the treatment. The authors help the patients to decide how *dire* they consider the outcome the authors are trying to prevent *compared to* the side effects that may be produced with treatment. Is the blindness that the treatment is intended to prevent 20 times worse than the constant discomfort or glare from a filtering bleb? Or 10 times as bad? Is it 10 times better than failure in the immediate postoperative period? Some patients may be able to directly express that the possible adverse outcome is (to them) 20 or 100 times worse (or better) than the side effect that the treatment may induce. Others may need a scale to rate and compare one versus the other. An example of such a scale is shown in (Fig. 45.1). Other examples are also available.[9] At one end it represents the worst-case scenario of losing vision completely (0.0 or 0%); at other end it has 1 (100%) representing perfect vision. The patient

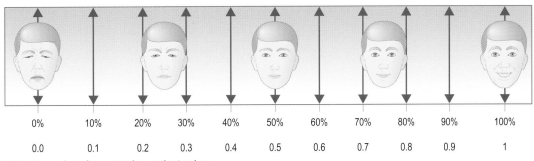

FIGURE 45.1 Rating values for assessing patient values.

is asked to place a mark where he or she considers the value of the event that is hoped to be prevented by the treatment is located. Assume this is placed at 0.1, indicating a 'low' or 'poor' value for the consequence of the disease to be prevented. The patient then places a second mark for his or her 'feeling' about the adverse events. Suppose this is placed at 0.9, indicating a high value (or minimal disability for the adverse event from therapy). It can then be concluded that the patient believes that blindness is 0.9/0.1 or 10 times worse compared to a complication of therapy. In other words, the patient believes the side effects are minor and that what the procedure is trying to prevent is 10 times worse. The process is repeated a couple of times to ensure that the patient actually understands what the authors are eliciting and is consistent in the responses.

REFERENCES

1. Thomas R, Padma P, Braganza A, et al. Assessment of clinical significance: the number needed to treat. Indian J Ophthalmol 1996; 44:113–115.

2. Sackett DL, Haynes RB, Guyatt GH, et al. Clinical epidemiology. A basic science for clinical medicine. New York: Little, Brown; 1991:199–215

3. Haynes RB, Sackett DL, Guyatt GH, et al. Clinical epidemiology. How to do clinical research. Philadelphia: Lippincott Williams & Williams; 2006: 129–132.

4. Kass MA, Heuer DK, Higginbotham EJ, et al. The Ocular Hypertension Treatment Study: a randomized trial determines that topical ocular hypotensive medication delays or prevents the onset of primary open-angle glaucoma. Arch Ophthalmol 2002; 120:701–713.

5. Cioffi GA, Liebmann JM. Translating the OHTS results into clinical practice. J Glaucoma 2002; 11:375–377.

6. Thomas R, Thomas R, Kumar RS, et al. Applying the recent clinical trials on primary open angle glaucoma: the developing world perspective. J Glaucoma 2005; 14:324–327.

7. Heijl A, Leske MC, Bengtsson B, et al. Early Manifest Glaucoma Trial Group. Reduction of intraocular pressure and glaucoma progression: results from the Early Manifest Glaucoma Trial. Arch Ophthalmol 2002; 120:1268–1279.

8. Feiner L, Piltz-Seymour JR. Collaborative Initial Glaucoma Treatment Study: a summary of results to date. Curr Opin Ophthalmol 2003; 14:106–111.

9. Sackett DL, Straus SE, Richardson WS, et al. Evidence-based medicine: how to practice and teach EBM. Toronto: Churchill Livingstone; 2000: 111–129.

10. Sackett DL, Haynes RB, Guyatt GH, et al. Clinical epidemiology. A basic science for clinical medicine. New York: Little, Brown; 1991: 238–244.

11. Reigelman RK. Studying a study and testing a test. How to read the medical evidence. Philadelphia: Lippincott, Williams and Wilkins; 2000: 40–54.

12. Asrani S, Zeimer R, Wilensky J, et al. Large diurnal fluctuations in intraocular pressure are an independent risk factor in patients with glaucoma. J Glaucoma 2000; 9:134–142.

MEDICAL THERAPY

CHAPTER 46

Parasympathomimetics

Lineu Shiroma and Vital Costa

INTRODUCTION

The class of drugs that mimics the effects of acetylcholine is known as cholinergic agents, miotics, or parasympathomimetics. Considered the first class of agents used for treating primary open-angle glaucoma (POAG) in the nineteenth century, the major problems of parasympathomimetics are the ocular side effects, which relegated them to a second-line position.

Cholinergic drugs mimic and amplify the parasympathetic nervous system, whose neurotransmitter is acetylcholine. They can be divided into two groups, based on the site of action. Pilocarpine, carbachol, and acetylcholine act directly at the neuromuscular junction. The indirect-acting parasympathomimetics, also knows as anticholinesterase agents, bind to acetylcholinesterase at the neuromuscular junction, resulting in a build-up of acetylcholine and stimulation of the parasympathetic nervous system.

Pilocarpine is the direct stimulator most commonly used in the treatment of glaucoma. Other parasympathomimetics, including direct-acting agents (carbachol, a synthetic derivative of choline) and the indirectly acting cholinesterase inhibitors (demecarium bromide and echothiophate iodide), are seldom used, but may be helpful in case a miotic is required in a patient allergic to pilocarpine.[1]

Despite the advent of new classes of drugs (β-blockers, prostaglandin analogues, and adrenergic agonists), parasympathomimetics may be important in selected patients.

CLASSIFICATION

DIRECT-ACTING DRUGS

Pilocarpine Pilocarpine, a colorless or yellow poisonous compound ($C_{11}H_{16}N_2O_2$; Fig. 46.1), is the most popular and most extensively studied miotic, produced under various formulations. It is a muscarinic alkaloid, obtained from the leaves of tropical American shrubs from the genus *Pilocarpus microphyllus* or *jaborandi*.

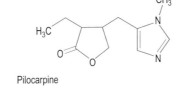

Pilocarpine
(3S,4R)-3-ethyl-4- [(3-methylimidazol-4-yl)methyl]oxolan-2-one

FIGURE 46.1 The chemical formula of pilocarpine.

The alkaloid was first isolated in 1875, and its muscarinic activity was described shortly thereafter.

Although pilocarpine is a direct-acting muscarinic agonist, it has been demonstrated that it also has an indirect effect by activating choline acetyltransferase synthesis of acetylcholine.[2]

Pilocarpine ophthalmic solutions have been used for treatment of some types of glaucoma for over a hundred years. Recently, an oral formulation of pilocarpine was approved by the United States Food and Drug Administration (FDA) for the treatment of dry mouth in 1994 and for Sjögren's syndrome in 1998.

Initially, pilocarpine has been used to treat both primary angle-closure and open-angle glaucomas, but recently its use has been limited to treat some special conditions, such as plateau iris, creeping angle closure, and during an episode of acute angle-closure glaucoma, once the intraocular pressure (IOP) has been reduced.

There are several preparations and brand names of pilocarpine available on the market, with concentrations varying from 0.25% to 10% (Table 46.1). The frequency of administration and drug concentration of pilocarpine are detailed below.

Carbachol Carbachol, also known as carbamylcholine, is classified as a cholinergic and acts as an acetylcholine receptor agonist. It is a dual-action parasympathomimetic that produces direct motor end plate stimulation, as well as an indirect parasympathomimetic effect by inhibition of acetylcholinesterase. It stimulates both muscarinic and nicotinic receptors.

Carbachol is the most potent parasympathetic agent with a longer duration of action, up to 8 hours with

TABLE 46.1 **Commercially available miotic preparations**

PREPARATIONS	BRAND NAMES	CONCENTRATIONS (%)
Pilocarpine hydrochlorides	Akarpine	1, 2, 4
	Isopto Carpine	0.25, 0.5, 1, 2, 3, 4, 6, 8, 10
	Pilocar	0.5, 1, 2, 3, 4, 6
	Piloptic	0.5, 1, 2, 3, 4, 6
	Pilostat	0.5, 1, 2, 3, 4, 6
Pilocarpine nitrate	Pilagan	2, 4
Pilocarpine gel	Pilopine HS Gel	4
Fixed combination*	Timpilo	2, 4 (+timolol 0.5%)
	Fotil	
Carbachol	Isopto Carbachol	0.75, 1.5, 2.25, 3.0
	Carboptic	
Echothiophate iodide	Phospholine Iodide	0.125
Intracameral injections		
Acetylcholine	Miochol	0.01 in 2 mL
Carbachol	Miostat	0.01 in 1.5 mL

*Not available in the United States.

topical administration and 24 hours for intraocular administration. Carbachol ophthalmic is available with a prescription under the brand names Isopto Carbachol Ophthalmic and Carbotic in 0.75%, 1.5%, 2.25, and 3% solutions. Since carbachol is poorly absorbed through topical administration, benzalkonium chloride is mixed in to promote absorption. It is recommended three times daily, and is indicated in patients who develop allergy to pilocarpine and require a miotic agent.

Compared to pilocarpine, carbachol produces more IOP reduction and more side effects. A study comparing 1.5% carbachol three times daily with 2% pilocarpine four times daily showed better IOP control with carbachol therapy. However, accommodative spasm and ocular pain were more frequent with carbachol.[3]

Intracameral carbachol has been used after cataract surgery to achieve miosis and has been shown to provide better IOP control in the early postoperative period than intracameral acetylcholine.

INDIRECT-ACTING DRUGS

Indirect acting parasympathomimetics inhibit the enzymatic destruction of acetylcholine by inactivating cholinesterase, leaving acetylcholine free to act on the effector cells of the iris sphincter and ciliary muscles, causing pupillary constriction and spasm of accommodation. Anticholinesterase agents are generally more potent than pilocarpine, but show more severe side effects, which led to the abandonment of these drugs for the past 20 years.

Echothiophate iodide Echothiophate is a parasympathomimetic and organophosphate that binds irreversibly to cholinesterase. Because of the very slow rate at which echothiophate is hydrolyzed by cholinesterase, its effects can last a week or more.

Echothiophate iodide 0.06% is more potent than pilocarpine 4%; its maximal effect occurs within 24 hours, lasts up to 2 weeks, and it causes intense and prolonged miosis.

It has been associated with anterior subcapsular cataracts and, because of the risk of prolonged apnea, should be stopped 6 weeks before general anesthesia with succinylcholine. The antidote for echothiophate iodide toxicity is pralidoxime chloride.

Physostigmine Physostigmine is one of the oldest drugs and was successfully used for the treatment of glaucoma in 1864. Also known as eserine, it is a parasympathomimetic, more specifically, a reversible cholinesterase inhibitor obtained from the Calabar bean. It helps prolong the activity of acetylcholine and, by interfering with the metabolism of acetylcholine, physostigmine indirectly stimulates both nicotinic and muscarinic receptors.

It causes a contraction of the pupil more marked than in the case of any other known drug and stimulates the fibers of the ciliary muscle. Considering that physostigmine is useful against toxic levels of atropine, toxic levels of physostigmine are conversely countered by atropine.

MECHANISM OF ACTION

Pilocarpine directly stimulates cholinergic receptors, acting on a subtype of muscarinic receptor (M_3) found on the iris sphincter muscle, causing the muscle to contract and produce miosis.[4] This effect is important in the short-term management of some angle-closure glaucomas. In these cases, pilocarpine-induced miosis relieves pupillary block, and opens the anterior chamber angle,

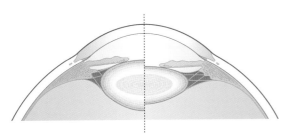

FIGURE 46.2 Schematic picture showing the ciliary muscle contraction in the left side, with slight decrease in the anterior chamber depth, thickening of the lens, and opening of the anterior chamber angle.

changing the anatomy of the peripheral iris (Fig. 46.2). In open-angle glaucoma, pilocarpine contracts the ciliary muscle, increasing the outflow of aqueous humor, which reduces intraocular pressure.

Acting on the parasympathetic nervous system, pilocarpine stimulates the sphincter pupillae in the iris and the ciliary muscle, resulting in displacement of the scleral spur, opening of the trabecular meshwork and/or Schlemm's canal, and enhancement of conventional aqueous outflow. When evaluating enucleated human eyes previously treated with pilocarpine, Grierson et al.[5] observed a posterior pull on the scleral spur, widening of trabecular space, endothelial meshwork distention, and an increase in the number of pores in the inner endothelium of Schlemm's canal.

It is known that the incidence of glaucoma increases with age, and aging seems to affect the efficacy of pilocarpine. In monkeys, the effect of pilocarpine in contracting the ciliary muscle has been shown to be directly proportional to the decline in accommodation.

Some studies have suggested that pilocarpine may decrease aqueous inflow.[6] In fact, in the rabbit's iris-ciliary body tissue preparation, the cholinergic system has been found to directly modulate adenylate cyclase and aqueous humor secretion.

Pilocarpine decreases uveoscleral outflow, an opposite mechanism of action to prostaglandin analogues, and may cause a paradoxical rise in IOP in patients who depend on the secondary drainage pathway.[7]

ADMINISTRATION

Pilocarpine is bound to ocular tissues. Whether it is distributed is not known, but it apparently does not accumulate in ocular tissues. Pilocarpine penetrates the eye through the cornea, where it is absorbed or degraded, with only a small percentage (<3%) entering the anterior chamber.[8] Metabolism has not been elucidated, but any systemic absorption can produce parasympathomimetic effects.

PHARMACOKINETICS

Pilocarpine can be administered topically or orally, but the most common formulation used is eyedrops.

The peak aqueous humor concentration occurs 20 minutes after dosing and lasts for 4 hours. The IOP-lowering effect in ocular hypertension individuals peaked approximately within 2 hours and lasted for at least 8 hours, with IOP reduction of 20% at 2–8 hours after dosing and 14–15% at 12–15 hours after dosing.[9]

The duration of action and the IOP-lowering effect are dose related up to a concentration of 4%.[9] Higher concentrations, such as 6%, may have additional IOP reduction in darkly pigmented eyes.

The recommended medical regimen is four times daily. However, Zimmerman et al. reported that two times daily instillation of 2% pilocarpine followed by nasolacrimal occlusion has had the same optimal ocular hypotensive effectiveness.[10]

DELIVERY SYSTEMS

Vehicles are polymers that reduce the initial rapid drainage and prolong the drug–cornea contact time, interfering with the amount of medication available for ocular penetration. It changes the duration of the effect, may reduce the number of instillations per day and, thereby, leads to a reduction in side effects and improvement in quality of life. However, none of the preparations described below is able to completely avoid the side effects of pilocarpine.

1. *Ointments*: increase drug bioavailability by reducing loss in tears, providing a higher effective concentration of the drug.
2. *Pilocarpine gel*: equivalent to 4% pilocarpine hydrochloride in a high-viscosity acrylic vehicle (Pilopine™). Generally used once daily at bedtime, it has been reported to reduce IOP significantly for 18–24 hours, with a similar IOP-lowering efficacy of pilocarpine hydrochloride eyedrops four times daily,[11] with less induced myopia and impaired nocturnal visual activity. Pilopine™ has been shown to cause fine corneal haze in 15 of 53 patients (28%) after long-term use.
3. *Membrane-controlled delivery system*: Ocusert-Pilo™ used to be a slow-release ophthalmic delivery system consisting of a reservoir of pilocarpine bordered by a semipermeable membrane. The small, elliptical device was placed under the upper or lower eyelid and left in place for 7 days. This system allowed a sustained release of pilocarpine over 7 days, with the maximal effect being achieved 1.5–2 hours after the system was applied. The system allowed two rates of release (20 µg or 40 µg/h), which reduced the intensity of the drug's side effects.[12] Ocusert-Pilo™ was a useful alternative for patients who could tolerate and retain the system, but it is no longer available.

Alternative approaches include soluble polymers (methylcellulose and polyvinyl alcohol), oily solutions, sodium hyaluronate, cyanoacrylate block copolymer, and poly (butyl cyanoacrylate) nanoparticles.

DRUG INTERACTIONS AND COMPARISON WITH OTHER AGENTS

OTHER MIOTICS

Echothiophate iodide is as effective alone as in combination with pilocarpine.[13] Furthermore, pretreating monkeys with echothiophate iodide demonstrated marked subsensitivity to pilocarpine, and required several weeks or months to recover normal pilocarpine sensitivity.

Physostigmine (eserine) is a reversible cholinesterase inhibitor that interferes with the metabolism of acetylcholine and indirectly stimulates both nicotinic and muscarinic receptors. It is a slightly weaker indirect-acting parasympathomimetic and has no addictive effect on tonographic values when added to pilocarpine therapy.

ADRENERGIC AGONISTS

Epinephrine compounds produce additional IOP reduction when combined with pilocarpine,[14] significantly greater than the effect of either drug given alone.

Ren and co-workers reported that pilocarpine 4% is at least as effective as apraclonidine 1% in post argon laser trabeculoplasty (ALT) IOP spike prophylaxis.[15]

The single-dose response of open-angle glaucoma eyes to pilocarpine 1%, clonidine 0.125%, a combination of pilocarpine 1% and clonidine 0.125%, and timolol 0.5% was studied in a double-blind, masked, crossover study. The combination of pilocarpine 1% and clonidine 0.125% was well tolerated, and the IOP-lowering efficacy was significantly greater than that of either drug alone. Years later, the same group compared the efficacy and safety of two drug combinations, pilocarpine 1%/clonidine 0.06% and pilocarpine 1%/clonidine 0.125%, with timolol 0.25%. They concluded that the combination of pilocarpine 1% and clonidine 0.125% produced an IOP reduction comparable to that achieved with timolol 0.25% drops twice daily (28.45% and 24.64%, respectively, $p < 0.05$) and did not result in any significant ocular and systemic adverse effects.[16]

BETA-BLOCKERS

Compared with timolol, pilocarpine has an equivalent or slightly weaker IOP-lowering effect. Vogel et al. compared the efficacy and safety of timolol 0.25% twice daily with pilocarpine 2% four times daily. The concentration of each antiglaucoma agent could be increased (to 0.5% for timolol or 4% for pilocarpine) if the initial IOP response was inadequate. After a follow-up of 24 months, a higher rate of patients in the pilocarpine group quit the study because of inadequate IOP control and or significantly greater visual field deterioration.[17] On the other hand, another study showed that pilocarpine gel was as effective as twice-daily timolol 0.5%.

Adrenergic antagonists have partially additive effects with pilocarpine. The effects of pilocarpine 4% alone, timolol 0.5% alone, and a combination of timolol 0.5% and pilocarpine 4% were compared in 43 glaucoma

patients. The mean IOP reduction from baseline was 17.6%, 21.2%, and 28.5%, respectively. Intraocular pressure was consistently lower with the combination treatment than with timolol or pilocarpine alone.[18]

In some parts of the world, two fixed combinations of timolol and pilocarpine (Timpilo™ and Fotil™) are available. Studies have revealed an equivalent IOP-lowering efficacy when the fixed combination is compared to both drugs given separately.

Bron and co-workers evaluated the efficacy and safety of fixed combinations of carteolol 2% and pilocarpine 2% versus timolol 0.5% and pilocarpine 2%. They concluded that the carteolol–pilocarpine combination appeared as safe and as effective as the timolol–pilocarpine combination (17.3% versus 19.5% IOP reduction, respectively) in the medical treatment of POAG or ocular hypertension.[19]

PROSTAGLANDIN ANALOGUES

The interaction between pilocarpine and prostaglandin (PG) analogues has been investigated by several authors. Pilocarpine contracts the ciliary muscle, leading to a decrease in uveoscleral outflow and an increase in trabecular outflow facility by pulling on the scleral spur. On the other hand, prostaglandin analogues improve uveoscleral outflow, relaxing the ciliary muscle and remodeling the extracellular matrix.[20]

An initial observation suggested that pilocarpine antagonized the effects of $PGF_{2\alpha}$ in monkeys. However, although these categories of drugs have opposite mechanisms of action, there is an additive IOP-lowering effect of the PG agents when added to pilocarpine.

In fact, Toris et al. showed that pilocarpine did not impair the action of latanoprost, and demonstrated an additive effect by fluorophotometry, tonometry, and venomanometry.[21] Another study evaluated the association of pilocarpine at various concentrations to bimatoprost, showing that it was neither additive nor antagonistic to the effect of bimatoprost. Hence, it is possible that the reduction in uveoscleral outflow promoted by pilocarpine is outweighed by the inverse effect of prostaglandin analogues.

One study tried to evaluate the optimal timing of using latanoprost and pilocarpine, showing that pilocarpine was most effective if administered four times daily and when the bedtime drop was instilled 1 hour after latanoprost.[22]

Two independent studies, with similar designs, compared the effect on intraocular pressure of latanoprost monotherapy and timolol–pilocarpine b.i.d. in patients with glaucoma not adequately controlled with timolol 0.5%. Latanoprost monotherapy was found to be at least as effective as the fixed combination of timolol–pilocarpine in reducing mean diurnal IOP.

CARBONIC ANHYDRASE INHIBITORS

Topical carbonic anhydrase inhibitors are a viable alternative to pilocarpine in the adjunctive therapy with β-blockers. One study compared the use of dorzolamide and pilocarpine as adjunctive therapy to timolol in patients with elevated intraocular pressure. Patients received 0.5% timolol twice daily plus either 0.7% dorzolamide twice daily (n = 83), 2% dorzolamide twice daily (n = 89), or 2% pilocarpine four times daily (n = 44). After 6 months, additional mean IOP reductions were 9%, 13%, and 10% for 0.7% dorzolamide, 2% dorzolamide, and 2% pilocarpine, respectively. However, the side effects of pilocarpine were more common and disturbing that those observed with dorzolamide.[23]

Kaluzny et al. compared the efficacy of two fixed combinations (timolol 0.5%/dorzolamide 2% (TDFC) versus timolol 0.5%/pilocarpine 2% (TPFC)) twice daily in 36 POAG or ocular hypertensive patients. Their mean baseline IOP with timolol was 22.3 mmHg. Following 6 weeks of treatment, the mean IOP was 18.0 mmHg for TDFC and 17.4 mmHg for TPFC (p = 0.22). The authors suggested that the timolol 0.5%/pilocarpine 2% fixed combination could provide at least similar IOP reduction as the timolol 0.5%/dorzolamide 2% fixed combination, but patients using pilocarpine complained more about the side effects.[24]

The IOP-lowering efficacy of pilocarpine 2% as initial therapy of primary open-angle glaucoma was compared with ALT in a prospective study. After 2 years of follow-up, no difference in efficacy was found between pilocarpine 2% and ALT.

CONTRAINDICATIONS AND PRECAUTIONS

Miotic therapy is associated with ciliary body congestion and breakdown of the blood–aqueous barrier, increasing the permeability to plasma proteins. These effects are dose dependent and have been demonstrated both with the laser flare cell meter and fluorophotometry.[25] For this reason, miotics should be avoided in uveitic glaucoma, neovascular glaucoma, or any other condition where the blood–aqueous barrier is already compromised.

Ciliary muscle contraction results in axial thickening of the lens, reducing the depth of the anterior chamber and, thereby, allowing a phacomorphic closure of the anterior chamber angle. Hence, pilocarpine is formally contraindicated in eyes with phacomorphic glaucoma or other conditions where the glaucoma is caused by anterior displacement of the iris–lens diaphragm.

The correlation between the onset of malignant glaucoma and treatment with miotics (either preoperative or postoperative) has been described long ago.[26] While this condition is relieved by cycloplegic–mydriatic therapy, miotics increase ciliary block, inducing the production of aqueous humor towards the vitreous. For this reason, miotics are formally contraindicated in eyes with aqueous misdirection.

There are no data evaluating the safety of pilocarpine in pregnant or breastfeeding women. Very high doses of the drug may be teratogenic in animals. Studies have also not been done to test the use of pilocarpine by children.

Pilocarpine should not be taken by people who are sensitive to this compound or who have uncontrolled asthma. It should be avoided by people with breathing problems, gallbladder disease, kidney problems, retinal disease, or heart disease.

SIDE EFFECTS

SYSTEMIC TOXICITY

Therapy with pilocarpine may result in a range of systemic adverse effects, most of them related to its action as a muscarinic receptor agonist. Pilocarpine has been known to cause excessive sweating, excessive salivation, bradycardia, hypotension, bronchospasm, and increased bronchial mucus secretion.[27] Symptoms of overdose include irregular heartbeat, chest pain, fainting, confusion, stomach cramps or pain, and trouble breathing. Blood pressure and pulse may rise or fall, depending on the degree of autonomic stimulation.

Pilocarpine also stimulates smooth muscles, such as those found in the gallbladder, ureters, bile ducts, capsular muscle of the spleen, and intestinal tracts, which may lead to nausea, vomiting, and diarrhea.[28]

The increment in bronchial mucus secretion, associated with the smooth muscle contraction, indicates that patients with pulmonary disease, such as asthma or chronic obstructive pulmonary disease, should not be treated with pilocarpine.

Progressive cognitive dysfunction has been associated with topical pilocarpine in patients with Alzheimer's disease. Patients with Alzheimer's disease are probably more sensitive to cholinergic drugs, because of lower levels of cholinesterase in their brain.

Patients with underlying conduction system disease (His-Purkinje conduction) are at risk from developing atrioventricular block if pilocarpine is used intensively.

As mentioned above, pilocarpine can produce systemic effects similar to those of muscarine, but these side effects are rare with the dosage used in the chronic management of glaucoma. However, it may be seen in patients receiving frequent instillations of the drug in the treatment of acute angle-closure glaucoma.

Parasympatholytics or cholinergic antagonists block the response of acetylcholine at the receptor. This class of medications includes tropicamide, cyclopentolate, and atropine, the latter being the antidote for systemic pilocarpine toxicity.

OCULAR SIDE EFFECTS

The use of pilocarpine is limited by its adverse effects, especially the ocular side effects, such as miosis and accommodative spasm, which, coupled with the high frequency of dosage, make it an unpopular drug, particularly in younger patients.

Local side effects are frequent and have two major consequences: they interfere with the patient's quality of life and reduce the compliance with therapy.[29]

The ocular side effects are due to the shared expression of muscarinic cholinergic receptor subtypes. Ciliary muscle spasm may cause brow ache, which usually gets better after a few weeks of continued therapy.

The most disturbing effect is the induced myopia, caused by the contraction of the ciliary muscle, which takes the tension off the zonules, resulting in an increase in axial lens diameter and shallowing of the anterior chamber.[30] After one drop of 2% pilocarpine, the diopter change begins in approximately 15 minutes, peaks in 45–60 minutes, and lasts for 1.5–2 hours. It is more noted in young patients, but also occurs in the elderly.

Miotics may contribute to functional disability, causing dim vision and constriction of visual field, especially if cortical or subcapsular lens opacities are present. An average deterioration of −1.49 dB in the mean deviation (MD) of automated visual field was documented in patients using pilocarpine.[31] Long-term use of pilocarpine can lead to permanent miosis, which reduces both the amount of light entering the eye and the visual field. On the other hand, the smaller pupil may act as a pinhole and improve visual acuity in some patients.

A cataractogenic effect has been suggested in patients on long-term miotic therapy.[32] A prospective study of uniocular miotic therapy using the fellow eye as a control was done with 30 patients using 2% pilocarpine and 29 patients on 0.125% echothiophate iodide. Pilocarpine was found to be cataractogenic, but the changes were less marked and required more time to develop than those induced by echothiophate iodide.

Retinal detachment[33] has been associated with miotic therapy, especially in eyes with other risk factors, such as myopia, aphakia, or lattice degeneration. It is presumed that vitreoretinal traction may occur as a result of ciliary muscle contraction, leading to retinal tears. A careful retinal examination is recommended before the initiation of therapy. Macular holes have been reported to develop within weeks after starting 2% pilocarpine, probably as a result of vitreoretinal traction.

Dose-dependent corneal endothelial toxicity has been reported in rabbit studies. However, a study performed in humans to evaluate the long-term effect of 4% pilocarpine gel on corneal transparency and endothelial cell count identified no adverse corneal effects.[34]

Miotic therapy was considered to be associated with allograft rejection, induced by intraocular inflammation or anatomical changes in the anterior chamber angle. In this series, each graft rejection episode resolved with discontinuation of pilocarpine and administration of a topical steroid.

Miotics may cause a transitory conjunctival hyperemia due to vasodilatation. Allergy and toxic conjunctival changes may occur due to the drug or the preservative. Allergic reactions usually involve eyelids and conjunctiva, often with giant papillary reaction, whereas a toxic reaction usually includes a follicular response in the conjunctiva.

Summary

Pilocarpine has been used in the treatment of glaucoma for over 100 years. It acts on the muscarinic receptors found on the iris sphincter and the ciliary muscle. The trabecular meshwork is opened through increased tension on the scleral spur, which facilitates conventional aqueous outflow and decreases IOP.

Pilocarpine has few systemic side effects and is relatively inexpensive. Nevertheless, the ocular side effects (miosis, myopia, brow ache, and dimming of vision) and the inconvenience of dosing four times daily make pilocarpine less popular than other categories of drugs used to treat glaucoma. Nevertheless, pilocarpine must still be considered in the treatment of some forms of angle-closure glaucoma, and as adjunctive therapy, providing additional IOP-lowering effect when associated with other medications.

Miotics should not be prescribed in patients with uveitic glaucoma, neovascular glaucoma, and conditions where the glaucoma is caused by anterior displacement of the iris–lens diaphragm. Echothiophate has to be stopped a few weeks before surgery if succinylcholine is going to be used as anesthetic.

REFERENCES

1. Taniguchi T, Kitazawa Y. A risk–benefit assessment of drugs used in the management of glaucoma. Drug Saf 1994; 11: 68–74.

2. Mindel JS, Kharlamb AB. Alteration of acetylcholine synthesis by pilocarpine. In vivo and in vitro studies. Arch Ophthalmol 1984; 102(10):1546–1549.

3. Francois J, Goes F. Ultrasonographic study of the effect of different miotics on the eye components. Ophthalmologica 1977; 175(6):328–338.

4. Nietgen GW, Schmidt J, Hesse L, et al. Muscarinic receptor functioning and distribution in the eye: molecular basis and implications for clinical diagnosis and therapy [Review]. Eye 1999; 13(Pt 3a):285–300.

5. Grierson I, Lee WR, Abraham S. Effects of pilocarpine on the morphology of the human outflow apparatus. Br J Ophthalmol 1978; 62(5):302–313.

6. Miichi H, Nagataki S. Effects of pilocarpine, salbutamol, and timolol on aqueous humor formation in cynomolgus monkeys. Invest Ophthalmol Vis Sci 1983; 24(9):1269–1275.

7. Bleiman BS, Schwartz AL. Paradoxical intraocular pressure response to pilocarpine. A proposed mechanism and treatment. Arch Ophthalmol 1979; 97(7):1305–1306.

8. Asseff CF, Weisman RL, Podos SM, et al. Ocular penetration of pilocarpine in primates. Am J Ophthalmol 1973; 75(2): 212–215.

9. Drance SM, Bensted M, Schulzer M. Pilocarpine and intraocular pressure. Duration of effectiveness of 4 percent and 8 percent pilocarpine instillation. Arch Ophthalmol 1974; 91(2):104–106.

10. Zimmerman TJ, Sharir M, Nardin GF, et al. Therapeutic index of pilocarpine, carbachol, and timolol with nasolacrimal occlusion. Am J Ophthalmol 1992; 114(1):1–7.

11. Goldberg I, Ashburn FS Jr, Kass MA, et al. Efficacy and patient acceptance of pilocarpine gel. Am J Ophthalmol 1979; 88(5):843–846.

12. François J, Goes F, Zagorski Z. Comparative ultrasonographic study of the effect of pilocarpine 2 per cent and Ocusert P 20 on the eye components. Am J Ophthalmol 1978; 86:233–238.

13. Kini MM, Dahl AA, Roberts CR, et al. Echothiophate, pilocarpine, and open-angle glaucoma. Arch Ophthalmol 1973; 89(3):190–192.

14. Harris LS, Mittag TW, Galin MA. Aqueous dynamics of pilocarpine-treated eyes. The influence of topically applied epinephrine. Arch Ophthalmol 1971; 86(1):1–4.

15. Ren J, Shin DH, Chung HS, et al. Efficacy of apraclonidine 1% versus pilocarpine 4% for prophylaxis of intraocular pressure spike after argon laser trabeculoplasty. Ophthalmology 1999; 106(6):1135–1139.

16. Sihota R, Rajashekhar YL, Venkatesh P, et al. A prospective, long-term, randomized study of the efficacy and safety of the drug combination pilocarpine 1% with clonidine 0.06% or clonidine 0.125% versus timolol 0.25%. J Ocul Pharmacol Ther 2002; 18(6):499–506.

17. Vogel R, Crick RP, Mills KB, et al. Effect of timolol versus pilocarpine on visual field progression in patients with primary open-angle glaucoma. Ophthalmology 1992; 99(10):1505–1511.

18. Zadok D, Geyer O, Zadok J, et al. Combined timolol and pilocarpine vs pilocarpine alone and timolol alone in the treatment of glaucoma. Am J Ophthalmol 1994; 117(6): 728–731.

19. Bron AM, Garcher CP, Sirbat D, et al. Comparison of two fixed beta-blocker-pilocarpine combinations. The Carteolol-Pilocarpine Study Group. Eur J Ophthalmol 1997; 7(4): 351–356.

20. Weinreb RN, Toris CB, Gabelt BT, et al. Effects of prostaglandins on the aqueous humor outflow pathways [Review]. Surv Ophthalmol 2002; 47(Suppl 1):S53–S64.

21. Toris CB, Zhan GL, Zhao J, et al. Potential mechanism for the additivity of pilocarpine and latanoprost. Am J Ophthalmol 2001; 131(6):722–728.

22. Kent AR, Vroman DT, Thomas TJ, et al. Interaction of pilocarpine with latanoprost in patients with glaucoma and ocular hypertension. J Glaucoma 1999; 8(4):257–262.

23. Strahlman ER, Vogel R, Tipping R, et al. The use of dorzolamide and pilocarpine as adjunctive therapy to timolol in patients with elevated intraocular pressure. The Dorzolamide Additivity Study Group. Ophthalmology 1996; 103(8): 1283–1293.

24. Kaluzny JJ, Szaflik J, Czechowicz-Janicka K, et al. Timolol 0.5%/dorzolamide 2% fixed combination versus timolol 0.5%/pilocarpine 2% fixed combination in primary open-angle glaucoma or ocular hypertensive patients. Acta Ophthalmol Scand 2003; 81(4):349–354.

25. Mori M, Araie M, Sakurai M, et al. Effects of pilocarpine and tropicamide on blood–aqueous barrier permeability in man. Invest Ophthalmol Vis Sci 1992; 33(2):416–423.

26. Merritt JC. Malignant glaucoma induced by miotics postoperatively in open-angle glaucoma. Arch Ophthalmol 1977; 95(11):1988–1989.

27. Curti PC, Renovanz HD. [The effect of unintentional overdoses of pilocarpine on pulmonary surfactant in mice]. Klin Monatsbl Augenheilkd 1981; 179(2):113–115.

28. Greco JJ, Kelman CD. Systemic pilocarpine toxicity in the treatment of angle closure glaucoma. Ann Ophthalmol 1973; 5(1):57–59.

29. Granstrom PA, Norell S. Visual ability and drug regimen: relation to compliance with glaucoma therapy. Acta Ophthalmol (Copenh) 1983; 61(2):206–219.

30. Abramson DH, Chang S, Coleman DJ, et al. Pilocarpine-induced lens changes. An ultrasonic biometric evaluation of dose response. Arch Ophthalmol 1974; 92(6):464–469.

31. Webster AR, Luff AJ, Canning CR, et al. The effect of pilocarpine on the glaucomatous visual field. Br J Ophthalmol 1993; 77(11):721–725.

32. Axelsson U. Glaucoma, miotic therapy and cataract. I. The frequency of anterior subcapsular vacuoles in glaucoma eyes treated with echothiophate (Phospholine Iodide), pilocarpine or pilocarpine-eserine, and in nonglaucomatous untreated eyes with common senile cataract. Acta Ophthalmol (Copenh) 1968; 46(1):83–98.

33. Beasley H, Fraunfelder FT. Retinal detachments and topical ocular miotics. Ophthalmology 1979; 86(1):95–98.

34. Nagasubramanian S, Stewart RH, Hitchings RA. Long-term effects of glaucoma therapy with 4% pilocarpine gel on corneal clarity and endothelial cell density. Int Ophthalmol 1994; 18(1):5–8.

CHAPTER 47

Beta-Blockers

Ann M Hoste

INTRODUCTION

The ocular hypotensive effects of β-blockers were originally demonstrated after oral administration of propranolol in 1967.[1] This drug was the first β-blocker to be introduced into therapy in 1965 and was soon widely used in the treatment of a variety of cardiovascular disorders. However, propranolol could not be commercialized in an ophthalmic solution because of its marked membrane stabilizing or local anesthetic properties due to its sodium (Na^+) channel blocking activity. Long-term topical application of the drug would thus inevitably have caused corneal damage.

The first β-blocker available in an ophthalmic solution was timolol.[2] Timolol was introduced on the market in 1978 (Fig. 47.1) and has since become the standard β-blocker in ophthalmology. In the 1980s, it was estimated that the use of timolol had increased to account for 70% of all glaucoma medications used.[3] Over time, various congeners of propranolol have been developed, some of which have also become available in ophthalmic solutions (Table 47.1). This development is typical of any drug group that has major therapeutic relevance and a relatively fixed active structure. The intraocular pressure (IOP)-lowering capacity of timolol has, however, never been surpassed by any congener, although some may have an added value such as neuroprotective properties or systemic tolerability profiles superior to timolol.

Three decades after its introduction on the market timolol is still by far the most studied of all glaucoma medications. It provides the reference against which other β-blockers and all newer glaucoma medications are evaluated. Timolol, being no longer protected by patent, is offered as a generic by different manufacturers under various proprietary names in different countries. The use of timolol (and of the other topical β-blockers) has declined since the arrival of newer agents, especially since that of the prostaglandin analogues. It is, however, likely to be on the rise again with the increased use of modern combination products, all of which contain timolol.

DRUG FORMULATIONS AND DOSING

OPHTHALMIC SOLUTIONS

All topical β-blockers are available in conventional ophthalmic solutions (see Table 47.1).

Dosing and time of administration The standard dosing of the ophthalmic solutions is twice daily. However, the long washout periods of timolol and levobunolol indicate that their ocular hypotensive effects persist for at least 24 hours once β-blockade has been achieved (see Washout Period, below). In accordance with this, several studies have shown that both β-blockers can indeed be used once daily with little difference in effect.[4–7]

The preferred timing of the single administration can be questioned. Since timolol is less effective at night (see Twenty-Four-Hour IOP Control, below), it has traditionally been recommended that the single dose be applied in the morning. However, once a steady state

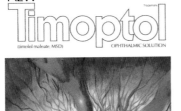

FIGURE 47.1 Launching the first topical β-blocker in 1978.

TABLE 47.1 Beta-blockers available in conventional ophthalmic solutions

β-BLOCKER	BRAND NAMES	MANUFACTURER	YEAR INTRODUCED IN THE USA	CONCENTRATIONS (%)	DOSING REGIMEN	BAC (%)*	NUMBER OF STUDIES**
Timolol	Timoptol Timoptic	MSD (Merck)	1978	0.25–0.5	1× or 2×	0.01	>3400
Betaxolol	Betoptic Betoptic S***	Alcon	1985	0.5 0.25	2×	0.01	>790
Levobunolol	Betagan	Allergan	1986	0.25–0.5	1× or 2×	0.004	>250
Metipranolol	OptiPranolol Beta-Ophtiole	Bausch & Lomb Dr. Mann	1990	0.1–0.3–0.6	2×	0.004	>290
Carteolol	Carteol Ocupress	Otsuka Novartis	1992	1–2	2×	0.005	>380

*Concentration of the preservative benzalkonium chloride.
**As estimated by the number of hits at PubMed.
***Suspension.

TABLE 47.2 Beta-blockers in gel-forming solutions

β-BLOCKER	BRAND NAMES	MANUFACTURER	CONCENTRATIONS (%)	DOSING REGIMEN
Timolol	Timoptic-XE Timoptolgel	MSD (Merck)	0.25–0.5	1×
	Nyogel	Novartis	0.1	
Carteolol	Arteoptic	Bausch & Lomb	1–2	

at the β-adrenoceptors is reached for at least 24 hours, one could expect the timing of the administration of the β-blocker to play only a minor role. In agreement with this, in a study specifically comparing the effects of morning versus evening instillation, the time of the single administration of timolol appeared not to make any difference.[7] Recent studies of the IOP-lowering effects of combination products containing timolol are in line with this. The time of the single application of DuoTrav® (fixed combination with travoprost) appears to play no role.[8] As for Xalacom®, evening rather than morning dosing is recommended, this timing probably having no impact on the effects of timolol but, on the other hand, possibly slightly optimizing the effects of the latanoprost in the solution.[9]

There are no studies of single dosing of the other β-blockers. Carteolol, betaxolol, and metipranolol ophthalmic solutions should thus always be administered twice daily.

Drug concentrations Most ophthalmic solutions are available in two drug concentrations; metipranolol is available in three (see Table 47.1). The higher concentration of timolol confers, however, little therapeutic advantage,[7,10] and this appears to also hold true for all other β-blockers.[11–15] As the use of higher drug concentrations might increase the risk of systemic toxicity, it

is justified to preferably use the solutions with the lowest effective drug concentrations available.

GEL-FORMING SOLUTIONS

Timolol has been marketed in gel-forming solutions to enhance the drug's delivery into the eye and to lower systemic absorption by providing a longer ocular contact time (Table 47.2). The efficacy of Timoptic XE administered once daily is comparable to conventional timolol solution twice daily.[16] Similarly, carteolol in gel form given once daily is as efficacious in decreasing IOP as standard carteolol given twice daily.[17] Nyogel is a generic gel-forming product with the lowest timolol concentration available (0.1%) to have an acceptable IOP-lowering effect.[18] For the preferred time of administration of the single dose, see Dosing and time of administration, above.

PRESERVATIVE-FREE PREPARATIONS

Glaucoma patients treated long term with timolol ophthalmic solution have an increased expression of immunoinflammatory markers by the conjunctival epithelium.[19] The same effect is observed after the use of topical drugs belonging to other classes of glaucoma medication such as Xalatan.[19] It appears, however, to be much less pronounced after the long-term

TABLE 47.3 Timolol in unpreserved solutions

BRAND NAMES	MANUFACTURER	TIMOLOL CONCENTRATION	DOSING REGIMEN
Timoptic in Ocudose (unit dose container)	MSD (Merck)		
Timabak (ABAK dispenser)	Thea		
Timo-Pos		0.25–0.5%	1× or 2×
Timo-Comod	Ursapharm		
(COMOD dispenser)			

TABLE 47.4 The modern combination products, all containing timolol 0.5%

BRAND NAME	MANUFACTURER	OTHER COMPONENT		DOSING REGIMEN
Cosopt	MSD	Carbonic anhydrase inhibitor	Dorzolamide	2×
Combigan	Allergan	α_2-adrenergic agonist	Brimonidine	2×
Xalacom	Pfizer		Latanoprost	1×*
DuoTrav	Alcon	Prostaglandin analogue	Travoprost	1×
Ganfort	Allergan		Bimatoprost	1×
*Preferably in the evening.				

use of unpreserved timolol, indicating that it is mainly due to the benzalkonium chloride used as the primary preservative agent in the ophthalmic solutions,[19] in weight-to-volume ratios ranging from 0.004% (Betagan, OptiPranolol) to 0.020% (Xalatan) (see Table 47.1).

Chronic subclinical conjunctival inflammation can have a major clinical impact, as it is associated with a fibrotic tissue response. It may be an important cause of failure of filtration surgery.[20] The use of preservative-free preparations in disposable, sterile, single-dose containers or more practical modern special dispensers could potentially raise filtration surgery success rates (Table 47.3).

COMBINATION PRODUCTS

All modern combination products contain timolol, demonstrating the major therapeutic relevance of the drug (Table 47.4). Since neither dosing regimen (once or twice daily) nor time of single application of timolol appears to be of great concern (see Dosing and time of administration, above), both factors are determined by the other drug in the combination product. For more information on the combination products, see Interactions with Topical Drugs – the Combination Products, below.

MECHANISM OF ACTION

PHARMACOLOGY

Adrenoceptors fall into three major groups, labeled α_1, α_2, and β. Currently, three subtypes of β-adrenoceptors have been identified in various organ tissues. Beta$_1$-adrenoceptors are mainly found in cardiac muscle and pacemaker fibers, stimulation of which augments all heart functions. Activation of the β_2-subtype accounts for the β-adrenergic response of smooth muscles. It dilates blood vessels and bronchioles and relaxes the muscles of the uterus, deferent and gastrointestinal duct, urinary bladder, and dilator pupillae. Further effects of β_2-adrenoceptor activation are decreased platelet aggregation and glycogenolysis in the liver (resulting in glucose release) and in skeletal muscle. Beta$_3$-adrenoceptors have metabolic effects as well since they have been found to mediate lipolysis in adipose tissue, resulting in free fatty acid release and increased body heat production. Receptors of this subtype have also been identified in the cardiovascular system but the physiological importance of these remains unclear.

The adrenergic pathways are well known. Adrenergics (catecholamines) bind to β-adrenoceptors to activate (via the stimulatory G_S protein) the membrane-bound enzyme adenylate cyclase (Fig. 47.2). This enzyme accelerates the conversion of adenosine triphosphate (ATP) to the second messenger cyclic adenosine 3',5'-monophosphate (cAMP). cAMP then activates protein kinase A (PKA), which phosphorylates different functional proteins, usually enzymes and membrane proteins dependent on the target cell type, to exert its various biological effects.

Beta-blockers compete with adrenoceptor agonists for β-adrenoceptors, their mode of action thus being from antagonism of endogenous adrenergic responses (see Fig. 47.2). Both adrenaline (epinephrine) and noradrenaline (norepinephrine) circulate in blood plasma. The latter hormone actually mainly serves as a neurotransmitter in the sympathetic nervous system. However, diffusion of part of the noradrenaline from the synaptic cleft into the blood raises noradrenaline plasma levels. Adrenaline is directly secreted into the blood by the adrenal medulla. All adrenoceptors respond to adrenaline, but noradrenaline has little effect on β_2-adrenoceptors (see Fig. 47.2). Timolol is a nonselective β-blocker with powerful β$_1$- and β$_2$-adrenoceptor binding capacity. At the β$_2$-adrenoceptors it thus mainly counteracts the effects of adrenaline. The other topical β-blockers have similar receptor affinities, except for betaxolol, which has a higher affinity for β$_1$-adrenoceptors than for β$_2$-adrenoceptors. Carteolol has intrinsic sympathomimetic activity (ISA): that is, it acts as a partial β-agonist.

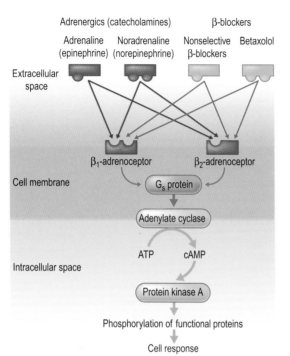

FIGURE 47.2 The adrenergic pathway and the sites of action of β-blockers. The nonselective β-blockers are timolol, levobunolol, metipranolol, and carteolol.

EFFECTS ON AQUEOUS HUMOR DYNAMICS

Timolol has no effect on outflow facility.[21] IOP reduction is achieved via suppressed aqueous humor production.[21,22] The mechanism underlying this effect has not been unquestionably demonstrated. It is generally believed that it is mainly due to interaction with β$_2$-adrenoceptors in the ciliary epithelium and antagonism of circulating adrenaline at this site, because the β-receptors found in the ciliary processes are mainly of the β$_2$-subtype (Fig. 47.3)[22,23] Beta-blockers might, however, additionally act on the β$_2$-adrenoceptors present in the ciliary arteries[24] to induce vasoconstriction, which in turn could contribute to the reduction of aqueous humor production.[25] Moreover, an additional effect, via antagonism of noradrenaline released from nerve endings in the proximity of the epithelial cells, can also not be excluded (Fig. 47.4). Further complicating the picture is the fact that the β$_2$-adrenoceptor binding capacity of β-blockers may not completely account for their therapeutic efficacy, as the β$_1$-selective β-blocker betaxolol is an effective IOP-lowering agent as well. Although the IOP-lowering efficacy of betaxolol might be due to greater betaxolol concentrations at the adrenoceptors making up for its lower β$_2$-adrenoceptor binding capacity, this hypothesis has not been fully substantiated in the literature.[26]

Part of the effects of the drugs may even be attributable to properties other than β-blockade (see Fig. 47.3). Because calcium (Ca^{2+}) channel blockers have been shown to have IOP-lowering effects,[27] the Ca^{2+} channel blocking activity of β-blockers, and especially that of betaxolol,[28] may be considered from this aspect (see also Direct vascular effects, below). Lastly, serotonergic

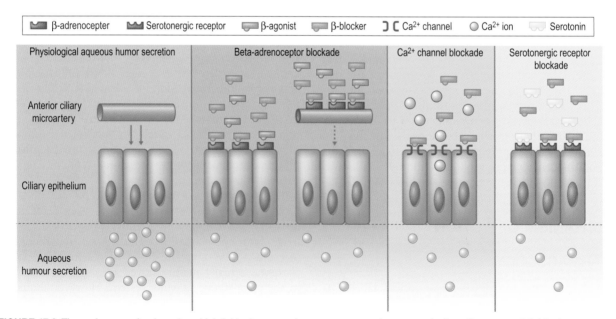

FIGURE 47.3 The various mechanisms by which β-blockers can decrease aqueous humor production. *Green panel*: β-blockers probably mainly exert their β-blocking effect directly at the ciliary epithelium. In addition, however, they could bind to β$_2$-adrenoceptors in the anterior ciliary artery wall, causing vasoconstriction and thus indirectly decreasing aqueous humor secretion. The Ca^{2+} channel blocking properties of β-blockers might add to their IOP-lowering effects (*orange panel*) as well as their ability to bind to serotonergic receptors (*yellow panel*).

receptors of the 5-HT$_{1A}$ type in the ciliary epithelium might be partly involved in the IOP-lowering effect of β-blockers.[29]

OTHER THERAPEUTIC EFFECTS

Glaucoma medications might further protect against visual disability through mechanisms other than IOP

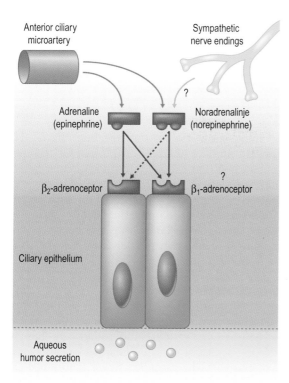

FIGURE 47.4 The possible adrenergic pathways inhibited by β-blockers. The general view is that β-blockers mainly interact with β$_2$-adrenoceptors on the ciliary epithelial cells, thus antagonizing the effects of circulating adrenaline. In addition, however, part of their IOP-lowering effect may be due to their β$_1$-adrenoceptor blocking capacity. Antagonism of noradrenaline released from sympathetic nerve endings in the proximity of the epithelial cells might play a role as well.

reduction. In recent years, attention has turned to the prevention of retinal cell loss by directly targeting (1) retinal and optic nerve blood vessels and/or (2) retinal neurons. In this respect, β-blockers should be evaluated for their possible vasoactivity and neuronal effects in the posterior portion of the eye.

Vascular effects in the posterior eye segment

Reduced blood flow in the back of the eye has been identified as a risk factor in the development of glaucoma.[30] This is probably all the more so in cases of normal-tension glaucoma where a clear association with vascular factors is found.[30]

Presence or absence of functional β-adrenoceptors

First of all, the question arises whether β-blockers might have any harmful vascular effects in the back of the eye. In general, β$_2$-adrenoceptor stimulation causes vasodilatation, whereas α$_1$-adrenoceptor stimulation causes vasoconstriction. Beta-blockers can induce vasoconstriction since during β$_2$-adrenoceptor blockade, α$_1$-mediated effects of endogenous adrenergics are no longer opposed (Fig. 47.5). Thus, it has widely been assumed that β-blockers reaching the posterior eye segment after topical application might, to some extent, cause vasoconstriction and negatively affect ocular blood flow. However, in vitro evidence shows that not enough functional β-adrenoceptors are present in the posterior ocular vasculature to mediate such effects. The *small vessel myograph* used in all these studies allows highly precise measurements of drug effects on isolated segments of microvessels, while conditions in the organ bath are perfectly controlled (Fig. 47.6).[31] Selective β-adrenergic agonists consistently failed to induce significant relaxation (i.e. vasodilatation) in bovine retinal, choroidal, short posterior ciliary, and ophthalmic artery alike.[24,31] Similar results were obtained in porcine and feline tissues, and a few experiments done on human arteries were also in line with this.[24,32] Thus, β-blockers should not be expected to have adverse vasoconstrictor effects in the back of

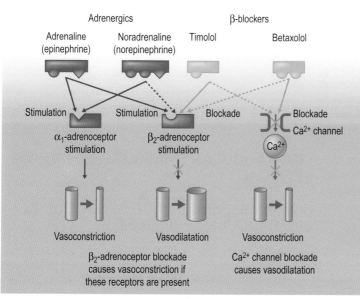

FIGURE 47.5 The vascular effects of adrenergics and β-blockers. Beta-blockers cause vasoconstriction from unopposed α$_1$-adrenergic vasoconstrictor effects only if functional β-adrenoceptors are present. As this appears not to be the case in much of the posterior ocular vasculature, β-blockers probably have no adverse effects on ocular blood flow through their β-adrenoceptor blocking capacity. On the other hand, they can have direct vasodilator effects via their Ca^{2+} channel blocking activity. Betaxolol is the most potent Ca^{2+} channel blocker of all topical β-blockers.

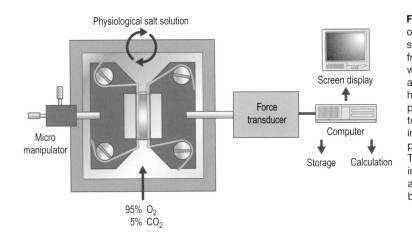

FIGURE 47.6 The small vessel myograph, top view of the organ bath, and experimental set-up. Ring segments of posterior ocular arteries are dissected free under a microscope, threaded on two thin wires (that usually have a diameter of only 40 μm) and mounted with these wires on two specimen holders. Because the holders are kept at a fixed position, the smooth muscle cells are not allowed to shorten when they contract. They develop force instead. Connection to a force transducer allows precise measurements of this force development. Thus, it is possible to directly observe and quantify in a highly precise manner the effects of drugs added to the physiological salt solution in the organ bath, under perfectly controlled conditions.

the eye through their β-adrenoceptor blocking activity, because such receptors are too few in number to affect vascular tone. Obviously, this holds true for all β-blockers. In the absence of a significant number of β-adrenoceptors, it is not important that the β-blocker has intrinsic sympathomimetic activity (carteolol), or that it might be metabolized in the anterior portion of the eye, thus diminishing diffusion into the posterior eye segment (levobunolol), or that it is β_1-selective (betaxolol).

The absence of functional β-adrenoceptors may well explain the highly conflicting results obtained with the in vivo studies of blood flow that are much less accurate than the in vitro technique described here.

Direct vascular effects In vitro studies have consistently demonstrated that β-blockers can act as vasodilators in retinal and posterior ciliary artery through their Ca^{2+} channel blocking activity. This activity is independent of a β-adrenoceptor mechanism, the site of action probably being the L-type voltage-gated Ca^{2+} channels in the cell membrane (see Fig. 47.5).[28,32–34] Propranolol (the standard β-blocker) and betaxolol both have significant Ca^{2+} channel blocking activity that is more powerful than that of timolol or carteolol.

Practically all research into possible clinically relevant implications of this activity has thus been directed to betaxolol. Although animal studies have been available for some time,[35] the question whether the drug could reach the back of the eye of glaucoma patients in concentrations high enough to exert a biological effect has only recently been answered positively.[36] Demonstration of in vivo effects of betaxolol, or any other glaucoma medication, on blood flow in the human eye, however, remains, to date a more difficult step to take. This is despite the many efforts that have been made and the abundant literature available on the subject. The accuracy and sensitivity of in vivo techniques remain limited up to now because of the small size of the vessels and vascular beds in question. Furthermore, it is impossible to perform such studies under controlled conditions. A major problem in this regard is the indirect effects on blood flow of the

drug under study via its IOP-lowering effects. Thus, although a number of studies using various techniques have indicated that betaxolol improves ocular hemodynamics, caution in the interpretation of these results is required.[37] Improved visual function with betaxolol compared to timolol, despite the slightly greater IOP-lowering effects of the latter drug, has been reported.[38] It remains difficult, however, to draw definite conclusions from these studies.

Neuroprotection Neuroprotection involves slowing down or preventing retinal cell death, mainly that of the ganglion cells. Again, most research into the possible neuroprotective effects of β-blockers has been directed to betaxolol. Its Ca^{2+} channel blocking activity demonstrated by the vascular studies mentioned above may indeed confer a neuroprotective effect by antagonism of the excitotoxic damage mediated by Ca^{2+} overload in neurons. Support for this comes from in vitro studies, which, in addition, showed that betaxolol can reduce Na^+ influx into neurons, the latter effect probably adding to its neuroprotective effects.[39] Furthermore, betaxolol appears to be an efficient neuroprotective agent in the in vivo situation against retinal ischemia in various animal models.[35] At present, however, there are no human data on the subject.

INDICATIONS

Beta-blockers are effective IOP-lowering agents in patients with ocular hypertension and they can be used in the treatment of all types of glaucoma.

INTRAOCULAR PRESSURE-LOWERING EFFICACY

AVERAGE PERCENTAGE REDUCTION IN INTRAOCULAR PRESSURE

Timolol exerts most of its IOP-lowering effects within 2 weeks of initiation of therapy.[40] The average percentage reduction in IOP induced by timolol 0.5% twice daily varies between clinical trials and is between 19%[10] and 29%.[41] A meta-analysis of 11 randomized, controlled trials revealed that the mean percentage reduction in IOP from baseline produced by timolol was 26.9% (SE, 3.4%) at 3 months.[42] This is in line with another recent meta-analysis comparing the average effects of most topical medications.[43] In this analysis, timolol reduced IOP by 27% at peak moment and 26% at through moment (at time of maximal and minimal drug effect, respectively). Timolol was the most effective IOP-lowering agent after the prostaglandin analogues. The latter drugs in this analysis induced IOP reductions of 31% to 33% at peak moment and 28% to 29% at through moment.

Timolol is as effective in reducing IOP as the other nonselective β-blockers levobunolol,[44] carteolol,[45] and metipranolol.[46] It is more potent than the β_1-selective drug betaxolol in most studies,[47] although in some, the two drugs were comparable with regard to efficacy in lowering IOP.[41]

TWENTY-FOUR-HOUR INTRAOCULAR PRESSURE CONTROL

Timolol appears to be less effective during the nighttime hours.[48,49] In the first place, β-blockers may have little inhibitory effect on nocturnal aqueous humor secretion because this secretion is already reduced as part of the diurnal cycle.[50] Moreover, sympathetic (adrenergic) activity is lower at night.[51] Because β-blockers act by competing with endogenous adrenergics for β-adrenoceptors, this may add to their lower efficacy during the nocturnal period. Incidentally, it has been hypothesized that the physiological reduced nocturnal aqueous humor secretion is due to the lower sympathetic activity at night.

NONRESPONDER RATE

The nonresponder rate depends on the definition of nonresponse. If patients are considered nonresponders when IOP reduction achieved by timolol is less than 6 mmHg, or measured IOP remains above 20 mmHg with timolol, the nonresponder rate is about 20%.[52]

LONG-TERM DRIFT

Long-term drift, that is, an increase in IOP after long-term application of timolol, may be attributable in part to progression of the glaucomatous disease.[53] A small loss of efficacy might be partly responsible for this phenomenon, as aqueous humor flow is somewhat higher after a year's treatment than it had been after a week.[54] In general, IOP control with timolol can be regarded as well maintained over several years.

WASHOUT PERIOD

If timolol is discontinued after long-term application, its effects will remain for at least 2 weeks[53,55] and the same holds true for levobunolol.[56] Discontinuation for up to 4 weeks may be required for complete disappearance of timolol effect.[55] Timolol appears to concentrate mainly in pigmented ocular tissues, where the drug is only slowly released and can still be present 42 days after its withdrawal.[57]

SIDE EFFECTS AND CONTRAINDICATIONS

LOCAL SIDE EFFECTS

There are no significant local side effects associated with the use of topical β-blockers. The drugs are generally well tolerated locally as punctuate keratopathy, dry eyes, and allergic reactions occur rarely.[58] As with other classes of glaucoma medications, some problems may arise from the benzalkonium chloride used as the preservative agent in the ophthalmic solutions (see Preservative-Free Preparations, above).

SYSTEMIC SIDE EFFECTS

Topical β-blockers are generally well tolerated. They undergo systemic absorption, however, and can thus have systemic side effects. Because topically applied drugs are directly absorbed into the venous circulation, they bypass hepatic metabolism. Therefore, the risk of systemic side effects is higher compared to the same drug dose taken orally.

Systemic absorption can be reduced by nasolacrimal duct occlusion (achieved by applying fingertip pressure to the nasal corner of the eye) and/or eyelid closure at the very least for 1 minute after the drop is instilled. A study reports that patients taking timolol showed reduced plasma levels by more than 60% with either method.[59] The use of the lowest doses of β-blockers, of timolol in gel-forming solution, or applying timolol or levobunolol ophthalmic solutions once daily instead of twice, might further reduce the risk of systemic side effects in patients with comorbidity (see Drug concentrations and Gel-Forming Solutions, above).

It is important to note that β-blockers are the class of glaucoma medications with which we have had the most experience. Moreover, it is the only class that is also widely used as oral medicine in the treatment of a wide variety of internal (mainly cardiovascular) disorders. This yields the important advantage over newer drugs in that side effects have long been identified and consequently can mostly be avoided by careful patient selection.

Respiratory effects The most serious side effects of β-blockers are the exacerbation of chronic obstructive airways disease and the precipitation of bronchospasm in some patients.[60] Beta$_2$-adrenoceptor blockade in bronchi and bronchioles can result in increased airway resistance from unopposed parasympathetic activity.

In patients (even older ones) without reactive airway disease, β-blockers should not worsen pulmonary function.[61,62] The drugs are, however, potentially dangerous in patients with existing respiratory disease. Patients with asthma or other bronchospastic conditions, or with chronic obstructive pulmonary disease (that is, chronic bronchitis or emphysema) even of mild severity, should not receive β-blockers.

Because these adverse respiratory effects are related to the β2-adrenoceptor blocking activity of the drugs, betaxolol (which is β1-selective) seems relatively free of it.[63] This may, however, be dose related and caution should nevertheless be exercised in patients with respiratory comorbidity.

Cardiovascular effects

Cardiac conduction defects Cardiac conduction defects are another category of strong contraindications to β-blocker therapy. The drugs can, through their β1-adrenoceptor blocking activity, elicit potentially dangerous alterations in heart rate and rhythm in patients with existing sinus bradycardia or arrhythmias (that is, second- or third-degree atrioventricular block).[60,62] Development of symptomatic bradycardia on topical β-blockers likely indicates underlying cardiac conduction defects.[62] In otherwise healthy patients, effects such as minor reduction in resting heart rate[64] or inhibition of exercise-induced tachycardia give little cause for concern. Betaxolol appears to have fewer effects on heart rate than timolol,[63] probably due to its pharmacokinetic properties.[26] The drug is more protein bound in blood plasma than timolol and is thus less available to the cardiac β1-adrenoceptors.

Heart failure Heart failure has traditionally been regarded as another contraindication for β-blockers[65,66] related to their β1-adrenoceptor blocking (i.e. depressant) effects on heart muscle. This, however, clearly needs reconsideration as in recent times cardiologists make increasingly more use of β-blockers in the treatment of this disease. It appears that contrary to long-held beliefs, systemic administration of β-blockers does not aggravate heart failure and is indeed effective for the management of the disease, even in the elderly.[62,66-68] Patients with heart failure have decreased cardiac output, and as a consequence increased sympathetic nervous system activity together with a greater release of adrenergics (Fig. 47.7). The resulting activation of cardiac β1-adrenoceptors leads to increased heart rate and contractility. This compensatory mechanism is primarily directed at restoring cardiac output. But over time it can lead to overexcitation of the heart, worsening of the disease, and sudden arrhythmic death. Beta-blockers can inhibit this downward spiral. They have been shown to reduce morbidity and mortality of patients with mild, moderate, and severe heart failure. The impressive survival data collected from several well-designed large randomized trials have made β-blockers a component of standard heart failure therapy.[66-68] In this regard β-blockers are also widely used to reduce the risk of reinfarction and mortality in both the immediate and long term after myocardial infarction.[69]

Miscellaneous Because oral β-blockers are commonly used in the treatment of arterial hypertension, the effects of topical β-blockers on blood pressure have been studied. It appears that topical β-blockers have a tendency to slightly decrease blood pressure, but they have no clinically meaningful effect on it.[64,70]

Nonselective β-blockers (timolol more so than carteolol) may unfavorably affect the lipid profile by reducing high-density lipoprotein (HDL) cholesterol levels in plasma.[45] There are currently, however, no indications that this affects the clinical outcome of the patient (see also Does the intrinsic sympathomimetic activity of carteolol matter?, below).

Negative effects on the peripheral circulation, such as worsening of Raynaud's phenomenon[71] or claudication, have sporadically been reported with the use of topical β-blockers. The drugs can indeed induce vasoconstriction from unopposed α1-mediated vasoconstrictor effects of endogenous adrenergics (see Presence or absence of functional β-adrenoceptors, above, and Fig. 47.5). The role of β-blockers in the induction of Raynaud's phenomenon has been questioned in the medical literature.[72] Although there are reports of digital vasospastic phenomena resulting from the use of oral β-blockers, well-designed studies could not corroborate this. For example, a study could not detect adverse effects after intravenous injection of the β-blocker propranolol on the peripheral circulation in patients with Raynaud's phenomenon or arterial hypertension. Neither could it demonstrate a favorable effect of β1-selectivity or ISA (see below) in comparison to the nonselective β-blocker propranolol without ISA.[73]

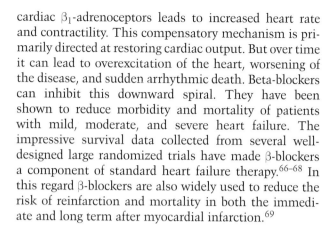

FIGURE 47.7 The vicious circle of heart failure that can be broken with β-blockers. In the past decade, concomitant sympathetic activation became recognized and validated as a self-perpetuating influence on chronic heart failure and progressive adverse events. This activation thus became an additional therapeutic target and led to the integration of β-blockade as a critical component of standard therapy for heart failure.

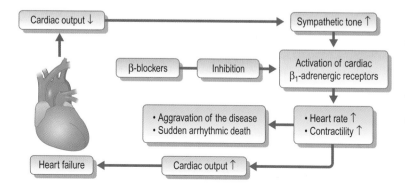

Interestingly, a low dosage of β-blockers has even been proposed as a therapeutic approach to Raynaud's disease, the beneficial effects having been attributed to a presynaptic β-adrenoceptor blockade effect.[74]

Does the intrinsic sympathomimetic activity of carteolol matter? Carteolol, which has intrinsic sympathomimetic activity (ISA; see Pharmacology, above) has theoretically less systemic β-blockade effect and thus might have cardiovascular tolerability profiles better than the other nonselective β-blockers.[45,75] However, the theoretical advantages of ISA have not been fully substantiated in the ophthalmologic literature for topically applied carteolol;[63] neither have they been so in the medical literature for systemically administered β-blockers with potent ISA such as pindolol. Carteolol can be preferably prescribed in patients with unfavorable lipid profiles as it does not alter the lipid profile to the same extent as timolol,[45] but whether this confers a therapeutic advantage remains, to date, an open question.

Other systemic side effects Depression, fatigue, anxiety, confusion, sexual dysfunction, and impaired neuromuscular transmission have occasionally been reported with the use of topical β-blockers.[76] An evidence-based assessment could, however, not identify studies supporting the development of most of these adverse events, neither with systemic nor with topically applied β-blockers.[62] According to this study, wide acceptance of such traditionally purported side effects has been largely due to propagation of isolated case reports and short series.

In agreement with this, a recent extensive study of the prevalence of depression among glaucoma patients showed that the use of topical β-blockers does not increase the risk of this condition.[77] Similarly, in the medical literature, the methodological quality of studies associating the use of systemic β-blockers and depression has been weak. A recent well-designed study could not demonstrate such association in postmyocardial infarction patients.[78]

PREGNANCY AND NURSING MOTHERS

Timolol should be used with caution by pregnant women, as fetal bradycardia and cardiac arrhythmia have been reported.[79] Furthermore, much higher concentrations of timolol can be retrieved in the milk of nursing mothers than in blood plasma.[80] Therefore, nursing should be avoided during timolol therapy.

DRUG INTERACTIONS

INTERACTIONS WITH SYSTEMICALLY ADMINISTERED DRUGS

Effects of orally administered β-blockers on the intraocular pressure-lowering efficacy of topical β-blockers Topical β-blockers can be less efficacious in patients on concomitant oral β-blocker therapy, because β-blockers administered systemically can lower IOP as well.[81]

Potentially hazardous combinations There are few reports of clinically important interactions with systemic drugs. The combinations that can potentially be hazardous can be predicted on the basis of the known contraindications to β-blocker therapy (see Systemic Side Effects, above). In practice, caution is required in patients who take medicine that can elicit bradycardia or cardiac arrhythmia. Topical β-blockers may augment these effects and might even cause cardiac arrest. Because of the narrow therapeutic index of antiarrhythmic agents, potential drug interactions with other medications such as β-blockers are indeed of major clinical importance. These agents mainly include cardiac glycosides (digitalis, digoxin), Na^+ channel blockers (quinidine, procainamide, lidocaine), and the Ca^{2+} channel blockers verapamil and diltiazem.[82] If a Ca^{2+} channel blocker needs to be used concomitantly with a topical β-blocker, the one used should have little effect on heart rate or conduction.

Beta-blockers can mask the symptoms of hypoglycemia in diabetics on hypoglycemic therapy.[62,75] When blood glucose levels fall below a critical level, adrenaline is released that acts on the β_2-adrenoceptor in the liver to release glucose in the blood (see Pharmacology, above). Beta-blockers inhibit this counter-regulation and in addition mask adrenaline-mediated warning signs of imminent hypoglycemia such as tachycardia. This does not, however, preclude the use of β-blockers in these patients and rather reinforces the need for good control of the disease itself.

Finally, one should remember that all of the side effects of β-blockers may be exacerbated with the concomitant use of topical and systemic β-blockers.

INTERACTIONS WITH TOPICAL DRUGS – THE COMBINATION PRODUCTS

Effects of topical drugs on the intraocular pressure-lowering efficacy of β-blockers The combined action of β-blockers with epinephrine (adrenaline) or dipivefrin is poor. The latter drugs belong to an old class of glaucoma medications, the nonselective α/β-adrenergic agonists, the use of which has become marginal.

Beta-blockers are effective and well tolerated when used in combination with any other glaucoma medication. Further IOP reductions are achieved by an additive effect: that is, by summation rather than synergy. In recent years, various fixed-combination products have been developed, potential benefits of which include convenience (fewer bottles and drops per day) and thus improved compliance, less application of the preservative benzalkonium chloride, cost savings based on fewer co-payments, and elimination of potential washout effects. The first combination products contained the parasympathetic drug pilocarpine, examples of which are Timpilo® or Normoglaucon®, i.e. combinations with timolol or metipranolol, respectively. As pilocarpine acts by a different mechanism (increasing trabecular outflow), the fixed combination with a β-blocker manifests additive effects on IOP. The prescription rates have obviously been in constant decline since the arrival of the newer agents, as the pilocarpine in the solution is often not well tolerated locally.

It is striking that all modern combination products contain timolol even when the manufacturer offers another topical β-blocker on the market (see Table 47.4). This development demonstrates the major therapeutic relevance of the drug, and it became possible after the expiration of the patent for timolol. The first modern product was Cosopt®, the fixed combination with the topical carbonic anhydrase inhibitor (CAI) dorzolamide. Timolol and dorzolamide are almost completely additive in their effects both on aqueous humor flow and on IOP, despite the fact that both drugs act by decreased aqueous humor production.[83] Consistent effects were observed in the 1980s with timolol and the oral CAI acetazolamide (Diamox®).[84]

In the past few years, fixed combinations with the α_2-adrenergic agonist brimonidine (Combigan®) and all of the prostaglandin analogues (Xalacom®, DuoTrav®, and Ganfort®) have become available (see Table 47.4).

All of these combination products work better than either constituent used alone, and there are no further safety issues with the combination product versus monotherapy. Xalacom®, however, is available worldwide but has not been approved by the FDA for use in the USA, because this combination was judged to have only modest additional efficacy over latanoprost alone.[85] Possible FDA approval for the newer products DuoTrav and Ganfort is still pending.

Effects of timolol on local tolerance of topical glaucoma medications
An unexpected finding with various combination products is that the timolol in the solution seems to protect some patients from local intolerance of the other constituent. Although there are no studies available corroborating (or contradicting) this, it is the strong impression of many an ophthalmologist that Cosopt® is better tolerated than Trusopt® (dorzolamide alone) in terms of stinging, conjunctival hyperemia, or ocular allergy. The same appears to hold true for Combigan® versus Alphagan® (brimonidine alone).[86] Moreover, results of a clinical trial indicate that Ganfort® has a superior local tolerability profile versus Lumigan® (bimatoprost monotherapy), as it induced 40% less conjunctival hyperemia.[87] Any explanations for these beneficial timolol effects are speculative at this time.

SPOTLIGHT: BETA-BLOCKERS

Tony Realini and TJ Zimmerman

Consider the history of medical therapy for glaucoma prior to 1978. Pilocarpine, extracted from *Pilocarpus jaborandi* (a flowering shrub native to South America), was first used to lower intraocular pressure in 1876. Within 1 year, the parasympathomimetic class of intraocular pressure (IOP)-lowering drugs expanded with the addition of physostigmine (derived from the bean of a flowering vine native to the Calabar region of Nigeria). Over the next 100 years, we gained two additional drug classes: the sympathomimetics and the systemic carbonic anhydrase inhibitors (CIAs). In 1977, first-line therapy for IOP reduction was pilocarpine dosed four times daily (with its attendant miosis), and maximal medical therapy consisted of pilocarpine, epinephrine or its prodrug dipivifrin, and an oral carbonic anhydrase inhibitor.

In this historical context, it is no wonder that the ophthalmology community greeted timolol's introduction in 1978 with a red-carpet welcome. Here was a drug offering both excellent IOP reduction and a more patient-friendly twice-daily (once in some patients!) dosing regimen. True, timolol had a long list of potential systemic side effects, but it was much better tolerated than the systemic CAIs and did not cause the pesky miosis that diminished quality of vision and made cataract surgery so challenging in patients using pilocarpine. Timolol rapidly became the first-line drug of choice for glaucoma management. As a testament to the benefits of β-blockers for glaucoma, four additional ophthalmic β-blockers were introduced into the United States marketplace in the 12 years following timolol's debut.

The development of timolol for ophthalmic use was a watershed moment that marked the beginning of the modern era of glaucoma pharmacology. Within just a few short years in the mid-1990s, two old drug classes became new again.

Carbonic anhydrase inhibitors moved from the drug of last resort to the preferred second-line class with the development of topical formulations. Apraclonidine and brimonidine elevated the sympathomimetic class to a higher adjunctive position in the stepped glaucoma treatment algorithm. And in 1996 came a second watershed moment in glaucoma drug development: the introduction of topical prostaglandins, which quickly and rightfully deposed β-blockers as preferred first-line therapy based on their superior safety profile and comparable to superior IOP-lowering efficacy.

Now, a decade later, prostaglandins still reign supreme as the preferred first-line therapy for IOP reduction. No new drug classes have emerged in nearly a dozen years. Interestingly, β-blockers are enjoying renewed relevance as components in various fixed combinations of IOP-lowering medications. Their once-daily dosing and complementary mechanism of action make them ideal partners for prostaglandins; however, the meager additional IOP reduction over prostaglandin monotherapy may not justify the additional β-blocker side effects in a fixed combination. These prostaglandin/β-blocker fixed combinations are available in several international markets, but to date, none has achieved regulatory approval in the United States.

In summary, timolol was the right drug at the right time in glaucoma. Beta-blockers offer excellent efficacy and safety with well-established contraindications. The superior safety profile of the prostaglandins in no way diminishes the fact that β-blockers are still good drugs in appropriately screened patients. While no longer the preferred first-line drug class, β-blockers will continue to be an important part of the ophthalmologist's pharmamentarium for the foreseeable future.

SPOTLIGHT: BETA-BLOCKERS

Josef Flammer

Beta-blockers (BBs) have been used systemically since 1964 and locally on the eye since 1978. BBs are powerful intraocular pressure (IOP)-lowering drugs even though they are less potent than prostaglandin analogues. They can be combined with any other glaucoma drug. The combination of BBs with carbonic anhydrase inhibitors, for example, is as effective as prostaglandin analogues.

Besides their IOP-lowering capacity, all β-blockers, in particular betaxolol, have a calcium channel blocking activity, which, in turn, stabilizes ocular perfusion[1] and protects neuronal cells.[2] Unfortunately, clinical studies evaluating these effects of BBs are limited. Glaucoma does not occur only in wealthy countries. Beta-blockers have a good 'value for many' and therefore should remain in the forefront of glaucoma drugs.

In the past, the main concerns regarding BBs were related to their side effects. These effects, however, were often rather overemphasized. The local tolerability is, on the average, good and can be further improved by using preservative-free preparations. BBs are systemically absorbed. When treating with BBs, we should therefore keep in mind the systemic contraindications (e.g. bronchial asthma). Recent studies in internal medicine and cardiology have revealed, however, that a systemic β-blockade is not only harmless for most subjects but even beneficial for most patients, including those with heart failure,[3] diabetes mellitus, migraine, arterial hypertension, and hypotension,[4] etc. We further learned that the frequency of many side effects, such as depression or sexual dysfunction, are in the same range as for placebo controls.[5]

In summary, β-blockers are potent, safe, and economical glaucoma drugs and should therefore not automatically be replaced with new classes of drugs.

References

1. Dong Y, Ishikawa H, Wu Y, et al. Effect and mechanism of betaxolol and timolol on vascular relaxation in isolated rabbit ciliary artery. Jpn J Ophthalmol 2006; 50:504–508.
2. Osborne NN, Wood JP, Chidlow G. Invited review: neuroprotective properties of certain beta-adrenoceptor antagonists used for the treatment of glaucoma. J Ocul Pharmacol Ther 2005; 21:175–181.
3. Gottlieb SS, McCarter RJ, Vogel RA. Effect of beta-blockade on mortality among high-risk and low risk patients after myocardial infarction. N Engl J Med 1998; 339:489–497.
4. Cleophas TJ, Grabowsky I, Niemeyer MG, et al. Paradoxical pressor effects of beta-blockers in standing elderly patients with mild hypertension: a beneficial side effect. Circulation 2002; 105:1669–1671.
5. Ko DT, Hebert PR, Coffey CS, et al. Beta-blocker therapy and symptoms of depression, fatigue, and sexual dysfunction. JAMA 2002; 288:351–357.

Summary

Beta-blockers have been around for three decades and have been the top prescribing drug class for a very long time. In view of the broad range of glaucoma medications currently available, we may never again use a particular drug class on such a scale. The experience we have had with the β-blockers may thus well remain unmatched. Furthermore, β-blockers are the only drugs used in the treatment of glaucoma that are also widely prescribed as oral medicine to treat a variety of internal (mainly cardiovascular) disorders. Thus, their potentially dangerous side effects have long been recognized. Ophthalmologists should be able to identify the vast majority of patients with cardiopulmonary contraindications. With careful patient selection, β-blockers do have a favorable tolerability profile. We may have been rather too cautious as in the past decade, it has become evident that heart failure can no longer be regarded as a contraindication to β-blocker therapy.

Beta-blockers have various strengths. The IOP-lowering efficacy of timolol has been surpassed only by the prostaglandin analogues. The drug can be combined with any of the newer glaucoma medications. Beta-blockers can be used in the treatment of all types of glaucoma. And last but not least, their local tolerability profile is better than that of most, if not all, other drug classes.

REFERENCES

1. Phillips CI, Howitt G, Rowlands DJ. Propranolol as ocular hypotensive agent. Br J Ophthalmol 1967; 51: 222–226.
2. Zimmerman TJ, Kaufman HE, Timolo S. A beta-adrenergic blocking agent for the treatment of glaucoma. Arch Ophthalmol 1977; 95:601–604.
3. Novack GD. Ophthalmic beta-blockers since timolol. Surv Ophthalmol 1987; 31:307–327.
4. Rakofsky SI, Lazar M, Almog Y, et al. Efficacy and safety of once-daily levobunolol for glaucoma therapy. Can J Ophthalmol 1989; 24:2–6.
5. Silverstone D, Zimmerman T, Choplin N, et al. Evaluation of once-daily levobunolol 0.25% and timolol 0.25% therapy for increased intraocular pressure. Am J Ophthalmol 1991; 112:56–60.
6. Derick RJ, Robin AL, Tielsch J, et al. Once-daily versus twice-daily levobunolol (0.5%) therapy. A crossover study. Ophthalmology 1992; 99:424–429.
7. Letchinger SL, Frohlichstein D, Glieser DK, et al. Can the concentration of timolol or the frequency of its administration be reduced? Ophthalmology 1993; 100:1259–1262.
8. Denis P, Andrew R, Wells D, et al. A comparison of morning and evening instillation of a combination travoprost 0.004%/timolol 0.5% ophthalmic solution. Eur J Ophthalmol 2006; 16:407–415.
9. Konstas AG, Nakos E, Tersis I, et al. A comparison of once-daily morning vs evening dosing of concomitant latanoprost/timolol. Am J Ophthalmol 2002; 133:753–757.
10. Mills KB. Blind randomised non-crossover long-term trial comparing topical timolol 0.25% with timolol 0.5% in the

treatment of simple chronic glaucoma. Br J Ophthalmol 1983; 67:216–219.

11. Battershill PE, Sorkin EM. Ocular metipranolol. A preliminary review of its pharmacodynamic and pharmacokinetic properties, and therapeutic efficacy in glaucoma and ocular hypertension. Drugs 1988; 36:601–615.

12. Serle JB, Lustgarten JS, Podos SM. A clinical trial of metipranolol, a noncardioselective beta-adrenergic antagonist, in ocular hypertension. Am J Ophthalmol 1991; 112:302–307.

13. Long DA, Johns GE, Mullen RS, et al. Levobunolol and betaxolol. A double-masked controlled comparison of efficacy and safety in patients with elevated intraocular pressure. Ophthalmology 1988; 95:735–741.

14. Weinreb RN, Caldwell DR, Goode SM, et al. A double-masked three-month comparison between 0.25% betaxolol suspension and 0.5% betaxolol ophthalmic solution. Am J Ophthalmol 1990; 110:189–192.

15. Stewart WC, Shields MB, Allen RC, et al. A 3-month comparison of 1% and 2% carteolol and 0.5% timolol in open-angle glaucoma. Graefe's Arch Clin Exp Ophthalmol 1991; 229:258–261.

16. Shedden A, Laurence J, Tipping R. Timoptic-XE 0.5% Study Group. Efficacy and tolerability of timolol maleate ophthalmic gel-forming solution versus timolol ophthalmic solution in adults with open-angle glaucoma or ocular hypertension: a six-month, double-masked, multicenter study. Clin Ther 2001; 23:440–450.

17. Trinquand C, Romanet JP, Nordmann JP, Allaire C; Groupe d'etude. [Efficacy and safety of long-acting carteolol 1% once daily. A double-masked, randomized study]. J Fr Ophtalmol 2003; 26:131–136.

18. Uusitalo H, Nino J, Tahvanainen K, et al. Efficacy and systemic side-effects of topical 0.5% timolol aqueous solution and 0.1% timolol hydrogel. Acta Ophthalmol Scand 2005; 83:723–728.

19. Baudouin C, Hamard P, Liang H. Conjunctival epithelial cell expression of interleukins and inflammatory markers in glaucoma patients treated over the long term. Ophthalmology 2004; 111:2186–2192.

20. Baudouin C. Side effects of antiglaucomatous drugs on the ocular surface. Curr Opin Ophthalmol 1996; 7:80–86.

21. Coakes RL, Brubaker RF. The mechanism of timolol in lowering intraocular pressure in the normal eye. Arch Ophthalmol 1978; 96:2045–2048.

22. Bromberg BB, Gregory DS, Sears ML. Beta-adrenergic receptors in ciliary processes of the rabbit. Invest Ophthalmol Vis Sci 1980; 19:203–207.

23. Nathanson JA. Human ciliary process adrenergic receptor: pharmacological characterization. Invest Ophthalmol Vis Sci 1981; 21:798–804.

24. Nyborg NC, Nielsen PJ. Beta-adrenergic receptors regulating vascular smooth muscle tone are only localized to the intraocular segment of the long posterior ciliary artery in bovine eye. Surv Ophthalmol 1995; 39:S66–S75.

25. Watanabe K, Chiou GC. Action mechanism of timolol to lower the intraocular pressure in rabbits. Ophthalmic Res 1983; 15:160–167.

26. Phan TM, Nguyen KP, Giacomini JC, et al. Ophthalmic beta-blockers: determination of plasma and aqueous humor levels by a radioreceptor assay following multiple doses. J Ocul Pharmacol 1991; 7:243–252.

27. Santafe J, Martinez de Ibarreta MJ, Segarra J, et al. A complex interaction between topical verapamil and timolol on intraocular pressure in conscious rabbits. Naunyn Schmiedebergs Arch Pharmacol 1996; 354:198–204.

28. Hoste AM, Sys SU. Ca^{2+} channel blocking activity of propranolol and betaxolol in isolated bovine retinal microartery. J Cardiovasc Pharmacol 1998; 32:390–396.

29. Osborne NN, Chidlow G. Do beta-adrenoceptors and serotonin 5-HT1A receptors have similar functions in the control of intraocular pressure in the rabbit? Ophthalmologica 1996; 210:308–314.

30. Flammer J, Orgül S, Costa VP, et al. The impact of ocular blood flow in glaucoma. Prog Retin Eye Res 2002; 21:359–393.

31. Hoste AM, Boels PJ, Brutsaert DL, et al. Effect of alpha-1 and beta agonists on contraction of bovine retinal resistance arteries in vitro. Invest Ophthalmol Vis Sci 1989; 30:44–50.

32. Hoste AM. In vitro studies of the effects of beta-adrenergic drugs on retinal and posterior ciliary microarteries. Surv Ophthalmol 1999; 43:S183–S190.

33. Yu DY, Su EN, Cringle SJ, et al. Effect of betaxolol, timolol and nimodipine on human and pig retinal arterioles. Exp Eye Res 1998; 67:73–81.

34. Hester RK, Chen Z, Becker EJ, et al. The direct vascular relaxing action of betaxolol, carteolol and timolol in porcine long posterior ciliary artery. Surv Ophthalmol 1994; 38: S125–S134.

35. Osborne NN, DeSantis L, Bae JH, et al. Topically applied betaxolol attenuates NMDA-induced toxicity to ganglion cells and the effects of ischaemia to the retina. Exp Eye Res 1999; 69:331–342.

36. Hollo G, Whitson JT, Faulkner R, et al. Concentrations of betaxolol in ocular tissues of patients with glaucoma and normal monkeys after 1 month of topical ocular administration. Invest Ophthalmol Vis Sci 2006; 47:235–240.

37. Costa VP, Harris A, Stefansson E, et al. The effects of antiglaucoma and systemic medications on ocular blood flow. Prog Retin Eye Res 2003; 22:769–805.

38. Kaiser HJ, Flammer J, Stumpfig D, et al. Long term visual field follow-up of glaucoma patients treated with beta-blockers. Surv Ophthalmol 1994; 38:S156–S159; discussion S160.

39. Chidlow G, Melena J, Osborne NN. Betaxolol, a beta(1)-adrenoceptor antagonist, reduces Na(+) influx into cortical synaptosomes by direct interaction with Na(+) channels: comparison with other beta-adrenoceptor antagonists. Br J Pharmacol 2000; 130:759–766.

40. Sherwood M, Brandt J; Bimatoprost Study Groups 1 and 2. Six-month comparison of bimatoprost once-daily and twice-daily with timolol twice-daily in patients with elevated intraocular pressure. Surv Ophthalmol 2001; 45:S361–S368.

41. Stewart RH, Kimbrough RL, Ward RL. Betaxolol vs timolol. A six-month double-blind comparison. Arch Ophthalmol 1986; 104:46–48.

42. Zhang WY, Po AL, Dua HS, et al. Meta-analysis of randomised controlled trials comparing latanoprost with timolol in the treatment of patients with open angle glaucoma or ocular hypertension. Br J Ophthalmol 2001; 85:890–983.

43. van der Valk R, Webers C, Schouten J, et al. Intraocular pressure lowering effects of all commonly used glaucoma drugs. Ophthalmology 2005; 112:1177–1185.

44. Boozman FW 3rd, Carriker R, Foerster R, et al. Long-term evaluation of 0.25% levobunolol and timolol for therapy for elevated intraocular pressure. Arch Ophthalmol 1988; 106:614–618.

45. Freedman SF, Freedman NJ, Shields MB, et al. Effects of ocular carteolol and timolol on plasma high-density lipoprotein cholesterol level. Am J Ophthalmol 1993; 116:600–611.

46. Merte HJ, Stryz JR, Mertz M. Comparative studies of initial pressure reduction using 0.3% metipranolol and 0.25% timolol in eyes with wide-angle glaucoma. Klin Monatsbl Augenheilkd 1983; 182:286–289.

47. Allen RC, Hertzmark E, Walker AM, et al. A double-masked comparison of betaxolol vs timolol in the treatment of open-angle glaucoma. Am J Ophthalmol 1986; 101:535–541.

48. Orzalesi N, Rossetti L, Invernizzi T, et al. Effect of timolol, latanoprost, and dorzolamide on circadian IOP in glaucoma or ocular hypertension. Invest Ophthalmol Vis Sci 2000; 41:2566–2573.

49. Liu JH, Kripke DF, Weinreb RN. Comparison of the nocturnal effects of once-daily timolol and latanoprost on intraocular pressure. Am J Ophthalmol 2004; 138:389–395.

50. Reiss GR, Lee DA, Topper JE, et al. Aqueous humor flow during sleep. Invest Ophthalmol Vis Sci 1984; 25:776–778.

51. Prinz PN, Halter J, Benedetti C, et al. Circadian variation of plasma catecholamines in young and old men: relation to rapid eye movement and slow wave sleep. J Clin Endocrinol Metab 1979; 49:300–304.

52. Goldberg I, Cunha-Vaz J, Jakobsen JE, et al. Comparison of topical travoprost eye drops given once daily and timolol 0.5% given twice daily in patients with open-angle glaucoma or ocular hypertension. J Glaucoma 2001; 10:414–422.

53. Steinert RF, Thomas JV, Boger WP 3rd. Long-term drift and continued efficacy after multiyear timolol therapy. Arch Ophthalmol 1981; 99:100–103.

54. Brubaker RF, Nagataki S, Bourne WM. Effect of chronically administered timolol on aqueous humor flow in patients with glaucoma. Ophthalmology 1982; 89:280–283.

55. Schlecht LP, Brubaker RF. The effects of withdrawal of timolol in chronically treated glaucoma patients. Ophthalmology 1988; 95:1212–1216.

56. Hong YJ, Shin DH, Ahn BH, et al. Intraocular pressure after a two-week washout following long-term timolol or levobunolol. J Ocul Pharmacol Ther 1995; 11:107–112.

57. Trope GE, Menon IA, Liu GS, et al. Ocular timolol levels after drug withdrawal: an experimental model. Can J Ophthalmol 1994; 29:217–219.

58. Van Buskirk EM. Adverse reactions from timolol administration. Ophthalmology 1980; 87:447–450.

59. Zimmerman TJ, Kooner KS, Kandarakis AS, et al. Improving the therapeutic index of topically applied ocular drugs. Arch Ophthalmol 1984; 102:551–553.

60. Nelson WL, Fraunfelder FT, Sills JM, et al. Adverse respiratory and cardiovascular events attributed to timolol ophthalmic solution, 1978–1985. Am J Ophthalmol 1986; 102:606–611.

61. Stewart WC, Day DG, Holmes KT, et al. Effect of timolol 0.5% gel and solution on pulmonary function in older glaucoma patients. J Glaucoma 2001; 10:227–232.

62. Lama PJ. Systemic adverse effects of beta-adrenergic blockers: an evidence-based assessment. Am J Ophthalmol 2002; 134:749–760.

63. Diggory P, Cassels-Brown A, Fernandez C. Topical beta-blockade with intrinsic sympathomimetic activity offers no advantage for the respiratory and cardiovascular function of elderly people. Age Ageing 1996; 25:424–428.

64. Berson FG, Cohen HB, Foerster RJ, et al. Levobunolol compared with timolol for the long-term control of elevated intraocular pressure. Arch Ophthalmol 1985; 103:379–382.

65. Sica DA. Pharmacotherapy in congestive heart failure: cardiopulmonary effects of ophthalmically administered beta-blockers. Congest Heart Fail 1999; 5:81–85.

66. Hermann DD. Beta-adrenergic blockade 2002: a pharmacologic odyssey in chronic heart failure. Congest Heart Fail 2002; 8:262–269; 283.

67. Sin DD, McAlister FA. The effects of beta-blockers on morbidity and mortality in a population-based cohort of 11,942 elderly patients with heart failure. Am J Med 2002; 113:650–656.

68. Fowler M. Beta-adrenergic blocking drugs in severe heart failure. Rev Cardiovasc Med 2002; 3:S20–S26.

69. Fonarow GC. Beta-blockers for the post-myocardial infarction patient: current clinical evidence and practical considerations. Rev Cardiovasc Med 2006; 7:1–9.

70. Atkins JM, Pugh BR Jr, Timewell RM. Cardiovascular effects of topical beta-blockers during exercise. Am J Ophthalmol 1985; 99:173–175.

71. Meuche C, Heidrich H, Bleckmann H. Raynaud syndrome following timolol-containing eyedrops. Fortschr Ophthalmol 1990; 87:45–47.

72. Wigley FM. Raynaud's phenomenon. Curr Opin Rheumatol 1993; 5:773–784.

73. Franssen C, Wollersheim H, de Haan A, et al. The influence of different beta-blocking drugs on the peripheral circulation in Raynaud's phenomenon and in hypertension. J Clin Pharmacol 1992; 32:652–659.

74. Brotzu G, Susanna F, Roberto M, et al. Beta-blockers: a new therapeutic approach to Raynaud's disease. Microvasc Res 1987; 33:283–288.

75. Zimmerman TJ. Topical ophthalmic beta blockers: a comparative review. J Ocul Pharmacol 1993; 9:373–384.

76. Munroe WP, Rindone JP, Kershner RM. Systemic side effects associated with the ophthalmic administration of timolol. Drug Intell Clin Pharm 1985; 19:85–89.

77. Kaiserman I, Kaiserman N, Elhayany A, et al. Topical beta-blockers are not associated with an increased risk of treatment for depression. Ophthalmology 2006; 113:1077–1080.

78. van Melle JP, Verbeek DE, van den Berg MP, et al. Beta-blockers and depression after myocardial infarction: a multicenter prospective study. J Am Coll Cardiol 2006; 48:2209–2214.

79. Wagenvoort AM, van Vugt JM, Sobotka M, et al. Topical timolol therapy in pregnancy: is it safe for the fetus? Teratology 1998; 58:258–262.

80. Lustgarten JS, Podos SM. Topical timolol and the nursing mother. Arch Ophthalmol 1983; 101:1381–1382.

81. Schuman JS. Effects of systemic beta-blocker therapy on the efficacy and safety of topical brimonidine and timolol. Brimonidine Study Groups 1 and 2. Ophthalmology 2000; 107:1171–1177.

82. Kinoshita H, Taniguchi T, Nishiguchi M, et al. An autopsy case of combined drug intoxication involving verapamil, metoprolol and digoxin. Forensic Sci Int 2003; 133:107–112.

83. Wayman L, Larsson LI, Maus T, et al. Comparison of dorzolamide and timolol as suppressors of aqueous humor flow in humans. Arch Ophthalmol 1997; 115:1368–1371.

84. Dailey RA, Brubaker RF, Bourne WM. The effects of timolol maleate and acetazolamide on the rate of aqueous formation in normal human subjects. Am J Ophthalmol 1982; 93:232–237.

85. Fechtner RD, Realini T. Fixed combinations of topical glaucoma medications. Curr Opin Ophthalmol 2004; 15:132–135.

86. Sherwood MB, Craven ER, Chou C, et al. Twice-daily 0.2% brimonidine-0.5% timolol fixed-combination therapy vs monotherapy with timolol or brimonidine in patients with glaucoma or ocular hypertension: a 12-month randomized trial. Arch Ophthalmol 2006; 124:1230–1238.

87. Hommer A; Ganfort Investigators Group I. A double-masked, randomized, parallel comparison of a fixed combination of bimatoprost 0.03%/timolol 0.5% with non-fixed combination use in patients with glaucoma or ocular hypertension. Eur J Ophthalmol 2007; 17:53–62.

CHAPTER 48

Carbonic Anhydrase Inhibitors

Gábor Holló

INTRODUCTION

Carbonic anhydrase (CA) is an enzyme which catalyzes the hydration and dehydration of carbon dioxide (Fig. 48.1). CA has many important functions in the body. It is present in the lung, brain, pancreas, liver, gallbladder, muscles, kidney, and red blood cells; and it also serves a number of different functions in the eye.[1,2] CA is, in fact, not a single enzyme but rather several isoenzymes with somewhat different characteristics, distributed in different proportions in the various tissues (Table 48.1). In the eye, CA is a key enzyme in aqueous humor production (Fig. 48.2). Thus, inhibition of its activity in the ciliary processes causes decreased aqueous humor secretion, which in turn leads to lowering of the intraocular pressure (IOP).[2,3] The site of aqueous humor secretion is the nonpigmented ciliary epithelial cell. In these cells two CA isoenzymes (isoenzyme II (CA II) and isoenzyme IV (CA IV)) are the predominant forms of CA. CA II is intracytoplasmic and can be blocked with both topical and systemic carbonic anhydrase inhibitors (CAIs). CA IV is membrane-bound and its activity is not influenced by topical CAIs. Since CA II is an especially active enzyme, in order to achieve a clinically significant IOP decrease it is necessary to achieve an almost total enzyme inhibition (99.9%) in the nonpigmented ciliary epithelial cells.[1,3]

DRUG FORMULATION: SYSTEMIC AND TOPICAL CARBONIC ANHYDRASE INHIBITORS

Five different CAI molecules have been used in clinical practice to reduce elevated IOP in glaucoma (Fig. 48.3). Three of them (acetazolamide, methazolamide,

$$CO_2 + H_2O \leftrightarrow H_2CO_3 \leftrightarrow H^+ + HCO_3^-$$

FIGURE 48.1 The hydration and dehydration of CO_2. Bicarbonate ion (HCO_3^-) secretion catalyzed by carbonic anhydrase (CA) in the nonpigmented ciliary epithelial cells is a key step in aqueous humor production. CA speeds up the process by a factor of 10 000 to 100 000.[1]

TABLE 48.1 Distribution of the CA isoenzymes in the human eye

Anterior segment of the eye	
Corneal endothelium	CA I, CA II
Lens	CA I, CA II
Posterior segment of the eye	
Nonpigmented ciliary epithelial cells	CA II, CA IV
Retinal pigment epithelium	CA II, CA IV
Parafoveal cones	CA II
Müller cells	CA II
Choriocapillaries	CA IV

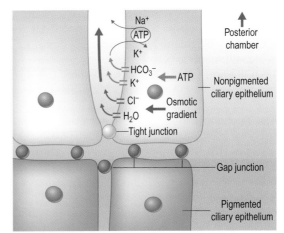

FIGURE 48.2 A simplified representation of the role of bicarbonate secretion in active aqueous humor production. (Adapted from Holló G. Glaucoma: pathophysiology and clinical practice. Budapest: Inthera AG, 1997, with permission.) Sodium and bicarbonate ions are secreted into the eye's posterior chamber via an ATP (energy)-dependent process. Water molecules follow sodium and bicarbonate passively due to the osmotic gradient. Thus, blocking CA reduces the quantity of bicarbonate ions available for the active transport, and consequently the number of the passively following H_2O molecules is also reduced. This decreases the volume of aqueous humor production.[1]

Systemic CAIs

Acetazolamide

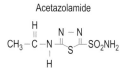

Methazolamide

Topical CAIs

Dorzolamide

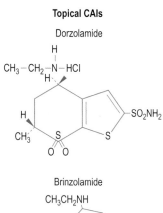

Brinzolamide

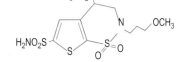

FIGURE 48.3 Molecular structure of the clinically widely used systemic and topical CA inhibitors.

and dichlorphenamide) are administered systemically (orally or intravenously).[2,3] The other two CAIs (brinzolamide and dorzolamide) are applied topically.[2] All CAIs are sulfonamide derivatives.

The IOP-lowering effect of acetazolamide was discovered by Becker in 1954,[4] and since that time it has been used in clinical practice, under various different trade names. Though the IOP reduction achieved with oral or intravenous acetazolamide is especially favorable, long-term use of this molecule is not favored because of its systemic side effects. Since absorption of acetazolamide from the ocular surface is minimal, formulation of this molecule for topical use proved unsuccessful. The topical CAIs were developed in order to provide clinically significant IOP reduction in glaucoma without the systemic side effects of acetazolamide.[2]

SYSTEMIC CARBONIC ANHYDRASE INHIBITORS: ACETAZOLAMIDE, METHAZOLAMIDE, AND DICHLORPHENAMIDE

The most frequently used systemic CAI is acetazolamide. Acetazolamide (e.g. Diamox™) is formulated for oral use (250 mg/tablet) and for intravenous administration

(500 mg/mL). It is also prepared in 500 mg slow-release capsules (Diamox Retard™) that can be given once daily. Methazolamide (Neptazane™) tablets (50 mg) are less frequently used than acetazolamide. The usual daily dosage of methazolamide varies between 100 and 150 mg. Dichlorphenamide (Daranide™) is produced in 50 mg tablets. The daily dosage of this rarely used molecule is 100–150 mg.[3]

TOPICAL CARBONIC ANHYDRASE INHIBITORS: DORZOLAMIDE AND BRINZOLAMIDE

Dorzolamide hydrochloride 2% (Trusopt™, Merck, Whitehouse Station, NJ, USA) was the first topically applied CAI, and was introduced in clinical practice in 1995.[2,5] Ocular penetration of topical dorzolamide (absorption from the ocular surface, transport through the cornea and then via the aqueous humor to the ciliary processes) requires a substance of an ampholytic character, meaning that the molecule contains both a cation and an anion group. The ampholytic character results in ionization in both acidic and basic environments, and also in increased lipid solubility between pH 7 and 8. Dorzolamide is formulated in a solution of acidic pH (pH = 5.6), which is necessary for good ocular absorption but which unfortunately seems to be responsible for the ocular pain frequently reported immediately after instillation. Cosopt™ (Merck, Whitehouse Station, NJ, USA) is the fixed combination of dorzolamide 2% and timolol 0.5%.

Brinzolamide 1% (Azopt™, Alcon, Fort Worth, TX, USA) was introduced in clinical practice in 1998.[2,5,6] For brinzolamide, the problem of ocular absorption has been solved in a different way than in the case of dorzolamide. Brinzolamide is highly lipophilic, which promotes its corneal penetration. In Azopt™ the active ingredient (brinzolamide) is dissolved in a viscous ophthalmic suspension (carbomer), which allows a long contact time with the ocular surface, with close to physiological values for pH (pH = 7.5) and osmolality (300 mOsm/kg). The clinically most important characteristics of the respective formulations of dorzolamide and brinzolamide are summarized in Table 48.2.

MECHANISM OF ACTION

All CAIs inhibit the active aqueous humor secretion by blocking CA in the nonpigmented ciliary epithelial cells in the ciliary processes. Systemic acetazolamide decreases aqueous humor secretion by 30%.[2] When given orally, the IOP decrease is already detectable at 30 minutes after administration, reaches its peak at 2 hours, and lasts at least for 6–8 hours. The washout time of the systemic CAIs is 3 days.[7] Acetazolamide binds to plasma proteins to the extent of 93%, and it is removed from the body via renal excretion without metabolism. The renal excretion of methazolamide is only 25%, and therefore its clinical use is less limited by impaired renal function.[1,3]

In contrast to the relatively nonselective acetazolamide, the topical CAIs (dorzolamide and brinzolamide)

TABLE 48.2 Comparison of the clinically most important characteristics of dorzolamide and brinzolamide

	DORZOLAMIDE	BRINZOLAMIDE
Formulation	Solution	Suspension
Concentration	2%	1%
Number of daily instillations	2–3	2
pH	5.6	7.5
Osmolality	Data not available	300 mOsm/kg
BAC concentration	0.0075%	0.01%
Site of the ocular absorption	Cornea	Cornea
Ocular absorption is due to	Ampholyte character	Lipophilic character
Washout duration	1 week	1 week

BAC, benzalkonium chloride.

TABLE 48.3 Influence of CAIs on the ocular perfusion and visual functions

TYPE OF PERFUSION CHANGE	ALTERATION INDUCED WITH CAI ADMINISTRATION	COMMENT
Arteriovenous transit time	Shortens	Short-term and medium-term observations
Optic nerve head capillary die transit	Accelerates	Short-term observation
Macular capillary perfusion	Hastens	Short-term observation
Pulsatile ocular blood flow	Increases	Short-term observation
Perfusion in the retrobulbar vessels	Inconsistent data	Short-term and medium-term observations
Optic nerve head oxygen tension	Increases	Data only from animal experiments
Optic nerve head capillary perfusion	Increases	Medium-term observation
Choroidal capillary perfusion	Increases	Medium-term observation
Capillary perfusion in the peripapillary retina	Increases or no change is detected	Medium-term observation

have a special affinity for CA II.[2,5,6] Their affinity is approximately 1000 times higher for CA II than for CA I, and approximately 40 times higher for CA II than for CA IV. The decrease of aqueous humor secretion induced by twice-daily instillation of a topical CAI in healthy volunteers is 13% in the daytime and 9% at night.[2] This significant decrease is clinically important since it shows that (in contrast to the topical beta-receptor blockers) topical CAIs work for 24 hours a day. The selectivity of the topical CAIs for CA II is considered to be the explanation for their smaller IOP-lowering efficacy as compared to that achieved by acetazolamide, which acts nonselectively on both CA II and IV isoenzymes.

INFLUENCE OF CARBONIC ANHYDRASE INHIBITORS ON OCULAR BLOOD FLOW AND VISUAL FUNCTIONS

Oral or intravenous acetazolamide and topically applied dorzolamide and brinzolamide have all been reported to shorten the arteriovenous transit time, accelerate macular and optic nerve head capillary dye transit, and increase the ocular pulse amplitude and the pulsatile ocular blood flow, both in glaucoma patients and in normal subjects.[8,9] However, influence on the ophthalmic artery and on the retrobulbar hemodynamics was not consistently found in the different studies.[8,10] In animal models, using intravitreal electrodes, increased optic nerve head oxygen tension was measured following intravenous dorzolamide injection.[11] It is important to emphasize that the above-mentioned perfusion changes are all short-term alterations, and are attributed to the increased CO_2 level caused by the CAIs.[11] The CAI-induced decrease of the pH (acidosis) cannot be considered the cause of the altered ocular perfusion.[8,11] The increase of intraocular perfusion induced by dorzolamide is maintained when dorzolamide is applied in combination with timolol (dorzalomide/timolol fixed combination).[8,12]

The above-mentioned short-term findings suggest that the topical CAIs in their approved clinical dosages may have some beneficial influence on the retinal ganglion cell function. In fact, in earlier short-term clinical investigations improvement of mean sensitivity of the central visual field and increase of contrast sensitivity were reported in healthy volunteers after topical CAI medication.[8] In more recent studies, however, these findings were not confirmed.[10]

Recently, clinical studies with up to 6 months' follow-up time have been published on blood flow changes induced by topical CAIs applied in the usual clinical dosage.[13,14] In these clinically more relevant investigations increased capillary perfusion was detected in the optic nerve head, choroid, and in some parts of the peripapillary retina, and a shortened arteriovenous transit time was measured. However, no change was found in the retrobulbar hemodynamics.[10] The perfusion changes induced by CAIs are summarized in Table 48.3.

For the clinician, the most important question regarding the effects of the topical CAIs on ocular blood flow is whether the alterations represent any real benefit for the long-term preservation of visual functions in glaucoma. At present, the answer to this cannot be given because of the lack of long-term clinical studies and, in particular, because of the difficulty of separating the presumed benefit caused by the CAI-induced lowering of IOP from the possible consequences of the CAI-induced perfusion changes.

INDICATION

In the treatment of the various types of glaucoma (primary open-angle, congenital, pediatric, juvenile, normal-tension, aphakic, exfoliative, aniridic, and trau-matic glaucoma), as well as in ocular hypertension, top-ical CAIs are usually used as adjunctive drugs, but they can be effective also in monotherapy.[15,16] The dorzola-mide/timolol fixed combination is frequently used as a medication of first choice. Since oral or intravenous acetazolamide induces a faster and larger IOP decrease than is produced by the topical CAIs, it is widely used to break acute angle-closure glaucoma, and also to prevent the IOP spikes induced by Nd:YAG laser iri-dotomy.[2] In cases of very high IOP (independent of the type of glaucoma) systemic acetazolamide can also be used to achieve temporary IOP lowering prior to filter-ing surgery.

INTRAOCULAR PRESSURE-LOWERING EFFICACY AND DOSAGE IN MONOTHERAPY AND IN COMBINED MEDICATION

Use of acetazolamide is generally restricted to the above-mentioned situations where it is necessary to achieve acute IOP reduction; however, in intractable glaucoma its long-term use may become necessary.[1,3] Since individual response to acetazolamide varies con-siderably, the required daily dosage varies between one and four tablets (up to 1000 mg per day). The maximum acetazolamide-induced IOP decrease is approximately 40%. To prevent systemic hypokalemia consequent on increased diuresis, acetazolamide is normally given together with oral potassium supplementation.

For long-term medication, topical CAIs are pre-ferred.[2] When used in monotherapy, dorzolamide is instilled three times daily, but as a part of combined medication dorzolamide can be administered both b.i.d. and t.i.d. (see also Ch. 51, Fixed-Combination Therapy in Glaucoma). The administration of dorzolamide/timolol fixed combination is always b.i.d., since this delivers the minimum effective daily dosage of dorzola-mide together with the maximum safe daily dosage of timolol. Administration of brinzolamide is b.i.d. both in monotherapy and in combination.

The IOP decrease provided by dorzolamide and brin-zolamide is very similar. In monotherapy the peak IOP reduction (at 2 hours after instillation) varies between 16.3% and 22.9%, and the 12-hour trough reduction is between 13.2% and 18.9% in primary open-angle glau-coma and ocular hypertension.[2] The long-term IOP-lowering efficacy of topical CAIs is stable; no long-term drift phenomenon has been reported.

Topical CAIs are most frequently used in combina-tion with topical β-receptor blockers.[2,3,17,18] In primary open-angle glaucoma and ocular hypertension, addition of b.i.d. dorzolamide or brinzolamide to b.i.d. timolol 0.5% results in a further IOP decrease of 11–22% at peak and 12–16.3% at trough. Dorzolamide/timolol fixed combination is equally effective in IOP reduction as compared to the concomitant administration of dor-zolamide and timolol.[19,20] The IOP decrease provided by the dorzolamide/timolol fixed combination is somewhat

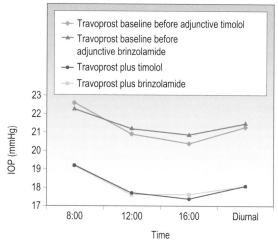

FIGURE 48.4 IOP-lowering efficacy of brinzolamide (b.i.d.) adjunctive to topical $PGF_{2\alpha}$ analogue travoprost (q.d.). (Adapted from Holló G et al. Eur J Ophthalmol 2006; 16:816–823, with permission.[23])

lower or similar to that seen with prostaglandin ana-logue monotherapy.[21,22]

In a recent multicentric, randomized, double-masked clinical study on primary open-angle glaucoma and ocu-lar hypertension patients, brinzolamide 1% and timolol 0.5% were equally effective as adjunctive medication as compared to travoprost.[23] From the travoprost baseline (22.3 mmHg for the brinzolamide arm and 22.6 mmHg for the timolol arm) the mean diurnal IOP decrease was 15.2% for brinzolamide and 14.1% for timolol after 3 months of treatment (Fig. 48.4). The result is espe-cially interesting since, in monotherapy, IOP reduc-tion induced by the nonselective β-receptor blockers is greater than that achieved with brinzolamide.[7] In a different investigation, when brinzolamide was added to latanoprost, the IOP decreased by a further 20%.[24] When dorzolamide was added to latanoprost, the addi-tional IOP decrease varied between 8% and 15%.[2,25]

Addition of a topical CAI to systemic acetazola-mide does not provide additional IOP reduction, but it is reported that further IOP decrease can be achieved when 250 mg acetazolamide is added to a single drop of topical CAI.[2] In clinical practice no combination within the CAI class is recommended. Addition of pilo-carpine 1% or 2% to dorzolamide monotherapy resulted in a further IOP decrease of 8.4%.[2] Published data on drug combinations containing CAIs are summarized in Table 48.4.

CONTRAINDICATIONS AND SYSTEMIC SIDE EFFECTS OF THE CARBONIC ANHYDRASE INHIBITORS

Since all CAIs are sulfonamide derivatives, cautions and contraindications against sulfonamides are relevant for CAIs.[2,3] Thus, CAIs are contraindicated in cases of known sulfonamide allergy. CAIs are excreted pre-dominantly by the kidney. Therefore, in patients with severe renal impairment (CrCl < 30 mL/min) caution

TABLE 48.4 Additive effects of topical CAIs used with other IOP-lowering drugs

TOPICAL CAI ADDED TO	ADDITIVITY	COMMENT
Topical β-receptor blockers	YES	Clinically useful combination
		Combined preparation available
PGF$_{2\alpha}$ analogues	YES	Clinically useful combination
Pilocarpine 1% or 2%	YES	Small additional IOP decrease
Systemic CAIs	NO	No additional IOP decrease

TABLE 48.5 Contraindications for topical and systemic CAIs

CONTRAINDICATION	TOPICAL CAIs	SYSTEMIC CAIs
Sulfonamide allergy	Yes	Yes
Previous contact dermatitis due to a topical CAI	Yes	Not known
Renal dysfunction (CrCl < 30mL/min)	Relative contraindication	Yes
Hepatic impairement	Not known	Not known
Pregnancy and lactation	Relative contraindication	Relative contraindication
Premature newborns	Yes	Yes

TABLE 48.6 Systemic side effects of the systemic and topical CAIs

TYPE OF SIDE EFFECT	SYSTEMIC CAIs	TOPICAL CAIs
Blood dyscrasia	Yes	Rare, less severe
Bitter taste	Yes	Yes
Gastrointestinal complaints	Yes	Rare, less severe
Paresthesia	Yes	Rare, less severe
Renal stone formation	Yes	Rare, less severe
Acidosis	Yes	Yes, on immature newborns

is indicated, especially when systemic CAIs are given.[1] Pregnancy and lactation represent a relative contraindication against the use of CAIs, since no adequate studies have been conducted on pregnant and nursing women. The CAIs are excreted with the milk,[2] and therefore they may influence the red blood cell CA activity in the newborn. The potential influence of severe hepatic impairment on the CAI metabolism needs to be clarified.[2] In conclusion, in the above-mentioned cases, individual judgment is necessary regarding the introduction or withdrawal of the CAI therapy: the potential benefit of the treatment must exceed the potential risks.

The systemic side effects of CAIs can appear in acute form due to hypersensitivity (e.g. Stevens–Johnson syndrome), or can develop gradually, due to dose-dependent systemic alterations which can be reversible after the CAI medication is stopped. CAI-induced severe blood dyscrasia (agranulocytosis, thrombocytopenia, aplastic anemia, or pancytopenia) has reportedly resulted in 120 lethal cases over 40 years.[2,26,27] These reactions are attributed to systemic CAIs, but thrombocytopenia has also been reported in a very small number of patients using topical dorzolamide.[28] In these cases the outcome was less severe than reported in connection with acetazolamide, and the thrombocyte production recovered after cessation of the topical CAI treatment. In order to be able to detect the above-mentioned potential side effects in good time, repeated hematological laboratory testing is recommended during chronic treatment with systemic CAIs.

The less serious adverse effects (tiredness, paresthesia, headache, gastrointestinal side effects, taste perversion, bitter taste feeling, decreased appetite, renal stone formation, malaise, and acidosis) are common during long-term systemic CAI medication, but are relatively rare and less severe under topical CAI treatment.[2,29] It is important to know that even topically applied CAIs accumulate in the red blood cells and inhibit approximately 21% of the CA II content of the cells.[2] This inhibition does not cause any clinically detectable side effects in adults, but in newborns or premature newborns who have fetal hemoglobin, it may lead to acidosis.[30] Thus, administration of topical CAIs in newborns requires special caution. In diabetes mellitus,

acetazolamide-induced acidosis may worsen the hyperosmolar status.[31] When dorzolamide is applied as a part of the fixed dorzolamide/timolol combination, the systemic side effects of the β-receptor component also have to be considered. The contraindications against the systemic and topical CAIs, and the systemic side effects of the CAIs, are summarized in Table 48.5 and Table 48.6.

OCULAR SIDE EFFECTS AND OCULAR TOLERANCE

Choroidal detachment and transient myopia are known infrequent side effects of the sulfonamide derivatives, which can occur under either systemic or topical CAIs medication. A rare allergic complication of topical dorzolamide is marginal keratitis, which resolves spontaneously after withdrawal of dorzolamide. Periorbital contact dermatitis and allergic conjunctivitis are much more common complications of topically applied dorzolamide.[32] Though periorbital dermatitis and allergic conjunctivitis recover soon after the dorzolamide exposition is stopped, it reappears if a CAI is later introduced in the topical medication. Thus, periocular CAI allergy in the history represents a contraindication against any topical CAI medication.

As shown in Table 48.1, the corneal endothelium contains CA II isoenzyme, which is blocked by the

TABLE 48.7 Ocular side effects of the topical CAIs

TYPE OF SIDE EFFECT	DORZOLAMIDE	BRINZOLAMIDE
Burning/itching after instillation	++	−/+
Bitter taste after instillation	++	+
Blurred vision after instillation	+	++
Periocular contact dermatitis	++	−/+
Allergic conjunctivitis	++	−/+
Decompensation of the compromised corneas	+	+

Increasing number of + symbols indicates increased frequency and severity.

TABLE 48.8 Drug interactions reported for the systemic and topical CAIs

DRUG EFFECT	INTERACTION
Ciclosporin toxicity	Increased
Digitalis toxicity	Increased
Lithium toxicity	Increased
Aspirin toxicity	Increased
Potassium loss due to diuretics	Increased
Diphenylhydantoin-induced osteoporosis	Increased
Effect of oral antidiabetics	Decreased
Effect of antihypertensive medications	Increased
Cholinesterase activity	Decreased

topically applied CAIs. Decreased function of the corneal CA II may cause hydration and thickening of the cornea, which may even lead to corneal decompensation. Clinical practice, however, has shown that in eyes with normal cornea the central cornea thickness does not change in a clinically significant manner even during 1 year of topical CAI medication,[2] and that the endothelial cell loss under topical CAI medication does not differ from that measured on β-blocker users.[2] In contrast, topical CAIs can worsen the status of the compromised corneas with decreased endothelial cell number and function (e.g. in Fuchs' dystrophy, decreased endothelial cell density due to complicated cataract surgery. This can lead to manifest corneal decompensation that is not necessarily reversible after the withdrawal of the CAI molecule from the treatment.[2]

Ocular tolerance and comfort are especially important points in chronic CAI administration, and may influence the compliance and therefore the IOP control achieved. Chronic use of topical dorzolamide has been consistently found associated with increased frequency of ocular burning, tearing, itching, irritation, and deep discomfort feeling compared with both placebo drops and brinzolamide.[2] The subjective complaints associated with dorzolamide can be explained by the relatively acidic pH of Trusopt™, which is necessary to the ocular absorption of dorzolamide. The pH and osmolality of Azopt™ are close to the physiological values; thus, ocular tolerance of brinzolamide has been consistently reported as being superior to that of dorzolamide.[2,17,18] On the other hand, transient blurred vision immediately after instillation is more frequent with brinzolamide than with dorzolamide, as a consequence of the viscous carbomer suspension used with the former.

It is interesting that in dorzolamide monotherapy the frequency of side effects was found to be twice as high in the first year as in the second year of the treatment.[2] This suggests that patients in whom dorzolamide is well tolerated have a probability for experiencing fewer side effects with increased length of dorzolamide use. In clinical practice, the side effects are less frequently seen when the dorzolamide/timolol fixed combination is used, though in randomized clinical trials the adverse-effect profile and frequency of dorzolamide and of dorzolamide/timolol fixed combination were found to be similar.[33] In clinical studies, discontinuation of the treatment because of side effects varied between 0.1% and 24.1% for dorzolamide, and between 0.03% and 17% for brinzolamide.[2,17,34] The ocular side effects of the topical CAIs are summarized in Table 48.7.

DRUG INTERACTIONS WITH THE CARBONIC ANHYDRASE INHIBITORS

The drug interactions involving CAIs are systemic interactions (Table 48.8). Additive side effects or increased toxicity have been reported for systemic CAIs taken together with systemically administered ciclosporin, digitalis, lithium, aspirin (increased toxicity), and diuretics (increased potassium loss). Systemic acetazolamide decreases the effects of oral antidiabetics, and diminishes cholinesterase activity.[1,35]

Summary

Carbonic anhydrase inhibitors are IOP-lowering sulfonamide derivatives which inhibit the activity of CA in the ciliary processes of the eye, thus reducing aqueous humor formation and consequently decreasing IOP. Systemic CAIs provide an approximately 40% IOP reduction, and their effect develops rapidly. Therefore, systemic CAIs (most frequently acetazolamide) are useful to break acute angle-closure glaucoma and to reduce high IOP prior to filtering surgery. However, when used chronically, systemic CAIs have many systemic side effects. Indeed, some side effects of acetazolamide can even be lethal. In contrast, the topical CAIs dorzolamide and brinzolamide are safe systemically, and their side effects are mostly local. In monotherapy, the IOP decrease achieved with either of these topical CAIs varies between 15% and 20%, a figure which is considerably less than the reduction produced by acetazolamide. In clinical practice, topical CAIs are mainly used as a part of a combined IOP-lowering medication. Their additional IOP-lowering efficacy is especially favorable when they are added to nonselective β-receptor blockers or prostaglandin analogues. The IOP reduction provided by the topical CAIs is stable over long usage, with no long-term drift phenomenon. In order to increase the ocular penetration, dorzolamide is formulated with an acidic pH, which may explain the more frequent and severe local side effects as compared to brinzolamide. All CAIs influence ocular perfusion, but the clinical significance of the CAI-induced increase of ocular blood flow remains to be specified. At present, the information on the altered ocular perfusion due to CAI administration cannot be interpreted as an evidence of IOP-independent retinal ganglion cell protection in glaucoma.

ACKNOWLEDGEMENTS

Supported by Hungarian National Health Grant no. ETT 001/2006.

REFERENCES

1. Pfeiffer N. Carbonic anhydrase: pharmacology and inhibition. In: Orgül S, Flammer J, eds. Pharmacotherapy in glaucoma. Bern: Hans Huber Verlag; 2000:137–143.

2. Holló G. The use of topical carbonic anhydrase inhibitors in glaucoma treatment. In: Orgül S, Flammer J, eds. Pharmacotherapy in glaucoma. Bern: Hans Huber Verlag; 2000:145–152.

3. Lippa EA. Carbonic anhydrase inhibitors. In: Ritch R, Shields MB, Krupin T, eds. The glaucomas. 2nd edn. St Louis: Mosby; 1996:1463–1481.

4. Becker B. Decrease in intraocular pressure in man by a carbonic anhydrase inhibitor, Diamox. Am J Ophthalmol 1954; 37:13–15.

5. Sugrue MF. Pharmacological and ocular hypotensive properties of topical carbonic anhydrase inhibitors. Prog Retin Eye Res 2000; 19:87–112.

6. DeSantis L. Preclinical overview of brinzolamide. Surv Ophthalmol 2000; 44(Suppl 2):S119–sS129.

7. European Glaucoma Society. Terminology and guidelines for glaucoma. 2nd edn. Savona: DOGMA s.r.l.; 2003.

8. Holló G. Influence of intraocular pressure lowering medication on vascular supply. In: Shaarawmy T, Flammer J, eds. Phrmacotherapy in glaucoma. London: Martin Dunitz; 2004:143–161.

9. Costa VP, Harris A, Stefansson E, et al. The effects of antiglaucoma and systemic medications on ocular blood flow. Prog Retin Eye Res 2003; 22:769–805.

10. Kaup M, Plange N, Niegel M, et al. Effects of brinzolamide on ocular haemodynamics in healthy volunteers. Br J Ophthalmol 2004; 88:257–262.

11. Stefansson E, Pedersen DB, Jensen PK, et al. Optic nerve oxygenation. Prog Retin Eye Res 2005; 24:307–332.

12. Uva MG, Longo A, Reibaldi M, et al. The effect of timolol–dorzolamide and timolol–pilocarpine combinations on ocular blood flow in patients with glaucoma. Am J Ophthalmol 2006; 141:1158–1160.

13. Fuchsjager-Mayrl G, Wally B, Rainer G, et al. Effect of dorzolamide and timolol on ocular blood flow in patients with primary open angle glaucoma and ocular hypertension. Br J Ophthalmol 2005; 89:1293–1297.

14. Iester M, Altieri M, Michelson G, et al. Retinal peripapillary blood flow before and after topical brinzolamide. Ophthalmologica 2004; 218:390–396.

15. Miglior S, Zeyen T, Pfeiffer N, et al. Results of the European Glaucoma Prevention Study. Ophthalmology 2005; 112:366–375.

16. Ott EZ, Mills MD, Arango S, et al. A randomized trial assessing dorzolamide in patients with glaucoma who are younger than 6 years. Arch Ophthalmol 2005; 123:1177–1186.

17. Michaud JE, Friren B. International Brinzolamide Adjunctive Study Group. Comparison of topical brinzolamide 1% and dorzolamide 2% eye drops given twice daily in addition to timolol 0.5% in patients with primary open-angle glaucoma or ocular hypertension. Am J Ophthalmol 2001; 132:235–243.

18. Shin D. Adjunctive therapy with brinzolamide 1% ophthalmic suspension (Azopt) in patients with open-angle glaucoma or ocular hypertension maintained on timolol therapy. Surv Ophthalmol 2000; 44(Suppl 2):S163–S168.

19. Hutzelmann J, Owens S, Shedden A, et al. Comparison of the safety and efficacy of the fixed combination of dorzolamide/timolol and the concomitant administration of dorzolamide and timolol: a clinical equivalence study. Br J Ophthalmol 1998; 82:1249–1253.

20. Strohmaier K, Snyder E, DuBiner H, et al. The efficacy and safety of the dorzolamide–timolol combination versus the concomitant administration of its components. Ophthalmology 1998; 105:1936–1944.

21. Coleman AL, Lerner F, Bernstein P, et al. A 3-month randomized controlled trial of bimatoprost (Lumigan) versus combined timolol and dorzolamide (Cosopt) in patients with glaucoma or ocular hypertension. Ophthalmology 2003; 110:2362–2368.

22. Konstas AG, Papapanos P, Tersis I, et al. Twenty-four-hour diurnal curve comparison of commercially available latanoprost 0.005% versus the timolol and dorzolamide fixed combination. Ophthalmology 2003; 110:1357–1360.

23. Holló G, Chiselita D, Petkova N, et al. The efficacy and safety of timolol maleate versus brinzolamide each given twice daily added to travoprost in patients with ocular hypertension or primary open-angle glaucoma. Eur J Ophthalmol 2006; 16:816–823.

24. Shoji N, Ogata H, Suyama H, et al. Intraocular pressure lowering effect of brinzolamide 1.0% as adjunctive therapy to latanoprost 0.005% in patients with open angle glaucoma or ocular hypertension: an uncontrolled, open-label study. Curr Med Res Opin 2005; 21:503–508.

25. Konstas AG, Karabatsas CH, Lallos N, et al. 24-hour intraocular pressures with brimonidine purite versus dorzolamide added to latanoprost in primary open-angle glaucoma subjects. Ophthalmology 2005; 112:603–608.

26. Kodjikian L, Durand B, Burillon C, et al. Acetazolamide-induced thrombocytopenia. Arch Ophthalmol 2004; 122:1543–1544.

27. Fraunfelder FT, Bagby GC. Monitoring patients taking oral carbonic anhydrase inhibitors. Am J Ophthalmol 2000; 130:221–223.

28. Martin XD, Danese M. Dorzolamide-induced immune thrombocytopenia: a case report and literature review. J Glaucoma 2001; 102:133–135.

29. Carlsen J, Durcan J, Zabriskie N, et al. Nephrolithiasis with dorzolamide. Arch Ophthalmol 1999; 117:1087–1088.

30. Morris S, Geh V, Nischal KK, et al. Topical dorzolamide and metabolic acidosis in a neonate. Br J Ophthalmol 2003; 87:1052–1053.

31. Zaidi FH, Kinnear PE. Acetazolamide, alternate carbonic anhydrase inhibitors and hypoglycaemic agents: comparing enzymatic with diuresis induced metabolic acidosis following intraocular surgery in diabetes. Br J Ophthalmol 2004; 88:714–715.

32. Delaney YM, Salmon JF, Mossa F, et al. Periorbital dermatitis as a side effect of topical dorzolamide. Br J Ophthalmol 2002; 86:378–380.

33. Clineschmidt CM, Williams RD, Snyder E, et al. A randomized trial in patients inadequately controlled with timolol alone comparing the dorzolamide–timolol combination to monotherapy with timolol or dorzolamide. Ophthalmology 1998; 105:1952–1959.

34. March WF, Ochsner KI. The long-term safety and efficacy of brinzolamide 1.0% (Azopt) in patients with primary open-angle glaucoma or ocular hypertension. Am J Ophthalmol 2000; 129:136–143.

35. Tabbara KF, Al-Faisal Z, Al-Rashed W. Interaction between acetazolamine and cyclosporine. Arch Ophthalmol 1998; 116:832–833.

CHAPTER 49

Alpha Agonists

Adam C Reynolds

INTRODUCTION

Adrenergic agonists have been used in the treatment of chronic glaucoma for decades. The discovery and delineation of distinct classes and subtypes of adrenergic receptors, specifically the α- and β-adrenergic receptors, has led to the development of several different strategies involving the adrenergic system to lower intraocular pressure. The β-adrenergic antagonists, timolol being the parent compound, will be discussed elsewhere. The development of agents specific to the α-adrenergic subtypes α-1, α-2, and imidazole receptors has resulted in several different very effective ocular hypotensive agents. The α-adrenergic agents in current use include clonidine, which is no longer used often in ophthalmic treatment, and its two derivatives, apraclonidine and the recently introduced derivative brimonidine.

Most use of alpha agonists for glaucoma treatment has gravitated toward brimonidine over the last decade for many different reasons, which will be discussed. However, most of the original studies of the mechanism of action and pharmacology involved clonidine and apraclonidine, making their discussion in that context imperative.

DRUG FORMULATIONS

Clonidine is the parent topical alpha agonist for topical ophthalmic use, and is still available as dichlorophenyl aminoimidazoline in a formulation called Isoglaucon in concentrations of 0.125%, 0.2%, and 0.5%. Apraclonidine is available as Iopidine in 0.5% and 1% formulations. Brimonidine tartrate is currently available in several different formulations. Alphagan was originally available in 0.2% and 0.5% formulations preserved with benzalkonium chloride. The 0.2% formulation is now available in several different generic forms and recently Alphagan-P has been introduced in 0.15% and 0.10% formulations, marketed by Allergan, preserved with Purite which is chlorine dioxide. An additional formulation of brimonidine 0.15% preserved with polyquaternium-1 is currently being considered for marketing as well. Fixed-combination formulations of 0.2% brimonidine with 0.5% timolol are available in Europe, Canada, and the USA.

MECHANISM OF ACTION

PHARMACOLOGY

Adrenergic stimulation in the eye is mediated by transmembrane receptors which activate quinine nucleotide-binding enzymes (G proteins). Each adrenergic receptor is associated with at least one unique G protein. Alpha-1 is associated with the Gq receptor and α-2 the Gi receptor. Numerous receptor subtypes have been identified and are currently being intensively studied as new, more specific targets.[1] Adrenergic receptor activation appears to regulate intraocular pressure (IOP) primarily via the levels of adenylate cyclase in the ciliary epithelium. Net inhibition of adenylate cyclase and reduction of intracellular cyclic adenosine monophosphate (cAMP) causes reduction of aqueous production and probably other related effects, namely the reduction of episcleral venous pressure. The second messengers for the intracellular effect of receptor stimulation appear to be prostaglandins in animal models but there have been problems proving this mechanism in human eyes. Several studies have shown that nonsteroidal anti-inflammatory medications such as flurbiprofen can block apraclonidine's IOP-lowering effect in cynomolgus monkeys but not in humans,[2–4] indicating unique effects on the human eye different from other primates.

Currently, the precise site of action of α-adrenergic stimulation in lowering of IOP in humans is unclear. These agents can occupy adrenergic and imidazole receptors in the brain, ciliary body, and possibly the trabecular meshwork. Unilateral application of apraclonidine or brimonidine can cause up to a 19% reduction in contralateral IOP and this effect appears to be greater with brimonidine.[5,6] This crossover effect varies among species and does not appear to be mediated by sympathetic nervous system input in humans or monkeys but is demonstrated in other nonprimate animal models. There are also possibilities that have been raised in more recent studies that alpha agonists

547

may have dual mechanisms of action lowering IOP by increasing trabecular outflow or nonpressure-dependent pathways such as uveal–scleral outflow,[7–9] which will be discussed more fully later.

Apraclonidine is a hydrophilic derivative of clonidine and achieves substantial IOP reduction without causing the centrally mediated side effects of hypotension and drowsiness that clonidine is particularly known for. Although structurally similar to clonidine, it has a hydrophilic amide group at the C4 position of the benzene ring. This modification makes apraclonidine more hydrophilic (less lipophilic) and therefore less able to have significant blood–brain barrier penetration. This makes its ability to penetrate the cornea more difficult, however. Corneal penetration of apraclonidine is six times slower than clonidine. Apraclonidine is a moderate α-2 selective agent, having 72 times more α-2 than α-1 affinity.[10] At 0.25%, α-1 activity is still sufficient to cause notable conjunctival blanching and eyelid retraction.

Brimonidine is a highly selective α-2 agonist. In rabbit models it appears to be 7–12 times more α-2 selective than clonidine and 23–32 times more selective than apraclonidine.[11] Human data suggest that this increased α-2 selective effect may not be as pronounced in humans as in animal models, as conjunctival blanching and lid retraction do occur in unilateral doses. Brimonidine is less lipophilic than clonidine but more than apraclonidine. Penetration of the cornea and therefore the blood–brain barrier is probably intermediate compared to the other two agents and sedation, hypotension, and other centrally mediated effects are probably more of an issue partly because of this. Central effects causing IOP lowering may be a more likely part of brimonidine's mechanism of action as well. In one study it is suggested that brimonidine may lower IOP in monkeys via nonadrenergic imidazole receptor agonism in the ciliary body.[12] This may in fact be the case and an important difference opposed to apraclonidine as other imidazole receptors located in the medulla are possibly involved in the central hypotensive response to clonidine. The molecular structures of clonidine, apraclonidine, and brimonidine are shown in Figure 49.1.

EFFECT ON AQUEOUS HUMOR DYNAMICS

Modern techniques to determine an ocular hypotensive drug's effect on aqueous humor dynamics rely on the understanding of aqueous physiology modeled by the Goldmann equation:

$$IOP = P_{ev} + (F - U)/C_{tm}$$

The variables are defined as:
   IOP = intraocular pressure
   P_{ev} = episcleral venous pressure
   F = aqueous flow
   U = uveoscleral outflow
   C_{tm} = trabecular outflow facility.
Conclusive statements about effects of different medication and interventions on aqueous humor dynamics

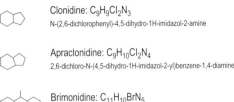

Clonidine: $C_9H_9Cl_2N_3$
N-(2,6-dichlorophenyl)-4,5-dihydro-1H-imidazol-2-amine

Apraclonidine: $C_9H_{10}Cl_2N_4$
2,6-dichloro-N-(4,5-dihydro-1H-imidazol-2-yl)benzene-1,4-diamine

Brimonidine: $C_{11}H_{10}BrN_5$
5-bromo-N-(4,5-dihydro-1H-imidazol-2-yl)quinoxaline-6-amine

FIGURE 49.1 Molecular formulations and structures for clonidine, apraclonidine, and brimonidine.

require measurement of at least three of the variables, which is often extremely difficult to determine during human in vivo studies. In early studies of apraclonidine it appeared that the majority of IOP reduction was through aqueous production decrease alone, but these early conclusions have been challenged. A more complete trial in ocular hypertensive patients suggests that longer-term use of apraclonidine lowers IOP through multiple mechanisms, primarily by increasing trabecular outflow facility.[8] In agreement with prior studies, apraclonidine has no apparent effect on tonographic outflow facility; however, IOP was lowered in this study by increasing fluorophotometric outflow facility (53%), and secondarily by decreasing episcleral venous pressure (10%) and decreasing aqueous flow (12%).

Similar studies of brimonidine's effect on aqueous dynamics have shown some important differences between it and apraclonidine as well. Aqueous inflow was shown to be reduced by 20% and increasing uveoscleral outflow apparently produced some IOP-lowering effect. However, the uveoscleral effect has now been challenged in subsequent studies.[13] It would also make sense that a central mechanism of brimonidine's IOP-lowering effect may be more likely than with apraclonidine, as shown by a larger contralateral IOP-lowering effect than with apraclonidine as well as more likelihood of centrally mediated effects on IOP due to more central nervous system (CNS) penetration.

ALTERATION OF OCULAR BLOOD FLOW

Perhaps no other category of medications for the treatment of glaucoma than the alpha agonists, in particular brimonidine, have come under more thorough scrutiny for possible other detrimental or additive effects involving neuroprotection or optic nerve microcirculation. There are multiple factors that led to the ongoing investigation and controversies of these issues with these medications.

Because of the centrally mediated systemic hypotensive and vascular constrictive effects of clonidine and the local effects of conjunctival, oral, and nasal vasoconstriction of apraclonidine, there were major safety concerns initially that constriction of optic nerve arterial circulation may occur. Obviously, concerns of exacerbation of compromised optic nerve microcirculation in patients with glaucoma using these medications, despite the lowering of IOP, were legitimate. Several investigations showed that topical apraclonidine therapy does cause an acute reduction in blood flow in the anterior segment of the eye, including the iris,[14] but no vascular effects of the optic nerve or peripapillary retina were identified in vivo. There is acknowledgment, however, that optic nerve blood flow is difficult to measure in humans and vascular effects of alpha agonists already have known species-specific effects on different vascular beds, making extrapolation to humans problematic. Several studies of Doppler ultrasonographic measurement of retinal and peripapillary blood flow in normal volunteers treated with apraclonidine failed to show any affect from treatment.[15] However, these studies involved treatment of one eye with measurements involving the other eye as the control. Central effects could still have been an issue in this study, confounding the results.

With its higher penetration of the blood–brain barrier and more centrally mediated side effects, this issue is possibly even more of a concern with brimonidine. However, some animal model studies have shown that brimonidine possibly actually increases retinal arteriolar blood flow.[16] Multiple studies using different parameters of measurement looking at brimonidine's effect on circulation in the posterior segment of the eye in humans, similar to previous studies with apraclonidine, have failed to show any effects, either vasoconstrictive or dilatory, using several different techniques.[17–20] Again, even with current technology, measuring blood flow changes in vivo in the vascular bed of the peripapillary choroid and the optic nerve itself in humans is still a technology in development.

NEUROPROTECTION

Recent efforts in research and development of neuroprotective treatment strategies for numerous neurodegenerative diseases, including glaucoma, have led to speculation that some treatments already approved for treatment of glaucoma via IOP-lowering effects may have other effects in protecting human optic nerve structure or function from glaucomatous optic neuropathy. The subject of neuroprotection in glaucoma is a subject far beyond the scope of this chapter and will no doubt be discussed elsewhere in depth. However, as this subject pertains to topical alpha agonists in particular, it should be discussed in this context.

Several animal studies of high doses of brimonidine used in models of acute optic nerve injury in the late 1990s apparently showed some protective effect having nothing to do with IOP lowering.[21,22] These results led to much speculation that brimonidine could possibly have other beneficial effects apart from IOP lowering in human glaucoma. It was also shown that receptors for brimonidine do exist in the retina. The last 5 years have seen several sophisticated studies in animal models, particularly in rats and mice, showing that in acute ischemic or glaucomatous injury to the optic nerve, brimonidine, in doses that produce equivalent concentrations in the posterior segment in humans with topical treatment, does indeed preserve optic nerve, optic tract, and ganglion cell structure and function compared to placebo.[23–25] Many

different theories have been proposed to explain this effect, including inhibition of excitatory neuropeptides, maintenance of antigrade axonal flow and neurotropic factors, or stabilization of the immunoreactivity of mitochondrial membranes, among them. The complexity of the different theories of possible neuroprotective strategies in many different disease models makes specific application even to these models of acute optic nerve injury difficult.

However, several elegant studies in humans have failed to show similar effects in acute optic nerve injury. Several studies of brimonidine's possible benefit in acute ischemic optic nerve injury in humans are ongoing and completed studies have failed to show a protective effect.[26] Acute angle-closure glaucoma would appear to provide a reasonable glaucomatous disease entity with an acute enough course to test the possible neuroprotective effects of brimonidine. In one randomized, controlled study of acute angle-closure glaucoma in humans, there was no difference in visual field preservation after treatment with either brimonidine or timolol.[27] Proving preservation of ganglion cell or other neural pathway functions in long-term studies in humans and separating IOP-lowering benefits of medications, even in well-designed prospective, randomized trials, is extremely difficult. Until direct measurements of ganglion cell function and apoptotic processes in humans become a way to assess effects separated from lowering IOP, or IOP fluctuations can be constantly monitored to eliminate possible undetected differences in IOP control, these questions may, in fact, be almost impossible to answer. Perhaps, once neuroprotection for glaucoma is a proven concept with medications in clinical trials now which have no affect on lowering IOP, possible neuroprotective benefits of alpha agonists, and other IOP-lowering medications, can be tested in a more reasonable and reproducible fashion.

INDICATIONS

PROPHYLAXIS OF INTRAOCULAR PRESSURE ELEVATIONS POST-PROCEDURES

Alpha agonists have indications for the prevention or treatment of elevated intraocular pressure in many different contexts. Originally, apraclonidine, because of its relatively rapid onset of action compared with other topical agents, became the standard of care to prevent acute IOP rise after various ophthalmic procedures. Argon laser trabeculoplasty (ALT), which is effective in lowering IOP chronically, is subject to causing significant IOP spikes initially after treatment. IOP elevations of at least 10 mmHg have been found in one-third of patients after 360° of ALT.[28] The Glaucoma Laser Trial (GLT) found that treating half of the trabecular meshwork still resulted in 21% of patients having an IOP rise of 6 mmHg or more. Several trials demonstrated the ability of apraclonidine to prevent these IOP spikes. In one trial, use of 1% apraclonidine decreased the incidence of any IOP rise after ALT from 59% to 21% and the percentage of eyes having an IOP rise higher than 10 mmHg fell from 18% to 0%.[29] Another randomized trail showed that apraclonidine was superior to pilocarpine 4%, timolol 0.5%, dipiverine 0.1%, and acetazolamide in preventing IOP spikes in this context.[30] The Food and Drug Administration (FDA) actually approved the use of 1% apraclonidine for the prevention of post-laser IOP spikes and the 0.5% solution has undergone several trials showing probable equivalency.[31,32] While apraclonidine's role in the prevention of acute IOP spikes after ALT is well documented, the long-term benefits of prevention of visual field loss, visual acuity, or optic nerve damage used in this context is not proven.

Apraclonidine's use to prevent IOP spikes in other procedures has been studied as well. Up to one-third of patients undergoing either Nd:YAG or argon laser iridotomy have an acute IOP rise of 10 mmHg or more. Apraclonidine 1% has been shown to be quite effective in preventing acute IOP rise after laser iridotomy in several different groups of patients.[33,34] Similarly, IOP rise after YAG laser capsulotomy, particularly in patients with glaucoma, has been well documented.[35] Several multicentered trials have found that use of apraclonidine 1% prophylactically eliminated nearly all significant IOP elevations after YAG capsulotomy.[32,35] Apraclonidine has also been shown to be effective in preventing IOP rise after cataract surgery. One trial showed that two drops of apraclonidine 1% before and one drop after cataract surgery prevented the early postoperative IOP rise better than placebo or oral acetazolamide.[36]

Several more recent trials have shown the equivalence of brimonidine 0.2% to apraclonidine 1% used to prevent IOP spikes of this type. In randomized trials comparing the two in ALT,[37] LPI,[38] and YAG capsulotomy[39] brimonidine 0.2% has shown equivalence, although, as expected, there were more centrally mediated side effects with brimonidine.

CHRONIC INTRAOCULAR PRESSURE ELEVATION

Although apraclonidine 0.5% use three times daily (t.i.d) has ample evidence that long-term administration does lower IOP in ocular hypertension and in different forms of chronic glaucoma, it has fallen out of favor for use in this context. Several factors have contributed to this, including the high incidence rate of local adverse reactions, including allergic follicular conjunctivitis and tachyphylaxis.[40] For chronic use of alpha agonists to lower IOP, brimonidine in its various formulations has become the much more commonly used agent. Several factors led to its popularity as a first-line agent in this context, including general lack of systemic side effects in most patients and better long-term tolerance. The initial interest and acceptance of brimonidine's potential neuroprotective properties may also have

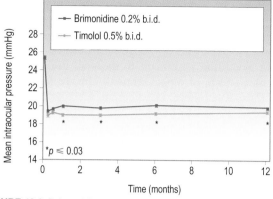

FIGURE 49.2 Brimonidine 0.2% b.i.d. vs timolol 0.5% b.i.d., mean intraocular pressure lowering shows small overall differences. (From Katz LJ. Am J Ophthalmol 1999; 127:1.)

contributed to its use in first-line monotherapy. However, the necessity of dosing three times a day as a single-use agent, questions of diurnal IOP variability, especially in more acceptable twice-daily (b.i.d.) dosing, as well as the lack proven validity of neuroprotective properties in patients with glaucoma, and the continued problems with the incidence of allergic reactions have been recent issues of concern.

In the 1-year randomized clinical trial for FDA approval in the USA comparing brimonidine 0.2% t.i.d. to timolol 0.5% b.i.d., the two medications lowered IOP in a similar fashion about 25% below baseline. More recent trials measuring mean IOP lowering of brimonidine 0.2% b.i.d. compared to timolol 0.5% b.i.d. show very little difference in mean IOP lowering (Fig. 49.2). However, like apraclonidine, brimonidine 0.2% loses more of its peak effect at trough compared to timolol, particularly in matched b.i.d. dosing. Several other long-term trials of b.i.d. treatment with brimonidine 0.2% compared to timolol 0.5% b.i.d. have been completed showing similar discontinuation rates from side effects and similar efficacy in terms of mean IOP control and visual field preservation.[41] However, as shown in Figures 49.3 and 49.4, with b.i.d. dosing there are significant differences in trough IOP effects. With the evolving understanding of diurnal IOP curve flattening being an important parameter to consider in preventing glaucoma progression, these issues have recently become a more important consideration and it has increased awareness of the need to use brimonidine in t.i.d. dosing for chronic treatment as monotherapy.

Several different formulations of brimonidine have been approved recently, including both an 0.15% and 0.10% formulation with a different preservative (Alphagan-P). Several 1-year studies of these formulations using them t.i.d. as monotherapy compared with the original formulations[42] have shown that both the 0.15% and 0.10% solutions are apparently equivalent in IOP reduction. Figures 49.5 and 49.6 show the results of these studies. It is particularly interesting that the

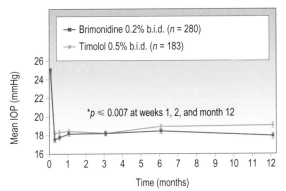

FIGURE 49.3 Brimonidine 0.2% b.i.d. vs timolol 0.5% b.i.d. Peak intraocular pressure lowering shows slight differences.

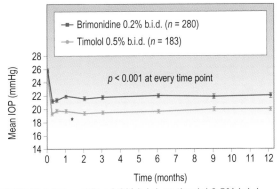
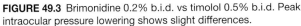

FIGURE 49.4 Brimonidine 0.2% b.i.d. vs timolol 0.5% b.i.d. Trough intraocular pressure lowering shows average differences of approximately 2 mmHg.

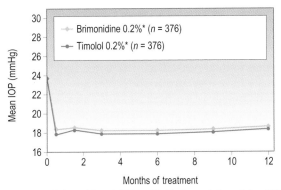

FIGURE 49.5 Brimonidine 0.15% with Purite vs brimonidine 0.2% with BAK. Pooled data show no significant differences in IOP lowering.

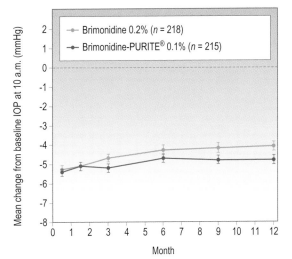

FIGURE 49.6 Brimonidine 0.2% vs brimonidine 0.1%, showing no significant difference in IOP lowering. Allergan file data from FDA approval trial not yet published. (From Cantor L. Ther Clin Risk Manag 2006; 2:4.)

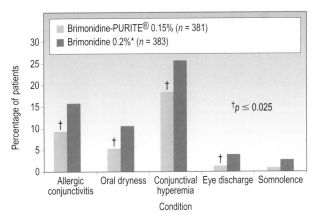

FIGURE 49.7 Brimonidine 0.2% preserved with BAK vs bromonidine 0.15% preserved with purite showing decreased side effects with the Purite-preserved formulation after 1 year of treatment.

0.10% formulations of brimonidine appear to be equal in efficacy, and there has been some discussion that even lower concentrations might be effective. It has also been shown, at least in 1-year studies, that the rates of follicular conjunctivitis and CNS effects of the lower concentrations are less and those with both different preservatives and lower concentrations appear to show lower rates of allergic conjunctivitis as well (Fig. 49.7).[42,43]

Currently there is one formulation of a fixed combination of brimonidine with timolol in use (see also Ch. 51, Fixed-Combination Therapies in Glaucoma). This fixed-combination eyedrop, marketed by Allergan and called Combigan™, is 0.2% brimonidine with 0.5% timolol. Several studies have been completed showing that this combination lowers IOP significantly better than either of the constituents used alone in b.i.d. dosing.[44] Importantly, diurnal variation is less with this combination used b.i.d. than with brimonidine 0.2% alone used t.i.d., as shown in two studies in the USA.[45,46] Results from one of these studies are shown in Figure 49.8. This study used four different time-point measurements throughout the day, resulting in a very good delineation of the differences in diurnal variation of IOP between timolol 0.5% b.i.d. and brimonidine

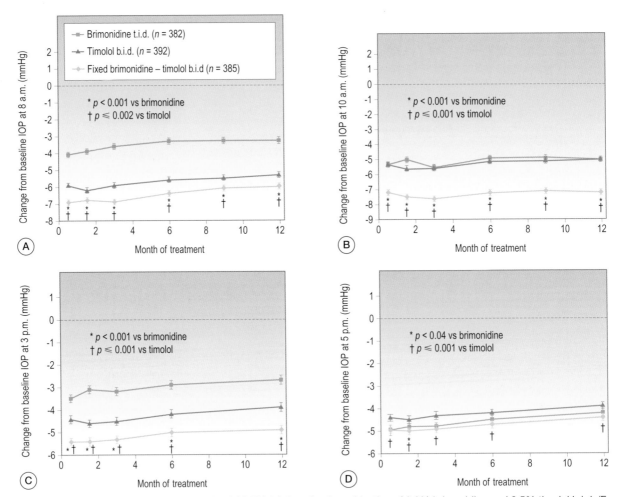

FIGURE 49.8 A–D Brimonidine 0.2% t.i.d. vs timolol 0.5% b.i.d. vs fixed combination of 0.2% brimonidine and 0.5% timolol b.i.d. (From Sherwood et al. Arch Ophthalmol 2006; 124:1230–1238.[45])

0.2% t.i.d. in glaucoma and ocular hypertensive patients. Obvious advantages of combination therapy include increased compliance and convenience as long as the combination is more effective than the single agents used alone. This fixed combination is now approved for use in the USA.

EFFICACY AND COMPARISON WITH OTHER AGENTS

Several factors in the principles of treatment of glaucoma in general have led to changes in the measurements of efficacy and goals of treatment and how they apply to topical medications to lower intraocular pressure. These changes will be discussed at length elsewhere, but how they specifically apply to the use of alpha agonists in particular in comparison to other agents will be discussed. As noted earlier, the principles of the possible neuroprotective properties of topical alpha agonists are the subject of much future and ongoing research, and proving efficacy in this area in an evidenced-based fashion in human studies of glaucoma has not yet occurred. Another major issue is the subject of diurnal variability of IOP as an important principle

in evaluating efficacy of IOP-lowering medications in addition to their peak effects. As noted earlier, the alpha agonists have a relatively short half-life of action from peak to trough when used as single agents, prompting FDA approval studies and recommendations for t.i.d. use. In light of compliance issues being a much more recognized part of real-world efficacy of glaucoma medications, this factor has become a much more important issue recently.

Many different studies of efficacy of IOP lowering among the different medications used as monotherapy for ocular hypertension and glaucoma have been completed over the last 10 years and a thorough discussion of all of the studies comparing alpha agonists to other medication classes is beyond the scope of this chapter. A very complete meta-analysis of 28 randomized clinical trials of all the commonly used glaucoma medications was completed in 2005.[47] For brimonidine 0.2% in this analysis, peak IOP lowering was −31% and trough was −28%. This was very comparable to latanoprost, which had a peak of −31% and a trough of −29%. Another very recently completed meta-analysis directly comparing latanoprost and brimonidine as primary medical therapy in glaucoma using 14 clinical

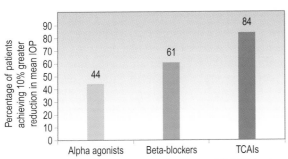

FIGURE 49.9 Adjunctive treatment to latanoprost 0.005% q.h.s. Percentage of patients on each different adjunctive regimen reaching an average of 10% or more IOP reduction.

trials showed that IOP reduction favored latanoprost by a mean weighted difference of 1.10 mmHg and the only significant difference in side-effect profile was a higher rate of fatigue associated with brimonidine as monotherapy.[48]

The use of alpha agonists as adjunctive therapy to prostaglandin analogues is another very important area of inquiry. As prostaglandin analogues have, in general, replaced most other medication classes as currently preferred monotherapy, and because IOP targets in many cases of glaucoma have been lowered significantly, this has resulted in the very common situation of combination therapy to achieve IOP targets. The comparison of alpha agonists in this role to other options is a subject of several recent clinical studies and intense interest. One of the first inquires into this question was a retrospective study looking at adjunctive therapy to latanoprost between dorzolamide, brimonidine, and timolol showing that dorzolamide showed better IOP-lowering results compared to the other two options (Fig. 49.9).[49] Several randomized trials have been completed in the last few years with differing results. One study found no significant difference in additional IOP lowering or side effects between brimonidine 0.15% b.i.d. preserved with purite and dorzolamide b.i.d. added to latanoprost,[50] while at least one other trial showed that brinzolamide, another topical carbonic anhydrase inhibitor, added more IOP lowering than either brimonidine or timolol added to travaprost.[51] Several other large-scale randomized trials of different options added to prostaglandin analogues are ongoing and will soon be published. However, it appears that all three of the major popular options of topical therapies adjunctive to prostaglandin analogues – beta-blockers, carbonic anhydrase inhibitors, and alpha agonists – are safe and effective to use in addition to prostaglandin analogues. Custom tailoring adjunctive therapies to a particular patient appears to be a reasonable current approach and alpha agonists are an effective option for adjunctive therapy with prostaglandin analogues.

CONTRAINDICATIONS

There are few true contraindications for the currently used topical alpha agonist medications.

Known sensitivity to systemic alpha agonists is a concern, probably more so with brimonidine secondary to its higher CNS side-effect profile when compared to apraclonidine. Related to this issue is the relative contraindication of the use of topical alpha agonists in pediatric populations. Brimonidine, in particular, probably because of its greater penetration of the blood–brain barrier, is associated with a high rate of CNS depression in children, particularly in infants. Several reviews and many case reports of this issue are in the relevant literature showing that this is a relatively common problem with these medications, which should be used with caution in pediatric populations.[52–54] One study characterizing these effects in children showed a definite relationship of these side effects to decreasing age and weight in children.[55] Currently, most clinicians generally avoid topical alpha agonists in young children and infants because of these CNS-mediated effects.

Although both apraclonidine and brimonidine have shown minimal effects on blood pressure, human clinical trials suggest that they should be used with caution in patients with severe cardio- and cerebrovascular disease as well as patients with hepatic or renal impairment. They also should probably be used with caution in patients with Raynaud's phenomenon or other peripheral circulatory insufficiency states. Because of the proven effect of decreasing anterior segment circulation, alpha agonists should be used with caution in patients with severe diabetic eye disease and anterior segment ischemic syndromes.

SIDE EFFECTS

The more common immediate side effects of topical alpha agonist treatment include conjunctival, oral, and nasal vasoconstriction, leading to dry nose and mouth symptoms. Conjunctival blanching and mild eyelid retraction can accompany these effects. Some of the dry nose and mouth symptoms can be modulated somewhat by punctal occlusion techniques. These symptoms typically diminish over length of treatment, especially in the first few weeks. Minimal mydriasis occurs sometimes with either apraclonidine or brimonidine and is a small enough effect as not to be an issue as a possible source of precipitation of angle-closure attacks.[56] Apraclonidine is probably associated with more of these localized acute symptoms than brimonidine due to the fact that it is relatively less α-2 selective.

Apraclonidine apparently has little if any effect on human cardiovascular physiology compared with clonidine. Clinical evidence appears to show that apraclonidine does not cause sedation,[7,57] but these studies are relatively small. Brimonidine has many more reports and evidence of these CNS and systemic side effects. In one study using brimonidine 0.5%, nearly 44% of study participants had a 20% decrease in resting systolic blood pressure. This same study showed use of topical brimonidine caused a dose-dependent fatigue or drowsiness in 6.7%, 10.4%, and 29.2% of participants using the 0.08%, 0.2%, and 0.5% concentrations,

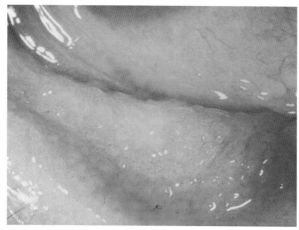

FIGURE 49.10 Typical delayed allergic reaction to brimonidine 0.2% after 8 months of monotherapy treatment. There is a large follicular conjunctivitis prominent in the inferior fornix.

respectively.[58] In another more recent prospective, randomized, placebo-controlled trial comparing apraclonidine to brimonidine, it was found that there were no blood pressure effects with apraclonidine compared to placebo but brimonidine 0.2% had small but significant effects of lowering systolic blood pressure and resting heart rate.[59] These related side effects are one of the reasons for development and study of the IOP-lowering equivalence of lower concentration formulations of topical brimonidine.

Probably the most bothersome and concerning side effect from the use of topical alpha agonists is the development of a sometimes severe allergic reaction. This presents usually as a delayed allergy-like reaction with prominent follicular conjunctivitis and periocular dermatitis, particularly of the lower lid (Fig. 49.10). The cause is unknown and appears to be either an increased sensitivity to external allergens or activation and antigen formation from a specific part of the drug itself. One theory is that adrenergically induced cell shrinkage may stress intracellular junctions, enabling the penetration of environmental allergens.[60] More recent investigations show that oxidation of a hydroquinone-like subunit, which apraclonidine shares with epinephrine but not brimonidine, may conjugate with thiol groups in ocular tissues, creating a potentially highly sensitizing hapten.[61] This may have some implications for lack of cross-reactivity between apraclonidine and brimonidine shown in some studies.

In previous studies with apraclonidine 1%, allergic conjunctivitis occurred in up to 48% of patients after a mean of 4.6 months.[60] A 90-day prospective trial comparing apraclonidine to timolol showed allergy rates of 9% with apraclonidine 0.25%, 36% with the 0.5% concentration, and none in the timolol 0.5% group. Several other studies show similar results with apraclonidine,[62–64] and time of therapy increases the chance of occurrence. This phenomenon, in addition to tachyphylaxis, has in general led to apraclonidine being used to treat or prevent acute rises in IOP and not to treat chronic IOP elevation. In general, studies of brimonidine show less development of allergic conjunctivitis but it is still a common occurrence. One large study of brimonidine 0.2% showed an allergy rate of 9.6% after 1 year.[65] Several longer-term studies of brimonidine 0.2% have found 1-year allergy rates as high as 25.7%[66] and as low as 4.7%.[67] Introduction of brimonidine with a different preservative apparently has some impact on the rate of allergic conjunctivitis. Pooled data of two studies involving about 700 patients randomized to treatment with either brimonidine 0.2% preserved with BAK vs Alphagan-P (purite) 0.15% preserved with chlorine dioxide found an allergy rate of 15% after 1 year of use in the brimonidine with BAK group vs 8.5% in the purite preserved group.[42] The lower concentration of brimonidine in the purite could also have contributed to this result.

With brimonidine now used so commonly as chronic treatment to lower intraocular pressure the allergic conjunctivitis has been further characterized in several studies. There has been an association made between the development of the allergic condition to brimonidine and the intraocular pressure rising[68] and the development of an associated anterior uveitis.[69] Previous allergic-like reactions to topical β-blockers as well as ocular surface disease are associated with a higher rate of the development of this problem.[70] Development of an allergic reaction to brimonidine was also associated with the development of subsequent allergic reactions to other topical ophthalmic medications.[71] One of the major areas of inquiry once brimonidine was introduced was whether there was significant cross-reactivity in patients with a known allergy to apraclonidine. Two studies apparently show a lack of crossover allergy in such patients with typical rates of allergy development in patients previously allergic to apraclonidine re-challenged with brimonidine.[72,73]

DRUG INTERACTIONS

In the literature there is a well-known contraindication for the use of topical alpha agonists in patients taking monoamine oxidase inhibitors. This contraindication is theoretical, with no case reports or controlled studies documenting adverse interactions between these two drug classes. Potentially, alpha agonists could potentiate the centrally mediated effects of monoamine oxidase inhibitors, in particular the side effect of hypotension. Norepinephrine, which is spared from metabolism centrally, by inhibition of monoamine oxidase, explaining monamine oxidase inhibition's therapeutic effect in treating depression, also stimulates α-2 receptors centrally, resulting in vasodilation and systolic blood pressure lowering. A bothersome side effect of monoamine oxidase inhibitors is orthostatic hypotension. It is thought that centrally acting alpha agonists, in particular clonidine and perhaps brimonidine, could produce a profound synergistic hypotensive effect used with monoamine oxidase inhibitors and cause cardiovascular collapse in sensitive patients.[74]

Summary

Alpha agonists lower intraocular pressure primarily through stimulation of α-2 receptors in the eye, which lowers adenylate cyclase activity, resulting in lower intracellular cAMP levels. Secondary prostaglandin mediators and central nervous system effects may be contributory as well. Exact mechanisms of effects on aqueous dynamics in humans are not well delineated; however, alpha agonists appear to decrease aqueous inflow as well as increasing aqueous outflow possibly involving the uveoscleral pathway or other nonpressure-dependent dynamics. Neuroprotective properties aside from IOP-lowering effects of alpha agonists are being intensively studied; however, it is premature to make any claims of neuroprotection in clinical use at this time.

Topical alpha agonists have become an important and commonly employed group of agents in the armamentarium to treat elevated intraocular pressure. Brimonidine, in particular, can be used as monotherapy for chronic treatment and adjunctively with other agents. Apraclonidine is not currently widely used for chronic treatment secondary to the higher incidence of allergic reactions and tachyphylaxis. Both apraclonidine and brimonidine are very effective and superior to other topical and even oral IOP-lowering agents in treating and preventing acute IOP elevation in acute glaucomas and after various ophthalmic procedures including laser trabeculoplasty, laser iridotomy, Nd:YAG capsulotomy, cataract surgery, and other interventions. Alpha agonists have been shown to be effective as adjunctive therapy to other classes of topical intraocular pressure-lowering agents, in particular the prostaglandin analogues. There is also a formulation now available in the USA with brimonidine in fixed combination for b.i.d. dosing with timolol.

Alpha agonists have a favorable safety index but there are well-known side effects. Apraclonidine has little if any associated CNS-mediated side effects of fatigue and hypotension but has a high rate of the development of associated delayed allergic responses. Brimonidine has a much lower rate of allergy but does have more CNS-mediated side effects, limiting its use, especially in pediatric populations. The side-effect profile of brimonidine has led to the development of formulations with different preservatives and lower concentrations that are apparently equal in efficacy to earlier formulations and appear to have less development of delayed allergic reactions and associated fatigue.

REFERENCES

1. Savage H, Robin AL. Adrenergic agents. In: Ophthalmology monograph 13, glaucoma principles and management. Netland P, ed. San Francisco, CA: American Academy of Ophthalmology; 1999:47–75.

2. Wang RF, Camras CB, Podos SM, et al. The role of prostaglandins in the para-aminoclonidine-induced reduction of intraocular pressure. Trans Am Ophthalmol Soc 1989; 87:94–104.

3. Sulewski ME, Robin AL, Cummings HL, et al. Effects of topical flurbiprofen on the intraocular pressure lowering of apraclonidine hydrochloride and timolol maleate. Arch Ophthalmol 1991; 109:807–809.

4. McCannel C, Koskela T, Brubaker RF. Topical flurbiprofen pretreatment does not block apraclonidine's effect on aqueous flow in humans. Arch Ophthalmol 1991; 109:810–811.

5. Jampel HD, Robin AL, Quigley HA, et al. Apraclonidine: a one week dose–response study. Arch Ophthalmol 1988; 106:1069–1073.

6. Gabelt BT, Robinson JC, Hubbard WC, et al. Apraclonidine and brimonidine effects on anterior ocular and cardiovascular physiology in normal and sympathectomized monkeys. Exp Eye Res 1994; 59:633–644.

7. Coleman AL, Robin AL, Pollack IP, et al. Cardiovascular and intraocular pressure effects and plasma concentrations of apraclonidine. Arch Ophthalmol 1990; 108:1264–1267.

8. Toris CB, Tafoya ME, Camras CB, et al. Effects of apraclonidine on aqueous humor dynamics in human eyes. Ophthalmology 1995; 102:456–461.

9. Toris CB, Gleason ML, Camras CB, et al. Effects of brimonidine on aqueous humor dynamics in human eyes. Arch Ophthalmol 1995; 113:1514–1517.

10. Coleman AL, Robin AL, Pollack IP. New ophthalmic drugs: apraclonidine hydrochloride. Ophthalmol Clin North Am 1989; 2:97–108.

11. Burke JA, Potter DE. Ocular effects of a relatively selective alpha 2 agonist (UK-14,304-18) in cats, rabbits and monkeys. Curr Eye Res 1986; 5:665–676.

12. Burke J, Padillo E, Shan T, et al. Adrenergic and imidazoline receptor-mediated responses to Uk-14,304-18 (brimonidine) in rabbits and monkeys. A species difference. Ann NY Acad Sci 1995; 763:78–95.

13. Maus TL, Nau C, Brubaker RF. Comparison of the early effects of brimonidine and apraclonidine as topical ocular hypotensive agents. Arch Ophthalmol 1999; 117:586–591.

14. Serdahl CL, Galustian J, Lewis RA. The effects of apraclonidine on conjunctival oxygen tension. Arch Ophthalmol 1989; 107:1777–1779.

15. Kim TW, Kim DM. Effects of 0.5% apraclonidine on optic nerve head and peripapillary retinal blood flow. Br J Ophthalmol 1997; 81:1070–1101.

16. Rosa RH, Hein TW, Yuan Z, et al. Brimonidine evokes heterogeneous vasomotor response of retinal arterioles: diminished nitric oxide-mediated vasodilatation when size goes small. Am J Physiol Heart Circ Physiol 2006; 291: H231–H238.

17. Simsek T, Yanik B, Conkbayir I, et al. Comparative analysis of the effects of brimonidine and dorzolamide on ocular blood flow velocity in patients with newly diagnosed primary open-angle glaucoma. J Ocul Pharmacol Ther 2006; 22:79–85.

18. Schmidt KG, Klingmuller V, Gouveia SM, et al. Short posterior ciliary artery, central retinal artery, and choroidal hemodynamics in brimonidine-treated primary open-angle glaucoma patients. Am J Ophthalmol 2003; 136:1038–1048.

19. Carlsson AM, Chauhan BC, Lee AA, et al. The effect of brimonidine tartrate on retinal blood flow in patients with ocular hypertension (corrected). Am J Ophthalmol 2000; 129:297–301.

20. Costagliola C, Parmeggiani F, Ciancaglini M, et al. Ocular perfusion pressure and visual field indices modifications induced by alpha-agonist compound (clonidine 0.125%, apraclonidine 1.0%, and brimonidine 0.2%) topical administration. An acute study on primary open-angle glaucoma patients. Ophthalmologica 2003; 217:39–44.

21. Burke J, Schwartz M. Preclinical evaluation of brimonidine. Surv Ophthalmol 1996; 41(Suppl 1):s9–s18.

22. Yoles E, Wheeler LA, Schwartz M. α2-Adrenorecptor agonists are neuroprotective in a rat model of optic nerve degeneration. Invest Ophthalmol Vis Sci 1999; 40:65–73.

23. Mayor-Torroglosa S, De la Villa P, Rodriquez ME, et al. Ischemia results 3 months later in altered ERG, degeneration of inner layers, and deafferented tectum: neuroprotection with brimonidine. Invest Ophthalmol Vis Sci 2005; 46:3825–3835.

24. Aviles-Trigueros M, Mayor-Torroglosa S, Garcia-Aviles A, et al. Transient ischemia of the retina results in massive degeneration of the retinotectal projection: long-term neuroprotection with brimonidine. Exp Neurol 2003; 184:767–777.

25. Vidal-Snaz M, Lafuente MP, Mayor-Torroglosa S, et al. Brimonidine's neuroprotective effects against transient ischaemia-induced retinal ganglion cell death. Ur J Ophthalmol 2001; 11(Suppl 2):s36–ss40.

26. The BRAION study group; Wilhelm B, Ludtke H, Wilhelm H. Efficacy and tolerability of 0.2% brimonidine tartrate for the treatment of acute non-arteritic anterior ischemic optic neuropathy (NAION): a 3-month, double-masked, randomized, placebo-controlled trial. Graefe's Arch Clin Exp Ophthalmol 2006; 244:551–558.

27. Aung T, Oen FT, Wong HT, et al. Randomized controlled trial comparing the effect of brimonidine and timolol on visual field loss after acute primary angle closure. Br J Ophthalmol 2004; 88:88–94.

28. Weinreb RN, Ruderman J, Juster R, et al. Immediate intraocular pressure response to argon laser trabeculoplasty. Am J Ophthalmol 1983; 7:279–286.

29. Robin AL, Pollack IP, House B, et al. Effects of ALO2145 on intraocular pressure following argon laser trabeculoplasty. Arch Ophthalmol 1987; 105:646–650.

30. Robin AL. Medical therapy to prevent the intraocular pressure rise associated with argon laser trabeculoplasty. Ophthalmic Surg 1991; 22:31–37.

31. Threlkeld AB, Assalian AA, Allingham RR, et al. Apraclonidine 0.5% versus 1% for controlling intraocular pressure elevation after argon laser trabeculoplasty. Ophthalmic Surg Lasers 1996; 27:657–660.

32. Rosenberg LF, Krupin T, Ruderman J, et al. Apraclonidine and anterior segment laser surgery: comparison of 0.5% versus 1.0% apraclonidine for prevention of postoperative intraocular pressure rise. Ophthalmology 1995; 102:1312–1318.

33. Robin AL, Pollack IP, deFaller JM. Effects of topical ALO 2145 (p-aminoclonidine hydrochloride) on the acute intraocular pressure rise after argon laser iridotomy. Arch Ophthalmol 1987; 105:1208–1211.

34. Ffernandez-Bahamonde JL, Alcaraz-Michelli V. The combined use of apraclonidine and pilocarpine during laser iridotomy in a Hispanic population. Ann Ophthalmol 1990; 22:446–449.

35. Cullam RD, Jr Schwartz LW. The effect of apraclonidine on the intraocular pressure of glaucoma patients following Nd:YAG laser posterior capsulotomy. Ophthalmic Surg Lasers 1993; 24:623–626.

36. Feist RM, Palmer DJ, Fiscella R, et al. Effectiveness of apraclonidine and acetazolamide in preventing postoperative intraocular pressure spikes after extracapsular cataract extraction. J Cataract Refract Surg 1995; 21:191–195.

37. Cevrier RL, Assalian A, Duperre J, et al. Apraclonidine 0.5% versus brimonidine 0.2% for the control of intraocular pressure elevation following anterior segment laser procedures. Ophthalmic Surg Lasers 1999; 30:199–204.

38. Yuen NS, Cheung P, Hui SP. Comparing brimonidine 0.2% to apraclonidine 1.0% in the prevention of intraocular pressure elevation and their papillary effects following laser peripheral iridotomy. Jpn J Ophthalmol 2005; 49:89–92.

39. Chen TC. Brimonidine 0.15% versus apraclonidine 0.5% for prevention of intraocular pressure elevation after anterior segment laser surgery. J Cataract Refract Surg 2005; 31:1710–1712.

40. Schuman JS, Horwitz B, Choplin NT, et al. A 1-year study of brimonidine twice daily in glaucoma and ocular hypertension. A controlled, randomized, multicenter clinical trial. Chronic Brimonidine Study Group. Arch Ophthalmol 1997; 115:847–852.

41. Cantor LB. The evolving pharmacotherapeutic profile of brimonidine, an alpha 2-adrenergic agonist, after four years of continuous use. Expert Opin Pharmacother 2000; 1:815–834.

42. Katz LJ. Twelve-month evaluation of brimonidine-purite versus brimonidine in patients with glaucoma or ocular hypertension. J Glaucoma 2002; 11:119–126.

43. Whitson JT, Ochsner KI, Moster MR, et al. The safety and intraocular pressure-lowering efficacy of brimonidine tartrate 0.15% preserved with polyquaternium-1. Ophthalmology 2006; 113:1333–1339.

44. Goni FJ. Brimonidine/Timolol Fixed Combination Study Group. 12-week study comparing the fixed combination of brimonidine and timolol with concomitant use of the individual components in patients with glaucoma and ocular hypertension. Eur J Ophthalmol 2005; 15:581–590.

45. Sherwood MB, Craven ER, Chou C, et al. Twice-daily 0.2% brimonidine–0.5% timolol fixed-combination therapy vs monotherapy with timolol or brimonidine in patients with glaucoma or ocular hypertension: a 12-month randomized trial. Arch Ophthalmol 2006; 124:1230–1238.

46. Craven ER, Walters TR, Williams R, et al. Brimonidine and timolol fixed-combination versus monotherapy: a 3 month randomized trial in patients with glaucoma or ocular hypertension. J Ocul Pharmacol Ther 2005; 21:337–348.

47. van der Valk R, Webers CA, Schouten JS, et al. Intraocular pressure-lowering effects of all commonly used glaucoma drugs: a meta-analysis of randomized clinical trials. Ophthalmology 2005; 12:1177–1185.

48. Fung AT, Reid SE, Jones MP, et al. Meta-analysis of randomized controlled trials comparing latanoprost with brimonidine in the treatment of open-angle glaucoma, ocular hypertension or normal-tension glaucoma. Br J Ophthalmol 2007; 91:62–68.

49. O'Connor DJ, Martone JF, Mead A. Additive intraocular pressure lowering effect of various medications with latanoprost. Am J Ophthalmol 2002; 133:836–837.

50. Konstas AG, Karabatsas CH, Lallos N, et al. 24-hour intraocular pressures with brimonidine purite versus dorzolamide added to latanoprost in primary open-angle glaucoma subjects. Ophthalmology 2005; 112:603–608.

51. Reis R, Queiroz CF, Santos LC, et al. A randomized investigator-masked, 4-week study comparing timolol maleate 0.5%, brinzolamide 1%, and brimonidine tartrate 0.2% as adjunctive therapies to travoprost 0.004% in adults with primary open-angle glaucoma or ocular hypertension. Clin Ther 2006; 28:552–559.

52. Bowman RJ, Cope J, Nischal KK. Ocular and systemic effects of brimonidine 0.2% eye drops (Alphagan) in children. Eye 2004; 18:24–26.

53. Talbot AW, Russell-Eggitt I. Pharmaceutical management of the childhood glaucomas. Expert Opin Pharmacother 2000; 1:697–711.

54. Enyedi LB, Freedman SF. Safety and efficacy of brimonidine in children with glaucoma. J AAPOS 2001; 5:281–284.

55. Al-Shahwan S, Al Torbak AA, Turkmani S. Side-effect profile of brimonidine tartrate in children. Ophthalmology 2005; 112:2143.

56. Krawitz PL, Podos SM. Use of apraclonidine in the treatment of acute angle closure glaucoma. Arch Ophthalmol 1989; 107:1777–1779.

57. Morrison JC, Robin AL. Adjunctive glaucoma therapy. A comparison of apraclonidine to dipivefrin when added to timolol maleate. Ophthalmology 1989; 96:3–7.

58. Derick RJ, Robin AL, Walters TR, et al. Brimonidine tartrate: a one-month dose–response study. Ophthalmology 1997; 104:131–136.

59. Yuksel N, Karabas L, Altintas O, et al. A comparison of the short-term hypotensive effects and side effects of unilateral brimonidine and apraclonidine in patients with elevated intraocular pressure. Ophthalmologica 2002; 216:45–49.

60. Butler P, Mannshreck M, Lin S, et al. Clinical experience with the long-term use of 1% apraclonidine: incidence of allergic reactions. Arch Ophthalmol 1995; 113:293–296.

61. Thompson CD, Macdonald TL, Garst ME, et al. Mechanisms of adrenergic agonist induced allergy bioactivation and antigen formation. Exp Eye Res 1997; 64:767–773.

62. Stewart WC, Ritch R, Shin DH, et al. The efficacy of apraclonidine as an adjunct to timolol therapy. Apraclonidine Adjunctive Therapy Study Group. Arch Ophthalmol 1995; 113:287–292.

63. Araujo SV, Bond JB, Wilson RP, et al. Long term effect of apraclonidine. Br J Ophthalmol 1995; 79:1098–1101.

64. Robin AL, Ritch R, Shin DH, et al. Short-term efficacy of apraclonidine hydrochloride added to maximum-tolerated medical therapy for glaucoma. Am J Ophthalmol 1995; 120:423–432.

65. Schuman JS. Clinical experience with brimonidine 0.2% and timolol 0.5% in glaucoma and ocular hypertension. Surv Ophthalmol 1996; 41(Suppl 1):s27–s37.

66. Blondeau P, Rousseau JA. Allergic reactions to brimonidine in patients treated for glaucoma. Can J Ophthalmol 2002; 37: 21–26.

67. Melamed S, David R. Ongoing clinical assessment of the safety profile and efficacy of brimonidine compared with timolol: year three results. Brimonidine Study Group II. Clin Ther 2000; 22:103–111.

68. Watts P, Hawksworth N. Delayed hypersensitivity to brimonidine tartrate 0.2% associated with high intraocular pressure. Eye 2002; 16:132–135.

69. Becker HI, Walton RC, Diamant JI, et al. Anterior uveitis and concurrent allergic conjunctivitis associated with long-term use of topical 0.2% brimonidine tartrate. Arch Ophthalmol 2004; 122:1063–1066.

70. Manni G, Centofanti M, Sacchetti M, et al. Demographic and clinical factors associated with development of brimonidine tartrate 0.2%-induced ocular allergy. J Glaucoma 2004; 13: 163–167.

71. Osborne SA, Montgomery DM, Morris D, et al. Alphagan allergy may increase the propensity for multiple eye-drop allergy. Eye 2005; 19:129–137.

72. Gordon RN, Liebmann JM, Greenfield DS, et al. Lack of cross-reactive allergic response to brimonidine in patients with known apraclonidine allergy. Eye 1998; 12(pt 4):697–700.

73. Williams GC, Orengo-Nania S, Gross RL. Incidence of brimonidine allergy in patients previously allergic to apraclonidine. J Glaucoma 2000; 9:235–238.

74. Thomson Healthcare Inc. Interaction effects of apraclonidine, brimonidine, and monoamine oxidase inhibitors. Micromedex 2007 and United States Pharmacopeia 2004.

CHAPTER 50

Prostaglandin Analogues

Norbert Pfeiffer and Hagen Thieme

INTRODUCTION

There is no doubt that prostaglandin analogues have tremendously enriched our armamentarium of medical glaucoma therapy in the past 10 years. Prostaglandin derivatives, sometimes referred to as hypotensive lipids, were introduced into medical glaucoma therapy in 1996, with the availability of latanoprost. Since then, these drugs have been used most successfully in the management of glaucoma, leading to enhanced medical treatment of the disease. Thus, patients can be kept on topical therapy for longer time periods. Furthermore, prostaglandin analogues led to a decreasing number of surgical interventions.

Initially, the prostaglandin effect on intraocular pressure (IOP) had been expected to be very small. This class of substances can lead to intraocular inflammation. To date, prostaglandin analogues are considered to be potent IOP-lowering drugs and may enhance patient compliance due to a once-daily application. Their IOP-lowering potency is superior to any other single drug formulation for the treatment of glaucoma. Also, their side-effect profile appears to be very mild, which explains why prostaglandin analogues have become the first-line choice and first-line therapy for the medical treatment of glaucoma in many countries. Therefore, they have become the most frequently used drugs for medical glaucoma treatment. Many patients who previously failed a medical therapy can now be controlled for longer. Recently, several fixed combinations appeared on the market combining β-blockers with prostaglandin analogues, enhancing efficacy and compliance.

DRUG FORMULATIONS

Prostaglandins are naturally occurring substances in the eye; they were first extracted from accessory gland secretions (prostate gland = prostaglandin) and in the eye from irides.[1] The word 'irine' was the German term used as a description for this group of substances. Prostaglandins are produced in many tissues, including the eye, from their precursor, arachidonic acid (Fig. 50.1).

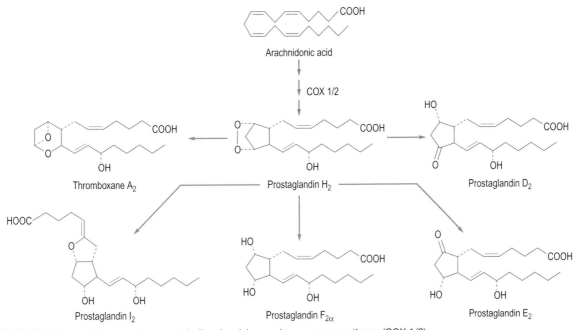

FIGURE 50.1 Arachnidonic pathway metabolism involving cyclooxygenase pathway (COX 1/2).

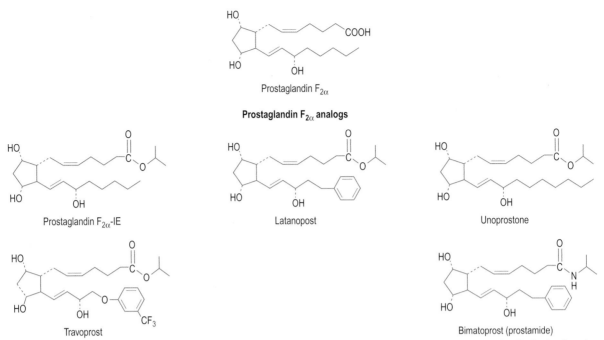

FIGURE 50.2 Chemical structure of the common prostaglandin analogues in use today. For comparison prostaglandin $F_{2\alpha}$ is also shown.

They act via G-protein-coupled prostaglandin receptors of which there are several different types, namely FP, EP_{1-4}, IP, TP, and DP. The variety of naturally occurring prostaglandins is large, their degradation is rather rapid, and their receptor specificity depends on whether or not the metabolites act on other receptors as well. Therefore, all currently available prostaglandin analogues have different receptor profiles, indicating that in the event of noneffectiveness of one drug a different one could be tried.

Prostaglandin analogues have generally been associated with intraocular inflammation. This observation dates back to animal experiments from the 1960s and 1970s when prostaglandins were administered in high concentrations to the eyes of test animals, usually by intraocular injection. However, it had previously been noted by clinicians that in an inflamed eye, such as in acute iritis, the IOP is usually lower than in the non-affected eye. Therefore, the search was intense to find prostaglandins which might exhibit pressure-lowering properties. Camras et al. showed a reduction in IOP after topical administration of prostaglandins to the rabbit eye, soon followed by similar observations in cats, dogs, and primates shown by other authors.[2] Thereafter, it was merely drug design which led to the application of these drugs in humans. However, naturally occurring prostaglandins (PGs) such as $PGF_{2\alpha}$ are not useful in clinical practice due to adverse effects such as irritation, conjunctival hyperemia, and even headache. Therefore, PG analogues of better tolerability were developed, at the same time keeping IOP-lowering properties. These are isopropyl unoprostone (a metabolite of $PGF_{2\alpha}$), latanoprost, bimatoprost (a prostamide), and travoprost (Fig. 50.2). Of those, only

bimatoprost was suggested not to bind to PG receptors. Unoprostone still bears the name of its inventor Ueno (trade name Rescula, Novartis). This docosanoid shows a weaker IOP-lowering effect than other PGs and needs to be administered twice daily. It was named docosanoid because of its increased numbers of carbon atoms. It was first introduced into clinical practice in Japan in 1993, where it still holds a place in the market today. In Europe and the USA, unoprostone was not quite as successful, mainly due to strong competition from the other prostaglandin analogues that appeared on the market shortly afterwards.[3]

Most of the information regarding drug formulation and alteration after administration has been obtained for latanoprost, which was the first commercially available true PG analogue and second after unoprostone. The drug is rapidly hydrolyzed in the cornea and its active metabolite, latanoprost free acid, reaches peak aqueous humor levels of 15–20 ng/mL 1–2 hours after topical administration. Penetration through the cornea is enhanced by a low pH of the formulations. This partly explains why prostaglandin analogues have the highest benzalkonium chloride concentration of all antiglaucomatous drugs currently available. Low pH is also achieved by addition of buffer solutions (phosphate buffer). Given once daily (in the evening) the IOP-lowering effect is maintained over 24 hours, with the onset of an IOP-reducing effect after 3–4 hours.[4]

MECHANISM OF ACTION

Intraocular pressure is determined by the production of aqueous humor in the ciliary body epithelium and by the rate this fluid is removed from the eye. There are two major routes for aqueous humor to exit the eye: (1) drainage through the trabecular meshwork into Schlemm's canal, and (2) through the uveoscleral route along the ciliary muscle into the subciliary space. It is believed that 80–85% of total flow is along the conventional (trabecular) route, whereas the nonconventional (uveoscleral) pathway accounts for 15–20%. In this context, the amount which is absorbed via the vitreous cavity is negligible.

It is the uveoscleral pathway that PG analogues effect, and by triggering a cascade of tissue remodeling enzymes, such as metalloproteinases and transcription factors such as c-fos, collagen is degraded. This opens the intercellular spaces for fluid drainage, ultimately leading to increased uveoscleral flow rates and hence lowered IOP.

An effect on the trabecular route has been proposed but is not proven yet. What is known from in vitro studies is the fact that intracellular calcium signaling pathways in human trabecular meshwork cells are affected by PG analogues. A direct affect on the conventional outflow pathway is currently under investigation.[5–7]

PHARMACOLOGY

The pharmacokinetics of prostaglandin analogues were investigated using radiolabeled latanoprost. With the exception of bimatoprost, all major clinically used PG analogues are prodrugs that undergo hydrolysis to their acid form after topical administration. This hydrolysis requires a low pH, which accounts for buffer solutions. Benzalkonium chloride is mainly used as a preservative which also enhances corneal uptake of the drugs due to its tensidic properties. In patients who underwent cataract surgery, latanoprost was found at its maximal concentration 2.5 hours after topical administration of the compound. Half-elimination time for the free acid (latanoprost acid) was at a rate of 2.5 hours within the eye. The compound is metabolized rapidly in the liver by beta-oxidation and finally eliminated through the feces and urine.[8,9]

EFFECT ON AQUEOUS HUMOR DYNAMICS

Prostaglandin analogues widen the spaces in the uveoscleral route, leading to increased aqueous humor passage. On a molecular level, c-fos and metalloproteinases (MMPs) are activated and collagen is degraded, resulting in increased permeability of the tissue.[10,11] Because of the rapid onset of IOP lowering after administration of the drugs there has been some speculation that PG analogues also exert an effect on the conventional outflow pathway by effects on the trabecular meshwork. For unoprostone and fluprostenol an antiendothelin effect (i.e. relaxation of the contractile trabecular meshwork) has been proposed; however, the basic data lack clinical proof.[12,13] From clinical observation, it seems quite obvious that an additional effect on the conventional pathway exists, as the onset of the drugs is within hours, and the increase in IOP after discontinuing the drugs is rather quick. These effects can hardly be explained by tissue remodeling in the uveoscleral pathway alone.

OTHER THERAPEUTIC EFFECTS (I.E. NEUROPROTECTION OR ALTERATION OF BLOOD FLOW)

There has been some speculation about blood flow impairment by prostaglandin analogues. At first glance, prostaglandin analogues appear to exert a vasodilatory effect on ocular vessels because of the observation of conjunctival and scleral hyperemia. This effect appears only on the surface area of the eye, whereas the effects on intraocular vessels appear to be quite the opposite. The first compound which was tested on isolated vessels was $PGF_{2\alpha}$. Its vasoconstrictory effects have been shown in many extraocular vessels.[14,15] It appears that the concentrations required for retinal vessel constriction are higher than those used in topical glaucoma treatment. In a special subpopulation of patients the compounds may reach the back of the eye in a sufficient concentration to exert a vasoconstrictor effect. Reports of patients suffering from cystoid macular edema after cataract removal underline the possibility that due to barrier breakdown diffusion of prostaglandin analogues and their free acids could be enhanced, causing side effects.[16] Therefore, caution is advised in glaucoma patients scheduled for cataract operation. Some cataract surgeons suggest that drugs should be discontinued at least 2 weeks prior to surgery.

INDICATIONS

Prostaglandin analogues are used for the treatment of most forms of glaucoma. The compounds should be used whenever low target pressures are called for in both normal-tension glaucoma or primary open-angle glaucoma (POAG), as well as ocular hypertensive (OHT) patients where treatment seems mandatory. Studies suggest that conversion from OHT to POAG is reduced or slowed by IOP lowering, including the use of PGs.[17] In most countries, prostaglandin analogues are prescribed as first-line and first-choice treatment for glaucoma patients. With patients' compliance issues becoming more and more important, these drugs offer high quality-of-life scores due to a once-daily and therefore very convenient application (usually in the evening). The drugs have also been approved for the treatment of pediatric and juvenile glaucoma where, naturally, compliance issues are even more pressing.[18]

EFFICACY AND COMPARISON WITH OTHER AGENTS

Nowadays, lower target pressures are aimed for in glaucoma patients, because large multicenter studies have shown the benefits of achieving very low IOP levels. This has led to a trend towards a more aggressive treatment of patients. According to various studies, listed prostaglandin analogues offer a range of 20–40% IOP reduction in POAG and OHT patients and can therefore be regarded as the most powerful compounds at present.

Prostaglandins can be effectively combined with other compounds, and fixed combinations with β-blockers are commercially available.[19] Pharmacodynamics appear to make the fixed combination of prostaglandin analogues and carbonic anhydrase less valuable, but the free combination is readily used.

Prostamides and prostaglandin analogues appear to be equally or more effective in lowering IOP compared to timolol. Unoprostone has less potency in this respect. Many comparative studies have been performed so far but, generally speaking, the three hypotensive lipids bimatoprost, latanoprost, and travoprost seem to have comparable efficacy.[20,21]

CONTRAINDICATIONS

Naturally, any patient suffering from hyperreactivity towards the compounds or its preservatives (benzalkonium chloride) should avoid the drugs. Furthermore, the drugs should be avoided in patients wearing contact lenses. Removing the lenses and refitting them after 15 minutes is permissible. Due to their possible inflammatory response, they should be used cautiously in all forms of inflammatory (secondary) glaucoma. Caution is advised in all patients suffering from elevated IOP due to uveitis and secondary glaucoma because of inflammation. This relates to the acute state and to chronic disease. Also, in acute angle-closure glaucoma in all situations where fibrinous reactions are present these compounds should be avoided, because the drugs might trigger further inflammatory responses. Many ophthalmologists discontinue PG analogues before cataract surgery because cases of cystoid macular edema have been reported following administration of prostaglandin analogues, particularly in patients undergoing cataract surgery. Also, many surgeons discontinue PGs in operated cataract patients in whom an intraoperative complication such as a rupture of the capsular bag has occurred.

Treating one eye only can result in iris color changes, which is then noticeable to the patient and to his or her relatives. This should best be avoided, especially in bright irides.[18]

SIDE EFFECTS

Data from numerous clinical trials confirm the ocular and systemic safety of prostaglandin analogues as well as their tolerability when used as first-line monotherapy or adjunctive therapy with other IOP-lowering agents in patients with POAG or OHT. However, one needs to differentiate between local and systemic effects.

LOCAL SIDE EFFECTS

The most frequent side effects are hyperemia (bimatoprost up to 44.7%, latanoprost up to 27.6%, travoprost up to 49.5%, and unoprostone up to 9%) and foreign

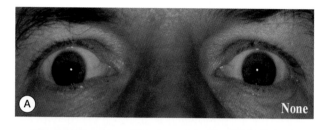
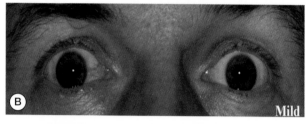
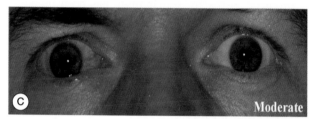
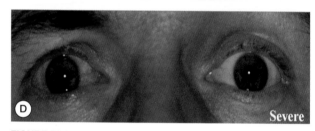

FIGURE 50.3 Redness grading scale showing increased prominent conjunctival vessels **A–D** as prostaglandin treatment continues.

body sensations as well as itching and stinging (Fig. 50.4). Generally speaking, these effects only seem to last for a short period of time, vanishing or becoming less severe in most cases.[22]

Long-lasting administration can lead to eye lash changes. They increase in thickness, count, and pigmentation.[23] This was observed to be a reversible effects once the drugs are discontinued. Additionally, an iris color change can occur, especially in patients with green-brown, blue/gray-brown, and brown irides (Fig. 50.3). Currently the long-term effect of these changes remains to be investigated.[24] Unoprostone is the only drug in this group which does not seem to lead to changes in iris color on long-term follow-up.

Prostamides and prostaglandin analogues can lead to the development and worsening of cystoid macular edema, especially in patients after cataract removal. Caution is suggested in these cases.[25]

Patients who had been suffering from herpes keratitis may develop a recurrence. Additionally, an anterior uveitis can develop. Again, caution in these cases is mandatory.[26]

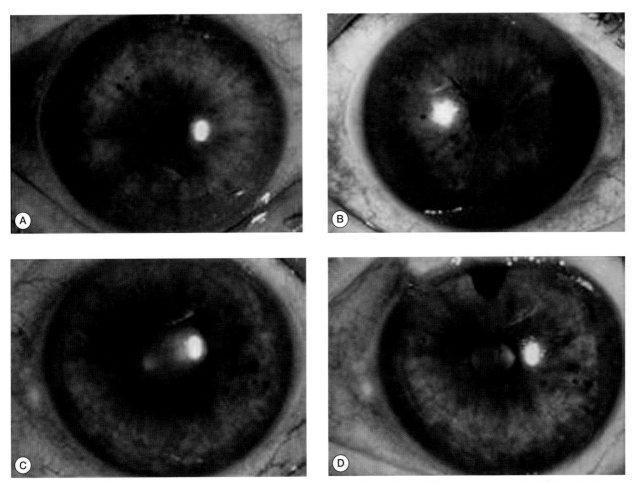

FIGURE 50.4 Discoloration of an iris in an eye which had received prostaglandin analogues. The two images on the left show before (**A**) and after (**B**) treatment with topical prostaglandin therapy. The yellow eye received surgical treatment; (**C**) before and (**D**) after trabeculectomy.

SYSTEMIC SIDE EFFECTS

Special attention is needed interpreting the following observations which were obtained during routine clinical use of the drugs. There can be no real estimate about how often these occur. Systemic side effects were dyspnea, asthma, and acute asthma.[27] Caution is also advised in pregnancy.

Supportive evidence for the tolerability of prostaglandin analogues also comes from studies investigating medication persistence. Patients were less likely to discontinue treatment compared to other treatment regimens and, of those who did discontinue treatment, the length of therapy was significantly longer with prostaglandin analogues compared to other drugs. This indicates that prostagladin analogues enhance patient compliance and quality of life. Both of these factors are essential and vital key points for a lifelong treatment of glaucoma.[28]

DRUG INTERACTIONS

Drug interactions are a key point to focus on when prostaglandin analogues should be combined with other compounds. Fixed combinations currently combine prostaglandin analogues with β-blockers. Prostaglandin analogues can be combined readily with almost all other antiglaucoma drugs currently available as they have a unique mode of action. All other compounds which lower aqueous humor secretion through the ciliary body can be combined. Thus, two separate modes of action are augmented: decreased production, and increased outflow.[18] There is one exception to this: pilocarpine. Pilocarpine induces ciliary muscle contraction, leading to decreased flow through the uveoscleral pathways. Prostaglandin analogues act in an antagonistic manner, opening the spaces of this very pathway.[29] This approach, however, appears to be quite academic as clinical experience shows a small additive effect of pilocarpine with prostaglandin analogues.[30] As pilocarpine nowadays is no longer first-choice medical treatment, the necessity for a combination therapy of prostaglandin analogues with pilocarpine becomes less important.

A significant number of patients show a poor response to treatment with prostaglandin analogues. Individual studies show that their rate varies between 4% to almost 50% of study patients. Due to their differences in pharmacokinetics and receptor binding it appears warranted to switch from one prostaglandin analogue to another if one does not show an effect on IOP.[31]

Summary

Recent landmark studies have suggested that lower IOPs are beneficial for the course of glaucoma. Due to the introduction of prostaglandin analogues, many patients who previously could not be treated adequately with topical medications can now be treated satisfactorily. Prostaglandin analogues are powerful and potent drugs which yield a 20–40% decrease in IOP. This is achieved by a once-daily application. By a unique mode of action (enhancing uveoscleral flow) these drugs lower IOP more than any other antiglaucoma drug. However, other mechanisms appear to play a role. Their safety and adverse side-effect profile is very good (usually mild hyperemia, iris pigment changes, and eyelash growth), making prostaglandin analogues the first choice and first-line therapy in many countries. Caution is advised in patients with an inflammatory history such as uveitis, herpes keratitis, and in patients in whom cataract extraction is planned. In patients with intraoperative complications (rupture of capsular bag) prostaglandin analogues may be causative for the development of cystic macular edema.

New drug formulations offer combination therapies in which β-blockers are combined with prostagladin analogues. In summary, prostaglandin analogues offer an important option in terms of both cost-efficiency and quality of life.

REFERENCES

1. Ventura WP, Freund M. Evidence for a new class of uterine stimulants in rat semen and male accessory gland secretions. J Reprod Fertil 1973; 33:507–511.

2. Camras CB, Bito LZ, Eakins KE. Reduction in intraocular pressure by prostaglandins applied topically to the eyes of conscious rabbits. Invest Ophthalmol Vis Sci 1977; 16: 1125–1134.

3. Alexander CL, Miller SJ, Abel SR. Prostaglandin analog treatment of glaucoma and ocular hypertension. Ann Pharmacother 2002; 36:504–511.

4. Alm A, Stjernschantz J. The Scandinavian Latanoprost Study Group. Effect on intraocular pressure and side effects of 0.005% latanoprost applied once daily, evening or morning: a comparison with timolol. Ophthalmology 1995; 102: 1743–1752.

5. Bill A. Some aspects of aqueous humor drainage. Eye 1993; 7(pt 1):14–19.

6. Nilsson SF. The uveoscleral outflow routes. Eye 1997; 11(pt2):149–154.

7. Toris CB, Zhan G, Fan S, et al. Effects of travorprost on aqueous humor dynamics in patients with elevated intraocular pressure. J Glaucoma 2007; 16(2):189–195.

8. Alm A. Prostaglandin derivates as ocular hypotensive agents. Prog Ret Eye Res 1997; 17:291–312.

9. Sjöquist B, Stjernschantz J. Ocular and systemic pharmacokinetics of latanoprost in humans. Surv Ophthalmol 2002; 47(Suppl 1):S6–S12.

10. Lindsey JD, Kashiwagi K, Boyle D, et al. Prostaglandins increase proMMP-1 and proMMP-3 secretion by human ciliary smooth muscle cells. Curr Eye Res 1996; 15:869–875.

11. Lindsey JD, Kashiwagi K, Kashiwagi F, et al. Prostaglandins alter extracellular matrix adjacent to human ciliary muscle cells in vitro. Invest Ophthalmol Vis Sci 1997; 38:2214–2223.

12. Thieme H, Stumpff F, Ottlecz A, et al. Mechanism of action of unoprostone on trabecular meshwork contractility. Invest Ophthalmol Vis Sci 2001; 42:3193–3201.

13. Thieme H, Schimmat C, Boxberger M, et al. Endothelin-antagonism: effects of FP receptor agonists F2alpha and fluprostenol on trabecular meshwork contractility. Invest Ophthalmol Vis Sci 2006; 47(3):938–945.

14. Astim M. Effects of prostaglandin E2; F2alpha and latanoprost acid on isolated ocular blood vessels in vitro. J Ocul Pharmacol Ther 1998; 14:119–128.

15. Hoste A. Cosopt® versus Xalatan®. In: Shaarawy T, Flammer J, eds. Glaucoma therapy 'current issues and controversies.' London: Martin Dunitz; 2004:123–142.

16. Schumer RA, Camras CB, Mandahl AK. Latanoprost and cystoid macular edema: is there a causal relation? Curr Opin Ophthalmol 2000; 11:94–100.

17. Kass MA, Gordon MO, Hoff MR. Topical timolol administration reduces the incidence of glaucomatous damage in ocular hypertensive individuals. A randomized, double-masked, long-term clinical trial. Arch Ophthalmol 1989; 107:1590–1598.

18. No authors listed. Chapter 3: Treatment principles and options. Hitchings R, Traverso C, eds. Terminology and guidelines for glaucoma. 2nd edn. European Glaucoma Society. Italy: Editrice DOGMA S.r.l.; 2003.

19. Pfeiffer N. A comparison of the fixed combination of latanoprost and timolol with its individual components. Graefe's Arch Clin Exp Ophthalmol 2002; 240:893–899.

20. Netland PA, Landry T, Sullivan EK. Travoprost compared with latanoprost and timolol in patients with open-angle glaucoma or ocular hypertension. Am J Ophthalmol 2001; 131:472–484.

21. Kobayashi H, Kobayashi K, Okinami S. A comparison of intraocular pressure-lowering effect of prostaglandin $F_{2\alpha}$ analogues, latanoprost, and unoprostone isopropyl. J Glaucoma 2001; 10:487–492.

22. Stewart WC, Kolker AE, Stewart JA, et al. Conjunctival hyperemia in healthy subjects after short-term dosing with latanoprost, bimatoprost, and travoprost. Am J Ophthalmol 2003; 135:314–320.

23. Johnstone MA, Albert DM. Prostaglandin-induced hair growth. Surv Ophthalmol 2002; 47(Suppl 1):S185–S202.

24. Grierson I, Pfeiffer N, Cracknell KP, et al. Histology and fine structure of the iris and outflow system following latanoprost therapy. Surv Ophthalmol 2002; 47(Suppl 1):S176–S184.

25. Wand M, Shields BM. Cystoid maculalr edema in the era of ocular hypotensive lipids. Am J Ophthalmol 2002; 133:393–397.

26. Kroll DM, Schuman JS. Reactivation of herpes simplex virus keratitis after initiating bimatoprost treatment for glaucoma. Am J Ophthalmol 2002; 133:401–403.

27. Hedner J, Everts B, Moller CS. Latanoprost and respiratory function in asthmatic patients: randomized, double-masked, placebo-controlled crossover evaluation. Arch Ophthalmol 1999; 117:1305–1309.

28. Spooner JJ, Bullano M, Ikeda LI, et al. Rates of discontinuation and change of glaucoma therapy in a managed care setting. Am J Manag Care 2002; 8:S255–S261.

29. Crawford K, Kaufman PL. Pilocarpine antagonizes prostaglandin F_{2alpha}-induced ocular hypotension in monkeys. Evidence for enhancement of uveoscleral outflow by prostaglandin F_{2alpha}. Arch Ophthalmol 1987; 105:1112–1116.

30. Toris CB, Zhan GL. Xhao J Potential mechanism for the additivity of pilocarpine and latanoprost. Am J Ophthalmol 2001; 131:722–728.

31. Gandolfi SA. Bimatoprost. In: Shaarawy T, Flammer J, eds. Glaucoma therapy 'current issues and controversies'. London: Martin Dunitz; 2004.

CHAPTER 51

Fixed-Combination Therapy in Glaucoma

Anastasios GP Konstas, Dimitrios Mikropoulos, and William C Stewart

INTRODUCTION

The initial treatment of glaucoma typically is to prescribe a single ocular hypotensive medication to reduce the intraocular pressure (IOP). However, over time the pressure may again become elevated, requiring the addition of a second medication. Current evidence suggests that approximately 50% of patients with primary open-angle glaucoma in the USA require adjunctive therapy within 2 years.[1] Furthermore, in the Collaborative Initial Glaucoma Treatment Study,[2] after the first 2 years more that 75% of patients in the medically treated group required two or more medications to reach a target IOP (mean 35% reduction in IOP). Adjunctive therapy may even more frequently be needed in other types of glaucoma, or, in advanced disease, when a greater decrease in pressure (30–40%) might be required to prevent further glaucomatous progression. However, the need for adjunctive therapy may cause a dilemma for the clinician: whether to add a second drug or change to a fixed combination.

FIXED COMBINATIONS AND ADHERENCE

Orally administered fixed-dose combinations were introduced several years ago to improve adherence to chronic medical therapy for systemic diseases. Published evidence from several medical specialties suggests that almost half of patients with chronic, asymptomatic diseases do not take their medications as prescribed.[3,4] Unfortunately, inadequate adherence may diminish drug efficacy and lead to worsening of health problems. Furthermore, poor adherence may inflate the cost of healthcare by increasing the rate of complications, medical visits, and hospital admissions. In general medicine, a recent meta-analysis showed that nonadherence to medical therapy is reduced by 24–26% with fixed-dose combination regimens compared with unfixed concomitant therapies.[4]

Glaucoma patients also commonly demonstrate poor adherence with long-term therapy.[5,6] Published work has stressed that between 28% and 55% of patients do not adhere to their prescribed treatment regimen.[5] This poor adherence might contribute to the current incidence of blindness among glaucoma sufferers. Factors often associated with poor adherence with treatment in chronic diseases are frequent dosing and the complexity of the therapeutic regimen.[4,7,8] Importantly, the availability of oral fixed-dose combinations has simplified adjunctive medication regimens.[9] Recent reviews of the impact of oral fixed-dose combinations on systemic and chronic diseases have shown that they may improve adherence,[4,9] reduce costs, decrease adverse events, and improve clinical outcomes.[10–12]

Theoretically, topical fixed combinations may provide similar advantages in glaucoma treatment as in the other fields of medicine. Nevertheless, the precise impact on adherence of fixed-combination products in glaucoma therapy remains unclear. Although logical, there is as yet no solid scientific evidence to show that reduced dosing obtained with fixed combinations enhances adherence. Several studies have observed that patients taking glaucoma medications more than twice daily demonstrate worse adherence.[5,6,12] However, there is still no published evidence comparing adherence with twice-daily to once-daily dosing which is now available with prostaglandin/timolol fixed combinations. Importantly, a recent study by Robin and Covert[13] noted that glaucoma patients being treated with adjunctive unfixed glaucoma regimens show worse adherence compared to those on once-daily monotherapy. Future studies are needed to establish the precise impact of fixed combinations on adherence, specifically in glaucoma.

FIXED COMBINATIONS AND PRESERVATIVES

Preservatives are important components of ophthalmic preparations, suppressing microbial growth and preventing decomposition of the active drug. Benzalkonium chloride (BAC), a quaternary ammonium compound, is the most commonly used preservative in ophthalmic preparations (concentration range 0.004–0.02%).

However, BAC may have several adverse effects on the eye. First, on the precorneal tear film, it may reduce stability, turnover, and production and, in addition, BAC may create a detergent effect on the lipid layer, resulting in increased evaporation. Secondly, in the conjunctiva, BAC may affect the tear film indirectly by decreasing the density of goblet cells.[14] Furthermore, impression cytology studies have demonstrated inflammation, squamous metaplasia, and subconjunctival fibrosis in the conjunctiva and Tenon's capsule associated with the chronic exposure to BAC.[15] These side effects are dose dependent and therefore may worsen with increasing frequency of instillation.[16] Thirdly, on the cornea, BAC may reduce cell proliferation and viability and impair wound healing as well as disrupt the epithelial barrier. Lastly, BAC may induce allergy, usually a type IV cytotoxic reaction, and may result in contact allergies of the eyelid, which is often difficult to differentiate from other causes of periocular inflammation.[16]

The long-term use of BAC may occasionally result in drug-induced pemphigoid. This chronic condition is characterized by a marked and self-sustaining inflammatory process with cicatrizing conjunctivitis and fornical shortening. Furthermore, strong evidence suggests that the conjunctival inflammation associated with long-term topical treatment for glaucoma may constitute an important risk factor for failure of filtering surgery.[17,18] Therefore, physicians might benefit many patients by limiting their long-term exposure to BAC, as medically appropriate, by prescribing preparations without, or with lower concentrations of, this preservative, and reducing their number of daily doses.

Accordingly, when adjunctive therapy is indicated, prescribing a fixed combination may significantly reduce exposure to preservatives. Indeed, this may be partly the reason why in regulatory trials fixed combinations showed a reduced incidence of adverse events compared with unfixed therapy and almost the same prevalence with monotherapy.

The concentration of BAC in the various fixed combinations is shown in Table 51.1. Although preservative-free medications would be ideal, non-BAC preparations are available only in some markets (timolol in preservative-free single-dose units, travoprost preserved with sofZia® and brimonidine preserved with Purite®). Although few data are currently available, recently, dorzolamide/timolol fixed-combination preservative-free (Merck Inc, Whitehouse Station, NJ, USA) has been introduced in Canada (PF Cosopt, Merck Frosst, Canada) and a few European countries.

TABLE 51.1 **BAC concentration in commercially available fixed combinations**

FIXED COMBINATION	BAC CONCENTRATION
Latanoprost/timolol (Xalacom)	0.02%
Travoprost/timolol (DuoTrav)	0.015%
Dorzolamide/timolol (Cosopt)	0.0075%
Brimonidine/timolol (Combigan)	0.005%
Bimatoprost/timolol (Ganfort)	0.005%

ADVANTAGES OF FIXED COMBINATIONS IN CLINICAL PRACTICE

The primary importance of the development of fixed combinations for glaucoma is that by improving patient adherence they may also improve long-term prognosis. However, the relationship between fixed combinations and enhanced adherence has yet to be demonstrated in a controlled study. Certainly, fixed combinations improve the convenience of glaucoma therapy by reducing the number of eyedrops, as well as potentially decreasing the cost of therapy.[19]

Fixed combinations generally offer more IOP lowering than each of their components alone, whereas their safety profile is almost as good as their individual constituents.[19] More importantly, in routine practice, fixed combinations may provide better IOP control in some patients than unfixed concomitant therapy,[20] presumably due to the combined effects of enhanced convenience, elimination of the washout effect from the second drop, and improved adherence. A recent study[20] comparing the dorzolamide/timolol fixed combination to the concomitant administration of dorzolamide and timolol showed a significant advantage (1.7 mmHg) for the fixed combination. The amount of information on the effects of fixed combinations in glaucoma is increasing rapidly and the reader is referred to a recently published comprehensive review.[19]

LIMITATIONS OF FIXED COMBINATIONS IN CLINICAL PRACTICE

Although fixed combination therapy generally demonstrates greater treatment efficacy to each of its individual components, the enhanced reduction in pressure with some fixed combinations has been less than was originally anticipated.[21] This may be due at least in part to the potency of prostaglandin analogues when used as monotherapy and the use of timolol only once daily in the prostaglandin/timolol fixed combinations. However, all the potential reasons have not been clarified. As a consequence, most fixed combinations today have not yet received Food and Drug Administration (FDA) approval.

Furthermore, the unfixed combinations generally provide a small, but statistically nonsignificant, greater reduction in IOP compared to the fixed combination containing the same medicines. Even the dorzolamide/timolol fixed combination (Cosopt), when compared to its individual components (timolol dosed twice daily and dorzolamide dosed three times daily), manifested slightly reduced IOP efficacy (0.7 mmHg) at the morning trough level.

Fixed combinations may reduce flexibility of individualized patient care.[21] All available fixed combinations contain timolol 0.5% solution, which in some elderly patients may represent overtreatment. Similarly, the ideal administration time for prostaglandin/timolol fixed combinations can be difficult to determine in all patients.

Unfortunately, to date there is limited published information evaluating the new fixed combinations versus monotherapies, or unfixed therapy, beyond 2–3 time points in the daytime. In the future, it will be important to assess the therapeutic equivalence of fixed combinations versus unfixed therapy throughout the 24-hour period.

There is no perfect uniformity among registration trials and therefore it is sometimes difficult to compare the efficacy between fixed combinations in the same therapeutic category. For example, in the travoprost/timolol fixed combination trials the unfixed arm included timolol dosed once a day, whereas the unfixed therapy arm of the other two prostaglandin/timolol fixed combinations included timolol dosed twice daily. Further, the design of published studies typically includes only patients with ocular hypertension, or primary open-angle glaucoma. It is not known, therefore, how the new fixed combinations work in other glaucomas (e.g. closed-angle glaucoma).

Generally, the reported adverse events of fixed combinations are similar to those reported for individual components. It is fortunate that, so far, fixed combinations have not been associated with the emergence of unique adverse events.[19,21] More information is required, however, on the long-term efficacy, safety, and tolerability of fixed combinations versus unfixed concomitant therapies.

FUTURE ROLE OF FIXED COMBINATIONS IN GLAUCOMA

Currently available fixed-combination drugs include the dorzolamide/timolol fixed combination (Cosopt), which is available worldwide, and latanoprost/timolol (Xalacom), travoprost/timolol (DuoTrav), bimatoprost/timolol (Ganfort), and brimonidine/timolol (Combigan), which are available in Canada and most of Europe. These drugs are generally selected as second- or third-line therapy. Which fixed combination is superior in terms of efficacy and safety is not yet known. A new fixed combination that includes brinzolamide and timolol maleate (Azarga, Alcon, Inc., Fort Worth, Texas, USA), will become available within the next year in Europe. There are a number of pharmacological obstacles (dosage, differences in pharmacokinetics, potential drug interactions, instability of combined molecules, etc.) that do not currently allow the introduction of other conceptually attractive fixed combinations, e.g. combining prostaglandins and topical carbonic anhydrase inhibitors. Such a new fixed combination may however become avilable in the future.

It is not yet known if fixed-combination therapy is appropriate for initial glaucoma therapy. Oral fixed combinations have been found to be cost-efficient and improve clinical outcomes in several systemic chronic diseases when prescribed as initial therapy.[22] A fixed combination may have the advantage as initial therapy to more rapidly reduce IOP when the patient presents with an unusually high pressure (e.g. exfoliative or neovascular glaucoma), or with advanced damage. However, concern remains that a fixed combination might be prescribed in real-life practice, as initial therapy, without

a clear understanding of its efficacy and safety profile.[19] In addition, the therapeutic effect of the individual components cannot be confirmed, and any adverse event might not be ascribed to the correct component.

In summary, fixed combinations offer additional choices for the treatment of glaucoma. They combine standardized doses of two medications in a single bottle and may improve treatment adherence, efficacy, or tolerability through a variety of mechanisms. The value and future promise of fixed-dose medications remains to be determined. To date, regulatory approvals worldwide and published literature are based on efficacy and safety comparisons between the fixed combinations and the individual components, or the concomitant use of both constituents.[22] This approach, however, is not ideal since it does not take into account other important potential clinical benefits such as enhanced adherence, improved convenience, and reduced cost to patients. In the current management of glaucoma, inadequate adherence greatly diminishes drug efficacy in real life and may often lead to a worsening, or undertreatment of glaucoma. Further, the challenge in glaucoma management is to try to keep medical therapy practicable. This concept probably consists of up to two bottles, one of which can be a fixed-combination product.[21] The possibility exists that this relatively new and rapidly expanding class of medications may prove instrumental in improving the prognosis of glaucoma.

DRUG FORMULATIONS

The search to develop effective fixed combinations of glaucoma drugs has intensified over the last few years. A number of new combination therapies have been approved by various regulatory authorities in different countries and numerous studies have been published on the subject.[23–53] This section will not discuss fixed combinations of historical interest (e.g. timolol/pilocarpine). It aims to briefly review the key characteristics and the efficacy of those which are currently available.

DORZOLAMIDE/TIMOLOL MALEATE FIXED COMBINATION

Fixed-combination therapy in glaucoma has gained popularity in recent years principally due to the relative success of the dorzolamide/timolol fixed combination (Cosopt® Merck & Co Inc, Whitehouse Station, NJ, USA). This combination therapy was released commercially in the USA and in Europe in 1998. At present, this and the brimonidine/timolol (Combigan, Allergan), are the only fixed combinations approved by the FDA. The pharmacology of this product is related to its two active ingredients and it is prescribed for twice-daily dosing. The regulatory data showed that this fixed combination reduced the IOP by 9 mmHg (32.7%) at peak compared with 5.4 mmHg (19.8%) and 6.3 mmHg (22.6%) for dorzolamide and timolol monotherapy, respectively.[21] At trough, the IOP reduction was 7.7 mmHg (27%) for the fixed combination. These efficacy data demonstrated that the dorzolamide/timolol fixed combination decreases the pressure by a further 1.1–1.3 mmHg from timolol maleate at trough and by 2.8 mmHg at peak (2 hours after dosing).[23] The dorzolamide/timolol fixed combination demonstrated clinical equivalence to unfixed concomitant therapy with the largest, but nonsignificant, difference found at 16:00 hours (0.7 mmHg difference for unfixed therapy). Importantly, in real-life practice the dorzolamide/timolol fixed combination provides better IOP control compared with unfixed concomitant therapy,[20,21] owing to enhanced convenience, elimination of the washout effect from the second drop, and improved adherence. The safety and efficacy profile of this fixed combination has been reviewed by Frampton and Perry.[23] Common ocular side effects with this fixed combination have been mostly related to the dorzolamide component, including bitter taste and stinging/burning on instillation.

Fechtner and associates[24] evaluated daytime IOP of latanoprost dosed each evening versus the dorzolamide/timolol fixed combination and showed that the diurnal pressure control was similar with both these products (Table 51.2). However, Konstas and co-workers[25] found over 24 hours that the fixed combination provided better 24-hour pressure control (−0.6 mmHg) mainly due to greater efficacy at night (22:00) vs evening-dosed latanoprost (Fig. 51.1). Further, Orzalesi and associates[26] noted similar pressure control between these two products, except at 09:00, when the fixed combination was more effective. Nonetheless, despite these data, the above studies suffered from limited patient size and short-term follow-up. In a recent randomized, prospective, crossover 24-hour IOP study on 53 patients with primary open-angle glaucoma or ocular hypertension

Konstas and associates[27] compared the 24-hour IOP efficacy of the dorzolamide/timolol fixed combination vs latanoprost over 2 and 6 months (Fig. 51.2). After 2 months of therapy, the dorzolamide/timolol fixed combination provided significantly better control at 3 time-points (10:00, 18:00 and 22:00) and for the mean of 24-hour pressure (18.0 ± 1.8 vs 18.6 ± 1.9 mmHg; $p = 0.0002$). However, following 6 months of chronic treatment, the mean 24-hour IOP was similar between the two medications (18.1 ± 1.9 vs 18.3 ± 1.9 mmHg). The fixed combination still provided significantly better IOP at 2 timepoints (10:00 and 22:00; $p < 0.01$).[27] Compared to 2 months of therapy, at 6 months the fixed combination showed no significant change in the mean 24-hour IOP with no evidence of tachyphylaxis, whereas latanoprost manifested a further reduction of 0.3 mmHg.

Harris and co-workers[54] have demonstrated that dorzolamide/timolol fixed combination significantly increases superior retinal arteriovenous passage time, thus increasing blood flow rate and retinal perfusion. They documented that timolol had no adverse effects on the retinal circulation, but the dorzolamide component of the fixed combination improved hemodynamics by a direct or indirect mechanism of action. Further, in a recent comparison between the dorzolamide/timolol and the latanoprost/timolol fixed combinations in newly diagnosed open-angle glaucoma patients, Martinez and Sanchez[55] documented similar IOP lowering between the two fixed combinations but reported that only the dorzolamide/timolol fixed combination had an effect on the retrobulbar vessels in their glaucoma patients.

The dorzolamide/timolol fixed combination has been evaluated as initial therapy in glaucoma patients with

TABLE 51.2 Dorzolamide/timolol fixed combination (DTFC) vs latanoprost

TREATMENT	N	BASELINE	MONTH 3	CHANGE IN IOP	% CHANGE
DTFC	121	26.1 (4.2)	18.9 (3.0)	−7.1 (3.8)	−26.4 (11.4)
Latanoprost	125	25.6 (3.0)	18.4 (2.9)	−7.1 (3.3)	−27.3 (10.2)

Mean diurnal IOP (mmHg ± SD).
With permission from Fechtner RD, Airaskinen PJ, Getson AJ, et al. Acta Ophthalmol Scand 2004; 82:42–48.[24]

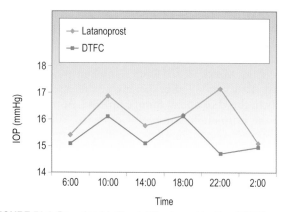

FIGURE 51.1 Dorzolamide/timolol fixed combination (DTFC) vs latanoprost. (From Konstas AG, Papapanos P, Tersis I, et al. Twenty-four-hour diurnal curve comparison of commercially available latanoprost 0.005% versus the timolol and dorzolamide fixed combination. Ophthalmology 2003; 110:1357–1360.[25])

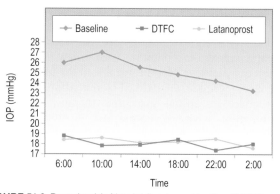

FIGURE 51.2 Dorzolamide/timolol fixed combination (DTFC) vs latanoprost. (From Konstas AGP, Kozobolis VP, Tsironi S, et al. Comparison of the 24-hour intraocular pressure-lowering effects of latanoprost and dorzolamide/timolol fixed combination after 2 and 6 months of treatment. Ophthalmology 2008; 115:99–103.[27])

high baseline pressures. It was found to be a viable option in these patients, demonstrating a significant IOP-lowering effect.[56,57] In a prospective study Henderer and associates[56] employed this combination as initial therapy in 18 patients with a mean pretreatment IOP of 37.5 mmHg. Two hours after the initial dose of the fixed combination the IOP fell to 18.2 mmHg, whereas after 2 months of therapy the treated IOP ranged between 21.1 mmHg at trough and 17.6 mmHg at peak (mean reduction of 40–49%).

LATANOPROST/TIMOLOL MALEATE FIXED COMBINATION

The latanoprost/timolol maleate fixed combination (Xalacom™, Pfizer, Inc., New York, NY, USA) was commercially released in Europe in 2001. The regulatory trials of Pfeiffer and associates and Higginbotham and co-workers showed that morning dosing of the fixed combination further reduced the IOP compared to both latanoprost dosed once daily (1.1 to 1.2 mmHg), or timolol dosed twice daily (1.9 to 2.9 mmHg, respectively) (Fig. 51.3).[28,29] Unfortunately, the extent of IOP reduction with the latanoprost/timolol fixed combination compared to latanoprost alone was less than anticipated during development. The reason for the relative lack of efficacy has not been explained. Preclinical data suggest that the combination of the two drugs in one formulation did not adversely affect the absorption of either drug.[29] The bioavailability of latanoprost and timolol into the aqueous with the fixed combination was at least as good as for the two drugs administered separately. However, it may be that the relative lack of efficacy is because the fixed combination was instilled in the morning in both regulatory trials, whereas latanoprost alone was dosed in the evening in the Higginbotham study.[29] Previously, Alm and associate[30] as well as Konstas, Stewart and co-workers[31–33] have demonstrated that night-time dosing of latanoprost provides lower daytime pressures than morning dosing (Figs 51.4–51.6).

Therefore, the study design of the regulatory trials itself may have limited both the daytime efficacy and the difference from the individual components of the latanoprost/timolol fixed combination. Accordingly, a study by Konstas and associates[33] showed that latanoprost/timolol

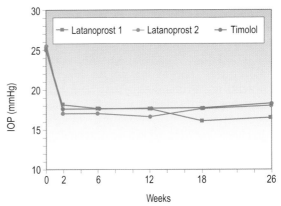

FIGURE 51.4 Latanoprost added to timolol b.i.d.. (From Alm A, Stjernschantz J; the Scandinavian Latanoprost Study Group. Effects on intraocular pressure and side effects of 0.005% latanoprost applied once daily, evening or morning: a comparison with timolol. Ophthalmology 1995; 102:1743–1752.[30])

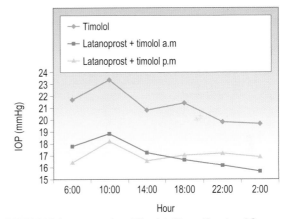

FIGURE 51.5 Latanoprost and timolol. (From Konstas AG, Nakos E, Stewart WC, et al. A comparison of once-daily morning vs evening dosing of concomitant latanoprost/timolol. Am J Ophthalmol 2002; 133:753–757.[31])

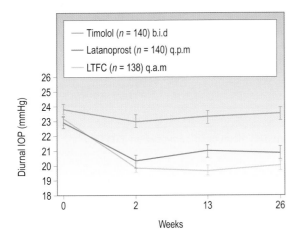

FIGURE 51.3 US experience. Latanoprost and timolol combination therapy (LTFC) vs timolol and latanoprost alone. (From Higginbotham EJ, Feldman R, Stiles M, et al. Latanoprost and timolol combination therapy vs monotherapy: one-year randomized trial. Arch Ophthalmol 2002; 120:915–922.[29])

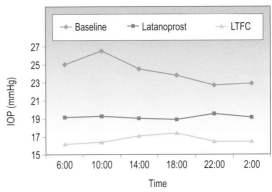

FIGURE 51.6 Latanoprost/timolol fixed combination (LTFC) vs latanoprost. (From Konstas AGP, Boboridis K, Stewart WC, et al. 24-hour intraocular pressure short-term control with the latanoprost/timolol maleate fixed combination versus latanoprost, both dosed once each evening, in primary open-angle glaucoma patients. Arch Ophthalmol 2005; 123:898–902.[33])

fixed combination compared to latanoprost alone, both dosed in the evening, provided a wider margin (2.5 mmHg more than latanoprost) over 24 hours than the morning dosing used in the regulatory trial. Furthermore, in a more recent, crossover study[53] the fluctuation of 24-hour IOP was significantly lower with the latanoprost/timolol fixed combination dosed in the evening (3.2 mmHg) compared with timolol alone (4.4 mmHg). This fluctuation was less than shown in past diurnal studies[31,40] evaluating this fixed combination with morning dosing (3.9–4.3 mmHg). The reason for the lower fluctuation of IOP with night-time dosing may have been because, again, latanoprost instilled at night has limited the pressure spikes typically seen during the daytime.

This effect was also shown in the trials comparing the fixed combination to the individual components in separate bottles by Diestelhorst and Larsson.[34,35] The original trial compared morning-dosed latanoprost/timolol fixed combination vs unfixed therapy (timolol dosed twice and latanoprost dosed in the evening) and showed a significant 1.1 mmHg difference for the benefit of unfixed therapy.[34] In contrast, a more recent study by the same group[35] compared the evening dosing of the latanoprost/timolol fixed combination vs the same unfixed therapy and found clinical equivalence between the two treatments with only a small difference between groups (0.3 mmHg). Nevertheless, to

date there is no direct comparison between morning and evening dosing of the latanoprost/timolol fixed combination.

Compared to other adjunctive treatments, Stewart and co-workers[36] noted that latanoprost/timolol fixed combination dosed in the evening was more effective at 6–12 hours after dosing, and for the end of the daytime diurnal curve, than brimonidine and timolol dosed concomitantly (Fig. 51.7). In addition, Garcia-Sanchez and associates[37] showed in a 6-month, multicentered, parallel study that latanoprost/timolol fixed combination reduced the pressure more than timolol and brimonidine given separately over a three-point diurnal curve (16.9 ± 2.8 vs 18.2 ± 3.1 mmHg). Further, Stewart and co-workers[38] found that the latanoprost-based fixed combination provided equal efficacy to latanoprost and brimonidine (dosed twice daily) in a three-point diurnal curve (Fig. 51.8).

Compared to dorzolamide/timolol fixed combination given twice daily, Shin and associates[39] demonstrated that the latanoprost/timolol fixed combination reduced the pressure 1.0 mmHg further over three daytime points (Table 51.3). In contrast, Konstas and co-workers showed that latanoprost/timolol fixed combination provided similar efficacy to dorzolamide/timolol fixed combination over a 12-hour diurnal curve measured every 2 hours (Fig. 51.9).[40]

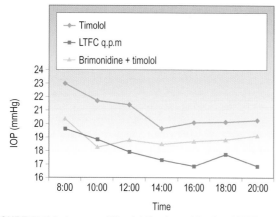

FIGURE 51.7 Latanoprost/timolol fixed combination (LTFC) vs timolol and brimonidine. (From Stewart WC, Stewart JA, Day D, et al. Efficacy and safety of latanoprost/timolol maleate fixed combination verses timolol maleate and brimonidine given twice daily. Acta Ophthalmol Scand 2003; 81:242–246.[36])

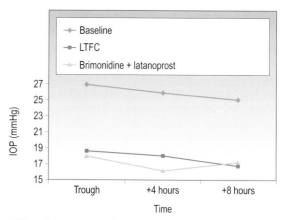

FIGURE 51.8 Latanoprost/timolol fixed combination (LTFC) vs brimonidine and latanoprost. (From Stewart WC, Stewart JA, Day DG, et al. Efficacy and safety of the latanoprost/timolol maleate fixed combination versus concomitant brimonidine and latanoprost therapy. Eye 2004; 18:990–995.[38])

TABLE 51.3 Latanoprost/timolol fixed combination (LTFC) vs dorzolamide/timolol fixed combination (DTFC)

	ESTIMATED MEAN IOP REDUCTION FOR LTFC	ESTIMATED MEAN IOP REDUCTION FOR DTFC	ESTIMATED DIFFERENCE IN IOP REDUCTION (LTFC − DTFC)	95% CONFIDENCE INTERVAL OF ESTIMATED DIFFERENCE
8 a.m.	9.59	8.37	1.22	0.33–2.12
12 p.m.	9.09	8.82	0.27	−0.49–1.03
4 p.m.	9.64	8.23	1.41	0.67–2.15
Diurnal	9.45	8.44	1.00	0.31–1.69

With permission from Shin DH, Feldman RM, Sheu WP. Ophthalmology 2004; 111:276–282.[39]

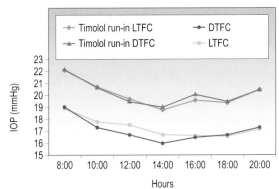

FIGURE 51.9 Latanoprost/timolol fixed combination (LTFC) q.a.m. vs dorzolamide/timolol fixed combination (DTFC) b.i.d. (From Konstas AGP, Kozobolis VP, Stewart WC, et al. Daytime diurnal curve comparison between the fixed combinations of latanoprost/timolol and dorzolamide/timolol. Eye 2005; 18:1264–1269.[40])

More recently Topouzis and associates[41] evaluated latanoprost/timolol fixed combination vs travoprost/timolol fixed combination, both dosed once daily in the morning, in a parallel, multicenter study. The treatments were found to be equivalent except the travoprost-based fixed combination was statistically more effective at 09:00 when all visits were considered across the 6-month study period.

TRAVOPROST/TIMOLOL MALEATE FIXED COMBINATION

Recently, the travoprost 0.004%/timolol maleate 0.5% fixed combination (DuoTrav™, Alcon, Inc., Fort Worth, Texas, USA) gained regulatory approval in Europe. This new fixed combination is indicated for the treatment of patients with open-angle glaucoma or ocular hypertension needing further intraocular pressure reduction from a β-blocker or prostaglandin analogue. Two randomized, controlled trials have compared the travoprost/timolol fixed combination with the use of its components. Barnebey and associates[42] showed that patients treated with the travoprost/timolol fixed combination dosed in the morning had a further reduction of IOP from baseline of 1.9–3.3 mmHg more than timolol monotherapy and 0.9–2.4 mmHg more than travoprost alone (Fig. 51.10). Furthemore, Schuman

and co-workers[43] demonstrated that the mean IOP was 16.2–17.4 mmHg with the travoprost/timolol fixed combination dosed in the morning compared with 15.4–16.8 mmHg with the concomitant travoprost and timolol group. In a similar study, Hughes and associates[44] noted the mean IOP was 15.2–16.5 mmHg in the patients using the travoprost/timolol fixed combination compared with 14.7–16.1 mmHg in the concomitant therapy group. Consequently, morning-dosed travoprost/timolol fixed combination should provide incrementally better pressure control than prior β-blocker or prostaglandin analogue monotherapy and almost similar control to concomitant therapy with these same products.

Despite the labeling in Europe for morning or evening dosing, little information is available evaluating the evening dosing of the travoprost/timolol maleate fixed combination. Previous research has suggested that prostaglandin analogues dosed in the evening may provide lower daytime mean IOP and 24-hour pressure fluctuation. In a recent crossover study, Konstas and co-workers[45] evaluated the 24-hour IOP control between morning and evening dosing of the travoprost/timolol fixed combination in primary open-angle or exfoliative glaucoma patients. This study showed that both morning and evening dosing of this fixed combination provided a statistically significant reduction from untreated baseline for each time point on the 24-hour pressure curve. However, when both treatment regimens were compared, evening dosing demonstrated a lower absolute IOP, and greater, significant, reduction from untreated baseline, for the 24-hour pressure curve and individual daytime time points at 10:00, 14:00, 18:00, and 06:00 hours.[45] In contrast, morning dosing provided a slightly lower, nonsignificant, reduction in pressure at 22:00 and 02:00 hours. This study was the first direct 24-hour IOP comparison between morning and evening dosing for any of the timolol/prostaglandin fixed combinations and suggests that both dosing regimens of travoprost/timolol fixed combination provide effective 24-hour IOP reduction. However, evening dosing demonstrates a narrower range of 24-hour IOP fluctuation and peak pressures as well as a lower mean 24-hour IOP and daytime pressures.

These results are consistent with past studies by Alm and Stjernschantz[30] and Konstas and co-workers[31–33]

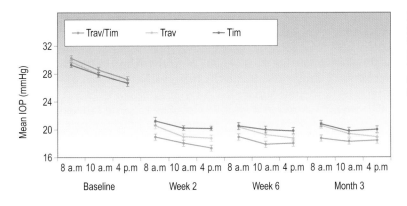

FIGURE 51.10 Mean intraocular pressure for patients on travoprost/timolol (Trav/Tim), travoprost (Trav), or timolol (Tim) therapy. (From Barnebey HS, Orengo-Nania S, Flowers BE, et al. The safety and efficacy of travoprost 0.004%/timolol 0.5% fixed combination ophthalmic solution. Am J Ophthalmol 2005; 140:1–7.[42])

that have indicated that prostaglandin (PG) analogues (latanoprost, travoprost, or latanoprost added to timolol) when dosed in the evening consistently provide lower daytime pressures when compared to morning dosing. This may be due to the fact that PGs demonstrate their peak efficacy 12–24 hours after dosing. Consequently, it can be expected that an evening-dosed prostaglandin/timolol fixed combination will generally provide its maximum pharmacologic effect, and its best ocular hypertensive control, in the daytime. This fact is clinically important because most 24-hour studies indicate that the IOP is usually higher in the morning and during the daytime. This dosing may maximize the treatment benefit of the new fixed combination and consequently may lead to greater separation between travoprost/timolol and travoprost.

The current literature has not yet offered controlled studies evaluating the efficacy and safety of the travoprost/timolol fixed combination vs most other available fixed combinations such as the dorzolamide/timolol, the bimatoprost/timolol, and the brimonidine/timolol fixed combinations. To date, only one parallel study[41] has evaluated this fixed combination vs the latanoprost/timolol fixed combination. As previously discussed, this study found the two fixed combinations to be clinically equivalent except for the 09:00 time point when the travoprost-based fixed combination was statistically more effective across the 6-month study period. Future, comparative studies may help the clinician to select the best fixed combination therapy for their patients. Furthermore, no controlled study has documented as yet the long-term pressure control of the travoprost/timolol fixed-combination therapy. Further research is required to determine the overall most efficacious, safe, and cost-efficient fixed-combination therapy for glaucoma.

BIMATOPROST/TIMOLOL MALEATE FIXED COMBINATION

Bimatoprost/timolol fixed-combination eyedrop solution (Ganfort™, Allergan, Inc., Irvine, CA, USA) is a new product composed of a synthetic prostamide, bimatoprost 0.3%, and a nonselective β-adrenergic blocker, timolol 0.5%. The new fixed combination is used as a once-daily topical ocular therapy for the reduction of elevated IOP in patients with open-angle glaucoma or ocular hypertension for whom monotherapies provide insufficient IOP control. The individual active components of this new fixed combination, bimatoprost and timolol maleate, are established therapeutic agents with well-documented IOP efficacy. Bimatoprost and timolol have complementary mechanisms of hypotensive action. Bimatoprost is believed to lower IOP mainly by increasing uveoscleral outflow, whereas timolol lowers IOP predominantly by reducing aqueous humor formation.

The overall development program for the bimatoprost/timolol fixed combination involved 1964 patients. In all four studies conducted and submitted to the European Medicines Agency for approval the administration of the new fixed combination has been in the morning. These studies consisted of two 12-month, three-arm, parallel designs in which the morning administration of this fixed combination was compared to once-daily evening dosing of bimatoprost and twice-daily dosing of timolol. In these trials the reduction provided by the bimatoprost/timolol fixed combination with morning dosing was less than might be anticipated vs bimatoprost monotherapy. The reasons for the relative lack of efficacy, with this new fixed combination, has not been fully explained as yet. However, as previously discussed, it may be because the fixed combination was instilled in the morning in these regulatory trials, whereas bimatoprost monotherapy was dosed in the evening. Bimatoprost, like all prostaglandin analogues, is generally dosed at night and previous data have demonstrated that the evening dosing provides lower daytime IOP.

Hommer and co-workers[46] reported the results of a double-masked, parallel, 3-week study where the bimatoprost/timolol fixed combination was not inferior to the unfixed therapy of bimatoprost and timolol dosed twice daily at all three time points measured. The mean diurnal IOP control obtained with the fixed combination after 3 weeks of therapy (16.1 mmHg) was similar in terms of hypotensive efficacy with the unfixed therapy (15.6 mmHg) and 1 mmHg better than bimatoprost monotherapy (17.1 mmHg). In this study the fixed combination therapy group manifested a lower propensity for conjunctival hyperemia (19.3% vs 25.6% for the unfixed therapy group and 27.8% for bimatoprost), although the among-group difference was not statistically significant. Interestingly, from the overall regulatory data, it is evident that the proportion of patients who reported at least one adverse reaction with the bimatoprost/timolol fixed combination was significantly lower than with bimatoprost monotherapy, i.e. 48% vs 60% ($p = 0.001$). Likewise, the rate of discontinuation because of adverse events was 3.6% in the fixed combination group as opposed to 7.9% in the bimatoprost monotherapy group ($p = 0.008$). These differences may be clinically relevant, and may lead to better adherence and persistence in those patients treated chronically with the fixed combination. The reasons for the decreased incidence of adverse events seen in the fixed combination group remain unclear. It may be due to the direct effect of timolol, which may reduce the development of hyperemia by reducing the vasodilatory effects of endogenous catecholamines at the relevant conjunctival β receptors. Further, there may also be a benefit from the reduction in the active drug amount and the preservative delivered to the ophthalmic surface.

A recent 4-week study[47] has suggested the possibility that the evening administration of bimatoprost/timolol may be more effective than the evening dosing of the latanoprost/timolol fixed combination, but this requires confirmation from a larger, adequately powered study.

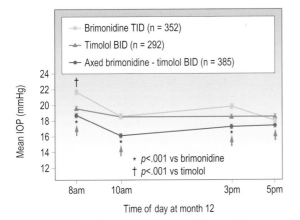

FIGURE 51.11 Mean intraocular pressure at 8 a.m., 10 a.m., 3 p.m., and 5 p.m. at month 12. (From Sherwood MB, Craven ER, Chou C, et al. Twice-daily 0.2% brimonidine–0.5% timolol fixed-combination therapy vs monotherapy with timolol or brimonidine in patients with glaucoma or ocular hypertension: a 12-month randomized trial. Arch Ophthalmol 2006; 124:1230–1238.[49])

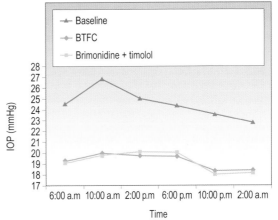

FIGURE 51.12 Brimonidine/timolol fixed combination (BTFC) vs brimonidine and timolol. (From Konstas AGP, Katsimpris IE, Kaltsos K, et al. Twenty-four-hour efficacy of the brimonidine/timolol fixed combination versus therapy with the unfixed components. Eye 2007 (Epub ahead of print).[51])

In the future it will be clinically important to compare the evening vs the morning dosing of the bimatoprost/timolol fixed combination to establish which dosing is more effective and to compare this fixed combination with the other available fixed combinations.

BRIMONIDINE/TIMOLOL MALEATE FIXED COMBINATION

The brimonidine/timolol fixed combination (Combigan™, Allergan, Inc., Irvine, CA, USA) has recently been approved by the FDA as well as in Canada and the European Union. Craven and co-workers[48] demonstrated that the brimonidine/timolol fixed combination, compared to each of its individual components, reduced the morning trough pressure by 28% from no treatment and 1.6 mmHg from timolol alone. However, the afternoon time point at 15:00 showed only a 0.6 mmHg further reduction in pressure while at 17:00 no additional decrease was observed, compared to timolol alone. Further, Sherwood and associates[49] recently showed, in a meta-analysis of the two regulatory trials, that brimonidine/timolol fixed combination reduced the pressure more than the individual components at all time points, except compared to brimonidine

at 17:00 (dosed three times daily) (Fig. 51.11). The range of reduction was 4.4–7.6 mmHg with brimonidine/timolol fixed combination, 2.7–5.5 mmHg with brimonidine, and 3.9–6.2 mmHg with timolol.

In another comparison, Goni and co-workers[50] showed that the brimonidine/timolol fixed combination provided almost equal efficacy (0.4 mmHg difference) to the unfixed combination of its individual components (brimonidine and timolol dosed twice daily) with reductions ranging from 4.4 to 5.3 mmHg in both groups at morning trough and peak time points. More recently, Konstas and associates[51] showed that the brimonidine/timolol fixed combination demonstrated equal 24-hour pressure control to the unfixed components, both dosed twice daily, in a crossover trial (Fig. 51.12). The range of pressure reduction from untreated baseline was 19–26% for both treatment groups.

Compared to another fixed-combination treatment, Arcieri and associates, in a 30-patient crossover study, found equivalent pressures between the brimonidine/timolol (15.0 ± 2.1 mmHg) and the dorzolamide/timolol fixed combinations (15.4 ± 2.1 mmHg) using a three-point diurnal curve.[52]

Summary

Fixed-combination drugs can provide effective IOP control, enhance adherence and convenience, eliminate the washout effect, and significantly reduce exposure to preservatives. In real-life practice, fixed combinations can often be superior to unfixed concomitant therapy. However, there is still limited verification for the benefits accrued and little is known concerning the comparative efficacy between the new fixed combinations. No studies have explored a number of clinically important issues between fixed and unfixed therapy: for

example, adherence, convenience, drug utilization, quality of life, and cost–benefit measures. Although a number of benefits can be assumed, only tentative conclusions can be drawn for their role in glaucoma therapy today. As yet, there is no information on whether fixed combinations improve long-term clinical outcome, and this will be a promising line of future research. The possibility exists that this relatively new and rapidly expanding class of medications may prove instrumental in improving management and prognosis in glaucoma.

REFERENCES

1. Kobelt-Nguyen G, Gerdtham UG, Alm A. Costs of treating primary open-angle glaucoma and ocular hypertension: a retrospective observational two-year chart review of newly diagnosed patients in Sweden and the United States. J Glaucoma 1998; 7:95–104.

2. Lichter P, Musch DC, Gillespie BW, et al. Interim clinical outcomes in the Collaborative Initial Glaucoma Treatment Study comparing initial treatment randomized to medications or surgery. Ophthalmology 2001; 108:1943–1953.

3. Schroeder K, Fahey T, Ebrahim S. How can we improve adherence to blood pressure-lowering medication in ambulatory care? Systematic review of randomized controlled trials. Arch Intern Med 2004; 164:722–732.

4. Bangalore S, Kamalakkannan G, Parkar S, et al. Fixed-dose combinations improve medication compliance: a meta-analysis. Am J Med 2007; 120:713–719.

5. Olthoffn CM, Schouten JSAG, Bornevander BW, et al. Noncompliance with ocular hypotensive treatment in patients with glaucoma or ocular hypertension. Ophthalmology 2005; 112:953–961.

6. Schwartz GF. Compliance and persistency in glaucoma follow-up treatment. Curr Opin Ophthalmol 2005; 16:114–121.

7. Claxton AJ, Cramer J, Pierce C. A systematic review of the association between dose regimens and medication compliance. Clin Ther 2001; 23:1296–1310.

8. Petrilla AA, Benner JS, Battleman DS, et al. Evidence-based interventions to improve patient compliance with antihypertensive and lipid-lowering medications. Int J Clin Pract 2005; 59:1441–1451.

9. Connor J, Rafter N, Rodgers A. Do fixed-dose combination pills or unit-of-use packaging improve adherence? A systematic review. Bull World Health Organ 2004; 82:935–939.

10. Sica DA. Rationale for fixed-dose combinations in the treatment of hypertension: the cycle repeats. Drugs 2002; 62:443–462.

11. Melikian C, White TJ, Vanderplas A, et al. Adherence to oral antidiabetic therapy in a managed care organization: a comparison of monotherapy, combination therapy, and fixed-dose combination therapy. Clin Ther 2002; 24:460–467.

12. Konstas AGP, Maskaleris G, Gratsonidis S, et al. Compliance and viewpoint of glaucoma patients in Greece. Eye 2000; 14:752–756.

13. Robin AL, Covert D. Does adjunctive glaucoma therapy affect adherence to the initial primary therapy? Ophthalmology 2005; 112:863–868.

14. Ishibashi T, Yokoi N, Kinoshita S. Comparison of the short-term effects on the human corneal surface of topical timolol maleate with and without benzalkonium chloride. J Glaucoma 2003; 12:486–490.

15. Broadway DC, Grierson I, O'Brien C, et al. Adverse effects of topical antiglaucoma medication. I. The conjunctival cell profile. Arch Ophthalmol 1994; 112:1437–1445.

16. Baudouin C. Allergic reaction to topical eyedrops. Curr Opin Allergy Clin Immunol 2005; 5:459–463.

17. Lavin MJ, Wormald RP, Migdal CS, et al. The influence of prior therapy on the success of trabeculectomy. Arch Ophthalmol 1990; 108:1543–1548.

18. Sherwood MB, Grierson I, Millar L, et al. Long-term morphologic effects of antiglaucoma drugs on the conjunctiva and Tenon's capsule in glaucomatous patients. Ophthalmology 1989; 96:327–335.

19. Fechtner RD, Realini T. Fixed combinations of topical glaucoma medications. Curr Opin Ophthalmol 2004; 15:132–135.

20. Francis BA, Du LT, Berke S, at al. and the Cosopt Study Group. Comparing the fixed combination dorzolamide-timolol (Cosopt®) to concomitant administration of 2% dorzolamide (Trusopt®) and 0.5% timolol – a randomized controlled study and a replacement study. J Clin Pharm Ther 2004; 29: 375–380.

21. Khouri AS, Realini T, Fechtner RD. Use of fixed-dose combination drugs for the treatment of glaucoma. Drugs Aging 2007; 24:1007–1016.

22. Elliott WJ. Is fixed combination therapy appropriate for initial hypertension treatment? Curr Hypertens Rep 2002; 4:278–285.

23. Frampton JE, Perry CM. Topical dorzolamide 2%/timolol 0.5% ophthalmic solution: a review of its use in the treatment of glaucoma and ocular hypertension. Drugs Aging 2006; 23:977–995.

24. Fechtner RD, Airaksinen PJ, Getson AJ, et al. Cosopt versus Xalatan Study Groups. Efficacy and tolerability of the dorzolamide 2%/timolol 0.5% combination (Cosopt) versus 0.005% (Xalatan) in the treatment of ocular hypertension or glaucoma: results from two randomized clinical trials. Acta Ophthalmol Scand 2004; 82:42–48.

25. Konstas AG, Papapanos P, Tersis I, et al. Twenty-four-hour diurnal curve comparison of commercially available latanoprost 0.005% versus the timolol and dorzolamide fixed combination. Ophthalmology 2003; 110:1357–1360.

26. Orzalesi N, Rossetti L, Bottoli A, et al. The effect of latanoprost, brimonidine, and a fixed combination of timolol and dorzolamide on circadian intraocular pressure in patients with glaucoma or ocular hypertension. Arch Ophthalmol 2003; 121:453–457.

27. Konstas AGP, Kozobolis VP, Tsironi S, et al. Comparison of the 24-hour intraocular pressure-lowering effects of latanoprost and dorzolamide/timolol fixed combination after 2 and 6 months of treatment. Ophthalmology 2008; 115:99–103.

28. Pfeiffer N; the German Latanoprost Fixed Combination Study Group. A comparison of the fixed combination of latanoprost and timolol with its individual components. Graefe's Arch Clin Exp Ophthalmol 2002; 240:893–899.

29. Higginbotham EJ, Feldman R, Stiles M, et al. Latanoprost and timolol combination therapy vs monotherapy: one-year randomized trial. Arch Ophthalmol 2002; 120:915–922.

30. Alm A, Stjernschantz J; Effects on intraocular pressure and side effects of 0.005% latanoprost applied once daily, evening or morning. A comparison with timolol. The Scandinavian Latanoprost Study Group. Ophthalmology 1995; 102:1743–1752.

31. Konstas AG, Nakos E, Stewart WC, et al. A comparison of once-daily morning vs evening dosing of concomitant latanoprost/timolol. Am J Ophthalmol 2002; 133:753–757.

32. Konstas AGP, Maltezos AC, Gandi S, et al. Comparison of the 24-hour intraocular pressure reduction with two dosing regimes of latanoprost and timolol in patients with open-angle glaucoma. Am J Ophthalmol 1999; 128:15–20.

33. Konstas AGP, Boboridis K, Stewart WC, et al. 24-hour intraocular pressure short-term control with the latanoprost/timolol maleate fixed combination versus latanoprost, both dosed once each evening, in primary open-angle glaucoma patients. Arch Ophthalmol 2005; 123:898–902.

34. Diestelhorst M, Larsson LI; European Latanoprost Fixed Combination Study Group. A 12 week study comparing the fixed combination of latanoprost and timolol with the concomitant use of the individual components in patients with open angle glaucoma and ocular hypertension. Br J Ophthalmol 2004; 88:199–203.

35. Diestelhorst M, Larsson LI; European-Canadian Latanoprost Fixed Combination Study Group. A 12-week, randomized, double-masked, multicenter study of the fixed combination of latanoprost and timolol in the evening versus the individual components. Ophthalmology 2006; 113:70–76.

36. Stewart WC, Stewart JA, Day D, et al. Efficacy and safety of latanoprost/timolol maleate fixed combination verses timolol maleate and brimonidine given twice daily. Acta Ophthalmol Scand 2003; 81:242–246.

37. Garcia-Sanchez J, Rouland JF, Spiegel D, et al. A comparison of the fixed combination of latanoprost and timolol with the unfixed combination of brimonidine and timolol in patients with elevated intraocular pressure. A six month, evaluator masked, multicentre study in Europe. Br J Ophthalmol 2004; 88:877–883.

38. Stewart WC, Stewart JA, Day DG, et al. Efficacy and safety of the latanoprost/timolol maleate fixed combination versus concomitant brimonidine and latanoprost therapy. Eye 2004; 18:990–995.

39. Shin DH, Feldman RM, Sheu WP. Efficacy and safety of the fixed combinations latanoprost/timolol versus dorzolamide/timolol in patients with elevated intraocular pressure. Ophthalmology 2004; 111:276–282.

40. Konstas AGP, Kozobolis VP, Stewart WC, et al. Daytime diurnal curve comparison between the fixed combinations of latanoprost/timolol and dorzolamide/timolol. Eye 2005; 18:1264–1269.

41. Topouzis F, Melamed S, Danesh-Meyer H, et al. A 1-year study to compare the efficacy and safety of once-daily travoprost 0.004%/timolol 0.5% to once-daily latanoprost 0.005%/timolol 0.5% in patients with open-angle glaucoma or ocular hypertension. Eur J Ophthalmol 2007; 17:183–190.

42. Barnebey HS, Orengo-Nania S, Flowers BE, et al. The safety and efficacy of travoprost 0.004%/timolol 0.5% fixed combination ophthalmic solution. Am J Ophthalmol 2005; 140:1–7.

43. Schuman JS, Katz GJ, Lewis RA, et al. Efficacy and safety of a fixed combination of travoprost 0.004%/timolol 0.5% ophthalmic solution once daily for open-angle glaucoma or ocular hypertension. Am J Ophthalmol 2005; 140:242–250.

44. Hughes BA, Bacharach J, Craven ER, et al. A three-month, multicenter, double-masked study of the safety and efficacy of travoprost 0.004%/timolol 0.5% ophthalmic solution compared to travoprost 0.004% ophthalmic solution and timolol 0.5% dosed concomitantly in subjects with open angle glaucoma or ocular hypertension. J Glaucoma 2005; 14:392–399.

45. Konstas AGP, Tsironi S Vakalis AN, et al. 24-hour intraocular pressure control obtained with evening dosed, versus morning dosed, travoprost/timolol fixed combination in open-angle glaucoma. Acta Ophthalmol Scand 2008 (in press).

46. Hommer A; Ganfort Investigators Group I. A double-masked randomized, parallel comparison of a fixed combination of bimatoprost 0.03%/timolol 0.5% with non-fixed combination use in patients with glaucoma or ocular hypertension. Eur J Ophthalmol 2007; 17:53–62.

47. Martinez A, Sanchez MA. Comparison of the safety and intraocular pressure lowering of bimatoprost/timolol fixed combination versus latanoprost/timolol fixed combination in patients with open-angle glaucoma. Curr Med Res Opin 2007; 23:1025–1032.

48. Craven ER, Walters TR, Williams R, et al. Brimonidine and timolol fixed-combination therapy versus monotherapy: a 3-month randomized trial in patients with glaucoma or ocular hypertension. J Ocul Pharmacol Ther 2005; 21:337–348.

49. Sherwood MB, Craven ER, Chou C, et al. Twice-daily 0.2% brimonidine–0.5% timolol fixed-combination therapy vs monotherapy with timolol or brimonidine in patients with glaucoma or ocular hypertension: a 12-month randomized trial. Arch Ophthalmol 2006; 124:1230–1238.

50. Goni FJ; Brimonidine/Timolol Fixed Combination Study Group. 12-week study comparing the fixed combination of brimonidine and timolol with concomitant use of the individual components in patients with glaucoma and ocular hypertension. Eur J Ophthalmol 2005; 15:581–590.

51. Konstas AGP, Katsimpris IE, Kaltsos K, et al. Twenty-four-hour efficacy of the brimonidine/timolol fixed combination versus therapy with the unfixed components. Eye 2007 Jun 15 (Epub ahead of print).

52. Arcieri ES, Arcieri RS, Pereira AC, et al. Comparing the fixed combination brimonidine-timolol versus fixed combination dorzolamide-timolol in patients with elevated intraocular pressure. Curr Med Res Opin 2007; 23:683–689.

53. Konstas AGP, Lake S, Economou AI, et al. 24-hour control with a latanoprost–timolol fixed combination vs timolol alone. Arch Ophthalmol 2006; 124:1553–1557.

54. Harris A, Jonescu-Cuypers CP, Kagemann L, et al. Effect of dorzolamide timolol combination versus timolol 0.5% on ocular blood flow in patients with primary open-angle glaucoma. Am J Ophthalmol 2001; 132:490–495.

55. Martinez A, Sanchez M. Retrobulbar haemodynamic effects of the latanoprost/timolol and the dorzolamide/timolol fixed combinations in newly diagnosed glaucoma patients. Int J Clin Pract 2007;61:815–825.

56. Henderer JD, Wilson RP, Moster MR, et al. Timolol/dorzolamide combination therapy as initial treatment for intraocular pressure over 30 mm Hg. J Glaucoma 2005; 14:267–270.

57. Konstas AGP, Kozobolis VP, Tersis I, et al. The efficacy and safety of the timolol/dorzolamide fixed combination versus latanoprost in exfoliation glaucoma. Eye 2003; 7:41–46.

NEW HORIZONS

CHAPTER 52

Neuroprotection and Neuroregeneration

Leonard A Levin

INTRODUCTION

Glaucoma is the most common optic neuropathy. It is also the only optic neuropathy distinguished by a highly characteristic morphology of the optic disc: namely, cupping with a relative absence of pallor. The distinctive appearance reflects the fact that the primary pathophysiology of the disease takes place at the optic disc itself. In fact, it has been suggested that change in the optic disc, such as stretching of axons,[1] ischemia of axons against the scleral edge,[2] or other mechanisms is the primary injury that causes the glaucomatous phenotype.

As with other optic neuropathies, glaucoma is manifested by death of retinal ganglion cells, loss of retinal ganglion cell axons, and loss of vision. For each of these neurobiological consequences there is a corresponding clinical manifestation. The loss of retinal ganglion cell axons results in decreased thickness of the nerve fiber layer, optic nerve atrophy, and a decrease in the size of the optic nerve on neuroimaging. The optic atrophy of glaucoma is virtually pathognomonic, being a morphological excavation without significant disc pallor, and is not seen in other optic neuropathies. The loss of retinal ganglion cells is not seen on clinical examination, but can be demonstrated by loss of the pattern electroretinogram (pattern ERG) and loss of the retinal ganglion cell components of the multifocal ERG. The loss of visual function is manifested by a variety of clinical measures, predominantly visual field loss in a nerve fiber bundle defect pattern, and late in the course of the disease, decreased visual acuity and color vision.

The recognition that glaucoma is an optic neuropathy (albeit often associated with an elevated intraocular pressure or a response to intraocular pressure lowering) suggested that therapies directed at preventing the neuronal loss may be efficacious for patients with the disease. In addition, the permanent loss of vision in glaucoma reflects the permanent loss of retinal ganglion cells and their axons. Therefore, visual restoration would require a restoration of retinal ganglion cells and their axons, i.e. neurorepair and neuroregeneration. This chapter reviews neuroprotection and regeneration with respect to glaucomatous optic neuropathy. Further elaboration of some of this material can be found in previously published materials.[3]

MECHANISMS OF RETINAL GANGLION CELL DEATH AND NEUROPROTECTION

The damage in glaucoma primarily occurs at the optic disc. It is through the disc that the axons of the retinal ganglion cells course. Therefore, the death of retinal ganglion cells is an irreversible consequence of axonal injury, the likely mechanism for injury in glaucomatous optic neuropathy.[4,5] Much is known about the effect of axonal injury on retinal ganglion cells, because of several years of research studying acute transection of the axons in experimental animals. Cutting the optic nerve within the orbit causes the retinal ganglion cells to die over the course of days to weeks.[6] The process of glaucomatous cell death involves apoptosis, a suicide-like process in which axonal injury apparently signals the retinal ganglion cell to die.[7] Blocking apoptosis (e.g. by blocking the expression of apoptosis-related proteins or using chemical inhibitors of apoptosis) increases cell survival. Similarly, there are survival factors that can be injected into the eye and which maintain retinal ganglion cell survival, despite a severe axonal injury. For example, researchers crushed the optic nerve of rats, injecting a survival factor called brain-derived neurotrophic factor (BDNF) into the vitreous.[6] In the control eyes, approximately 50% of the retinal ganglion cells died after 7 days, while in the BDNF-injected eyes, almost all of the cells survived. Combinations of survival factors, and expressing the receptors for the survival factors on retinal ganglion cells, can increase survival, so that a great number of retinal ganglion cells can be preserved.[8] One method for developing neuroprotective therapies for glaucoma is to better understand what happens within retinal ganglion cells to mediate the cell death process after optic nerve injury. For example, superoxide anion may serve as an intracellular signal for cell death.[9]

Neuroprotection is a therapy directed at neuronal loss, either prophylactic or after the insult has taken place. The

TABLE 52.1	**Methods for neuroprotection**
Pharmacological	
Glutamate receptor antagonists	
NMDA receptors	
AMPA/kainate antagonists	
Calcium channel blockade	
α_2-adrenergic agonists	
Neurotrophic factors	
Nitric oxide synthase inhibitors	
Inhibition of death signaling cascades	
Activation of survival signaling cascades	
Reactive oxygen species scavengers	
Apoptosis inhibitors	
Inhibition of cytochrome c release	
Caspase inhibitors	
Immune modulation	
Preconditioning	

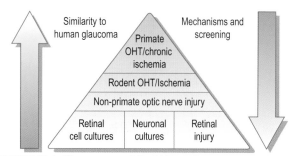

FIGURE 52.1 Glaucoma models. OHT, ocular hypertension.

loss of the cell is targeted, not the disease process by which the loss occurs. In glaucomatous optic neuropathy, the retinal ganglion cell is treated, and not the elevated intraocular pressure (or other etiology) that indirectly causes the death of the retinal ganglion cell. Although intraocular pressure lowering and other such therapies can be considered indirectly neuroprotective, by strict definition and by comparison with other cytoprotective therapies, a neuroprotective therapy is directed at the neuron itself. Strategies for neuroprotection are diverse (Table 52.1).

Neuroprotective therapies are therefore *downstream* therapies, while most standard therapies are *upstream* therapies. If one considers disease as a tissue insult resulting in injury or death of cells, therapies that address the process by which the cells are injured are upstream therapies, e.g. upstream of the cellular injury. Therapies that address the mechanism by which the cellular injury results in dysfunction or death of the cell are downstream therapies, and target the mechanism by which the injury results in loss of function or death. For example, lowering the intraocular pressure in glaucoma would be considered an upstream therapy, while neuroprotection of retinal ganglion cells would be a downstream therapy.

ASSESSMENT OF NEUROPROTECTIVE THERAPIES: THEORY

Current therapies of glaucoma are directed at lowering the intraocular pressure. The assessment of these therapies only requires demonstration that the intraocular pressure is lowered, and to what degree. With neuroprotection, the therapy is directed at neuronal death, and therefore the assessment of efficacy must reflect this end point. There are at least two different ways of looking at retinal ganglion cell end points: namely, functional and structural. Preclinical studies should use models that are useful for predicting the response when the therapy is applied to patients. Furthermore, if a drug is used, there must be evidence that it, or an indirect effector, is active at the retinal ganglion cell or its axon.

DOES THE MODEL IN WHICH THE THERAPY IS BEING TESTED MIMIC ASPECTS OF CLINICAL GLAUCOMA?

Glaucoma models can be represented in a pyramid, with the most applicable models at the top, and the relatively less applicable models at the bottom (Fig. 52.1). This does not mean that the top is 'better' than the bottom, as there is a role for each in terms of the similarity to human glaucoma with respect to morphology, time-course, cell biology, and how the model is carried out. A retinal ganglion cell culture cannot reflect the complicated pathophysiology that is far more closely reproduced in a nonhuman primate model. On the other hand, one cannot screen thousands of drugs in monkeys or even rats, but one can in a cell culture model.

Experimental paradigms of neuroprotective strategies in glaucoma include in vitro cell models, in vivo models of optic nerve injury and glaucoma in animals, and clinical trials in humans. Each has its advantages and disadvantages. The most important aspects to consider are the similarity to glaucoma and the utility for testing neuroprotection (Table 52.2).

Cultures of retinal ganglion cells are useful for understanding mechanisms of how axonal injuries cause cell death, but the culture itself as a disease model is very different from glaucoma. There are many animal models of central nervous system injury and disease or cultures of other neuronal cell types, but these are pathophysiologically distant from the glaucomatous process itself, and thus cannot be used to provide good evidence of therapeutic efficacy for neuroprotection in glaucoma. Other helpful, but less extrapolative models, include those where the intraocular pressure (IOP) is raised to higher than the systolic blood pressure, causing retinal ischemia, or models where N-methyl-D-aspartate (NMDA) or other excitotoxic chemicals are injected into the eye, killing retinal ganglion cells.[10,11]

Further up the pyramid are optic nerve injuries (e.g. optic nerve transection or optic nerve crush). This is an acute injury of the optic nerve, different from glaucoma, but sharing the characteristics of optic neuropathy. The model's usefulness is the ability to study signaling mechanisms of retinal ganglion cell death, in this case after axonal injury.[9] The next higher level on the pyramid are experimental glaucoma models, particularly where the IOP is chronically raised, simulating the effect of higher IOP in humans. A parallel model

TABLE 52.2 Neuroprotection models

MODEL	SIMILARITY TO GLAUCOMA	UTILITY FOR TESTING NEUROPROTECTION
Neuronal culture models other than retinal ganglion cells	Low	Good for understanding mechanisms of neuronal death
Retinal ganglion cell culture models	Common feature is retinal ganglion cell death	Good for understanding mechanisms of retinal ganglion cell death
Retinal photic injury	Not an optic neuropathy	May be good test of whether a drug is neuroprotective for retinal cells (e.g. photoreceptors) other than retinal ganglion cells
Retinal ischemia	Causes retinal ganglion cell and axonal ischemia, and therefore indirectly causes an optic neuropathy, but not cupping	Good for testing neuroprotection of cell body injuries
Optic nerve head ischemia	Causes optic neuropathy with cupping	Good for testing neuroprotection of axonal injuries
Crush or other mechanical insult to the optic nerve	Causes axonal damage with consequent effects on the retinal ganglion cell; no cupping	Good for testing neuroprotection of axonal injuries
Animal ocular hypertension	Causes axonal damage and cupping; also can cause cell body injury if intraocular pressure is too high	Good for testing neuroprotection of glaucoma

is that of chronic disc ischemia, induced by infusing vasoconstrictive endothelin-1[12] into the subarachnoid space. Often, the morphological functional and histological features of these animal models closely match those of the human disease, although taking place over a shorter time period. Rodent models of ocular hypertension have become well characterized, but the primate model of ocular hypertension after argon laser damage to the trabecular meshwork represents the closest model akin to human glaucoma. The randomized, controlled clinical trial in patients remains the gold standard for assessing efficacy.

HOW IS THE EFFECT OF NEUROPROTECTION ASSESSED?

Functional assessment The functional assessment of the retinal ganglion cell and its axon is reflected in the ability: (1) to generate action potentials based on incoming information generated from its synapses with bipolar and amacrine cells; (2) to conduct these impulses down the optic nerve toward cells in the lateral geniculate nucleus and other targets within the central nervous system; and (3) to be relayed to processing neurons of the visual cortex within the occipital lobe. At the highest level, this pathway can be assessed with visual function measures, particularly the visual field. A wide variety of measurements of visual fields have been developed, with the most common being white-on-white automated perimetry, as well as short-wave (blue on yellow) automated perimetry, frequency doubling perimetry, high pass perimetry, and several other techniques.

There are also several methods for assessing whether or not there is progression in the visual field. Some are based on looking at single points, others on clusters of points, and others on summation of the entire visual field. These range from techniques as simple as looking at the mean deviation of the visual field, compared with an age-matched normal control group, to complex techniques, assessing the border of the increasing scotoma or other techniques.[13]

Some visual parameters are less sensitive for assessing neuroprotection in glaucoma because they are only affected late in the course of the disease. These include visual acuity and color vision measures. Mass measures of optic nerve function such as the afferent papillary defect are useful only when there is significant asymmetrical optic neuropathy.

The summation of the electrical generation of action potentials within the retinal ganglion cell can be determined with the pattern ERG. More recently, there has been success in using late components of the multifocal ERG to detect retinal ganglion cell outputs.[14] The latter has the advantage of generating a retinotopic mapping, with the focal loss of retinal ganglion cell function in a specific area depicted in a manner similar to that used for visual fields. Conduction down the optic nerve can be measured with the visually evoked response to a contrast-reversing checkerboard pattern, or as a retinotopic map from a multifocal visually evoked response. These techniques, which in humans rely on measurements made at the cortex, actually reflect not just the conduction down the optic nerve, but also the geniculocortical connection. In animals, electrodes can be placed at the superior colliculus (the target for most retinal ganglion cell axons in lower animals), thereby isolating the function of the anterior visual pathways.

The analysis of retinal ganglion cell and axonal function on a single cell basis is important for preclinical study and evaluation of neuroprotective techniques, even if it is currently inapplicable to routine clinical use. Animal retinas can be dissociated and retinal ganglion cells cultured. This allows study of multiple retinal ganglion cell functions, e.g. electrical activity and calcium influx.[15] Retinal ganglion cells within the living animal can also be imaged and studied. For example, Cordeiro and colleagues described the use of annexin V, which binds exposed phosphatidylserine on apoptotic cells, as a measure of an early step in apoptosis.[16]

Structural assessment As retinal ganglion cells and their axons disappear in glaucoma, the nerve fiber layer thins, and this can be detected on the fundus examination, especially when there is focal thinning. Examination of the nerve fiber layer is aided by red-free photography. The size of the nerve fiber layer can be assessed more precisely with optical coherence tomography (OCT), which directly measures the thickness, or with nerve fiber layer polarimetry, which measures the amount of birefringence from microtubules within the axons contained in the nerve fiber layer. If there is microtubule dysfunction or destruction independent of loss of retinal ganglion cell axons, then there may be a discrepancy between the OCT and polarimetry measurements.

In glaucoma, changes in the morphology of the optic nerve head reflect the number of remaining retinal ganglion cell axons. As glaucoma progresses, the size of the cup increases (more accurately, the size of the neuroretinal rim decreases). The change in the disc can be assessed by observation, with stereophotography, or with specialized instruments, e.g. Heidelberg retinal tomography or OCT.

The number of retinal ganglion cell axons within the optic nerve decreases in glaucoma, and this causes a smaller optic nerve, which can be studied by neuroimaging. Magnetic resonance imaging (MRI), computed tomography, and ultrasonography have all been used for this purpose. For MRI, the appropriate pulse sequences are necessary in order to avoid problems in discriminating the optic nerve from orbital fat, e.g. the use of fat suppression in T1-weighted MRI. The inherent contrast between fat and the optic nerve makes computed tomography particularly straightforward for assessing the optic nerve, although the discrimination between a large amount of subarachnoid cerebrospinal fluid in an atrophic nerve and a large number of axons in a normal nerve may be difficult. Specific MRI sequences for analyzing optic nerve axons have been developed.[17,18] Ultrasonography also can be used. It does not require complex instrumentation but is highly operator dependent.

Neuroprotective strategies addressed at maintaining ganglion cell viability can be assessed by counting the number of living retinal ganglion cells after an experimental intervention. Most commonly these are done on either retinal whole-mounts or optic nerve cross-sections. In a whole-mount the entire retina is flattened out onto a microscope slide. Retinal ganglion cells are identified by retrograde labeling with a fluorescent dye that had previously been injected into one of the targets of retinal ganglion cells, e.g. the superior colliculus, by immunohistochemistry, or with ganglion cell-specific promoters driving a fluorescent dye.[19] The optic nerve can also be sectioned and the number of retinal ganglion cell axons counted. Each axon corresponds to a living retinal ganglion cell.

The number of neurons within the *targets* of the retinal ganglion cell is also important for studying neuroprotective therapies. There is loss or dysfunction of lateral geniculate nucleus neurons in glaucoma.[20-23] Even if a neuroprotective therapy rescues a retinal ganglion cell and its axon, if the process which causes the lateral geniculate neuron (or its target in the cortex) to die is not halted, then visual function may not be spared. The techniques for counting lateral geniculate neurons are stereological, i.e. require corrections for the number and thickness of the tissue slices and other factors. Therefore, lateral geniculate nucleus assessment is not as simple as counting retinal whole-mounts or optic nerve cross-sections.

Preservation of a retinal ganglion cell and its axon is ineffective if the cell is not connected to those cells in the retina that excite or inhibit it. These connections occur via the dendritic tree and the cell body. The nature of the dendritic tree of retinal ganglion cells, which retracts in glaucoma,[24] can be studied by electrophysiologically identifying retinal ganglion cells and directly injecting Lucifer yellow or other dyes into the ganglion cell body.[24]

Does the concentration of the drug at its target match the concentration needed to be neuroprotective? There have been many attempts at producing comparable concentrations of ocular neuroprotectants in both in vivo and in vitro models. Although it is often difficult to extrapolate drug dosing and intraocular concentrations from the in vivo model to the human model, this helps in determining whether a neuroprotective therapy is likely to be effective. Table 52.3 lists several potential neuroprotective drugs extrapolated from several studies, their primary targets, and pharmacological data from animal and human studies. The calculated intravitreal concentrations achieved with clinical dosing for several studies are described.

ASSESSMENT OF NEUROPROTECTIVE THERAPIES: PRACTICE

PRECLINICAL STUDIES OF NEUROPROTECTION FOR GLAUCOMA

In the past, the evidence for neuroprotection was mostly generated by preclinical data from the bottom two layers of the pyramid (see Fig. 52.1). Models of ocular hypertension have recently provided more evidence, one layer higher in the pyramid. Compounds tested include 2-aminoguanidine,[25] brimonidine,[26] Cop-1 vaccine,[27] erythropoietin,[28,29] memantine,[30] brain-derived neurotrophic factor,[31] and many others. The randomized, controlled trial is the gold standard for deciding whether a therapy is truly efficacious. The variability in disease progression and the inherent variability in measuring visual function or optic nerve structure has implications for the study of glaucoma, necessitating

TABLE 52.3 Pharmacology of some ocular neuroprotectants

DRUG	TARGET	DOSE OR CONCENTRATION PROTECTIVE OF RETINAL GANGLION CELLS IN ANIMAL STUDIES	SIDE EFFECTS	DOSE IN CLINICAL TRIALS OR CLINICAL USE	ACHIEVABLE INTRAVITREAL CONCENTRATION WITH CLINICAL DOSING
2-aminoguanidine	Inducible nitric oxide synthase inhibition	60 mg daily in rat cautery ocular hypertension model[25] Not seen with rat hypertonic saline ocular hypertension model[84]	?	300–600 mg p.o. daily	?
Brain-derived neurotrophic factor	TrkB receptor	1 μg intravitreal[85]	Injection site reaction, diarrhea	25–100 μg/kg[86]	?
Betaxolol	β_1-adrenergic receptor (antagonist) and calcium influx	10–235 μM (culture)[87-89] 0.25% topical b.i.d.[90,91]	Stinging	0.25% topical bid	0.48 μg/g retina (rabbit)[90] (approx 1.3 μM)
Brimonidine	α_2-adrenergic receptor (agonist)	1 mg/kg daily s.c. infusion[26] 0.5% topical[92]	Conjunctival injection, drowsiness	0.15–0.2% topical b.i.d. –t.i.d.	82 nM (monkey)[93] 1.4–1836 nM (human)[94]
Eliprodil	NMDA receptor	1 nM (culture)[95] 20 nmol intravitreal[96] 10 mg/kg i.p.[96]	Few	2.5–10 mg p.o. daily[97]	?
Memantine	NMDA receptor	4 mg/kg p.o. daily[40,41] 10 mg/kg i.p.[30]	Dizziness, headache, constipation	20 mg p.o. daily	0.3–1.8 μM (monkey vitreous)[41]

Examples of neuroprotective drugs, their primary targets, and some pharmacological data from animal and human studies. No distinction is made between the various types of animal studies, particularly with respect to ability to extrapolate results to human glaucoma.

that good randomized, controlled trials require somewhere in the region of hundreds of patients.

In the early years of studying neuroprotection in retinal ganglion cells, most studies focused either on survival of retinal ganglion cells in culture or survival after severe injuries such as optic nerve crush. More recently, the focus has shifted to animal models of glaucoma that are closer to the human disease. These are usually intraocular hypertension models. Rodents are most commonly used, but nonhuman primates are also employed.

The main interventions for neuroprotection that have been studied in preclinical research are pharmacological, preconditioning, and immune-based therapies. The vast majority are pharmacological. The following section discusses some seminal studies of neuroprotection in animal models of glaucoma.

NONHUMAN PRIMATE GLAUCOMA

The nonhuman primate model of glaucoma,[32] based on trabecular meshwork ablation with the argon laser, is the closest to the human disease in terms of disc morphology and relationship of progression with intraocular pressure. This model has been used to study memantine, an NMDA antagonist. The original rationale for studying NMDA antagonists in glaucoma was the activity of NMDA receptor-mediated excitotoxicity of retinal ganglion cells,[33] by analogy to how neurons die by

excitotoxicity from glutamate in stroke, and early studies demonstrated elevated intraocular glutamate levels in experimental primate and human glaucoma[34] and rodent optic nerve crush.[35] Subsequently, large increases in levels of extracellular glutamate in glaucoma were not confirmed,[36,37] and the nature of glutamate excitotoxicity in retinal ganglion cells was questioned.[38,39]

In a small but long-term monkey study, memantine reduced the functional loss associated with glaucoma, as measured by multifocal ERG and visual-evoked responses,[40] maintained disc structural integrity,[41] and partly decreased retinal ganglion cell death.[41] Significantly, memantine also reduced glaucoma-induced changes in the brain, i.e. cell shrinkage in the lateral geniculate nucleus.[42]

Although it is highly controversial how much glutamate excitotoxicity actually occurs in glaucoma, there appears to be less progression of structural and functional measures of glaucomatous optic neuropathy in monkeys treated with memantine. This suggests the possibility that memantine, and probably other NMDA antagonists, might preserve visual function and structure in glaucoma not by blocking excitotoxicity, but by another means, perhaps decreasing metabolic load or similar mechanism. Drug concentrations of systemically delivered memantine appear to be similar to that necessary for inhibiting NMDA receptor activation.[43] In monkeys treated with 4 mg/kg/day,[44] the plasma levels of memantine reached the same concentration as that

TABLE 52.4 Drugs that are neuroprotective in animal models of glaucoma	
DRUG OR OTHER THERAPY	**MECHANISM**
2-aminoguanidine[25] (conflicting results[84])	iNOS inhibitor
Brain-derived neurotrophic factor (BDNF)/SPBN[31]	Neurotrophin / reactive oxygen species scavenger
Brimonidine[26]	α_2-agonist
Ciliary neurotrophic factor (CNTF)[98]	Neurotrophin
Electroacupuncture[99]	Unknown
Erythropoietin[28,29]	PI3 kinase/Akt kinase activator
Geranylgeranylacetone; heat stress[100,101]	Heat shock protein activator
Glatiramer acetate[27] (conflicting results[102])	T-cell activator
Glial cell line-derived neurotrophic factor (GDNF)[103]	Neurotrophin
L-N[6]-(1-iminoethyl)lysine 5-tetrazole amide[45]	Prodrug for iNOS inhibitor
Lycium barbarum Lynn[104]	Medicinal herb
Memantine[30]	NMDA antagonist
Minocycline[105]	Antiapoptosis (blocks cytochrome *c* release)
Phenytoin[106]	Sodium channel blocker
R(-)-1-(benzo [b] thiophen-5-yl)-2-[2-(N, N-diethylamino) ethoxy] ethanol hydrochloride (T-588)[107]	Upregulation of MAP kinase pathways

measured in human subjects treated for Parkinson's disease.

RODENT OCULAR HYPERTENSION

Several drugs have been studied in rat and mouse models of ocular hypertension. Mechanisms include blockade of nitric oxide synthase with two antagonists, aminoguanidine and L-N(6)-(1-iminoethyl)lysine 5-tetrazole amide[25,45] activation of the α_2-adrenergic receptor with brimonidine,[26] and memantine.[30] These and other drugs are summarized in Table 52.4.

IMMUNE MECHANISMS

Focal activation of the immune system in the optic nerve and/or retina is a way of preserving retinal ganglion cells and their functions in the face of optic neuropathy. Activated T lymphocytes primed to optic nerve constituents, e.g. myelin basic protein, home to sites of injury and release factors which are neuroprotective.[46] This was first demonstrated with optic nerve crush models, where the crush was partial, and thus there were several marginally injured axons.[47] Similar findings were seen in a laser ocular hypertension model in the rat.[27] Not only was generation of an immune response to myelin basic protein a mechanism for inducing this immune-mediated neuroprotection but also to copolymer-1,[48] a synthetic polypeptide which is also used for the treatment of multiple sclerosis.

CLINICAL TRIALS IN NEUROPROTECTION

The biggest concern regarding neuroprotection as a therapy for glaucoma is the substantial history of clinical trials in stroke that failed to show efficacy.[49] No neuroprotective drug has been approved by the United States Food and Drug Administration for the treatment of stroke, despite dozens of drugs being successful in animal models of stroke and hundreds of millions of dollars being spent on randomized clinical trials.[50] In one case, a drug was effective in one large phase III study[51] but not in a second and larger study.[52] Yet, in every case the decision to go to clinical trial was based on preclinical studies showing that the drugs worked very well.

The discrepancy between the preclinical and clinical results could result from several causes: (1) the model did not properly simulate the human disease; (2) the variability in patients was much higher than the variability of the disease in laboratory animals; or (3) the pathophysiology of the disease in humans is intrinsically different from that in animals. Most laboratory animals are small and their brains not as highly developed as humans. It is possible that the ratio of axonal damage to neuronal damage differs in human versus animal studies, and this may be one of the reasons why human neuroprotective studies of stroke have in general failed to show efficacy. Interestingly, studies of Alzheimer's disease,[53] and to a lesser extent amyotrophic lateral sclerosis,[54] have shown efficacy for presumed neuroprotective agents (memantine and riluzole, respectively). These are chronic degenerative diseases, for which it is likely that direct axonal damage plays less of a role.

Is the failure of neuroprotection in stroke relevant to neuroprotection in glaucoma? There is a wealth of studies demonstrating that various pharmacological agents and other agents are neuroprotective for retinal ganglion cells in optic nerve injuries, including ocular hypertension models that simulate human glaucoma. In stroke, drugs that were neuroprotective in the laboratory failed to show efficacy in patients. Therefore, animal data of neuroprotection in glaucoma are insufficient for deciding whether a drug is effective in patients. It is therefore crucial that well-designed randomized, controlled trials of potential neuroprotective agents be performed, and used to guide therapy. Although several small studies have been published on neuroprotective agents in patients with glaucoma, none is of sufficient quality to guide clinical decision-making.

LOW-PRESSURE GLAUCOMA TREATMENT STUDY

The Low-Pressure Glaucoma Treatment Study (LoGTS) randomized 190 patients between 1998 and 2000 who had normal-tension glaucoma and were 30 years of age or older to either brimonidine 0.2% or timolol 0.5%. These drugs were chosen because they have equivalent pressure-lowering effects, and therefore the neuroprotective effects of brimonidine could be tested independent of intraocular pressure lowering. All patients completed enrollment and were followed for a minimum of 4 years. Patients had to have intraocular pressures less than or equal to 21 mgHg on a diurnal curve. Patients, physicians, technicians, and the reading centers for visual fields and optic disc photographs were masked. The outcome measure was defined on the basis of visual fields as a 'significant progression of the same two or more points, on a Humphrey Glaucoma change probability map or by Progressor linear regression analysis, in three consecutive (over an 8-month period) Humphrey 24-2 full-threshold fields.'[55]

The design of the LoGTS study was published in early 2005.[55] As of the time of writing of this chapter, the results have not been published.

MEMANTINE IN OPEN-ANGLE GLAUCOMA

Memantine, an NMDA receptor antagonist, was studied in two industry-supported (Allergan, Irvine, CA) phase III studies, each with approximately 1000 patients and lasting multiple years. Patients received standard management of their glaucoma and were randomized to receive oral memantine or placebo. The primary outcome measure was visual function. This was probably the largest study of neuroprotection in an ophthalmic disease.

As of the time of writing of this chapter, the results of the memantine studies have not been published. A press release from the study sponsor stated that one of the two trials was analyzed in part, with the following preliminary outcome: 'Two measures of visual function were selected in the statistical analysis plan to assess the efficacy of memantine in glaucoma. The functional measure chosen as the primary end point did not show a benefit of memantine in preserving visual function. In a number of analyses using the secondary functional measure, memantine demonstrated a statistically significant benefit of the high dose compared to placebo.' A second announcement stated that the other trial also did not meet its primary end point.

AXOPROTECTION

As mentioned earlier, several treatments are successful for preventing the death of retinal ganglion cells in experimental models of glaucoma. However, treatments that maintain retinal ganglion cell viability without taking into account the functional consequences are unlikely to have a positive clinical outcome when translated to human use. For patients, visual function is the end point that is relevant to the patient's quality of life, and therefore the value of neuroprotection directed at retinal ganglion cell soma survival alone has been questioned.

If the optic nerve is transected, maintaining the viability of a retinal ganglion cell despite a damaged axon will not prevent visual loss. Even if the retinal ganglion cell can send impulses through the nerve fiber layer towards the optic disc, if the axon is damaged or transected the impulse will never reach the brain, and the patient will not be able to see using that axon. It is not know whether axonal damage alone from glaucoma is irreversible, or whether it relies on the death of the retinal ganglion cell as well. However, from studies of other optic nerve injuries, it appears that once axonal injury has occurred that is sufficient to disrupt the structure of the axon, the axon will not be regenerated or maintained for the life of the animal. Therefore, a different strategy should be considered, one in which preservation of the axon is necessary. This strategy is called 'axoprotection,' and is a theoretical protection of axonal integrity and function in the face of damage.

There are two types of axonal processes that occur after a focal injury to an axon. Degeneration distal to the site of injury is called 'wallerian degeneration,' while degeneration proximal to the site of injury is called retrograde degeneration. Much of the understanding of axonal protection relies on data from either ischemic injuries to the rodent optic nerve[56] or strains of mutant mice or rats in which a mutant gene called WldS (wallerian degeneration slow) causes the distal part of the axon to maintain its integrity despite a transection proximal to the site of injury.[57] There is little known about how best to protect an axon in glaucoma. The most investigated area is ischemia of the isolated optic nerve, with work by Waxman and colleagues dating back to the 1990s. They and others showed that calcium and sodium influx mediate ischemic or anoxic damage to retinal ganglion cell axons,[58] and that this can be ameliorated by drugs that block sodium channels.[59] This area has been comprehensively reviewed.[60]

Although the concept of axoprotection is in its very early stages, it is likely that understanding axonal death and injury and how axons can be maintained will lead to advances in therapies for diseases such as glaucoma.

NEUROREGENERATION

Neuroprotection is a strategy for preventing the death of neurons; however, once the neuron has died and the axon disappeared, visual function cannot be restored unless a new neuron is delivered and connected to the appropriate afferent and efferent targets. Regeneration (or neuroregeneration) of the optic nerve requires the production and differentiation of new retinal ganglion cells from stem cells, connection to bipolar and amacrine cells, and extension of their axons to their appropriate targets in the brain.

DIFFERENTIATION OF STEM CELLS INTO RETINAL GANGLION CELLS

Differentiating neural stem cells into specific classes of retinal neurons is a first step in repopulating the neurons lost in glaucoma. Transplantation studies with stem cells have been increasingly used in attempts to repopulate neurons lost in degenerative or traumatic disease. A wide variety of stem cells have been studied for this purpose, e.g. embryonic stem cells,[61] brain-derived precursor cells,[62] hippocampal-derived neural stem cells,[63] and bone marrow-derived stem cells.[64] Retinal stem cells have been demonstrated in the ciliary marginal zone (CMZ) of adult vertebrate eyes.[65,66] However, the fact that visual loss from most optic nerve diseases does not spontaneously improve implies that CMZ stem cells do not normally divide, differentiate into retinal ganglion cells (RGCs), or repopulate the retina.

Although stem cell transplantation of brain-derived, hippocampal-derived, and bone marrow-derived stem cells into the retina leads to integration of these stem cells,[61,62,67] the majority do not differentiate into RGCs, even after RGC depletion.[68] Instead, they mostly develop into amacrine and horizontal cells.[63] Müller glia can induce neural progenitor cells to differentiate into RGCs,[69] and in vitro conditions can induce release of excitatory neurotransmitters from newly produced RGCs.[70]

A major goal is therefore to find ways of directing the differentiation of stem cells into specific retinal neurons, and thereby replacing those lost due to pathology. The most complete data for retinal neuronal development exist for the RGC. It is known that several signals are involved in the developmental differentiation of progenitor cells into mature RGCs. This differentiation is paralleled by the expression of specific developmentally regulated genes.[71]

AXONAL REGENERATION

Regeneration of axons from retinal ganglion cells is a scientific problem that has been studied for many years. The mammalian optic nerve does not regenerate after it is transected, unlike that in lower animals such as the goldfish, which readily regenerate and form appropriate connections to targets in the brain. Nerves in the peripheral nervous system are also able to regenerate once transected, but mammalian central nerves cannot. Two decades ago, Aguayo and colleagues demonstrated that transection of the optic nerve, followed by replacement of part of the optic nerve with a sciatic (peripheral) nerve graft allowed limited regeneration.[72]

Regenerating axons are derived from retinal ganglion cells that express growth-associated protein-43 (GAP-43).[73] Subsequently, studies of the factors which prevent regeneration in the central nervous system focused on the role of myelin-associated substances[74] (e.g. myelin-associated glycoprotein[75]) and glial (astrocyte-derived) scarring (e.g. proteoglycans[76]) as inhibitory factors. Downregulation of the receptor for Nogo, a myelin-associated protein,[77,78] enables regeneration of retinal ganglion cell axons when appropriately sensitized.[79] Instead of targeting the receptors by which the inhibition of axonal extension is signaled, some groups have focused on the subcellular transduction pathways for inhibition. For example, upregulation of cyclic adenosine monophosphate allows regeneration of spinal cord[80] and retinal ganglion cell[81] axons, and mice lacking receptor protein tyrosine phosphatase sigma have increased retinal ganglion cell axon regeneration past a glial scar.[82] Finally, there is a dramatic reduction in the axonal extension rate of retinal ganglion cells around the time of birth. This switch appears to be signaled by contact with amacrine cells,[83] and the nature of the signal and how it is transduced is being studied.

Regeneration of optic nerve axons is one component of the challenge of regenerating the optic nerve. A greater problem is the guidance of extending axons along the complex path to the target. This trajectory begins at the retinal ganglion cell body within the inner retina to the optic nerve head, through the optic nerve, then crossing (of nasal fibers) at the chiasm, and continuing along the optic track to the retinotopic map within the lateral geniculate nucleus within the appropriate layer. In development, this complex pathway is determined by cell surface molecules and secreted chemotactic gradients. In many cases it is not known whether the same set of molecules is present in the adult organism. If not, those molecules would have to be recreated in order to allow an extending axon to find its appropriate target.

ASSESSMENT OF NEUROREGENERATION

Assessment of replacement and regeneration of RGCs requires demonstration that its axon has extended out of the retina and, ideally, to its target. This is usually done with orthograde labeling of axons, by injecting a dye or other marker into the eye, making sagittal or coronal sections of the optic nerve, and assessing the degree of axonal extension and connectivity. Assessment of RGC replacement in the retina, e.g. with stem cells, requires identification that the cells truly are RGCs, that they connect to neighboring neurons, and that they at least partially extend an axon towards the optic nerve. Functional assessment of stem cell replacement would require demonstration that the cells fire action potentials in an appropriate pattern corresponding to light input to photoreceptors in the immediate area of the RGC. Functional assessment of regeneration would require electrophysiological evidence of activation of target areas within the central nervous system, e.g. the superior colliculus or the pretectal nuclei for the pupil. The pupil can also be used as a functional measure, as the pretectal nuclei synapse on neurons within the Edinger-Westphal nuclei, and send efferents which, after synapsing in the ciliary ganglion, cause the pupil to constrict.

The complexity of the stem cell replacement and reconnection process for glaucoma is clearly immense. But even if replacement and regeneration could be achieved, without appropriate mapping to retinotopic targets, vision would be coarse and low resolution.

Summary

Glaucoma is a distinctive optic nerve disease in which the primary damage occurs to the retinal ganglion cell axon. The loss of either the retinal ganglion cell or its axon is sufficient to cause visual loss. Therapies that prevent death of the retinal ganglion cell (neuroprotection) or its axon (axoprotection), or that regenerate retinal ganglion cells and their axons, should theoretically be useful in treating glaucoma. At present, all data are derived from animal studies. Randomized clinical trials are crucial for assessing whether these strategies are useful for treating patients with glaucoma.

ACKNOWLEDGEMENTS

Grant Support: Canada Research Chair Program, National Institutes of Health, Research to Prevent Blindness, Retina Research Foundation.

REFERENCES

1. Levin LA. Pathophysiology of the progressive optic neuropathy of glaucoma. Ophthalmol Clin North Am 2005; 18:355–364.

2. Hasnain SS. Scleral edge, not optic disc or retina, is the primary site of injury in chronic glaucoma. Med Hypotheses 2006; 67:1320–1325.

3. Levin LA. Neuroprotection and regeneration in glaucoma. Ophthalmol Clin North Am 2005; 18:585–596.

4. Boden C, Sample PA, Boehm AG, et al. The structure–function relationship in eyes with glaucomatous visual field loss that crosses the horizontal meridian. Arch Ophthalmol 2002; 120:907–912.

5. Levin LA. Relevance of the site of injury of glaucoma to neuroprotective strategies. Surv Ophthalmol 2001; 45: S243–S249.

6. Mansour-Robaey S, Clarke DB, Wang YC, et al. Effects of ocular injury and administration of brain-derived neurotrophic factor on survival and regrowth of axotomized retinal ganglion cells. Proc Natl Acad Sci USA 1994; 91:1632–1636.

7. Quigley HA, Nickells RW, Kerrigan LA, et al. Retinal ganglion cell death in experimental glaucoma and after axotomy occurs by apoptosis. Invest Ophthalmol Vis Sci 1995; 36:774–786.

8. Di Polo A, Aigner LJ, Dunn RJ, et al. Prolonged delivery of brain-derived neurotrophic factor by adenovirus-infected Muller cells temporarily rescues injured retinal ganglion cells. Proc Natl Acad Sci USA 1998; 95:3978–3983.

9. Lieven CJ, Schlieve CR, Hoegger MJ, et al. Retinal ganglion cell axotomy induces an increase in intracellular superoxide anion. Invest Ophthalmol Vis Sci 2006; 47:1477–1485.

10. Siliprandi R, Canella R, Carmignoto G, et al. N-methyl-D-aspartate-induced neurotoxicity in the adult rat retina. Vis Neurosci 1992; 8:567–573.

11. Schlamp CL, Johnson EC, Li Y, et al. Changes in Thy1 gene expression associated with damaged retinal ganglion cells. Mol Vis 2001; 7:192–201.

12. Cioffi GA, Orgul S, Onda E, et al. An in vivo model of chronic optic nerve ischemia: the dose-dependent effects of endothelin-1 on the optic nerve microvasculature. Curr Eye Res 1995; 14:1147–1153.

13. Schiefer U, Flad M, Stumpp F, et al. Increased detection rate of glaucomatous visual field damage with locally condensed grids: a comparison between fundus-oriented perimetry and conventional visual field examination. Arch Ophthalmol 2003; 121:458–465.

14. Hood DC, Greenstein V, Frishman L, et al. Identifying inner retinal contributions to the human multifocal ERG. Vision Res 1999; 39:2285–2291.

15. Levin LA. Retinal ganglion cells and supporting elements in culture. J Glaucoma 2005; 14:305–307.

16. Cordeiro M, Guo L, Luong V, et al. Real-time imaging of single nerve cell apoptosis in retinal neurodegeneration. Proc Natl Acad Sci USA 2004; 101:13352–13356.

17. Wheeler-Kingshott CA, Trip SA, Symms MR, et al. In vivo diffusion tensor imaging of the human optic nerve: pilot study in normal controls. Magn Reson Med 2006; 56:446–451.

18. Ueki S, Fujii Y, Matsuzawa H, et al. Assessment of axonal degeneration along the human visual pathway using diffusion trace analysis. Am J Ophthalmol 2006; 142:591–596.

19. Bernstein SL, Koo JH, Slater BJ, et al. Analysis of optic nerve stroke by retinal Bex expression. Mol Vis 2006; 12:147–155.

20. Chaturvedi N, Hedley-Whyte ET, Dreyer EB. Lateral geniculate nucleus in glaucoma. Am J Ophthalmol 1993; 116:182–188.

21. Vickersn JC, Hof PR, Schumer RA, et al. Magnocellular and parvocellular visual pathways are both affected in a macaque monkey model of glaucoma. Aust NZ J Ophthalmol 1997; 25:239–243.

22. Yücel YH, Zhang Q, Gupta N, et al. Loss of neurons in magnocellular and parvocellular layers of the lateral geniculate nucleus in glaucoma. Arch Ophthalmol 2000; 118:378–384.

23. Weber AJ, Chen H, Hubbard WC, et al. Experimental glaucoma and cell size, density, and number in the primate lateral geniculate nucleus. Invest Ophthalmol Vis Sci 2000; 41: 1370–1379.

24. Weber AJ, Kaufman PL, Hubbard WC. Morphology of single ganglion cells in the glaucomatous primate retina. Invest Ophthalmol Vis Sci 1998; 39:2304–2320.

25. Neufeld AH, Sawada A, Becker B. Inhibition of nitric-oxide synthase 2 by aminoguanidine provides neuroprotection of retinal ganglion cells in a rat model of chronic glaucoma. Proc Natl Acad Sci USA 1999; 96:9944–9948.

26. WoldeMussie E, Ruiz G, Wijono M, et al. Neuroprotection of retinal ganglion cells by brimonidine in rats with laser-induced chronic ocular hypertension. Invest Ophthalmol Vis Sci 2001; 42:2849–2855.

27. Schori H, Kipnis J, Yoles E, et al. Vaccination for protection of retinal ganglion cells against death from glutamate cytotoxicity and ocular hypertension: implications for glaucoma. Proc Natl Acad Sci USA 2001; 98:3398–3403.

28. Tsai JC, Wu L, Worgul B, et al. Intravitreal administration of erythropoietin and preservation of retinal ganglion cells in an experimental rat model of glaucoma. Curr Eye Res 2005; 30:1025–1031.

29. Zhong L, Bradley J, Schubert W, et al. Erythropoietin promotes survival of retinal ganglion cells in DBA/2J glaucoma mice. Invest Ophthalmol Vis Sci 2007; 48:1212–1218.

30. WoldeMussie E, Yoles E, Schwartz M, et al. Neuroprotective effect of memantine in different retinal injury models in rats. J Glaucoma 2002; 11:474–480.

31. Ko ML, Hu DN, Ritch R, et al. The combined effect of brain-derived neurotrophic factor and a free radical scavenger in experimental glaucoma. Invest Ophthalmol Vis Sci 2000; 41:2967–2971.

32. Gaasterland D, Kupfer C. Experimental glaucoma in the rhesus monkey. Invest Ophthalmol 1974; 13:455–457.

33. Hahn JS, Aizenman E, Lipton SA. Central mammalian neurons normally resistant to glutamate toxicity are made sensitive by elevated extracellular Ca^{2+}: toxicity is blocked by the N-methyl-D-aspartate antagonist MK-801. Proc Natl Acad Sci USA 1988; 85:6556–6560.

34. Dreyer EB, Zurakowski D, Schumer RA, et al. Elevated glutamate levels in the vitreous body of humans and monkeys with glaucoma. Arch Ophthalmol 1996; 114:299–305.

35. Yoles E, Schwartz M. Elevation of intraocular glutamate levels in rats with partial lesion of the optic nerve. Arch Ophthalmol 1998; 116:906–910.

36. Wamsley S, Gabelt BT, Dahl DB, et al. Vitreous glutamate concentration and axon loss in monkeys with experimental glaucoma. Arch Ophthalmol 2005; 123:64–70.

37. Honkanen RA, Baruah S, Zimmerman MB, et al. Vitreous amino acid concentrations in patients with glaucoma undergoing vitrectomy. Arch Ophthalmol 2003; 121:183–188.

38. Luo X, Baba A, Matsuda T, et al. Susceptibilities to and mechanisms of excitotoxic cell death of adult mouse inner retinal neurons in dissociated culture. Invest Ophthalmol Vis Sci 2004; 45:4576–4582.

39. Ullian EM, Barkis WB, Chen S, et al. Invulnerability of retinal ganglion cells to NMDA excitotoxicity. Mol Cell Neurosci 2004; 26:544–557.

40. Hare WA, WoldeMussie E, Lai RK, et al. Efficacy and safety of memantine treatment for reduction of changes associated with experimental glaucoma in monkey, I: functional measures. Invest Ophthalmol Vis Sci 2004; 45:2625–2639.

41. Hare WA, WoldeMussie E, Weinreb RN, et al. Efficacy and safety of memantine treatment for reduction of changes associated with experimental glaucoma in monkey, II: structural measures. Invest Ophthalmol Vis Sci 2004; 45:2640–2651.

42. Yucel YH, Gupta N, Zhang Q, et al. Memantine protects neurons from shrinkage in the lateral geniculate nucleus in experimental glaucoma. Arch Ophthalmol 2006; 124:217–225.

43. Chen HS, Lipton SA. Mechanism of memantine block of NMDA-activated channels in rat retinal ganglion cells: uncompetitive antagonism. J Physiol 1997; 499(Pt 1):27–46.

44. Hare W, WoldeMussie E, Lai R, et al. Efficacy and safety of memantine, an NMDA-type open-channel blocker, for reduction of retinal injury associated with experimental glaucoma in rat and monkey. Surv Ophthalmol 2001; 45(Suppl 3):S284–S289; discussion S295–S286.

45. Neufeld AH, Das S, Vora S, et al. A prodrug of a selective inhibitor of inducible nitric oxide synthase is neuroprotective in the rat model of glaucoma. J Glaucoma 2002; 11: 221–225.

46. Moalem G, Gdalyahu A, Shani Y, et al. Production of neurotrophins by activated T cells: implications for neuroprotective autoimmunity. J Autoimmun 2000; 15: 331–345.

47. Moalem G, Leibowitz-Amit R, Yoles E, et al. Autoimmune T cells protect neurons from secondary degeneration after central nervous system axotomy. Nat Med 1999; 5:49–55.

48. Kipnis J, Yoles E, Porat Z, et al. T cell immunity to copolymer 1 confers neuroprotection on the damaged optic nerve: possible therapy for optic neuropathies. Proc Natl Acad Sci USA 2000; 97:7446–7451.

49. Hill MD. Stroke: the dashed hopes of neuroprotection. Lancet Neurol 2007; 6:2–3.

50. Liebeskind DS, Kasner SE. Neuroprotection for ischaemic stroke: an unattainable goal? CNS Drugs 2001; 15:165–174.

51. Lees KR, Zivin JA, Ashwood T, et al. NXY-059 for acute ischemic stroke. N Engl J Med 2006; 354:588–600.

52. Shuaib A, Lees KR, Lyden P, et al. NXY-059 for the treatment of acute ischemic stroke. N Engl J Med 2007; 357:562–571.

53. Reisberg B, Doody R, Stoffler A, et al. Memantine in moderate-to-severe Alzheimer's disease. N Engl J Med 2003; 348: 1333–1341.

54. Bensimon G, Lacomblez L, Meininger V. A controlled trial of riluzole in amyotrophic lateral sclerosis ALS/Riluzole Study Group. N Engl J Med 1994; 330:585–591.

55. Krupin T, Liebmann JM, Greenfield DS, et al. The Low-pressure Glaucoma Treatment Study (LoGTS) study design and baseline characteristics of enrolled patients. Ophthalmology 2005; 112:376–385.

56. Stys PK, Lesiuk H. Correlation between electrophysiological effects of mexiletine and ischemic protection in central nervous system white matter. Neuroscience 1996; 71:27–36.

57. Araki T, Sasaki Y, Milbrandt J. Increased nuclear NAD biosynthesis and SIRT1 activation prevent axonal degeneration. Science 2004; 305:1010–1013.

58. Waxman SG, Black JA, Ransom BR, et al. Protection of the axonal cytoskeleton in anoxic optic nerve by decreased extracellular calcium. Brain Res 1993; 614:137–145.

59. Fern R, Ransom BR, Stys PK, et al. Pharmacological protection of CNS white matter during anoxia: actions of phenytoin, carbamazepine and diazepam. J Pharmacol Exp Ther 1993; 266:1549–1555.

60. Stys PK. White matter injury mechanisms. Curr Mol Med 2004; 4:113–130.

61. Zhao X, Liu J, Ahmad I. Differentiation of embryonic stem cells into retinal neurons. Biochem Biophys Res Commun 2002; 297:177.

62. Warfvinge K, Kamme C, Englund U, et al. Retinal integration of grafts of brain-derived precursor cell lines implanted subretinally into adult, normal rats. Exp Neurol 2001; 169:1–12.

63. Nishida A, Takahashi M, Tanihara H, et al. Incorporation and differentiation of hippocampus-derived neural stem cells transplanted in injured adult rat retina. Invest Ophthalmol Vis Sci 2000; 41:4268–4274.

64. Tomita M, Adachi Y, Yamada H, et al. Bone marrow-derived stem cells can differentiate into retinal cells in injured rat retina. Stem Cells 2002; 20:279–283.

65. Tropepe V, Coles BL, Chiasson BJ, et al. Retinal stem cells in the adult mammalian eye. Science 2000; 287:2032–2036.

66. Reh TA, Levine EM. Multipotential stem cells and progenitors in the vertebrate retina. J Neurobiol 1998; 36:206–220.

67. Sakaguchi DS, Van Hoffelen SJ, Grozdanic SD, et al. Neural progenitor cell transplants into the developing and mature central nervous system. Ann NY Acad Sci 2005; 1049: 118–134.

68. Mellough CB, Cui Q, Spalding KL, et al. Fate of multipotent neural precursor cells transplanted into mouse retina selectively depleted of retinal ganglion cells. Exp Neurol 2004; 186:6–19.

69. Yao J, Sun X, Wang Y, et al. Muller glia induce retinal progenitor cells to differentiate into retinal ganglion cells. Neuroreport 2006; 17:1263–1267.

70. Rowe EW, Jeftinija DM, Jeftinija K, et al. Development of functional neurons from postnatal stem cells in vitro. Stem Cells 2005; 23:1044–1049.

71. Mu X, Klein WH. A gene regulatory hierarchy for retinal ganglion cell specification and differentiation. Semin Cell Dev Biol 2004; 15:115–123.

72. Aguayo AJ, Vidal-Sanz M, Villegas-Perez MP, et al. Growth and connectivity of axotomized retinal neurons in adult rats with optic nerves substituted by PNS grafts linking the eye and the midbrain. Ann NY Acad Sci 1987; 495:1–9.

73. Schaden H, Stuermer CA, Bahr M. GAP-43 immunoreactivity and axon regeneration in retinal ganglion cells of the rat. J Neurobiol 1994; 25:1570–1578.

74. Caroni P, Schwab ME. Antibody against myelin-associated inhibitor of neurite growth neutralizes nonpermissive substrate properties of CNS white matter. Neuron 1988; 1:85–96.

75. McKerracher L, David S, Jackson DL, et al. Identification of myelin-associated glycoprotein as a major myelin-derived inhibitor of neurite growth. Neuron 1994; 13:805–811.

76. McKeon RJ, Hoke A, Silver J. Injury-induced proteoglycans inhibit the potential for laminin-mediated axon growth on astrocytic scars. Exp Neurol 1995; 136:32–43.

77. Chen MS, Huber AB, van der Haar ME, et al. Nogo-A is a myelin-associated neurite outgrowth inhibitor and an antigen for monoclonal antibody IN-1. Nature 2000; 403:434–439.

78. GrandPré T, Nakamura F, Vartanian T, et al. Identification of the Nogo inhibitor of axon regeneration as a Reticulon protein. Nature 2000; 403:439–444.

79. Fischer D, He Z, Benowitz LI. Counteracting the Nogo receptor enhances optic nerve regeneration if retinal ganglion cells are in an active growth state. J Neurosci 2004; 24:1646–1651.

80. Neumann S, Bradke F, Tessier-Lavigne M, et al. Regeneration of sensory axons within the injured spinal cord induced by intraganglionic cAMP elevation. Neuron 2002; 34:885–893.

81. Monsul NT, Geisendorfer AR, Han PJ, et al. Intraocular injection of dibutyryl cyclic AMP promotes axon regeneration in rat optic nerve. Exp Neurol 2004; 186:4–133.

82. Sapieha S, Duplan L, Uetani N, et al. Receptor protein tyrosine phosphatase sigma inhibits axon regrowth in the adult injured CNS. Mol Cell Neurosci 2005; 28:625–635.

83. Goldberg JL, Klassen MP, Hua Y, et al. Amacrine-signaled loss of intrinsic axon growth ability by retinal ganglion cells. Science 2002; 296:1860–1864.

84. Pang IH, Johnson EC, Jia L, et al. Evaluation of inducible nitric oxide synthase in glaucomatous optic neuropathy and pressure-induced optic nerve damage. Invest Ophthalmol Vis Sci 2005; 46:1313–1321.

85. Ko ML, Hu DN, Ritch R, et al. Patterns of retinal ganglion cell survival after brain-derived neurotrophic factor administration in hypertensive eyes of rats. Neurosci Lett 2001; 305:139–142.

86. No authors listed. A controlled trial of recombinant methionyl human BDNF in ALS: The BDNF Study Group (Phase III). Neurology 1999; 52:1427–1433.

87. Gross RL, Hensley SH, Gao F, et al. Retinal ganglion cell dysfunction induced by hypoxia and glutamate: potential neuroprotective effects of beta-blockers. Surv Ophthalmol 1999; 43(Suppl 1):S162–S170.

88. Gross RL, Hensley SH, Gao F, et al. Effects of betaxolol on light responses and membrane conductance in retinal ganglion cells. Invest Ophthalmol Vis Sci 2000; 41:722–728.

89. Zhang J, Wu SM, Gross RL. Effects of beta-adrenergic blockers on glutamate-induced calcium signals in adult mouse retinal ganglion cells. Brain Res 2003; 959:111–119.

90. Osborne NN, DeSantis L, Bae JH, et al. Topically applied betaxolol attenuates NMDA-induced toxicity to ganglion cells and the effects of ischaemia to the retina. Exp Eye Res 1999; 69:331–342.

91. Wood JP, DeSantis L, Chao HM, et al. Topically applied betaxolol attenuates ischaemia-induced effects to the rat retina and stimulates BDNF mRNA. Exp Eye Res 2001; 72:79–86.

92. Aviles-Trigueros M, Mayor-Torroglosa S, Garcia-Aviles A, et al. Transient ischemia of the retina results in massive degeneration of the retinotectal projection: long-term neuroprotection with brimonidine. Exp Neurol 2003; 184:767–777.

93. Acheampong AA, Shackleton M, John B, et al. Distribution of brimonidine into anterior and posterior tissues of monkey, rabbit, and rat eyes. Drug Metab Dispos 2002; 30:421–429.

94. Kent AR, Nussdorf JD, David R, et al. Vitreous concentration of topically applied brimonidine tartrate 0.2%. Ophthalmology 2001; 108:784–787.

95. Pang IH, Wexler EM, Nawy S, et al. Protection by eliprodil against excitotoxicity in cultured rat retinal ganglion cells. Invest Ophthalmol Vis Sci 1999; 40:1170–1176.

96. Kapin MA, Doshi R, Scatton B, et al. Neuroprotective effects of eliprodil in retinal excitotoxicity and ischemia. Invest Ophthalmol Vis Sci 1999; 40:1177–1182.

97. Modell S, Naber D, Holzbach R. Efficacy and safety of an opiate sigma-receptor antagonist (SL 82.0715) in schizophrenic patients with negative symptoms: an open dose-range study. Pharmacopsychiatry 1996; 29:63–66.

98. Ji JZ, Elyaman W, Yip HK, et al. CNTF promotes survival of retinal ganglion cells after induction of ocular hypertension in rats: the possible involvement of STAT3 pathway. Eur J Neurosci 2004; 19:265–272.

99. Chan HH, Leung MC, So KF. Electroacupuncture provides a new approach to neuroprotection in rats with induced glaucoma. J Altern Complement Med 2005; 11:315–322.

100. Park KH, Cozier F, Ong OC, et al. Induction of heat shock protein 72 protects retinal ganglion cells in a rat glaucoma model. Invest Ophthalmol Vis Sci 2001; 42:1522–1530.

101. Ishii Y, Kwong JM, Caprioli J. Retinal ganglion cell protection with geranylgeranylacetone, a heat shock protein inducer, in a rat glaucoma model. Invest Ophthalmol Vis Sci 2003; 44:1982–1992.

102. Blair M, Pease ME, Hammond J, et al. Effect of glatiramer acetate on primary and secondary degeneration of retinal ganglion cells in the rat. Invest Ophthalmol Vis Sci 2005; 46:884–890.

103. Ward MS, Khoobehi A, Lavik EB, et al. Neuroprotection of retinal ganglion cells in DBA/2J mice with GDNF-loaded biodegradable microspheres. J Pharm Sci 2007; 96:558–568.

104. Chan HC, Chang RC, Koon-Ching Ip A, et al. Neuroprotective effects of Lycium barbarum Lynn on protecting retinal ganglion cells in an ocular hypertension model of glaucoma. Exp Neurol 2007; 203:269–273.

105. Levkovitch-Verbin H, Kalev-Landoy M, Habot-Wilner Z, et al. Minocycline delays death of retinal ganglion cells in experimental glaucoma and after optic nerve transection. Arch Ophthalmol 2006; 124:520–526.

106. Hains BC, Waxman SG. Neuroprotection by sodium channel blockade with phenytoin in an experimental model of glaucoma. Invest Ophthalmol Vis Sci 2005; 46:4164–4169.

107. Maeda K, Sawada A, Matsubara M, et al. A novel neuroprotectant against retinal ganglion cell damage in a glaucoma model and an optic nerve crush model in the rat. Invest Ophthalmol Vis Sci 2004; 45:851–856.

CHAPTER 53

Interpreting Clinical Studies on Glaucoma Neuroprotection

Robert N Weinreb and Anne L Coleman

INTRODUCTION

Particularly because it is an emerging area for glaucoma intervention, critical assessment of clinical studies of glaucoma neuroprotection will be needed before deciding whether to prescribe a neuroprotective drug to an individual patient. Although this assessment is similar to that which is necessary before prescribing any new therapeutic intervention, there are several caveats that also are relevant specifically to neuroprotective studies.

It is noteworthy that there has not yet been even a single drug that has demonstrated glaucoma neuroprotection and obtained regulatory approval for clinical use. Until recently, studies that have been performed have not had appropriate methodology to demonstrate glaucoma neuroprotection. Some of these trials have been subject to bias, which results in unreliable estimates of treatment effect, and others have had inadequate numbers of patients to detect whether the rate of glaucoma progression has been slowed. Still others have lacked detailed methodology, and have not explicitly and accurately described specific aspects of the study design, conduct, and analysis.

OVERVIEW OF STUDY METHODOLOGY

Consideration of the design and conduct of a clinical trial of neuroprotection provides an overview of the appropriateness of the study. Randomized assignment and masking of the treatments should be a sine qua non of any such trial. Despite randomization, sometimes there are differences in a measured parameter between treatment groups at baseline. These differences potentially can affect the study results because the main reason for randomizing subjects to treatment and for masking treatments is to preserve the study intervention as the only difference in patient care among treatment groups. For example, if the baseline intraocular pressure of two treatment groups is different, it may not be possible to sensitively ascertain whether a neuroprotective agent is effective, since the subjects with lower intraocular pressure have a lower risk of glaucoma progression. Similarly, if intraocular pressure is significantly lower in one group during the course of the study, it also may not be possible to determine the effectiveness of a neuroprotective agent. As another example, if one of two treatment groups has visual fields that are significantly more damaged than another group, it may not be possible to ascertain whether the neuroprotective treatment is any different than the treatment to which it is being compared, since changes in the more damaged visual field may be more difficult to detect.[1]

A plethora of original articles on evidence-based medicine have proposed a hierarchy for the strength of clinical study outcomes (Fig. 53.1). Ideally, the benefit of a treatment for a particular patient would be assessed directly in that individual patient. The patient would be followed for response to the treatment that was initiated. If that treatment was ineffective, it would be discontinued and a new treatment would be initiated to test for a satisfactory treatment response in that individual patient. This treatment paradigm is only ideal for an individual patient, and not practical for most patients or generalizable to other patients. A systematic review of randomized clinical trials provides a less ideal, but more practical, approach to predicting the response to treatment in a patient. Such a review should include the results of a thorough search of national and international peer-reviewed publications. Unfortunately for

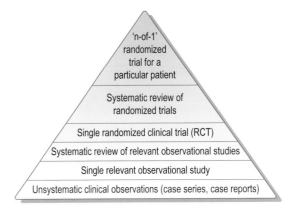

FIGURE 53.1 Proposed hierarchy of strength of evidence for treatment decisions ranges from lowest (case series, case reports) to highest ('n-of-1') trial.

glaucoma neuroprotection, there are no high-quality studies available at the current time that would qualify for inclusion in such a review.

What exactly is a high-quality clinical study? A high-quality clinical study is one designed to directly address whether a treatment prevents or ameliorates glaucomatous neurodegeneration, independently of intraocular pressure, by evaluating both visual function and optic nerve structure. Needless to say, the study should have produced reliable and accurate data, and should have been analyzed using appropriate statistical methods. There should be an adequate control group, sufficiently long follow-up, good compliance with therapy, and acceptable loss to follow-up.

THE RANDOMIZED CLINICAL TRIAL

In practice, the randomized clinical trial (RCT) has become the most practical means for assessing treatment effectiveness and inferring causation. In general, outcomes of RCTs are more robust than those reported from observational studies of a similar size because all known and unknown confounders or variables are more likely to be randomly distributed between the treatment groups in RCTs while in observational studies the distribution of unknown confounders is unknown.

A report of an RCT should transparently convey to the clinician why the study was undertaken and how it was conducted and analyzed. To assess the strengths and limitations of an RCT, a clinician needs to determine the quality of its methods. In a well-designed RCT, the allocated intervention should be the only major difference between groups, treatments should be administered in a masked fashion, the certainty of delivery of interventions in treatment groups should be documented, and complete follow-up for each study participant should be recorded. The reported results should be reviewed carefully to ascertain whether efficacy was reported among all subjects who were randomized to the treatment whether or not they received the treatment (the 'intent to treat' population).

EVALUATION OF A RANDOMIZED CLINICAL TRIAL

When evaluating the results of RCTs, sample size and/or power determinations need to be assessed. The power of the study to detect a specific effect size should have been calculated prior to the enrollment of the first subject in the study by the investigators. When a result of no statistical significance is reported, failure to report the power of the study to detect a specific effect size should raise concern, as it may not be possible to ascertain whether there truly was no difference between treatments or the study sample size was simply too small for the investigators to detect a difference.

Another important factor to consider is the number of clinical sites in the clinical trial. Although multiple sites can increase enrollment and enhance the generalizability of the study, it is important for the investigators to control for the sites in the analyses, since equipment, examiners, and subjects may vary at the different sites.

In 1996, the Consolidating Standards of Reporting Trials (CONSORT) Group created guidelines with specific criteria designed to improve reporting of RCTs (Table 53.1).[2] The guidelines consist of a checklist and flow diagram for reporting an RCT. They are primarily intended for use in writing, reviewing, or evaluating reports of simple two-group parallel RCTs. Most major journals now require adaptation of these guidelines as a prerequisite for acceptance of RCT manuscripts. Although CONSORT guidelines encourage accurate and thorough reporting in publications, their use does not ensure validity of results and so it is important for readers of the literature to be knowledgeable and critical about study design and analysis.[3]

OTHER TYPES OF STUDIES

Consensus or individual opinions, small noncomparative case series (with or without controls), and individual case reports generally should be considered to provide weak evidence for or against a neuroprotective agent. Chart reviews and randomized controlled trials evaluating highly subjective outcome data should be considered to provide weak evidence.

GENERALIZABILITY OF STUDY RESULTS

The generalizability of the results from a study of glaucoma neuroprotection also needs to be considered. If study conditions were not similar to those encountered in clinic practice, the results may not be applicable to patient care. Characteristics that are related to the patient, including age, gender, race, or specific type and severity of glaucoma, are important to report because it is these characteristics which can aid the clinician in determining whether the study results are applicable to an individual patient. As an example, results from a trial of glaucoma neuroprotection conducted in Asian angle-closure glaucoma patients may not be relevant to a group of patients of African ancestry with primary open-angle glaucoma. As another example, the external validity of a study conducted in glaucoma patients with frequent disc hemorrhages and rapid progression may not be relevant to glaucoma patients with few glaucoma risk factors and slowly progressive disease. Another characteristic is the drug regimen, including the specific drugs being administered, as well as their dosing and method of delivery. The study design also affects the generalizability of the results because of the potential biases inherent in subject selection or the tests used for assessing the efficacy and safety of the neuroprotective agent. Regardless of the results of a single study, one should keep in mind the importance of confirming them and gaining clinical experience in a broader population before the efficacy and safety of the investigational neuroprotective drug are established.

TABLE 53.1 Items to consider when evaluating a randomized trial

SELECTION AND TOPIC	ITEM#	DESCRIPTOR
Title and abstract	1	How participants were allocated to interventions (e.g. 'random allocation,' 'randomized,' or 'randomly assigned')
Background	2	Scientific background and explanation of rationale
Participants	3	Eligibility criteria for participants and the settings and locations where the data were collected
Interventions	4	Precise details of the interventions intended for each group and how and when they were actually administered
Objectives	5	Specific objectives and hypotheses
Outcomes	6	Clearly defined primary and secondary outcome measures and, when applicable, any methods used to enhance the quality of measurements (e.g. multiple observations, training of assessors)
Sample size	7	How sample size was determined and, when applicable, explanation of any interim analyses and stopping rules
Randomization Sequence generation	8	Method used to generate the random allocation sequence, including details of any restriction (e.g. blocking, stratification)
Allocation concealment	9	Method used to implement the random allocation sequence (e.g. numbered containers or central telephone), clarifying whether the sequence was concealed until interventions were assigned
Implementation	10	Who generated the allocation sequence, who enrolled participants, and who assigned participants to their groups
Masking (blinding)	11	Whether or not participants, those administering the interventions, and those assessing the outcomes were masked to group assignment. If done, how the success of masking was evaluated
Statistical methods	12	Statistical methods used to compare groups for primary outcome(s); methods for additional analyses, such as subgroup analyses and adjusted analyses
Participant flow	13	Flow of participants through each stage (a diagram is strongly recommended). Specifically, for each group report the numbers of participants randomly assigned, receiving intended treatment, completing the study protocol, and analyzed for the primary outcome. Describe protocol deviations from study as planned, together with reasons
Recruitment	14	Dates defining the periods of recruitment and follow-up
Baseline data	15	Baseline demographic and clinical characteristics of each group
Numbers analyzed	16	Number of participants (denominator) in each group included in each analysis and whether the analysis was by 'intention-to-treat.' State the results in absolute numbers when feasible (e.g. 10/20, not 50%)
Outcomes and estimation	17	For each primary and secondary outcome, a summary of results for each group, and the estimated effect size and its precision (e.g. 95% confidence interval)
Ancillary analyses	18	Address multiplicity by reporting any other analyses performed, including subgroup analyses and adjusted analyses, indicating those prespecified and those exploratory
Adverse events	19	All important adverse events or side effects in each intervention group
Interpretation	20	Interpretation of the results, taking into account study hypotheses, sources of potential bias or imprecision, and the dangers associated with multiplicity of analyses and outcomes
Generalizability	21	Generalizability (external validity) of the trial findings
Overall evidence	22	General interpretation of the results in the context of current evidence

Adapted from Moher D, Schulz KF, Altman D. The CONSORT Statement: revised recommendations for improving the quality of reports of parallel-group randomized trials. JAMA 2001; 285:1987–1991.[2]

SPECIAL CONSIDERATIONS FOR NEUROPROTECTION TRIALS

A neuroprotective agent needs to prevent and/or ameliorate the neurodegenerative process secondary to glaucoma beyond that of intraocular pressure-reducing agents. Detection of a neuroprotective effect beyond that obtained with intraocular pressure reduction is challenging because it is likely that the additive effect is smaller, since the subjects already have some protection from the reduction of their intraocular pressures. This means that more subjects are needed in order to have enough statistical power to detect this smaller effect size, even if the tests used to detect the protection are more robust and less affected by random noise. Unfortunately, diagnostic testing always has random noise and measurement errors, so currently the focus is to enroll enough subjects for the detection of a small effect size.

Another challenge for neuroprotective trials is that important confounders for glaucoma progression should be controlled in the study design, if possible, or in the statistical analysis. In this regard, the current clinical practice of measuring and recording intraocular pressure at a single point in time is problematic. Although it is widely accepted that intraocular pressure is the most important risk factor for glaucoma, it varies throughout the day and over long durations even when the subject is under treatment for glaucoma. When controlling for the effect of intraocular pressure in a neuroprotection trial, decisions will need to be made on how frequently to measure the intraocular pressure, under what experimental conditions this measurement occurs, whether the actual measurement of the intraocular pressure is made by one or two observers, how many baseline intraocular pressures are obtained, and whether the mean, median, range, standard deviation, area under the curve, peak or trough intraocular pressure are the most important intraocular pressure factors to be included in statistical models. All of these study design issues and statistical summaries may greatly influence the results and the conclusions.

Trials of glaucoma neuroprotection should be designed to control not only for intraocular pressure but also for the amount of glaucomatous damage. The severity of glaucomatous damage influences the amount of prevention or amelioration that can be detected in individual subjects. Eyes with advanced glaucomatous damage may have too much damage present to detect progressive worsening or prevention (a ceiling effect). In addition, the rate of damage in eyes may differ greatly among eyes since a variable number of retinal ganglion cells may be damaged or lost among subjects with similar-appearing visual fields, even when those fields appear to be normal. Because the severity of glaucoma is assessed not only by visual fields or other psychophysical tests but also by the appearance of the optic nerve head and retinal nerve fiber layer, it is important to assess the structure of the optic nerve in any neuroprotective trial. Although there may not be a one-to-one correlation in the appearance of the optic nerve and the number of remaining ganglion cells, the appearance of the optic nerve may serve as a surrogate for the presence of retinal ganglion cells. There are several devices that are available for documenting and assessing the appearance of the optic nerve head and retinal nerve fiber layer. Each of these devices has limitations and accompanying measurement errors, which also influences the effect size that can be measured in a neuroprotective trial.

Summary

Evidence-based medicine seeks to improve, not replace, patient-based medicine by encouraging clinicians to verify the validity, precision, and applicability of research findings before applying them to the care of individual patients.

While the peer-review process remains the most successful method of ensuring the validity of published studies and reviews, the reader is still required to make judgments about study validity, particularly with respect to how the study applies to the care of their individual patients. There are unique aspects of trial design, analyses, and interpretations that need to be considered when assessing clinical studies of glaucoma neuroprotection.[4]

REFERENCES

1. Coleman AL, Singh K, Wilson R, et al. Applying an evidence-based approach to the management of patients with ocular hypertension: evaluating and synthesizing published evidence. Am J Ophthalmol 2004; 138:S3–S10.

2. Moher D, Schulz KF, Altman D. The CONSORT Statement: revised recommendations for improving the quality of reports of parallel-group randomized trials. JAMA 2001; 285:1987–1991.

3. Plint AC, Moher D, Morrison A, et al. Does the CONSORT checklist improve the quality of reports of randomized controlled trials? A systematic review. Med J Aust 2006; 185:263–267.

4. Levin LA, Weinreb RN, Di Polo A, eds. A pocket guide of neuroprotection in glaucoma. New York: Ethis Communications; 2007.

CHAPTER 54

Stem Cells: A Future Glaucoma Therapy?

Thomas V Johnson, Natalie D Bull, and Keith R Martin

INTRODUCTION

Current therapy for glaucoma involves pharmacologically or surgically lowering the intraocular pressure (IOP), an intervention that can dramatically slow disease progression and delay functional damage. Treatment modalities for glaucoma have improved dramatically but many patients suffer irreversible visual loss due to extensive retinal ganglion cell (RGC) death prior to diagnosis. Other patients progress to blindness despite seemingly adequate IOP control. Thus, there is a pressing need to develop new treatments to enable restoration of visual function.

Stem cell therapy is currently a field of intense scientific and clinical interest, particularly in the central nervous system (CNS) where inherent repair is inadequate and functional damage is often permanent. The prospective therapeutic power of stem cells lies in their ability to generate new cells of many types and to effect tissue repair. By definition, a stem cell is multipotent, with the capacity to self-renew and to produce daughter cells capable of differentiating into multiple mature cell types. However, progenitor cells, which possess the ability to generate a more limited range of adult cell types, may also contribute to tissue repair. Thus, stem and/or progenitor cells offer new hope for treating historically incurable diseases, such as glaucoma, via the selective replacement of degenerated cells to restore function.[1–5]

In this chapter, the authors discuss research relevant to the use of stem cell therapy for glaucoma treatment. Potential stem cell sources and therapeutic targets are considered, and potential barriers to progress are discussed.

OBJECTIVES FOR STEM CELL THERAPY IN GLAUCOMA

RETINAL GANGLION CELL REPLACEMENT

The clinical end point for uncontrolled glaucoma is total visual field loss as a result of progressive RGC death. Despite aggressive treatment, a significant proportion of glaucoma patients experience considerable visual field reduction within their lifetimes. Theoretically, the most direct approach to treating these patients would be to stimulate endogenous repair mechanisms within the retina. In fish and amphibians, retinal regeneration is an automatic process that proceeds via differentiation of ocular stem cells located in the ciliary marginal zone. In adult mammals, however, retinal regeneration after injury or in neurodegenerative disease does not occur. While mammalian retinal progenitor cells have been identified in vitro, they appear to remain quiescent in vivo. Within the adult mammalian CNS, neurogenesis is limited to discrete regions (for example, the hippocampus) and outside these areas the environment is notoriously resistant to the generation and integration of new neurons.

Alternatively, degenerated retinal neurons could be replaced via transplantation of suitable precursor cells. It has been demonstrated that neural precursor cells derived from embryonic stem cells, when transplanted into the eye, can migrate into the retina and express markers of mature retinal neurons.[6] In addition, retinal progenitor cells derived from neonatal animals have been shown to achieve retinal integration, to exhibit photoreceptor differentiation, and to provide some functional benefit to animals with retinal dystrophy.[7] Transplanted fetal-derived hippocampal progenitors also demonstrate the ability to localize to the retinal ganglion cell layer, from whence they may extend neurites into the inner plexiform layer and towards the optic nerve head.[8] Despite these initial successes, the migration and incorporation of transplanted cells is difficult to achieve in the adult mammalian retina. Furthermore, the challenge of glaucomatous retinal regeneration does not end at the optic disc. In order to achieve complete functional repair in glaucoma, transplanted cells would not only need to integrate into the existing retinal circuitry but also to reestablish functional connections with target neurons in the brain. This would involve the extension of RGC axons through the optic nerve to the lateral geniculate nucleus (a matter of several centimeters in the human) and the precise regeneration of the retinotopic map. Furthermore, new axons need to be myelinated within the optic nerve to allow signal conduction at the appropriate velocity. Obviously, significant progress must be made before stem cell therapy can be used to repair the visual pathway so comprehensively. However, the hope is that even a small functional benefit in patients with severe visual loss could translate into a meaningful improvement in quality of life. Whether this hope is realistic remains to be seen.

While RGC replacement and optic nerve regeneration are key areas of research at present, it is worth highlighting three other possible contexts for stem cell therapy in the treatment of glaucoma: the optic nerve head, the trabecular meshwork, and in glaucoma filtering surgery.

OPTIC NERVE HEAD RESTORATION

The optic nerve head (ONH) is the origin of the optic nerve within the eye. Important changes to the ONH and the surrounding extracellular matrix occur as a result of glaucoma. Structural alterations include excavation of the optic disc, loss of elastin fibers, and changes in collagen regulation.[9] In addition, glaucoma has been found to stimulate activation of resident astrocytes, increase nitric oxide secretion, and induce vascular changes.[10] These changes place biomechanical, toxic, and ischemic stress on RGCs. Stem cell therapy directed toward repairing the structure and function of the ONH has been proposed as a possible way to slow disease progression. For example, given that fibroblast cells are responsible for maintaining the ONH extracellular matrix, it is conceivable that fibroblast precursor cells could modulate the environment of the glaucomatous ONH to enhance RGC survival. Indeed, such cells have been shown to benefit some models of wound healing. Alternatively, transplantation of neural or glial progenitor cells could have a modulatory effect on the immune system[11] or provide neurotrophic support, both of which could ameliorate local neurotoxicity.

TRABECULAR MESHWORK RESTORATION

Glaucoma often involves disruption to aqueous outflow through the trabecular pathway, which contributes to elevated IOP. Outflow resistance is increased by a reduction in the clearance of fibrillar material and sheath-derived plaques by trabecular meshwork cells.[12] In addition, age-related loss of trabecular meshwork cells seems to be exaggerated in glaucoma. Restoration of trabecular meshwork function is, therefore, also a potential target for stem cell transplantation. While progenitor cell populations isolated from the trabecular meshwork can be expanded in culture,[13] it remains to be established whether such a cell population is capable of improving the conventional outflow pathway in glaucoma patients.

CONJUNCTIVAL RESTORATION AND GLAUCOMA FILTERING SURGERY

A relatively common complication of glaucoma filtering surgery is the development of a thin, cystic bleb at the surgical site, which increases the risk of infection and hypotony. Although good surgical technique

and the application of antiproliferative agents to a wide treatment area can dramatically reduce the incidence of such leaking blebs, this surgical complication remains a significant problem for many ophthalmologists. One emerging technique to repair leaky blebs is through ocular surface grafting of tissue equivalents. Tissue equivalents can be generated by the isolation and in vitro expansion of conjunctival specimens isolated from the superior fornix, which contains a population of conjunctival progenitor cells. Engraftment of conjunctival progenitor cells to repair and replace damaged conjunctival tissue around the bleb has been found to reduce leakage.[14] Expansion of this technique may help to reduce a major complication of glaucoma surgery.

SOURCES AND DIFFERENTIATION OF STEM CELLS

EMBRYONIC STEM CELLS

Embryonic stem (ES) cells are derived from the inner cell mass of the developing blastocyst and are capable of indefinite self-renewal and proliferation in culture (Fig. 54.1A). They are also pluripotent, meaning that they can generate all cell types of the body. As such, ES cells are a powerful transplantation source for stem cell therapy and, consequently, are the subject of intense research in many different medical fields, including neurodegeneration.

To date, transplantation of ES cells into the mammalian retina has yielded mixed results. While engrafted ES cells have demonstrated some potential for survival within the retina, they have yet to achieve robust retinal integration or neuronal differentiation, and may be tumorigenic.[15] Lineage restriction of ES cells towards a particular cell class prior to transplantation may offer a more controlled cell source. In the context of glaucoma, differentiation of ES cells in vitro has yielded both glial and neuronal cell types.[16–18] Differentiation may be accomplished in vitro by mimicking the molecular events that occur during development via exposure of cells to signaling molecules. Thus, ES cells have been differentiated into retinal precursor cells that express markers of retinal development, including Pax6, Lhx2, Rx/Rax, and Six3/6.[16,18] Furthermore, terminal differentiation of these cells can produce progeny with characteristics of various mature retinal neurons. This includes RGC-like cells as evidenced by the expression of RGC markers (HuC/D, Neurofilament-M, and Tuj-1) and the generation of glutamate-induced calcium fluxes.[16,18] Ectopically induced gene expression offers an alternative technique to manipulate ES cell fate in vitro. This approach has yielded retinal progenitor cells with the ability to produce RGC-like cells as assessed phenotypically and electrophysiologically.[17]

The use of ES cells also has important limitations. The ethical issues surrounding the isolation of ES cells from human embryos are well publicized and a matter of intense debate. In addition, ES cell transplants are necessarily allogeneic and therefore carry

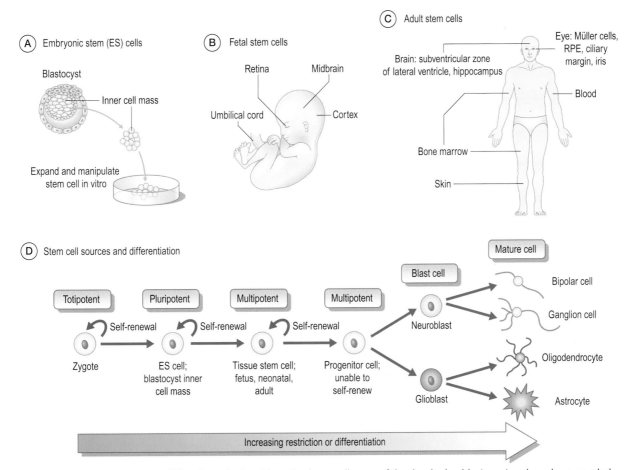

FIGURE 54.1 **(A)** Embryonic stem (ES) cells are isolated from the inner cell mass of the developing blastocyst and can be expanded indefinitely in culture. ES cells can also be manipulated in vitro to limit their fate and trigger their differentiation into potentially all cell types. **(B)** During development, stem cells with the potential to differentiate into neural cells can be isolated from many tissues, including the brain, retina, and umbilical cord. **(C)** In the adult body, stem cell populations can be found within various tissues and many of these stem cells, including those from the CNS, blood, bone marrow, and skin, are reportedly potential sources of neural precursor cells. **(D)** Stem cells can be found throughout development from the zygote to the adult; however, the potential of stem cells is inversely related to their stage of differentiation. Thus, stem cells isolated from the zygote or blastocyst display the greatest plasticity and have the potential to generate all cell types. In contrast, stem cells isolated from the adult animal are more restricted and can normally only generate cell components of the tissue type they were isolated from. In addition, stem cells may divide asymmetrically (as opposed to symmetrically to generate more stem cells) to produce progenitor cells, which are subject to further restrictions. These, in turn, differentiate into blast cells and finally mature cells, such as neurons or glia.

the risk of graft rejection. This is particularly important when the transplant is placed in a location such as the vitreous, which is less immune privileged than the brain. Furthermore, tissue sources are limited and ES cell transplants potentially carry a risk of malignant transformation.

SOMATIC STEM CELLS

Adult tissues that require constant replenishment possess discrete niches where their stem cells, termed somatic stem cells, reside and divide to generate cells required for tissue maintenance (Fig. 54.1C). This has been particularly well characterized in tissues such as the skin and bone marrow. In vivo, somatic stem cells are restricted, perhaps by their environment, to the production of cell types native to the tissue in which they dwell. Therefore, their applicability for therapy in other tissue types needs to be established. Interestingly,

somatic stem cells derived from the blood, skin, bone marrow, and umbilical cord may all have neural potential. For instance, bone marrow- and blood-derived mesenchymal stem cells have been shown to express neural cell markers such as nestin, βIII-tubulin, and glial fibrillary acidic protein (GFAP) following neural induction. Transplantation of these cells into the injured CNS has also conferred functional improvement.[19] Furthermore, intraocular implantation of mesenchymal- and umbilical cord-derived stem cells into a degenerative photoreceptor model has demonstrated an ability to improve retinal structure and function. However, the mechanism responsible for the observed improvement may have been via trophic support, as opposed to functional integration, as neuronal differentiation was not confirmed.

Somatic stem cells are an attractive transplantation source for regenerative stem cell therapy for a number of reasons. Significantly, many types of somatic stem cells can be relatively easily obtained from the recipient prior to transplantation. This would facilitate autologous grafting and avoid the ethical concerns surrounding other sources, such as ES cells. In addition, an autologous source avoids graft rejection and negates the need for immune suppression. Such benefits sustain research into the difficult task of determining how to reprogram somatic stem cells in order to exploit them for repair of different tissue types.

NEURAL STEM CELLS

Neural stem (NS) cells are somatic stem cells that give rise to neurons, astrocytes, and oligodendrocytes in the CNS. A number of phenotypic markers are used to identify NS cells, including nestin (an intermediate filament), Sox2, Notch, and CD133.[5] NS cells can be isolated and expanded in vitro from various neural tissues throughout development, from embryonic stages through to adulthood, although their proliferative potential decreases with age. The developing cerebral cortex, midbrain, and retina have been identified as sources of fetal NS cells (Fig. 54.1B). In adult animals, NS cells are commonly isolated from the subventricular zone of the lateral ventricle. In this region in vivo, NS cells continually proliferate in order to repopulate olfactory bulb neurons. The hippocampal dentate gyrus also exhibits extensive neurogenesis throughout life and NS cells may also be isolated from this CNS region. Outside these well-documented adult neurogenic regions the presence of NS cells is more controversial; however, it has also been reported that NS cells may be cultured from various cortical regions and the spinal cord.

Despite demonstrated potential in vitro, so far there is little direct evidence that transplantation of NS cells or their progeny into the eye can achieve functional improvement. This is especially true of adult NS cells, which do not assimilate into healthy adult retinas but can show a modest level of retinal integration in damaged tissue with concomitant expression of early neuronal cell markers.[20] In vitro modulation of differentiation conditions may be necessary to guide NS cell differentiation toward a retinal fate. Indeed, treatment of cultured NS cells with transforming growth factor (TGF)-β_3 can induce opsin expression and a photoreceptor-like phenotype. However, in vitro differentiation of NS cells into mature RGCs has yet to be achieved.

ADULT OCULAR CELLS

The adult eye contains a number of potential somatic stem cell niches. Cells located in the basal limbal area undergo continuous differentiation and migration to support corneal epithelial maintenance. As mentioned above, a population of cells in the trabecular meshwork has been isolated and expanded in culture.[13] Genetic analysis suggests these trabecular meshwork cells exhibit an undifferentiated, progenitor phenotype.

A number of cell types have also been isolated from the posterior segment that exhibit neural potential in vitro, although these cells appear quiescent in vivo.[21]

Progenitor cells have been isolated from the pigmented epithelium at the ciliary margin and induced to differentiate into neural retinal cell types.[22] Proliferative cells capable of generating neural retinal cells have also been cultured from the pigmented ciliary body[23] and the pigmented iris epithelium.[24] Interestingly, the pigmented iris epithelium shares developmental origins with the pigmented ciliary body and neural retina. This suggests the possibility that these cells, under the correct conditions, may possess the potential to generate cells for each tissue type.

Müller glia within the neural retina may also possess the ability to produce new neuronal cells. In chicks, injury induced Müller cells to reenter the cell cycle in order to proliferate and dedifferentiate; that is, they stopped expressing mature Müller cell proteins and instead expressed classical markers of developmental retinal progenitor cells such as Pax6 and Chx10. Such Müller cell-derived progenitor cells can generate neuronal-like cells, which express Hu, calretinin, or cellular retinoic acid-binding protein. Interestingly, induction of RGC-specific death promotes the synthesis of cells morphologically similar to RGCs that express RGC-type cell markers such as Brn3, Islet 1, RPF1, and neurofilament-M.[25] This observation suggests that lesions which target specific neuronal classes may provoke an environment that is permissive for regeneration of that particular cell type. In adult mammals, Müller cells also display some stem cell-like properties. For example, when cultured in vitro they can self-renew and differentiate into phenotypically neural cell types. Furthermore, when transplanted in vivo they can generate new neurons within lesioned retinas.[26] Recent evidence reveals that Müller cells can also be stimulated to divide in vivo following the intraocular application of appropriate mitogenic factors, which hints at the possibility of endogenous retinal repair. As such, the potential of Müller cells for retinal repair appears promising. In addition, using adult ocular stem cells as a source for stem cell therapy could facilitate autologous transplantation with the attendant benefit that these cells may be inherently restricted to an ocular fate.

STRATEGIES FOR STEM CELL THERAPY IN GLAUCOMA

TRANSPLANTATION

The possible replacement of photoreceptors by transplantation in diseases such as macular degeneration and retinitis pigmentosa has received much recent attention.[7] Restoration of photoreceptors by transplantation has several advantages not shared by RGC transplantation. In particular, the only afferent input to photoreceptors is light, and the target neurons to which connections must be established are in close proximity within the retina. In contrast, the complete functional replacement of RGCs requires the establishment of appropriate local afferent connections within the inner retina and also long-range efferent connections to the brain. Another important consideration for transplantation approaches is graft location. Some studies have suggested that the subretinal environment favors the selective differentiation of grafted cells into a photoreceptor phenotype.[6] Subretinal transplants enjoy a more immune-privileged milieu than those in the vitreous, and subretinal placement also ensures that the engrafted cells are held in close proximity to the retina. Alternatively, intravitreal introduction theoretically provides the transplanted cells with direct access to the inner retina. This route may, therefore, prove to be more appropriate for glaucoma-directed therapy, as opposed to outer retinal therapy. Further research on this topic is required to determine the superior transplantation technique.

MORPHOLOGICAL INTEGRATION

One of the first tasks transplanted cells must accomplish is morphological integration into the host tissue (Fig. 54.2). In studies on the Brazilian opossum, for example, exogenous stem cells readily integrated into the retina of early postnatal animals, but this amalgamation decreased as the eye developed. By 35 days after birth, little incorporation of transplanted cells was observed.[3] Similarly, integration into the intact rodent retina occurs much more readily in young animals than in adults, although the cells can survive in the posterior segment of adult eyes for weeks.[27] This lack of integration may be partially overcome by injuring the adult retina.[20] Many different disease models, including mechanical injury to the retina or optic nerve, chemical toxicity, ischemia, and inherited retinal degeneration, have all demonstrated an ability to enhance graft integration into adult retinas. Furthermore, degeneration of a specific neuronal type tends to trigger donor cell migration to the site of neurodegeneration, an effect that has also been observed in the brain. Thus, it appears that endogenous signals from the injured retina play a key role in determining the potential for integration of engrafted cells.

NEURONAL DIFFERENTIATION

Transplantation of highly undifferentiated stem cells into the intact or lesioned mammalian retina has yielded limited success with regard to the production of appropriate retinal cell types. This may be due, in part, to molecular suppression of RGC differentiation in the mature retina. In addition, highly undifferentiated cells, such as ES cells, may not detect all of the necessary RGC differentiative cues due to an absence of receptor expression. In contrast, directing differentiation toward a particular cell lineage prior to transplantation may enhance generation of the desired cellular identity. Neural stem cells, and even retinal-specific neural progenitors, have been derived from ES cells in vitro.[16–18] In addition, neural stem cells derived from the brain have been guided towards a retinal fate,[28] while some ocular stem cells also possess retinal neural potential.[22–26] Transplantation of lineage-restricted cells has shown that grafted cells can differentiate and express some RGC-specific markers in vivo.

The ideal stage of differentiation for cellular transplants remains uncertain and it is likely that a compromise between plasticity and maturity will be required. It may not be necessary to create fully differentiated RGCs in vitro for transplantation as it is possible that some of the required signals may remain endogenous to the adult retina, allowing less mature cells to be used. For instance, grafted cells that migrate to different layers of the retina tend to express markers specific to local cell types. This suggests that differentiation may be modulated by indigenous factors within the retina. A key to directed in vivo differentiation may be cell-specific depletion, and subsequent induction of a microenvironment conducive to the generation of that particular cell class. Whether the glaucomatous retina can provide the necessary cues to guide the migration, differentiation, and integration of transplanted cells remains to be established.

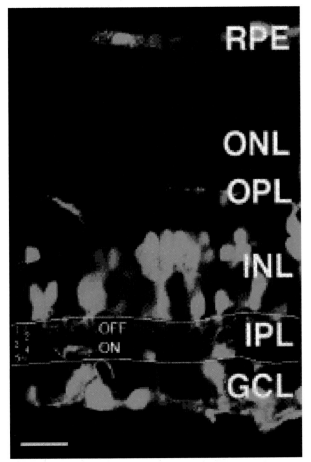

FIGURE 54.2 Neural progenitor cells transplanted into a host retina integrate throughout all layers but mainly localize to the nuclear layers. Neurites extend into the plexiform layers and respect the 'on' and 'off' sublamina. RPE, retinal pigmented epithelium; ONL, outer nuclear layer; OPL, outer plexiform layer; INL, inner nuclear layer; IPL, inner plexiform layer; GCL, ganglion cell layer. (Reprinted from Klassen et al.[3])

FUNCTIONAL INTEGRATION

To the authors' knowledge, the establishment of functional connections by grafted cells in the glaucomatous eye is yet to be demonstrated. Interestingly, hippocampal-derived neural precursor cells have been observed to populate all retinal layers when transplanted into the vitreous of neonatal rats suffering inherited photoreceptor degeneration (see Fig. 54.2).[8] In the ganglion cell layer, new neurons sent neurites into the inner plexiform layer where they associated closely with host dendrites, although functional synapse formation was not confirmed (Fig. 54.3). Grafted cells in the ganglion cell layer also extended processes through the nerve fiber layer and into the optic nerve head. Despite these promising results in neonatal rats, very little retinal integration of hippocampal-derived neural precursor cells was observed in adult animals and this was only achieved following injury. Thus, how to achieve an environment conducive to dendrite/axon extension and connection in the adult retina remains to be elucidated.

This is not to say that functional connectivity is impossible. Recently, an investigation of photoreceptor replacement has demonstrated an impressive level of functional integration in the adult retina.[7] In this study, retinal precursor cells were isolated from neonatal retinas and transplanted into a mouse model for photoreceptor degeneration. Following migration and integration, new neurons extended neurites from the outer nuclear layer into the outer plexiform layer, where they established functional connections with bipolar cells. Stem cell therapy in this context provided measurable functional benefit in these animals. These results provide hope that the generation of functional connections for RGCs is possible, albeit much more complicated than for photoreceptors.

A further challenge to the complete functional integration of transplanted cells within the visual system will be directing growing axons through the optic nerve and into the brain. Furthermore, the development of meaningful synaptic connections within the lateral geniculate nucleus must be addressed. The challenge of establishing functional connections in the brain is increased by the fact that glaucomatous damage extends beyond RGC axons to their target neurons. It has been observed that raised IOP and subsequent RGC loss in a

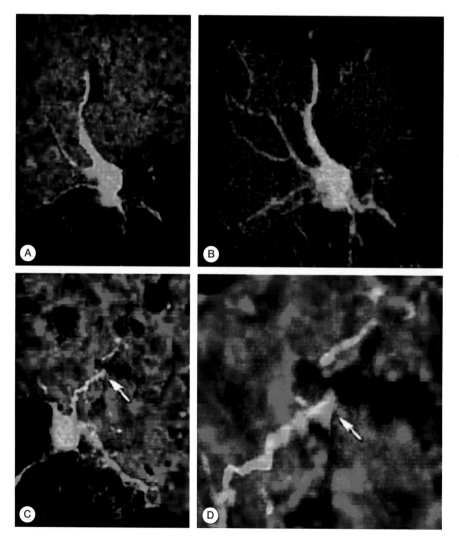

FIGURE 54.3 Transplanted neural progenitor cells localized to nuclear layers in the retina and extending neurites (arrows) into the plexiform layers. A grafted cell extending a large projection **(A)** is shown in higher power and reconstructed to demonstrate the extent of neuritic branching **(B)**. The extended process of a grafted cell **(C)** is shown under higher power **(D)**. (Reprinted from Young et al.[8])

primate glaucoma model correlate with magno-, parvo-, and koniocellular loss in the lateral geniculate nucleus. In addition, pathological changes to the visual cortex were observed.[29] Therefore, the development of neuroprotective strategies in glaucoma will need to consider the entire visual pathway as higher-level visual processing must be preserved in order to ameliorate blindness using a stem cell-based therapy.

TRANSDIFFERENTIATION AND ENDOGENOUS REPAIR

An alternative to transplantation-based approaches to stem cell therapy would be the activation of endogenous retinal repair mechanisms. Endogenous repair may proceed in two ways: transdifferentiation of mature cells or proliferation of a resident precursor cell population. Transdifferentiation is a process whereby fully committed somatic cells dedifferentiate to produce cells with a phenotype resembling that of an immature cell (that is, cells stop expressing mature cell markers and begin expressing immature markers). The newly formed precursor cells may then redifferentiate, often after first proliferating, into a new cell type that is different from the original cellular identity. Transdifferentiation seems to play a role in retinal repair in some animals and may be a target for clinical modulation in order to treat neurodegenerative retinal disease.[30] As discussed earlier, there are a number of cell types within the mammalian eye that retain the ability to proliferate. For instance, a quiescent population of proliferative cells exits in the peripheral retina, which may be analogous to the regenerative cells of the ciliary marginal zone in fish and amphibians, although their ability to differentiate in response to injury in vivo appears to have been lost during evolution. Furthermore, in chicks, injury-triggered transdifferentiation of Müller cells leads to the generation of new cells that differentiate into cell types similar to those lost due to pathology.[25] In mammals, signaling through the Notch and Wnt pathways may perpetuate the dormancy of these cells, as stimulating either of these pathways increases the proliferation of Müller cells isolated from the retina.[26] Little is known about what signaling pathways control activation of other proliferative ocular cells, such as those residing in the iris and ciliary body. Conceivably, therapy aimed at modulating the activity of these endogenous proliferative cell populations may provide an avenue for retinal repair. Alternatively, in vitro transdifferentiation of ocular precursor cells may provide donor cells that are appropriate for transplantation.

STEM CELL-MEDIATED TROPHIC SUPPORT

Recent research suggests that transplantation of stem cells within the CNS can provide neuroprotection or support to surviving neurons proximal to the graft site.[31] Transplanted cells have also demonstrated an ability to modulate immune cell behavior to reduce tissue damage.[11] Most studies to date have involved transplantation into the injured brain; however, it is conceivable that such protection may also translate to the retina. This raises the possibility that stem cell therapy may offer functional benefit to glaucoma patients, without specifically replacing lost RGCs, by protecting the inner retina from further neuronal loss.

Alternatively, neurite sprouting by engrafted cells could form local connections within the inner retina that theoretically might increase the receptive field of surviving cells with a concomitant improvement in vision.

INFLAMMATION

The role of inflammation in glaucoma progression and retinal repair must necessarily be examined as both surgical intervention and preexisting disease conditions stimulate immune reactivity. The contribution of inflammation to injury, neuroprotection, and regeneration of the CNS is emerging as a very complex question. On the one hand, the immune system and regeneration may be in opposition as inflammation has been shown to suppress neurogenesis that occurs naturally in the adult brain.[32] Conceivably, inflammation may also hamper attempts at therapeutic induction of neurogenesis in nonregenerative CNS regions. Additionally, abnormal immune activity within the CNS contributes pathologically to a variety of neurodegenerative disorders, including multiple sclerosis, Alzheimer's disease, and Parkinson's disease. Conversely, inflammation may be beneficial to CNS regeneration. Immune cells which infiltrate the site of a CNS injury can release chemokines that attract transplanted progenitor cells to the damaged area.[33] Furthermore, it has been suggested that inflammation may also be neuroprotective in certain circumstances. For example, the induction of a controlled autoimmune response specific for CNS self-antigen may be neuroprotective following CNS injury.[34] Therefore, precise inflammatory modulation may be required to achieve maximal benefit from stem cell therapy in the retina, and in the CNS in general.

POTENTIAL HURDLES

REJECTION

A major complication of allogeneic transplantation is the potential for graft rejection by the host. Immune-suppressant drugs can alleviate graft rejection; however, long-term therapy with these drugs carries its own risks. Preferentially, autologous transplantation of the recipient's own somatic stem cells (either from the eye or elsewhere) would be a desirable future therapy. While autologous stem cell therapy is currently less advanced than ES- or fetal-derived stem cell therapy, the clinical potential for autologous stem cell transplantation necessitates further research.

REACTIVE GLIOSIS

Following neural injury, reactive gliosis, and subsequent glial scarring, erects physical and environmental barriers between healthy and diseased CNS tissue. These barriers obstruct endogenous neurite regrowth and can impede the migration and integration of engrafted stem cells. The potency of the inhibitory milieu created by gliosis was recently demonstrated by comparing the integration of transplanted cells transplanted into the retina of normal mice compared to those with suppressed glial reactivity. Grafts into mice lacking the GFAP and/or vimentin genes (both involved in reactive gliosis) demonstrated greater neuronal integration into the ganglion cell layer when compared to control eyes. Furthermore, new neurons in the retinas of these knockout animals extended processes further into both the nerve fiber layer and inner plexiform layer than those implanted into normal eyes.[35]

AXONAL GUIDANCE AND MYELINATION

The adult CNS environment, outside regions of continued neurongenesis, is inherently inhibitory to the integration of new neurons. This provides a challenge for stem cell therapy, especially in diseases where the replacement of functional neurons requires considerable neurite outgrowth. For example, in glaucoma the strict replacement of RGCs will require extension of dendrites into the inner nuclear layer and axons from the inner retina through the optic nerve and into the lateral geniculate nucleus. In culture, many CNS neurons possess the ability to generate quite long processes; therefore, it appears that the main antagonist of in vivo neurite extension lies in the environment. Furthermore, in vivo adult mammalian RGCs retain the ability to regenerate an axon through the more permissive environment of a peripheral nerve graft.[36] Such grafts have been used as a conduit between the eye and the brain, following optic nerve transection, to achieve functional recovery revealed by restoration of the pupillary light reflex. This result suggests the possibility of using conduits permissive to axonal growth to guide reconnections between RGCs and the brain. This conduit could be tissue borrowed from another part of the body or perhaps a bioengineered prosthetic.

An alternative approach would be to enhance the permissiveness of the host retina and optic nerve to neurite extension. One possible mechanism involves the downregulation of growth inhibitory molecules such as myelin-associated protein (MAG), oligodendrocyte-myelin glycoprotein or Nogo. All of these proteins are associated with CNS myelin and act directly on neurons to prevent neurite outgrowth. Indeed, Nogo receptor antagonization has demonstrated efficacy in optic nerve repair following axon regeneration signaling to RGCs.[37] Heparin and chondroitin sulfate proteoglycans have also been revealed as potential barriers to CNS regeneration. These proteoglycans encapsulate mature neurons and their synapses within the brain, contribute to glial scar formation, and inhibit neurite growth.[38] Such proteoglycans are present in the retina and, thus, enzymes that digest them may facilitate optic nerve regeneration. In addition, a wide variety of other potential signaling factors, such as cyclic adenosine monophosphate (cAMP), have been identified as axonal growth promoters and could be used therapeutically to enhance neurite extension. Taken together, these observations suggest that modulation of the CNS regenerative blockade may enhance the integration of grafted cells in the glaucomatous retina.

Should RGC axonal extension from the eye to the brain be achieved, myelination of the optic nerve fibers will be essential in order to maintain physiological conduction velocities. Research focused on demyelinating diseases, such as multiple sclerosis, may provide clues as to possible mechanisms for triggering remyelination. Inflammation is known to play a positive role in remyelination of damaged CNS neurons by oligodendrocyte precursor cells. It is possible that modulation of endogenous oligodendrocytes or transplantation of oligodendrocyte precursor cells will be required to complete the functional integration of new RGCs.

ASSESSING VISUAL IMPROVEMENT IN ANIMAL MODELS

Assessing functional improvement in animal models of glaucoma presents a particular challenge. Some clinical methodologies for measuring general visual function have been adapted to many different species, including electroretinography, visual evoked potential measurement, and pupillometry. In addition, behavioral tests, such as observing head tracking responses to visual targets, have also been exploited. Unfortunately, the sensitivity of these tests is relatively low and a visual benefit that may be clinically relevant to a human patient may currently be below the threshold for detection in animal models. Thus, efforts to develop more sensitive and reliable visual function assessments for experimental models are required.

CONTINUED DISEASE PROGRESSION

While stem cell therapy may offer the hope of restoring visual field function in glaucoma, one must remember that the pathology itself will not be 'cured' by such treatment. Thus, clinical management of the disease would necessarily continue to prevent renewed neurodegeneration. Presumably, the new neurons would be as vulnerable to the pathophysiological conditions of glaucoma as their predecessors. Furthermore, depletion of endogenous RGCs will also likely persist. As such, glaucoma may require lifelong ocular hypotensive, and possibly neuroprotective, treatment, even after stem cell therapy. Perhaps new advances in neuroprotection and/or gene therapy will offer additional tools to the glaucoma specialist.

Summary

Stem cells offer the potential to develop powerful new therapies for treating historically incurable neurodegenerative diseases, such as glaucoma, by providing a possible means of replacing dead cells to effect functional recovery. In addition, stem cell therapy may possess other less direct therapeutic benefits such as providing trophic support for remaining neurons, modulating immune responses, and generating local neuronal networks.

Stem cell therapy could be achieved via the transplantation of cultured stem cells or by manipulating endogenous repair mechanisms. A variety of potential stem or progenitor cell sources, each with inherent strengths and weaknesses, are available for transplantation-based therapies. In order to cure glaucoma completely, stem cell therapy would necessarily replace degenerated retinal neurons and reestablish the visual pathway. This means stem cells would ideally integrate into the retinal ganglion cell layer, differentiate into mature RGCs, establish connections with appropriate afferent neurons, extend axons through the optic nerve to the lateral geniculate nucleus, and make functional connections within the brain to preserve the retinotopic map. Such complete RGC replacement is likely to remain a formidable challenge. However, it is also possible that the survival and partial integration of transplanted cells within the retina may provide alternative benefits by enhancing the survival and function of host RGCs. In addition, glaucoma stem cell therapy could be used to treat other complications of glaucoma, including reversal of optic nerve head pathology, restoration of the trabecular outflow pathway, or to heal leaky blebs following surgery.

There are also a number of possible obstacles to the development of a successful stem cell-based therapy for glaucoma. Given that allogeneic transplantation would necessitate long-term immune suppression in order to avoid graft rejection, it would be highly desirable to develop autologous stem cell therapies. In addition, techniques to promote RGC axon extension, connection, and myelination may need to be developed to achieve significant visual field restoration. Finally, the issue of continued disease progression will need to be addressed in order to protect new and host neurons.

As with many new approaches in medicine, there is the danger that advocates of stem cell research may promise more than can conceivably be delivered in a realistic timeframe, leading to disappointment, disillusionment, and a loss of confidence in the potential of the approach. We must acknowledge that the technology and understanding needed to achieve functional improvement in glaucoma using stem cell therapy is in its infancy. However, in the absence of any other treatment with the potential to restore vision in glaucoma, further research on the therapeutic use of stem cells in glaucoma remains both justifiable and eagerly awaited.

REFERENCES

1. Quigley HA, Iglesia DS. Stem cells to replace the optic nerve. Eye 2004; 18:1085–1088.

2. Levin LA, Ritch R, Richards JE, et al. Stem cell therapy for ocular disorders. Arch Ophthalmol 2004; 122:621–627.

3. Klassen H, Sakaguchi DS, Young MJ. Stem cells and retinal repair. Prog Retin Eye Res 2004; 23:149–181.

4. Limb GA, Daniels JT, Cambrey AD, et al. Current prospects for adult stem cell-based therapies in ocular repair and regeneration. Curr Eye Res 2006; 31:381–390.

5. Young MJ. Stem cells in the mammalian eye: a tool for retinal repair. APMIS 2005; 113:845–857.

6. Banin E, Obolensky A, Idelson M, et al. Retinal incorporation and differentiation of neural precursors derived from human embryonic stem cells. Stem Cells 2006; 24:246–257.

7. MacLaren RE, Pearson RA, MacNeil A, et al. Retinal repair by transplantation of photoreceptor precursors. Nature 2006; 444:203–207.

8. Young MJ, Ray J, Whiteley SJ, et al. Neuronal differentiation and morphological integration of hippocampal progenitor cells transplanted to the retina of immature and mature dystrophic rats. Mol Cell Neurosci 2000; 16:197–205.

9. Hernandez MR, Andrzejewska WM, Neufeld AH. Changes in the extracellular matrix of the human optic nerve head in primary open-angle glaucoma. Am J Ophthalmol 1990; 109:180–188.

10. Neufeld AH, Liu B. Glaucomatous optic neuropathy: when glia misbehave. Neuroscientist 2003; 9:485–495.

11. Pluchino S, Zanotti L, Rossi B, et al. Neurosphere-derived multipotent precursors promote neuroprotection by an immunomodulatory mechanism. Nature 2005; 436:266–271.

12. Gabelt BT, Kaufman PL. Changes in aqueous humor dynamics with age and glaucoma. Prog Retin Eye Res 2005; 24:612–637.

13. Gonzalez P, Epstein DL, Luna C, et al. Characterization of free-floating spheres from human trabecular meshwork (HTM) cell culture in vitro. Exp Eye Res 2006; 82:959–967.

14. Hwang JM, Kee C. Injection of cultured autologous fibroblasts into the subconjunctival space of rabbits treated with mitomycin C. Am J Ophthalmol 2006; 142:259–263.

15. Arnhold S, Klein H, Semkova I, et al. Neurally selected embryonic stem cells induce tumor formation after long-term survival following engraftment into the subretinal space. Invest Ophthalmol Vis Sci 2004; 45:4251–4255.

16. Ikeda H, Osakada F, Watanabe K, et al. Generation of $Rx^+/Pax6^+$ neural retinal precursors from embryonic stem cells. Proc Natl Acad Sci USA 2005; 102:11331–11336.

17. Tabata Y, Ouchi Y, Kamiya H, et al. Specification of the retinal fate of mouse embryonic stem cells by ectopic expression of Rx/rax, a homeobox gene. Mol Cell Biol 2004; 24:4513–4521.

18. Lamba DA, Karl MO, Ware CB, et al. Efficient generation of retinal progenitor cells from human embryonic stem cells. Proc Natl Acad Sci USA 2006; 103:12769–12774.

19. Kim S, Honmou O, Kato K, et al. Neural differentiation potential of peripheral blood- and bone-marrow-derived precursor cells. Brain Res 2006; 1123:27–33.

20. Nishida A, Takahashi M, Tanihara H, et al. Incorporation and differentiation of hippocampus-derived neural stem cells transplanted in injured adult rat retina. Invest Ophthalmol Vis Sci 2000; 41:4268–4274.

21. Reh TA, Levine EM. Multipotential stem cells and progenitors in the vertebrate retina. J Neurobiol 1998; 36:206–220.

22. Tropepe V, Coles BL, Chiasson BJ, et al. Retinal stem cells in the adult mammalian eye. Science 2000; 287:2032–2036.

23. Ahmad I, Tang L, Pham H. Identification of neural progenitors in the adult mammalian eye. Biochem Biophys Res Commun 2000; 270:517–521.

24. Haruta M, Kosaka M, Kanegae Y, et al. Induction of photoreceptor-specific phenotypes in adult mammalian iris tissue. Nat Neurosci 2001; 4:1163–1164.

25. Fischer AJ, Reh TA. Potential of Müller glia to become neurogenic retinal progenitor cells. Glia 2003; 43:70–76.

26. Das AV, Mallya KB, Zhao X, et al. Neural stem cell properties of Müller glia in the mammalian retina: regulation by Notch and Wnt signaling. Dev Biol 2006; 299:283–302.

27. Takahashi M, Palmer TD, Takahashi J, et al. Widespread integration and survival of adult-derived neural progenitor

cells in the developing optic retina. Mol Cell Neurosci 1998; 12:340–348.

28. Dong X, Pulido JS, Qu T, et al. Differentiation of human neural stem cells into retinal cells. Neuroreport 2003; 14:143–146.

29. Yucel YH, Zhang Q, Weinreb RN, et al. Effects of retinal ganglion cell loss on magno-, parvo-, koniocellular pathways in the lateral geniculate nucleus and visual cortex in glaucoma. Prog Retin Eye Res 2003; 22:465–481.

30. Tsonis PA, Del Rio-Tsonis K. Lens and retina regeneration: transdifferentiation, stem cells and clinical applications. Exp Eye Res 2004; 78:161–172.

31. Meyer JS, Katz ML, Maruniak JA, et al. Embryonic stem cell-derived neural progenitors incorporate into degenerating retina and enhance survival of host photoreceptors. Stem Cells 2006; 24:274–283.

32. Ekdahl CT, Claasen JH, Bonde S, et al. Inflammation is detrimental for neurogenesis in adult brain. Proc Natl Acad Sci USA 2003; 100:13632–13637.

33. Belmadani A, Tran PB, Ren D, et al. Chemokines regulate the migration of neural progenitors to sites of neuroinflammation. J Neurosci 2006; 26:3182–3191.

34. Schwartz M, Kipnis J. Protective autoimmunity: regulation and prospects for vaccination after brain and spinal cord injuries. Trends Mol Med 2001; 7:252–258.

35. Kinouchi R, Takeda M, Yang L, et al. Robust neural integration from retinal transplants in mice deficient in GFAP and vimentin. Nat Neurosci 2003; 6:863–868.

36. Aguayo AJ, Vidal-Sanz M, Villegas-Perez MP, et al. Growth and connectivity of axotomized retinal neurons in adult rats with optic nerves substituted by PNS grafts linking the eye and the midbrain. Ann NY Acad Sci 1987; 495:1–9.

37. Fischer D, He Z, Benowitz LI. Counteracting the Nogo receptor enhances optic nerve regeneration if retinal ganglion cells are in an active growth state. J Neurosci 2004; 24:1646–1651.

38. Carulli D, Laabs T, Geller HM, et al. Chondroitin sulfate proteoglycans in neural development and regeneration. Curr Opin Neurobiol 2005; 15:116–120.

CHAPTER 55

Gene Therapy in Glaucoma

Stuart J McKinnon

INTRODUCTION

Genetic manipulation of the mammalian central nervous system has progressed rapidly over the past two decades. Gene transfer has been a well-characterized technique in molecular and cellular biology for many years, and the ability to express a protein in mammalian cell culture has given us a great deal of information concerning both normal and pathological cellular processes. The use of transgenic animals has extended this approach, but the use of these animals is time-consuming and subject to difficulties in interpretation. To allow more controlled genetic manipulations, neurobiologists have taken advantage of pathogenic viruses to develop systems to deliver genes of interest (transgenes) to specific neuronal cell populations. For glaucoma, targets of gene therapy approaches include aqueous humor outflow modification in the trabecular meshwork (TM), and neuroprotection of retinal ganglion cells (RGCs) and the optic nerve.

VIRUS CLASSIFICATION

Viruses are small, infectious, intracellular parasites characterized by their simple organization, mode of replication, and nucleic acid composition. Viruses intrinsically lack the ability to produce energy or synthesize proteins and enzymes, and therefore invade a host cell to obtain access to these functions. Rather than dividing as most microorganisms do, viruses reproduce in host cells by assembling subunits into infectious particles, consisting of DNA or RNA surrounded by a symmetric protein coat (capsid). The capsid protects the internal nucleic acids from the external environment, confers antigenicity, and mediates attachment to susceptible cells. The viral life cycle consists of two phases: the intracellular phase in which the viral nucleic acids are replicated and packaged within the capsid to form the virion, and the infectious extracellular phase in which the virion invades the host causing cellular alteration or death. Viruses are classified according to the type of nucleic acid (DNA or RNA), the secondary structure of the nucleic acid (single-stranded, double-stranded, circular, or coiled), the symmetry of the capsid (icosahedral or helical), and the presence of a cell-derived envelope (naked or enveloped).[1] The author will limit this review to the common viral vector types that have been employed in ocular gene therapy, specifically adenovirus, adeno-associated virus (AAV), and retroviruses such as lentivirus.

ADENOVIRUS

One of the first viruses to be employed as a vector for gene transfer is adenovirus, which in its native form causes respiratory tract and ocular infections in humans. Adenovirus has been well characterized as to genetic make-up, gene functions, and interactions with the infected host cell. Adenovirus consists of a 36 kilobase (kb) linear double-stranded DNA genome surrounded by a nonenveloped (naked) icosahedral capsid. Adsorption of adenovirus to the host cell involves binding of fiber proteins that project from each of the 20 vertices of the icosahedral capsid to a coxsackievirus adenovirus receptor (CAR).[2] This receptor is present in a wide range of cell types, but when absent leads to viral toxicity and resistance to transgene expression. Recently, several CAR-independent adenovirus vectors that incorporate different capsid proteins have been generated to improve adenoviral vector transduction. Restricting viral tropism to selected cell types has also been furthered by altering viral genomes to produce virions with modified capsids (pseudotyping).[3]

The first generation of adenoviral vectors was engineered to render the virus replication defective, by deleting the E1A, E1B, and E3 genes. E1A proteins are the first viral proteins to be expressed after transduction, and activate transcription by modifying transcription factors and transcriptional regulators. E1A proteins also interact with the retinoblastoma protein (pRB) to induce quiescent cells to enter the S phase of the cell cycle.[4] The E1B protein is required for efficient accumulation of viral messenger RNA (mRNA), and is also expressed early. E1B modulates cell cycle progression by

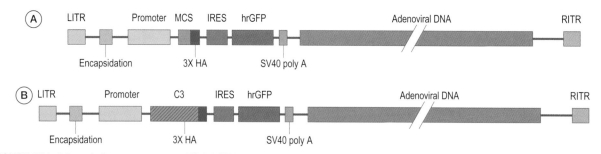

FIGURE 55.1 Adenoviral vector structure. **(A)** Ad-GFP incorporating IRES expressing human recombinant GFP. **(B)** Ad-C3-GFP, which has the C3 gene cloned into the multiple cloning site of the backbone, expresses C3 transferase and human recombinant GFP. LITR, left inverted terminal repeat; MCS, multiple cloning site; IRES, internal ribosome entry site; hrGFP, human recombinant green fluorescent protein; RITR, right inverted terminal repeat; C3, C3 transferase. (Redrawn from Liu X, Hu Y, Filla MS, et al. The effect of C3 transgene expression on actin and cellular adhesions in cultured human trabecular meshwork cells and on outflow facility in organ cultured monkey eyes. Mol Vis 2005; 11:1112–1121.[44])

targeting p53, a DNA-binding tumor-suppressor protein.[5] Both E1A and E1B proteins also block apoptosis, and prevent the host cell from activating intrinsic cell death machinery before virion replication can occur. E3 proteins protect the infected cell from host immune responses by preventing lysis from cytotoxic T lymphocytes and tumor necrosis factor.[6] These first-generation adenovirus vectors caused inflammation due to low-level expression of viral genes, because viral transcription still occurs despite the absence of E1A and E1B genes.[2] Further generations of adenovirus have incorporated a mutated E2A gene, which is required for adenoviral DNA replication, and have demonstrated reduced cytotoxic T-lymphocyte infiltration.[7] Despite these improvements, a human gene therapy trial involving adenovirus vectors to treat ornithine transcarbamylase deficiency resulted in the death of 18-year-old Jesse Gelsinger from a severe immune system reaction and multiple organ system failure. As a result, the Food and Drug Administration suspended human gene therapy experiments at the University of Pennsylvania in 2000.

Prior to 1996, recombinant (E1A, E1B, E3-deleted) adenovirus vectors were generated by homologous recombination of plasmids and digested adenoviral DNA in human embryonic kidney cells (HEK 293). Vector clones were isolated by amplifying individual plaques, a time-consuming process. This method has been replaced by engineering a recombinant plasmid containing the DNA transgene of interest, featuring an adenoviral inverted terminal repeat (ITR) sequence that is sufficient for packaging and integration, a multiple cloning site (MCS), and adenoviral E2B sequence (Fig. 55.1). The adenoviral vectors are then generated by homologous recombination of plasmid in *Escherichia coli* strains, followed by isolation and purification of the recombinant adenovirus.

ADENO-ASSOCIATED VIRUS

Adeno-associated viruses (AAVs) were first noticed in the late 1960s as a contaminant of adenovirus stocks.[8]

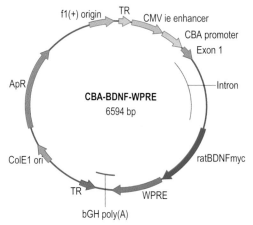

FIGURE 55.2 Map of the AAV-CBA -BDNF-WPRE virus. f1(+) origin, f1 bacteriophage origin of replication; TR, terminal repeats; CMV ie enhancer, cytomegalovirus immediate early enhancer; CBA promoter, chicken β-actin promoter; ratBDNFmyc, myc-tagged rat brain-derived neurotrophic factor sequence; WPRE, woodchuck hepatitis post-transcriptional regulatory element; bGH poly(A), bovine growth hormone polyA sequence; ColE1 ori, *Escherichia coli* origin of replication; ApR, ampicillin resistance sequence. (Redrawn from Martin KR, Quigley HA, Zack DJ, et al. Gene therapy with brain-derived neurotrophic factor as a protection: retinal ganglion cells in a rat glaucoma model. Invest Ophthalmol Vis Sci 2003; 44:4357–4365.[54])

AAV is a small, helper-dependent parvovirus consisting of a single-stranded 4.7 kb DNA genome surrounded by a simple, naked icosahedral capsid. The AAV vector is attractive for use in gene therapy because it is efficient, long lived, and nontoxic. No human pathology has been reported from AAV, although approximately 85% of adult humans are seropositive for AAV. Wild-type (wt) AAV requires a helper virus (adenovirus, herpesvirus, or vaccinia virus) to establish infectivity. In the absence of helper virus or toxic challenge, wtAAV integrates into chromosome 19 of the human genome. Recombinant AAV (rAAV) vectors have 96% of the viral genome removed, leaving only the two 145 base-pair ITRs. Deleted portions of the AAV genome code for structural capsid (Cap) proteins and nonstructural replication (Rep) proteins (Fig. 55.2). The advantage of AAV for use as vectors lies in the fact that the

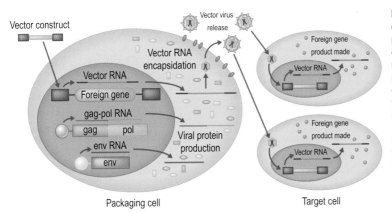

FIGURE 55.3 Retroviral vector production. A retroviral construct is introduced into a packaging cell, producing RNA coding for the foreign transgene of interest. Separate viral constructs produce the retroviral structural and enzymatic proteins gag, pol, and env. Foreign transgene RNA is packaged, encapsidated, and released. The resulting retrovirus vector does not express viral packaging proteins, and the vector will not be replicated further in infected target cells. (Redrawn from Buchschacher GL Jr, Wong-Staal F. Development of lentiviral vectors for gene therapy for human diseases. Blood 2000; 95:2499–2504).

absence of *Rep* and *Cap* viral sequences means that no viral protein synthesis occurs following transduction, minimizing the amount of foreign protein available to trigger immune responses. Therefore, rAAV vectors are considered to have one of the highest biosafety ratings among all viral vectors. Another beneficial feature of AAV for gene transfer is its ability to infect both dividing and nondividing cells.[9] Due to the small size of the AAV genome, the amount of DNA that can be inserted is limited to less than 5 kb.[10] Because rAAV vectors lack the *Rep* sequences responsible for integration into chromosomal DNA, the AAV genome exists autonomously in the cytoplasm in an episomal form[11] and has demonstrated stable transgene expression for over 1 year.[12]

Currently, 10 different AAV serotypes (AAV-1 through AAV-10) have been classified according to differences in *Cap* gene sequences, conferring varying host cell binding and tropism behaviors.[13] Pseudotyping has also been employed, generating hybrid rAAV vectors that contain the genome of one serotype (typically AAV-2) packaged into the capsid of another serotype, improving cellular tropism and the onset and the intensity of gene expression.[14] As mentioned above, AAV depends on cotransfection with a helper virus for efficient replication. Recombinant AAV vectors have the *Rep* and *Cap* sequences replaced by the transgene of interest, so replication and packaging of AAV relies on similar sequences derived from helper viruses such as the adenovirus sequences E1A, E1B, E2A, and E4.

In the past, rAAV was produced by calcium phosphate cotransfection of adenovirus-infected 293 cells with a rAAV vector plasmid and a wild-type AAV helper plasmid. The rAAV was then purified by stepwise precipitation of rAAV with ammonium sulfate, followed by two or three rounds of CsCl density gradient centrifugation. Each gradient required fractionation and identification of the virus-containing regions by dot-blot hybridization or by polymerase chain reaction (PCR) analysis. This required up to 2 weeks for completion, and often resulted in poor recovery and poor-quality virus.[15] Because of the potential for contamination with unwanted adenovirus, 'mini-adenovirus' helper plasmids have been engineered to contain only the adenoviral genes necessary for helper function and by omitting the structural and replication adenoviral genes. Further refinements in the purification process employ heparin sulfate affinity chromatography columns that improve rAAV binding, and nonionic iodixanol step gradient purification, which allows more rapid and efficient separation of rAAV. Virus stocks are titrated by a quantitative PCR assay and typically yield an average of $1–4 \times 10^{13}$ viral particles.[10,15]

LENTIVIRUS

Retroviruses are RNA-containing viruses that are known to infect a wide variety of species, and use a unique method of replication. Specific viral coat proteins, encoded by the viral *env* gene, enable the retrovirus to interact with a receptor on the host cell membrane.[16] Once inside the cell cytoplasm, uncoating of the virion occurs. A unique retroviral RNA-dependent DNA polymerase, reverse transcriptase, encoded by the *pol* gene, transcribes a double-stranded DNA complementary to the viral RNA, and the complementary DNA moves into the nucleus where it is incorporated into the host cell's chromosome.[17] The integrated DNA is then used as a template for transcription of retroviral RNA and translation into required viral proteins.[1] The newly synthesized viral proteins gag (capsid), pol (reverse transcriptase), and env (envelope glycoprotein) associate with viral genomic RNA via the export and packaging sequences, *rev* and *psi*. The packaged proteins and RNA then interact with the host cell membrane, resulting in encapsulation and release by budding from the cell surface of mature infectious virions (Fig. 55.3).[18]

Tumor-producing retroviruses such as Maloney murine leukemia virus achieve stable integration into the host cell genome, but only in dividing cells. Lentiviruses such as human immunodeficiency virus (HIV) and feline immunodeficiency virus (FIV) offer the advantage of stable incorporation into both dividing and nondividing cell genomes, making them excellent vectors for use in gene therapy. Lentiviruses are nononcogenic retroviruses that produce multiorgan diseases characterized by long incubation periods and persistent infection. Five serotypes have been discovered, characterized by the mammalian hosts with which they are associated. It is imperative that the use of lentiviral vectors such as HIV for gene therapy does not cause reconstitution of a replication-competent retrovirus. To eliminate this possibility, lentiviral vectors are produced by transient cotransfection of separate plasmids that express the lentiviral transfer genome containing the transgene of interest, the lentiviral structural components gag, pol, and rev, and a heterologous env protein that confers stability and broad cell tropism. Another significant modification to the transfer vector construct has been the deletion in the long terminal repeat (LTR) region, rendering the LTR transcriptionally inactive. These self-inactivating (SIN) vectors increase biosafety by decreasing insertional mutagenesis due to transcription from the 3' LTR of the integrated provirus, and by decreased production of vector transcripts that contain the packaging signal psi.[19]

MODULATION OF VIRAL VECTOR EXPRESSION

In order to initiate transcription, a DNA sequence exists upstream of the gene of interest to which the enzyme RNA polymerase binds. In viral vectors, these 'promoter' sequences have been incorporated to insure efficiency of gene expression in specific cell populations. The most common promoter is derived from cytomegalovirus (CMV), and drives expression in multiple neuronal and vascular cell types. The CMV promoter is small in size (700 bp), which makes it ideal for use in size-limited vectors such as rAAV. In ocular applications, the CMV promoter is efficient in driving expression in TM cells, but is relatively inefficient in driving expression in RGCs.[20] Another commonly used promoter is the CMV enhancer/chicken β-actin (CBA) promoter. The CBA promoter enables high levels of long-term rAAV-mediated gene expression in neurons,[21] and particularly in RGCs.[22] Neuronal promoters such as human platelet-derived growth factor (PDGF) and neuron-specific enolase (NSE), and glia-specific promoters such as glial fibrillary acidic protein (GFAP) have promise for use in ocular gene therapy applications but have not been widely tested. Promoters have also been identified that target gene expression to TM or Schlemm's canal (SC). Studies of TM gene expression by sequencing of cDNA clones identified the matrix Gla protein, a member of a potassium-dependent protein that is widely expressed in bone, heart, kidney, and lung.[23] VE-cadherin, which modulates cell–cell adhesion between vascular endothelial cells, was identified using specific antibodies to be a marker for SC cells, but not TM cells.[24]

DNA sequence elements can be incorporated into the viral vector backbone as 'enhancers' of translation of proteins coded by the inserted transgene of interest. For example, hepatitis B viruses are known to regulate and enhance levels of protein synthesis in infected cells due to a post-transcriptional regulatory element in the 3' untranslated region of the hepatitis viral genome. A similar sequence has been isolated from woodchuck hepatitis virus, termed the woodchuck post-transcriptional regulatory element (WPRE). WPRE increases viral RNA stability and is required for the cytoplasmic accumulation of viral RNAs.[25] Incorporation of the WPRE enhancer into rAAV vectors causes approximate 10-fold increases in the number of transfected neuronal cells and in protein expression as measured by Western blot, when compared to vectors without WPRE.[26,27]

The gene therapy approaches detailed above rely on transfection of a host cell by the viral vector, and expression of the transgene of interest relies on the host cell to modulate release of the gene product. The laminar protein fibronectin is secreted through a non-regulated constitutively active pathway, and inclusion of the fibronectin secretory signal sequence (FIB) in an AAV vector caused significant gene product secretion in vitro.[28] A novel secretion strategy has been developed in which the FIB secretion signal sequence is fused with a transgene coding for a therapeutic peptide, causing marked enhancement of protein expression and positive therapeutic effect in a rat seizure model.[29]

Once viral DNA is transcribed by RNA polymerase into mRNA, protein translation by the ribosome begins at a unique site bound to the 5'-end of the mRNA, termed the 5' cap. Viral vectors have been designed to express two proteins (bicistronic expression) by incorporating an internal ribosome entry site (IRES) element that provides an additional ribosomal translation site. In this way, a second protein such as the reporter protein's green fluorescent protein (GFP) or lacZ can be coexpressed from the same viral vector. Efficiency of viral vector transduction can be assessed when reporter protein expression is noted in cells due to the IRES-dependent mechanism, therefore implying that the same cell is also expressing the transgene of interest due to the cap-dependent mechanism.[30]

In contrast to gene therapy techniques that are designed to enhance protein expression, it is sometimes necessary to temporally regulate protein expression or to prevent toxicity from overexpression. Such inducible gene expression systems take advantage of the tetracycline or doxycycline antibiotics, which are small lipophilic drugs that enter eukaryotic cells by passive diffusion. They are attractive as gene expression modulators because they are routinely used in both human and veterinary medicine with negligible side effects.[31] In a typical 'Tet-Off' application, expression of two vectors is necessary. The first vector expresses a tetracycline-controlled transactivator (tTA). The second vector expresses a tetracycline-response element (TRE) that activates transcription of a transgene under the control of the TRE. Upon doxycycline treatment, the target gene is conditionally turned off because tTA bound with doxycycline cannot bind to the TRE, and transcription is repressed.[32] 'Tet-On' systems can also be designed where genes are conditionally turned on by administration of doxycycline, but these are limited by the need for use of much higher levels of doxycycline.[31]

DOWNREGULATION OF GENE EXPRESSION USING ANTISENSE OLIGONUCLEOTIDES AND siRNA

Antisense therapy involves downregulation of gene expression by complementary oligonucleotide binding to target mRNA. Antisense oligonucleotides are short, single-stranded DNA sequences engineered to be complementary to the specific 'sense' (5' to 3') orientation of mRNA coding for the targeted protein. After introduction into a host cell, the antisense oligonucleotide hybridizes to the complementary mRNA sequence, forming a heteroduplex. This causes mRNA degradation by RNase H, an endoribonuclease that hydrolyzes phosphodiester bonds of RNA hybridized to DNA. Antisense oligonucleotides offer the benefit of rapid manufacture, on the order of days to weeks. However, antisense oligonucleotides made from native nucleotides are prone to degradation from endogenous nucleases. To increase resistance to degradation, synthetic oligonucleotides can be designed that commonly modify the ribose-phosphate backbone. A sulfur atom can be substituted for oxygen in the bridging phosphate group in the nucleotide linkages of the synthesized chain. This provides a phosphorothioate oligonucleotide backbone that prevents ubiquitous nuclease degradation while still allowing RNase H degradation.[33] A nitrogen atom can be substituted for oxygen at the 3' position in the bridging phosphate group, providing a phosphoramidate oligonucleotide with increased target affinity and nuclease stability.[34] Morpholinos are antisense oligonucleotides with modified backbones, with nucleic acid bases bound to six-member morpholine rings instead of five-member deoxyribose rings and linked through phosphorodiamidate groups instead of phosphates.[35] Advantages of morpholino antisense oligonucleotides are high affinity, nuclease resistance, and ease of permeating cell membranes.[36]

Short interfering or silencing RNAs (siRNAs) are small (20–25 bp) double-stranded RNA molecules that are currently being explored for use in a gene therapy. RNA interference (RNAi) is an evolutionarily conserved pathway whereby siRNA silences gene expression post-transcriptionally. In the cytoplasm, siRNAs interact with a nuclease-containing, RNA-induced silencing complex (RISC). Upon binding to RISC, the double-stranded siRNA unwinds, pairs with its complementary target mRNA, and allows the RISC complex to cleave the mRNA strand within the target site. This cleavage causes degradation of the mRNA molecule, preventing protein translation.[37] Standard transfection methods can be employed to introduce exogenous siRNAs into cells to allow silencing of a specific gene of interest. As siRNA gene silencing is transient, the siRNA can be continuously expressed by an engineered plasmid vector. Drawbacks of the siRNA technique include immune responses due to siRNA overexpression and mistaken host recognition as a viral sequence. Treatments of ocular disease have shown promise, as adenovirus vectors coding for siRNA targeting vascular endothelial growth factor (VEGF) have been shown to reduce choroidal neovascularization in a mouse model of age-related macular degeneration (AMD) and are currently in phase 1 trials in humans.[38]

MODULATION OF AQUEOUS OUTFLOW

Injection of viral vectors into the anterior chamber is an efficient technique to express transgenes, specifically in the TM, because aqueous outflow causes deposition of vector primarily in this location. Gene delivery primarily using adenoviral or lentiviral vectors has demonstrated success in TM transfection and in modulation in aqueous outflow, usually by targeting extracellular matrix or cytoskeleton proteins. Recent success using siRNA therapy to target TM gene expression is an exciting development as well.

Anterior chambers of perfused porcine and human anterior segment cultures were injected with replication-deficient adenoviral constructs coding for reporter genes such as lacZ, luciferase, or GFP (Fig. 55.4).[39,40] Transduction of all layers of the TM (uveal, corneoscleral, and juxtacanalicular) and inner wall of SC was noted. Injections of high titers of vector were noted to cause an increase in outflow facility, possibly due to constipation of outflow channels with viral particles.[39] TM cultures were transduced by adenovirus coding for aquaporin-1, an integral membrane protein that functions as a channel for water and ion transport. Increases in mean resting cell volumes and paracellular permeability were seen in monolayers of TM cells, suggesting that aquaporin-1 is a modulator of outflow facility in vivo.[41]

Human TM cultures and rat anterior segments were noted to be efficiently transduced with replication-deficient adenovirus coding for stromelysin, a connective tissue-degrading enzyme of the matrix metalloproteinase (MMP) family.[42] Human TM and SC cell cultures as well as perfused human anterior segment cultures were transduced with an adenoviral construct coding for RhoA, a member of the Ras superfamily of GTP-binding proteins known to regulate cytoskeleton–cell interactions and endothelial barrier functions. Histological evidence of disruption of cytoskeleton components and endothelial cell adhesions was noted in cell culture, as well as a significant 32.5% mean increase of outflow facility in anterior segment culture after 72 h.[43]

Human TM cell cultures and perfused monkey eye anterior segments were transduced with adenovirus delivering exoenzyme C3 transferase, a member of the Rho GTPase family derived from *Clostridium botulinum*. Alterations in the cytoskeleton components actin, vinculin, and β-catenin were noted in cell culture, as well as a mean 90% increase in outflow facility in monkey anterior segment culture.[44] Human TM cell cultures and perfused monkey and human eye anterior segment cultures were transduced with adenovirus delivering caldesmon, a regulator of myosin activity in smooth muscle cells. Changes in actin cytoskeleton

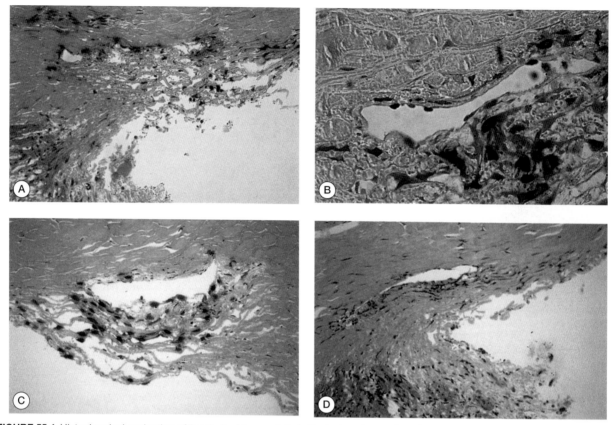

FIGURE 55.4 Histochemical evaluation of β-galactosidase activity in the trabecular meshwork of perfused human anterior segment cultures. **(A)** Trabecular meshwork cells 48 h after transfection stain with Ad-lacZ. **(B, C)** Juxtacanalicular trabecular meshwork cells transfected with Ad-lacZ stain with X-gal (*large dark areas*). **(D)** Trabecular meshwork cells treated with control vehicle do not stain with X-gal. (From Borras T, Rowlette LL, Erzurum SC, et al. Adenoviral reporter gene transfer to the human trabecular meshwork does not alter aqueous humor outflow. Relevance for potential gene therapy of glaucoma. Gene Ther 1999; 6:515–524.[39])

and matrix adhesions were noted in TM cultures, and outflow facility was increased in anterior segment cultures of human eyes by a mean of 43% and in monkey eyes by a mean of 35% at 3 days and 66% at 6 days.[45]

Lentiviral vectors derived from feline immunodeficiency virus (FIV) have been shown to efficiently transduce TM cells for up to 10 months after anterior chamber injection, with minimal inflammation and cell loss.[46,47] The same group of researchers also showed that a second-generation FIV vector caused an approximate 80% transduction of TM cells in perfused human anterior segment cultures, with a transient 30% decrease of outflow facility that resolved after 72 h.[48] Lentiviral gene therapy to increase outflow facility has great potential to lower intraocular pressure (IOP), and such studies are currently ongoing but have yet to be published.

Human perfused anterior segments were perfused with short interfering RNA (siRNA) targeting matrix Gla protein (MGP). MGP transcripts as measured by reverse transcriptase-PCR (RT-PCR) were reduced by at least 93% in these eyes.[37] In a separate experiment, glucocorticoid receptor (GR) siRNA was perfused for 48 h, followed by perfusion with dexamethasone for 24 h. Dexamethasone is a potent steroid known to bind to GR and induce expression of myocilin, a gene associated with juvenile open-angle glaucoma.[49] A reduction of MGP and myocilin gene expression was noted by RT-PCR, and protein expression downregulation was confirmed by Western blot.[37] This experiment suggests that the IOP-elevating effects of steroids could be blocked by pretreatment with GR siRNA.

NEUROPROTECTION OF RETINAL GANGLION CELLS

Due to the high efficiency of AAV vectors to transduce RGCs after intravitreal injection, the majority of studies attempting neuroprotection have employed AAV to deliver transgenes of interest to the retina. Initial studies using AAV to deliver reporter genes such as GFP or lacZ demonstrated no inflammation and persistence of transgene expression for up to 12 months.[50,51] Neurotrophins and their receptors were among the first transgenes explored in neuroprotective gene therapy experiments. TrkB is a receptor for the neurotrophin brain-derived neurotrophic factor (BDNF), which is important for RGC homeostasis. In an experimental monkey glaucoma model, interruption of BDNF retrograde transport and accumulation of TrkB at the optic nerve head was noted, suggesting a role for neurotrophin deprivation in the pathogenesis of RGC death

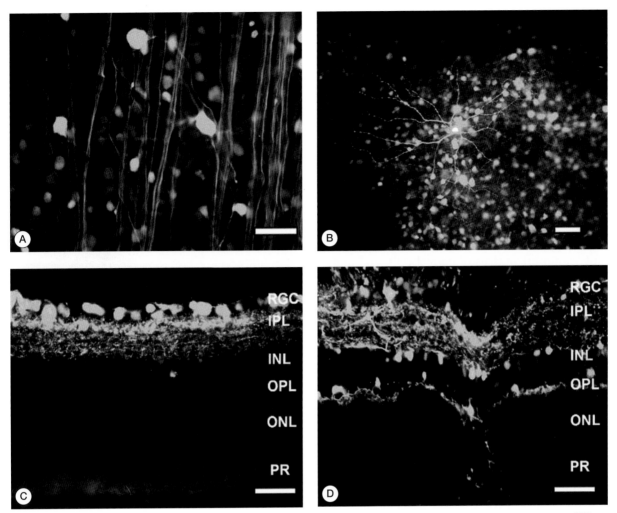

FIGURE 55.5 Transfection of rat retina with AAV-CBA-GFP-WPRE vector. **(A)** Individual RGCs and their axons clearly express GFP. **(B)** Dendritic trees of RGCs are also clearly seen. **(C)** GFP-labeled cells are localized almost exclusively to the RGC layer in retinal cross-sections. **(D)** In the immediate vicinity of the injection site, inner retinal cells are also transfected. RGC, retinal ganglion cell; IPL, inner plexiform layer; INL, inner nuclear layer; OPL, outer plexiform layer; ONL, outer nuclear layer; PR, photoreceptors. Bars, 50 μm (From Martin KR, Klein RL, Quigley HA. Gene delivery to the eye using adeno-associated viral vectors. Methods 2002; 28:267–275.[20])

in glaucoma.[52] After optic nerve axotomy (an acute injury model in which 90% of RGCs die by 2 weeks), TrkB mRNA was noted to decrease to approximately 50% of levels seen in intact retinas.[53] AAV vector incorporating a CMV promoter was used to direct expression of either TrkB or GFP (control) in RGCs after intravitreal injection in rats. One week later, the optic nerves of the treated eyes were axotomized. Two weeks after axotomy, RGC survival was compared between the control AAV-GFP eyes and the AAV-TrkB eyes augmented with exogenous BDNF administration. Survival in the AAV-TrkB/BDNF group was 76%, compared to less than 10% in the AAV-GFP group.[53] In a similar experiment, AAV incorporating the CBA promoter and WPRE was used to direct expression of BDNF or GFP in RGCs after intravitreal injection in rats (Fig. 55.5). Two weeks later, argon laser was applied to the trabecular meshwork, causing aqueous humor outflow obstruction and subsequent IOP elevation. After 4 weeks of elevated IOP exposure, RGC survival was assessed by axon counting of optic nerve cross-sections. Mean axon

survival was significantly increased in the AAV-BDNF-WPRE group (67.7%) when compared to the control AAV-GFP-WPRE group (47.7%).[54] These studies show the potential for neuroprotection of injured RGCs using neurotrophin replacement by AAV gene therapy.

Modulation of programmed cell death, or 'apoptosis,' is an attractive strategy for neuroprotection, as RGCs are known to die by apoptosis in human glaucoma.[55] Endogenous inhibitors of apoptosis proteins (IAPs) are evolutionarily conserved proteins known to directly inhibit caspases, the effector proteases of the apoptotic cascade.[56] Rats were given unilateral intravitreal injections of AAV-CBA vector coding for human baculoviral IAP repeat-containing protein-4 (BIRC4), a potent caspase inhibitor. Ocular hypertension was induced in the same eye by sclerosis of aqueous humor outflow channels with hypertonic saline.[57] After 12 weeks of chronic exposure to elevated IOP, optic nerve axon counts were performed to determine the neuroprotective effects of retinal BIRC4 expression, and axon survival was compared between AAV-BIRC4 and control AAV-GFP groups. AAV-BIRC4 gene therapy significantly promoted mean optic nerve axon survival (49.7%) when compared AAV-GFP (22.3%).[22] Following optic nerve axotomy in rats, RGC death is preceded by an early upregulation of the pro-apoptotic protein Bax.[58] After injection of antisense Bax oligonucleotides in the temporal superior retina of rats, the number of RGCs surviving 8 days after optic nerve transection was increased when compared to eyes receiving control oligonucleotides. However, this neuroprotective effect was not seen at 14 days, suggesting that limitations in transfection efficiency and short half-lives limit the use of antisense oligonucleotides for neuroprotection of RGCs.[59]

Intracellular signaling pathways involved in cell death are also targets for neuroprotection of RGCs using AAV gene therapy. The transcription factor Max is found mostly within the nucleus of normal cells, and undergoes exclusion from the nucleus early in the apoptotic cascade in RGCs.[60] AAV was used to overexpress Max in rat RGCs after intravitreal injection. Cell morphology was preserved in retinal explants from eyes treated with AAV-Max, when compared to retinal explants from uninjected control eyes.[61] The extracellular signal-regulated kinase (Erk)1/2 pathway is an evolutionarily conserved mechanism used by several peptide factors to promote cell survival. AAV coding for MEK1, an upstream activator of Erk1/2, was injected into rat eyes 3 weeks prior to IOP elevation induced by episcleral injection of hypertonic saline. After 7 weeks of exposure to chronic IOP elevation, AAV-MEK treatment significantly increased mean RGC survival (1366 RGCs/mm^2 retina) when compared to AAV-GFP treatment (680 RGCs/mm^2).[62] Basic fibroblast growth factor (FGF-2) is a member of the fibroblast growth factor (FGF) family of neurotrophic factors that are involved in neuronal survival and synaptic plasticity. FGF-1 is known to be a potent stimulator of developmental RGC axon growth and is correlated with activation of the Erk1/2 pathway. Adult rat eyes were given intravitreal injections of AAV coding for FGF-2, followed by partial optic nerve crush injury. Although only transient neuroprotection of RGCs was noted, FGF-2 gene transfer led to a 10-fold increase in the number of axons extending 0.5 mm distal to the lesion site when compared to control nerves. These exciting findings show that factors mediating axon outgrowth during development may promote regeneration of injured adult RGC axons.[63,64]

Summary

Glaucoma is uniquely well suited to gene therapy. The trabecular meshwork or Schlemm's canal can be targeted by anterior chamber injection due to aqueous humor outflow, and RGCs can be targeted with intravitreal injection due to their proximal inner retinal location to the vitreous. Although these efforts are still in their relative infancy, successful gene therapy experiments have been directed toward modification of trabecular meshwork extracellular matrix and cytoskeleton components using adenovirus and lentivirus constructs, and modulation of apoptosis and intracellular signaling pathways in RGCs has been achieved with AAV constructs. However, idiosyncratic immune responses leading to human deaths have been reported using systemic administration of both adenoviral and AAV vectors. The decreased amount of viral vector used for ocular administration should reduce this risk considerably, but caution is certainly warranted with any human gene therapy that is undertaken. Nonviral techniques are also being employed for gene transfer, using cationic lipid delivery systems (lipofection) or the use of electric current (electroporation) to deliver DNA sequences into target cells. These nonviral techniques provide a complementary approach that could minimize the immune responses that can limit therapeutic viral vector gene transfer trials.[65]

REFERENCES

1. Rapp F. Nature and classification of viruses. In: Stringfellow DA, ed. Virology. Kalamazoo, MI: Upjohn; 1986:9–20.

2. Shenk T. Group C adenoviruses as vectors for gene therapy. In: Kaplitt MG, Loewy AD, eds. Viral vectors. Gene therapy and neuroscience applications. San Diego, CA: Academic Press; 1995:43–55.

3. Borras T. Recent developments in ocular gene therapy. Exp Eye Res 2003; 76:643–652.

4. Nevins JR. E2F: a link between the Rb tumor suppressor protein and viral oncoproteins. Science 1992; 258:424–429.

5. Sarnow P, Ho YS, Williams J, et al. Adenovirus E1b-58kd tumor antigen and SV40 large tumor antigen are physically associated with the same 54 kd cellular protein in transformed cells. Cell 1982; 28:387–394.

6. Wold WS, Gooding LR. Region E3 of adenovirus: a cassette of genes involved in host immunosurveillance and virus-cell interactions. Virology 1991; 184:1–8.

7. Engelhardt JF, Ye X, Doranz B, et al. Ablation of E2A in recombinant adenoviruses improves transgene persistence and decreases inflammatory response in mouse liver. Proc Natl Acad Sci USA 1994; 91:6196–6200.

8. Snyder RO, Flotte TR. Production of clinical-grade recombinant adeno-associated virus vectors. Curr Opin Biotechnol 2002; 13:418–423.

9. Flotte TR, Afione SA, Zeitlin PL. Adeno-associated virus vector gene expression occurs in nondividing cells in the absence of vector DNA integration. Am J Respir Cell Mol Biol 1994; 11:517–521.

10. Peel AL, Klein RL. Adeno-associated virus vectors: activity and applications in the CNS. J Neurosci Methods 2000; 98:95–104.

11. Duan D, Sharma P, Yang J, et al. Circular intermediates of recombinant adeno-associated virus have defined structural characteristics responsible for long-term episomal persistence in muscle tissue. J Virol 1998; 72:8568–8577.

12. Woo YJ, Zhang JC, Taylor MD, et al. One year transgene expression with adeno-associated virus cardiac gene transfer. Int J Cardiol 2005; 100:421–426.

13. Cearley CN, Wolfe JH. Transduction characteristics of adeno-associated virus vectors expressing cap serotypes 7, 8, 9, and Rh10 in the mouse brain. Mol Ther 2006; 13:528–537.

14. Duan D, Yue Y, Engelhardt JF. Expanding AAV packaging capacity with trans-splicing or overlapping vectors: a quantitative comparison. Mol Ther 2001; 4:383–391.

15. Hauswirth WW, Lewin AS, Zolotukhin S, et al. Production and purification of recombinant adeno-associated virus. Methods Enzymol 2000; 316:743–761.

16. White JM. Viral and cellular membrane fusion proteins. Annu Rev Physiol 1990; 52:675–697.

17. Baltimore D. RNA-dependent DNA polymerase in virions of RNA tumour viruses. Nature 1970; 226:1209–1211.

18. McDermott KW, Luskin MB. The use of retroviral vectors in the study of cell lineage and migration during the development of the mammalian central nervous system. In: Kaplitt MG, Loewy AD, eds. Viral vectors. Gene therapy and neuroscience applications. San Diego, CA: Academic Press; 1995:411–433.

19. Logan AC, Lutzko C, Kohn DB. Advances in lentiviral vector design for gene-modification of hematopoietic stem cells. Curr Opin Biotechnol 2002; 13:429–436.

20. Martin KR, Klein RL, Quigley HA. Gene delivery to the eye using adeno-associated viral vectors. Methods 2002; 28:267–275.

21. Fitzsimons HL, Bland RJ, During MJ. Promoters and regulatory elements that improve adeno-associated virus transgene expression in the brain. Methods 2002; 28:227–236.

22. McKinnon SJ, Lehman DM, Tahzib NG, et al. Baculoviral IAP repeat-containing-4 protects optic nerve axons in a rat glaucoma model. Mol Ther 2002; 5:780–787.

23. Gonzalez P, Caballero M, Liton PB, et al. Expression analysis of the matrix GLA protein and VE-cadherin gene promoters in the outflow pathway. Invest Ophthalmol Vis Sci 2004; 45:1389–1395.

24. Heimark RL, Kaochar S, Stamer WD. Human Schlemm's canal cells express the endothelial adherens proteins, VE-cadherin and PECAM-1. Curr Eye Res 2002; 25:299–308.

25. Donello JE, Loeb JE, Hope TJ. Woodchuck hepatitis virus contains a tripartite posttranscriptional regulatory element. J Virol 1998; 72:5085–5092.

26. Paterna JC, Moccetti T, Mura A, et al. Influence of promoter and WHV post-transcriptional regulatory element on AAV-mediated transgene expression in the rat brain. Gene Ther 2000; 7:1304–1311.

27. Klein RL, Hamby ME, Gong Y, et al. Dose and promoter effects of adeno-associated viral vector for green fluorescent protein expression in the rat brain. Exp Neurol 2002; 176:66–74.

28. Schwarzbauer JE, Patel RS, Fonda D, et al. Multiple sites of alternative splicing of the rat fibronectin gene transcript. EMBO J 1987; 6:2573–2580.

29. Haberman RP, Samulski RJ, McCown TJ. Attenuation of seizures and neuronal death by adeno-associated virus vector galanin expression and secretion. Nat Med 2003; 9:1076–1080.

30. Martinez-Salas E. Internal ribosome entry site biology and its use in expression vectors. Curr Opin Biotechnol 1999; 10:458–464.

31. Corbel SY, Rossi FM. Latest developments and in vivo use of the Tet system: ex vivo and in vivo delivery of tetracycline-regulated genes. Curr Opin Biotechnol 2002; 13:448–452.

32. Baron U, Bujard H. Tet repressor-based system for regulated gene expression in eukaryotic cells: principles and advances. Methods Enzymol 2000; 327:401–421.

33. Crooke ST. Progress in antisense technology: the end of the beginning. Methods Enzymol 2000; 313:3–45.

34. Sazani P, Vacek MM, Kole R. Short-term and long-term modulation of gene expression by antisense therapeutics. Curr Opin Biotechnol 2002; 13:468–472.

35. Summerton J, Weller D. Morpholino antisense oligomers: design, preparation, and properties. Antisense Nucleic Acid Drug Dev 1997; 7:187–195.

36. Summerton J. Morpholino antisense oligomers: the case for an RNase H-independent structural type. Biochim Biophys Acta 1999; 1489:141–158.

37. Comes N, Borras T. Functional delivery of synthetic naked siRNA to the human trabecular meshwork in perfused organ cultures. Mol Vis 2007; 13:1363–1374.

38. Cashman SM, Bowman L, Christofferson J, et al. Inhibition of choroidal neovascularization by adenovirus-mediated delivery of short hairpin RNAs targeting VEGF as a potential therapy for AMD. Invest Ophthalmol Vis Sci 2006; 47:3496–3504.

39. Borras T, Rowlette LL, Erzurum SC, et al. Adenoviral reporter gene transfer to the human trabecular meshwork does not alter aqueous humor outflow. Relevance for potential gene therapy of glaucoma. Gene Ther 1999; 6:515–524.

40. Borras T, Gabelt BT, Klintworth GK, et al. Non-invasive observation of repeated adenoviral GFP gene delivery to the anterior segment of the monkey eye in vivo. J Gene Med 2001; 3:437–449.

41. Stamer WD, Peppel K, O'Donnell ME, et al. Expression of aquaporin-1 in human trabecular meshwork cells: role in resting cell volume. Invest Ophthalmol Vis Sci 2001; 42:1803–1811.

42. Kee C, Sohn S, Hwang JM. Stromelysin gene transfer into cultured human trabecular cells and rat trabecular meshwork in vivo. Invest Ophthalmol Vis Sci 2001; 42:2856–2860.

43. Vittitow JL, Garg R, Rowlette LL, et al. Gene transfer of dominant-negative RhoA increases outflow facility in perfused human anterior segment cultures. Mol Vis 2002; 8:32–44.

44. Liu X, Hu Y, Filla MS, et al. The effect of C3 transgene expression on actin and cellular adhesions in cultured human trabecular meshwork cells and on outflow facility in organ cultured monkey eyes. Mol Vis 2005; 11:1112–1121.

45. Gabelt BT, Hu Y, Vittitow JL, et al. Caldesmon transgene expression disrupts focal adhesions in HTM cells and increases outflow facility in organ-cultured human and monkey anterior segments. Exp Eye Res 2006; 82:935–944.

46. Loewen N, Fautsch MP, Peretz M, et al. Genetic modification of human trabecular meshwork with lentiviral vectors. Hum Gene Ther 2001; 12:2109–2119.

47. Loewen N, Fautsch MP, Teo WL, et al. Long-term, targeted genetic modification of the aqueous humor outflow tract coupled with noninvasive imaging of gene expression in vivo. Invest Ophthalmol Vis Sci 2004; 45:3091–3098.

48. Loewen N, Bahler C, Teo WL, et al. Preservation of aqueous outflow facility after second-generation FIV vector-mediated expression of marker genes in anterior segments of human eyes. Invest Ophthalmol Vis Sci 2002; 43:3686–3690.

49. Nguyen TD, Chen P, Huang WD, et al. Gene structure and properties of TIGR, an olfactomedin-related glycoprotein cloned from glucocorticoid-induced trabecular meshwork cells. J Biol Chem 1998; 273:6341–6350.

50. Dudus L, Anand V, Acland GM, et al. Persistent transgene product in retina, optic nerve and brain after intraocular injection of rAAV. Vision Res 1999; 39:2545–2553.

51. Guy J, Qi X, Muzyczka N, et al. Reporter expression persists 1 year after adeno-associated virus-mediated gene transfer to the optic nerve. Arch Ophthalmol 1999; 117:929–937.

52. Pease ME, McKinnon SJ, Quigley HA, et al. Obstructed axonal transport of BDNF and its receptor TrkB in experimental glaucoma. Invest Ophthalmol Vis Sci 2000; 41:764–774.

53. Cheng L, Sapieha P, Kittlerova P, et al. TrkB gene transfer protects retinal ganglion cells from axotomy-induced death in vivo. J Neurosci 2002; 22:3977–3986.

54. Martin KR, Quigley HA, Zack DJ, et al. Gene therapy with brain-derived neurotrophic factor as a protection: retinal ganglion cells in a rat glaucoma model. Invest Ophthalmol Vis Sci 2003; 44:4357–4365.

55. Kerrigan LA, Zack DJ, Quigley HA, et al. TUNEL-positive ganglion cells in human primary open-angle glaucoma. Arch Ophthalmol 1997; 115:1031–1035.

56. Takahashi R, Deveraux Q, Tamm I, et al. A single BIR domain of XIAP sufficient for inhibiting caspases. J Biol Chem 1998; 273:7787–7790.

57. Morrison JC, Moore CG, Deppmeier LM, et al. A rat model of chronic pressure-induced optic nerve damage. Exp Eye Res 1997; 64:85–96.

58. Isenmann S, Wahl C, Krajewski S, et al. Up-regulation of Bax protein in degenerating retinal ganglion cells precedes apoptotic cell death after optic nerve lesion in the rat. Eur J Neurosci 1997; 9:1763–1772.

59. Isenmann S, Engel S, Gillardon F, et al. Bax antisense oligonucleotides reduce axotomy-induced retinal ganglion cell death in vivo by reduction of Bax protein expression. Cell Death Differ 1999; 6:673–682.

60. Petrs-Silva H, de Freitas FG, Linden R, et al. Early nuclear exclusion of the transcription factor max is associated with retinal ganglion cell death independent of caspase activity. J Cell Physiol 2004; 198:179–187.

61. Petrs-Silva H, Chiodo V, Chiarini LB, et al. Modulation of the expression of the transcription factor Max in rat retinal ganglion cells by a recombinant adeno-associated viral vector. Braz J Med Biol Res 2005; 38:375–379.

62. Zhou Y, Pernet V, Hauswirth WW, et al. Activation of the extracellular signal-regulated kinase 1/2 pathway by AAV gene transfer protects retinal ganglion cells in glaucoma. Mol Ther 2005; 12:402–412.

63. Sapieha PS, Peltier M, Rendahl KG, et al. Fibroblast growth factor-2 gene delivery stimulates axon growth by adult retinal ganglion cells after acute optic nerve injury. Mol Cell Neurosci 2003; 24:656–672.

64. Sapieha PS, Hauswirth WW, Di Polo A. Extracellular signal-regulated kinases 1/2 are required for adult retinal ganglion cell axon regeneration induced by fibroblast growth factor-2. J Neurosci Res 2006; 83:985–995.

65. Kachi S, Oshima Y, Esumi N, et al. Nonviral ocular gene transfer. Gene Ther 2005; 12:843–851.

Ultrastructural Imaging

Aachal Kotecha and Frederick W Fitzke

INTRODUCTION

The eyes are often seen as the windows to the soul, but they are also portals that enable a view of the complex internal structures of one of the primary sense organs of the human body. The advances in computer and laser technology that have emerged in the last two decades of twentieth century have led to the development of devices that can image microscopic details of the internal ocular structures in vivo in real time.

These technological advances offer an unprecedented opportunity to develop methods to assess the structure and function of individual retinal cells and their connections in vivo, having implications for the development of new treatments for hitherto irreversible blinding conditions. But that lies in the future. The purpose of this chapter is to review the current instrumentation that provides a high-resolution, or ultrastructural, view of fundal features, with specific reference to developments in scanning laser ophthalmoscopy and optical coherence tomography technologies.

A BRIEF HISTORY OF FUNDAL IMAGING

Leonardo da Vinci is credited with the discovery that it was the retina and optic nerve, not the crystalline lens, that facilitated vision.[1] However, it was over 300 years after this 'discovery' that it became possible to view these structures in vivo following the development of the direct ophthalmoscope in the mid-nineteenth century.[2,3] Although initially poorly received by the ophthalmological community, within a decade of its introduction the ophthalmoscope revolutionized the specialty and had a major impact on the understanding of many eye diseases. Von Jaeger published the first atlas of fundus drawings in 1869, with particular reference to fundal changes observed in glaucoma.[4,5] Attempts were made to produce permanent records of fundal appearance in the late nineteenth century, and the first commercially available fundus camera was introduced in the early twentieth century by Nordeson.[6] In 1949, a team led by Harold Ridley at St. Thomas' Hospital in London attempted to produce televised ophthalmoscopy. The

system, developed with the help of Marconi Engineering, was based on an indirect ophthalmoscope and, while successful, it proved impractical to use routinely.[7]

LIMITATIONS OF FUNDAL VIEWING USING CONVENTIONAL OPHTHALMOSCOPY

When viewing the fundus, the pupil is used to both illuminate and view the area of interest. The incident and reflected light pass through a series of ocular tissues of different refractive indices, the value of which varies with changes in tissue hydration. Refraction, reflection, and absorption of light occur at tissue interfaces, significantly attenuating rays. This is particularly apparent when using polychromatic light, such as white light, as each wavelength will be altered by different amplitudes at each interface. Thus, the traditional view of the fundus using the conventional ophthalmoscope is limited and requires a dilated pupil for optimum viewing.

Some of these limitations are overcome by using monochromatic light for fundal imaging. The stratified layers of the fundus have different absorption and reflection characteristics, therefore details of individual layers are better seen using light of a single wavelength.[8] Shorter-wavelength light is predominantly reflected by the superficial retinal layers and is used to view macula pigmentation and arcuate nerve fiber bundles. The deeper retinal and choroidal vasculature become visible with the use of longer-wavelength light, particularly in lightly pigmented fundi. With wavelengths of 600 nm or more there is an increase in light penetration and choroidal vasculature becomes visible in highly pigmented eyes, while near-infrared imaging is most useful for investigating subretinal structures.[9,10]

ULTRASTRUCTURAL IMAGING WITH THE SCANNING LASER OPHTHALMOSCOPE

INTRODUCTION

Developed in 1980, the scanning laser ophthalmoscope (SLO) provides a high-quality image of the fundus using

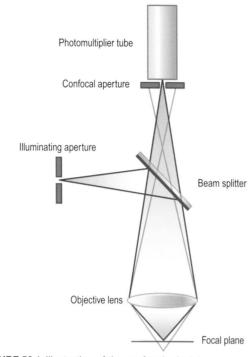

Photomultiplier tube

Confocal aperture

Illuminating aperture

Beam splitter

Objective lens

Focal plane

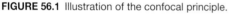

FIGURE 56.1 Illustration of the confocal principle.

a fraction of the light required to illuminate the fundus with conventional light ophthalmoscopy.[11] The fundus is illuminated with a small spot of monochromatic laser light that sweeps across it in a raster fashion. Reflected light is collected by a light detector and a real-time, piece-by-piece image of the fundus is produced on a digital monitor. As the SLO only illuminates a small area of the fundus at any one time, only a small amount of the patient's pupil is used for illumination, allowing the rest of it to be available for light collection. This is quite different from conventional indirect ophthalmoscopy, where almost the whole pupil is used for illumination and approximately one-tenth of the pupil is used for fundal viewing.

Most SLO systems are confocal, whereby a pinhole is placed in front of the detector, conjugate to the laser plane of focus. In this confocal mode, light that is reflected or scattered by structures at different depths and lateral locations is blocked by the pinhole, thus removing the masking reflections that would otherwise degrade the final image (Fig. 56.1). The size of the pinhole determines the degree of confocality, such that a small pinhole aperture will give a highly confocal image, although the minimum aperture size is restricted by diffraction limits.[12] The image produced is a narrow optical section of the area of fundus under investigation. Unlike conventional ophthalmic imaging, where objects outside the plane of interest contribute to the final image, in the confocal SLO (cSLO) the contrast is improved. However, due to the diffraction limits of the eye, axial resolution with the cSLO is limited to approximately 300 μm.[13] Because of this, cSLO cannot be used for true axial sectioning of the fundus.[14]

IMPROVING THE RESOLUTION OF CONFOCAL SCANNING LASER OPHTHALMOSCOPE IMAGES (I): IMAGE PROCESSING METHODS

In a perfect optical imaging system, the image of a point object would be a point. However, due to the diffraction of light at the edges of the optical system, in reality the image is a pattern that spreads over a finite area. The optics of the cSLO are designed to compensate for most aberrations but a number remain which affect image resolution. However, following capture it is possible to improve the detail within the image using image processing methods.

Image processing methods can improve the quality of images by either:

1. Recovering original information about the area of interest by improving the signal-to-noise ratio,
2. Extending the effective resolution of the image by using deconvolution methods, or
3. Enhancing the image by improving its esthetic appearance without actually increasing the amount of available information.

In vivo images of the human foveal photoreceptor mosaic and optic nerve lamina cribrosa have been obtained using the cSLO. In cSLO imaging, pixels that should have relatively uniform reflectance in regions of the image may appear to vary in value due to electronic noise within the imaging system. This variation in pixel value is known as *noise* and the ratio of the contrast within an image that is due to actual difference within the object scene and the contrast caused by the noise level is termed the *signal-to-noise ratio* (SNR). When the SNR is low, features within the image may appear almost invisible to the observer. By adding together frames of the same object scene, there is an improvement in the quality of the image that is proportional to the square root of the number of frames.[15] This technique is termed *averaging*. With averaging, it is important that the pixels within the object scene are in the same position in each frame. The living human eye is not perfectly stable, even in subjects with excellent fixation, and is prone to involuntary, saccadic eye movements. With ocular imaging it is therefore necessary to align individual frames to each other before the averaging process.

Ultrastructural imaging with the confocal scanning laser ophthalmoscope using image processing methods Figures 56.2 and 56.3 are images taken using a prototype Carl Zeiss (Jena GmbH) SLO at the UCL Institute of Ophthalmology, London, using a helium neon laser light source of wavelength 633 nm. Photoreceptors (see Fig. 56.2) were imaged using a micro-scanning attachment fixed to the front of the cSLO which generated a 2.5° scan angle. Sixty-four scans taken at a single retinal plane and location were aligned and averaged to produce the final image. The figure shown is a montage of averaged images from different retinal eccentricities. Lamina cribrosa images (see Fig. 56.3) were acquired

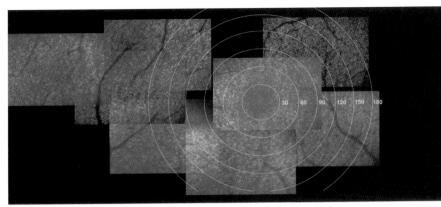

FIGURE 56.2 Retinal foveal photoreceptor mosaic taken with the cSLO.

using a 20° scan angle. The upper figure (Fig. 56.3A) is produced from the alignment and averaging of 32 individual frames, while the lower figure (Fig. 56.3B) is a result of further image processing of the averaged image, using a 'blind' deconvolution techique.

A more recent application of the cSLO in experimental models has been in imaging retinal ganglion cells (RGCs). Studies have suggested that RGC death in glaucoma involves the apoptosis pathway and excessive activation of glutamate receptors on cell membranes is greatly implicated in the apoptotic process.[16] The use of the fluorescent-labeled protein marker annexin-5 has been employed to view the RGC apoptotic process in vivo. Annexin-5 has a high affinity for the phospholipid phosphatidylserine (PS) found on the inner cell membrane of RCGs. In the early stages of the apoptotic process, PS becomes externalized and it is possible that this may be visualized in vivo by annexin-5 labeling techniques, using appropriate imaging wavelengths and pass-filters in the cSLO. This technique for imaging apoptotic cells has been applied only to animal models and has yet to be verified in humans.

IMPROVING THE RESOLUTION OF CONFOCAL SCANNING LASER OPHTHALMOSCOPE IMAGES (II): ADAPTIVE OPTICS SCANNING LASER OPHTHALMOSCOPE

Image processing techniques can restore information within the image that may have been lost in the image capturing technique but they cannot compensate for the ocular aberrations that degrade the image. Adaptive optics (AO) is a technology initially developed for the field of astronomics and improves the performance of optical systems by compensating for the effects of rapidly changing aberrations. In astronomical imaging using Earth-based telescopic systems, turbulence in the Earth's atmosphere produce inhomogeneities in the air refractive index that results in a distortion of the final image. AO works by measuring and rapidly compensating for atmospheric changes on image quality by either using deformable mirrors or materials with variable refractive properties. Although the technique of AO was theoretically understood for many years it was only

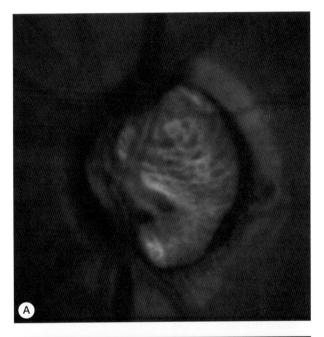

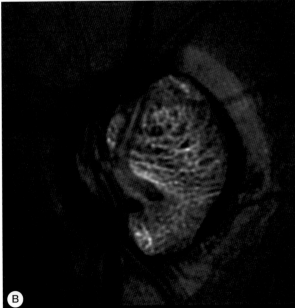

FIGURE 56.3 Lamina cribrosa images **(A)** after averaging and **(B)** after further image processing.

advances in computer technology during the 1990s that finally made the technique practical.

A form of AO was first used in cSLO retinal imaging by Dreher and colleagues who used *active optics* to correct for aberrations induced by the cornea and lens when imaging the fundus with a dilated pupil.[12] In their system, collimated laser light was passed into the eye and the reflected light was relayed to a 13-segment adjustable mirror. Using this set-up, aberrations were measured and compensated in the same way as that used for astronomical imaging. However, this method of optical compensation works on a much longer time scale than true AO and only really corrects for corneal and lenticular astigmatism. However, with this set-up the axial resolution of their cSLO system improved from 400 μm to approximately 200 μm.

Measurement of ocular aberrations was greatly improved with the development of the Hartmann-Shack wavefront sensor in 1994.[17] The design of the sensor was first proposed in 1900 by a German astronomer, Johannes Franz Hartmann, and built in 1971 by Shack

and Platt.[18] The sensor consists of an array of lenses (called lenslets) of equal focal length, each focused onto a charge-coupled device (CCD) array (Fig 56.4). As a waveform passes across the lenslets, the relative tilt of the waveform across each lens can be calculated from the position of the focal spot on the CCD. Any phase shift in the waveform can be approximated to a set of discrete tilts. By sampling an array of lenslets, all of these tilts can be measured and the whole wavefront approximated.

Ultrastructural imaging with the adaptive optics scanning laser ophthalmoscope

A Hartmann-Shack wavefront sensor was first used in retinal imaging in 1997.[19] A laser light source was used to illuminate the fundus and the reflected waveform was analyzed by the wavefront sensor. High-order aberrations caused by the eye's optics were compensated by a deformable mirror. The set-up not only allowed photographic images of the retinal cone mosaic, but it also improved the functional vision of the subjects assessed, allowing them to resolve fine gratings that were otherwise invisible in the non-AO compensated eye.

The use of the Hartmann-Shack sensor and deformable mirror compensation in SLO imaging was first described in 2002 by Austin Roorda et al.[20] Compensation of aberrations was achieved at a frequency of 5 MHz. The set-up enabled high-resolution axial retinal scanning from the nerve fiber layer through to the retinal cone mosaic. Real-time high-resolution imaging of retinal blood flow through the capillaries adjacent to the foveal avascular zone was also permitted. The AO compensation improved SLO axial resolution to approximately 2.5 μm and transverse resolution to 100 μm. Recently, the Roorda group has used the adaptive optics scanning laser ophthalmoscope (AOSLO) to image the lamina cribrosa. Figure 56.5 shows images of the lamina cribrosa acquired with the AOSLO.

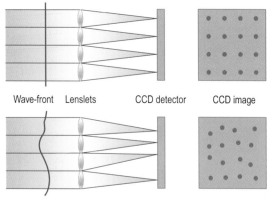

FIGURE 56.4 Principal of the Hartmann–Shack wavefront sensor. (With kind permission from Andrei Tokovinin, Cerro Tololo Inter-American Observatory, La Serena, Chile.)

Experimental Glaucoma

Normal

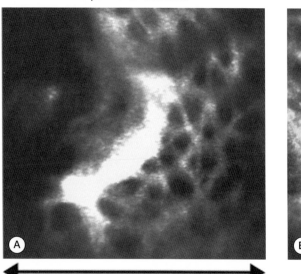

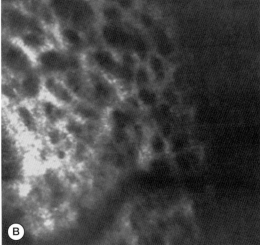

2.5 degrees, ~600 microns

FIGURE 56.5 Lamina cribrosa images of 2 monkey eyes taken using AOSLO (reproduced from Vilipuru AS, Rangaswamy NV, Frishman LJ. An adaptive optics scanning to laser ophthalmoscopy for in vivo imaging of lamina cribrosa. J Opt Soc Am A Opt image Sci Vis 2007; 24:1417–1425. With kind permission of the Optical Society of America)

ULTRASTRUCTURAL IMAGING WITH OPTICAL COHERENCE TOMOGRAPHY

INTRODUCTION

Optical coherence tomography (OCT) was first described for use in retinal imaging in 1991.[21] The principle behind OCT is analogous to ultrasound imaging, a widely used technique that allows visualization of internal structures and pathologies of the body by observing the acoustic echo of internally projected sound waves. Ultrasound imaging requires direct contact of the measuring device onto the area of interest. Typical diagnostic ultrasound scanners operate in the frequency range of 2–13 MHz; sound wave frequencies of 10 MHz yield spatial resolutions of 150 μm. The choice of frequency determines both the depth of tissue penetration and the resolution of the image obtained. Lower frequencies give less resolution but greater imaging depth, while higher frequencies are strongly attenuated by biological tissues, limiting their use to imaging the anterior segment of the eye.[22]

With OCT, instead of observing acoustic echoes from internal structures, the magnitude and time delay of light reflected from microstructures is assessed. The OCT system uses *low coherence interferometry* to make micron (μm)-depth measurements of the structure under observation. 'Coherence' describes the correlation between waveforms. When two perfectly coherent, anti-phase waveforms are combined, they will exhibit complete destructive interference (Fig. 56.6). Waveforms of different frequencies with a fixed relative-phase relationship, otherwise known as having 'low coherence,' will partially interfere to produce a waveform akin to a short 'pulse' of light (Fig. 56.7). The length of the pulse is also known as the 'coherence length.'

In time-domain OCT, a partially reflecting mirror splits incident low-coherent light into two paths (Fig. 56.8). One path is directed to the structure under investigation (in the case of fundal OCT imaging, this will be the retina) and the other to a scanning reference mirror. Light reflected from the fundus will consist of multiple 'echos' corresponding to the various retinal layers, while light reflected from the reference mirror will be at a known spatial position at any one point in time. The reflected light from the retina and the reference mirror will only coincide if they both arrive simultaneously at the detector within the coherence length,

which will only occur when they have both traveled the same distance. This will produce a phenomenon known as *interference*. The position of the reference mirror is altered so that the time delay from the mirror coincides with light reflected from the different structures within the eye. The position of the reference mirror is known and from this the relative depth of each reflective layer within the retina can be determined. Highly reflective areas will create large interference patterns; light scattered or reflected outside the coherence length will not interfere. The resultant reflectivity profile is an axial scan similar to the A-scan produced in ultrasound measurements. By mechanically scanning the reference mirror, a reflectivity profile of the sample can be obtained, similar to a B-scan. The resulting two-dimensional reflectivity profile is digitally processed and displayed as a gray-scale or false color image.

ADVANCES IN OPTICAL COHERENCE TOMOGRAPHY TECHNOLOGY

Ultra-high resolution optical coherence tomography

The axial resolution of OCT is determined by the coherence length of the light source and this is inversely proportional to the bandwidth of the light source. Light sources within the band 600 nm to 2000 nm are used as these are least affected by absorption by ocular structures.[13] Standard OCT systems use a superluminescent diode (SLD) source, which is relatively inexpensive but has limited axial resolution of the order of 10–15 μm.

Recent advances in laser technology have produced short-pulse, or *femtosecond*, solid-state lasers which generate ultra-broad bandwidth light.[23] The titanium sapphire (Ti:Al$_2$O$_3$) laser is an example of a broadband laser used in OCT imaging and generates pulses as short as 5.4 femtoseconds. This results in an axial

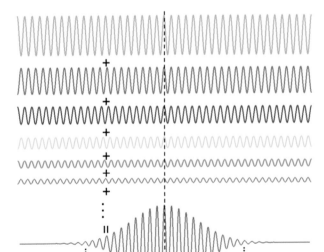

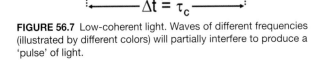

FIGURE 56.7 Low-coherent light. Waves of different frequencies (illustrated by different colors) will partially interfere to produce a 'pulse' of light.

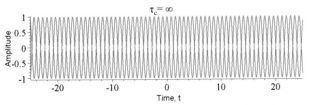

FIGURE 56.6 Perfectly coherent light. The two waveforms have exactly the same amplitude and frequency. When combined as shown, they will exhibit complete destructive interference.

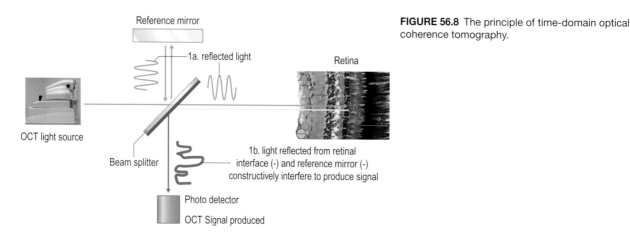

FIGURE 56.8 The principle of time-domain optical coherence tomography.

resolution of 2–3 μm,[23] enabling visualization of the individual corneal and intraretinal layers.[24,25] However, despite this vast improvement in axial resolution, image acquisition takes approximately 4 seconds. Therefore, image quality may be degraded by microsaccadic eye movements.

Ultra-high speed spectral domain optical coherence tomography

Frequency domain/spectral OCT (also known as Fourier-domain OCT) represents a further advance in OCT technology. In time-domain OCT, the speed at which an image is acquired is determined by the scanning speed of the reference mirror. However, in frequency-domain OCT the interference pattern generated by the light reflected from the reference mirror and retina is acquired with spectrally separated detectors. No mechanical scanning of the reference mirror is required as all the light reflected back from the internal eye is collected simultaneously. As a result, the time for image acquisition is dramatically increased; using a Ti:Al$_2$O$_3$ femtosecond laser a 2 μm axial resolution image can be obtained in 0.13 seconds, thereby virtually eliminating any motion artifacts from the scan.[26] A spectrometer within the detector of the interferometer measures the spectrum of reflected/backscattered light. This undergoes Fourier transformation to generate axial measurements of reflected light delay and magnitude. Fourier-domain OCT has been shown to be sensitive to even the weakest reflected light signals and therefore imaging can be performed with extremely low light level exposures.

Transverse resolution is determined by the smallest spot-size on the retina, which, when taking into account the diffraction limits of the eye, can theoretically approximate 10 μm. However, this value is never achieved, as scattering of light in deeper retinal structures will further degrade the image.

Three-dimensional retinal imaging with high-speed ultra-high resolution optical coherence tomography

Using OCT with Fourier-domain OCT it is possible to acquire three-dimensional datasets, generating volumetric images of the retina. Wojtkowski et al. have described a prototype system that has a PC-controlled galvanometer-actuated steering mirror to scan across the retina. The high-speed ultra-high resolution optical coherence tomography (UHROCT) acquires up to 16 000 axial scans per second, which corresponds to more than 30 images per second. As images are acquired so rapidly, they are relatively free from motion artifacts (Fig. 56.9).[26]

Polarization-sensitive optical coherence tomography

Light passing through the retinal nerve fiber layer (RNFL) will exhibit birefringence due to the regular, parallel arrangement of the RNFL microtubules. Scanning laser polarimetry techniques exploit this property of the RNFL and measure the retardation of reflected polarized light to identify areas of glaucomatous RNFL thinning around the optic nerve head. This technique is discussed in detail in Chapter 19. Polarization-sensitive OCT (PS-OCT) combines the high-resolution cross-sectional imaging capabilities of OCT with information on RNFL birefringence using polarized light. PS-OCT may provide a better contrast between the birefringent RNFL layer and other retinal layers and give a more accurate measure of RNFL thinning compared with standard scanning laser polarimetry techniques. In addition, because the RNFL is used as a reference, this method of measuring RNFL thickness is unaffected by corneal birefringence. This technique is still in its embryonic form and needs to be validated on larger numbers of normal and glaucomatous subjects before its role in the early detection of glaucoma can be elucidated.[27]

Optical Doppler tomography

Optical Doppler tomography (ODT) is an extension of OCT that is capable of high-resolution imaging and quantification of blood flow through the retinal vasculature. Both time- and spectral-domain OCT can provide a real-time measure of human retinal blood flow and flow dynamics in larger vessels. Ren and co-workers[28] have recently described a spectral-domain moving-scatterer-sensitive (MSS) technique for Doppler flow imaging, which suppresses the stationary scatterers on blood vessel walls to allow optical imaging of blood flow. The technique uses a Ti:Al$_2$O$_3$ laser light source and in flow phantom experiments the technique was shown to accurately measure flow in a capillary tube of 75 μm diameter. However, the technique still needs to be validated in vivo in humans.

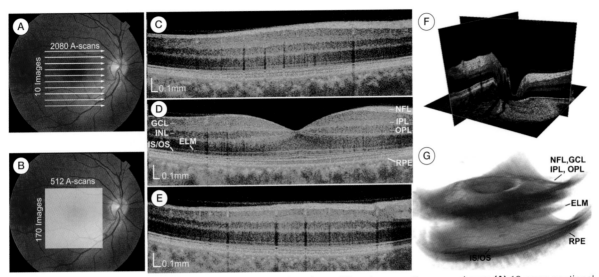

FIGURE 56.9 Ultra-fast ultra-high resolution OCT images. Examples of two different scan patterns are shown: **(A)** 10 cross-sectional images with 2048 transverse scans each, and **(B)** 170 images with 512 axial scans. **(C–E)** High-resolution scans of the macula. **(F)** Cross-sectional images along orthogonal planes of the optic disc generated from the 3-D OCT dataset. **(G)** Volume rendering of the macula from the 3-D data. Key: ELM, external limiting membrane; GCL, ganglion cell layer; INL, inner nuclear layer; IPL, inner plexiform layer; IS/OS, boundary between the inner and outer segments of the photoreceptors; NFL, nerve fiber layer; OPL, outer plexiform layer; RPE, retinal pigment epithelium. (Courtesy Professor James Fujimoto.[26])

Anterior segment optical coherence tomography

Imaging the anterior segment using OCT technology (ASOCT) was first described in 1994, when a modified posterior segment OCT was used to image the cornea and iris structures.[29] Recent advances in high-speed scanning and Fourier-domain image acquisition techniques, coupled with the use of longer wavelength light sources (1310 nm) that facilitate transscleral imaging, have enabled real-time, in vivo anterior chamber angle imaging (Figs 56.10 and 56.11).[30,31] This technique offers several advantages over traditional methods of viewing the anterior angle structures, primarily due to the noncontact nature and speedy image acquisition of the technique. This technique is covered in detail in Chapter 15.

THE FUTURE

Current techniques for fundal imaging have made a significant contribution to our understanding of the pathophysiology of many ocular diseases. Research within the area is advancing at a tremendous pace, from investigations into the use of adaptive optics OCT to provide volumetric measurements of photoreceptors in vivo to the use of functional ultra-fast, ultra-high resolution OCT as a noninvasive, noncontact analogue of electrophysiology, so termed 'optophysiology.' In the not so distant future, imaging techniques will be used as a substitute for histopathological analysis in determining the etiology of disease processes as well as the cellular nature of mass lesions. Indeed, research has already begun into the development of OCT methods to provide a noninvasive in vivo 'optical biopsy' for detection of early neoplastic changes at a subcellular level for earlier cancer diagnosis.

With advances in the field of nanotechnology, the future of ophthalmic imaging will have no boundaries. The use of nanotechnology molecular contrast agents

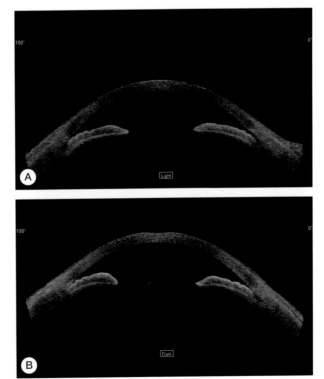

FIGURE 56.10 (A) ASOCT: narrow anterior chamber angle in light conditions. With the pupil constricted, the angles are clearly open, but narrow. (Taken with the Visante TM OCT; courtesy Andrew Scott, Research Fellow, Moorfields Eye Hospital.) **(B)** ASOCT: narrow anterior chamber angle in dark conditions. As the pupil dilates, the angle is obstructed by the peripheral iris. (Taken with the Visante TM OCT; courtesy Andrew Scott, Research Fellow, Moorfields Eye Hospital.)

in magnetic resonance and computed tomography imaging has enabled detailed assessments of the integrity of the blood–brain barrier and the perfusion of cerebral vasculature. Gold nanorods have been injected into the bloodstream and fluoresce when excited by infrared

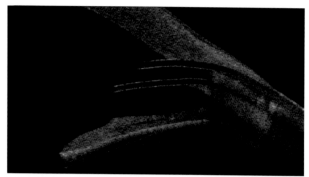

FIGURE 56.11 ASOCT image of aqueous shunt implant. (Taken with the Visante™ OCT; courtesy Andrew Scott, Research Fellow, Moorfields Eye Hospital.)

light (which has better penetration through skin), making it possible to visualize vasculature of the mouse earlobe in vivo.[32] The ability to observe the microcirculation in such detail holds possibilities for early cancer diagnosis. In the future, it may even be possible to develop miniscule remote controlled vehicles to be injected into the eye to image anterior and posterior segments in vivo in real time, enabling the visualization of normal anatomy, the progress of infectious agents, and disease processes. The advancements in technology appear almost unstoppable. With them will come an extraordinary evolution in methods to image the structure and function of the human body. The possibilities are endless.

REFERENCES

1. Wheeler JR. History of ophthalmology through the ages. Br J Ophthalmol 1946; 30:264–275.

2. Mark HH. The first ophthalmoscope? Adolf Kussmaul 1845. Arch Ophthalmol 1970; 84(4):520–521.

3. Chance B. The early years of Helmholtz: In: Commemoration of the centenary of the invention of the ophthalmoscope. Trans Am Ophthalmol Soc 1950; 48:23-35

4. Blanchard DL. Jaeger, about glaucoma. Doc Ophthalmol 1995; 89(1–2):185–191.

5. von Jaeger E. Ophthaloskopischer Handatlas. Vienna: Druck und Verlag der KK Hof und Staatsdruckerei; 1869.

6. Masters BR. Non-invasive diagnostic techniques in ophthalmology. In: Masters BR, ed. New York: Springer-Verlag; 1990.

7. Ridley H. Television in ophthalmology. XVI Concilium Ophthalmologicum Brittania Acta 1950; 2:1397–1404.

8. Delori FC, Gragoudas ES, Francisco R, et al. Monochromatic ophthalmoscopy and fundus photography The normal fundus. Arch Ophthalmol 1977; 95(5):861–868.

9. Delori FC, Gragoudas ES. Light source for monochromatic ophthalmoscopy and fluorescein angiography. Arch Ophthalmol 1979; 97(7):1349–1350.

10. Elsner AE, Burns SA, Weiter JJ, et al. Infrared imaging of subretinal structures in the human ocular fundus. Vision Res 1996; 36(1):191–205.

11. Webb RH, Hughes GW. Scanning laser ophthalmoscope. IEEE Trans Biomed Eng 1981; 28(7):488–492.

12. Dreher AW, Bille JF, Weinreb RN. Active optical depth resolution improvement of the laser tomographic scanner. Appl Optics 1989; 28(4):804–808.

13. Podoleanu AG. Optical coherence tomography. Br J Radiol. 2005; 79(935):976–988.

14. Weinreb RN, Dreher AW. Reproducibility and accuracy of topographic measurements of the optic nerve head with the laser tomographic scanner. In: Nasemann JE, Burk RO, eds. Laser scanning ophthalmoscopy and tomography. Berlin: Quintessenz; 1990.

15. Russ JC. The image processing handbook. 3rd edn. Boca Raton, FLA: CRC and IEEE Press; 1998.

16. Kaushik S, Pandav SS, Ram J. Neuroprotection in glaucoma. J Postgrad Med. 2003; 49(1):90–95.

17. Liang J, Grimm B, Goelz S, et al. Objective measurement of wave aberrations of the human eye with the use of a Hartmann-Shack wave-front sensor. J Opt Soc Am A Opt Image Sci Vis. 1994; 11(7):1949–1957.

18. Platt BC, Shack R. History and principles of Shack-Hartmann wavefront sensing. J Refract Surg. 2001; 17(5):S573–S577.

19. Liang J, Williams DR, Miller DT. Supernormal vision and high-resolution retinal imaging through adaptive optics. J Opt Soc Am A. 1997; 14(11):2884–2892.

20. Roorda A, Romero-Borja F, Donnelly WJ, et al. Adaptive optics scanning laser ophthalmoscopy. Optics Express. 2002; 10(9):405–412.

21. Huang D, Swanson EA, Lin CP, et al. Optical coherence tomography. Science 1991; 254(5035):1178–1181.

22. Pavlin CJ, McWhae JA, McGowan HD, et al. Ultrasound biomicroscopy of anterior segment tumors. Ophthalmology 1992; 99(8):1220–1228.

23. Drexler W, Morgner U, Ghanta RK, et al. Ultrahigh-resolution ophthalmic optical coherence tomography. Nat Med. 2001; 7(4):502–507.

24. Drexler W, Sattmann H, Hermann B, et al. Enhanced visualization of macular pathology with the use of ultrahigh-resolution optical coherence tomography. Arch Ophthalmol. 2003; 121(5):695–706.

25. Ko TH, Fujimoto JG, Schuman JS, et al. Comparison of ultrahigh- and standard-resolution optical coherence tomography for imaging macular pathology. Ophthalmology 2005; 112(11):1922.

26. Wojtkowski M, Srinivasan V, Fujimoto JG, et al. Three-dimensional retinal imaging with high-speed ultrahigh-resolution optical coherence tomography. Ophthalmology 2005; 112(10):1734–1746.

27. Cense B, Chen TC, Park BH, et al. Thickness and birefringence of healthy retinal nerve fiber layer tissue measured with polarization-sensitive optical coherence tomography. Invest Ophthalmol Vis Sci. 2004; 45(8):2012–2606.

28. Ren H, Sun T, MacDonald DJ, et al. Real-time in vivo blood-flow imaging by moving-scatterer-sensitive spectral-domain optical Doppler tomography. Opt Lett. 2006; 31(7):927–929.

29. Izatt JA, Hee MR, Swanson EA, et al. Micrometer-scale resolution imaging of the anterior eye in vivo with optical coherence tomography. Arch Ophthalmol. 1994; 112(12):1584–1589.

30. Radhakrishnan S, Rollins AM, Roth JE, et al. Real-time optical coherence tomography of the anterior segment at 1310 nm. Arch Ophthalmol. 2001; 119(8):1179–1185.

31. Radhakrishnan S, Goldsmith J, Huang D, et al. Comparison of optical coherence tomography and ultrasound biomicroscopy for detection of narrow anterior chamber angles. Arch Ophthalmol. 2005; 123(8):1053–1059.

32. Wang H, Huff TB, Zweifel DA, et al. In vitro and in vivo two-photon luminescence imaging of single gold nanorods. Proc Natl Acad Sci USA 2005; 102(44):15752–15756.

EMERGENCY CARE MANAGEMENT

CHAPTER 57

Acute Intraocular Pressure Rise

Prin Rojanapongpun

INTRODUCTION

Acute glaucoma is a non-specific clinical term used to describe a sudden and severe increase of intraocular pressure (IOP). This is commonly seen in acute angle closure (AAC), especially in Asians and certain other ethnic groups, though there are a few other conditions that also lead to a similar acute rise of IOP.

In general, acute glaucoma occurs less frequently than chronic glaucoma. However, it is usually very serious as it can lead to rapid optic nerve damage and intense pain. The degree of damage depends on the magnitude, the rapidity, and the duration of IOP rise. If the IOP is very high, the ganglion cell and retinal nerve fiber will be damaged immediately. The hemodynamic status and other weaknesses of the optic nerve must also be taken into account (see Chapter 27 'Primary Angle Closure Glaucoma' for a fuller discussion an definitions and diagnosis). This chapter will retain the term 'acute angle closure glaucoma' even though it includes the clinical entities 'acute angle closure', 'and acute angle closure glaucoma' as, from a therapeutic point of view, management of both conditions is very similar.

There are two main clinical entities that lead to acute glaucoma. One is 'acute primary angle closure' that is characterized by a sudden blockage of the drainage angle, usually in an eye with an anatomical narrow angle. The condition is known to most clinicians as 'acute angle-closure glaucoma' (AACG), though there may not yet be any detectable changes at the optic nerve head or in visual function. The World Glaucoma Association (WGA) suggests using the term 'acute angle closure' (AAC), as this may be more accurate.

Another clinical entity is grouped as 'acute secondary glaucoma.' Rapid IOP rise is actually a complication of one of several other eye conditions, such as an inflammation, trauma, hemorrhage, infection, cataract, or drug induction. The mechanism of glaucoma can be either open or angle closure based upon the primary pathology and its stage. The diagnosis and treatment has to be directed to detect and correct the underlying pathology together with the reduction of IOP.

Reduction of IOP by medical, laser, and/or surgery continues to be the mainstay of therapy for glaucoma. Despite successful treatment to lower IOP, some individuals still experience continued progression of glaucomatous optic neuropathy (GON) and associated visual field loss.[1]

ACUTE PRIMARY ANGLE CLOSURE

Angle closure is a condition in which the trabecular meshwork is blocked by peripheral iris. The prerequisites are anatomical disorder of the anterior segments and the angle-closure mechanism(s) that induce an apposition or closure of peripheral iris to trabecular meshwork to the point that the drainage of aqueous humor is critically compromised. In the case of acute primary angle closure the complete blockage occurs abruptly and thus IOP rises acutely. The process of angle closure is dynamic (see Ch. 27).

EPIDEMIOLOGY

The prevalence of primary angle-closure glaucoma (PACG) varies among different racial and ethnic groups. It is more common among Asians than Caucasians or Africans. The highest rates are reported in Inuit[2] and Asian populations.[3–5] Lower rates are reported in African- and European-derived populations.[6] By and large, angle-closure glaucoma (ACG) is a more severe form of glaucoma when compared to open-angle glaucoma (OAG). Half of all glaucoma blindness is caused by ACG, although OAG is more prevalent than ACG worldwide.

The prevalence of PACG increases with age in both sexes. Women are affected four times more often than men and the sex difference persists across all age groups. In general, AACG is not the most common form of PACG, as the majority of sufferers present with asymptomatic disease (66–75% of cases). Chronic angle-closure glaucoma is thus a more common form of PACG. However, in less developed societies, acute symptomatic angle-closure glaucoma (AACG) can be a more common form of PACG.[7] In one high-risk population of untreated Greenland Inuit with narrow, potentially occludable, angles the prevalence of definite PACG after 10 years of follow-up was 16%.

The incidence of acute primary angle-closure glaucoma varies from 2.9 to 12.2 per 100 000 per year.[8] Half of those affected were seen 3 days or more after the onset of symptoms. The probability of monocular blindness associated with PACG at the time of diagnosis was 14%.[9]

RISK FACTORS

There are demographic and ocular risk factors. The major demographic risk factors are:
- advancing age
- female sex
- Asian ancestry.[10–13]

Major risk factors identified were age of 60 years or older (relative risk, 9.1), female sex (relative risk, 2.4), and Chinese ethnic origin (relative risk, 2.8). Seasonal variations in the occurrence of AACG were reported, with preponderance of attacks occurring during summer and winter.[14] Family history of angle closure has been suggested as a risk factor, but is not consistently recognized. No genetic associations have yet been proven, although there may be a potential linkage with certain gene loci.

Reported ocular risk factors include:
- shallower limbal[15] and axial anterior chamber depth[16]
- narrower drainage angles
- thicker lens
- shorter axial length
- more anteriorly positioned lens
- hyperopia
- smaller corneal diameter.

These relevant ocular risk factors are found in both affected eyes and the contralateral eyes of patients with AACG.[17] Among these, the major ocular risk factors are mainly limbal and axial anterior chamber depth. The shallower the anterior chambers, the higher the rates of angle closure.[18,19] There are associations between the anterior segment biometry and advancing age or female gender. These are explainable on the basis of differences in biometry. Older people have a shallower anterior chamber than younger people, and women have a shallower anterior chamber than men.[20] But the reason for higher rates of angle closure in Asians remains controversial.

ETIOLOGY AND PATHOGENESIS

There are three or more approaches to classify angle-closure mechanisms. The most widely used classification is the 'anatomical level' scheme, which identifies obstructions to aqueous flow at four different levels from anterior to posterior:[21]
- pupillary block (aqueous pressure)
- plateau iris (ciliary pressure)
- lens-induced/lens mechanism (lens pressure)
- causes behind the lens (vitreous pressure).

Angle-closure mechanisms can also be classified using pupillary block as a main denominator:
- pupillary block mechanism
- nonpupillary block mechanism.

While pupil block is a well-defined and well-understood entity, the definition of nonpupil block mechanism is not so clearly established. Nonpupillary block includes mechanisms such as plateau iris, prominent last row iris, lens related, and ciliary block mechanisms.

A third classification is to use the forces that act on the iris and conceptually classify angle-closure mechanisms into:
- mechanisms that push the iris forward from behind
- mechanisms that pull the iris forward into contact with the trabecular meshwork.

The first two classifications seem to be more practical, as they guide the clinician in the management of angle-closure glaucoma, because identification and removal of the underlying angle-closure mechanism(s) is the principle of management before one can reestablish the natural drainage of the trabecular meshwork. There may be more than one mechanism operating in each eye. In any case, all identified mechanisms must be corrected.

In general, pupillary block is the most common mechanism.[22] It may present as a sole mechanism or mixed with others. For example, relative pupillary block can be a consequence of an anteriorly displaced lens coupled with a relatively thick iris or plateau iris resulting in an increased area of contact between the lens and iris. In East Asia, mixed-mechanism angle closure is believed to be especially prevalent and pure pupillary block mechanism may account for only one-third of cases.[23,24]

Pupil block results in an increase in pressure within the posterior chamber, this causes the iris to bow forward, which occludes the angle and blocks aqueous drainage. This condition is known as 'iris bombe.' Iris bombe further closes the already narrow angle and compromises aqueous drainage, thus further increasing IOP. Synechiae or adhesions may develop if closure is prolonged or sustained, which can result in further damage to the trabecular meshwork.

In plateau iris, anterior rotation and elongation of ciliary processes have been described as underlying pathology.[25] The peripheral iris is supported by the anterior positioning of ciliary processes and presses up against the trabecular meshwork. On gonioscopy, the peripheral iris angulates forward and then flat down centrally, causing a plateau iris configuration with apparent apposition of peripheral iris to the drainage angle. With indentation gonioscopy, a 'double-hump sign' can be demonstrated. This is caused by the iris draping over the lens; the deepest point of indentation is at the site of the small posterior chamber, and then the beam curves up again over the ciliary processes and the angle opens only slightly.

The diagnosis of plateau iris is usually made after iridotomy and is based on qualitative assessment. There is no precise quantitative definition of how narrow the angle has to be or how anteriorly positioned the ciliary processes must be. A more definite diagnosis can be made with imaging devices. Although there is a suggested classification of different heights of blockage by plateau iris, no precise cutoff is defined and thus the description is mainly qualitative. Not all cases can be documented with such anterior positioning of the ciliary process as there may be many other causes.[26]

Crowding of the angle is a broad clinical term to describe findings that may result from an anterior placement of the lens due to either an increase in thickness or anterior displacement of the lens, anterior rotation of the ciliary body, or perhaps iris anatomical factors such as smaller anterior chamber angle dimensions and a thicker iris[27] or plateau iris.[28] This often coexists with pupillary block and can also cause angle-closure glaucoma by itself. Thus, detail mechanism(s) should be identified to guide treatment. This often needs the assistance of imaging devices.

SIGNS AND SYMPTOMS

Acute glaucoma classically presents with sudden onset of a severely painful, red eye with reduced visual acuity and hazy cornea. Severe cases can also have systemic symptoms such as headache, malaise, or gastrointestinal disturbance. Some patients may present with mild symptoms and vague headache. Occasionally, sweating and abdominal or chest pain may be present, causing confusion with the diagnosis.

Eye examinations have demonstrated ocular signs that relate to three main disease processes, namely: angle closure (high IOP and corneal edema), inflammation (ciliary injection and engorged iris vessels), and ischemic sequelae (fixed mid-dilated pupil, iris atrophy, iris whirling, and glaukomflecken) (Fig. 57.1). However, as with any other disease, these findings can be quite variable. Other findings include:
- Decreased corneal endothelial cell density.
- Peripheral anterior synechiae (PAS): compression (indentation) gonioscopy with a four-mirror or similar lens is particularly helpful to evaluate for appositional closure vs synechial angle closure and for extent of PAS.
- Retinal nerve fiber layer (RNFL) change: recent studies showed that superior and inferior average RNFL thickness from scanning laser polarimetry was found to decrease significantly from week 2 to week 16, after an episode of AAC.[29] This is also confirmed with optical coherence tomography (OCT) that demonstrated significant reduction of RNFL at 3 months post acute attack.[30,31]
- Optic disc change: Shen et al. demonstrated that the mean cup-to-disc ratio increased and the mean neuroretinal rim area decreased from week 2 to week 16 after an episode of AAC. Quadrantic and sector

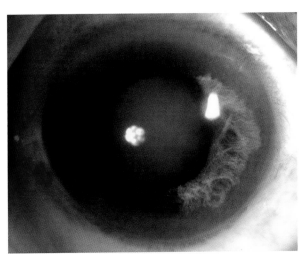

FIGURE 57.1 APAC eye with ischemic sequel of the iris.

analysis showed preferential loss of neuroretinal rim area at the superotemporal and inferotemporal areas.[32]
- Visual field change: an isolated attack of acute glaucoma produces in most cases a perimetric defect of generalized or mixed type. This may be reversible. The most affected zones were the upper half (upper nasal) of the visual field and the 9–21° area.[33]

TREATMENT PRINCIPLES AND OPTIONS IN ACUTE PRIMARY ANGLE CLOSURE

This section will focus on the treatment of primary angle-closure glaucoma. There are three basic principles of treatment in acute angle closure (AAC):
- Rapid reduction and control of IOP and inflammation
- Modification of angle configuration to correct the mechanical blockage
- Institution of definitive treatment to maintain IOP control and prevent recurrence of angle closure based on mechanism(s).

The IOP must be brought down as soon as possible to limit damage to the nerve and anterior segment structures (ischemic sequel), as well as for symptomatic relief. Besides medication, there are other alternatives such as immediate laser iridoplasty[34–37] and paracentesis[38] to rapidly decrease IOP. Studies have shown that these interventions reduce IOP more effectively in the first 24 hours when compared to conventional medical treatment (Fig. 57.2). A recent study suggested that after lowering IOP for only 1 hour, there was a significant decrease in mean cup volume and mean cup depth, there being a corresponding increase in mean rim area.[39]

Iridotomy must be performed whenever possible to remove pupillary block, as it is always present in AAC.

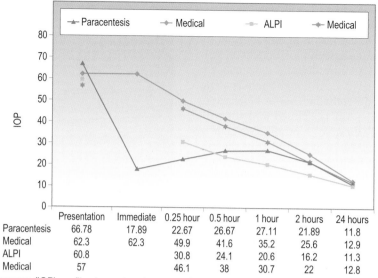

	Presentation	Immediate	0.25 hour	0.5 hour	1 hour	2 hours	24 hours
Paracentesis	66.78	17.89	22.67	26.67	27.11	21.89	11.8
Medical	62.3	62.3	49.9	41.6	35.2	25.6	12.9
ALPI	60.8		30.8	24.1	20.6	16.2	11.3
Medical	57		46.1	38	30.7	22	12.8

FIGURE 57.2 Intraocular pressure (IOP) profiles in acute primary angle closure (APAC) from two randomized controlled trials comparing paracentesis with conventional medical treatment and argon laser peripheral iridoplasty (ALPI) with conventional treatment as first-line treatment of APAC. (With data from references 35 and 38.)

Laser iridoplasty can be performed before or after iridotomy. In principle, all angle-closure mechanisms must be identified and removed at an appropriate time.

The final step is to monitor and maintain the structural and functional integrity of the optic disc and the retinal nerve fiber layer similar to treating other types of glaucomatous optic neuropathy. But attention must be paid to maintaining angle opening by identification and removal of any residual angle-closure mechanism that may be contributing to further closure of the drainage angle.

A marked inflammatory reaction is usually associated with AAC. The administration of steroid in the form of topical 1% prednisolone or 0.1% dexamethasone is desirable from the start to reduce inflammation before laser or surgery. Severe pain may be treated with analgesics, and vomiting may be treated with antiemetics.

MEDICATION

Medical therapy has been a conventional treatment and is usually initiated first because of its simplicity and relative safety. Medication includes some or all of the following:

- topical β-blockers
- topical α_2-adrenergic agonists
- systemic carbonic anhydrase inhibitors (CAIS)
- systemic hyperosmotic agents
- topical miotics.

A combination of different medical agents usually reduces pain and clears up the corneal edema in preparation for iridotomy. Systemic CAI (i.e. acetazolamide 500 mg intravenous or oral) should be given with topical β-blocker. Intravenous acetazolamide has a much faster onset of action, 15 minutes, when compared to the 1–2 hours of the oral form.

Oral osmotic agents, such as glycerin, are effective in reducing intraocular pressure. Peak action of oral glyc-

erin is 30–90 minutes and the duration of IOP reduction is 5–6 hours. Oral glycerin should be used with caution in patients with diabetes, renal failure, or cardiovascular disease. Intravenous mannitol can be used to reduce intraocular pressure. Peak IOP reduction is 1 hour after administration. Extra care must be exercised when giving mannitol.

Miotic drugs such as pilocarpine should be used selectively and as a second-line drug after initiation of the aqueous suppressant and hyperosmotic agents. There is a theoretical risk that miotics may further shallow the anterior chamber (paradoxical shallowing), induce uveal congestion, and cause an inflammatory reaction. A pupil that is unresponsive to the first few drops suggests iris sphincter ischemia and should alarm the physician to hold back a stronger dose of pilocarpine. If miasis does occur, treatment with miotics may open the angle and enhance further IOP lowering. There has been a suggestion that pilocarpine should be administered only after 45–60 minutes of first-line medication or when the IOP has been brought down to relieve sphincter ischemia.

An α-agonist (i.e. brimonidine) can also decrease IOP in AAC. However, the potential neuroprotective effect cannot be demonstrated in the first 16 weeks after AAC. There was no difference in the prevalence of visual field defects or rate of visual field progression between brimonidine- and timolol-treated groups.[40]

LASER

There are two laser procedures that are often used in the treatment of APAC, laser iridotomy and iridoplasty.

Laser peripheral iridotomy Laser peripheral iridotomy (LPI) is the treatment of pupillary block, which is the most common mechanism of AAC. It is effective

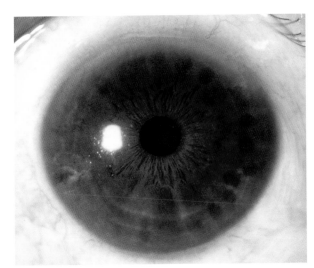

FIGURE 57.3 APAC eye shows with patent iridotomy at 8:15 o'clock position and multiple laser spots in the peripheral iris from ALPI. ALPI burns may be placed more centrally in areas where clearance between corneal endothelium and iris are limited or dense arcus senilis.

for both the affected and contralateral eyes of AAC. However, its effectiveness in preventing long-term rise of IOP depends on the stage of angle closure[41] and whether there is the presence of glaucomatous optic neuropathy.[42] LPI is effective for preventing increased IOP in eyes of angle-closure suspects (97%)[42] and fellow eyes of those with AAC (91%),[43] but is less effective for eyes with AAC (42%).[44] But once glaucomatous optic neuropathy associated with synechial angle closure has occurred, LPI alone is less effective at controlling IOP (6%).[42,45]

LPI modifies the angle anatomy. The angle widens in the first 2 weeks after LPI, but will not change thereafter. Gonioscopic grading of the angle opening significantly increases in all four quadrants. The amount of PAS remains stable throughout 12 months' follow-up, which indicates the effectiveness of LPI in preventing progressive closure of the angle in the first year after APAC.[46] However, LPI corrects only pupillary block and not other angle-closure mechanism. Nonpupil block mechanisms may contribute to the failure of LPI in controlling IOP.[47] In essence, LPI is best effective when the eye has only pupillary block mechanism and is still at an early stage of primary angle-closure.

Performing LPI in eyes with an edematous cornea can be challenging. Topical glycerin drops can help clear up the epithelial edema and may allow peripheral iridotomy. A combination of argon laser prior to Nd:YAG laser reduces hemorrhage[48] and enhances successful LPI in the thick and dark iris commonly seen in African and Asian patients.[49,50] Diode laser may have advantages over the argon blue-green laser for iridotomy/iridoplasty because of better diode laser tissue penetration in opaque media.[51]

Laser iridoplasty Argon laser peripheral iridoplasty (ALPI) is a useful procedure to eliminate appositional

angle closure. This procedure creates contracting burns placed at the iris periphery in order to pull the iris root away from the angle (Fig. 57.3).

Iridoplasty is effective for AAC,[34,35,37,52,53] but has no proven efficacy for CACG. Recent studies showed that ALPI was more effective than conventional treatment with medications in acute APAC. ALPI can also be used as initial treatment for acute phacomorphic glaucoma before cataract extraction.[54]

The main use of iridoplasty in APAC is when the response to intensive medical therapy is poor. The author has performed the procedure in over 60 cases of angle closure unresponsive to medical therapy (unpublished data), even after several days. All eyes but one, which had total synechial angle closure, responded with normalization of IOP and opening of the angle to a certain extent. However, iridoplasty is not a replacement of LPI but is a useful adjunct when there is severe corneal edema and LPI is difficult. Iridoplasty will not break permanent synechiae.

Iridoplasty has, additionally, been used to relieve appositional angle closure secondary to plateau iris syndrome, or lens-related angle closure, and to widen the angle prior to argon laser trabeculoplasty. There is also evidence to suggest that it is highly effective for pure plateau iris syndrome in Caucasians.[55]

ANTERIOR CHAMBER PARACENTESIS

Immediate paracentesis has been proposed as an alternative procedure to rapidly lower the IOP in AAC.[38] It has shown that IOP decreased from 53 mmHg to 24 mmHg at 10 minutes and to 18.2 mmHg at 24 hours.[56] The unique advantage of immediate paracentesis lies in the rapidity of IOP control and almost instantaneous relief of the severe symptoms. Rapid IOP control may limit the extent of ocular tissue damage[57] and result in less ischemia that might be responsible for both the focal endothelial damage and in the retinal nerve fiber.[58]

Because this procedure reduces IOP and clears corneal edema so rapidly, it may allow LPI to be performed earlier than conventionally possible. However, this technique should only remain an add-on therapy to usual treatments due to its relatively invasive nature. The IOP reduction is only temporary and a more definitive procedure must be undertaken.

LEN EXTRACTION

The role of lens extraction as a treatment for angle closure has been debated for many years. With the knowledge that the lens could be the single most important contributing factor to the development of angle-closure and having acquired the technology and skills to perform relatively safe small-incision cataract surgery, lens extraction in angle-closure patients has been proposed with the aim of preventing the development of glaucomatous optic neuropathy at a later stage. This is because removing the lens creates more space in the anterior chamber and widens the angle, which helps

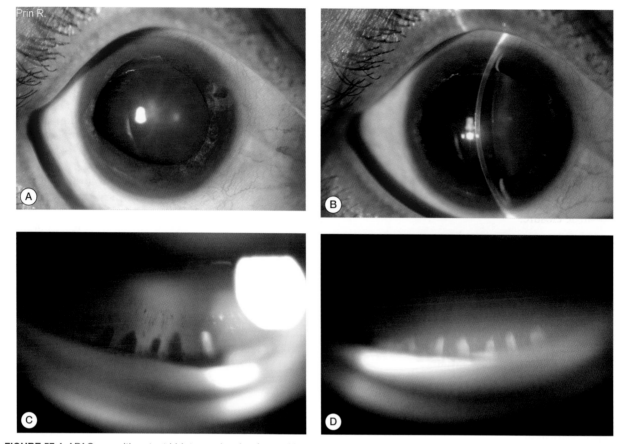

FIGURE 57.4 APAC eye with patent iridotomy showing forward lens position causing shallowing of the anterior chamber, both centrally and peripherally. The ciliary processes can be visualized through gonioscopy.

achieving IOP control.[59] This can significantly reduce both intraocular pressure and the requirement for glaucoma drugs.[60] Some studies suggest that cataract surgery may be as effective as filtering surgery in controlling IOP in angle-closure glaucoma cases.[61,62] However, any discussion of early lens extraction does not in any way imply that ophthalmologists should deviate from current protocols for the management of AAC.[63]

Since most patients with AAC will have a significant degree of improvement in visual acuity following an acute attack, it may not be justifiable to propose primary lens extraction instead of iridotomy as treatment for acute angle closure.[64] There are ongoing trials aimed at looking into the role of primary lens extraction in AAC. They are designed to see whether such an approach will result in better outcome as a reduction in further medical or surgical glaucoma treatment and improved visual performance. Until this is proven, lens extraction, which is often technically challenging in AAC patients and may have more complications when compared to simple cataract surgery, should be reserved for cases in which the acute attack is not responding to conventional medical and laser treatment or in cases with clinical signs demonstrating the presence of a lens mechanism (Fig. 57.4). However, when selected appropriately, lens removal may be an effective means of achieving rapid control of the IOP.[65]

GONIOSYNECHIALYSIS

Goniosynechialysis (GSL) is a surgical procedure designed to break peripheral anterior synechiae (PAS) from the angle wall.[66] Earlier studies have shown that in patients with angle closure of less than 6 months' duration it may be an effective means of reducing PAS and lowering IOP.[67] When combined with phacoemulsification and posterior chamber intraocular lens (IOL) implantation and performed within 6 months of an attack of APAC, it can be effective in reducing PAS, improving visual acuity, and controlling IOP.[68] A significant reduction of the number of postoperative glaucoma medications and further surgical intervention has also been reported in AAC cases unresponsive to conventional treatment.[69]

Viscogonioplasty is a procedure for injecting heavy viscoelastic into the angle for 360°, aiming to break the PAS from the trabecular meshwork and deepen the anterior chamber. It may have a role in controlling IOP effectively and safely in patients with refractory acute APAC by producing a large drop in IOP and opening of the angle.[70]

FILTERING SURGERY

Filtering surgery is not the procedure of choice in treating AAC. Incisional surgery for angle-closure glaucoma is typically required when laser surgery and/or medical therapy fail to control IOP. Emergency trabeculectomy in the modern management of acute angle-closure glaucoma is not advocated for these eyes are ('hot'), inflamed. Primary trabeculectomy in medically unresponsive cases of APAC may result in higher risk of peri and postoperative complications as well as surgical failure.[71]

PRACTICAL APPROACH TO ACUTE ANGLE CLOSURE

The following is a suggested approach to a patient with acute angle closure:

1. Obtain a careful history of symptoms relating to intermittent angle-closure attacks, attacks in the fellow eye, prescription or nonprescription medications that may precipitate attacks, and the type of activity preceding the attack.
2. Examine the affected eye and fellow eye with attention to both the central and peripheral anterior chamber depth and the shape of the peripheral iris.
3. Administer oral acetazolamide and a topical β-blocker. Intravenous acetazolamide may be given, if available. A hyperosmotic agent such as 50% glycerin solution orally or intravenous mannitol should be administered should there is no contraindication or if the patient cannot take an oral medication without vomiting.
4. Have the patient lie supine to permit the lens to fall backward with vitreous dehydration.
5. Reassess ocular findings after 1 hour. The IOP is usually decreased, but the angle usually remains appositionally closed. Give 1 drop of 2% or 4% pilocarpine and reexamine the patient 30 minutes later.
   - If the IOP is reduced and the angle is open, the patient may be treated medically with topical low-dose pilocarpine, β-blockers and steroids, and oral acetazolamide, if necessary, until the eye quiets and laser iridotomy can be performed.
   - If the IOP is unchanged or elevated and the angle remains closed, lens-related angle closure should be suspected, further pilocarpine withheld, and the attack broken by argon laser peripheral iridoplasty. Paracentesis can also be considered to rapidly reduce the IOP.

LONG-TERM OUTCOMES AND PROGNOSIS

Glaucomatous optic neuropathy can occur rapidly (within days) or gradually (over years) in AAC eyes if high IOP cannot be reduced and controlled well enough. A study found that 17.8% of subjects after being seen with AAC were blind in the attack eye, almost half had glaucomatous optic nerve damage, and 15.5% having markedly cupped optic discs (cup-to-disc ratio > 0.9) after being followed for 6 years.[72]

In a study with a mean follow-up period of 6 years, all of the patients with a history of an episode of AAC that had resolved after LPI required further treatment with antiglaucoma medications. Sixty-three percent of patients eventually underwent filtering surgery at a mean of 7.3 months.[45]

Untreated fellow phakic eyes are at increased risk for developing an acute attack. Prophylactic LPI prevents long-term rise in IOP in 88.8% of fellow eyes at 4 years' follow-up. However, because a small proportion of fellow eyes did experience a rise in IOP within the first year despite the presence of a patent LPI, close monitoring is still advised.[43] Even at presentation, definite or probable glaucoma was present in 2.5% of fellow eyes. An additional 6.5% developed glaucoma with a mean follow-up of 6 years. More than 80% of this cohort retained good vision in contrast to the eye that developed APAC.[73]

ACUTE SECONDARY GLAUCOMA

Acute rise of IOP may also be seen with other forms of glaucoma. These secondary glaucomas must be differentiated from AAC. Acute secondary glaucoma may have open- or closed-angle mechanisms as follows:

- Open-angle mechanisms: mostly associated with inflammation, hemorrhage, rubeosis iridis, and drug-induced.
- Angle-closure mechanisms: either anterior pulling or posterior pushing mechanism, such as ciliary body swelling or inflammation, malignant glaucoma, posterior segment tumors, contracting retrolental tissue, post laser or surgery, nanophthalmos, lens induced, or drug-induced.

In open-angle glaucoma, there are several mechanisms which lead to increased IOP, including clogging of TM (red blood cells, macrophages, neoplastic cells, pigment, lens protein, photoreceptor outer segment, viscoelastic), inflammation (edema of trabecular meshwork, trabecular meshwork endothelial cell dysfunction), trauma, toxin or medication, and increased episcleral venous pressure.

Secondary angle-closure glaucoma is an angle closure secondary to a pathologic process in the eye which can be from an anterior pulling or a posterior pushing mechanism.

Some of these conditions will be described briefly in this section, particularly those that are more commonly seen in the clinic.

AQUEOUS MISDIRECTION SYNDROME

The aqueous misdirection syndrome (malignant glaucoma, ciliary block glaucoma) (see Ch. 78) presents with elevated IOP and flat or shallow anterior chamber following intraocular surgery without pupillary block. It can also occur following laser iridotomy,[74] laser suture lysis after trabeculectomy,[75] and transscleral Nd:YAG[76] or diode laser cyclophotocoagulation.[77]

Hyperopia, narrow iridocorneal angle, and ciliary sulcus as well as plateau iris configuration and a history of miotics are predisposing risk factors for aqueous misdirection.

The fellow eye is also at risk. Therefore, prophylactic YAG iridotomy should be considered.

Diagnosis Aqueous misdirection usually follows intraocular surgery or a laser procedure. The diagnositc criteria can include the following:

- axial shallow to flat anterior chamber, usually with a marked forward movement of the anterior lens capsule (phakia).
- Raised IOP of a variable amount, however post-filtration surgery this could be initially low to normal IOP; or
- the presence of a patent iridotomy.

Mechanism Aqueous misdirection occurs with an abnormal relationship between the anterior vitreous, ciliary process, and lens periphery. The precise mechanism is still unclear but the most widely accepted explanation is that there is a diversion of aqueous flow from the posterior chamber into the vitreous instead of the normal route from posterior to anterior chamber. Coincidental accumulation of fluid in the supraciliary space moves the ciliary process closer to the lens equator; especially if the lens is relatively large.

Ultrasound biomicroscopy is a valuable instrument for differentiating pupillary block glaucoma from aqueous misdirection.

It has been proposed that aqueous misdirection be separated into: a) ciliary block, which is concerned with the narrow and small structure of the anterior segment of the eye, and b) lens–iris block, caused by anterior displacement of the iris–lens diaphragam. Both types have the same clinical features.[78]

Treatment Treatment is still controversial but generally starts with medical therapy before surgical intervention(s). If the condition is recognized and treated at an early stage, the chance of relieving the attack with medical treatment is high. Combination therapy with cycloplegics (atropine), systemic carbonic anhydrase inhibitors, hyperosmotic agents concomitant with topical β-blockers, α_2-agonists, and possibly topical carbonic anhydrase inhibitors, is considered optimal medical therapy for malignant glaucoma.

If medications fail to control IOP, argon laser of ciliary processes (if visible) and Nd:YAG anterior hyaloidotomy are suggested.

If the eye does not respond to laser treatment, a surgical approach involving lensectomy and pars plana (partial) vitreo-capsulo-iridectomy has been reported to be a good alternative in treating malignant glaucoma.[79]

POSNER-SCHLOSSMAN SYNDROME (GLAUCOMATOCYCLITIC CRISIS)

Posner-Schlossman syndrome (PSS) was originally described in 1948 by Posner and Schlossman as a self-limiting and benign condition. It is also known as glaucomatocyclitic crisis characterized by unilateral, recurrent attacks of mild, nongranulomatous iritis with elevated IOP (30–70 mmHg) during the acute attack,

open angles, normal visual fields and optic discs. In between the attacks, the IOP, tonography, and provocative tests are within normal limits.

Diagnosis The diagnostic features of PSS are:

- typically unilateral
- mild symptoms of discomfort, slightly blurred vision, and halos
- mild nongranulomatous cyclitis, usually few to no cells in anterior chamber, and trace flare
- mild mydriasis
- markedly elevated IOP during acute attack but minimal or no corneal edema
- fine to medium-sized keratic precipitates (Fig. 57.5).

Posner-Schlossman syndrome normally occurs in younger individuals between the third to sixth decades of life. The condition usually recurs with variable frequency. However, the magnitude of IOP elevation is not proportional to the level of inflammation.

Though not all PSS develops glaucomatous optic neuropathy, it should not be viewed as a benign condition.

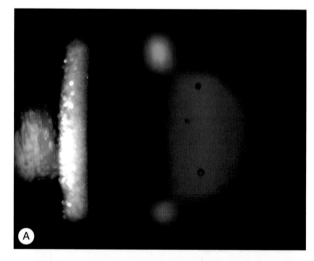

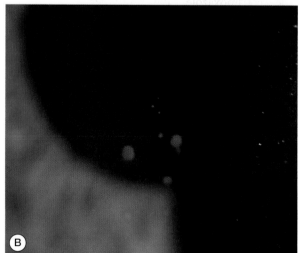

FIGURE 57.5 Keratic precipitates in Posner-Schlossman syndrome consisting of fine to medium-sized nonpigment, located in the central to inferior corneal endothelium.

A recent long-term study reported approximately one-fourth of patients developed glaucoma as a result of repeated attacks. Patients with 10 years or more of PSS have a 2.8 times higher risk (95% confidence interval, 1.19–6.52) of developing glaucoma compared with patients with less than 10 years' duration of the disease. Glaucoma filtering surgery was necessary in 17% of patients. In essence, PSS patients should be monitored for any structural and functional change.

Mechanism The etiology of PSS is unknown. Cytomegalovirus and herpes simplex virus may be a cause of this disease. Acute rise of IOP is thought to be a result of trabecular inflammation.

Treatment Medical treatment is indicated to reduce inflammation with corticosteroid and to reduce IOP in acute phase. Topical hypotensive agents such as β-blockers, α-agonists, and carbonic anhydrase inhibitors are useful in controlling intraocular pressure. If intraocular pressure is not controlled with medication, trabeculectomy can be performed.

DRUG-INDUCED GLAUCOMA

At least one-third of AACG cases are related to an over-the-counter or prescription drug. The mechanism of acute AACG can be from pupillary block or ciliochoroidal effusion without pupillary block.[80]

Acute angle-closure glaucoma due to pupillary block can be caused by adrenergic agents, either local (phenylephrine drops, nasal ephedrine, or nebulized salbutamol) or systemic (epinephrine for anaphylactic shock), drugs with anticholinergic effects including tropicamide and atropine drops, tri- and tetracyclic antidepressants, and cholinergic agents such as pilocarpine.

Sulfa-based drugs (acetazolamide, hydrochlorothiazide, cotrimoxazole, and topiramate) lead to ciliary body edema that causes relaxation of the zonules, which allows lens thickening. Anterolateral rotation of the ciliary body leads to anterior displacement of the lens and iris and concomitant shallowing of the anterior chamber. Choroidal detachment and supraciliary effusion are frequently present.

Acute secondary angle-closure glaucoma after massive vitreous, choroidal, or subretinal hemorrhage is a rare complication of anticoagulant therapy. Risk factors are overtreatment with anticoagulants, exudative age-related macular degeneration, and nanophthalmos. Both heparin and low molecular weight heparin (enoxaparin, warfarin) have been reported to cause AACG.

Many inhalational agents should be used with caution in patients with a narrow angle. There are some reports of nebulized salbutamol, nebulized albuterol, nebulized ipratropium bromide, and local tiotropium which may cause acute angle-closure glaucoma in susceptible patients.

Corticosteroids can also induced acute glaucoma but in open-angle mechanisms. It can be caused by prolonged use of topical, periocular, inhaled, or systemic formulations. The type and potency of the agent, the means and frequency of its administration, and the susceptibility of the patient all affect the duration of the time before IOP rises and the extent of this rise.

HERPES SIMPLEX KERATOUVEITIS

Herpes simplex keratitis is probably the most common ocular disease associated with uveitis. Patients with stromal keratitis often have a concurrent anterior uveitis. Uveitis associated with herpetic lesions accounts for about 5% of all uveitis seen in adults. The incidence of increased IOP in herpetic keratouveitis varies from 28% to 40%. In severe cases of herpetic keratouveitis complicated by anterior segment ischemia, secondary glaucoma can develop in up to 83% of cases. The IOP usually remains elevated for 3–10 weeks.

The elevated IOP may be caused by trabeculitis, inflammatory obstruction of the trabecular meshwork, and angle closure in severe keratouveitis.

The management of elevated IOP is initially directed toward controlling the viral replication and inflammation. Some topical antiviral drugs can penetrate the deep cornea and are effective in controlling viral replication. The associated intraocular inflammation should be treated with topical corticosteroids. Antiglaucoma therapy must be given when IOP elevation persists.

The IOP usually returns to normal levels as the inflammation subsides. Approximately 10% of patients have persistently elevated IOP, requiring prolonged antiglaucoma therapy and even filtering surgery.[81]

Summary

- Acute glaucoma is characterized by a sudden and severe increase in pressure within the eye. It occurs when the internal fluid drainage system in the eye suddenly becomes blocked.

- Acute glaucoma can be primary or secondary; primary involves angle closure, secondary can be either with an open or closed angle.

- Treatment is an emergency as the high pressure in the eye can rapidly result in optic nerve damage and loss of vision.

- Laser peripheral iridotomy is still the primary treatment in acute angle closure due to pupillary block.

- The fellow eye of a patient with acute pupillary block glaucoma should be evaluated since it is at high risk for a similar event. The fellow eye usually need a prophylactic iridotomy.

- Not every acute glaucoma is primary in origin.

- In secondary glaucoma, the type of treatment prescribed depends on the cause. Treatment should be directed to correct the primary cause as well as control the raised intraocular pressure.

REFERENCES

1. Gordon MO, Beiser JA, et al. The Ocular Hypertension Treatment Study: baseline factors that predict the onset of primary open-angle glaucoma. Arch Ophthalmol 2002; 120(6):714–720; discussion 829–830.

2. Arkell SM, Lightman DA, et al. The prevalence of glaucoma among Eskimos of northwest Alaska. Arch Ophthalmol 1987; 105(4):482–485.

3. Dandona L, Dandona R, et al. Angle-closure glaucoma in an urban population in southern India. The Andhra Pradesh eye disease study. Ophthalmology 2000; 107(9):1710–1716.

4. Jacob A, Thomas R, et al. Prevalence of primary glaucoma in an urban south Indian population. Indian J Ophthalmol 1998; 46(2):81–86.

5. Foster PJ, Johnson GJ. Glaucoma in China: how big is the problem? Br J Ophthalmol 2001; 85(11):1277–1282.

6. Tielsch JM, Katz J, et al. A population-based evaluation of glaucoma screening: the Baltimore Eye Survey. Am J Epidemiol 1991; 134(10):1102–1110.

7. Casson RJ, Newland HS, et al. Prevalence of glaucoma in rural Myanmar: the Meiktila Eye Study. Br J Ophthalmol 2007; 91(6):710–714.

8. Seah SK, Foster PJ, et al. Incidence of acute primary angle-closure glaucoma in Singapore. An island-wide survey. Arch Ophthalmol 1997; 115(11):1436–1440.

9. Erie JC, Hodge DO, et al. The incidence of primary angle-closure glaucoma in Olmsted County, Minnesota. Arch Ophthalmol 1997; 115(2):177–181.

10. Vijaya L, George R, et al. Prevalence of angle-closure disease in a rural southern Indian population. Arch Ophthalmol 2006; 124(3):403–409.

11. Foster PJ, Baasanhu J, et al. Glaucoma in Mongolia. A population-based survey in Hovsgol province, northern Mongolia. Arch Ophthalmol 1996; 114(10):1235–1241.

12. Foster PJ, Oen FT, et al. The prevalence of glaucoma in Chinese residents of Singapore: a cross-sectional population survey of the Tanjong Pagar district. Arch Ophthalmol 2000; 118(8):1105–1111.

13. Alsbirk PH. Primary angle-closure glaucoma. Oculometry, epidemiology, and genetics in a high risk population. Acta Ophthalmol 1976; 127(Suppl):5–31.

14. David R, Tessler Z, et al. Epidemiology of acute angle-closure glaucoma: incidence and seasonal variations. Ophthalmologica 1985; 191(1):4–7.

15. Foster PJ, Devereux JG, et al. Detection of gonioscopically occludable angles and primary angle closure glaucoma by estimation of limbal chamber depth in Asians: modified grading scheme. Br J Ophthalmol 2000; 84(2):186–192.

16. Devereux JG, Foster PJ, et al. Anterior chamber depth measurement as a screening tool for primary angle-closure glaucoma in an East Asian population. Arch Ophthalmol 2000; 118(2):257–263.

17. Friedman DS, Gazzard G, et al. Ultrasonographic biomicroscopy, Scheimpflug photography, and novel provocative tests in contralateral eyes of Chinese patients initially seen with acute angle closure. Arch Ophthalmol 2003; 121(5):633–642.

18. Congdon NG, Youlin Q, et al. Biometry and primary angle-closure glaucoma among Chinese, white, and black populations. Ophthalmology 1997; 104(9):1489–1495.

19. Aung T, Nolan WP, et al. Anterior chamber depth and the risk of primary angle closure in 2 East Asian populations. Arch Ophthalmol 2005; 123(4):527–532.

20. Foster PJ, Alsbirk PH, et al. Anterior chamber depth in Mongolians: variation with age, sex, and method of measurement. Am J Ophthalmol 1997; 124(1):53–60.

21. Ritch R, Shields MB, Krupin T, eds. The Glaucomas. 2nd edn. St. Louis: Mosby; 1996:801.

22. Nolan WP, Foster PJ, et al. YAG laser iridotomy treatment for primary angle closure in east Asian eyes. Br J Ophthalmol 2000; 84(11):1255–1259.

23. Wang N, Zhou W, et al. Clinical studies of primary angle closure glaucoma. Zhonghua Yan Ke Za Zhi 1995; 31(2):133–134.

24. Wang N, Wu H, et al. Primary angle closure glaucoma in Chinese and Western populations. Chin Med J (Engl) 2002; 115(11):1706–1715.

25. Garudadri CS, Chelerkar V, et al. An ultrasound biomicroscopic study of the anterior segment in Indian eyes with primary angle-closure glaucoma. J Glaucoma 2002; 11(6):502–507.

26. He M, Foster PJ, et al. Angle-closure glaucoma in East Asian and European people. Different diseases? Eye 2006; 20(1):3–12.

27. He M, Friedman DS, et al. Laser peripheral iridotomy in eyes with narrow drainage angles: ultrasound biomicroscopy outcomes. The Liwan Eye Study. Ophthalmology 2007; 114(8):1513–1519.

28. Ritch R, Chang BM, et al. Angle closure in younger patients. Ophthalmology 2003; 110(10):1880–1889.

29. Aung T, Husain R, et al. Changes in retinal nerve fiber layer thickness after acute primary angle closure. Ophthalmology 2004; 111(8):1475–1479.

30. Tsai JC, Lin PW, et al. Longitudinal changes in retinal nerve fiber layer thickness after acute primary angle closure measured with optical coherence tomography. Invest Ophthalmol Vis Sci 2007; 48(4):1659–1664.

31. Fang AW, Qu J, et al. Measurement of retinal nerve fiber layer in primary acute angle closure glaucoma by optical coherence tomography. J Glaucoma 2007; 16(2):178–184.

32. Shen SY, Baskaran M, et al. Changes in the optic disc after acute primary angle closure. Ophthalmology 2006; 113(6):924–929.

33. Bonomi L, Marraffa M, et al. Perimetric defects after a single acute angle-closure glaucoma attack. Graefe's Arch Clin Exp Ophthalmol 1999; 237(11):908–914.

34. Lam DS, Lai JS, et al. Immediate argon laser peripheral iridoplasty as treatment for acute attack of primary angle-closure glaucoma: a preliminary study. Ophthalmology 1998; 105(12):2231–2236.

35. Lam DS, Lai JS, et al. Argon laser peripheral iridoplasty versus conventional systemic medical therapy in treatment of acute primary angle-closure glaucoma : a prospective, randomized, controlled trial. Ophthalmology 2002; 109(9):1591–1596.

36. Lai JS, Tham CC, et al. Immediate diode laser peripheral iridoplasty as treatment of acute attack of primary angle closure glaucoma: a preliminary study. J Glaucoma 2001; 10(2):89–94.

37. Lam DS, Lai JS, et al. Argon laser peripheral iridoplasty versus conventional systemic medical therapy in treatment of acute primary angle-closure glaucoma: a prospective, randomized, controlled trial. Ophthalmology 2002; 109(9):1591–1596.

38. Lam DS, Chua JK, et al. Efficacy and safety of immediate anterior chamber paracentesis in the treatment of acute primary angle-closure glaucoma: a pilot study. Ophthalmology 2002; 109(1):64–70.

39. Meredith SP, Swift L, et al. The acute morphologic changes that occur at the optic nerve head induced by medical reduction of intraocular pressure. J Glaucoma 2007; 16(6):556–561.

40. Aung T, Oen FT, et al. Randomised controlled trial comparing the effect of brimonidine and timolol on visual field loss after acute primary angle closure. Br J Ophthalmol 2004; 88(1):88–94.

41. Yamamoto T, Shirato S, et al. Treatment of primary angle-closure glaucoma by argon laser iridotomy: a long-term follow-up. Jpn J Ophthalmol 1985; 29(1):1–12.

42. Nolan WP, Foster PJ, et al. YAG laser iridotomy treatment for primary angle closure in east Asian eyes. Br J Ophthalmol 2000; 84(11):1255–1259.

43. Ang LP, Aung T, et al. Acute primary angle closure in an Asian population: long-term outcome of the fellow eye after prophylactic laser peripheral iridotomy. Ophthalmology 2000; 107(11):2092–2096.

44. Aung T, Ang LP, et al. Acute primary angle-closure: long-term intraocular pressure outcome in Asian eyes. Am J Ophthalmol 2001; 131(1):7–12.

45. Alsagoff Z, Aung T, et al. Long-term clinical course of primary angle-closure glaucoma in an Asian population. Ophthalmology 2000; 107(12):2300–2304.

46. Lim LS, Aung T, et al. Acute primary angle closure: configuration of the drainage angle in the first year after laser peripheral iridotomy. Ophthalmology 2004; 111(8):1470–1474.

47. Hung PT, Chou LH. Provocation mechanism of angle-closure glaucoma after iridectomy. Arch Ophthalmol 1979; 97(10):1862–1864.

48. Goins K, Schmeisser E, et al. Argon laser pretreatment in Nd:YAG iridotomy. Ophthalmic Surg 1990; 21(7):497–500.

49. Ho T, Fan R. Sequential argon-YAG laser iridotomies in dark irides. Br J Ophthalmol 1992; 76(6):329–331.

50. de Silva DJ, Gazzard G, et al. Laser iridotomy in dark irides. Br J Ophthalmol 2007; 91(2):222–225.

51. Chew PT, Wong JS, et al. Corneal transmissibility of diode versus argon lasers and their photothermal effects on the cornea and iris. Clin Experiment Ophthalmol 2000; 28(1):53–57.

52. Lim AS, Tan A, et al. Laser iridoplasty in the treatment of severe acute angle closure glaucoma. Int Ophthalmol 1993; 17(1):33–36.

53. Lai JS, Tham CC, et al. Laser peripheral iridoplasty as initial treatment of acute attack of primary angle-closure: a long-term follow-up study. J Glaucoma 2002; 11(6):484–487.

54. Tham CC, Lai JS, et al. Immediate argon laser peripheral iridoplasty (ALPI) as initial treatment for acute phacomorphic angle-closure (phacomorphic glaucoma) before cataract extraction: a preliminary study. Eye 2005; 19(7):778–783.

55. Ritch R, Tham CC, et al. Long-term success of argon laser peripheral iridoplasty in the management of plateau iris syndrome. Ophthalmology 2004; 111(1):104–108.

56. Arnavielle S, Creuzot-Garcher C, et al. Anterior chamber paracentesis in patients with acute elevation of intraocular pressure. Graefe's Arch Clin Exp Ophthalmol 2007; 245(3):345–350.

57. Bigar F, Witmer R. Corneal endothelial changes in primary acute angle-closure glaucoma. Ophthalmology 1982; 89(6):596–599.

58. Radius RL, Anderson DR. Breakdown of the normal optic nerve head blood–brain barrier following acute elevation of intraocular pressure in experimental animals. Invest Ophthalmol Vis Sci 1980; 19(3):244–255.

59. Hayashi K, Hayashi H, et al. Changes in anterior chamber angle width and depth after intraocular lens implantation in eyes with glaucoma. Ophthalmology 2000; 107(4):698–703.

60. Hayashi K, Hayashi H, et al. Effect of cataract surgery on intraocular pressure control in glaucoma patients. J Cataract Refract Surg 2001; 27(11):1779–1786.

61. Greve EL. Primary angle closure glaucoma: extracapsular cataract extraction or filtering procedure? Int Ophthalmol 1988; 12(3):157–162.

62. Gunning FP, Greve EL. Lens extraction for uncontrolled angle-closure glaucoma: long-term follow-up. J Cataract Refract Surg 1998; 24(10):1347–1356.

63. Nolan W. Lens extraction in primary angle closure. Br J Ophthalmol 2006; 90(1):1–2.

64. Tan GS, Hoh ST, et al. Visual acuity after acute primary angle closure and considerations for primary lens extraction. Br J Ophthalmol 2006; 90(1):14–16.

65. Roberts TV, Francis IC, et al. Primary phacoemulsification for uncontrolled angle-closure glaucoma. J Cataract Refract Surg 2000; 26(7):1012–1016.

66. Campbell DG, Vela A. Modern goniosynechialysis for the treatment of synechial angle-closure glaucoma. Ophthalmology 1984; 91(9):1052–1060.

67. Shingleton BJ, Chang MA, et al. Surgical goniosynechialysis for angle-closure glaucoma. Ophthalmology 1990; 97(5):551–556.

68. Teekhasaenee C, Ritch R. Combined phacoemulsification and goniosynechialysis for uncontrolled chronic angle-closure glaucoma after acute angle-closure glaucoma. Ophthalmology 1999; 106(4):669–674; discussion 674–675.

69. Harasymowycz PJ, Papamatheakis DG, et al. Phacoemulsification and goniosynechialysis in the management of unresponsive primary angle closure. J Glaucoma 2005; 14(3):186–189.

70. Varma D, Adams WE, et al. Viscogonioplasty in patients with chronic narrow angle glaucoma. Br J Ophthalmol 2006; 90(5):648–649.

71. Aung T, Tow SL, et al. Trabeculectomy for acute primary angle closure. Ophthalmology 2000; 107(7):1298–1302.

72. Aung T, Friedman DS, et al. Long-term outcomes in Asians after acute primary angle closure. Ophthalmology 2004; 111(8):1464–1469.

73. Friedman DS, Chew PT, et al. Long-term outcomes in fellow eyes after acute primary angle closure in the contralateral eye. Ophthalmology 2006; 113(7):1087–1091.

74. Cashwell LF, Martin TJ. Malignant glaucoma after laser iridotomy. Ophthalmology 1992; 99(5):651–658; discussion 658–659..

75. Macken P, Buys Y, et al. Glaucoma laser suture lysis. Br J Ophthalmol 1996; 80(5):398–401.

76. Hardten DR, Brown JD. Malignant glaucoma after Nd:YAG cyclophotocoagulation. Am J Ophthalmol 1991; 111(2):245–247.

77. Azuara-Blanco A, Dua HS. Malignant glaucoma after diode laser cyclophotocoagulation. Am J Ophthalmol 1999; 127(4):467–469.

78. Wang N, Zhou W, et al. [Pathogenesis and clinical classification of the malignant glaucoma]. Yan Ke Xue Bao 1999; 15(4):238–241; 252.

79. Schroeder W, Fischer K, et al. [Ultrasound biomicroscopy and therapy of malignant glaucoma]. Klin Monatsbl Augenheilkd 1999; 215(1):19–27.

80. Lachkar Y, Bouassida W. Drug-induced acute angle closure glaucoma. Curr Opin Ophthalmol 2007; 18(2):129–133.

81. Moorthy RS, Mermoud A, et al. Glaucoma associated with uveitis. Surv Ophthalmol 1997; 41(5):361–394.

CHAPTER 58

Glaucoma Secondary to Trauma

Baha' N Noureddin and Karim Tomey

INTRODUCTION

Ocular trauma is the most frequent cause of monocular blindness in the USA, and ranks second to cataract as the reason behind visual impairment.[1] Glaucoma associated with trauma may play a leading role in causing blindness, as it is sometimes overlooked in the presence of severe acute injury or during chronic follow-up.[2]

The management of this type of secondary glaucoma poses a serious challenge, as the pathogenesis is often multifactorial, and because the final outcome of treatment can be disappointing. What increases the complexity of this preventable complication is the fact that intraocular pressure (IOP) elevation frequently sets in years after the initial trauma.[3] Secondly, the various modalities of medical and surgical treatment that are employed in the management of injured eyes can, in themselves, lead to IOP elevation. Moreover, some of the more potent ocular hypotensive medications are contraindicated when trauma is associated with inflammation, which is often the case.

PREVALENCE AND EPIDEMIOLOGY

In the USA, close to 2.5 million ocular injuries occur every year,[4] resulting in an average annual hospitalization rate of 13.2 per 100 000 according to Klopfer et al.[5] A higher figure of 18.0 per 100 000 was reported in more recent studies,[6] and, as expected, significantly more in military reviews.[7,8] In other parts of the world, the rate is as low as 8.1 in Scotland,[9] and as high as 23.9 in Croatia,[10] with Singapore ranking in between at 12.6 per 100 000.[11]

Males are usually affected more frequently than females, with the ratios ranging from 3:1 to as high as 13:1.[12–15] Most of the injuries occur in the young,[1,13,16] with children constituting 25–50% of the total number.[1]

The causes of injury vary according to the age group. Whereas play is the most common in children, sports and assaults are predominant in young adults.[1] Domestic and occupational accidents are the usual causes in older adults.[1,17] Finally, ocular trauma tends to be more prevalent and more severe in the low socio-economic groups.[1,15]

RISK FACTORS LEADING TO GLAUCOMA IN TRAUMATIZED EYES

Each year, around 2.5 million eye injuries are reported.[18] This may be due to the inherent vulnerability of the eye owing to its prominent anatomic position, and because the act of vision necessitates that the eyes be directed toward the field of activity.

Ocular trauma falls into two large categories: blunt (nonpenetrating), which can be associated with hyphema (Fig. 58.1), and penetrating, where there may be retention of a foreign body (Fig. 58.2). In addition to the impact location, and the status of the globe before the trauma, several factors related to the injuring object determine the outcome: size, speed, shape, weight, composition, and direction.

Chemical (acid, alkali, etc.), electric, and radiation exposures are less common causes of ocular injury.

Irrespective of the type of injury, the dynamic and delicate balance between aqueous production and outflow is very frequently disrupted, resulting in IOP elevation.

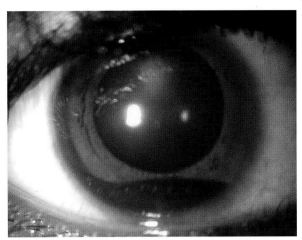

FIGURE 58.1 Traumatic hyphema.

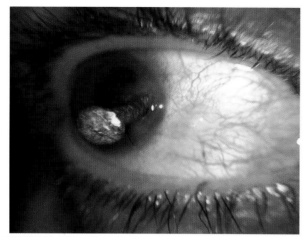

FIGURE 58.2 Metallic nail going through the cornea, right eye. (Courtesy of Dr George Cherfan.)

In nonpenetrating trauma, the impact of the moving object causes sudden, transient posterior displacement of the cornea and anterior sclera, with a compensatory expansion of the globe at the equator. Consequently, some of the sensitive and vital intraocular tissues may be torn under the impact of this sudden expansion, especially since both aqueous and vitreous are relatively incompressible. In 1991, Campbell[19] elegantly described seven anterior tissue rings where tears can occur as a result of blunt injury:

1. the sphincter pupillae (pupillary sphincter tears)
2. the peripheral iris attachment or iris root (iridodialysis, a traumatic separation between the iris and the ciliary body)
3. the anterior ciliary body (angle recession, a tear in the face of the ciliary body between the scleral spur and the ciliary body band, frequently occurring between the circular and longitudinal muscles of the ciliary body)
4. the ciliary body attachment to the scleral spur (cyclodialysis cleft, which allows passage of aqueous humor from the anterior chamber into the suprachoroidal space and may cause temporary or permanent hypotony)
5. the trabecular meshwork (trabecular dialysis)
6. the lens zonules (phacodonesis, subluxation, or lens dislocation)
7. the retinal attachment to the ora serrata (retinal dialysis and detachment).

PATHOGENESIS OF GLAUCOMA IN TRAUMATIZED EYES

BLUNT TRAUMA

Traumatic iritis Inflammation of the iris and/or ciliary body can occur as a direct consequence of trauma. The secondary inflammatory debris and proteins that are liberated into the anterior chamber can mechanically block the trabecular meshwork, causing a decrease in aqueous outflow and an increase in IOP. The meshwork itself can also become inflamed (trabeculitis) and swollen as a direct result of the trauma.[2] This rise in IOP can occur without hyphema, angle recession, or any visible physical disruption of the trabecular meshwork. While prostaglandins were thought to be instrumental in causing inflammation and secondary IOP rise by being released in blunt trauma in some studies, other studies failed to demonstrate any increase in their vitreous concentrations.[1]

Depending on the severity of the condition, slit lamp examination usually reveals inflammatory cells circulating in the anterior chamber, with or without ciliary injection. The anterior chamber is deep, and the angle is normal and wide.

In most cases, the IOP elevation is transient and responds well to treatment with topical aqueous suppressants. Topical corticosteroids are beneficial in controlling the inflammation and speeding up its resolution, and cycloplegics alleviate the pain caused by ciliary body spasm.[2]

Angle contusion Trauma may cause tears in the trabecular meshwork, which can be very subtle findings initially, and hence are often overlooked. Therefore, it is important to perform gonioscopy on both eyes, starting with the nontraumatized one.

Superficial tears manifest as trabecular flaps, often hinged at the level of the scleral spur.[2] In full-thickness tears, the outer wall of a blood-filled Schlemm's canal can be visualized, often together with some torn iris processes.[2] In either type of tear, the scleral spur is prominent and excessively white.

While these tears are probably the most common cause of early IOP rise in blunt trauma, they eventually heal in their original position without decreasing the outflow facility. Consequently, simple medical treatment can be sufficient to control the IOP in most instances. However, if significant scarring results from the healing process, chronic outflow obstruction occurs, and the secondary IOP rise might require filtering surgery later.[1] Following trauma, some eyes are found to have very low IOPs. This is thought to be secondary to ciliary body shock, which causes a temporary decrease in aqueous production.

Hyphema Hyphema is an accumulation of erythrocytes that disperse and layer in the anterior chamber, which is normally devoid of any kind of cells. Microhyphema refers to the situation where erythrocytes are suspended but no visible layering is seen by slit lamp microscopy.[20]

Traumatic hyphema is a frequent sequel of blunt and penetrating ocular injury. Its incidence has been recorded to be 12.2 per 100 000 of population, with 20.2 for males, 4.1 for females, and a prevalence of 70% in the pediatric population.[18] The peak incidence is between ages 10 to 20 years, with the average age being less than 25 years.[21] The causes are usually a high-energy blow to the orbit (61–66%), a strike from a missile or projectile (30.2–36%), or injury secondary to an explosion (2.4–3%).[18] The proportion of assaults, sports, and work accidents vary according to the specifically studied society and race.[21]

Blunt injury is associated with anteroposterior compression of the globe with simultaneous equatorial globe expansion.[21] As a result, the stromal iris and/or ciliary blood vessels are stretched and torn due to the displacement of the iris and lens.[18,22]

A second source of the initial hemorrhage is rupture of the fragile angle and iris vasculature due to an initial acute increase in IOP following the contusive trauma.[18] Bleeding will stop as a result of a fibrin-platelet clot, vascular spasm, and/or IOP tamponade. The clot may actually extend from the anterior into the posterior chamber and sometimes into the vitreous, reaching its maximal stabilization in 4–7 days.[20] These clots do not show fibroblastic activity or neovascularization, unlike other clots in the body.[23] Histologically, hyphema clots are an erythrocyte aggregate enveloped by a pseudocapsule of fibrin-plated coagulum.[18]

Hyphemas break down in the anterior chamber via the fibrinolytic system. The latter is activated by the conversion of plasminogen into plasmin.[20] As a result, free red blood cells and the breakdown products leave through the trabecular meshwork and Schlemm's canal.[18]

Secondary hemorrhage or re-bleeding may occur as a result of clot lysis and retraction from traumatized vessels.[21] It is the most common complication of traumatic hyphema, and usually occurs 2–5 days after the injury, at a rate of 22% (range 3.5–38%).[18,23] Re-bleeds are usually more severe than primary hemorrhages and more associated with complications such as glaucoma, corneal endothelial staining, and vitreous hemorrhage.[1] The risk factors for re-bleeds are 50% or more hyphema, ocular hypotony or hypertension, aspirin intake, black race,[20] sickle cell trait,[18] and poor vision on presentation.[1,20]

Hyphemas are universally graded on the basis of the volume of blood in the anterior chamber (Fig. 58.3). A grade I hyphema occupies less than one-third of the chamber, grade II is between one-third and one-half, grade III is more than one-half, and grade IV is a total hyphema.[18] The diagnosis of hyphema is strictly clinical, and usually there is a clear history of trauma, decreased vision, and pain. Abuse should be suspected in children whenever the reported circumstances are vague (Fig. 58.4).[20]

It is imperative to perform a complete eye examination, including tonometry and dilated funduscopy. However, both gonioscopy and ophthalmoscopy with scleral depression should be deferred, as such maneuvers may trigger re-bleeding. By the end of the first month, a careful gonioscopic examination should be done to rule out angle recession or other angle abnormalities. The same applies to the full retinal assessment.

The goal of management of traumatic hyphema is to minimize the chances of occurrence of complications such as re-bleeding, secondary glaucoma, and corneal endothelial blood staining.

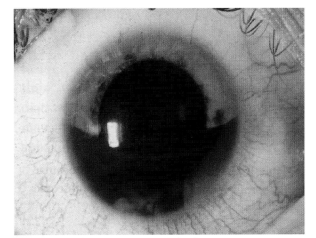

FIGURE 58.3 Fifty percent traumatic hyphema.

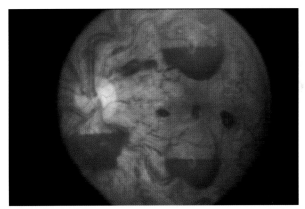

FIGURE 58.4 Preretinal boat-shaped hemorrhages and retinal venous congestion in a battered child.

In the past, hyphema patients used to be routinely admitted to hospital. Nowadays, the trend has changed to outpatient treatment, as studies have shown better cost-effectiveness of the latter, and that the rates of re-bleeding and of other complications were similar in the two treatments.[20] However, hospital admission is still indicated in specific cases, such as when the hyphema is larger than 50%, in re-bleeds, in cases with intractable glaucoma or sickle cell trait or anemia, and whenever child abuse is suspected.[18]

Similarly, and based on comparative studies, strict bed rest has been replaced by moderate activity.[20] Head elevation assists the hyphema to gravitate inferiorly, thus clearing the visual axis. Eye protection with a shield is indicated, usually without patching, unless there is an associated corneal abrasion, in which case topical antimicrobial therapy would also be required.[18] It is generally recommended that medications such as aspirin and nonsteroidal antiinflammatory agents be discontinued, although this issue has been controversial in some studies.[20]

Cycloplegics and topical corticosteroids have also been recommended in the majority of studies, to increase patient comfort and to decrease the inflammation that accompanies hyphema.[18,20] Posterior synechia formation is also decreased.

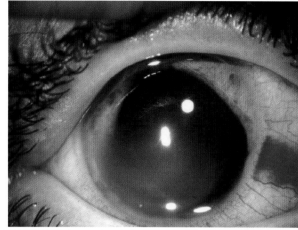

FIGURE 58.5 Corneal endothelial staining following traumatic hyphema.

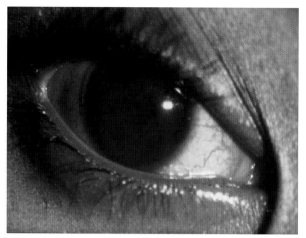

FIGURE 58.6 Eight-ball traumatic hyphema.

Systemic corticosteroid treatment (40 mg/day for adults and 0.6 mg/kg/day for children), given in divided doses, has been found to be associated with a lower rate of re-bleeding.[18,20]

Aminocaproic acid (ACA) is an antifibrinolytic agent that inhibits the conversion of plasminogen to plasmin, hence stabilizing the clot and preventing secondary hemorrhages. The recommended oral dose is 50 mg/kg every 4 hours for 5 days.[18] It should be started in hospital because of its frequent side effects; its topical use also seems promising.[20] Tranexamic acid has a similar mechanism of action to ACA, but is more potent and has fewer side effects.[20] Intracameral tissue plasminogen activator is indicated in hyphemas that end up being large, long-standing clots, with uncontrollable IOP.[18,20] Transcorneal oxygen therapy has been recommended in hyphema patients with sickle cell trait.[20]

The main cause of IOP increase in hyphema is thought to be the obstruction of the trabecular meshwork by erythrocytes and inflammatory debris.[20] Direct trauma to the angle may also play a role, as a significantly higher incidence of angle recession in hyphema patients with IOP increase has been reported.[24] Intraocular pressure elevation occurs in roughly 25% of hyphema patients, with sickle cell[20] and a large clot[21] being the most common risk factors. One must be aware that a component of pupillary block may be present if the clot occupies the whole pupillary aperture, thus preventing the normal passage of aqueous from the posterior to the anterior chamber.

The treatment of glaucoma secondary to hyphema is primarily medical, with topical agents such as β-blockers, α2-agonists, and carbonic anhydrase inhibitors (or a combination) being the most commonly used medications. Quite often, however, it is also necessary to use oral carbonic anhydrase inhibitors. In sicklers and in children it is preferable to use methazolamide rather than acetazolamide, as the latter lowers plasma pH, which promotes sickling of erythrocytes. Intravenous osmotic diuretics such as mannitol may also have to be used, kidney function permitting, in cases where rapid

IOP lowering is required.[18] Miotics and prostaglandin analogues should not be used, as they do cause an increase in the inflammatory response.[20]

Laser trabeculoplasty and filtering surgery have no role in the early management of IOP elevation in traumatic hyphema.

Beside glaucoma, the two other major complications of hyphema are the above-mentioned secondary bleeding and corneal endothelial staining (Fig. 58.5). Minor complications include peripheral anterior synechiae, posterior synechiae, cataract formation, and angle-recession glaucoma.[20]

Five percent to 7.2% of hyphema patients require surgical evacuation of the blood clot.[18] The classic indications for surgical treatment include a 100% hyphema (Fig. 58.6), early corneal blood staining, sickle cell trait/anemia, detection of active bleeding, and uncontrolled IOP despite maximally tolerated medical therapy.[18] One final indication would be the persistence of a hyphema that is more than 50% for more than 10 days.

Seventy-five percent of all hyphema patients are said to regain a final visual acuity of 20/50 or better.[20]

Angle recession Recession of the anterior chamber angle is extraordinarily common after blunt ocular trauma (Fig. 58.7).[2] The reported types of trauma causing angle recession include sports/recreational accidents in some studies[25] and assault in others.[26]

A spectrum of injuries to the outflow system ranging from isolated trabecular meshwork damage to frank angle recession has been reported in 60–94% of patients exposed to blunt ocular trauma.[1,25,26] Although recession can occur without bleeding in the anterior chamber, a strong correlation has been established between the former and hyphema. Several studies have demonstrated gonioscopically that 55–100% of patients with traumatic hyphema have some degree of angle recession.[25]

Although angle recession is a common finding after blunt trauma, only 7–9% of patients with recession will develop glaucoma, which usually appears years or even

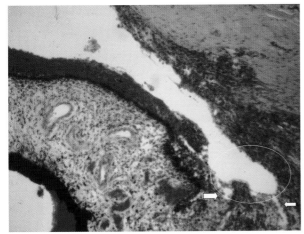

FIGURE 58.7 Traumatic angle recession. Circle outlines the amount of recession. Also tear in the ciliary body is observed (*arrows*).

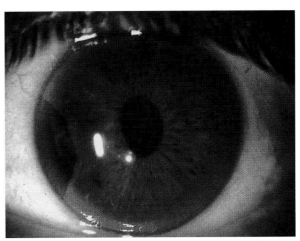

FIGURE 58.9 Traumatic iridodialysis between 7:00 and 10:00 o'clock.

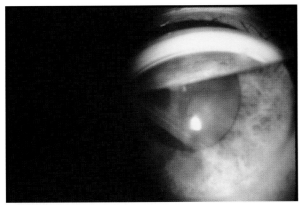

FIGURE 58.8 Angle recession apparent through the superior slit lamp goniophotograph.

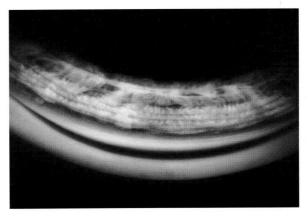

FIGURE 58.10 Slit lamp goniophotograph of inferior angle recession.

decades after the trauma.[2] Additionally, there appear to be two peak incidences for the glaucoma after recession: the first peak occurs within the first weeks to years after the trauma, while the second occurs 10 or more years after the injury.[25]

There is also an association between the extent of angle recession and the development of glaucoma. Patients with 180–360° of angle recession have a high risk of developing late-onset glaucoma, whereas those with less than 180° have a significantly lower risk.[25]

In 50% of patients with angle-recession glaucoma, the contralateral eye has been shown to develop open-angle glaucoma, sometimes years after the IOP rise in the traumatized eye.[25] These contralateral eyes were also positive for the topical corticosteroid provocative testing.[25] Consequently, it is speculated that there might be a genetic predisposition for developing glaucoma in some patients where angle recession occurs following trauma; angle recession seems to accelerate the appearance of glaucoma rather than being the cause in itself.[25]

Immediately after the injury, angle recession may not be apparent on gonioscopic examination, as blood, inflammatory cells, or corneal haze can obscure it. Great care must be taken while doing gonioscopy on eyes with a recent hyphema, for fear of triggering re-bleeding.[2] The contralateral uninjured eye should be examined first for comparison, and the appearance of the angle depends on the degree and extent of recession. With minor angle damage, there is disruption of the regular pattern of insertion of the iris fibers, widening of the ciliary body band, and whitening of the scleral spur (Fig. 58.8). Some iris processes might be torn, and some uveal tissue tufts might be seen overriding the iris root and trabecular meshwork.[25] Other accompanying features might be tears in the meshwork, iridodialysis (Fig. 58.9), and cyclodialysis.[25] In localized recession, there is deepening of the corresponding anterior chamber angle with change in its color and texture. In eyes with a 360° recession, comparison with the contralateral eye is what makes the diagnosis in many cases. Howard et al. used the depth of the ciliary muscle tears to classify angle recession into shallow, moderate (Fig. 58.10), and deep.[25] Soon after the injury, the ciliary body tear might scar, with the formation of peripheral anterior synechiae, which makes it difficult to assess the original depth and extent of the recession in future examinations. Consequently, critical search for one or more of the following associated findings should be undertaken: lid scars, very deep anterior chamber, ruptured pupillary sphincter, torn iris processes,

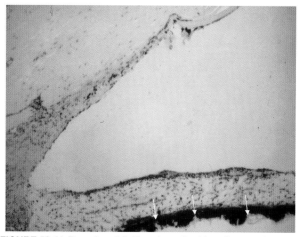

FIGURE 58.11 Pseudoexfoliation deposits. Note the prominent periodic acid-Schiff (PAS)-positive material on the iris pigment pithelium (*arrows*), which is irregular as a consequence.

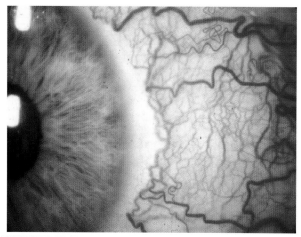

FIGURE 58.12 Engorged veins in an eye that has increased episcleral venous pressure glaucoma.

iridoschisis, irido/phacodenesis, and the presence of a Vossius' ring.[1]

The differential diagnosis for angle recession includes cyclodialysis, where the separation is between the longitudinal muscles of the ciliary body and the sclera rather than between the longitudinal and circular muscles of the ciliary body;[25] other entities include iridodialysis, trabecular tears, and other preexisting angle anomalies.[25] As unilateral and asymmetrical open-angle glaucoma is very uncommon, the following entities should also be ruled out: pseudoexfoliation (Fig. 58.11), uveitic, lens-induced, increased episcleral venous pressure (Fig. 58.12), and tumors.[25]

When corneal opacification prevents clear visualization of the angle structures, ultrasound biomicroscopy might be helpful in detecting moderate to significant angle recession.[25]

With respect to the mechanism of glaucoma, the finding of a ciliary body tear speaks for previous trauma, but might not be the cause of IOP increase.[25] Several experimental and animal-model studies have shown that blunt trauma forces the aqueous posteriorly and

laterally, and this in itself can create the tear in the ciliary body, and can also injure the anterior and posterior ciliary arteries resulting in hyphema when it happens.[25] The same traumatic force can cause direct damage to the meshwork, which explains the early IOP increase in some cases. The latter is also caused by the loss of the tension normally exerted by the longitudinal ciliary muscle over the trabecular meshwork and scleral spur.[25]

The more frequent and aggressive late glaucoma is due to degeneration, atrophy, fibrosis, and scarring of both the meshwork and Schlemm's canal.[25] Some studies have incriminated the growth of a Descemet's-like hyaline membrane that covers the iridocorneal angle, also contributing to the decrease in aqueous outflow.[25]

Attempting to increase outflow through the conventional (trabecular) and uveoscleral pathways by medical treatment is usually not very successful.[2] Miotics are also contraindicated as they have caused a paradoxical IOP increase in some cases, through impairing the uveoscleral outflow.[1] Prostaglandin analogues may be beneficial, as well as the aqueous suppressants (β-blockers, α_2-agonists, and carbonic anhydrase inhibitors).[25] While medical therapy may control the early IOP rise, it is usually not very effective in late-onset glaucoma.[25] Both argon laser trabeculoplasty[25] and Nd:YAG laser trabeculopuncture have been found to be unsatisfactory in controlling the IOP.[1] Trabeculectomy without antimetabolites has a lower rate of success in angle recession (43%) compared to primary open-angle glaucoma (75%).[25] Increased fibroblast proliferation, change in aqueous humor properties secondary to increase in the stimulatory and decrease in the inhibitory (fibroblast) growth factors have all been incriminated in the decreased surgical success rate.[25] On the other hand, when mitomycin C is used, the success rate of trabeculectomy was seen to increase to 77% in some studies.[16,25] Setons also have a favorable outcome, especially following failed filtering surgery.[25] Cyclodestructive procedures, especially diode laser cyclophotocoagulation, may be considered in intractable cases.[25]

Lens subluxation/pupil block Subluxation or total dislocation of the lens can occur secondary to traumatic zonular rupture (Fig. 58.13).[1,2] Lens injury (including subluxation/dislocation) has been found to be a risk factor for developing glaucoma 6 months following blunt trauma (Fig. 58.14).[27]

Partial anterior displacement of the lens can cause pupillary block and secondary angle closure. Occasionally, the vitreous itself may cause pupillary block as it prolapses through ruptured zonules. The rise in IOP is frequently acute in such cases, and is associated with anterior chamber shallowing, decreased acuity, acquired myopia, and a closed angle by gonioscopy. Laser iridotomy might be initially beneficial in relatively quiet eyes.

With total dislocation of the lens into the anterior chamber, there may be pupillary block and secondary

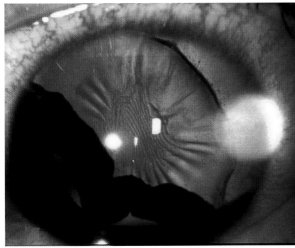

FIGURE 58.13 Slit lamp photograph of a subluxated lens and a superior and nasal iridodialysis.

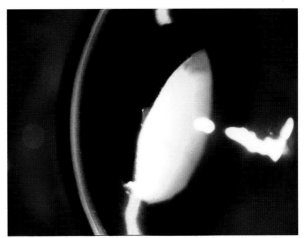

FIGURE 58.15 Traumatic posterior lens subluxation (slit lamp photograph).

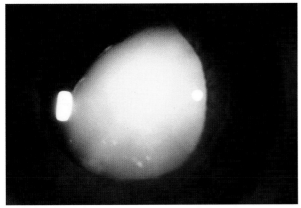

FIGURE 58.14 Traumatic inferonasal subluxation of the lens.

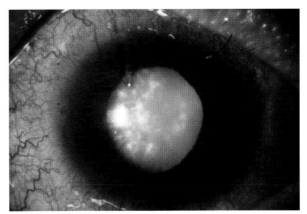

FIGURE 58.16 Phacolytic glaucoma.

angle closure, or the IOP might increase because of direct angle obstruction by the lens or its fragments. With either partial or total anterior lens displacement, corneal decompensation can occur, which necessitates urgent lens removal.[2]

With posterior lens displacement (Fig. 58.15), vitreous prolapse may be the cause of pupillary block, although the angle appears to be open, with peripheral anterior synechiae seen only occasionally.[2] Laser iridotomy is indicated, even if the lens is thrown far back in the vitreous cavity. Close follow-up is required as the lens may eventually need to be removed through a pars plana approach if it becomes hypermature and starts causing phacolytic glaucoma, or if it causes lens-particle glaucoma.[28]

An understanding of the mechanism of glaucoma in traumatic lens subluxation is essential for planning the correct therapeutic approach. Lensectomy is one of the obvious choices whenever secondary angle closure is causing an increase in IOP.

Depending on the anatomic logistics of the subluxation, lensectomy procedures vary from intracapsular to extracapsular, including phacoemulsification when enough zonular support is present, or most commonly pars plana lensectomy and vitrectomy.[29]

Lens-induced (phacolytic) glaucoma Phacolytic glaucoma is a secondary type of open-angle glaucoma that occurs mainly in developing countries, where there is usually a high incidence of hypermature cataracts. The second main cause is nonpenetrating ocular trauma. Microscopic leakage of high molecular weight lens proteins through an intact anterior capsule causes a severe inflammatory reaction, characterized by the presence of cells, flare, and white particles in a deep anterior chamber (Fig. 58.16).[30] The angle is wide open by gonioscopy, the cornea may be edematous, and occasionally a hypopyon may be seen.

The IOP rise is acute, because of blockage of the trabecular meshwork channels by proteins, protein-laden macrophages, and inflammatory debris (Fig. 58.17).[30] The trabecular blockage as well as the high IOP are both reversible when lens extraction is performed directly following the onset of symptoms, and the eye is treated with topical corticosteroids.[30] On the other hand, in cases that present late, cataract extraction alone may not be sufficient for adequate IOP control, because there may be permanent trabecular damage caused by the chronic inflammatory process. In such cases, it is recommended that cataract extraction be combined with filtering surgery.

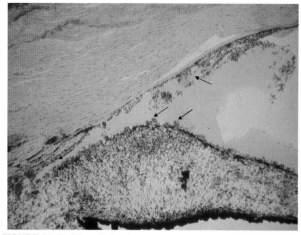

FIGURE 58.17 Phacolytic glaucoma. Protein-laden macrophages are seen in the anterior chamber angle and on the anterior iris surface (*arrows*).

Ghost-cell glaucoma Ghost-cell glaucoma is a type of secondary open-angle glaucoma that occurs in some cases where trauma has caused bleeding in the vitreous. One to three weeks following the hemorrhage, the fresh, pliable, and biconcave erythrocytes degenerate into smaller forms called ghost cells. The latter are rigid, spherical, khaki-colored, and contain denatured hemoglobin that is adherent to the cell membrane (Heinz bodies).[31]

The ghost cells pass into the anterior chamber through the disrupted anterior hyaloid face, and may remain there for months. Being more rigid and less pliable than red blood cells, ghost cells pass through the trabecular meshwork with significant difficulty, and can thus cause a threefold decrease in outflow facility; hence the rise in IOP.[31]

Observing the small tan-colored cells in a typically deep anterior chamber makes the clinical diagnosis. The angle is wide open by gonioscopy, and the meshwork is discolored due to the presence of the khaki-colored layer. The latter layer, when thick and settled inferiorly, has been confused with a hypopyon[1] in some instances, and the whole condition mistaken for endophthalmitis in others. The candy-stripe sign refers to the khaki layer on top of another red one, when fresh erythrocytes coexist with the ghost cells.

The histologic diagnosis is made by routine light microscopy of cytopsin and paraffin-embedded anterior chamber aspirates.[32] Staining with 1% methyl violet is another option, while phase-contrast microscopy of unstained aspirates is disappointing.[31]

The increase in the IOP is usually short-lived, except in some rare instances where it might take months for the denatured cells to disappear. The response to topical medical treatment with β-blockers, α$_2$-agonists, and carbonic anhydrase inhibitors is satisfactory in most patients. Resistant cases might require anterior chamber washout, or pars plana vitrectomy to remove the reservoir of ghost cells.[1]

Hemolytic glaucoma Traumatic vitreous hemorrhage is a prerequisite for causing this rare type of secondary open-angle glaucoma, and the similar pathophysiology to phacolytic glaucoma is responsible for the name.

Reddish-brown blood cells are seen in the anterior chamber, as well as on the trabecular meshwork, especially inferiorly. The increase in IOP is caused by the obstruction of the trabecular meshwork by red blood cell debris, free hemoglobin, and hemoglobin-laden macrophages.[31]

The clinical picture is similar to that of ghost-cell glaucoma. However, anterior chamber aspirates show macrophages containing golden-brown pigment, but no ghost cells.[1] Other histologic studies show degenerative changes in the trabecular endothelial cells, which also have phagocytosed blood.[1]

The IOP increase is transient, occurring days to weeks following the trauma, and usually responds well to medical treatment with topical β-blockers, α$_2$-agonists, and carbonic anhydrase inhibitors. Only rarely does anterior chamber washout or vitrectomy become indicated.[1]

Hemosiderotic glaucoma This is a rare type of glaucoma that presents many years after trauma, resulting either from long-lasting vitreous hemorrhage or from a retained iron-containing foreign body.[31] In either case, the iron from the disintegrating hemoglobin or from the foreign body itself will find its way into the anterior chamber, being helped by the liquefied vitreous in such cases.[31]

The mucopolysaccharides of the trabecular meshwork have a high affinity for iron, which will be phagocytosed by the endothelial cells.[31] The latter cells will be damaged, with secondary degenerative changes in the meshwork, including siderosis, sclerosis, and obliteration of the intertrabecular spaces.[1] The resulting decrease in aqueous outflow is responsible for the IOP rise. Treatment is the same as for ghost-cell glaucoma, and the clinical picture is similar except for the additional findings of ocular hemosiderosis, such as opacification of the lens, change in the iris color, and electroretinographic abnormalities.[31]

Corticosteroid-induced glaucoma Corticosteroids are often used to combat the inflammation that is associated with blunt and penetrating ocular trauma. The routes of administration can be topical, periocular, intravitreal, intravenous, or oral. It is conceivable that some cases requiring prolonged corticosteroid therapy, by any route, may turn out to be positive steroid responders and end up with secondary glaucoma.[33] Depending on the magnitude of IOP increase, 5–30% of the general population are steroid responders.[33] Primary open-angle glaucoma patients, their first-degree relatives, and ocular hypertensives are also at increased risk of being steroid responders.[33]

Age itself has been shown to be a risk factor with a bimodal distribution, the first being at the age of 6 years, and the second during adulthood.[33] The same applies to patients with high myopia, connective tissue disease, and type 1 diabetes mellitus.[33]

Increased aqueous outflow resistance is the mechanism by which steroids cause an increase in the IOP.

Increased resistance is partially caused by changes in the microstructure of the trabecular meshwork: actin stress fibers are reorganized into polygonal lattices in meshwork cells cultured with dexamethasone.[33]

The second mechanism by which the outflow facility is decreased is the deposition of extracellular matrix (ECM) in the trabecular meshwork. Glycosaminoglycan in elastin, fibronectin, and myocilin are all increased in trabecular meshwork cells cultured with dexamethasone.[33]

The last mechanism by which outflow facility is decreased is the lowered functional activity in the meshwork secondary to the reduced degradation and phagocytosis of substances in it. This has been confirmed when trabecular meshwork cultures were treated with dexamethasone: tissue plasminogen activator, stromelysin, metalloproteases, and arachidonic acid metabolism were all found to be decreased.[33]

The amount of IOP increase is proportional to the steroid's potency, and its intraocular availability; dexamethasone heads the list and is followed by prednisolone, medrysone, and fluorometholone.

The time span between steroid administration and IOP increase is usually days to months, with topical and intravitreal[33] being the fastest routes of delivery. The diagnosis requires a high index of suspicion, especially in ocular trauma where other serious findings might be confusing the picture.[34] The logical treatment is to stop, taper, or shift to a less potent steroid, while trying to lower the IOP. All the known antiglaucoma medications can be used, and the IOP usually returns to normal within weeks to months.[34] Laser trabeculoplasty has not been found to be effective, and filtering surgery is sometimes needed for intractable cases.[34]

PENETRATING INJURIES

Without intraocular foreign body Corneal wounds, especially if neglected for some time before being repaired, may cause secondary angle-closure glaucoma, due to the formation of extensive peripheral anterior synechiae as a result of prolonged anterior chamber flattening and chronic inflammation.[34] A second cause of glaucoma following corneal wounds is the formation of posterior synechiae secondary to inflammation, seclusion of the pupil, and iris bombe, leading itself to angle closure.[2] Consequently, prompt reformation of the anterior chamber through adequate wound closure is essential to prevent angle closure. Topical, and occasionally systemic, corticosteroids are indicated to control the inflammation postoperatively, and mydriasis is recommended. Laser peripheral iridotomy may also be performed to break the pupillary block, causing the iris to fall back from its bombe configuration, and thus preventing secondary angle closure.

Secondary glaucoma in penetrating injuries can also be caused by hyphema or by lens dislocation, as discussed above under blunt trauma.

Occasionally, phacomorphic, phacolytic, or ghost-cell glaucoma (discussed above) may also be seen following penetrating eye injuries.

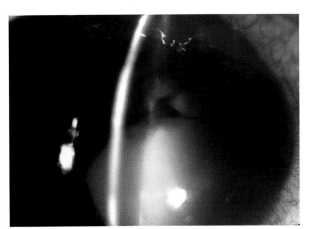

FIGURE 58.18 Slit lamp photograph of traumatic lens-particle glaucoma.

Lens-particle glaucoma Lens-particle glaucoma can occur in blunt ocular injury, but is more common in penetrating ones. It is not to be confused with phacolytic glaucoma, which is secondary open-angle glaucoma, related to a hypermature or mature cataract (discussed above).

True traumatic disruption of the lens capsule releases lens particles into the anterior chamber (Fig. 58.18). The former are accompanied in the chamber with white flakes, and seen also at the anterior vitreous. Anterior chamber aspirates are present together with lenticular cortical fibers. Peripheral anterior as well as posterior synechiae are formed by the secondary inflammation.[2]

Corticosteroids and cycloplegics are used to control the inflammation and prevent complications.

Glaucoma is acutely due to the lens particles physically obstructing the trabecular meshwork, and chronically is secondary to one or two types of synechiae.

Aqueous suppressants can control the IOP in most instances, but occasionally lens extraction becomes mandatory in intractable cases.

Sympathetic ophthalmia Sympathetic ophthalmia can be associated with glaucoma. The former is a very rare bilateral granulomatous panuveitis that occurs after penetrating ocular injury associated with uveal tissue prolapse. It is usually mild and self-limited. However, the inflammation can become chronic, with iris nodules, mutton-fat keratic precipitates, optic disc swelling, and multifocal choroiditis; it is under these conditions that the IOP is seen to increase.[35] The treatment is naturally directed towards controlling the inflammation with steroids, and sometimes immunosuppressive agents. Aqueous suppressants are the main antiglaucoma agents to be used.

Fibrous ingrowth/epithelial downgrowth Following penetrating injury, the external ocular epithelial surface is interrupted and might grow inside the eye, where it becomes implanted. The outcome is fibrous ingrowth, or epithelial downgrowth (Fig. 58.19), and glaucoma due to trabecular meshwork mechanical obstruction can occur with either one. Epithelial downgrowth is the

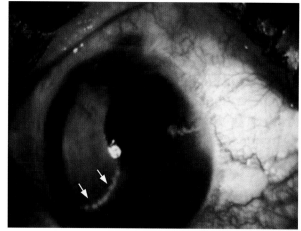

FIGURE 58.19 Arrows indicating the anterior edge of epithelial downgrowth following penetrating ocular injury.

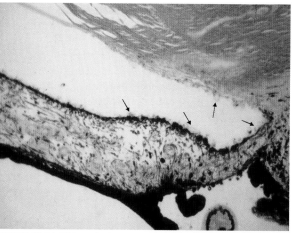

FIGURE 58.21 Siderosis. Iron material is deposited over the anterior iris surface, the angle, and the trabecular meshwork (*arrows*).

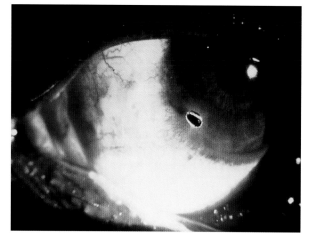

FIGURE 58.20 Metallic foreign body injury, left eye.

more aggressive, due to the extensive proliferation of the implanted cells.[2]

With intraocular foreign body Once inside the eye, a foreign body may lodge itself anywhere from the cornea and chamber anteriorly back to the choroid and retina posteriorly (Fig. 58.20). Common sequels are cataract formation due to capsule rupture, vitreous liquefaction/hemorrhage, and retinal bleeding and tears. Infections are common with stones and organic material, but not with inert materials such as glass, plastic, gold, or silver.[35]

The mechanisms responsible for IOP increase in blunt and penetrating injuries also apply to cases of penetrating trauma with retained intraocular foreign bodies.

Siderosis A specific late elevation of IOP is related to iron toxicity of a metallic foreign body, siderosis (Fig. 58.21). The pathogenesis of this glaucoma is trabecular meshwork damage.

Steel is probably the most common foreign body, and, upon its disintegration, iron gets deposited in the epithelial surfaces of mainly the lens and retina, where it exerts toxic effects on the cellular enzyme systems. Slit lamp findings include reddish-brownish iris heterochromia, mydriasis, and rust-like discoloration of the anterior lens surface.[34] Pigmentary retinopathy might be present, and electroretinography might be required to confirm the diagnosis, by showing progressive attenuation of the b wave.

Chalcosis Foreign bodies with a high copper content can cause a severe endophthalmitis-like reaction that might result in phthisis bulbi. Fortunately, however, brass and bronze have a relatively low copper content and when inside the eye might cause only chalcosis. This refers to the tissue damage caused by oxidized copper similar to that seen in Wilson's disease.[35] Slit lamp examination might reveal the Kayser-Fleischer ring, and the anterior sunflower cataract. Golden plaques are seen when retinal deposition occurs, but degenerative retinopathy is very rare as copper is less retinotoxic than iron. Chalcosis is also less frequently associated with glaucoma.[34]

Even if not done at the time of the first emergency surgery, prompt assessment and surgical removal of retained foreign bodies is associated with a better visual outcome and a reduced rate of complications, especially glaucoma.

CHEMICAL INJURIES

In the United States, 7–10% of all ocular injuries presenting to emergency departments are ocular burns, and 84% of those are chemical burns.[34] The ratio of the frequency of acids to alkalis has a mean of 1:4 in most studies, as alkalis are more widely used at home and in industry. In developing countries, 80% of ocular chemical burns are due to industrial and/or occupational exposure.[35]

Chemical injuries can cause extensive damage to the ocular surface and anterior segment, resulting in unilateral (and occasionally bilateral) permanent loss of vision. The most common alkalis involved are ammonia, sodium hydrochloride, and lime. Alkalis are lipophilic, and saponification of cell membrane fatty acids causes collagen denaturation, cell disruption, and death. The subsequent inflammation ends up in liquefaction necrosis through the release of proteolytic enzymes. Being very efficient in rapidly reaching the anterior chamber (10–15 minutes), the iris, ciliary body, lens, and trabecular meshwork are exposed to direct damage.[36]

Transient secondary glaucoma is most likely due to a short-lived trabeculitis as part of the generalized inflammation that accompanies mild alkali burns. In more severe cases, irreversible damage to the meshwork explains the intractable glaucoma that is resistant to medical therapy.

Acid burns cause protein coagulation in the corneal epithelium, which limits further penetration, and consequently makes the burns superficial and nonprogressive. The most implicated acids are sulfuric, sulfurous, hydrofluoric, acetic, chromic, and hydrochloric.[36]

With both acids and alkali, the severity of the burn depends on the duration and degree of penetration, the ocular surface area of exposure, and toxicity of the implicated substance.

The most critical step in the management is copious irrigation for up to 15 minutes, with removal of any retained material in the conjunctival fornices.

The IOP is usually initially increased secondary to anterior segment inflammation, shrinkage, and prostaglandin-mediated increased uveal blood flow. Hypotony occurs only if the ciliary body is severely damaged. Beta-blockers, α_2-agonists, and carbonic anhydrase inhibitors are recommended, but not miotics or prostaglandin analogues. While corticosteroids are theoretically needed at this stage, the increased predisposition to secondary infections makes their use controversial.[1]

The intermediate phase is characterized by attempts at reepithelialization and repair. In this stage the IOP is increased due to the persistent trabeculitis, and sometimes to pupillary block secondary to posterior synechia formation. A third mechanism would be trabecular meshwork damage due to either direct exposure or peripheral anterior synechia formation. Systemic corticosteroids are invariably needed to control the inflammation, but not topical ones because of the danger of corneal stromal melting. Cycloplegic/mydriatic therapy is used for pupillary block, and if it fails laser iridotomy should be attempted. The same antiglaucoma regimen as in the acute phase is usually used.[36]

Glaucoma occurring in the late and most severe stages of chemical injuries is the most intractable to treat. This is due to it being secondary to a closed angle with peripheral anterior synechiae, and to an irreversibly scarred trabecular meshwork. Corneal opacification that characterizes these stages makes routine applanation IOP measurements a problem (Fig. 58.22). Under such circumstances, the Tono-Pen or the pneumatonometer may be more useful and accurate. Conservative medical antiglaucoma therapy is rarely sufficient, and filtering surgery with antimetabolites is

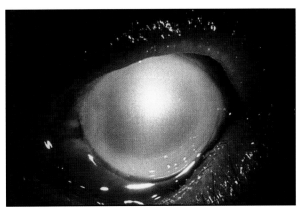

FIGURE 58.22 Stage IV corneal scar following severe thermal injury.

recommended, if there is enough viable conjunctiva. If this is not the case, then glaucoma drainage implantation or diode laser cyclodestruction will be the final option.[1]

THERMAL OCULAR BURNS

Ocular burns occur in 7–27% of thermal injuries admitted to burn units, and they account for 7–10% of ocular trauma cases presenting to emergency units.[37] They are more common in males, and the average age is 30 years. They usually result from accidents associated with firework explosions, steam, boiling water/liquids, hot gases, or molten metal.[38]

Thermal burns may produce extensive damage to the ocular surface epithelium and anterior segment, resulting in permanent unilateral or bilateral visual impairment.

Tissues are damaged by denaturation and coagulation of cellular proteins, and secondary vascular ischemia.

The lids are naturally the most affected because of their forward position and exposure, and their involvement follows a prognostic classification.[38]

Grading the degree of limbal stem cell loss is also of prognostic and therapeutic benefit. In general, the management should aim at controlling the inflammation, promoting ocular surface epithelial recovery, and increasing keratocyte collagen production. Amniotic membrane and limbal cell transplantation has come a long way in the management of advanced and severe cases.

The IOP is initially increased following a biphasic response: the first results from contraction of collagen with shrinkage of the outer coats of the eye, including the trabecular meshwork; the second is caused by the release of prostaglandins and is more sustained. This early IOP rise is transient and responds rather well to antiinflammatory therapy alone. It is the secondary glaucoma resulting from scarring of the meshwork and closure of the angle by peripheral synechiae that requires hypotensive therapy. Aqueous suppressants, topical and systemic, are tried first, and filtering surgery with antimetabolites, or setons are indicated in cases that are resistant to treatment.

ELECTRICAL INJURIES

The extent of ocular tissue damage caused by electrical injuries depends on the intensity and duration of the current, the retina and optic nerve being the most vulnerable structures.[39] The causes of injury are either accidental, such as in industrial exposure, or therapy-related, such as with cardioversion or electroshock treatment.[1]

Mydriasis ipsilateral to the side of injury is a transient finding that occurs secondary to temporary autonomic dysfunction.

Cataract formation is the most common sequel, occurring anywhere between 1 month and 2 years after the injury. Opacities start as anterior subcapsular vacuoles, to be replaced gradually by fine linear opacities, which eventually progress to the visual axis.[39]

Intraocular inflammation, specifically iritis, also occurs, but mainly in eyes that develop cataracts. Transient IOP elevation has also been observed in some of these cases and in cases where there is significant loss of iris pigment epithelium. Consequently, it is speculated that this short-lived glaucoma is inflammation related, while venous dilation and extraocular muscle contraction play a less important role in its pathogenesis.[1] Treatment is rarely needed, because of the transient nature of the IOP spike.

Finally, macular changes in the form of edema or hole formation have been observed in some cases.

RADIATION INJURIES

Injury to the visual system can occur as a complication of radiotherapy of intracranial, intraorbital, periocular, or intraocular neoplasms. Radiotherapy has become much safer, as minimal effective Gy dosages are currently being used for the various tumors, and because of the development of new techniques for optimal patient positioning, field reproducibility, unconventional angles of beam entry, and geometric shaping of the radiation vectors.[40]

But despite all the attention to detail, radiation-induced ocular injury still occurs. If the orbital contents are irradiated, lacrimal tissue injury is common, with secondary dry eye, and the sequelae of corneal edema, ulceration, infection, vascularization, and opacification. Consequently, shielding of the lacrimal apparatus during treatment is mandatory.

Radiation retinopathy is the second most common complication, occurring usually 2–3 years after radiation therapy, and is associated with rubeosis iridis and neovascular glaucoma in 50% of cases. Old age, chemotherapy, diabetes, and high-dose radiation are all risk factors for the occurrence of glaucoma. Treating the retinopathy by panretinal photocoagulation may be protective.[40] Other mechanisms of IOP increase include hemolytic changes associated with intraocular hemorrhage, and increased episcleral venous pressure caused by irradiation of the anterior segment.[1] Finally, blindness may occur in cases where there is direct radiation injury to the optic nerve or chiasm.

DIAGNOSTIC FEATURES

CLINICAL HISTORY AND EXAMINATION

In almost all cases of ocular trauma, the eye abnormalities can be attributed directly to the injury, based on a clear history given by the patient, or by the family in cases where the patient is a child or infant. Occasionally, such a link may not be obvious, for more than one reason:

1. The trauma may have occurred such a long time ago that the patient does not even recall it ever happening, or does not mention it because he or she does not appreciate its significance; for example, angle-recession glaucoma detected 10 years after a long-forgotten and overlooked blunt tennis ball injury.

2. The patient may never be aware of the trauma. Occasionally, very tiny, high-speed foreign bodies can penetrate the cornea and lodge anywhere within the eye without causing any immediate signs or symptoms. For example, the authors have seen localized lens opacities that remain stationary (and unnoticed by the patient, mostly because of their peripheral location) for long periods of time. These may be discovered long after the trauma, but only if and when lens proteins start leaking again from the initially self-sealing anterior capsular break, inducing inflammation, progression of cataract, or lens-induced glaucoma. When the eye is examined carefully, one can often detect the scar of a tiny corneal entry wound, and possibly also a tiny iridotomy. The foreign body itself may never be detected, either because it is extremely small, or engulfed within intraocular structures, such as iris or lens, or it may even be lodged in the angle.

3. The patient may be hiding or altering some facts because of certain medicolegal considerations. History taking in cases of intentional or unintentional ocular injuries inflicted by other individuals, or sustained at work, must be handled and interpreted with extreme caution. The patient may elect to change the facts in order to incriminate a presumed assailant or to obtain financial compensation from his or her employer or insurance company. The intricacies of medicolegal trauma cases are beyond the scope of this chapter.

OCULAR IMAGING

Various imaging techniques can be useful in evaluating the anterior and posterior segments of a traumatized eye if clinical examination is not possible or nonrevealing. Classical ultrasonography (A and B scan), ultrasound biomicroscopy (UBM), anterior-segment optical coherence tomography (OCT), and computed tomography (CT) scanning or magnetic resonance imaging (MRI) can all provide useful information about the integrity of intraocular structures if the view is obscured, for example, by hyphema or vitreous hemorrhage.

GONIOSCOPY

The importance of gonioscopy in elucidating the mechanism of glaucoma in a traumatized eye cannot be overemphasized. Angle recession is often missed if the treating ophthalmologist fails to look carefully at the angle. Other stigmata of trauma in the angle include iris or ciliary body dialysis, trabecular meshwork tears, and occasionally the presence of a foreign body (see sections on hyphema and angle recession above).

DIAGNOSTIC TAPS

Occasionally, when the clinical picture is not very clear as to the exact etiology of glaucoma, microscopic examination of aqueous or vitreous aspirates can be helpful. Examples of such situations include ghost-cell and lens-particle or phacolytic glaucoma.

TREATMENT OPTIONS

As with other types of glaucoma, there are three possible treatment modalities that can be resorted to in glaucoma secondary to trauma: medical, surgical, and cyclodestructive.

MEDICAL TREATMENT

Although most eyes that develop glaucoma as a result of trauma end up requiring surgical treatment, medical therapy is still useful, either in preparation for surgery or for the chronic treatment of those difficult cases that cannot be controlled fully by surgery. The treatment regimen should be individualized depending on the condition of the eye, the age of the patient, and the patient's general health. Eyes that harbor any degree of inflammation should not be given prostaglandin analogues or miotics. The latter should also be avoided in the young age groups. Alpha$_2$-adrenergic agonists, and to a lesser extent β-blockers, can have morbid or even fatal side effects in infants. Sometimes, desperate cases may require chronic treatment with systemic carbonic anhydrase inhibitors. If such treatment is inevitable, one may be able to reduce some of the side effects by giving doses smaller than what is generally recommended. Often, 125 mg of oral acetazolamide given twice daily may be sufficient. Alternatively, using slow-release acetazolamide capsules or other preparations such as methazolamide may improve tolerance. Of course, patients on such chronic systemic treatment should be monitored periodically for any serum electrolyte imbalance or blood dyscrasias.

SURGICAL TREATMENT

Filtering procedures Trabeculectomy is generally not very successful in traumatized eyes, especially in the presence of significant conjunctival scarring and/or anterior segment distortion, and following prior surgery

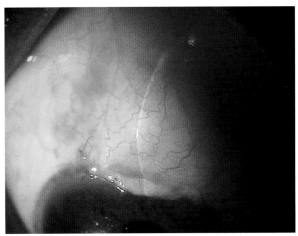

FIGURE 58.23 Elevated vascularized bleb.

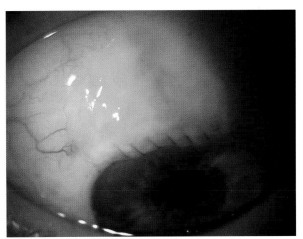

FIGURE 58.24 Elevated, avascular, Mitomycin C bleb.

(Fig. 58.23). The chances of success may be improved by the use of adjunctive antifibrotic agents during and after surgery (Fig. 58.24). It is a must to use such agents in high-risk eyes, unless there is an absolute contraindication, such as conjunctival or scleral thinning. Aphakic and pseudophakic eyes and those with distorted anterior segments are not good candidates for trabeculectomy, and hence other procedures need to be considered.

Glaucoma drainage devices Glaucoma drainage devices should be considered in eyes not suitable for trabeculectomy, the best example being aphakic eyes (Fig. 58.25). It is important to have enough space in the anterior segment that allows proper positioning of the tube. Occasionally, in eyes with totally obliterated chambers (for example, following penetrating keratoplasty), the tube may be introduced through iris tissue to lodge in the posterior chamber. Some devices can be adapted for pars plana implantation. However, this approach entails a very thorough vitrectomy, which in itself increases the morbidity of the procedure. Nevertheless, the long-term safety and efficacy of pars plana tube implantation remains questionable.

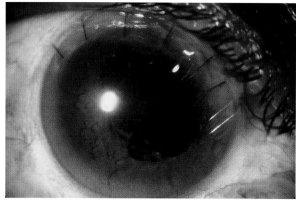

FIGURE 58.25 Glaucoma implant tip apparent in the anterior chamber of an eye that had undergone lensectomy-vitrectomy and suturing of a large corneoscleral laceration.

The specific type of device utilized does not make a lot of difference as far as the final outcome. The surgeon should choose the device that he or she is most familiar with and which gives the best results in his or her hands.

CYCLODESTRUCTIVE PROCEDURES

Cyclodestructive procedures have generally been reserved for eyes that are not suitable for filtering surgery or for tube implants, and mostly for those with poor visual prognosis. While this may apply to procedures such as cyclodiathermy (nowadays totally abandoned) or cyclocryotherapy, it may not necessarily be true when it comes to modern, less traumatic cyclodestructive techniques, such as diode laser (contact or endo-) cyclophotocoagulation. These modern techniques are nowadays being used more and more liberally, even on eyes with good visual potential. The precise and selective nature of modern-day laser cyclodestruction seems to have a much less negative impact on visual acuity and on the eye as a whole. However, eyes exposed to trauma, and often to repeated surgical procedures, are by definition at a relatively higher risk of developing phthisis following cyclodestruction. Therefore, it behooves the treating ophthalmologist to exercise great caution in selecting the proper candidates for cyclodestruction, as well as in performing and titrating the procedure.

LONG-TERM PROGNOSIS

Traumatized eyes that have been treated for glaucoma need regular, periodic, lifelong follow-up, even if the glaucoma treatment has been completely successful. Eyes that are under medical IOP control obviously need to be checked periodically to ensure continued efficacy of the treatment regimen. By the same argument, any type of surgical procedure needs periodic assessment, no matter how successful initially. Finally, the long-term outcome of any traumatized eye depends on the severity of the initial trauma itself, any additional damage incurred by treatment, especially surgical, secondary complications such as glaucoma, and other late-occurring complications such as retinal detachment, or even glaucoma appearing very late following the original trauma.

Summary

- Secondary glaucoma is one of the significant complications of blunt and penetrating ocular trauma.

- Acute IOP elevation may occur immediately after blunt injuries, caused by hemorrhage, inflammation, or contusion of the outflow mechanism.

- With penetrating injuries, there is usually a more severe degree of associated inflammation, caused by disruption of intraocular tissues, and possibly also by the retention of intraocular foreign bodies. The outflow channels are thus more likely to be damaged, either because of direct injury or by extensive synechiae that often form as a result of prolonged inflammation and/or anterior chamber flattening.

- Angle recession, a common complication of blunt ocular trauma, often results in intractable glaucoma that can appear even many years after the injury. Unfortunately, ophthalmologists can easily overlook this entity if they fail to evaluate the angle gonioscopically.

- Careful history taking and eye examination usually establish the diagnosis easily. Typical ocular findings denoting trauma may be seen in the iris, lens, angle, ciliary body, or retina.

- Medical therapy is required either in preparation for surgery or on a chronic basis in cases that cannot be controlled surgically. Treatment regimens must be individualized according to the condition of the eye itself, and to minimize the systemic side effects of certain medications.

- Successful filtering surgery requires a relatively healthy conjunctiva and an undistorted anterior segment, plus the use of adjunctive antifibrotic agents intra- and postoperatively, in most if not all cases.

- Glaucoma drainage devices are very useful whenever filtering surgery is not feasible. Here, too, a relatively intact anterior segment is required to allow enough space for tube insertion.

- Cyclodestruction nowadays carries lower morbidity with the use of the diode laser (as opposed to cryo). Laser energy can be delivered to the ciliary body either transsclerally or endoscopically, using a special probe for each approach. Great caution must be exercised in lasering severely traumatized eyes or those previously subjected to repeated operations, as such eyes can easily go into phthisis as a result of aggressive laser cyclophotocoagulation.

REFERENCES

1. Ritch R, Shields B, Krupin T. The glaucomas: clinical science. 2nd edn, vol II. St. Louis: Mosby; 1996.

2. De Leon-Ortega JE, Girkin CA. Ocular trauma-related glaucoma. Ophthalmol Clin North Am 2002; 15(2): 215–223.

3. Schlote T, Rohrbach M. [Traumatic glaucoma – a survey]. Klin Monatsbl Augenheilkd 2005; 222(10):772–782.

4. Kujn F, Morris R, Witherspoom CD, et al. Epidemiology of blinding trauma in the United States Eye Injury Registry. Ophthalmic Epidemiol 2006; 13(3):209–216.

5. Klopfer J, et al. Ocular trauma in the United States. Eye injuries resulting in hospitalization, 1984 throughout 1987. Arch Ophthalmol 1992; 110:838.

6. McGwin G Jr, Xie A, Owsley C. Rate of eye injury in the United States. Arch Ophthalmol 2005; 123(7):970–976.

7. Hsieh DA, Stout JW, Lee RB, et al. The incidence of eye injuries at three U.S. Army installations. Mil Med 2003; 168:101–105.

8. Wong TY, Smith GS, Lincoln AE, et al. Ocular trauma in the United States Army: hospitalization records from 1985 through 1994. Am J Ophthalmol 2000; 129(5):645–650.

9. Desai P, MacEwen CJ, Baines P, et al. Incidence of cases of ocular trauma admitted to hospital and incidence of blinding outcome. Br J Ophthalmol 1996; 80(7):592–596.

10. Karaman K, Gverovic-Antunica A, Rogosic V, et al. Epidemiology of adult eye injuries in Split-Dalmation County. Croat Med J 2004; 45(3):304–309.

11. Wong TY, Tielsch JM. A population-based study on the incidence of severe ocular trauma in Singapore. Am J Ophthalmol 1999; 128(3):345–351.

12. Moreira CA Jr, Deberet-Ribeiro M, Belfort R Jr. Epidemiological study of eye injuries in Brazilian children. Arch Ophthalmol 1986; 51:315.

13. Girkin CA, McGwin G Jr, McNeal SF, et al. Hypothyroidism and the development of open-angle glaucoma in a male population. Ophthalmology 2004; 111(9):1649–1652.

14. Sihota R, Sood NN, Agarwal HC. Traumatic glaucoma. Acta Ophthalmol Scand 1995; 73:252–254.

15. Chen G, Sinclair SA, Smith GA, et al. Hospitalized ocular injuries among persons with low socioeconomic status: a Medicaid enrollees-based study. Ophthalmic Epidemiol 2006; 13(3):199–207.

16. Manners T, Salmon JF, Barron A, et al. Trabeculectomy with mitomycin C in the treatment of post-traumatic angle recession glaucoma. Br J Ophthalmol 2001; 85(2):159–163.

17. Wong TY, Tielsch JM. A population-based study on the incidence of severe ocular trauma in Singapore. Am J Ophthalmol 1999; 128(3):345–351.

18. Brandt MT, Haug RH. Traumatic hyphema: a comprehensive review. J Oral Maxillofac Surg 2001; 59(12):1462–1470.

19. Campbell DJ. Traumatic glaucoma. In: Shingleton BJ, Hersh PS, Kenyon KR, eds. Eye trauma. St. Louis: Mosby; 1991.

20. Sankar PS, Chen TC, Grosskreutz CL, et al. Traumatic hyphema. Int Ophthalmol Clin 2002; 42(3):57–68.

21. Walton W, Von Hagen S, Grigorian R, et al. Management of traumatic hyphema. Surv Ophthalmol 2002; 47(4):297–334.

22. Spoor TC. Anterior segment injuries: blunt ocular trauma: what happens when the eye is struck by a blunt object? In: Spoor TC, ed. An atlas of ophthalmic trauma. London: Mosby; 1997: 35–49.

23. Albert DM, Jakobiec FA. Traumatic hyphema. Principles and practice of ophthalmology. Philadelphia: WB Saunders; 2000; 5203–5208.

24. Recchia FM, Saluja RK, Hammel K, et al. Outpatient management of traumatic microhyphema. Ophthalmology 2002; 109(8):1465–1470.

25. Tumbocon J, Latina M. Angle recession glaucoma. Int Ophthalmol Clin 2002; 42(3):69–78.

26. Mermoud A, Salmon JF, Barron A, et al. Surgical management of post-traumatic glaucoma. Ophthalmology 1993; 100: 634–642.

27. Girkin CA, McGwin G, Long C, et al. Glaucoma after ocular contusion: a cohort study of the United States Eye Injury Registry. J Glaucoma 2005; 14:470–473.

28. Synder A, Latecka-Krajewska B, Omulecki W. [Secondary glaucoma in patients with lens subluxation or luxation]. Klin Oczna 2000; 102(6):409–412.

29. Shields M. Glaucoma associated with disorders of the lens. In: Shields M, ed. Textbook of glaucoma. 4th edn. Baltimore: Williams and Wilkins; 1998.

30. Braganza A, Thomas R, George T, et al. Management of phacolytic glaucoma: experience of 135 cases. Indian J Ophthalmol 1998; 46(3):139–143.

31. Spraul C, Grossniklaus H. Vitreous hemorrhage. Surv Ophthalmol 1997; 42(1):3–39.

32. Bailez C, Pastor JC, Martin F, et al. [Ghost cell detection in vitreous cytology: clinico-pathological correlation]. Arch Soc Esp Oftalmol 2002; 77(7):369–375.

33. Jones R, Rhee D. Corticosteroid-induced ocular hypertension and glaucoma: a brief review and update of the literature. Curr Opin Ophthalmol 2006; 17(2):163–167.

34. Collignon NJ. Emergencies in glaucoma: a review. Bull Soc Belge Ophtalmol 2005; 296:71–81.

35. Kanski J. Clinical ophthalmology. 5th edn. London: Butterworth-Heinmann, International Editions; 2003.

36. Cheh A. Reenstra-Buras W. Rosen C. et al. Burns, ocular. 2006. Online. Available: http://www.emedicine.com/EMERG/topic736.htm

37. Bouchard CS, Morno K, Perkins J, et al. Ocular complications of thermal injury: a 3-year retrospective. J Trauma 2001; 50(1):79–82.

38. Spencer T, Hall AJ, Stawell RJ. Ophthalmologic sequelae of thermal burns over ten years at the Alfred Hospital. Ophthal Plast Reconstr Surg 2002; 18(3):196–201.

39. Miller B, Goldstein M, Monshizadeh R, et al. Ocular manifestations of electrical injury: a case report and review of the literature. CLAO J 2002; 28(4):224–227.

40. Parsons J. Radiation toxicity to the visual system. J Neuro-ophthalmol 2004; 24(3):193–194.

INDEX

A

absolute risk (AR), 509–10
absolute risk increase (ARI), 510
absolute risk reduction (ARR), 510
accommodation, pigment dispersion
    syndrome, 351
AccuMap system, 159
    artifacts, 165
    printouts and interpretation, 163, 164, 166
acetazolamide, 539–40
    acute angle closure, 628, 631
    childhood glaucoma, 374
    indications, 542
    IOP-lowering efficacy, 542
    mechanism of action, 540, 541
    post-traumatic glaucoma, 649
    side effects, 543
    uveitic glaucoma, 402
acid burns, 438, 647
active optics technology, 617
Activities of Daily Vision Scale (ADVS),
    472–3, 482
acute angle closure (AAC), 625
    drug-induced, 633
    primary see acute primary angle closure
    secondary, 631–3
acute angle closure glaucoma (AACG), 625
acute intraocular pressure rise
    biomechanical effects, 73–87
        engineering models, 77–9
        optic nerve head, 73–6
        role of sclera, 76–7
        tissue restructuring and remodeling, 84,
           85–6
    management, 625–33
    ocular blood flow changes, 79, 95
    see also specific conditions
acute primary angle closure (APAC), 328,
    455, 625–31
    epidemiology, 328, 329, 625–6
    etiology and pathogenesis, 626–7
    fellow eye management, 456, 631
    IOP reduction, 455–6, 627, 628
    laser iridotomy, 456–7, 628–9
    laser peripheral iridoplasty, 457, 629
    lens extraction, 457–8, 629–30
    practical management, 631
    prognosis, 329, 335, 631
    risk factors, 626
    signs and symptoms, 334, 627
    treatment, 627–31
    ultrasound biomicroscopy, 189–90
    undue emphasis, 327
acute secondary glaucoma, 625, 631–3

adaptive optics (AO) scanning laser
    ophthalmoscope, 617–18
additive genetic variance, 278
adeno-associated virus (AAV) vectors, 606–7,
    608, 610–12
adenovirus vectors, 605–6, 609–10
adherence and persistence, medication, 489–93
    developing countries, 34–5
    extent of problem, 489–91
    fixed-dose combinations, 565
    identifying problems, 491–2
    improving, 492–3
    primary open-angle glaucoma, 323, 452
adrenaline (epinephrine), 527–8
adrenergic agents, 527, 528
    angle closure induced by, 331, 633
    normal-tension glaucoma, 366
adrenergic agonists, 547
    vs parasympathomimetics, 520
    see also α agonists
adrenoceptors, 527–8, 547
Advanced Glaucoma Intervention Study
    (AGIS), 112, 323, 324
    end points, 497, 500, 502
    target IOP, 465, 466
adverse treatment outcomes, 503, 504
affected relative pair analyses, 281–2
Africa, 301–2
    management of glaucoma, 36–7
    North, 301–2
    prevalence and burden, 5, 6, 8, 36
    sub-Saharan, 36–7, 302
African-Americans
    central corneal thickness, 208
    risk of glaucoma, 316–17
Afro-Caribbeans, 297
age
    acute angle closure and, 625, 626
    as glaucoma risk factor, 316, 331
    of onset, congenital glaucoma, 371
    POAG prevalence and, 315
    target IOP and, 466–7
    see also children
aging
    aqueous humor dynamics, 59, 60
    lamina cribrosa changes, 49, 82
    optic nerve head remodeling and
        restructuring, 79–82
    see also elderly
AGIS see Advanced Glaucoma Intervention
    Study
alkali burns, 437–8, 646–7
allergic reactions, α agonists, 554
α agonists, 547–55

acute angle closure, 628
    childhood glaucoma, 374
    contraindications, 553
    drug interactions, 554
    efficacy and comparisons, 552–3
    formulations, 547
    indications, 549–52
    mechanisms of action, 547–9
    normal-tension glaucoma, 366
    pharmacology, 547–8
    prostaglandin analogue combination
        therapy, 553
    side effects, 553–4
    uveitic glaucoma, 402
α rhythm, artifact, 165
α_1-receptor antagonists, pigmentary
    glaucoma, 357
α-adrenoceptors, 547
α-fodrin autoantibodies, 365
amblyopia, optic disc shape, 215
American Academy of Ophthalmology
    assessing functional disabilities, 504
    grading of glaucoma severity, 323
    target IOP, 463, 468
aminocaproic acid, traumatic hyphema,
    434, 640
2-aminoguanidine, 583, 584
Amsler's sign, 398
amyloidosis, localized, 425
Andhra Pradesh Eye Disease Study (APEDS),
    299–300
angle, anterior chamber see anterior chamber
    angle
angle closure, 383
    acute see acute angle closure
    latent, 328
    mechanisms in uveitis, 395–8
    primary see primary angle closure
    provocation tests, 333–4
    screening, 20
angle opening distance (AOD 250 and AOD
    500), 186, 187, 200
    angle-closure glaucoma, 190
    anterior segment optical coherence
        tomography, 203
    clinical applications, 188
angle recess, 176, 177
angle recess area (ARA), 187, 200
    anterior segment optical coherence
        tomography, 203
angle recession, traumatic, 432–3, 640–2
    differential diagnosis, 642
    gonioscopy, 181, 182, 433, 641
    long-term prognosis, 436

angle-closure glaucoma, 383
    ciliary block, 191–2, 386, 387
    at ciliary body level, 384–5
    ciliochoroidal effusion/swelling, 192–3,
        386–7
    classification, 383
    definition, 295
    developing countries, 34, 35, 39
    diagnosis, 387–8
    economics, 25, 27
    elevated episcleral venous pressure, 426
    etiology and mechanisms, 383–7, 626–7
    genetics, 274
    goniosynechialysis see goniosynechialysis
    intraocular tumors, 441
    lens-induced, 385–6, 390
    malignant glaucoma, 191–2, 386, 387
    management, 389–91, 455–9
    neovascular, 387, 413
    plateau iris see plateau iris
    primary see primary angle-closure
        glaucoma
    pupillary block see pupillary block
    screening, 16
    secondary, 327, 383–91
        acute, 631–3
    signs and symptoms, 388–9
    systemic inflammatory diseases, 387
    ultrasound biomicroscopy, 189–93, 388
    uveitis, 395–8, 403
    vitreoretinal and retinal disorders, 427
angle-recession glaucoma, 181, 436, 640–2
    management, 436, 642
animal models, 580–1
    assessing visual function, 602
    neuroprotection studies, 582–4
aniridia, 273, 274, 377–8
anisotropic materials, 70–1
annexin-5, 582, 617
anterior chamber (AC)
    paracentesis, acute primary angle closure,
        456, 629
    washout, traumatic hyphema, 434–5
anterior chamber angle (ACA), 173
    anterior segment optical coherence
        tomography (AS-OCT), 198, 201–4
    blood vessels, 178
    contusion, 638
    crowding, 191, 627
    gonioscopy see gonioscopy
    imaging, 197–204
    new vessel formation see
        neovascularization of angle
    normal anatomy, 177–8
    occludable see primary angle-closure
        suspect
    pigment deposition syndrome/pigmentary
        glaucoma, 354, 355, 356
    traumatic injuries, 432–3
    tumors infiltrating, 441, 443
    ultrasound biomicroscopy, 185–95, 197,
        198–201
    uveitis-related changes, 395
anterior chamber angle (ACA) width
    angle-closure glaucoma, 189–90
    gonioscopic grading, 178–9
    optical coherence tomography, 203
    ultrasound biomicroscopy, 187
anterior chamber depth (ACD)
    angle closure risk and, 11, 331–2
    pigment deposition syndrome/pigmentary
        glaucoma, 354, 355
    ultrasound biomicroscopy, 186, 187
    van Herick technique, 204, 332, 333
anterior segment
    birefringence, scanning laser polarimetry,
        241–2

childhood glaucoma, 370
    pigment deposition, 354, 355, 356
    surgery, epithelial ingrowth complicating,
        428–9
anterior segment dysgenesis (ASD), 273
anterior segment optical coherence
        tomography (AS-OCT), 201–4, 621,
        622
    angle-closure glaucoma, 334, 388
    artifacts and technical tips, 203–4
    clinical applications, 197, 198, 202
    image analysis, 203
    mode of action, 201–2
    strengths and limitations, 202–3
    uveitic glaucoma, 400
    vs ultrasound biomicroscopy, 204
anticholinesterase agents, 518
anticoagulants, causing acute angle closure,
        633
antifibrotic therapy
    sub-Saharan Africa, 37
    see also mitomycin C
antisense oligonucleotides, 609
apoptosis
    gene therapy targeting, 611–12
    retinal ganglion cells, 579, 617
applanation tonometry, 103–6, 107–8, 207
    see also Goldmann applanation tonometry
apraclonidine, 547
    childhood glaucoma, 374
    contraindications, 553
    formulations, 547
    indications, 549–50
    mechanism of action, 547–9
    pharmacology, 547–8
    side effects, 553–4
aquaporin-1 gene therapy, 609
aqueous flow (rate) (Fa), 55–8
    fluctuations, 56, 109
    measurement, 56–8
    normal rates, 56, 57
    specific syndromes, 61, 62, 63, 64
aqueous humor
    dynamics, 55–64
        α agonist effects, 548
        β-blocker actions, 528–9
        fluctuations, 109–10
        healthy human eye, 55–61
        prostaglandin analogue actions, 561
        syndromes affecting IOP, 61–4
        uveitis, 394
    flow rate see aqueous flow
    production, 55–6
aqueous humor outflow, 58–9
    gene therapy targeting, 609–10
    resistance, 59
        factors affecting, 59
        primary open-angle glaucoma, 61–3
        see also trabecular outflow facility
    see also trabecular outflow pathways;
        uveoscleral outflow
aqueous misdirection (malignant glaucoma),
        386, 631–2
    diagnosis, 632
    mechanism, 632
    treatment, 390–1, 632
    ultrasound biomicroscopy, 191–2, 386, 387
arachidonic acid metabolism, 559
Aravind Comprehensive Eye Care Study, 34
arcuate scotomas, 120
area under the receiver operating
        characteristic curve (AUROC), 228–9,
        233, 236
argon laser trabeculoplasty (ALT), α agonist
        therapy after, 549–50
arteriosclerosis, 93
arteriovenous fistulas, 425, 426

arthro-ophthalmopathy, hereditary, 427
Asia
    prevalence and burden, 5, 6, 8, 9
    primary angle-closure glaucoma, 329–30,
        331–2
    risk factors, 10
AS-OCT see anterior segment optical
        coherence tomography
Assessment of Function Related to Vision
        (AFREV), 476, 504–5
association studies
    genetic, 277, 283–5
    genome-wide, 284
asthma, prostaglandin analogue-induced, 563
astrocytes
    glaucomatous changes, 85
    in vitro studies, 86
    role in axon damage, 50, 68
atherosclerosis, 93
Australia
    economic analyses, 28–9, 30
    epidemiology, 5, 8, 9, 11
autoimmunity, normal-tension glaucoma
        and, 365
autoradiographic methods, ocular blood flow
        measurement, 266
autoregulation, ocular blood flow, 93, 95–6
Avastin see bevacizumab
averaging technique, image processing, 616
Axenfeld anomaly, 376
Axenfeld-Reiger syndrome, 274, 376
axial length (of globe)
    childhood glaucomas, 370
    primary angle-closure glaucoma and, 331
axons, retinal ganglion cell see retinal
        ganglion cell (RGC) axons
axoplasmic transport
    blockage, 91
    changes in glaucoma, 84–6
    IOP-related changes, 79
    normal aging, 82
axoprotection, 585
Azarga see brinzolamide/timolol

B

baculoviral IAP repeat-containing protein-4
        (BIRC4) gene therapy, 611–12
Baltimore Eye Survey
    glaucoma risk factors, 10, 317, 467
    ocular perfusion pressure, 92
    prevalence, 315, 329, 361
    visual impairment, 29
Barbados Eye Study (BES), 10, 29, 208, 307
Barbados Family Study of Open-Angle
        Glaucoma (BFSG), 282
BDNF see brain-derived neurotrophic factor
Beaver Dam Eye Study, 282, 318
Bebie curve, 124
benefits and risks of treatment, 509–13
benzalkonium chloride (BAC; BAK)
    β-blocker preparations, 526, 527
    fixed-dose combinations, 566
    prostaglandin analogues, 560, 561
    side effects, 531, 554, 565–6
R(-)-1-(benzo [b] thiophen-5-yl)-2-[2-(N,
        N-diethylamino) ethoxy] ethanol,
        hydrochloride, 583
β-adrenergic agonists, aqueous flow and, 56
β-adrenoceptors, 527–8, 529–30
β-blockers, 525–35
    acute angle closure, 628, 631
    childhood glaucoma, 374
    combination products, 527, 533–4, 542
    drug interactions, 533–4
    formulations and dosing, 525–7
    history of development, 525, 534

indications, 530
IOP-lowering efficacy, 530–1
mechanisms of action, 527–30
normal-tension glaucoma, 366
pharmacology, 527–8
pilocarpine combinations, 520, 534
side effects and contraindications, 531–3, 535
spotlight, 534–5
uveitic glaucoma, 402
vs parasympathomimetics, 520
betaxolol, 526
IOP-lowering efficacy, 531
mechanisms of action, 528, 530
pharmacology, 583
side effects, 532
bevacizumab (Avastin), 414, 415
bias, epidemiological studies, 4
bimatoprost, 560
exfoliative glaucoma, 344–5
side effects, 562
bimatoprost/timolol (GANfort™), 527, 572
clinical role, 567
preservatives, 566
biomechanics see cornea, biomechanics; optic nerve head (ONH), biomechanics
bipolar cells, 133
bleb(s)
classification, 194
leaks, conjunctival tissue grafting, 596
ultrasound biomicroscopy, 194, 195
bleb-related endophthalmitis, 38
blepharospasm, 372
blind spot
baring or enlargement, 120
physiological, 115
blindness, 297–9, 502–3
definitions, 481, 502–3
economic analyses, 29–30
patient's viewpoint, 504
prevention
benefits, 298–9
developing countries, 37–9
ease of, 297–8
significance, 293, 299–303
see also low vision; visual impairment
blinking
automated perimetry, 129
pigment dispersion syndrome, 351
blood flow
ocular see ocular blood flow
peripheral, 265–6
blood pressure, systemic
β-blockers and, 532
nocturnal dips, 92, 93
normal-tension glaucoma, 364
optic nerve blood flow and, 51, 93
blood viscosity, increased, 93
blue field entoptics, 265
Blue Mountains Eye Study, 19, 279, 307, 317, 467
blunt ocular trauma, 431–6, 638–45
body mass index (BMI), 10
brain-derived neurotrophic factor (BDNF), 583, 584
gene therapy targeting, 610–11
retinal ganglion cell survival and, 51–2, 579
branch retinal artery occlusion, 362, 363
branch retinal vein occlusion, exfoliation syndrome, 344
Brazil, 299
breastfeeding
β-blockers, 533
carbonic anhydrase inhibitors, 543
brimonidine, 547
acute angle closure, 628

childhood glaucoma, 374
contraindications, 553
formulations, 547
indications, 550–2
IOP-lowering efficacy, 552–3
mechanism of action, 547–9
neuroprotection studies, 583, 584, 585
normal-tension glaucoma, 366, 585
pharmacology, 547–8, 583
side effects, 553–4
brimonidine/timolol (Combigan™), 527, 547, 572–3
clinical role, 567
IOP-lowering efficacy, 534, 551–2, 573
preservatives, 566
brinzolamide, 540, 541
IOP-lowering efficacy, 542
mechanism of action, 540–1
side effects, 544
vs α agonists, 553
brinzolamide/timolol (Azarga), 542, 567
buphthalmos, 372, 373
burns
chemical, 437–8, 646–7
thermal, 647

C

café au lait spots, 377
calcium channel blockers, 97
caldesmon gene therapy, 609–10
candidate gene analyses, 283–4
Canon laser blood flowmeter (CLBF), 264–5
carbachol, 517–18
carbon dioxide (CO_2), retrobulbar vascular responses, 96
carbonic anhydrase (CA), 539
carbonic anhydrase inhibitors (CAIs), 539–45
acute angle closure, 628
childhood glaucoma, 374
combination products, 542, 543
contraindications, 543
drug interactions, 544
formulations, 539–40
history of use, 534, 540
indications, 541–2
IOP-lowering efficacy, 542
mechanism of action, 540–1
post-traumatic glaucoma, 649
side effects and contraindications, 542–4
uveitic glaucoma, 402
vs α agonists, 553
vs parasympathomimetics, 520–1
carcinoma, metastatic intraocular, 441
cardiac conduction defects, 532
cardiac cycle, 258
cardiovascular disease, 10
carotid artery occlusion, 410
carotid–cavernous sinus fistulas, 425, 426
carteolol
formulations and dosing, 526
IOP-lowering efficacy, 531
mechanism of action, 528
pilocarpine combination, 520
side effects, 533
case detection, 15
cataract
after trabeculectomy, developing countries, 35, 38
congenital, glaucoma after surgery for, 379
developing countries, 37
electrophysiological measures and, 160, 162
exfoliation syndrome association, 343–4
phacolytic glaucoma, 419
scanning laser polarimetry, 245
SWAP testing and, 139

uveitis-associated, 404
cataract surgery
congenital cataract, 379
developing countries, 33–4, 36–7, 38
exfoliation syndrome, 343
neovascular glaucoma, 413
postoperative IOP rise, 550
primary angle-closure glaucoma, 334
prostaglandin analogues and, 561
retained lens fragment, 420
uveitic glaucoma, 404
see also intraocular lenses; lens extraction; phacoemulsification
causal associations, artifactual, 4
cavernous sinus thrombosis, 425
CCT see central corneal thickness
central corneal thickness (CCT), 207–11
clinical usefulness, 209–10, 211
genetic contribution, 278
impact on tonometry, 207–11
linkage studies, 283
measurement, 186
ocular hypertension risk of progression, 309–10
racial differences, 10, 208
target IOP and, 467
tonometry assumptions, 103, 207
variability, 10, 207–8
central retinal artery (CRA)
blood flow velocity, 257, 258
hemodynamics, 95
occlusion (CRAO), neovascular glaucoma, 410
central retinal vein occlusion (CRVO)
exfoliation syndrome, 344
neovascular glaucoma, 409–10
treatment, 413
central retinal vessel, lamina cribrosa surface, 217, 218–19
chalcosis, 437, 646
Chandler's syndrome, 420, 421
Charles Bonnet syndrome, 482
chemical burns, 437–8, 646–7
chicken β-actin (CBA) promoter, 608
child abuse, 639
childhood glaucomas, 369–80
classification, 371
evaluation, 369–70
intraocular tumors, 443–5
primary, 371–9
associated with ocular anomalies, 377–9
associated with systemic syndromes, 375–7
quality of life assessment, 484
secondary, 371, 372, 379
see also congenital glaucoma
children
α agonist side effects, 553
low-vision services, 484
ocular trauma, 431, 637
uveitic glaucoma, 393–4
China
costs of care, 35
primary angle-closure glaucoma, 329–30, 331
cholinergic agents see parasympathomimetics
choroidal blood flow
glaucoma, 94
impaired autoregulation, 96
chronic intraocular pressure elevation, α agonists, 550–2
chronic primary angle closure, 328, 455
laser iridotomy, 457
laser peripheral iridoplasty, 457
medical therapy, 456
prevalence in India, 330
ultrasound biomicroscopy, 189–90

CIGTS *see* Collaborative Initial Glaucoma Treatment Study
ciliary block glaucoma *see* malignant glaucoma
ciliary body
　anterior rotation, 396, 633
　band, gonioscopy, 177
　cysts
　　pigment dispersion, 356
　　pseudoplateau iris, 385
　　treatment, 390
　tumors, 441, 445
　　angle closure, 385
　　neovascular glaucoma, 410–11
ciliary neurotrophic factor (CNTF), 583
ciliochoroidal effusion/swelling, angle closure, 192–3, 386–7
cilioretinal artery, temporal, 219
circadian rhythm
　aqueous flow, 56, 109
　IOP, 109, 110–12
circle of Zinn-Haller, 50, 51, 68
citalopram, 331
classical test theory (CTT), 475
classification of glaucoma, ISGEO, 3, 5
clinical epidemiology, 12–13
clinical trials
　evaluation, 592, 593
　methodology, 591–2
clonidine, 547, 548
　formulations, 547
　pilocarpine combination, 520
closed-form solutions, optic nerve head biomechanics, 77
cloverleaf pattern, visual field, 129
CNTGS *see* Collaborative Normal Tension Glaucoma Study
coagulable state, 93
Cogan-Reese syndrome, 420, 421, 422, 423
Collaborative Initial Glaucoma Treatment Study (CIGTS), 323, 324
　benefit vs risk of treatment, 510–11
　end points, 497, 500, 502
　quality of life assessment, 472, 474–5
　target IOP, 465, 466, 468–9
Collaborative Normal Tension Glaucoma Study (CNTGS), 92, 324, 365–6, 452
　benefits of IOP lowering, 464–5, 466
　end points, 497, 500, 502
　risk factors for progression, 316
collagen XVIII deficiency, 353
color Doppler imaging (CDI), 257–8
　limitations, 266
　studies in glaucoma, 94–5, 257
color vision
　abnormal, 362
　short-wavelength sensitive, 135
　system overview, 133–4
Combigan™ *see* brimonidine/timolol
combination medical therapy, fixed *see* fixed-combination medical therapy
commingling analysis, 279
complement pathway, 52–3
compliance *see* adherence and persistence, medication
compressive stress, 70
computers, 484, 485
cones, 133
　short-wavelength (blue), 135
confocal scanning laser ophthalmoscopy (CSLO), 616–18
　adaptive optics (AO) technology, 617–18
　imaging processing methods, 616–17
　primary open-angle glaucoma, 322
　retinal nerve fiber layer, 239, 245–7
　structural–function correlation, 252, 254

see also Heidelberg Retina Tomograph
confounding, genetic association studies, 284
congenital glaucoma, 369–80
　age of presentation, 371
　differential diagnosis, 372, 373
　drainage implant surgery, 374
　genetics, 272–3, 371
　goniotomy and trabeculotomy, 372–4
　outcomes and prognosis, 374–5
　pathogenesis, 371–2
　prevalence, 371
　primary, 371–5
　risk factors, 371
　signs and symptoms, 372
　treatment, 372–4
congestive glaucoma *see* neovascular glaucoma
conjunctival tissue grafts, after filtering surgery, 596
connective tissue, optic nerve head, 67–8
　age-related changes, 79–82
　biomechanics, 73, 78–9
　remodeling and restructuring, 84–6, 87
consent, informed, failure to obtain, 300
CONSORT guidelines, 592, 593
contact lenses, 562
contusion trauma, 431
copper-containing foreign bodies, 437, 646
corectopia
　Axenfeld-Reiger syndrome, 271, 376
　iridocorneal endothelial syndrome, 421, 422
cornea
　biomechanics, 72, 209
　　after refractive surgery, 209
　　impact on tonometry, 207, 209, 210–11
　　measurement, 105, 209
　central leukoma, 378, 379
　elasticity, 209, 210
　enlargement, congenital glaucoma, 372, 373
　examination, childhood glaucoma, 370
　penetrating injuries, 645
　pigment deposits, 354, 356
　viscoelasticity, 209
corneal astigmatism, optic disc shape, 215
corneal compensation
　enhanced (ECC), 245
　variable (VCC), 241, 245
corneal dystrophy, posterior polymorphous, 422–3
corneal edema/decompensation
　angle-closure glaucoma, 388
　congenital glaucoma, 372, 373
　iridocorneal endothelial syndrome, 421
　laser iridotomy during, 629
corneal endothelium
　cell loss in primary angle-closure glaucoma, 334
　disorders causing glaucoma, 420–3
　staining after traumatic hyphema, 640
corneal hysteresis (CH), 105, 106, 209
corneal response (or resistance) factor (CRF), 105, 209
corneal thickness, central *see* central corneal thickness
corticosteroid-induced ocular hypertension/glaucoma, 307, 423–4
　acute angle closure, 633
　etiology/pathogenesis, 395, 423–4
　post-traumatic, 644–5
　treatment, 424
　uveitis, 393–4
corticosteroids
　acute angle closure, 628
　alkali burns, 438

aqueous flow effects, 56
　traumatic hyphema, 639–40
　uveitis, 401–2, 403
Cosopt® *see* dorzolamide/timolol
cost-benefit analysis (CBA), 26, 27
　glaucoma care, 30
cost-effectiveness analysis (CEA), 26, 31
cost-minimization analysis (CMA), 26–7
　glaucoma care, 30
costs
　of blindness/visual impairment, 29–30, 300
　disease related, 25–6
　of illness, 25–6, 28–9, 505
　medication adherence and, 34–5, 492
　to patients, 482
　screening for glaucoma, 16
　treatment interventions, 26, 34–5, 505
cost-utility analysis (CUA), 26, 31
　glaucoma care, 30
　ocular hypertension treatment, 312
　quality of life component, 472, 477–8
　utility measures, 476–7
coupling medium, ultrasound biomicroscopy, 186, 199, 201
coxsackievirus adenovirus receptor (CAR), 605
creep, 71–2
cross-sectional surveys, 3–4
cryoglobulinemia, systemic, 411
CSLO *see* confocal scanning laser ophthalmoscopy
cultural differences
　low-vision rehabilitation, 483–4
　significance of glaucoma, 297–303
　see also geographic variations; racial/ethnic variations
cup-to-disc ratio
　definition of glaucoma and, 296
　genetic contribution, 278
　glaucoma risk and, 309–10, 316
　horizontal, 218, 233
　linear, 226
　measurement
　　Heidelberg Retina Tomograph, 226
　　methods compared, 235–6
　　ocular hypertension, 308
　　optic disc photography, 218
　　optical coherence tomography, 233
　　variability, 236, 308
　neuroretinal rim blood flow and, 95
　vertical, 218, 233
cyclic adenosine monophosphate (cAMP)
　adrenergic pathways, 527, 547
　axonal regeneration and, 586, 602
cyclodestructive procedures
　neovascular glaucoma, 414
　post-traumatic glaucoma, 650
cyclodialysis cleft
　differential diagnosis, 642
　post-traumatic, 181–2, 433
cyclophotocoagulation
　neovascular glaucoma, 414
　ultrasound biomicroscopy, 194
　uveitic glaucoma, 404
CYP1B1 gene, 273, 284, 371
cystoid macular edema (CMO)
　prostaglandin analogue-induced, 562
　uveitic glaucoma, 402
cytokines, in uveitic glaucoma, 394–5
cytomegalovirus (CMV) promoter, 608

D

dapiprazole, pigmentary glaucoma, 357
DBA/2J mouse, 272, 352
decibels (dB), 117
deep sclerectomy (DS)

exfoliative glaucoma, 345
ultrasound biomicroscopy, 194–5
definition of glaucoma, 293–303, 496
epidemiological surveys, 3, 5, 12
terminology and, 293–6
delay time, 17
depression, β-blocker-treated patients, 533
developing countries, 33–9
glaucoma services, 39
nongovernmental organizations, 37–9
developmental glaucomas, genetics, 273–4
deviation map, 242, 243
diabetes mellitus, 10
β-blockers, 533
POAG risk, 317
type 1, aqueous humor dynamics, 62, 63–4
diabetic retinopathy, proliferative (PDR)
neovascular glaucoma, 409, 410
treatment, 413
diagnosis of glaucoma
anterior segment optical coherence
tomography, 201–4
developing countries, 34, 36, 38–9
early, 18
electrophysiological measures, 151–67
gonioscopy, 173–82
ocular blood flow evaluation, 257–65
optic disc imaging, 225–36
optic disc photography, 213–22
outcome measures and, 496–502
perimetry see perimetry
retinal nerve fiber layer photography and
computer analysis, 239–49
structure–function relationships, 251–4
tonometry see tonometry
ultrasound biomicroscopy, 185–95,
198–201
ultrastructural imaging, 615–22
visual fields, 115–30
see also screening
diagnostic tests, evaluating, 496–7
dichlorphenamide, 540
diode laser cyclophotocoagulation
developing countries, 35
traumatic glaucoma, 650
disability, visual see visual disability
disability-adjusted life year (DALY), 478
Disc Damage Likelihood Scale, 296, 498, 500
diurnal variation, IOP, 110–12
dominance, 278
Doppler effect, 259, 260
dorzolamide, 540, 541
IOP-lowering efficacy, 542
mechanism of action, 540–1
side effects, 543, 544
vs α agonists, 553
vs pilocarpine, 521
dorzolamide/timolol (Cosopt®), 527, 567–9
efficacy, 534, 542, 566, 567–9
side effects, 544
double-hump sign, plateau iris, 384, 626
drainage implant surgery
congenital glaucoma, 374
developing countries, 35
neovascular glaucoma, 414
post-traumatic glaucoma, 649–50
sub-Saharan Africa, 37
ultrasound biomicroscopy, 195
uveitic glaucoma, 404
driving fitness, 504
assessment, 119
drug-induced glaucoma, 331, 386–7, 633
DuoTrav™ see travoprost/timolol
Dynamic Contour Tonometer (DCT),
Pascal®, 106–7
dyschromatopsia, acquired, 362

early diagnosis, 18
see also screening
Early Manifest Glaucoma Study (EMGT),
323, 324, 452
benefit vs risk of treatment, 510, 512
benefits of IOP lowering, 464, 466
central corneal thickness, 208–9
end points, 497, 498, 500, 502
glaucoma screening and, 18, 19
IOP fluctuation, 112
normal-tension glaucoma, 365, 366
risk factors for glaucoma, 316
echothiophate iodide, 518, 520
economics
blindness in India, 300
glaucoma care, 25–31
current studies, 27–30
future research needs, 30–1
methods, 25–7
perspectives used, 27
impact of glaucoma on patients, 482
see also costs
ectopia lentis, 385–6
ectropion uvea, 377
EGPS see European Glaucoma Prevention
Study
Egypt, 301
elastic fibers, juxtacanalicular meshwork, 59
elastic materials, 72
elderly
limitations of perimetry, 129, 160
target IOP, 466–7
undetected glaucoma, 33
uveitic glaucoma, 394
see also aging
electrical injuries, 648
electroacupuncture, 583
electrocardiogram (ECG), artifacts, 165
electrophysiology, 151–67
electroretinogram (ERG), 151–4
full-field flash, 151–2
multifocal flash (mfERG), 156–7
multifocal recording techniques, 155–6
pattern (PERG), 153–4
artifacts and prevention, 164–6
data storage and retrieval, 162–3
multifocal (mfERG), 156
neuroprotection studies, 581
printouts and interpretation, 163–4
recording technique, 159
reference population, 161
strengths and limitations, 160
vs other tests, 161–2
pattern reversal, 157
photopic negative response (PhNR), 153
scotopic threshold response (STR), 152–3
eliprodil, 583
Elschnig's rim, 46
embryonic stem (ES) cells, 596–7
EMGT see Early Manifest Glaucoma Study
emotional factors, assessing, 482–3
endophthalmitis, bleb-related (BRE), 38
endothelin-1 (ET-1), 51, 344, 364
enhanced cornea compensation (ECC), 245
environmental factors, 285
epidemiology, 3–13
applications, 5
artifacts, 4
definitions and diagnostic criteria, 3,
4–5, 12
genetic, 277–86
interpretation of findings, 4
methods, 3–4
spotlights, 12–13

study designs, 3–4
epinephrine (adrenaline), 527–8
epiphora, 372
episcleral venous pressure (Pev), 57, 59–60
elevated, 425–7
fluctuation, 59–60, 109–10
measurement, 60
specific syndromes, 62
epistasis, 278
epithelial inclusion cysts, 429
epithelial ingrowth, 428–9
post-traumatic, 428–9, 437, 645–6
Epstein-Barr virus, 420–1
erythropoietin, 583
eserine see physostigmine
Esterman Test, binocular, 119
ethnic variations see racial/ethnic variations
Europe, 302–3
numbers affected, 8
prevalence, 5–6
European Glaucoma Prevention Study
(EGPS), 112, 208, 451
benefits of IOP lowering, 464, 466
end points, 497, 500
risk of progression to glaucoma, 309, 310
structure–function relationships, 251
European Glaucoma Society (EGS), 303, 463
Europeans, 297
evidence-based medicine, 591–2
exercise, inducing pigment dispersion,
350, 351
exfoliation material (XFM), 340–2, 343
exfoliation suspects, 342–3
exfoliation (pseudoexfoliation) syndrome
(XFS), 339–45
aqueous humor dynamics, 62, 63
diagnosis and testing, 342–3
differential diagnosis, 342–3, 356
epidemiology, 10–11, 339–40
etiology and pathogenesis, 272, 340–2
glaucoma risk, 317, 340
gonioscopy, 180–1
ocular associations, 343–4
systemic associations, 344
target IOP and, 467
ultrasound biomicroscopy, 189
exfoliative glaucoma (XFG), 339–45
etiology and pathogenesis, 272, 340–2
prognosis, 340
risk factors, 112, 340
treatment, 344–5
ultrasound biomicroscopy, 189
exoenzyme C3 transferase gene therapy, 609
experimental glaucoma models, 580–1
extracellular matrix (ECM)
abnormalities, exfoliation syndrome,
340–1
lamina cribrosa, 68
aging changes, 82
glaucomatous changes, 84, 85
trabecular meshwork, 59, 61–3
eye movements
monitoring, automated perimetry, 125
scanning laser polarimetry (SLP), 245
eyedrops
assessing ability to instill, 492
instructions for patients, 492
eyelid artifacts, diagnostic techniques,
129, 203

failure, mechanical, 72
false negatives (FN)
automated perimetry, 125, 135–6
screening, 20

false positives (FP)
    automated perimetry, 125, 135–6
    screening, 20
Fanconi anemia, 411
FASTPAC perimetry, 118, 119
fatigue effect, perimetry, 120, 129
FDT *see* frequency doubling technology
feline immunodeficiency virus (FIV) vectors, 607, 610
fibrinolytic agents, traumatic hyphema, 434, 640
fibroblast growth factor (FGF)
    acidic (aFGF; FGF-1), 612
    basic (bFGF; FGF-2), 612
fibroblast growth factor-2 (FGF-2) gene therapy, 612
fibronectin secretory signal sequence (FIB), 608
fibrous ingrowth, 429
    post-traumatic, 645–6
filtering blebs *see* bleb(s)
filtering surgery
    acute primary angle closure, 630–1
    angle-recession glaucoma, 436, 642
    conjunctival restoration after, 596
    in developing countries, 35–6
    neovascular glaucoma, 413–14
    post-traumatic glaucoma, 649
    primary angle closure, 458–9
    traumatic hyphema, 435
    ultrasound biomicroscopy, 194
    uveitic glaucoma, 403–4
    see also nonpenetrating glaucoma surgery; trabeculectomy
finite element (FE) models, optic nerve head, 71, 77–9, 86
    individual-specific, 78–9, 80, 81, 82
    parametric, 77–8
fixation losses (FL), automated perimetry, 125, 135
fixed-combination medical therapy, 565–73
    adherence, 565
    advantages, 566
    formulations, 567–73
    future role, 567
    limitations, 566–7
    preservatives, 565–6
    see also specific combinations
floaters
    Heidelberg Retina Tomograph, 231
    scanning laser polarimetry, 245
fluorescein, aqueous flow rate measurement, 56–8
fluorescein angiography (FA), 259, 266
    iris neovascularization, 411
fluorophotometry, 56–8, 59
5-fluorouracil (5-FU), sub-Saharan Africa, 37
α-fodrin autoantibodies, 365
foreign bodies, retained intraocular, 437, 646
frequency doubling technology (FDT) perimetry, 134, 139–44
    clinical interpretation, 141–2
    comparative studies, 146–7
    FDT Matrix instrument, 143–4, 145
    mode of action, 140–1
    primary open-angle glaucoma, 321
    strengths and limitations, 142–3
    structural correlation, 252
Friedenwald equation, 109
Fuch's adenoma, 445
Fuch's heterochromic iridocyclitis, 398
    aqueous humor dynamics, 62, 64
    diagnostic features, 399, 401
    differential diagnosis, 411
    gonioscopy, 181
functional abilities, assessing, 476, 482, 504–5

fundoscopy *see* ophthalmoscopy
fundus pulsation amplitude (FPA), 258–9, 266

G

GANfort™ *see* bimatoprost/timolol
gaze tracking, automated perimetry, 125
GDx VCC scanning laser polarimeter, 241–5
    change over time, 242, 498
    measuring outcomes, 498
    see also scanning laser polarimetry (SLP)
gender differences
    acute angle closure, 625, 626
    ocular trauma, 431, 637
    pigmentation dispersion syndrome, 349
    primary angle-closure glaucoma, 331
gene–environmental interactions, 285
gene–gene interactions, 285
gene therapy, 605–12
    antisense therapy, 609
    aqueous outflow modulation, 609–10
    neuroprotection strategies, 610–12
    short interfering (silencing) RNAs, 609
    virus vectors, 605–8
generic medications, variations in quality, 35
genetic epidemiology, 277–86
genetic variants, 283
genetics, 269–74
genome-wide association studies, 284
geographic variations
    exfoliation syndrome, 10–11, 340
    glaucoma care, 33–9
    glaucoma prevalence and numbers, 5–9
    risk factors, 9–11
    significance of glaucoma, 299–303
    see also cultural differences
geranylgeranylacetone, 583
Ghana, glaucoma care, 36–7
ghost-cell glaucoma, 427, 435, 644
glatiramer acetate, 583
glaucoma, definition *see* definition of glaucoma
Glaucoma Adherence and Persistency Study (GAPS), 491–2
Glaucoma Graph, 295–6
Glaucoma Health Perceptions Index (GHPI), 474–5
Glaucoma Hemifield Test (GHT), 124, 125
    SWAP, 136
glaucoma progression analysis (GPA), 127, 128
Glaucoma Quality of Life (GQL-15) questionnaire, 473–4, 475
Glaucoma Staging System, 500, 501
Glaucoma Symptom Scale (GSS), 473, 474, 482
glaucomatocyclitic crisis (Posner-Schlossman syndrome), 632–3
    aqueous humor dynamics, 62, 64
    diagnosis, 400, 632–3
    mechanism, 395, 633
    treatment, 633
glaukomflecken, 334, 389
GLC1 loci, 269, 281
glial cell line-derived neurotrophic factor (GDNF), 583
glial cells
    lamina cribrosa, 50
    role in axon damage, 50, 51
    see also astrocytes
glial fibrillary acid protein (GFAP), 50
gliosis, reactive, 602
global positioning systems, 484
glucocorticoid receptor (GR), short interfering RNA, 610
glutamate excitotoxicity, 52, 583

glycerin, acute angle closure, 628, 631
gold standard test, 497
Goldmann applanation tonometry (GAT), 103–4
    central corneal thickness and, 103, 207–11
    corneal biomechanics and, 207, 209–11
    principle, 103–4
    sources of error, 104, 105, 107, 207
Goldmann equation, 109, 425, 548
Goldmann goniolens, 173, 174
Goldmann gonioscopy, 175–6
Goldmann perimeter scale, 116
Goldmann perimetry, 116
goniolenses, 173–5
    sterilization, 176
gonioscopy, 173–82
    angle-closure glaucoma, 387–8
    children, 370
    failure to use, 300
    grading of angle width, 178–9
    historical background, 173
    indentation, 176
    normal angle anatomy, 177–8
    ocular trauma, 181–2, 433, 649
    optical principles, 173, 174
    pathological findings, 179–82
    primary angle-closure glaucoma, 333
    techniques, 175–6
goniosynechialysis (GSL)
    acute primary angle closure, 630
    phacoemulsification with (phaco-GSL), 458
    primary angle closure, 458
    secondary angle-closure glaucoma, 390
goniotomy
    congenital glaucoma, 372–4
    uveitic glaucoma, 404
GPNMB (glycoprotein NMB), 272, 352–3
graft rejection, transplanted stem cells, 601
Graves disease, 425
gray scale plots, automated perimetry, 121, 136
growth-associated protein-43 (GAP-43), 586

H

Haab's striae, 372, 373
hallucinations, visual, 482
halo glaucomatosus, 220
handicap, visual, 503
Hartmann-Shack wavefront sensor, 618
Haseman-Elston regression method, 282
heart failure, β-blockers and, 532
Heidelberg Retina Tomograph (HRT), 225–31
    analyses, printouts and interpretation, 225–8
    artifacts and prevention, 230–1
    change over time, 227–8, 229, 236, 498
    Cluster Change Analysis, 228, 229
    diagnostic accuracy, 228–30, 236
    Glaucoma Probability Score (GPS), 226–7, 228, 229–30, 236, 247
    mode of action, 225
    Moorfields Regression Analysis (MRA), 226, 227, 229–30, 231, 236, 247
    OU report, 226, 227, 246
    reproducibility, 225
    retinal nerve fiber layer (RNFL), 239, 245–7
    statistical image mapping (SIM), 228
    stereometric parameters, 225–6, 227
    strengths and limitations, 231
    Topographic Change Analysis (TCA), 227, 228, 229, 230, 236
    vs multifocal visual evoked potentials, 162, 163
    vs other imaging techniques, 235–6
    see also confocal scanning laser ophthalmoscopy

Heidelberg retinal flowmeter (HRF), 260–2
height variation contour, 226
Heijl-Krakau method, fixation monitoring, 125
Helen Keller International, 37
hemolytic glaucoma, 435, 644
hemorrhagic glaucoma *see* neovascular glaucoma
hemosiderotic glaucoma, 644
Henson perimeter, 117
  interpretation of results, 123
  spatial grid, 120
heritability, 278
herpes simplex keratouveitis, 395, 399, 402, 633
herpes simplex virus, 421
high-pass resolution perimetry (HPRP), 134, 145–6, 147
hill of vision, 115
Hispanic populations, 36, 297
home tonometry, 108–9
homocysteine, elevated levels, 344, 345
hoop stress, 72–3
horizontal integrated rim area (HIRW), 233
HRT *see* Heidelberg Retina Tomograph
human immunodeficiency virus (HIV), 607–8
Humphrey Field Analyzer (HFA) (perimeter), 117, 118
  reliability indices, 124–5
  short-wavelength automated perimetry, 135
  single field analysis, 121–4
  spatial grid, 120
  visual field progression, 125–9, 502
hydrogen clearance method, ocular blood flow measurement, 266
hypercapnia, retrobulbar vascular responses, 96
hypercoagulability, 93
hypermetropia, angle closure risk, 333
hypertension, systemic
  normal-tension glaucoma, 364
  ocular blood flow and, 93
  primary open-angle glaucoma, 317
hyphema
  eight-ball, 432, 434, 435, 640
  grading, 432, 639
  management, 434–5
  neovascular glaucoma, 412–13
  traumatic, 431–2, 637, 638–40
    complications, 432, 639, 640
    management, 434–5, 639–40
    mechanisms of glaucoma, 434, 640
hypotension, systemic, 93, 364

I

ICare tonometer, 108
ICE syndrome *see* iridocorneal endothelial syndrome
Imbert-Fick principle, 103
L-N^6-(1-iminoethyl)lysine 5-tetrazole amide, 583
immunological factors, glaucomatous optic neuropathy, 52–3
Impact of Vision Impairment (IVI), 473, 483
  children's version (IVI_C), 484
  Melanesian version (IVI_M), 484
incidence
  defined, 3
  measuring, 4
Indian subcontinent, 299–301
  primary angle-closure glaucoma, 330, 331
indocyanine green (ICG) angiography, 259
infantile glaucoma, 371
inflammation
  acute angle closure, 628
  pigment dispersion syndrome, 353

post-traumatic, 433
  prostaglandin analogues and, 560, 562
  stem cell therapy and, 601
inflammatory diseases, systemic, 387
inflammatory mediators, role in uveitic glaucoma, 394–5
inhibitors of apoptosis proteins (IAPs), 611–12
insulin, aqueous humor dynamics and, 64
insurance companies, 298
integrins, 85–6
interferometry, pulsatile ocular blood flow, 258
interleukin-1 (IL-1), 394–5
interleukin-18 (IL-18), 353
International Classification of Functioning (ICF), 482–3
International Society of Geographical and Epidemiological Ophthalmology (ISGEO)
  classification of glaucoma, 3, 5
  guidelines, 4
intraocular lenses (IOL)
  malignant glaucoma secondary to, 386
  pigmentary glaucoma secondary to, 356
intraocular pressure (IOP)
  aqueous humor dynamics and, 55–64
  axon loss and, 51
  baseline, target IOP and, 467
  biomechanical effects, 68–70, 72–3, 79–82
  control, acute angle closure, 455–6, 627, 628
  defining glaucoma, 293–4
  defining ocular hypertension, 307
  early post-traumatic period, 434, 436–7
  elevated *see* ocular hypertension
  fluctuation, 103, 109–12
    long-term, 112
    progression of glaucoma and, 51, 112
    short-term, 110–12
    target IOP and, 468
    ultra-short-term, 109, 110
  genetic contribution, 278, 279
  geographic variations, 10
  HRT accuracy and, 231
  linkage analysis, 282
  long-term drift, 531
  lowering efficacy
    α agonists, 552–3
    β-blockers, 530–1
    carbonic anhydrase inhibitors, 542
    fixed-dose combinations, 566
    prostaglandin analogues, 561–2
  measurement, 103–9
    accuracy and precision, 103
    failure to perform, 300
    neuroprotection trials, 594
    target IOP and, 467
    see also tonometry
  normal, 57, 294, 361
  ocular blood flow and, 94–5
  as outcome measure, 497–8
  peak, 110–12
  progression of glaucoma and, 316
  prophylaxis of post-procedure rises, 549–50
  screening, 18–19
  target, 463–9
    definition, 463
    factors influencing, 465–7
    limitations, 467–8
    ocular hypertension, 312, 463–4
    primary open-angle glaucoma, 322–3
    rationale, 463–5
    setting, 468–9
    very low, 468
intrinsic sympathomimetic activity (ISA), 528, 533

iodoantipyrine, ocular blood flow measurement, 266
IOL *see* intraocular lenses
IOP *see* intraocular pressure
iridectomy
  primary angle-closure glaucoma, 327, 334
  uveitic glaucoma, 403
iridocorneal endothelial (ICE) syndrome, 420–2
  gonioscopy, 180
  signs and symptoms, 421, 422, 423
iridodialysis, traumatic, 433, 641
iridoplasty, laser peripheral *see* laser peripheral iridoplasty
iridotomy, laser peripheral *see* laser peripheral iridotomy
iridotrabecular contact (ITC), 327
  diagnosis, 333, 387–8
  mechanisms, 330–1, 332, 383–7
iris
  appearances
    exfoliation syndrome, 342, 343
    pigment dispersion syndrome, 354, 356
    uveitis, 399, 401
  atrophy, progressive, 420, 421, 422
  color change, prostaglandin analogues, 562, 563
  heterochromia, 354
  high insertion, congenital glaucoma, 372, 373
  ischemia, exfoliation syndrome, 344
  neovascularization *see* neovascularization of iris
  plateau *see* plateau iris
  posterior bowing, pigment dispersion syndrome, 188, 350–1, 352
  processes, gonioscopy, 177–8
  pseudoplateau, 191, 192, 385
  texture and thickness, angle-closure glaucoma, 384
  transillumination defects, 354, 356
iris bombe
  acute angle closure, 626
  secondary angle closure, 389
  uveitic glaucoma, 396, 397
iris–ciliary body complex neoplasms, pigment dispersion, 356
iris ciliary process distance (ICPD), 186, 187
  angle-closure glaucoma, 190
iris cysts (iridociliary cysts), 445
  pigment dispersion, 356
  pseudoplateau iris, 191, 192, 385
iris distance (ID1, ID2, ID3), 186, 187
iris–lens angle (ILA), 187
iris–lens contact distance (ILCD), 186, 187
  angle-closure glaucoma, 190
  pigmentary dispersion syndrome, 188, 189
iris–lens diaphragm, forward movement in uveitic glaucoma, 396, 397
iris nevus syndrome, 423
  see also Cogan-Reese syndrome
iris zonule distance (IZD), 186, 187
  angle-closure glaucoma, 190
iris-chafing syndrome, 356
iritis, traumatic, 638
iron-containing foreign bodies, 437, 644, 646
ischemia, ocular
  exfoliation syndrome, 344
  neovascular glaucoma, 409–11
  see also ocular blood flow; retinal ischemia
ischemic optic neuropathy, nonarteritic anterior (NAION), 221, 362
ISGEO *see* International Society of Geographical and Epidemiological Ophthalmology
ISNT rule, 216
isopters, 116

isotropic materials, 70–1
item response theory (IRT), 476

J

Jampel formula, target IOP, 468, 469
Japan
  genetic epidemiology, 284, 285
  normal-tension glaucoma, 10, 362
  significance of glaucoma, 303
judgment, clinical
  treatment decisions, 509
  visual field progression, 125–6, 501
juvenile idiopathic arthritis (JIA), uveitic
    glaucoma, 393–4, 399
juvenile open-angle glaucoma, 371, 375
  genetics, 273, 281, 375
juvenile xanthogranuloma, 441, 444
juxtacanalicular tissue (JCT), 59

K

K cells, 134, 135
Koeppe goniolens, 174–5
Koeppe gonioscopy, 176
koniocellular retinal ganglion cells (K cells;
    bistratified cells), 134, 135
Korea, 303
Krukenberg spindle, 349, 354
krypton washout method, ocular blood flow
    measurement, 266

L

labile liposomes method, ocular blood flow
    measurement, 266
lamina cribrosa
  aging changes, 49, 82
  astrocytes mediating axon damage, 50, 68
  axon organization in relation to damage,
    46–8
  biomechanics
    engineering models, 78–9, 80, 81, 82
    IOP-related stress, 49, 73
    response to acute IOP elevations, 73–6
  glial cells, 50
  normal organization, 45–6, 47, 67–8
  position of central retinal vessel exit, 217,
    218–19
  remodeling and restructuring, 68–9, 84–6,
    87
  risk factors for glaucoma, 217
  ultrastructural imaging, 616–17, 618
  see also optic nerve head
Langham pulsatile ocular blood flow (POBF)
    technique, 258
Laplace's Law, 73
laser capsulotomy, prophylaxis of IOP rise
    after, 550
laser Doppler flowmetry (LDF)
  ocular blood flow, 260, 266
  peripheral blood flow, 265–6
laser Doppler velocimetry (LDV), 259–60
laser peripheral iridoplasty (LPI)
  acute angle closure, 456, 457, 629
  chronic angle closure, 457
  indications, 334–5
  lens-induced glaucoma, 390
  plateau iris, 457
  plateau iris syndrome, 389, 390
  secondary angle-closure glaucoma, 389–90
  ultrasound biomicroscopy, 194
laser peripheral iridotomy (LPI)
  acute angle closure, 456–7, 628–9
  anterior segment optical coherence
    tomography, 202
  chronic angle closure, 457
  developing countries, 38, 39

indications, 334–5
  malignant glaucoma, 391
  pigmentary glaucoma, 357–8
  postoperative management, 550
  prophylactic, 631
  secondary angle-closure glaucoma, 389–90
  ultrasound biomicroscopy, 193
  uveitic glaucoma, 403
laser speckle flowgraphy, 263
laser therapy
  acute angle closure, 628–9
  secondary angle-closure glaucoma, 389–90
  see also specific techniques
laser trabeculoplasty
  α agonist therapy after, 549–50
  in developing countries, 35
  exfoliative glaucoma, 345
  pigmentary glaucoma, 357
  primary open-angle glaucoma, 323
  uveitic glaucoma, 404
latanoprost, 560
  childhood glaucoma, 374
  exfoliative glaucoma, 344–5
  pharmacology, 561
  pigmentary glaucoma, 357
  side effects, 562
  uveitic glaucoma, 402
latanoprost/timolol (Xalacom™), 527, 569–70
  efficacy, 534, 569–70
  preservatives, 566
lateral geniculate nucleus (LGN)
  neurons, counting, 582
  retinal ganglion cell projections, 133–4
Latin America, 6, 8
lead time, 17, 18
learning effect, perimetry, 120–1
lens
  exfoliation material deposits, 342
  opacities, anterior subcapsular
    (glaukomfleken), 334, 389
  position and thickness, angle closure risk,
    332–3
  retained fragment, 420
  subluxation or dislocation
    exfoliation syndrome, 343, 344
    lens-induced angle closure, 385–6
    traumatic, 433, 435–6, 642–3
lens extraction, 335
  acute primary angle closure, 458, 629–30
  primary angle closure, 457–8
  uveitic glaucoma, 403
  see also cataract surgery
lens zonules
  fragility, exfoliation syndrome, 343, 344
  pigment deposition, 354, 356
lens-induced glaucoma
  closed angle, 385–6, 390
  open angle, 419–20
  post-traumatic, 643
  uveitis, 396, 397
lens-particle glaucoma, 419, 420
  post-traumatic, 436, 645
lentivirus vectors, 607–8, 610
leukemia, 441, 445
leukoma, central corneal, 378, 379
levobunolol, 526, 531
liability threshold model, complex diseases,
    278
lid artifacts, diagnostic techniques, 129, 203
life expectancy, 503–4
light-difference sensitivity, 115
likelihood of help versus harm (LHH), 509,
    511
likelihood ratio, 496, 497
Likert scales, 475–6
linear materials, 71
Linear Scale Thermometer, 477

linkage analysis, 277, 279–83, 285
  association analyses following, 284
  complex forms of glaucoma, 281–2
  monogenic glaucomas, 279–81
  nonparametric, 281–2
  parametric (model-based), 279, 281
  quantitative traits, 282–3
linkage disequilibrium, 283
Lisch nodules, 377
Liwan Eye Study, 20
load–deformation relationships, 70–2
  linear and nonlinear, 71
LOD scores, 280, 281–2
LogMAR chart, 481–2
long short posterior ciliary arteries, 50
low coherence interferometry, 619
low vision, 481–6
  assessing consequences, 481–3
  contextual factors, 483–4
  definition, 481, 503
  devices, 484, 485–6
  new technology, 484
  services, 484
  see also blindness; visual impairment
Lowe syndrome, 377, 378
Low-pressure Glaucoma Treatment Study
    (LoGTS), 364, 585
low-tension glaucoma see normal-tension
    glaucoma
LOXL1 gene, 272, 340
Lycium barbarum Lynn, 583
lymphoma, 441, 445
lysil oxidase-like 1 (LOXL1) gene, 272, 340

M

M cells, 133, 134
macrophages, phacolytic glaucoma, 419
macula
  cystoid edema see cystoid macular edema
  optical coherence tomography (OCT),
    248–9
magnetic resonance imaging (MRI),
    neuroprotection studies, 582
magnifiers, 484, 485–6
magnocellular retinal ganglion cells (M cells),
    133, 134
  My subset, 142, 143
Maklakov tonometer, 207
malignant glaucoma see aqueous
    misdirection
Maloney murine leukemia virus, 607
management
  angle closure, 455–9
  benefits and risks, 509–13
  different societies, 33–9
  economics, 25–31
  low-vision rehabilitation, 481–6
  medication adherence and persistence,
    489–93
  ocular hypertension and primary open-
    angle glaucoma, 451–3
  outcomes, 495–506
  target IOP see intraocular pressure (IOP),
    target
  see also treatment
mannitol, acute angle closure, 628, 631
Marfan's syndrome, 356, 386
material properties, tissue, 70–1
matrix G1a protein (MGP), short interfering
    RNA, 610
Max gene therapy, 612
mean deviation (MD), visual fields, 122
mechanical failure, 72
mechanical strain, 70
  engineering models, 77–9
  induced by elevated IOP, 76

lamina cribrosa, 49
tissue remodeling and restructuring, 84–6
mechanical stress, 70
  engineering models, 77–9
  hoop, 72–3
  IOP-generated, 49, 72–3
  lamina cribrosa, 49
  tissue remodeling and restructuring, 84–6
mechanical yield, 72
mechanics
  basic concepts, 70–2
  see also cornea, biomechanics; optic nerve
    head (ONH), biomechanics
Medical Outcomes Study Short-Form Health
    Survey (SF-36), 472
medical therapy
  acute primary angle closure, 456, 628
  adherence and persistence see adherence
    and persistence, medication
  adjunctive, 565
  chronic primary angle closure, 456
  congenital glaucoma, 374
  corticosteroid-induced ocular hypertension,
    424
  costs, 28, 29
    adherence and, 34–5, 492
    in developing countries, 34–5, 36, 38
  exfoliative glaucoma, 344–5
  fixed combination see fixed-combination
    medical therapy
  historical development, 534
  iridocorneal endothelial syndrome, 421–2
  neovascular glaucoma, 413
  normal-tension glaucoma, 365–6
  ocular hypertension, 311–12
  pigmentary glaucoma, 357
  post-traumatic glaucoma, 649
  primary angle-closure glaucoma, 335
  primary open-angle glaucoma, 323
  quality issues, 35
  secondary angle-closure glaucoma, 389
  uveitic glaucoma, 402–3
  see also α agonists; β-blockers;
    carbonic anhydrase inhibitors;
    parasympathomimetics; prostaglandin
    analogues individual agents
medulloepithelioma, 441, 443, 444
megalocornea, 372
MEK1 gene therapy, 612
melanin
  pigment dispersion see pigment dispersion
    syndrome
  trabecular deposition, 353–4
melanocytoma, 445
melanoma
  choroidal, 441, 442, 445
  iris or ciliary body, 441, 443, 445
  ring, 445, 446
  tapioca, 445
  uveal, 441, 445, 446
melanomalytic glaucoma, 441
melanosomal proteins, 352–3
melatonin, aqueous flow and, 56
Melbourne Low Vision ADL Index (MLVAI),
    482
memantine, 583–4, 585
membrane attack complex (MAC), 52–3
metallic foreign bodies, 437, 646
metastatic tumors, intraocular, 441, 445
methazolamide, 539–40
  post-traumatic glaucoma, 640
methylcellulose coupling medium, 186
metipranolol, 526, 531
microglia, optic nerve head, 52
microhyphema, 638
microscopy
  peripheral blood flow, 265

see also ultrasound biomicroscopy;
    ultrastructural imaging
microsphere method, ocular blood flow
    measurement, 266
migraine, 96
  glaucoma risk, 317
  normal-tension glaucoma and, 364
minocycline, 52, 583
miotics see parasympathomimetics
mitochondria, retinal ganglion cells, 45, 46–7
mitomycin C (MMC)
  angle-recession glaucoma, 642
  neovascular glaucoma, 413–14
  normal-tension glaucoma, 366
  sub-Saharan Africa, 37
  uveitic glaucoma, 403–4
MMC see mitomycin C
MMP-9 gene polymorphism, 274
models, experimental glaucoma, 580–1
'More Flow' (Moorfields/UK MRC) Study, 465
Müller cells, 598, 601
My cells, 142, 143
mydriasis, pharmacological
  pigment dispersion caused by, 350
  triggering angle closure, 331
  uveitic glaucoma, 403
myelodysplastic syndrome, 445
myeloma, multiple, 445
myocilin (MYOC) gene, 269–70, 281, 318,
    375
  corticosteroid-induced ocular hypertension
    and, 395, 424
  gene therapy targeting, 610
  interactions, 273, 282, 283, 285
  olfactomedin domain, 284
myocilin protein, 270
myofibroblasts, 411
myopia
  angle closure risk, 333
  differential diagnosis, 362–3
  glaucoma risk, 317
  optic disc shape, 215
  optic disc size, 213, 214
  pigmentary glaucoma, 349–50
  scleral crescent, 220

N

nail-fold capillary blood flow, 265–6
nail-patella syndrome (NPS), 273
nanophthalmos, autosomal dominant, 274
nanotechnology, 621
narrow angle see primary angle-closure
    suspect
narrow-angle glaucoma (NAG), 383
  see also angle-closure glaucoma
nasal step defect, 120
National Eye Institute, 323
  Visual Function Questionnaire (NEI-VFQ),
    473, 483
negative predictive value, 496
neovascular glaucoma (NVG), 409–15
  angle closure, 387, 413
  diagnosis and ancillary tests, 411
  differential diagnosis, 411
  elevated episcleral venous pressure, 426
  etiology and pathogenesis, 411
  future treatment options, 414–15
  intraocular tumors, 410–11, 443, 444
  prevalence, 409
  risk factors, 409–11
  signs and symptoms, 411–12
  stages, 412–13
  treatment, 413–14
neovascularization of angle (NVA), 412
  diagnosis, 411
  gonioscopy, 181

pathogenesis, 411
  treatment, 413, 414–15
  uveitis, 398
neovascularization of iris (NVI) (rubeosis
    iridis), 412
  angle-closure glaucoma, 413
  diagnosis, 411
  intraocular tumors, 444
  pathogenesis, 411
  risk factors, 409–11
  treatment, 413, 414–15
nerve fiber indicator (NFI), 242, 243, 244
neural cell adhesion molecule (NCAM), 49
neural progenitor cells, 599, 600
neural stem (NS) cells, 597, 598
neurofibromatosis type, 1, 369, 376–7, 444
neuroprotection, 579–85
  α agonists, 549
  assessing effect, 581–2
  β-blockers, 530
  clinical trials, 584–5
    critical assessment, 591–4
    generalizability of results, 592
    study methodology, 591–2
  experimental models, 580–1
  gene therapy approaches, 610–12
  immune mechanisms, 584
  mechanisms, 579–80
  methods, 580
  normal-tension glaucoma, 366, 585
  pharmacology, 582, 583
  preclinical studies, 582–4
  prostaglandin analogues, 561
  stem cell-mediated, 601
neuroregeneration, 585–7
  see also stem cell therapy
neuroretinal rim
  area, 215–16, 226, 233
    measurement methods compared, 235–6
    ocular hypertension, 308
  blood flow, cup-to-disc ratio and, 95
  ISNT rule, 216
  optical coherence tomography, 232
  pallor, 217, 362
  patterns of glaucomatous loss, 216–17
  shape, 213, 214, 216–17
  size, 215–16
  thinning, 308
  volume, 226
neurotrophins, retinal ganglion cell survival
    and, 51–2
nevus flammeus, 369, 375–6
NFI (nerve fiber indicator), 242, 243, 244
nitric oxide (NO), 50
nitric oxide synthase-2 (NOS-2), 50
N-methyl-D-aspartate (NMDA) receptor
    antagonists
  clinical studies, 366, 585
  preclinical studies, 583–4
NNO1 locus, 274
Noelin 1 and 2 genes, 284
Nogo receptor, 586, 602
nonarteritic anterior ischemic optic
    neuropathy (NAION), 221, 362
noncontact tonometer (NCT), 104, 105, 207
nongovernmental organizations (NGOs),
    37–9
nonlinear materials, 71
nonpenetrating glaucoma surgery (NPGS)
  ultrasound biomicroscopy, 194–5
  uveitic glaucoma, 404
norepinephrine (noradrenaline), 527–8
normal-tension glaucoma (NTG), 361–6
  aqueous humor dynamics, 62, 63
  differential diagnosis, 362–3
  familial, 270
  genetic variants, 284, 285–6

normal-tension glaucoma (NTG) (continued)
  geographic variations, 10, 362
  neuroprotection, 366, 585
  ocular blood flow, 91, 93, 96–7
  pathogenesis and systemic evaluation, 363–5
  prevalence, 361–2
  prognosis, 366
  target IOP, 468
  treatment, 365–6
  vascular changes, 92
  vasospastic changes, 96–7, 364
North Africa, 301–2
North America, glaucoma prevalence, 5–6
number needed to be treated to produce harm (NNH), 509–11
number needed to screen, 19–20
number needed to treat (NNT), 509–11
numerical solutions, optic nerve head biomechanics, 77–9

O

OAG see open-angle glaucoma
obesity, 10
obstructive sleep apnea syndrome, 363
occludable angle see primary angle-closure suspect
OCT see optical coherence tomography
Octopus perimeter, 117, 118, 119
  interpretation of results, 122, 124, 125
  short-wavelength automated perimetry, 135
  spatial grid, 120
ocular blood flow (OBF), 91–7
  α agonist actions, 548–9
  animal experimental methods, 266
  autoregulation, 93, 95–6
  carbonic anhydrase inhibitors and, 541
  current evidence of abnormal, 94–7
  effect of therapeutic IOP reduction, 94–5
  evaluation, 94, 257–65
    blue field entoptics, 265
    Canon laser blood flowmeter, 264–5
    color Doppler imaging, 257–8
    fluorescein and indocyanine green angiography, 259
    interpretation, 266
    laser Doppler flowmetry, 260
    laser Doppler velocimetry, 259–60
    laser speckle technique, 262
    limitations, 266
    pneumatonometry, 108
    retinal vessel analyzer, 263–4
    scanning laser Doppler flowmetry, 260–2
  exfoliation syndrome, 344
  glaucoma, 84–6, 91–2
  increased local resistance, 92, 93
  IOP-related changes, 68, 79, 94–5
  mechanisms of reduction, 92–3
  prostaglandin analogue actions, 561
  pulsatile (POBF), 258–9, 266
ocular hypertension (OHT), 307–13
  acute, 625–33
  animal models, 581
  aqueous humor dynamics, 61, 62
  benefit vs risk of treatment, 510
  corticosteroid-induced see corticosteroid-induced ocular hypertension/glaucoma
  definition, 307, 451
  detecting progression, 310–11
  electrophysiological measures, 154, 155
  follow-up, 312
  IOP fluctuation, 111–12
  management, 311–12, 451–2
  mechanisms of axon loss, 51
  neuroprotection studies, 584
  ocular blood flow, 94, 95

patient assessment, 307–9
prevalence, 307
risk of progression to glaucoma, 309–10, 316
screening, 18–19
SWAP testing, 137–8
target IOP, 312, 463–4
uveitis, 393–4, 399
Ocular Hypertension Treatment Study (OHTS), 323, 324, 451
  benefits and risks of treatment, 510
  central corneal thickness, 10, 208
  cost-utility analysis, 30
  end points, 497, 498, 500
  frequency of follow-up, 312
  glaucoma screening and, 18, 19
  optic disc imaging, 236
  risk factors for progression, 309, 310, 316, 317
  signs of progression, 310
  structure–function relationships, 251
  target IOP, 312, 463–4, 466
ocular ischemia see ischemia, ocular
ocular ischemic syndrome, neovascular glaucoma, 410
ocular perfusion pressure (OPP), 92–3
  autoregulatory defects, 95–6
ocular pulse amplitude (OPA), 107, 108
Ocular Response Analyzer (ORA), 104–5, 106, 209
oculocerebrorenal (Lowe) syndrome, 377, 378
Ocusert-Pilo™, 519
OHT see ocular hypertension
OHTS see Ocular Hypertension Treatment Study
OPA1 gene, 284
open-angle glaucoma (OAG)
  in developing countries, 34–5
  economics, 25, 27–30
  electrophysiological measures, 155, 158
  juvenile see juvenile open-angle glaucoma
  lens-induced, 419–20
  neovascular, 412–13
  neuroprotection studies, 585
  with normal IOP, 361
  ocular blood flow, 94, 95, 96, 97
  primary see primary open-angle glaucoma
  screening, 16, 20
  secondary, 631
    intraocular tumors, 441
    optic disc size, 214
    uveitis, 394–5, 403–4
    see also exfoliative glaucoma; pigmentary glaucoma
  vasospasm, 97
  vitreoretinal and retinal disorders, 427–8
ophthalmic artery (OA), blood flow velocity, 257, 258
ophthalmologists
  developing countries, 33, 39
  different societies, 299, 300, 302
  see also physicians
ophthalmoscopy, 615
  childhood glaucomas, 370
  confocal scanning laser see confocal scanning laser ophthalmoscopy
  limitations of conventional, 615
  optic nerve head, 213–22
  retinal nerve fiber layer, 221–2, 239–41
  scanning laser (SLO), 615–18
Ophthimus system, 145
optic atrophy, autosomal dominant, 284
optic cup
  area, 226, 233
  configuration, 218
  depth, 218, 226
  shape, 226

size in relation to disc size, 217–18
volume, 226
see also cup-to-disc ratio; optic disc, cupping
optic disc
  area, 213–14, 226, 233
  cupping
    biomechanical aspects, 84–6
    childhood glaucoma, 370
    differential diagnosis, 362, 372, 373
    normal-tension glaucoma, 361
    photography, 213–18
    see also cup-to-disc ratio; optic cup
  damage likelihood scale, 296, 498, 500
  hemorrhages, 219
    normal-tension glaucoma, 364–5, 366
    ocular hypertension, 311
    risk for progression to glaucoma, 316
  imaging, 225–36
    measuring outcomes, 498, 500
    methods compared, 235–6
    ocular hypertension, 308, 311, 312
    technological advances, 615–22
  ophthalmoscopy, 213–22
  outcome measures, 498
  photography, 213–22
    measuring outcomes, 498, 500
    ocular hypertension, 308, 311, 312
    primary open-angle glaucoma, 321–2
    vs other imaging methods, 235–6
  rim see neuroretinal rim
  shape, 214–15
  size, 213–14
    cup size in relation to, 217–18
    HRT accuracy and, 230
    see also cup-to-disc ratio
  staging systems, 498, 499
  structural changes
    acute angle closure, 627
    biomechanical aspects, 84–6
    early glaucoma, 308
    measurement, 498
    neuroprotection studies, 582
    normal-tension glaucoma, 362
    primary open-angle glaucoma, 318–19
    risk factors for progression, 316
  structural–function relationships, 251–4
  tilted, 215, 362
  very large (macrodisc), 214
    acquired or secondary, 214, 215
    primary, 214
  very small (microdisc), 214
optic nerve
  changes defining glaucoma, 294, 296
  experimental injury models, 580, 581
  fibers see retinal ganglion cell (RGC) axons
  neuroprotection studies, 582
  regeneration, 585–7
optic nerve head (ONH)
  astrocytes mediating axon damage, 50
  axon organization in relation to damage, 46–8
  biomechanics, 49, 67–79
    acute IOP elevations, 73–6, 79
    basic engineering concepts, 70–2
    conceptual framework, 67–70
    contribution of sclera, 76–7
    engineering models, 77–9
    finite element (FE) models, 71, 77–9, 80, 81, 82
    future directions, 86–7
    in vitro studies, 86
    overview, 72–3
  blood flow, 50–1, 67
    after therapeutic IOP reduction, 95
    autoregulation, 95–6
    glaucoma, 84–6, 94

IOP-related reduction, 68, 79
see also ocular blood flow
component (ONHC), multifocal
electroretinogram, 156
ophthalmoscopic examination, 213–22
optical coherence tomography (OCT),
232–5, 248–9
remodeling and restructuring, 69, 79–86
early glaucoma, 82–4, 85, 86, 87
later-stage glaucoma, 84–6
normal aging, 79–82
stem cell-mediated restoration, 596
structure–function relationships, 251–4
see also lamina cribrosa
optic neuropathy, glaucomatous
acute primary angle closure, 631
differential diagnosis, 362
early signs, 308
measurements, 496–502
neuroprotection and neuroregeneration,
579–87
pathogenesis, 45–53, 579–80
optical coherence tomography (OCT), 201,
619–21
advances in technology, 619–21
anterior segment *see* anterior segment
optical coherence tomography
macula, 248–9
neuroprotection studies, 582
optic nerve head (OHN), 232–5, 248–9
analyses, printouts and interpretation,
232–3
artifacts and prevention, 234–5
diagnostic accuracy, 233, 236
mode of action, 232
reproducibility, 232
strengths and limitations, 235
vs other imaging techniques, 235–6
polarization-sensitive, 620
primary open-angle glaucoma, 322
retinal nerve fiber layer (RNFL), 239,
247–9, 620
structural–function correlation, 252
time-domain, 619
ultra-high resolution (UHROCT), 619–20,
621
ultra-high speed spectral domain (Fourier-
domain), 620
optical Doppler tomography (ODT), 620
optineurin (OPTN) gene, 269, 270–1, 285–6
optophysiology, 621
orbital varices, 425
oscillatory potentials (OPs), 151–2
osmotic agents, acute angle closure,
628, 631
outcomes, glaucoma, 495–506
classification, 495
clinical, 496–504
patient's viewpoint, 504–5
quality of life, 504, 505–6
societal viewpoint, 505
spotlight, 505–6
oxygen tension method, ocular blood flow
measurement, 266

P

P cells, 133, 134, 145
PACG *see* primary angle-closure glaucoma
panretinal photocoagulation (PRP)
glaucoma caused by, 428
neovascularization, 413
paracentesis, acute primary angle closure,
456, 629
paracentral field defects, 120
parapapillary atrophy, optical coherence
tomography and, 235

parasympathomimetics (cholinergic agents;
miotics), 517–22
acute angle closure, 628
childhood glaucoma, 374
classification, 517–18
contraindications and precautions, 521
delivery systems, 519
drug interactions, 520–1
exfoliative glaucoma, 345
mechanism of action, 518–19
pharmacokinetics, 519
pigmentary glaucoma, 357
preparations available, 518
secondary angle-closure glaucoma, 389
side effects, 521–2
uveitic glaucoma, 402
vs other agents, 520–1
paroxetine, 331
parvocellular retinal ganglion cells (P cells),
133, 134, 145
Pascal® Dynamic Contour Tonometer
(DCT), 106–7
pathogenesis of glaucoma, 45–53, 579–80
aqueous humor dynamics and IOP
elevation, 55–64
mechanical strain and restructuring of
optic nerve head, 67–87
pressure theory, 91
role of ocular blood flow, 91–7
vascular theory, 91
patient(s)
adherence to medication *see* adherence and
persistence, medication
assessing values, 512–13
different societies, 299, 300–1
glaucoma outcomes, 504–5
reliability, automated perimetry, 120–1,
125
patient instructions
automated perimetry, 129
medical therapy, 492
patient-centered care, 471
pattern deviation plots, 122, 124, 136
pattern electroretinogram (PERG) *see*
electroretinogram (ERG), pattern
pattern standard deviation (PSD), 122–4,
136–7
pediatric glaucomas *see* childhood glaucomas
penetrating ocular injuries, 436–8, 645–6
Pentacam photography, 204
perfusion pressure, ocular *see* ocular
perfusion pressure
perimetry, 115–30
automated, 116–19
interpretation, 121–9
measurement variability, 120–1
patient instructions, 129
statistical analysis, 121–9
technical tips, 129
blue-yellow *see* short-wavelength
automated perimetry
failure to use, 300
frequency doubling technology *see*
frequency doubling technology (FDT)
perimetry
function-specific, 133–47, 252
high-pass resolution (HPRP), 134, 145–6,
147
history, 115–16
kinetic, 116
manual (Goldmann), 116
short-wavelength automated (SWAP) *see*
short-wavelength automated perimetry
standard automated (achromatic) *see*
standard automated perimetry
static, 116
structure–function relationships, 251–4

vs electrophysiological measures, 162, 163
white-on-white *see* standard automated
perimetry
see also visual evoked cortical potential;
visual field(s)
peripapillary chorioretinal atrophy, 219–20
α zone, 219, 220
β zone, 219–20
scanning laser polarimetry, 245
peripapillary sclera *see* sclera, peripapillary
peripheral anterior synechiae (PAS)
acute angle closure, 627
bridging, 396, 397
gonioscopy, 179–80, 388
goniosynechialysis *see* goniosynechialysis
inflammatory, 180
iridocorneal endothelial syndrome, 180,
421
post-traumatic, 437, 645
primary angle-closure glaucoma, 333, 455
uveitic glaucoma, 396–8
peripheral blood flow, 265–6
Perkins tonometer, 103
persistence, medication *see* adherence and
persistence, medication
Peter's anomaly, 273, 274, 378–9
phacoanaphylactic glaucoma, 419, 420
phacoantigenic uveitis, 420
phacoemulsification (PE)
plus goniosynechialysis (phaco-GSL), 458
primary angle closure, 458
phacolytic glaucoma, 419, 643, 644
phacomorphic glaucoma, 385–6
treatment, 390
uveitis, 396, 397
phakomatoses, 444
pharmaceutical industry, 298, 493
phenytoin, 583
phosphene tonometer, Proview, 108–9
photodynamic therapy, neovascular
glaucoma, 414
photography
optic disc *see* optic disc, photography
retinal nerve fiber layer, 221–2, 239–41
photophobia, 372
photopic a-wave, 151, 152
photopic b-wave, 151, 152
photopic negative response (PhNR), 153
photoreceptors, 133
transplantation, 598–9, 600
ultrastructural imaging, 616–17
physicians
glaucoma outcomes, 496–504
responsibility towards patients, 298–9
see also ophthalmologists
physostigmine, 518, 520
pigment dispersion syndrome (PDS), 349–59
aqueous humor dynamics, 62, 63
differential diagnosis, 355–6
etiology and pathogenesis, 350–4
exfoliation syndrome, 342–3, 356
genetics, 271–2, 351–3
gonioscopy, 180–1
natural history, 350
prevalence, 349–50
signs and symptoms, 354–5
ultrasound biomicroscopy, 188, 189,
350–1, 356
uveitis, 356, 399, 400
pigment reversal sign, 350
pigmentary glaucoma (PG), 349–59
differential diagnosis, 355–6
etiology and pathogenesis, 188, 350–4
genetics, 271–2, 351–3
laser trabeculoplasty, 357
natural history and risk factors, 350
prevalence, 349–50

pigmentary glaucoma (PG) (continued)
  prognosis, 358–9
  regression, 350
  secondary, 356
  signs and symptoms, 354–5
  treatment, 356–8
pigment-epithelium-derived factor (PEDF), 415
pilocarpine, 517
  acute angle closure, 628, 631
  β-blocker combinations, 520, 534
  contraindications and precautions, 521
  drug interactions, 520–1, 563
  exfoliative glaucoma, 345
  mechanism of action, 518–19
  pigment dispersion syndrome, 351, 352
  pigmentary glaucoma, 357
  plateau iris syndrome, 390
  preparations, 518
  side effects, 521–2
  vs other agents, 520–1
plateau iris (configuration), 331, 332, 384
  acute angle closure, 626–7
  laser peripheral iridoplasty, 457
  secondary (pseudo-), 191, 192, 385
  treatment, 389, 390
  ultrasound biomicroscopy, 191
plateau iris syndrome, 191, 384–5
  laser peripheral iridoplasty, 389, 390
  treatment, 389, 390
pneumatonometry, 107–8
POAG see primary open-angle glaucoma
polycoria
  Axenfeld-Reiger syndrome, 376
  iridocorneal endothelial syndrome, 421, 422
port-wine stain (nevus flammeus), 369, 375–6
position, body
  episcleral venous pressure and, 59, 110
  IOP variation with, 110
positive predictive value, 496
Posner-Schlossman syndrome see glaucomatocyclitic crisis
posterior block glaucoma see malignant glaucoma
posterior embryotoxon, 376
posterior polymorphous corneal dystrophy, 422–3
posterior segment
  pigment dispersion syndrome/pigmentary glaucoma, 355, 356
  vascular effects of β-blockers, 529–30
post-test odds, 496
post-test probability, 496
post-traumatic glaucoma, 431–8, 637–50
  diagnostic features, 648–9
  gonioscopy, 181–2
  long-term prognosis, 650
  pathogenesis, 434–8, 638–48
  risk factors, 637–8
  treatment, 649–50
  see also trauma
prednisone/prednisolone see corticosteroids
pregnancy
  β-blockers, 533
  carbonic anhydrase inhibitors, 543
prescriptions, unfilled, 489
preservative-free preparations
  β-blockers, 526–7
  fixed-dose combinations, 566
preservatives
  fixed-dose combinations, 565–6
  see also benzalkonium chloride
pressure theory, pathogenesis of glaucoma, 91
pre-test odds, 496
pre-test probability, 496

prevalence
  data applications, 5
  defined, 3
  glaucoma, 5–9
  measuring, 4
  undetected glaucoma, 11
prevention
  primary, 15
  secondary, 15
primary angle closure (PAC), 5, 383, 455
  acute see acute primary angle closure
  chronic see chronic primary angle closure
  filtering surgery, 458–9
  goniosynechialysis, 458
primary angle-closure glaucoma (PACG), 327–35, 383
  acute see acute primary angle closure
  anterior segment optical coherence tomography, 202
  chronic see chronic primary angle closure
  classification, 328
  clinical features, 334
  definition, 328
  diagnosis and testing, 333–4
  epidemiology, 328–30
    definitions used, 4, 5, 12
    geographic variations, 5–6, 8, 329–30
    incidence, 328–9
    prevalence and numbers affected, 8–9, 329–30
    undiagnosed cases, 11
  etiology and mechanisms, 11, 327, 330–1
  gonioscopy, 180
  management, 334–5, 455–9
  prevention of visual loss, 297
  prognosis, 335
  risk factors, 11, 331–3
  ultrasound biomicroscopy, 189–90
primary angle-closure suspect (PACS), 5, 455
  laser iridotomy, 456–7
primary open-angle glaucoma (POAG), 315–24
  aqueous humor dynamics, 61–3
  assessment, 452–3
  clinical trials, 323–4
  diagnosis, 318–22, 452
    functional defects, 320–1
    presumptive vs definitive, 318
    structural abnormalities, 318–20
  differential diagnosis, 362
  electrophysiological measures, 155, 158
  epidemiology, 6, 7, 8, 315
    definition used, 5, 12
    geographic variations, 5–6, 8
  family history, 317
  genetic epidemiology, 277–86, 318
    association studies, 283–4
    future perspectives, 285–6
    genetic susceptibility, 277–9
    linkage studies, 279–83
  genetics, 269–71, 318
  IOP variation and progression, 112
  management, 322–3, 451, 452–3
  monitoring, 453
  with normal IOP, 361
    see also normal-tension glaucoma
  ocular hypertension and, 307, 309–10
  optic disc size, 214
  pathogenesis, 317–18
  prevention of visual loss, 297–8
  quantitative traits
    genetic contribution, 278–9
    linkage analysis, 282–3
  racial variations, 6, 7, 277–8, 315, 316–17
  risk factors, 10, 316–17
  ultrasound biomicroscopy, 188
primate glaucoma, nonhuman, 581

neuroprotection studies, 583–4
progenitor cells, 595, 598
  transplantation, 599
progression of glaucoma
  defining disease, 295–6
  definition, 496
  frequency doubling technology (FDT), 143
  Heidelberg Retina Tomograph (HRT), 227–8, 229, 498
  IOP fluctuation and, 51, 112
  measurement, 496–502
    neuroprotection studies, 581, 582, 594
  optic disc imaging, 236, 498
  perimetry, 125–9, 500–2
  staging system, 500, 501
  structure–function relationships, 254, 502
  SWAP, 138
PROGRESSOR visual field analysis software, 127–8, 502
promoters, viral vectors, 608
propranolol, 525
prostaglandin analogues, 559–64
  adherence with therapy, 489–90, 491
  childhood glaucoma, 374
  combination therapy, 553, 563
  contraindications, 562
  drug interactions, 563
  efficacy and comparisons, 561–2
  exfoliative glaucoma, 344–5
  formulations, 559–60
  history of development, 534, 560
  indications, 561
  mechanism of action, 560–1
  normal-tension glaucoma, 366
  pigmentary glaucoma, 357
  pilocarpine interaction, 520, 563
  side effects, 562–3
  uveitic glaucoma, 402
  vs parasympathomimetics, 520
prostaglandins, 64, 559
proteoglycans, 602
Proview phosphene tonometer, 108–9
pseudoexfoliation syndrome see exfoliation syndrome
pseudoplateau iris, 191, 192, 385
psychosocial factors, assessing, 482–3
pulsatile ocular blood flow (POBF), 258–9, 266
pupillary block
  acute angle closure, 626
  after retinal surgery, 428
  drug induced, 633
  lens-induced, 385
  post-traumatic, 434, 642–3
  primary angle closure, 331, 383
  reverse see reverse pupillary block
  ultrasound biomicroscopy, 190, 191
  uveitis, 396, 397, 403

Q

quality of life (QOL), 30, 471–8
  assessment, 472–7
  definition, 471
  dimensions, 481
  impact of visual loss, 481–3
  importance, 471–2
  optimization, 481–7
  as outcome measure, 504, 505–6
  performance-based visual assessment, 476
  questionnaires, 472–6
    general health-related, 472
    glaucoma-specific, 473–5
    limitations, 476
    scoring systems, 475–6
    vision-specific, 472–3, 483
  utility measures, 476–7

quality-adjusted life year (QALY), 26, 477–8
quantitative trait loci (QTL), 282

R

racial/ethnic variations, 9, 297
  acute angle closure, 625, 626
  central corneal thickness (CCT), 10, 208
  exfoliation syndrome, 340–1
  ocular hypertension, 307
  optic disc size, 213–14
  pigmentary glaucoma, 349
  primary angle-closure glaucoma, 329, 331–2
  primary open-angle glaucoma, 6, 7, 277–8, 315, 316–17
  risk factors, 10
  target IOP, 467
  see also cultural differences; geographic variations
radiation injuries, 648
radiation-induced neovascular glaucoma, 443
randomized clinical trials (RCT), 592
  evaluation, 592, 593
  study design, 591
Rasch analysis, 475–6
Raynaud's phenomenon
  medical therapy and, 532–3, 553
  normal-tension glaucoma and, 364
Raynaud's syndrome, glaucoma risk, 51
rebound tonometry, 108
reference height, 226
reflectance image, 242–3
refractive error
  angle closure risk, 333
  optic disc size and, 213, 214
  scanning laser polarimetry, 245
refractive surgery, tonometry after, 209
refractory glaucoma, drainage implant surgery, 414
rehabilitation, low-vision, 481–7
  assessing need, 481–3
  context, 483–4
  equipment, 484–7
  services, 484
Reiger anomaly, 376
Reiger syndrome, 376
rejection, grafted stem cells, 601
relative afferent pupillary defect, 362
relative risk (RR), 511–12
relative risk reduction (RRR), 511–12
reliability indices
  automated perimetry, 124–5
  short-wavelength automated perimetry, 135–6
reliability of patients, automated perimetry, 120–1, 125
respiratory disease, β-blocker side-effects, 531–2
retardation image, 242–3
retina, 133
  endogenous repair and transdifferentiation, 601
  factors initiating retinal ganglion cell death, 52
  pigment dispersion syndrome/pigmentary glaucoma, 355
  ultrastructural imaging, 615–22
retinal arterioles, diameter, 220–1
retinal blood flow
  after therapeutic IOP reduction, 95
  glaucoma, 94
  see also retinal ischemia
retinal detachment (RD), Schwartz syndrome, 427–8
retinal disorders, causing glaucoma, 427–8
retinal ganglion cell (RGC) axons

age-related reduction, 221
damage/loss, 45, 222, 579
  axoprotection concept, 585
  mechanisms, 45–51
  retinal ganglion cell death after, 51–2
lamina cribrosa, 45, 46–8, 67
optic nerve head, 46–8, 67–8
regeneration, 586, 602
regional distribution, 217
transport see axoplasmic transport
retinal ganglion cells (RGC)
  bistratified (K cells), 134, 135
  cultures, 580, 581
  differentiation of stem cells into, 586, 599
  electroretinography, 151, 152–3, 156
  function-specific perimetry, 133–47
  gene therapy targeting, 610–12
  imaging, 617
  loss/death
    insensitivity of perimetry to early, 133–4
    mechanisms, 45, 51–3, 579–80
    see also optic neuropathy, glaucomatous
  methods of assessing, 581–2
  midget (P cells), 133, 134, 145
  mitochondria, 45, 46–7
  parasol (M cells) see magnocellular retinal ganglion cells
  protection see neuroprotection
  regeneration, 585–7, 595–6
  stem cell replacement, 586, 595–6, 599–601
  subpopulations, 133–4
retinal ischemia
  experimental models, 581
  neovascular glaucoma, 409–11
  treatment, 413
  see also retinal blood flow
retinal nerve fiber layer (RNFL)
  assessment in neuroprotection studies, 582
  confocal scanning laser ophthalmoscopy, 239, 245–7
  cross-sectional area, 226
  defects
    acute angle closure, 627
    diffuse (generalized), 222, 240–1
    localized (focal), 221–2, 240–1
    ocular hypertension, 311, 312
    primary angle-closure glaucoma, 334
    primary open-angle glaucoma, 318–19
  height variation, 246
  methods of analysis, 239–49
  ophthalmoscopy and photography, 221–2, 239–41
  optical coherence tomography, 239, 247–9, 620
  profile graph, 246
  scanning laser polarimetry, 239, 241–5
  structure–function relationships, 251–4
  thickness, 247–9
    genetic contribution, 278
    mean, 226, 246
retinal pigment epithelium (RPE), optical coherence tomography, 232, 234, 235
retinal progenitor cells
  generation from embryonic stem cells, 596
  transplantation, 595
retinal surgery, glaucoma complicating, 428
retinal vasculitis, 398
retinal vein occlusion, exfoliation syndrome, 344
Retinal Vessel Analyzer (RVA), 263–4
retinoblastoma, 441, 444, 446
retinopathies, causing glaucoma, 427–8
retinopexy, pneumatic, glaucoma complicating, 428
retinoschisis, X-linked juvenile, 411
Retiscan system, 159

retrobulbar tumors, 425
retroviral vectors, 607–8
reverse pupillary block, 188, 351
  laser iridotomy, 357–8
RGCs see retinal ganglion cells
RhoA gene therapy, 609
rim, neuroretinal see neuroretinal rim
rimexolone, 394
risk factors
  artifactual associations, 4
  exfoliative glaucoma, 340
  geographic variations, 9–11
  ocular hypertension progression, 309–10
  pigmentary glaucoma, 350
  post-traumatic glaucoma, 637–8
  primary angle-closure glaucoma, 11, 331–3
  primary open-angle glaucoma, 10, 316–17
  screening, 18–19, 20
  vascular, 91, 93
risks of treatment
  target IOP, 467
  vs benefits, 509–13
Ritch classification of angle-closure glaucoma, 383
RNA interference (RNAi), 609
RNFL see retinal nerve fiber layer
rodent ocular hypertension, 581
  neuroprotection studies, 584
rubeosis iridis see neovascularization of iris
rubeotic glaucoma see neovascular glaucoma

S

Salisbury Eye Evaluation Glaucoma Study, 29, 33, 315
Sampaolesi line, 181, 356
SAP see standard automated perimetry
sarcoidosis
  neovascular glaucoma, 411
  uveitic glaucoma, 399, 400
Saudi Arabia, 301–2
scanning laser Doppler flowmetry (SLDF), 260–2
  automatic full-field perfusion image analysis (AFFPIA), 262
  glaucoma studies, 94, 95, 262
  limitations, 266
scanning laser ophthalmoscope (SLO), 615–18
  see also confocal scanning laser ophthalmoscopy
scanning laser polarimetry (SLP), 239, 241–5
  changes over time, 242
  data printouts and interpretation, 242–4
  diagnostic accuracy, 236, 242
  factors affecting image quality, 244–5
  neuroprotection studies, 582
  primary open-angle glaucoma, 322
  structural–function correlation, 252
scanning peripheral anterior chamber (SPAC) depth analyzer, 204
Scheie grading system, 178
Scheimpflug photography, 204
Schlemm's canal
  aqueous outflow resistance, 59
  blood in, 181
  gonioscopy, 177
Schwalbe's line
  gonioscopy, 177
  pigment deposition, 180, 354, 355
Schwartz syndrome, 427–8
Schwartz-Matsuo syndrome, 436
sclera
  peripapillary, 67–8
    engineering models of stress and strain, 77–9
    geometry, 72, 76

sclera (*continued*)
    in vitro studies, 86
    IOP-related stress, 72–3
    material properties, 71, 76–7
    restructuring and remodeling, 84–6
    role in optic nerve head biomechanics, 76–7
    rigidity, IOP spike height and, 110
scleral buckling procedures, glaucoma complicating, 428
scleral canal
    biomechanics
        engineering models, 78–9
        IOP-related stress, 72, 73
        response to acute IOP elevations, 74–6
    changes in glaucoma, 84
scleral ciliary process angle (SCPA), 187
    angle-closure glaucoma, 190
scleral distance (SD), measurement, 186
scleral–iris angle (SIA), 187
    angle-closure glaucoma, 190
scleral spur, gonioscopy, 177
scotomas, arcuate, 120
scotopic a-wave, 151, 152
scotopic b-wave, 151, 152
scotopic threshold response (STR), 152–3
screening
    angle closure, 20
    criteria, 15–16
    glaucoma, 15–21
        concepts, 17–18
        costs, 16
        current status, 20–1
        developing countries, 34, 37–8, 39
        frequency doubling technology (FDT), 140–1, 143
        important questions, 18–20
        mass or community-based, 15
        number needed to screen, 19–20
        opportunistic, 15, 21
        risk factors, 18–19, 20
        tests, 16
    see also diagnosis of glaucoma
seclusio pupillae, 396, 397
    see also pupillary block
secondary glaucomas, 419–29
    acute, 625, 631–3
    angle closure, 327, 383–91
    childhood, 371, 372, 379
    corneal endothelial disorders, 420–3
    definition, 5, 399
    elevated episcleral venous pressure, 425–7
    epidemiology, 9
    epithelial and fibrous ingrowth, 428–9
    intraocular tumors, 441–6
    open angle *see* open-angle glaucoma (OAG), secondary
    retinal surgery-associated, 428
    vitreoretinal and retinal disorders, 427–8
    see also specific types
sensitivity, 496
services, glaucoma, in developing countries, 39
severity of glaucoma
    American Academy of Ophthalmology classification, 323
    disc damage grading systems, 498, 499
    target IOP and, 466
    visual field grading systems, 500, 501
sex differences *see* gender differences
Shaffer grading system, 178
shear strain, 70
shear stress, 70
short interfering RNAs (siRNAs), 609, 610
short posterior ciliary arteries (SPCA), 50, 51, 67, 68
    blood flow velocity, 257, 258

hemodynamics, 95
pathogenesis of glaucoma and, 51
Short-Form Health Survey (SF-36), 472
short-term fluctuation (SF) index, 125
short-wavelength automated perimetry (SWAP), 134, 135–9
    clinical interpretation, 135–7
    mode of action, 135
    primary open-angle glaucoma, 321
    SITA-SWAP, 139, 140, 147
    strengths and limitations, 137–9
    structural correlation, 252
shunt surgery *see* drainage implant surgery
sib pair analysis, 281–2
sickle cell anemia, traumatic hyphema, 432, 434, 435
Sickness Impact Profile (SIP), 472
siderosis, 437, 644, 646
signal-to-noise ratio (SNR), 616
silencing RNAs (siRNAs), 609, 610
silicone oil, as cause of glaucoma, 428
single nucleotide polymorphisms (SNPs), 284
SITA *see* Swedish Interactive Testing Algorithm
sleep apnea syndrome, 363
slit lamp OCT (SL-OCT), 201–2, 203–4
small vessel myograph, 529, 530
social factors, assessing, 482–3
social marketing, negative, 35, 37, 38
society, glaucoma outcomes, 505
sojourn time, 17, 18
somatic stem cells, 596–7
Spaeth grading system, 178–9
specificity, 496
spectacles, 484
staircase technique, perimetry, 118
standard automated perimetry (SAP), 116–18
    full-threshold techniques, 117, 118
    limitations, 133, 134
    measuring outcomes, 498–502
    primary open-angle glaucoma, 320–1
    structural correlation, 252, 253, 254
    suprathreshold techniques, 117–18
    vs electrophysiological measures, 162, 163
    vs FDT, 142, 143, 144, 145
    vs function-specific tests, 146–7
    vs HPRP, 146
    vs SWAP, 135, 136, 137–9
Standard Gamble (SG) method, 477
stem cell therapy, 595–603
    objectives, 595–6
    potential hurdles, 601–2
    providing trophic support, 601
    retinal ganglion cell replacement, 586, 595–6
    sources and differentiation, 596–8
    strategies, 598–601
    transdifferentiation and endogenous repair, 601
    transplantation, 586, 598–601
stem cells, 596–8
    adult ocular, 597
    neural, 597, 598
    somatic, 596–7
    see also embryonic stem (ES) cells
stereophotography, optic disc *see* optic disc, photography
steroid-induced ocular hypertension/glaucoma *see* corticosteroid-induced ocular hypertension/glaucoma
steroids *see* corticosteroids
Stickler's syndrome, 427
stiffness, structural, 72
strain, mechanical *see* mechanical strain
Stratus Optical Coherence Tomograph (OCT), 232–5, 247
stress, mechanical *see* mechanical stress

stress relaxation, 71–2
stress–strain relationships, 70–2
stroke, neuroprotection, 584–5
stromelysin, gene therapy, 609
structural changes *see* optic disc, cupping; optic disc, structural changes
structural stiffness, 72
structure–function relationships, 251–4
    automated imaging techniques, 252
    conventional testing, 251–2
    measurement, 502
    scaling issue, 253–4
    selective functional tests, 252
    strength, 253–4
    topographic, 253
Sturge-Weber syndrome, 375–6, 425, 444
    management of glaucoma, 445–6
    signs and symptoms, 369, 375–6
suction cup-induced IOP elevation, ocular blood flow changes, 95
sulfonamide allergy, 542
sunspots, 331
superior vena cava syndrome, 425
surgery, glaucoma
    congenital glaucoma, 372–4
    developing countries, 35–6, 38, 39
    exfoliative glaucoma, 345
    neovascular glaucoma, 413–14
    normal-tension glaucoma, 366
    pigmentary glaucoma, 358
    post-traumatic glaucoma, 649–50
    primary angle-closure glaucoma, 334–5
    primary open-angle glaucoma, 323
    sub-Saharan Africa, 36–7
    ultrasound biomicroscopy, 194–5
    uveitic glaucoma, 403–4
    see also drainage implant surgery; filtering surgery *specific procedures*
surgical management, traumatic hyphema, 434–5
surgical skills, in developing countries, 36
survival analysis, medication adherence, 490, 491
SWAP *see* short-wavelength automated perimetry
Swedish Interactive Testing Algorithm (SITA) perimetry, 118–19
    compared to FDT perimetry, 144, 145
    compared to function-specific tests, 146–7
    reliability indices, 125
    SITA Fast, 119
    SITA-SWAP, 139, 140
sympathetic agents *see* adrenergic agents
sympathetic ophthalmia, 398, 437, 645
Symptom Impact Glaucoma (SIG) questionnaire, 474–5
systematic reviews, 591–2
systemic disease, target IOP and, 467
systemic lupus erythematosus (SLE), 387

T

target intraocular pressure *see* intraocular pressure (IOP), target
telemedicine, 34
tensile stress, 70
tests, evaluating, 496–7
tetracycline-regulated gene expression system, 608
TGF-β *see* transforming growth factor-β
third-party payers, 298
thresholds, perimetry, 116–17, 118
thrombotic glaucoma *see* neovascular glaucoma
thymoxamine, pigmentary glaucoma, 357
thyroid ophthalmopathy, 425
TIGR gene *see* myocilin (MYOC) gene

time trade-off (TTO), 476–7
timolol, 525
  combination products, 520, 527, 534, 542, 567–73 *specific combinations*
  formulations and dosing, 526–7
  history of development, 525, 534
  IOP-lowering efficacy, 530–1
  mechanism of action, 528
  side effects, 531, 532, 533
  vs brimonidine, 550, 551
  vs pilocarpine, 520
tissue plasminogen activator (TPA)
  traumatic hyphema, 640
  uveitic glaucoma, 403
tonography, 59
tonometry, 103–9
  after refractive surgery, 209
  central corneal thickness and, 103, 207–11
  children, 369–70
  corneal biomechanics and, 207, 209, 210–11
  Goldmann applanation *see* Goldmann applanation tonometry
  home, 108–9
  noncontact, 104–5
  rebound, 108
Tonopen, 105–6, 207
TOP perimetry, 118, 119
topiramate, 386–7
topographic structure–function maps, 253
total deviation plots, 122, 124, 136
trabecular aspiration, pigmentary glaucoma, 358
trabecular ciliary process distance (TCPD), 186, 187
  angle-closure glaucoma, 190
  plateau iris syndrome, 191
trabecular meshwork (TM)
  corneoscleral, 59
  corticosteroid-induced changes, 395, 423–4
  cultured progenitor cells, 596, 598
  exfoliation material (XFM) deposits, 180–1, 341–2
  gene therapy targeting, 608, 609–10
  gonioscopic visualization, 176, 177
  juxtacanalicular tissue, 59
  pigment deposition, 353–4, 355
  stem cell-mediated restoration, 596
  traumatic injuries, 638
  tumors infiltrating, 441, 442
  uveal, 58–9
  uveitic changes, 394, 395
trabecular meshwork glucocorticoid response (TIGR) gene *see* myocilin (MYOC) gene
trabecular outflow facility (C), 59
  conditions affecting IOP, 61, 62, 63, 64
  fluctuation, 110
  healthy human eyes, 57
  measurement, 59
  see also aqueous humor outflow, resistance
trabecular outflow pathways, 58–9
trabeculectomy
  acute primary angle closure, 630–1
  angle-recession glaucoma, 642
  cataract progression after, 35, 38
  developing countries, 36–7, 38, 39
  exfoliative glaucoma, 345
  neovascular glaucoma, 413–14
  normal-tension glaucoma, 366
  pigmentary glaucoma, 358
  post-traumatic glaucoma, 649
  primary angle closure, 458–9
  primary angle-closure glaucoma, 327–8
  primary open-angle glaucoma, 323
  ultrasound biomicroscopy, 194
  uveitic glaucoma, 403–4

trabeculitis, 395
  chemical injuries, 647
  traumatic, 433, 638
trabeculotomy
  congenital glaucoma, 373–4
  exfoliative glaucoma, 345
training
  in developing countries, 33, 39
  ophthalmologists, 300
tranexamic acid, traumatic hyphema, 434, 640
transdifferentiation, and retinal repair, 601
transforming growth factor-β (TGF-β)
  optic nerve head remodeling and, 84
  uveitis, 395
transmission disequilibrium test (TDT), 284
transplantation, stem cell, 586, 598–601
  see also stem cell therapy
trauma, 431–8, 637–48
  blunt, 431–6, 638–45
  chemical burns, 437–8, 646–7
  electrical injuries, 648
  epidemiology, 431, 637
  epithelial ingrowth, 428–9, 437
  gonioscopy, 181–2, 433, 649
  penetrating, 436–8, 645–6
  pigmentary glaucoma, 356
  previous history, 307
  radiation injuries, 648
  retained lens fragment, 420
  thermal burns, 647
  see also post-traumatic glaucoma
travoprost, 560, 562
  chronic primary angle closure, 456
  exfoliative glaucoma, 344–5
travoprost/timolol (DuoTrav™), 527, 567, 571–2
  preservatives, 566
treatment
  adverse outcomes, 503, 504
  benefit vs risk, 509–13
  costs, 28–9, 505
    in different societies, 34–5
  in developing countries, 34–7, 38
  see also management; medical therapy; surgery, glaucoma
triamcinolone, intravitreal
  IOP elevation, 424, 428
  neovascular glaucoma, 414
tricyclic antidepressants, 331
TrkB, 51, 583
  gene transfer studies, 610–11
TSNIT parameters, 243
TSNIT plots, 243, 244, 247, 248
tumor necrosis factor-α (TNF-α) gene, 285
tumors, intraocular, 441–6
  diagnostic evaluation, 443
  differential diagnosis, 443–5
  glaucoma management, 445–6
  mechanisms of glaucoma, 441–3
  neovascular glaucoma, 410–11, 443, 444
  prognosis, 446
tyrosinase, 273
tyrosinase-related protein 1 (TYRP1), 272, 352–3
tyrosine kinase B receptors *see* TrkB

U

ultrasonography, childhood glaucomas, 370
ultrasound biomicroscopy (UBM), 185–95, 198–201
  after laser peripheral iridotomy, 193
  angle-closure glaucoma, 189–93, 388
  artifacts and technical tips, 200–1
  clinical applications, 194–5, 197
  data interpretation and storage, 199–200

examination techniques, 185–6
  instrumentation/mode of action, 185, 198–9
  measurement parameters, 186–8, 200
  mechanisms of glaucoma, 188–93
  mode of action, 198–9
  ocular blood flow measurement, 266
  pigment dispersion syndrome/pigmentary glaucoma, 188, 189, 350–1, 356
  primary angle-closure glaucoma, 334
  research applications, 193–4
  strengths and limitations, 199
  surgical treatment of glaucoma, 194–5
  vs anterior segment optical coherence tomography, 204
ultrastructural imaging, 615–22
  future advances, 621–2
  optic coherence tomography, 619–21
  scanning laser ophthalmoscope, 615–18
undetected glaucoma, 11, 33
unfolded protein response (UPR), 270
United States
  economic analyses, 28–9, 31
  epidemiology, 5–6, 8, 11
United States Preventive Services Task Force (UPSTF), 20–1
unoprostone, 560, 562
untreated glaucoma, costs, 29
utility measures, 476–7
uveitic glaucoma, 393–405
  clinical features, 399–400
  diagnosis and classification, 398–9
  epidemiology, 393–4
  etiology and pathogenesis, 394–8
  goniotomy, 404
  investigations, 400
  management, 401–4
uveitis
  hypertensive, 333
  phacoantigenic, 420
  pigment deposition, 356, 399, 400
  treatment, 401–2
uveoscleral outflow (Fu), 57, 60–1
  fluctuation, 110
  measurement, 60–1
  syndromes affecting IOP, 61, 62, 63

V

variable corneal compensation (VCC), 241, 245
variance component analyses, 278, 282
varices, orbital, 425
vascular changes
  exfoliation syndrome, 344
  ocular, 92
  systemic, 92
vascular disorders, systemic, 93
vascular effects
  α agonists, 548–9
  β-blockers, 529–30
  carbonic anhydrase inhibitors, 541
  prostaglandin analogues, 561
vascular endothelial growth factor (VEGF), 411, 414
  antagonists, 414, 415
vascular theory, pathogenesis of glaucoma, 91
vasoconstriction, retrobulbar, 96
vasodilators, systemic, 96–7
vasospasm, 10, 93, 96–7
  methods of assessment, 265–6
  normal-tension glaucoma and, 96–7, 364
VECP *see* visual evoked cortical potential
venomanometry, 60
venous obstruction, elevated episcleral venous pressure, 425
VEP *see* visual evoked cortical potential

VERIS Scientific™ system, 156, 159, 164
verteporfin, neovascular glaucoma, 414
vertical integrated rim area (VIRA), 233
Veteran Affairs Low Visual Functioning (VA
LV VFQ-48), 483
viral vectors
  gene transfer, 605–8
  modulating expression, 608
Visante™ OCT machine, 201–2, 203–4
viscoelastic materials, 71–2
viscogonioplasty, 630
vision, assessment, 481–2
Visual Activities Questionnaire (VAQ), 473
visual acuity (VA), testing, 481–2
  childhood glaucoma, 369
visual disability, 502–3
  assessing, 476, 482, 504–5
visual evoked cortical potential (VECP or
VEP), 151
  flicker, 155
  latency, 155
  multifocal pattern (mfVEP), 157–8
    artifacts and prevention, 164–6
    data storage and retrieval, 163
    method, 159–60
    printouts and interpretation, 164, 166
    reference population, 161
    strengths and limitations, 160–1
    technical tips, 166
    vs other tests, 162, 163
  multifocal recording techniques, 155–6
  neuroprotection studies, 581
  pattern (flash), 154–5
visual field(s), 115–30
  Glaucoma Hemifield Test (GHT), 124, 125
  indices, 122–4
    SWAP, 136
  mean deviation (MD), 122
  pattern deviation, 122
  pattern standard deviation (PSD), 122–4
  progression, 125–9
  reliability indices, 124–5

short-term fluctuation (SF) index, 125
single field analysis, 121–4
structural relationships, 251–4
visual field defects, 115, 120
  acute angle closure, 627
  defining glaucoma, 294
  diagnostic criteria, 500
  grading systems, 500, 501
  primary open-angle glaucoma, 320–1
visual field testing, 115–30
  automated, 116–19
  binocular, 119
  children, 370
  developing countries, 36, 38
  history, 115–16
  manual, 116
  measurement variability, 120–1
  measuring outcomes, 498–502
  neuroprotection studies, 581
  ocular hypertension, 309, 311
  see also perimetry
visual function
  assessment in animal models, 602
  measurement, 496–502
  performance-based testing, 476, 482,
504–5
  quality of life questionnaires, 472–6
  structural relationships see structure–
function relationships
Visual Function Index (VF-14), 473
visual hallucinations, 482
visual impairment, 502–3
  definitions, 481, 503
  economic analyses, 29–30
  patient's viewpoint, 504
  see also blindness; low vision
visual system, human, 133–4
Viswanathan Questionnaire, 473, 474
vitamin A deficiency, 37
vitrectomy
  glaucoma complicating, 428
  neovascular glaucoma, 413, 414

vitreoretinal disorders, causing glaucoma,
427–8
vitreoretinal surgery, glaucoma complicating,
428
vitreous hemorrhage
  ghost cells, 644
  hemolytic glaucoma after, 435, 644
VMD2 gene, 274
Vogt-Koyanagi-Harada (VKH) syndrome, 387,
398, 400
von Recklinghausen's disease see
neurofibromatosis type 1
von-Hippel-Lindau disease, 444

W

water bath, ultrasound biomicroscopy, 198,
199
WD repeat domain 36 (WDR36), 269, 271,
286
Weill-Marchesani syndrome (WMS), 385–6
white coat adherence, 492
woodchuck post-translational regulatory
element (WPRE), 608
worldwide significance of glaucoma, 297–303

X

Xalacom™ see latanoprost/timolol
xanthogranuloma, juvenile, 441, 444

Y

yield, mechanical, 72
Young's modulus of elasticity, 71, 209

Z

Zeiss goniolens, 174
Zeiss gonioscopy, 176
Zeyen formula, target IOP, 468
Zinn-Haller, circle of, 50, 51, 68
Zippy estimation of sequential testing (ZEST)
strategy, 143